HODGKIN LYMPHOMA

SECOND EDITION

HODGKIN LYMPHOMA

SECOND EDITION

Editors

Richard T. Hoppe, M.D.

Henry S. Kaplan-Harry Lebeson Professor in Cancer Biology
Chairman,
Department of Radiation Oncology
Stanford University School of Medicine
Stanford, California

Peter M. Mauch, M.D.

Professor, Department of Radiation Oncology
Harvard Medical School
Professor, Department of Radiation Oncology
Brigham and Women's Hospital
Dana-Farber Cancer Institute
Boston, Massachusetts

James O. Armitage, M.D.

Professor, Section of Hematology and Oncology
Department of Internal Medicine
University of Nebraska Medical Center
Omaha, Nebraska

Volker Diehl, M.D.

Professor, Department of Internal Medicine
Director, Clinic I for Internal Medicine
University of Cologne
Cologne, Germany

Lawrence M. Weiss, M.D.

Chairman, Division of Pathology
City of Hope National Medical Center
Duarte, California

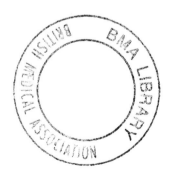

Wolters Kluwer | Lippincott Williams & Wilkins
Health
Philadelphia · Baltimore · New York · London
Buenos Aires · Hong Kong · Sydney · Tokyo

Acquisitions Editor: Jonathan W. Pine, Jr.
Managing Editor: Anne E. Jacobs
Project Manager: Alicia Jackson
Manufacturing Manager: Kathleen Brown
Associate Director of Marketing: Adam Glazer
Creative Director: Doug Smock
Cover Designer: Andrew Gatto
Production Service: International Typesetting and Composition
Printer: RR Donnelley-Willard

© 2007 by LIPPINCOTT WILLIAMS & WILKINS, a WOLTERS KLUWER business
530 Walnut Street
Philadelphia, PA 19106 USA
LWW.com

First Edition © 1999 Lippincott Williams & Wilkins

Library of Congress Cataloging-in-Publication Data

Hodgkin lymphoma / editors, Richard T. Hoppe . . . [et al.].—2nd ed.
   p. ; cm.
   Rev. ed. of: Hodgkin's disease / editors, Peter M. Mauch . . . [et al.]. c1999.
   Includes bibliographical references and index.
   ISBN-13: 978-0-7817-6422-3
   ISBN-10: 0-7817-6422-X
   1. Hodgkin's disease. I. Hoppe, R. (Richard) II. Hodgkin's disease.
   [DNLM: 1. Hodgkin Disease. WH 500 H6883 2007]
   RC644.H622 2007
   616.99'446—dc22

                                                        2007004416

Care has been taken to confirm the accuracy of the information presented and to describe generally accepted practices. However, the authors, editors, and publisher are not responsible for errors or omissions or for any consequences from application of the information in this book and make no warranty, expressed or implied, with respect to the currency, completeness, or accuracy of the contents of the publication. Application of the information in a particular situation remains the professional responsibility of the practitioner.

The authors, editors, and publisher have exerted every effort to ensure that drug selection and dosage set forth in this text are in accordance with current recommendations and practice at the time of publication. However, in view of ongoing research, changes in government regulations, and the constant flow of information relating to drug therapy and drug reactions, the reader is urged to check the package insert for each drug for any change in indications and dosage and for added warnings and precautions. This is particularly important when the recommended agent is a new or infrequently employed drug.

Some drugs and medical devices presented in the publication have Food and Drug Administration (FDA) clearance for limited use in restricted research settings. It is the responsibility of the health care provider to ascertain the FDA status of each drug or device planned for use in their clinical practice.

To purchase additional copies of this book, call our customer service department at (800) 638-3030 or fax orders to (301) 223-2320. International customers should call (301) 223-2300.

Visit Lippincott Williams & Wilkins on the Internet: at LWW.com. Lippincott Williams & Wilkins customer service representatives are available from 8:30 am to 6 pm, EST.

10 9 8 7 6 5 4 3 2 1

Richard F. Ambinder, M.D.
Department of Oncology,
*   Pharmacology, and Pathology*
Johns Hopkins University School
*   of Medicine*
Baltimore, Maryland

Ranjana Advani, M.D.
Associate Professor
Department of Medicine
Stanford University
Stanford, California

Cigdem Atayar, M.D., Ph.D.
Department of Pathology
University Medical Center
Groningen, The Netherlands

James O. Armitage, M.D.
Professor and Chairman
Department of Internal Medicine
Section of Oncology and Hematology
University of Nebraska
Omaha, Nebraska

Karolin Behringer
Department of Internal Medicine
Klinik I für Innere Medizin
der Universität zu Köln
Köln, Germany

Philip J. Bierman, M.D.
Associate Professor
Department of Internal Medicine
Section of Oncology and Hematology
University of Nebraska
Omaha, Nebraska

Peter Borchmann
Department of Internal Medicine
Klinik I für Innere Medizin
der Universität zu Köln
Köln, Germany

George P. Canellos, M.D., F.R.C.P. (Hon.),
DRs. (Hon.)
William Rosenberg Professor
Department of Medicine
Harvard Medical School;
Senior Physician
Department of Medical Oncology
Dana-Farber Cancer Institute
Boston, Massachusetts

Patrice Carde, M.D.
Professor, Chief of Service
Department of Medicine Oncology/Hematology
Institute Gustave-Roussy
Villejuif, France

Angelo M. Carella, M.D., Ph.D.
Coordinator
Department of Hematology
Azienda Ospedale/Università
Genova, Italy

Franco Cavalli, M.D.
Division of Oncology
Ospedale San Giovanni
Bellinzona, Switzerland

John K.C. Chan, M.D.
Consultant Pathologist
Department of Pathology
Queen Elizabeth Hospital
Kowloon, Hong Kong

Ellen T. Chang, Sc.D.
Research Scientist
Northern California Cancer Center
Fremont, California

Joseph M. Connors, M.D.
Clinical Professor of Medicine
Division of Medical Oncology
University of British Columbia
Vancouver, British Columbia

Louis S. Constine, M.D.
Professor
Department of Radiation Oncology and Pediatrics
University of Rochester Medical Center
Rochester, New York

Vincent T. DeVita, M.D.
Amy and Joseph Perella Professor
*   of Medicine*
Yale Cancer Center
Yale University School of Medicine
New Haven, Connecticut

Volker Diehl, M.D.
Professor
Department of Internal Medicine
Klinik I für Innere Medizin
der Universität zu Köln
Köln, Germany

Sarah S. Donaldson, M.D., F.A.C.R.
Catharine and Howard Avery Professor
Associate Chair
Department of Radiation Oncology
Stanford University School of Medicine
Stanford, California

Andreas Engert, M.D.
Klinik I für Innere Medizin
der Universität zu Köln
Köln, Germany

Sukru Mehmet Erturk, M.D.
Attending Radiologist
Division of Abdominal Radiology
Department of Radiology
Sisli Etfal Training and Research Hospital
Istanbul, Turkey

Henning Flechtner, M.D.
Associate Professor and Director
Department of Child and Adolescent
  Psychiatry
Otto-von-Guericke-University
Magdeburg, Germany

Patricia Fobair, M.P.H.
Clinical Social Worker
Department of Radiation Oncology
Stanford University School of Medicine
Stanford, California

Jeremy Franklin, M.Sc.
Statistician
Klinik I für Innere Medizin
der Universität zu Köln
Köln, Germany

Axel Gossmann, M.D.
Vice President
Department of Radiology
University of Cologne
Cologne, Germany

Mary K. Gospodarowicz, M.D., F.R.C.P.C.
Professor
Department of Radiation Oncology
University of Toronto;
Director of Clinical Programs
Department of Radiation Oncology
Princess Margaret Hospital
Toronto, Canada

Theodore Girinsky, M.D.
Department of Radiation Oncology
Institute Gustave-Roussy
Villejuif, France

Seymour Grufferman, M.D., Dr.P.H.
Research Professor
Department of Internal Medicine, Division of Epidemiology
  and Biostatistics
University of New Mexico School of Medicine
Albuquerque, New Mexico

Barry W. Hancock, M.D., F.R.C.P., F.R.C.R.
Professor
Clinical Oncology
University of Sheffield
United Kingdom

Steven L. Hancock, M.D., F.A.C.R.
Professor
Department of Radiation Oncology
Stanford University School of
  Medicine
Stanford, California

Martin-Leo Hansmann, M.D.
Head
Department of Pathology
University of Frankfurt
Frankfurt, Germany

Nancy Lee Harris, M.D.
Professor of Pathology
Harvard Medical School;
Director of Anatomic Pathology
Massachusetts General Hospital
Boston, Massachusetts

Dirk Hasenclever, M.D.
Senior Biomertician
Institut für Medizinische Informatik,
  Statistik und Epidemiologie
Universität Leipzig
Leipzig, Germany

Samuel Hellman, M.D., F.A.C.R.
A.N. Pritzker Distinguished Service Professor
Department of Radiation and Cellular
  Oncology
University of Chicago
Chicago, Illinois

Michel Henry-Amar, M.Sc., M.D.
Senior Scientist
Department of Clinical Research
Centre François Baclesse
Caen, France

Richard T. Hoppe, M.D., F.A.C.R.
Henry S. Kaplan—Harry Lebeson Professor
  in Cancer Biology
Chairman
Department of Radiation Oncology
Stanford University School of Medicine
Stanford, California

David C. Hodgson M.D. M.P.H.,
  F.R.C.P.C.
Assistant Professor
Department of Radiation Oncology
Department of Health Policy, Management,
  and Evaluation
University of Toronto;
Department of Radiation Oncology
Princess Margaret Hospital
Toronto, Canada

Sandra J. Horning, M.D.
Professor
Department of Medicine
Stanford University School of Medicine
Stanford, California

Rachel E. Hough, B.Med.Sci., B.M.B.S., M.R.C.P., M.R.C.Path., M.D.
Honarary Senior Lecturer
Hematology
University College London
United Kingdom

Melissa M. Hudson, M.D.
Member, Department of
 Hematology-Oncology
Director, After Completion of Therapy Clinic
St. Jude Children's Research Hospital
Memphis, Tennessee

Peter Jacobs, M.D., Ph.D.
Professor and Head
Division of Clinical Haematology
Department of Internal Medicine
Faculty of Health Sciences
Stellenbosch University
Tygerberg Academic Hospital;
Director
Department of Haematology and Bone Marrow
 Transplant Unit
Constantiaberg Medi Clinic
Cape Town, South Africa

Elaine S. Jaffe, M.D.
Chief, Hematopathology Section
Department of Pathology
National Cancer Institute
National Institutes of Health
Bethesda, Maryland

Florence Joly, M.D.
Medical Oncologist
Department of Medicine
Centre François Baclesse
Caen, France

Stefan Joos
Professor
German Cancer Research Center
Division of Molecular Genetics
Heidelberg Germany

Andreas Josting
Department of Internal Medicine
Klinik I für Innere Medizin
der Universität zu Köln
Köln, Germany

Armand Keating, M.D.
Princess Margaret Hospital
Medical Oncology and Hematology
Toronto, Canada

Dieter Körholz
Department of Pediatric Hematology
 and Oncology
Heinrich-Heine University Medical Center
Düsseldorf, Germany

Ralf Küppers, Ph.D.
Professor
Institute for Cell Biology (Tumor Research)
University of Duisburg-Essen, Medical School
Essen, Germany

Yue Ma, M.Sc.
Department of Pathology
University Medical Center Groningen
Groningen, The Netherlands

Peter M. Mauch, M.D.
Professor of Radiation Oncology
Harvard Medical School
Associate Chief
Department of Radiation
 Oncology
Brigham and Women's Hospital
Dana-Farber Cancer Institute
Boston, Massachusetts

Nancy E. Mueller, Sc.D.
Professor of Epidemiology
Harvard University School of
 Public Health
Boston, Massachusetts

Hans Konrad Mueller-Hermelink, M.D.
Professor of Pathology
Institute of Pathology
University of Wurzburg
Wurzburg, Germany

Andrea K. Ng, M.D., M.P.H.
Associate Professor
Department of Radiation Oncology
Brigham and Women's Hospital
Harvard Medical School
Boston, Massachusetts

Lucia Nogová
Department of Internal Medicine
Klinik I für Innere Medizin
der Universität zu Köln
Köln, Germany

Evert M. Noordijk, M.D., Ph.D.
Professor in Clinical Radiotherapy
Head, Department of Clinical Oncology
Leiden University Medical Center
Leiden, The Netherlands

Santiago Pavlovsky, M.D.
Medical Director
Angelica Ocampo Hospital and Research
 Center-Fundaleu
Buenos Aires, Argentina

Sibrand Poppema, M.D., Ph.D., F.R.C.P.C.
Professor of Pathology
Dean and Vice President
University Medical Center Groningen
Groningen, The Netherlands

Carol S. Portlock, M.D.
Professor of Clinical Medicine
New York Weill Cornell University
*   Medical College;*
Attending Physician
Lymphoma Service
Department of Medicine
Memorial Sloan-Kettering
*   Cancer Center*
New York, New York

John Raemaekers, M.D., Ph.D.
Associate Professor
Department of Medicine
Division of Hematology
University Hospital of Nijmegen
Nijmegen, The Netherlands

Daniel Re, M.D.
University Hospital of Cologne
Hematology and Medical
*   Oncology*
Cologne, Germany

Saul A. Rosenberg, M.D.
Professor Emeritus
Department of Medicine and Radiation
*   Oncology*
Stanford University School of Medicine
Stanford, California

Jens-Ulrich Rueffer, M.D.
Department of Hematology/Oncology
Klinik I für Innere Medizin
der Universität zu Köln
Köln, Germany

Paul Ruff
Department of Medicine
Division of Haematology/Oncology
Hillbrow Hospital and University of the
*   Witwatersrand*
Johannesburg, South Africa

Norbert Schmitz, M.D.
Associate Professor
Head, BMT Unit
Department of Internal Medicine II
Christian-Albrechts-University
Kiel, Germany

Roland Schnell
Department of Internal Medicine
Klinik I für Innere Medizin
der Universität zu Köln
Köln, Germany

Reiner Siebert
Professor
Institut für Humangenetik
Christian-Albrechts-Universität Kiel
Kiel, Germany

Lena Specht M.D., Ph.D
Associate Professor, Chief Oncologist
Departments of Oncology and Hematology
The Finsen Centre
Rigshospitalet, Copenhagen
*   University Hospital*
Copenhagen, Denmark

Jan Oliver Staak
Department of Internal Medicine
Klinik I für Innere Medizin
der Universität zu Köln
Köln, Germany

Harald Stein, M.D.
Professor and Head
Institute of Pathology
Universitätsklinikum Freien
*   Universität Berlin*
Berlin, Germany

Simon B. Sutcliffe, B.Sc., M.D.
Vancouver Cancer Center
Vancouver, British Columbia
Canada

Anthony J. Swerdlow, D.Sc.,
Section of Epidemiology
Institute of Cancer Research
Sutton, United Kingdom

Lois B. Travis, M.D., Sc.D.
Radiation Epidemiology Branch
Division of Cancer Epidemiology
*   and Genetics*
National Cancer Institute, NIH, DHHS
Bethesda, Maryland

Maurice Tubiana, M.D., Ph.D.
Emeritus Professor
Paris-Sud University
Paris, France;
Honorary Director
Institut Gustave-Roussy
Villejuif, France

Annick D. van den Abbeele, M.D.
Associate Professor of Radiology
Harvard Medical School
Chief, Department of Radiology
Dana-Farber Cancer Institute
Boston, Massachusetts

Anke van den Berg, Ph.D.
Department of Pathology
University Medical Center
*   Groningen*
Groningen, The Netherlands

Flora E. van Leeuwen, Ph.D.
Professor
Department of Epidemiology
The Netherlands Cancer Institute
Amsterdam, The Netherlands

Lydia Visser, Ph.D.
Department of Pathology
University Medical Center Groningen
Groningen, The Netherlands

Julie M. Vose, M.D.
Neumann M. and Mildred E. Harris Professor
Chief, Section of Hematology/Oncology
Professor of Medicine
University of Nebraska Medical Center
Omaha, Nebraska

Roger A. Warnke, M.D.
Professor
Department of Pathology
Stanford University School of Medicine
Stanford, California

Lawrence M. Weiss, M.D.
Chairman
Department of Pathology
City of Hope National Medical
Center
Duarte, California

Lucille Wood, B.A., M.Sc.
Medical Natural Scientist
Haematology Coordinator
Department of Haematology and
Bone Marrow Transplant Unit
Constantiaberg Medi Clinic
Cape Town, South Africa

Joachim Yahalom, M.D.
Professor of Radiation Oncology
Cornell University Medical
College;
Member and Attending
Department of Radiation Oncology
Memorial Sloan-Kettering Cancer Center
New York, New York

Saul A. Rosenberg

It has been my unique privilege and experience to be involved in the clinical investigation and care of patients with Hodgkin's disease for the past 50 years. The changes and advances in the management of the disease have been remarkable, and one of the major success stories in modern medicine.

As a commentary and introduction to the readers of this comprehensive textbook, written by most of the major experts who study Hodgkin's disease, it is of value to give a brief historical review of the major accomplishments and evolution of the management of the disease as they have occurred. Many of the initial advances of the understanding and treatment of Hodgkin's disease have been gradually changing over this time period, so that the dogmas and certainties of the early years are now rejected.

Fifty years ago, Hodgkin's disease was considered a "systemic" malignancy, much like leukemia, and almost universally fatal. A few radiotherapists felt otherwise, and reported improved survival of patients, if treated as if they had a neoplasm, which began in a limited site and "spread" to nearby or predictable regions.

When supervoltage irradiation equipment became available, radiotherapists were better able to treat greater areas with higher doses of irradiation, without undue acute toxicity. Prolonged disease-free survival was achieved for an increasing number of patients with the early and intermediate stages of disease. The radiotherapists' results were further improved when aggressive diagnostic staging techniques were employed, primarily lower extremity lymphography and exploratory laparotomy with splenectomy.

It was not until more effective chemotherapy agents and regimens became available, and the late effects of radiotherapy were documented, that the primary radiotherapy management of Hodgkin's disease was challenged, and has gradually been abandoned. The dogma and certainty of experienced investigators that very detailed staging and wide-field, high-dose irradiation were required is now rejected, even by those who developed these techniques.

Similarly, the discoveries of effective chemotherapy, primarily the alkylating agents, the vinca alkaloids and anthracyclines, led to controversies, and dogmas, as to which regimen was most valuable and whether chemotherapy should be the primary management, an adjuvant, or a component of combined-modality approaches. Some of these controversies continue to date. But there is now general agreement that combination chemotherapy should be the primary and initial treatment for virtually all patients with Hodgkin's disease. Additionally, despite the breakthrough success of the MOPP- and MVPP-type regimens, restricting the cumulative dose of the leukemogenic and sterility-inducing alkylating agents has been accepted.

The clinical investigators of Hodgkin's disease management have gone through a cycle of increasing aggressiveness in diagnostic and treatment modalities, with improved cure rates, to a more selective use of effective therapies and elimination of the most aggressive, often toxic and morbid, management methods. Yet prolonged survivals and probable cures are increasing worldwide, in all major and community centers.

Current challenges for clinical investigators are to maintain the very high cure and survival rates for patients with the more favorable settings of the disease, and to reduce acute and late treatment toxicities. Patients with less favorable prognostic factors, though still curable in the majority of cases, require more successful and tolerable management programs to further improve their length and quality of survival.

As in science and medicine in general, what have been thought to be truths and certainties in the past are often modified or disproved with further understanding and advances. This has been dramatically true for Hodgkin's disease. These dogmas of the past are no longer acceptable:

Hodgkin's disease is a systemic disease and invariably fatal.

Meticulous diagnostic studies, especially laparotomy and splenectomy, are required for best results.

Wide-field, high-dose irradiation is the treatment of choice for stages I, II, and IIIA Hodgkin's disease.

Chemotherapy should be reserved for patients with more advanced Hodgkin's disease, and those who recur after irradiation.

MOPP-like chemotherapy is the regimen of choice for Hodgkin's disease.

Sterility, chemotherapy-induced myelodysplasia and leukemia, and radiation-induced malignancies and cardiac damage are acceptable toxicities of the curative treatment of Hodgkin's disease.

Finally, it is a pity that pathologists and journal editors are determined to change the name of this unique disease, from Hodgkin's disease to some other term. The literature of over 150 years, thousands of articles, numerous books and innumerable clinical records have used the term Hodgkin's disease; it is time honored. The purists who would remove the apostrophe from the name, reject medical history and the literature, when many investigators were honored and remembered for their perception and insight, in recognizing new entities. Illnesses such as Waldenström's, Parkinson's, Alzheimer's, and many others remain in our medical usage and literature, with a very clear understanding of what these diseases are.

Moreover, Hodgkin's disease is not just another "lymphoma." There are so many unique features of this remarkable illness—including the often dramatic systemic symptoms, unique histology combining inflammation with neoplasia, unique paraneoplastic signs and syndromes of the disease, familial incidence, unique epidemiology, and especially its very high responsiveness to therapy—which separates Hodgkin's disease from the diverse groups of other lymphomas.

Pathologists and editors have no right to ignore the long history and name of this very special illness, which I will always call Hodgkin's disease.

Maurice Tubiana and Patrice Carde

The treatment of Hodgkin's disease in the early 1960s was only palliative. Aggressive treatments were avoided to spare patient discomfort. However a few radiotherapists, René Gilbert in particular, advocated extended-field radiation therapy with doses as high as possible. But poor tolerance to 200 kV x-rays barely allowed doses higher than 20 to 25 Gy. High-energy radiation therapy increased tolerance, and in the early 1960s higher doses started to be delivered. However, Hodgkin's disease was still believed always fatal. The first remissions with single-agent chemotherapy were spectacular but disappointing, because short-lived.

In this context, Easson's claim in 1963 that Hodgkin's disease was a curable disease met with great skepticism. Long remissions were known following extensive radiotherapy, but recurrence was believed inevitable because Hodgkin's disease was considered to be multifocal from the outset. In view of the controversy, we organized a symposium in Paris in 1965 that aimed at discussing the curability of Hodgkin's disease. A panel of pathologists reviewed the slides of all the patients apparently cured in the Manchester, Stanford, and Toronto studies and concluded that they did have Hodgkin's disease.

From 1965 to the late 1980s, spectacular progress in treatment made Hodgkin's disease one of the most fascinating stories of modern medicine. In 1964, survival increase was sought by attempting to improve the techniques of irradiation or by combining radiation therapy with chemotherapy. The first European Organization for Research and Treatment of Cancer (EORTC) controlled trial on Hodgkin's disease (H1 trial, 1964–1970) was the first to investigate whether chemotherapy (weekly vinblastine for 2 years) could improve the survival results over radiotherapy alone. A long-lasting relapse-free survival advantage was seen in the radiotherapy/chemotherapy arm (at 15 years 60% versus 38%, $p < 0.001$). The advantage in overall survival (at 15 years 65% versus 58%) was significant only in the unfavorable prognostic subgroup. In the 1970s, severe late effects, such as leukemia, started to be reported in more aggressively treated patients. Late effects gained importance with longer follow-up, as evidenced by the symposium and workshop organized in Paris through the EORTC. This inspired a new EORTC strategy: a) a less aggressive initial treatment in order to spare most late effects among nonrelapsing patients; and b) in relapsing patients, an aggressive salvage treatment to achieve a high overall survival rate. However, this strategy could only be successful if the relapse-free survival achieved with minimal treatment was sufficiently high. Otherwise a reduction in the side effects for the entire cohort of patients was not achievable.

Another important observation about the H1 trial and similar trials was the impact on the relapse rate of such factors as histologic subtype or systemic symptoms. This strategy required a good knowledge of prognostic factors to delineate the favorable and unfavorable subgroups.

The H2 trial had two goals. The first was to investigate the usefulness of staging laparotomy for the delineation of the favorable group. CS I and II patients were randomly assigned whether to undergo a staging laparotomy and splenectomy. In the arm without laparotomy, the spleen was irradiated. The relapse-free survival was higher in patients staged with laparotomy (68% and 76%) but overall survival (77% and 79%) was not different. The second goal was to introduce histologic subtype as a prognostic factor. In the following H5 trial (1977–1982), the use of prognostic factors was enlarged and it became systematic in subsequent trials. Accordingly, two or three therapeutic subgroups were distinguished for tailoring the treatment to the risk of relapse. The EORTC challenged the usefulness of staging laparotomy for the further delineation of favorable subgroups of patients; the H6-F randomized the staging procedure to investigate whether a mixture of prognostic factors could provide information as useful as laparotomy: survival was actually lower in the laparotomy arm, due to laparotomy-related mortality. Staging laparotomy was abandoned.

In the 1970s, it was anticipated that treatment-related adverse effects would stem mainly from chemotherapy, because the risk of leukemia was correlated with the amount of alkylating agents administered to patients. Thus the aim was to restrict drug exposure to those expected to be at higher risk of death due to Hodgkin's disease. Follow-up showed later that most late complications stemmed from radiotherapy.

In the 1960s, radiotherapy had become more extensive. In order to reduce side effects several avenues were explored. First, in favorable subgroups reduction of the number of irradiated nodal areas. In the H5 trial, favorable subgroups PS I-II stages were randomized between mantle field or mantle field plus paraaortic irradiation; there was no difference in relapse-free or total survival. In the H6 and H7 EORTC trials, the dose to the uninvolved area was reduced to 36 Gy without any increase in the incidence of recurrence. In the HD4 German study, patients with PS IA and II$_2$ A or B without mediastinal mass were randomized between 40 Gy to a wide field or 40 Gy to the involved areas plus 30 Gy to uninvolved areas. In the following HD5 trial, similar results were obtained using extensive-field 30 Gy + 10 Gy on bulky sites. The BNLI compared limited to more extensive irradiation. No difference in 10-year survival was detected. In another avenue of exploration, several trials showed that when RT was combined with CT that the number of irradiated areas and the dose could be reduced, provided that the aggressiveness of chemotherapy was adapted to that of the disease. This approach was pioneered in children because the severe bone growth arrest produced by conventional irradiation was not tolerable. Several groups extended this strategy to adults. Regimens less toxic than MOPP were investigated. The EORTC H7-F trial (1988–1993) showed for the first time that an abbreviated course of chemotherapy (EBVP × 6 = 3.5 months), combined with irradiation restricted to the involved nodal areas was superior to STNI. A confirmatory trial, H8-F (1993–1999), with MOPP/ABV × 3 (instead of EBVP) brought an additional overall survival advantage of the combined modality against STNI.

In the unfavorable subgroup, staging laparotomy was never performed in the EORTC trials, because these patients were to receive a strong treatment. The program of mantle-field irradiation between two courses of 3 × MOPP proved superior to STNI in the H5-U trial. In the H7-U trial, only involved fields were irradiated, sparing mediastinal irradiation in about 25% of the patients. However, in unfavorable patients, a concomitant reduction in chemotherapy strength (EBVP × 6 instead of MOPP/ABV × 6) with involved-field RT, compromised the outcome. The addition of STNI to a full CT course (MOPP/ABV × 4 months) in the H8-U trial brought no benefit but additional toxicity, a result confirmed by the GHSG HD8 trial. The GHSG HD10 compared IF RT 30 or 20 Gy after ABVD (× 4 or × 2): the 4-year freedom from treatment failure (FFTF) and OS were similar in all groups. The EORTC/GELA H10 study adopts more stringent irradiation field reduction using the "involved-node radiation therapy" technique.

In advanced Hodgkin's disease, the need for additional irradiation after CT had remained uncertain until the results of the EORTC H3-4 trial. A parallel GELA trial (H89) showed that consolidative irradiation (S)TNI in CR or good PR after 6 cycles of CT provided no advantage over consolidative CT with two additional cycles. In the EORTC trial, involved-field RT 20 Gy was randomized versus no irradiation after six or eight cycles of MOPP/ABV in patients who had achieved a stable CR/CRu: irradiation proved not beneficial but detrimental with higher survival in nonirradiated patients due to toxic deaths (mainly secondary tumors).

In 1975, Bonadonna introduced ABVD (adriamycin, bleomycin, vinblastine, dacarbazine), which had a greater therapeutic efficacy but was less toxic and carcinogenic than MOPP. Despite its cardiac and lung toxicities, ABVD is now standard treatment for both localized and disseminated disease.

Although retrospective studies suggested a chemotherapy dose-intensity response relationship, testing the concept failed until the German HD9 trial, which was built on three data sets: a predictive model of the effective dose/outcome relationship according to existing randomized trials, use of hematopoietic growth factors, and a large phase II clinical trial.

In disseminated Hodgkin's disease, a meta-analysis launched by the German group identified seven factors for patient stratification, the "International Prognostic Score" (IPS). This index indirectly reflects tumor burden, but is insufficient. Early tumor response has been reported to have high predictive value since 1983, has been confirmed prospectively, and has been used successfully to adapt treatment by the EORTC. Replacement of conventional imaging by ^{18}F-FDG-PET, as in the H10 EORTC/GELA trial, may further enhance the usefulness of early response assessment.

Improvement in Hodgkin's disease control makes treatment-related deaths, which now exceed those due to Hodgkin's disease progression, less acceptable. Late effects of chemotherapy, although less serious than those of RT, are not negligible. The relative importance of each of the late effects, the risk factors (smoking for bronchial and bladder carcinoma, younger age for breast cancer) suggest preventive measures (field and dose reduction for radiotherapy, alkylating agent and anthracycline reduction for chemotherapy). Individual factors, studied prior treatment, strongly suggest that shorter telomeres and increased in-vitro radiation-sensitivity of the peripheral lymphocytes may help one to detect patients prone to late complications.

Since the early 1960s, several tests have been used as prognostic factors or for patient monitoring, notably the erythrocyte sedimentation rate. The search for other biologic-related factors continues and is promising. Europeans have investigated the biology of Hodgkin's disease. The development of microdissection techniques facilitated the microscopic isolation of single CD30-positive RS cells and enabled the demonstration of monoclonality and the B-cell origin of RS cells. The establishment of Hodgkin-derived cell lines by European teams contributes to clarify the contrast between the intense inflammatory reaction and the absence of effective immune response, particularly against the HRS cell. The survival of RS cells through multiple activations of antiapoptotic pathways had been correlated to the amplifications of the chromosome regions 2p and 9p, respectively, both frequent in Hodgkin's disease tumor cells. The autocrine/paracrine cytokines released through the interaction between the Reed-Sternberg (RS) cell and its cellular environment, as well as retrieving peripheral lymphocyte and tumor DNAs, are being explored. The virus "JCV" may play a role in RS cell chromosomal instability. EBV has been found in the RS cell at initial diagnosis and along the successive relapses and its role may be linked to genetic susceptibility. Nevertheless, the immune escape that favors RS cell survival and the immunosuppression associated with this disease may explain the difficulties of immunotherapy, although the CD30 antigen has long been used as a tool to pinpoint RS cells.

In summary, prognostic factors and predictors for early tumor response have been of paramount importance to reduce the aggressiveness of treatment and, hopefully, late effects, a major task in the therapeutic strategy. As Hodgkin's disease and patient populations are heterogeneous, treatment should be adapted accordingly.

In the early 1970s, many oncologists believed that a therapeutic strategy could be assessed by the analysis of the 5-year survival. Hodgkin's disease, with its high incidence of severe late effects, showed the need for very long follow-up (15 to 30 years). It also emphasized the usefulness of international cooperation on controlled trials, quality assurance, and continued medical education.

Vincent T. DeVita, Jr.

I like textbooks. I always have. I have been known to read a textbook of medicine from cover to cover, and am actually reading a new textbook on cancer biology from cover to cover at the moment of this writing. I highly recommend the practice. When well done, and by that I mean carefully edited, written by experts in the field and kept up to date, a good textbook is like a foundation stone. It can give the reader a genuine feeling for the field, in a format that allows one to get his or her arms around the subject.

It can also serve as a launching pad in the sense that by collecting all the relevant wisdom on the subject in one place, a good textbook also exposes the gaps in a field and can lead inquisitive investigators down new paths.

So it should come as no surprise that I like this textbook, as it is timely, written by experts, and collects all the relevant information on a single disease, Hodgkin's disease, in a readable text. I can say this with some certainty, as the editors were kind enough to provide me with the proofs of most of the chapters in advance of writing this foreword.

Of course I have a bias, as I have worked with and studied this disease myself for over 43 years and published the definitive work showing advanced Hodgkin's disease could be cured by combination chemotherapy 36 years ago. As an indication of the excitement caused by that work at the time, that article still remains the most cited article in the history of the *Annals of Internal Medicine*. That was because Hodgkin's disease was the first tumor of a major organ system in adults shown to be curable by chemotherapy, so it holds a major place in the history of cancer treatment and the birth of the field of medical oncology, which followed shortly thereafter. The sequence of events that led to the current state of affairs were recounted in the previous edition of this text in a chapter on the history of the treatment of Hodgkin's disease written by me and my long-time colleague and friend, Gianni Bonadonna.

The importance of the paradigm provided by the evolution of Hodgkin's disease from incurable to curable goes beyond the impact of the current treatments on patients with this disease. I try to point this out at every opportunity I get. The cure of Hodgkin's disease, and its companion tumor at the time, childhood acute lymphatic leukemia, led to the passage of the National Cancer Act of 1971, which in turn led to expansion and refinement of all modalities used for cancer treatment, worldwide, and the revolution in molecular biology that has made the field of cancer research so exciting today. The question really addressed in the 1960s was not could you cure these diseases with drugs, but could cancer ever be cured by drugs. Most people at the time thought not. The work with Hodgkin's disease and leukemia proved otherwise. For physician–scientists it is a human model of a human disease.

And, because we had proof that drugs could cure cancer, they were added effectively as adjuvant treatment for common cancers, and the early and dramatic declines in mortality rates in the United States for both Hodgkin's disease and childhood leukemia (greater than 75%) have been followed by a sustained decline in incidence and mortality rates for all cancers starting in 1990 and (what most critics thought was impossible, given the increasing size and age of the U.S. population) a decline in overall deaths from cancer starting in 2005. So, many more people who are afflicted with cancer are alive today as a consequence of the cure of Hodgkin's disease and childhood leukemia than the rather small number of patients afflicted with these diseases. Early in my career, I was often accused of working on a "boutique cancer." Because of its rarity, the model it provided was not clearly understood.

Another impact that the study and management of Hodgkin's disease had on cancer medicine is the model it provided for collaboration across specialties. From the beginning, radiotherapists, chemotherapists, pathologists, and surgeons worked together. It was sometimes a strained relationship, but it grew to the most prominent example of the benefits of specialty collaboration in cancer medicine that exists today, and patients have benefited greatly from those collaborations.

This is very apparent when one reads this text. Strained relationships have yielded to rigorous and productive debate among interested parties. Curing the disease, which occurred well before we understood the biology of the Reed-Sternberg cell, also enhanced the interest of researchers in studying the cell of origin and today, as pointed out in the text, we know the origin of the cell and have a workable understanding of its aberrant biology, which has identified new potential targets for treatment. That's the foundation stone provide by this book. It is all here in one convenient location.

The information provided in this text also identifies the gaps in the field. In this sense the book is a launching pad. For despite the dramatic advances in treatment and reduced toxicity, we are in some ways victims of our own success. Today, 40 years after the development of curative combination chemotherapy, and its coupling to radiotherapy, Hodgkin's disease patients are cured in approximately 80% of cases. But, at 15 years from the end of treatment, a patient has a greater risk today of dying of a complication of treatment than of Hodgkin's disease itself. Most patients, regardless of stage, receive combination chemotherapy and radiotherapy, and those that fail, especially those with long first remissions, are often salvaged with intensive treatment programs, coupled with autologous stem cell transplantation as support for marrow suppression. The search for newer combinations of more effective and /or less toxic drug combinations goes on, but, as is apparent when one reads this text, the major effort has been to find some way to reduce toxicity of treatment, while retaining both radiation therapy and combination chemotherapy in the mixture.

We know that the Reed-Sternberg cell is a crippled B-cell, although this has not helped us yet therapeutically. Markers expressed by the Reed-Sternberg cell, and aberrant molecular pathways, are now targets for either monoclonal antibodies or recombinant immunotoxins derived from them, or small molecules to attack the pathways important to the growth of the Reed-Sternberg cell, like the NF kappa B pathway, but the latter methods have not advanced rapidly in a clinical situation crowded by a bewildering array of treatment options. We don't quite know where or how to test new therapies. The highly resistant malignant cell in any cancer, including the Reed-Sternberg cell, in vivo, is no better as a model than cells grown in vitro and is as likely to mislead us as to enlighten us. We are more likely to discard good therapies tested in heavily pretreated, terminal patients, than to discover their benefits. Patients who have not been previously treated are, therefore, the best experimental model for testing new approaches, but can we include new treatments early in any curable cancer without facing an ethical dilemma?

Because the salvage treatments are so successful, it is not even possible to design a trial to test new treatment in previously untreated patients and expect to see a survival advantage. In fact, despite the dramatic improvement in overall survival of patients with this disease, it has been a rare study that has shown improved survival as a result of any new treatment and the different approaches we are using today have been added together almost intuitively.

Also, our success in translating empiric treatments into practice, by training legions of oncologists, especially in the United States, has proven a handicap to testing and adopting new methods. Many practicing oncologists are conservative. They tend to use tried and tested treatments in newly diagnosed patients, rather than enter them into clinical studies. The fact that a significant fraction of patients with these diseases may be cured with the existing regimens has frozen our management in time. Childhood leukemia shares the same fate, once again, with Hodgkin's disease. I like to refer to it as "the curse of the cure." Once a high percentage of patients are cured by existing treatments it becomes extraordinarily difficult to design trials to test new agents. We become pinioned to our old approaches like a butterfly under glass.

Thus, we need both new ways to test novel treatments in treatable malignancies like Hodgkin's disease and a willingness to consider change by participating in clinical trials driven only by a hypothesis, not specialty competition. We owe future patients an approach to improving the quality of their lives as novel as the new targets we now know exist, to overcome "the curse of the cure." By treating us to a rich panoply of information about this disease, this text provides very interesting food for thought on how Hodgkin's disease, this human model of a human disease, can once again lead the way in the management of other tumor types when we are fortunate enough to cure most cancer patients.

It's not likely that Thomas Hodgkin ever anticipated the intense interest that was to develop around the disease that now bears his name. Indeed, that interest far exceeds the actual impact of Hodgkin lymphoma on the human population. It is relatively uncommon, accounting for less than 0.6% of cancers in the United States, and a much smaller proportion worldwide. But it has served as a model for the introduction of new treatment approaches for cancer including radical radiation therapy, combination chemotherapy, and combined-modality therapy. At the same time, the excellent prognosis and long survival of patients treated for Hodgkin lymphoma and the careful study of their late complications have stimulated the "survivorship" movement among people who have been treated for all forms of cancer. More recently, biological concepts related to the potential etiology of the disease have fascinated scientists and opened new doors to potential therapies.

This is the second edition of a multi-authored international text on this subject that the editors have published. A notable change from the first edition (1999) is the title, which previously was *Hodgkin's Disease*. At the time, that title was chosen to create continuity and association with the seminal texts of that name authored by Henry S. Kaplan. For this edition, the editors have decided to adopt the now more standard nomenclature of Hodgkin lymphoma, as proposed by the World Health Organization Classification. This change has been incorporated throughout the chapters of the text, except in certain cases of historical context, and in the Forewords, at the request of those contributors.

In this edition, many chapters have been radically revised and others have been updated, a reflection of new biological insights and changes in management. Except for the story of Thomas Hodgkin, the chapters on history have been deleted, which actually provides enduring value to the first edition. As an alternative, Professors Vincent DeVita, Saul Rosenberg, and Maurice Tubiana have each contributed Forewords that include their personal reflections on the disease that has defined their careers.

In Section I, the chapters on epidemiology and association with the Epstein-Barr virus have been changed extensively. Virtually all of the chapters in Section II, Biology and Pathology, have been rewritten to include notable advances in our understanding of the biology of the disease. In Section III, separate chapters on surgical procedures and staging laparotomy have been deleted and the coverage of staging has been expanded to include separate chapters on anatomic and functional imaging. Section IV, Treatment Principles and Techniques, and Section V, Selection of Treatment, have been updated carefully and include summaries of all recent clinical trials. Section VI, Late Effects, includes results of new studies of cardiovascular disease, secondary cancers, and general survivorship issues.

This edition includes 30 new contributors, a reflection of the dynamic nature of research and treatment of Hodgkin lymphoma. The editors are grateful to all of the authors who have contributed to this effort, a commitment based on their desire to disseminate knowledge about Hodgkin lymphoma to scientists and practitioners worldwide. Our personal participation in this effort has been immensely rewarding.

Richard T. Hoppe
Peter M. Mauch
James O. Armitage
Volker Diehl
Lawrence M. Weiss

Hodgkin's disease and childhood leukemia, both uniformly fatal prior to 1960, were the first cancers discovered to be highly curable with the development of multi-agent chemotherapy and modern radiation therapy. The outgrowth of the successful treatment of these diseases has provided a prototype for strategies for the curative treatment of other cancers over the past 30 years.

The last definitive text on Hodgkin's disease was published in 1980 by Harvard University Press. Dr. Henry S. Kaplan, a clinician and researcher whose many seminal contributions greatly improved our understanding and treatment of Hodgkin's disease, wrote editions of this book in 1972 and 1980. The text had no co-authors or co-editors, an amazing feat by today's standards. We have retained the original title of his book to credit and honor his work.

In designing the current text, we choose to be as inclusive as possible. We wanted a broad representation of the knowledge and treatment of Hodgkin's disease, and we wished to credit those who have made important contributions to our understanding of the disease. As a result the editors represent the disciplines of radiation oncology, medical oncology, molecular biology, and pathology. There are over 100 contributors from all parts of the world. In trying to be as representative as possible we apologize to those we may have inadvertently omitted in the process.

Hodgkin's Disease is divided into eight sections to represent the many advances in this disease that have occurred since 1980. Each chapter has been designed to stand alone and to comprehensively cover a topic. By intent a topic may be covered in several different chapters. Hodgkin's disease was felt to be an incurable illness by most physicians until the mid 1960s. Many of the physicians whose work was instrumental in developing a curative approach to this disease have generously contributed their perspectives to Section I.

Advances in the etiology and epidemiology of Hodgkin's disease, especially for the emerging role of the Epstein-Barr virus, are covered in Section II. Section III, composed of eight chapters on biology and pathology, presents the many new and exciting advances in our knowledge of the pathogenesis of Hodgkin's disease.

Sections IV (Staging and Initial Evaluation, V (Treatment Principles and Techniques), and VI (Selection of Treatment) outline the current treatment options and ongoing trials for patients with Hodgkin's disease. These chapters should prove to be a valuable resource to physicians, nurses, medical students, and patients.

The late effects of treatment are covered in Section VII. Increasing knowledge of these effects has dramatically changed our approach to the treatment of patients with Hodgkin's disease. Finally, special topics are covered in Section VIII.

We had several goals in designing this book. We wanted to provide a reference text for training programs and researchers. We wanted to provide information and guidance for practicing physicians. Finally we hoped to provide a foundation for new ideas in laboratory and clinical investigation.

The treatment of Hodgkin's disease is sufficiently effective that now we have the luxury of reducing treatment intensity to avoid late complications. We look forward to advances that will enable us to better understand the pathophysiology and etiology of Hodgkin's disease. These advances should aid in its prevention and in the development of safer treatment approaches.

Peter Mauch
James Armitage
Volker Diehl
Richard Hoppe
Lawrence Weiss

CONTENTS

SECTION I: HISTORICAL ASPECTS, ETIOLOGY, AND EPIDEMIOLOGY

SECTION II: BIOLOGY AND PATHOLOGY

SECTION III: STAGING AND INITIAL EVALUATION

SECTION IV: TREATMENT PRINCIPLES AND TECHNIQUES

SECTION V: SELECTION OF TREATMENT

SECTION VI: LATE EFFECTS

SECTION VII: SPECIAL TOPICS

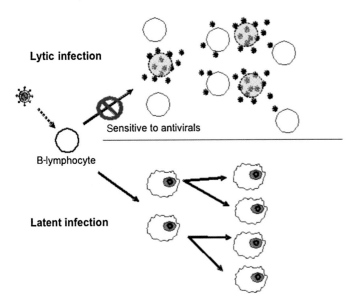

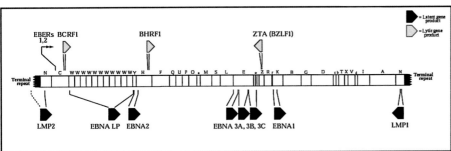

FIGURE 3.1. EBV infection of a B-lymphocyte. **Top:** When a virion harboring double-stranded linear DNA infects a B-lymphocyte, the lymphocyte may support the production of new virions, leading to the infection of other cells (lytic infection); or the viral genome may form an episome, express viral latency proteins that drive cell proliferation, and be passed on from mother to daughter cell without production of new virions. Replication of the viral genome and production of new virions can be inhibited by antivirals such as acyclovir and ganciclovir, but these agents have no effect on proliferation of infected cells. **Bottom:** Schematic map of the linear viral genome. Proteins discussed in the text are indicated. Vertical lines indicate Bam HI restriction sites. Restriction fragments are designated by letters. A variable number of terminal repeats are present at either end of the genome. (Artwork courtesy of M. Victor Lemas.)

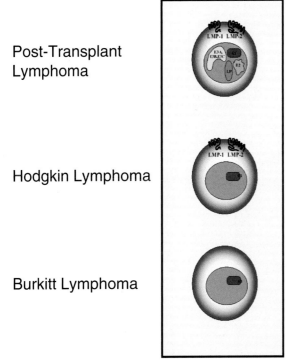

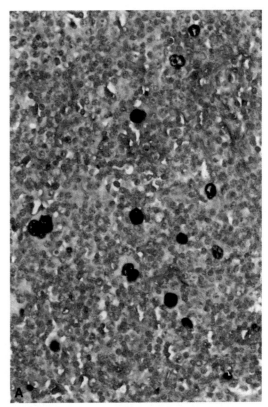

FIGURE 3.3. Epstein-Barr virus (EBV) in three types of lymphoma. Post-transplant lymphoproliferative disease is associated with expression of the full range of viral latency antigens in immortalized B-cells (latency I). Hodgkin lymphoma is associated with a more restricted pattern (latency II). Burkitt lymphoma is associated with the most restricted pattern (latency III). In Burkitt lymphoma, MHC class I molecules are often downregulated, and antigens are not processed for presentation. (Artwork courtesy of M. Victor Lemas.)

FIGURE 3.4A. EBV gene expression in Reed-Sternberg cells. A: Polymerase III transcript (EBER) in situ hybridization.

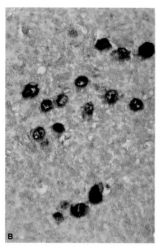

FIGURE 3.4B. EBV gene expression in Reed-Sternberg cells. **B:** EBER in situ hybridization with CD15 labeling of Hodgkin cells.

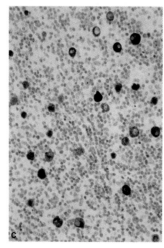

FIGURE 3.4C. EBV gene expression in Reed-Sternberg cells. **C:** Latent membrane protein 1 (LMP1) immunohistochemistry.

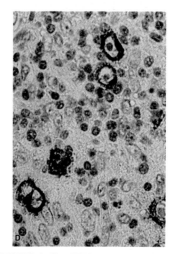

FIGURE 3.4D. EBV gene expression in Reed-Sternberg cells. **D:** LMP2 immuno-histochemistry.

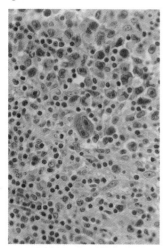

FIGURE 4.1. A diagnostic Reed-Sternberg cell with two nuclei is seen in the center, with a prominent eosinophilic nucleolus present in each nucleus. There is some chromatin clearing around each nucleolus. Several mononuclear Reed-Sternberg variants are also present in the upper half of the field.

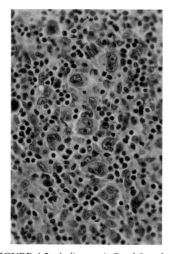

FIGURE 4.2. A diagnostic Reed-Sternberg cell is seen in the center, and many mononucleated and multinucleated Reed-Sternberg variants are seen throughout the field.

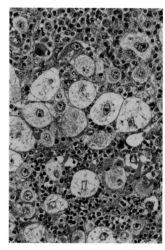

FIGURE 4.3. Several lacunar cells are present. A "mummified" Reed-Sternberg cell is in the upper left corner.

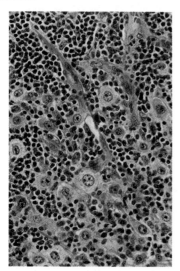

FIGURE 4.4. The background cells consist predominantly of small lymphocytes, along with scattered eosinophils, histiocytes, and plasma cells.

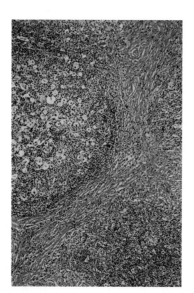

FIGURE 4.5. Nodular sclerosis Hodgkin lymphoma. Broad bands of fibrosis separate several nodules.

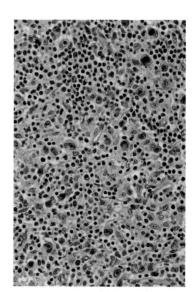

FIGURE 4.6. Mixed-cellularity Hodgkin lymphoma. There is an absence of fibrous bands.

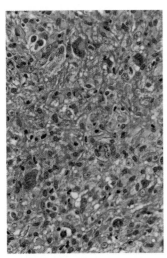

FIGURE 4.7. Lymphocyte depletion, diffuse fibrosis type. There is a reticulin collagen fibrosis around single cells. Although the Hodgkin cells appear atypical, results of immunophenotyping studies were characteristic of Hodgkin lymphoma in this case.

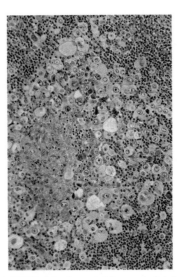

FIGURE 4.8. Syncytial form of nodular sclerosis Hodgkin lymphoma; sheets of lacunar cells are clustered around a central area of necrosis.

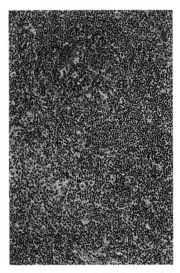

FIGURE 4.9. Interfollicular Hodgkin lymphoma. At the top is a reactive follicle. Several Hodgkin cells are seen in the interfollicular region in the bottom half of the field.

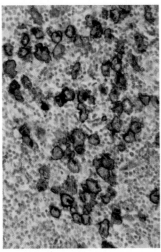

FIGURE 4.10. Immunostaining for CD30. There is strong membrane and paranuclear staining, and weaker cytoplasmic staining, of the Hodgkin cells.

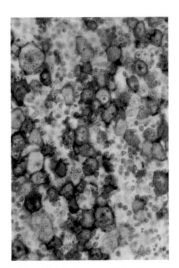

FIGURE 4.11. Immunostaining for CD15. There is strong membrane and paranuclear staining of the Hodgkin cells.

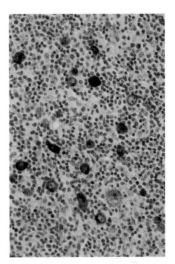

FIGURE 4.12. Immunostaining for Epstein-Barr virus (EBV) latent membrane protein (LMP) in a case of EBV-associated Hodgkin lymphoma. There is strong cytoplasmic staining, with paranuclear accentuation in the Hodgkin cells. EBV-positive small lymphocytes do not stain for LMP in Hodgkin lymphoma.

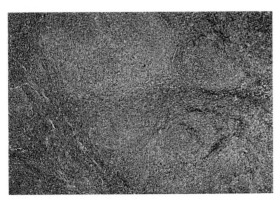

FIGURE 4.13. Nodular lymphocyte-predominanct Hodgkin lymphoma showing large irregular nodules, which are closely packed (hematoxylin and eosin).

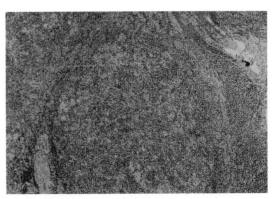

FIGURE 4.14. A nodule of nodular lymphocyte-predominant Hodgkin lymphoma is shown, composed mostly of small lymphocytes with scattered epithelioid histiocytes (hematoxylin and eosin).

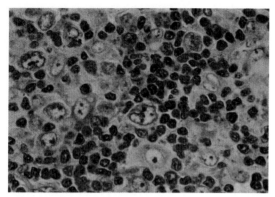

FIGURE 4.15. High magnification, showing characteristic L&H or "popcorn" cells (Giemsa stain).

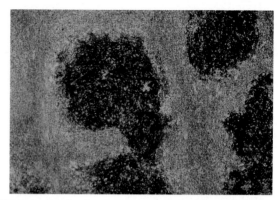

FIGURE 4.16. Follicular dendritic cells form large networks in nodular lymphocyte-predominant Hodgkin lymphoma (immuno-alkaline phosphatase, CD21).

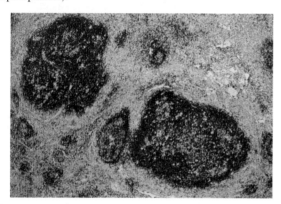

FIGURE 4.17. In addition to small lymphocytes, several L&H cells show a membrane-bound immunoreaction for CD20 (immuno-alkaline phosphatase).

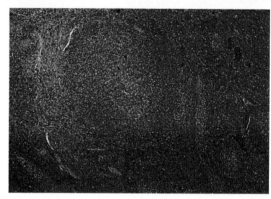

FIGURE 4.18. A large progressively transformed germinal center is surrounded by several small germinal centers (Giemsa stain).

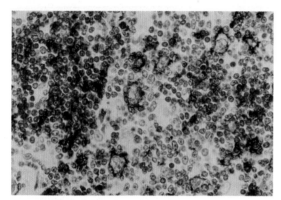

FIGURE 4.19. The progressively transformed germinal centers are composed mainly of B-cells, similar to the surrounding reactive follicles (immuno-alkaline phosphatase, CD20).

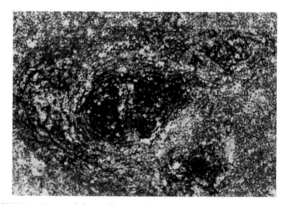

FIGURE 4.20. Nodular infiltrate of lymphocyte-rich classical Hodgkin lymphoma. Eccentrically localized remnants of germinal centers are visualized by immunostaining for follicular dendritic cells (immuno-alkaline phosphatase, CD21).

FIGURE 7.1. Immune response towards Epstein-Barr virus-infected cells in infectious mononucleosis and in Hodgkin lymphoma. In infectious mononucleosis, virus antigens are presented by HLA class I to CD8+ T-cells, which results in stimulation and co-stimulation, followed by proliferation and a cytotoxic response toward the virus-infected cells. The CD4+ T$_H$1-cells are activated by antigen-presenting cells and can give CD8+ T-cells help by producing IL-2 and several other T$_H$1-associated cytokines. In Hodgkin lymphoma there are only CD4+ T$_H$-cells present in the vicinity of the Hodgkin and Reed-Sternberg cells, and no CD8+ T-cells. This could be the result of a polymorphism or of absence of HLA class I molecules on the Hodgkin and Reed-Sternberg cells. Moreover, the CD4+ cells that surround the Hodgkin and Reed-Sternberg cells produce T$_H$2-associated cytokine IL-13, T$_H$3-associated cytokine TGF-β and T$_R$-associated cytokine IL-10. In addition, CD4/CD25 as well as Foxp3-positive regulatory T-cells are present. These cytokines (IL-13) may support the growth of the Hodgkin and Reed-Sternberg cells and further suppress a Th1-type cytotoxic response (IL-10, TGF-β).

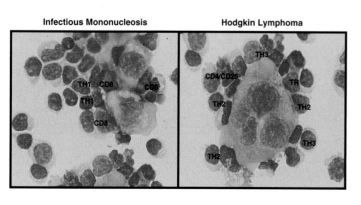

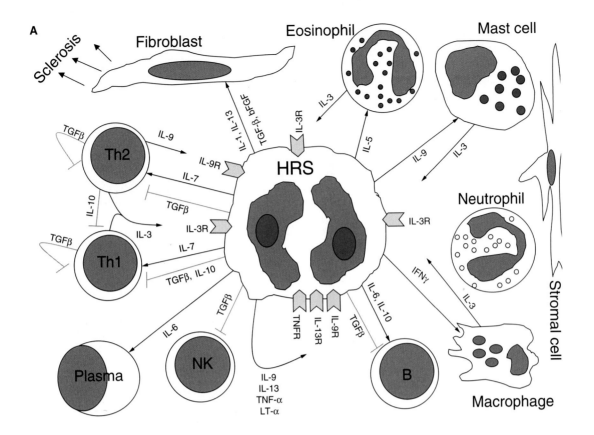

FIGURE 6.1A. Schematic representation of effects of cytokines and chemokines on Hodgkin and Reed-Sternberg cells and infiltrating cells. **A:** Schematic presentation of the cytokine effects. Black arrows represent positive/stimulating effects of cytokines and gray arrows represent negative/blocking effects.

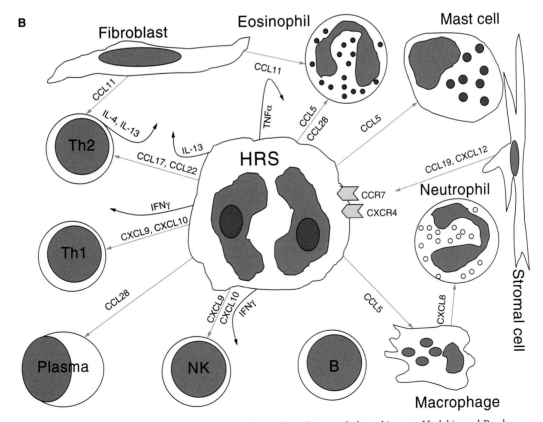

FIGURE 6.1B. Schematic representation of effects of cytokines and chemokines on Hodgkin and Reed-Sternberg cells and infiltrating cells. **B:** Schematic presentation of chemokine effects. Gray arrows present the chemokine attracting effects. Black arrows present the stimulatory effects of cytokines on chemokine production.

A) Microdissection

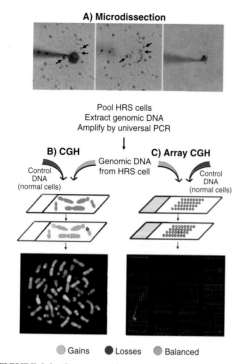

Pool HRS cells
Extract genomic DNA
Amplify by universal PCR

B) CGH

Control DNA (normal cells) → Genomic DNA from HRS cell → **C) Array CGH** ← Control DNA (normal cells)

○ Gains   ● Losses   ○ Balanced

FIGURE 8.2. Genome-wide screening for chromosomal imbalances by CGH and array CGH. **A:** Before CGH-analysis, HRS cells have to be enriched, for example, by microdissection using glass needles. Subsequently, the genomic DNA is amplified by universal PCR and labeled with suitable fluorochromes. **B:** In chromosomal CGH, the labeled probe is hybridized together with a differentially labeled genomic DNA probe from normal cells against metaphase chromosomes prepared from normal peripheral blood cells. Gains *(green)* and losses *(red)* within the tumor genome are recognized by different signal intensity ratios on the corresponding chromosomal target sequences of the hybridized chromosomes. **C:** In array CGH, arrays of genomic sequences (oligonucleotides, BAC clones) are hybridized instead of metaphase chromosomes. This allows the detection of chromosomal imbalances with higher resolution (~50 kb) as compared to chromosomal CGH (~5 Mb).

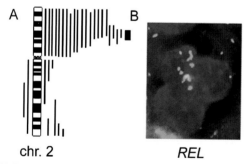

chr. 2   *REL*

FIGURE 8.5. Copy number gains of the short arm of chromosome 2 in primary Hodgkin lymphoma. **A:** Results from CGH analysis performed on pools of HRS cells derived from 40 different cHLs.[51] Gain of 2p or parts of it occur in more than half of the cases, while losses were never observed. The consensus region of these aberrations was defined by a distinct high-level amplification, which affects subband 2p15-16, where, for example, the *REL* gene is located. **B:** FISH analysis of a single HRS cell showing multiple *REL* signals *(green)* but only two signals of the centromere of chromosome 2 *(red)*.

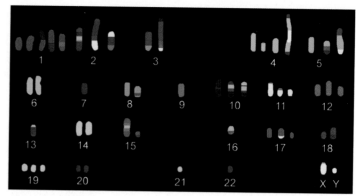

FIGURE 8.3. M-FISH analysis of HRS-derived cell line KM-H2. Individual chromosomes are differentially colored, making it possible to visualize the multiple rearrangements present in HRS cells. Note the complex composition of several translocated chromosomes and the frequently small size of translocated chromosomal bands, which are difficult to identify (e.g., by chromosomal banding analysis). (Image was provided by Dr. Anna Jauch, Human Genetics Department, University of Heidelberg, Germany.)

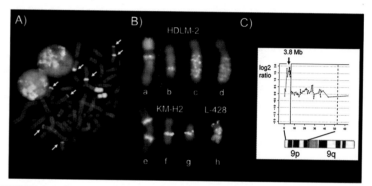

FIGURE 8.4. Segmental chromosome aberrations in HRS cell lines. **A:** Metaphase spread derived from cell line KM-H2 hybridized with a chromosome 7-specific painting probe. A number of segments inserted into different chromosomes *(arrows)* are visible, which are all derived from the distal part of chromosome 7q as demonstrated by the array CGH experiment (data not shown). **B:** Segmental chromosome aberrations of chromosomal region 9p24 in three different cHL cell lines. In *red*, the signal of a chromosome 9-specific painting probe is visible, while the *green* signal corresponds to a probe representing the *JAK2* locus on 9p24. a–c: Segmental chromosome aberrations of band 9p24 in three different chromosomes of cell line HDLM-2. In one chromosome, multiple insertions occurred. Segmental chromosome aberrations are flanked by r-DNA sequences, as shown in **(d)**, where an r-DNA-specific probe *(blue)* has been used for FISH. g–h: Three segmental chromosome aberrations of 9p24 in cell line KM-H2 and one in cell line L-428. **C:** Array CGH analysis of chromosome 9 in cell line HDLM-2. The hybridization intensity ratios (log2 ratio) of HDLM-2 DNA and normal DNA are shown for BAC clones distributed from the telomere to the centromere of chromsome 9p. As expected from the M-FISH results, the distal 9p region is strongly amplified. The size of this segmental chromosome aberration is 3.8 Mb and harbors *JAK2* as well as a number of other candidate genes like *PD-L1* and *PD-L2*. (From B. Radlwimmer, S. Ohl, P. Lichter, and S. Joos, unpublished data.)

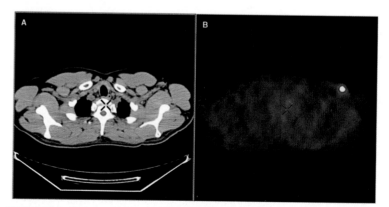

FIGURE 9.5. Patient with classical Hodgkin lymphoma with clinical involvement of left supraclavicular area. CT scan **(A)** showed small adenopathy in left axilla (did not meet size criteria), but the node was PET+ **(B)**. Radiation field was extended to include the left axilla.

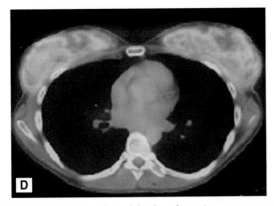

FIGURE 11.2D. Patient with Hodgkin lymphoma in recent postpartum status undergoing FDG-PET/CT scan for staging. Fused PET/CT (D) images clearly demonstrate the FDG-uptake in the breast tissue.

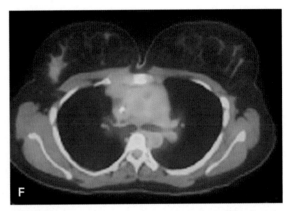

FIGURE 11.6C. PET/CT scans of a patient with Hodgkin lymphoma. Fused PET/CT (C) images demonstrate a large FDG-avid anterior mediastinal mass.

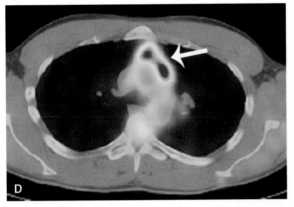

FIGURE 11.3D. PET/CT scan of a patient with Hodgkin lymphoma at the end of therapy. Fused PET/CT (D) images demonstrate that this uptake is within the thymus gland.

FIGURE 11.6F. PET/CT scans of a patient with Hodgkin lymphoma. Fused PET/CT image (F) confirms the diagnosis of complete resolution.

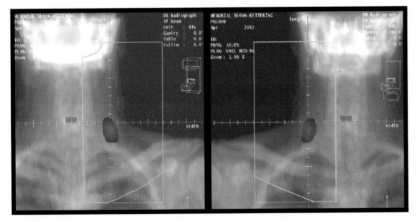

FIGURE 13.1. Involved-field irradiation for a patient with stage I Hodgkin lymphoma involving the left neck. The GTV (PET+ node) is displayed in red.

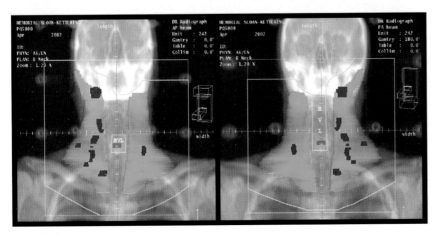

FIGURE 13.2. Involved-field irradiation for a patient with stage II Hodgkin lymphoma extensively involving the right neck and with a solitary node in the left neck. The GTV (PET+ disease) is displayed in red; the CTV (involved lymph node regions) is displayed in green.

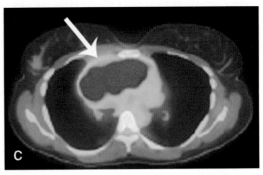

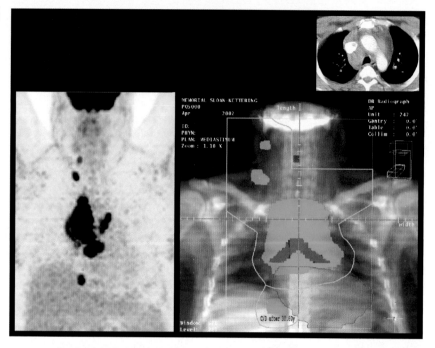

FIGURE 13.3. Involved-field irradiation for a patient with stage II Hodgkin lymphoma who has a large mediastinal mass and involvement of the right neck, right hilum, and right cardiophrenic region. The image at the left shows the FDG-PET localization of disease. The image at the top is an axial CT slice through the mediastinum. The GTV (PET+ disease) is displayed in green.

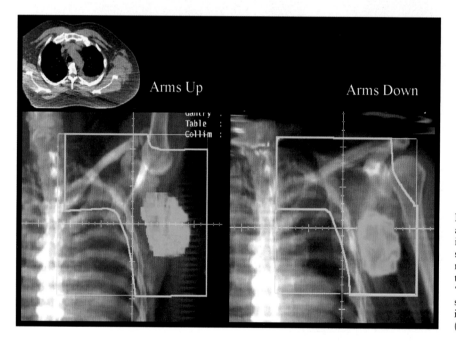

FIGURE 13.4. Involved-field irradiation for a patient with stage I Hodgkin lymphoma involving the left axilla. The image at the top shows an axial CT cut with the involved node outlined. The image on the left shows the field configuration with patient in an "arms-up" position. The image on the right shows the field configuration with the patient in an "arms-akimbo" position. The GTV (PET+ node) is displayed in green.

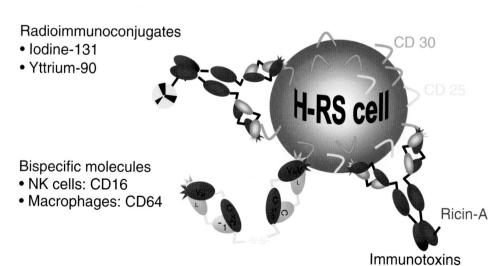

FIGURE 15.1. Examples of Mab-based constructs for immunotherapy of Hodgkin lymphoma.

HISTORICAL ASPECTS, ETIOLOGY, AND EPIDEMIOLOGY

CHAPTER 1 ■ BRIEF CONSIDERATION OF THOMAS HODGKIN AND HIS TIMES

SAMUEL HELLMAN

It is difficult to describe this complicated man and the world in which he lived in a brief chapter. To readers who are interested in a more detailed account, I recommend *Perfecting the World*, by Amalie and Edward Kass, and *Curator of the Dead*, by Michael Rose. The latter book title is an amalgamation of Hodgkin's official positions at Guy's Hospital, where he served as "Inspector of the Dead" and "Curator of the Museum," and although brief, the monograph gives the flavor of the man, which is more fully explicated in *Perfecting the World*.

Born August 17, 1798, to a family of staunch Quakers, Hodgkin was educated in and fully embraced the Quaker religion and worldview as a guide for his activities. This religious man was a major academic force despite spending most of his time in meliorist activities. A true Victorian, he was committed to the superiority of his civilization but also to the obligations required by noblesse oblige and his strong religious convictions. These missions informed much of his life. This chapter begins with a brief biographical sketch followed by an overview of his medical accomplishments and then some reflections on his social conscience.

Following a brief period as an apothecary's apprentice, Hodgkin chose a career in medicine and enrolled as a pupil able to walk the wards at Guy's Hospital. Because at that time Guy's and St. Thomas's had a close relationship, he was allowed to observe the clinical activity at both institutions. St. Thomas's is a venerable institution begun in the 12th century and named for Thomas à Becket. Much later, Thomas Guy, Jr., a wealthy benefactor, provided funds to build a new hospital related to St. Thomas's but devoted to investigation of new treatments for serious and incurable disease. Guy's Hospital opened in 1726 directly across from St. Thomas's. Essential to the development of Guy's into a leading world medical center was the extremely long tenure of Benjamin Harrison, Jr., who at age 26, succeeding his father in 1797, became the treasurer. He lived at the hospital and served for over 50 years. Although he was a despot who affected Thomas Hodgkin's life in important and unfortunate ways, he was strongly evangelical and a member of the Clapham sect, which encouraged religious piety by the poor and extensive evangelical missionary works abroad. We will return to Hodgkin's encounter with this man later.

Because Hodgkin was a Quaker, he was unable to enter the English universities of Oxford and Cambridge. Physicians were required to complete a university course of study; about one-quarter of the physicians in Britain went to those venerable institutions, while the remaining three-quarters studied in Edinburgh, Scotland, or on the continent. Hodgkin went to Edinburgh, accepted largely on the basis of the recommendation of the distinguished surgeon Astley Cooper, whose acquaintance he had made while walking the wards at Guy's

Hospital. It was at Edinburgh while still a medical student that he wrote his first paper, "On the Uses of the Spleen." This subject presages the description of the disease that bears his name. The Greeks believed the spleen to be a seat of laughter, and there was still a significant influence of Aristotelian and Hippocratic medicine on British physicians of the day. Hodgkin believed that the spleen's purpose was to regulate fluid volume within the body, clean impurities from the body, serve as a reservoir for excess nutrients coming from the gastrointestinal tract to the liver, and store and dispose of black bile (melancholy). He suggested that the spleen supplied expandability to the portal system. He noted that it was enlarged in many diseases but decreased in size with hemorrhage.

He interrupted his studies at Edinburgh to spend a year in Paris, then the center of medicine and intellectual life. In the 18th century, medicine was primarily an intellectual exercise based on logic and studies of the Greek scholars; but gradually in the beginning of the 19th century, it began to be based more on extensive observation; and later in the century, on experimentation. Medicine was considered to be a part of a broader intellectual universe, and British physicians were expected to have had a general education. While in Paris Hodgkin met with Laennec, who greatly influenced his approach to medicine. Laennec was among the most astute clinicians of the time, a careful observer who, among his many contributions, developed the stethoscope. But perhaps the most influential of the people Hodgkin met during that year was Baron von Humboldt, whom Hodgkin describes as the "hero of my youth," because of his interests in anthropology, particularly ethnography, a field for which Hodgkin had a great affinity. He also met Baron Cuvier, the distinguished anatomist and paleontologist whose Saturday soirees on both scientific and broadly intellectual subjects were often attended by the young medical student. A close contemporary was Thomas A. Bowditch, whose expeditions to Africa, concerned primarily with the ethnography of the natives, also greatly influenced Hodgkin's future activities. After this formative year in Paris, Hodgkin returned to Edinburgh to complete his studies. Following graduation from medical school, he returned to Paris to be the companion and traveling physician to Abraham Montefiore, a distinguished Jewish philanthropist who at that time was suffering from tuberculosis. Although Montefiore was dissatisfied with Hodgkin as a physician, they remained very good friends, and Hodgkin developed a lifelong friendship with Moses Montefiore, Abraham's older brother.

Hodgkin returned to London in 1825 to join the staff at Guy's Hospital, which had recently separated from St. Thomas's, to form a new medical school. In 1826 he was made "Inspector of the Dead" and "Curator of the Museum."

He also worked as a physician to the London Dispensary, a medical facility dealing with medical problems of the indigent, for which he received no fee but left after 2 years under acrimonious circumstances. During those years at Guy's Hospital, some of the leading doctors of the time were in active medical practice, including not only the surgeon Astley Cooper but the great physicians Richard Bright and Thomas Addison. And so, by his late 20s, Hodgkin had met many of the intellectual and medical giants of the time: Laennec, Humboldt, Cuvier, Bright, Cooper, and Addison. In addition, he became interested in the microscope and had a close association with Joseph Jackson Lister, who developed the achromatic microscope and was the father of the more famous Joseph Lister, who was responsible for aseptic surgery. This role of morbid anatomist provided the opportunity for the clinicopathologic correlations central to Hodgkin's career. In addition to this activity he greatly desired appointment as physician to Guy's Hospital.

In 1837, disaster struck Hodgkin; he ran afoul of Benjamin Harrison. The number of appointed physicians at Guy's Hospital was limited, and so his appointment required the death or retirement of an incumbent. With the retirement of James Cholmeley, Addison, an assistant physician, was expected to succeed Cholmeley, thereby providing a vacant assistant physician position. Hodgkin was felt to be next in line for such a position, and he was quite optimistic that he would be appointed. Unfortunately, his nonmedical activities had caused him to have some differences with Harrison. Hodgkin was distressed by the way the Hudson Bay Company was treating natives of western Canada. It was trading guns and alcohol for furs, and thus the traditional way of life was being destroyed but not replaced by that of a Western society. Harrison was one of seven members of the Grand Committee of the Hudson Bay Company, and Hodgkin was convinced that Harrison was sympathetic to his own values concerning the treatment of native populations. He wrote to Harrison, "I cannot believe that Benjamin Harrison, whose life is almost entirely devoted to institutions which have for their object the relief and amelioration of his fellow creatures, will either regard the subject with indifference, or have his attention fixed upon it without conceiving the means which may correct and retrieve the evil, or that he would advocate the cause in vain, were he to undertake it." Harrison was affronted by this letter, while Hodgkin, largely naive and unaware of how he was viewed, expected his support. When the opportunity to appoint an assistant physician occurred, Harrison effectively prevented the appointment, resulting in Hodgkin resigning from all positions at Guy's Hospital.

His activities in medicine, including a small and largely unsuccessful private practice as well as involvement in a number of medical and public health activities, continued until his death in 1866. In 1842, he briefly joined St. Thomas's Hospital, which had fallen considerably as a medical school when Guy's Hospital separated. Hodgkin was asked to design a new medical curriculum and to revive the museum. Again his naiveté caused him to be shocked and disappointed when he was not reappointed, largely because it was felt he had spent excessive funds on the museum. The remainder of his medical activities were limited to his small practice and to lecturing and writing on issues of public health, while his major efforts were with the betterment of aboriginal populations abroad as well as the poor of England.

From 1857 through 1866, with his friend Moses Montefiore, Hodgkin was involved in five journeys primarily concerned with helping Jews and Christians in Moslem lands. The relationship between the two friends was interesting; Montefiore, an observant Sephardic Jew, and Hodgkin, a religious Quaker, respected each other's religious views and were attracted to each other by their common adherence to religion and their actions on behalf of their fellow man consistent with their religious beliefs. On April 4, 1866, during the last of these trips, Hodgkin died of an unknown but lengthy illness and was buried in Jaffa. His brother John had inscribed upon the gravestone "Nothing of humanity was foreign to him." This was used earlier by Hodgkin when he dedicated his medical thesis to Humboldt. The quotation comes from the Roman slave Torrence: "He always thought that among all things nothing belonging to man was foreign to him." Unfortunately, this gravestone has been replaced with one much simpler and without this quotation.

MEDICAL ACCOMPLISHMENTS

Hodgkin played an important role in bringing the stethoscope to Great Britain while he was still a medical student. After spending a year as a medical student in Paris, he delivered a major lecture on the uses of the stethoscope devised by Laennec. This lecture at Guy's Hospital was considered to have been of major importance in the acceptance of the stethoscope in England, although there remained a significant number of practitioners who failed to appreciate its importance. As the Inspector of the Dead and Curator of the Museum of Morbid Anatomy, Thomas Hodgkin was in the vanguard of medical science. The correlation of clinical disease to pathologic material was quite new, and Hodgkin was the leading morbid anatomist of his day. Clinicopathologic correlation owes a great deal to Hodgkin, who in developing the museum at Guy's Hospital, had by 1829 over 1,600 specimens demonstrating the effects of disease. He taught the first core course in pathologic anatomy in Great Britain. He was critical of the vitalism of the time and emphasized the importance of the chemical nature of the body. From analysis of pathologic specimens, he described appendicitis with perforation and peritonitis. He described the local spread of cancer to draining lymph nodes, noting that the tumor at both sites had similar characteristics. All this was accomplished well before the microscope was used in pathology.

Hodgkin was also quite interested in microscopy and recognized the importance of the achromatic microscope devised by Joseph Jackson Lister. With Lister, the senior, he described the biconcave nature of the erythrocyte and the fibrillar and striated nature of muscle. They provided detailed descriptions of nerves and the three layers of arterial walls. They demonstrated that the globular theory of disease was false because the globules, due to aberrations in microscopy, were not present with the achromatic microscope. Although Dominic Corrigan is usually credited with first describing aortic insufficiency, it was Hodgkin who described the disease fully 20 years earlier. Using clinicopathologic correlation, he identified the valvular insufficiency and the bruit and murmur associated with this abnormality. Well before the separation of public health from clinical medicine in universities, physicians made contributions to both. These two areas of physician responsibility epitomized by the daughters of Aesculapius—Panacea and Hygeia—are both realized in Hodgkin; Panacea in the clinicopathologic descriptions of disease and Hygeia in his concerns for public health. He emphasized the dangers of lead pipes and proposed coating them with tin. He suggested that excessive cream and butter were harmful, and that wheat, to be fully nutritious, required the husk to be present. He recognized, probably for the first time, the importance of fiber in the diet, because he indicated that the consumption of the husk avoided the constipation associated with eating refined wheat. He recommended a decrease of sugar and meats in the diet and an increase in vegetables. He cautioned against both tobacco and alcohol.

Perhaps Hodgkin's major influences on public health were through his lectures on sanitation and adequate food and housing for the poor. As Asiatic cholera began creeping across Europe toward England, Hodgkin suggested that its effects could be limited by improving the conditions of the poor. He also recognized the contagious nature of the disease. Despite these efforts, there were about 80,000 cases of cholera in Britain during that epidemic, with an approximately 40% mortality. Both of these important clinical and public health contributions were central to the contemporary reputation of Hodgkin. They represent the essence of the man much more than that for which he is remembered in posterity.

He described in 1832 the eponymous disease for which he is known, in a paper entitled, "On Some Morbid Appearances of the Absorbent Glands and Spleen" that was presented and subsequently published in the *Medical-Chirurgical Society Transactions*. It was known at that time that cancer, inflammation, tuberculosis, and syphilis could cause lymph node enlargement. He separated six cases from the experience at Guy's Hospital as different, and added one sent to him in a detailed drawing by his friend Carswell. It is of interest that two of the six cases were patients of Bright and one of Addison. Subsequent histopathologic examination revealed that three of the cases, in fact, were Hodgkin lymphoma, which Hodgkin described from the gross anatomy because microscopic anatomy was not used until three decades later. He considered this lymph node enlargement different because it was not associated with pain or heat nor was it due to metastases from adjacent malignant tumors. This 1832 article was not widely recognized, although Bright in 1838 reported on the disease, emphasizing Hodgkin's original contributions. Samuel Wilks, in 1856, described the disease, quoting Bright and indicating he had thought that the observation was original until Bright had directed him to Hodgkin's original paper. In 1865, Wilks described the disease in further detail and attached the name Hodgkin's disease to this lymph node and splenic enlargement. It was also Wilks who in 1877 published "Historical Notes on Bright's Disease, Addison's Disease and Hodgkin's Disease," referring to these physicians as the three great men of Guy's, an appellation that has continued to this time. Although Wilks did not know of Hodgkin's priority until it was pointed out to him by Bright, Hodgkin mentions that the first reference that he could find to this or a similar disease was in fact by Malpighi in 1666. Hodgkin recognized that the disease spread primarily by contiguity of adjacent lymph nodes and that splenic involvement occurred late in the course of the disease. Nuland, in an interesting paper, has suggested that perhaps Wilks's generosity toward Hodgkin was not completely without pressure from Bright, although later Wilks and Betany, in *A Biological History of Guy's Hospital*, wrote "It must be said that in Hodgkin, Guy's Hospital lost one of its greatest ornaments and the profession in England one who was destined to add luster to its ranks." Before leaving the medical contributions of Hodgkin, I must cite his efforts in creating the University of London and its medical schools, the first in Britain requiring no affiliation with the Church of England. Both University College and King's College are a part of this university.

In June 1840, the 18-year-old Edward Oxford attempted to assassinate Queen Victoria and Prince Albert. Hodgkin appeared at the trial as an expert witness in his defense, supporting the view of moral insanity, which he explained as the inability to understand the significance of one's deeds or to refrain from criminal acts, despite appearing normal under many other circumstances. This carried the day, augmented by Oxford's seeming nonchalance and eagerness to accept responsibility as well as a strong family history of mental illness. It was the first successful use of this concept in English law.

NONMEDICAL INTERESTS

Hodgkin's involvement in the Quaker movement is central to understanding him and his activities. Not only was he born to a devout family, but he remained a devout member of the Society of Friends throughout his life. Deeply in love with his first cousin, he petitioned the society to allow the marriage of first cousins. Because of its refusal the cousins did not marry, and he remained a bachelor until 1850.

He was a strong and committed abolitionist whose animus toward slavery was a defining part of his life. This stemmed from his religion, but added to that, I believe, were the general meliorist views of some Victorian English. The dislocations produced by colonialism and the Industrial Revolution produced a great sense of responsibility to native peoples and the poor. This sense of noblesse oblige had a certain condescending tone based on the implicitly felt superiority of the English and of evangelical Protestant Christianity. The meliorist aspect of these goals also was consistent with Hodgkin's long-standing interest in ethnography, the latter enlarged by his association with Humboldt. Antislavery, concern for native people throughout the world including Africa, North America, New Zealand, and Australia, as well as a strong sense of responsibility, defined his life following his separation from Guy's Hospital. This was the time of extensive publicity and civic pride in the great English explorers, including Livingstone, Speck, Grant, and Burton in Africa; Palliser in the Canadian Rockies; as well as others in Australia. Livingstone, a medical missionary, embodied the many goals and responsibilities of mid–19th century Britain: civilizing, converting to Christianity, eliminating slavery, and exploring the world by the then dominant country. All those engaged in these explorations enjoyed wide publicity and public approbation, bringing to the British an awareness of indigenous civilizations. Many Victorians felt a responsibility to improve the plight of the natives, which included bettering their health, as a justification for imperialist goals. Hodgkin, although not particularly evangelical, was concerned with the well-being of the indigenous people. He founded and was the long-time president of the Aborigines Protection Society as well as a founder and long-term supporter of the Ethnological Society of London. The combination of his ethnologic interests and concerns for the welfare of indigenous civilizations was infused with his strong public health interests. Traveling with Moses Montefiore provided him opportunities for advocating public health measures not only in Britain but in North Africa, southern Europe, and the Middle East. Unfortunately, it was these very views that did not allow his advancement at Guy's Hospital.

SOME LESSONS FROM HODGKIN AND HIS TIMES

We cannot help but be awed by the prodigious accomplishments of this man. His medical accomplishments were primarily during the brief period (1825–1837) that he served at Guy's Hospital. Although his accomplishments continued after 1837, he became more enamored of his meliorist interests. The very breadth of his interests was grounded in an underlying worldview that many in the Victorian Age shared. This was still a time when medicine was considered a part of general intellectual activity, and physicians were expected to be broadly educated. Hodgkin is a paradigm of the best of Victorians and of physicians.

Hodgkin's success and his disappointment were due to his focus, drive, and naiveté as well as his prickly personality. Cameron, in *My Guy's Hospital* (1954), states that there was in Hodgkin's nature that which made it hard for him to obtain ultimate success in life, some perverse spirit that seemed always to place him in opposition. Although I believe that this characterization is neither accurate nor charitable, it does emphasize the way in which reformers and those who deviate from common practice are regarded.

Review of his scientific accomplishments reveals a mix of the prescient and what appears today to be ridiculous. His views must be considered in light of the then-contemporary state of medicine, with the continuing influence of the classic scholars and with the scientific method in its infancy. Systematic observation was just being appreciated as a requirement for acquiring new medical information, and the experimental method did not become widely used until later in the 19th century. Also remarkable is his close contact with the medical and intellectual leaders of the time. Hodgkin's acquaintance with Addison, Bright, Cooper, Humboldt, Laennec, Lister, and Montefiore is truly remarkable. All of these figures have had their names attached to diseases or entities that make them familiar well beyond their years. Addison's disease—adrenal insufficiency; Bright's disease—those several renal diseases associated with albuminurea; Cooper's ligament; Cuvier's duct; Humboldt's current; Laennec's cirrhosis. Even Lister and Montefiore have eponymous representations today—Lister through his son of aseptic surgery fame and for whom the genus *Listeria* is named; and Montefiore for the many monuments recognizing his philanthropic efforts, including the Montefiore hospitals. One lesson from Hodgkin's eponymous recognition is that it often does not represent the discoverer's major accomplishment. Hodgkin, were he alive today, would be surprised, I believe, that it is for Hodgkin lymphoma that he is remembered. Few recognize Laennec for the breadth of his clinical contributions or for the stethoscope; rather it is by the liver disease that his name continues to be familiar to physicians. Hodgkin lymphoma also teaches us something about the accuracy of medical attribution. Although the disease is associated with Hodgkin, he fully appreciated Malpighi's priority. Rene Gilbert, Vera Peters, and Henry Kaplan are associated with the notion of lymph node contiguity, but this was clearly described in Hodgkin's original article. The Reed-Sternberg cell was first described by Greenfield. Although Hodgkin described aortic insufficiency, Corrigan gets the credit.

From Hodgkin we also learn of the breadth of contribution possible, and of the extent to which a physician can extend his or her influence. He was concerned with individual patient care, medical research, and public health. But his commitments and contribution extended far beyond that to his obligations as a civilized human being. These latter were based on a particular and strongly felt worldview. This estimable person should serve as an exemplar for us all.

Bibliography

Bright R. Observations on abdominal tumors and intumescence, illustrated by cases of disease of the spleen. *Guy's Hosp Rep* 1838;3:401–409.

Cameron HC. *My Guy's Hospital.* London: Longman, 1954:154.

Hellman S. Thomas Hodgkin and Hodgkin's disease. Two paradigms appropriate to medicine today. *JAMA* 1991;265:1007–1010.

Hodgkin T. On the object of post-mortem examinations. *Lond Med Gaz* 1828;2:423–431.

Hodgkin T. *A catalogue of the preparations of the anatomical museum of Guy's Hospital.* London: R. Watts, 1829.

Hodgkin T. On the retroversion of the valves of the aorta. *Lond Med Gaz* 1829;3:433–442.

Hodgkin T. On some morbid experiences of the absorbent glands and spleen. *Med Chir Trans* 1832;17:69–97.

Hodgkin T. *Promoting and preserving health.* London: Cornhill Darton & Harvey Highley Fry, 1835.

Kass A, Kass E. *Perfecting the world: the life and times of Thomas Hodgkin (1798–1866).* New York: Harcourt Brace Jovanovich, 1988.

Kass EH, Carey AB, Kass AM. Thomas Hodgkin and Benjamin Harrison: crises and promotion in academia. *Med Hist* 1980;24:197–208.

Malpighi M. De viscerum structura exexcitato anatomica bononiae. *J Montij* 125–156. (Translated in *Ann Med Hist* 1925;7:245–263.)

Nuland SB. The lymphatic contiguity of Hodgkin's disease: a historical study. *Bull NY Acad Med* 1981;57:766–786.

Rose M. *Curator of the dead: Thomas Hodgkin (1798–1866).* London: Peter Owen, 1981.

Rosenblum J. An interesting friendship—Thomas Hodgkin, M.D., and Sir Moses Montefiore Bart. *Ann Med Hist* 1921;3:381–386.

Rosenfeld LR. *Thomas Hodgkin, Morbid Anatomist and Social Activist.* Lanham, Marytand, Madison Books, 1993.

Sakula S. Dr. Thomas Hodgkin and Sir Moses Montefiore Bart—the friendship of two remarkable men. *J R Soc Med* 1979;72:382–387.

Wilks S. Cases of lardaceous disease and some allied affections with remarks. *Guy's Hosp Rep* 1856;2:103–132.

Wilks S. Cases of enlargement of the lymphatic glands and spleen (or Hodgkin's disease), with remarks. *Guy's Hosp Rep* 1865;11:56–67.

Wilks S. Historical notes on Bright's disease, Addison's disease and Hodgkin's disease. *Guy's Hosp Rep* 1877;22:259–261,270–274.

CHAPTER 2 ■ THE EPIDEMIOLOGY OF HODGKIN LYMPHOMA

NANCY E. MUELLER, SEYMOUR GRUFFERMAN, AND ELLEN T. CHANG

HISTORICAL PERSPECTIVE

The early history of Hodgkin lymphoma is immensely rich, as documented in an extensive and comprehensive literature. In 1948, Hoster and Dratman[1,2] wrote one of the most extensive and thorough early reviews of the disease, which covered a bibliography of 572 late 19th to mid–20th century publications, clearly indicating that numerous physicians and scientists shared a great interest in the disease. Why has this disease, which is relatively uncommon, been of such great interest to generations of pathologists, oncologists, epidemiologists, and other researchers?

A large part of this interest has been focused on the long-suspected infectious etiology of the disease and the many curious epidemiologic observations about the disease. Several clinical features of the disease, such as fever, night sweats, and lymphadenopathy, have suggested an infectious etiology to investigators from the time of its first description. As a result, the literature is replete with scientific publications on suspected infectious causes of Hodgkin lymphoma. In the first part of the 20th century, there were reports of bacterial agents such as *Bacillus hodgkini* and *Corynebacterium granulomatis maligni*.[3,4] As late as the 1940s, Hodgkin lymphoma was classified in the category of infectious diseases in the International List of Causes of Death (4th edition) the precursor to the International Classification of Disease (ICD).[5]

The epidemiology of Hodgkin lymphoma is another source of fascination to students of the disease and also points to an infectious etiology. The landmark observations of MacMahon[6] regarding the bimodality of Hodgkin lymphoma age-specific incidence launched a whole new era of epidemiologic investigation of cancer causation. He was the first to recognize the bimodality in age-incidence patterns of the disease, and suggested that the young-adult form of the disease may be the result of an infectious process. Other investigators went on to liken the epidemiologic features of the disease to paralytic poliomyelitis and hypothesized that Hodgkin lymphoma was due to late age of first infection with a common infectious agent.[7–10] Two studies have provided confirmation of this hypothesis.[11,12] The notion of an infectious etiology for the disease was accelerated by two startling reports that suggested that the disease might be transmitted from person to person in schools.[13,14] Although these findings could not be confirmed by others, they led to another outpouring of publications on the possibly infectious nature of the disease.[15–17]

More recently, great interest in the disease has been generated by the use of molecular methods to identify the frequent presence of the Epstein-Barr virus genetic material in tumor specimens from patients with Hodgkin lymphoma.[18] The Epstein-Barr virus, a human herpesvirus that is the cause of infectious mononucleosis, was first isolated from a Burkitt lymphoma tumor specimen. The scientific data causally linking the Epstein-Barr virus with Hodgkin lymphoma have become compelling enough for the International Agency for Research on Cancer (IARC) in 1997 to classify the Epstein-Barr virus as a group 1 carcinogen (that is, "the agent is carcinogenic to humans") for Hodgkin lymphoma.[19] Thus, the intuition of generations of scientific investigators has finally been validated.

DESCRIPTIVE EPIDEMIOLOGY

Incidence, Mortality, and Variation with Age

The distinguishing epidemiologic feature of Hodgkin lymphoma is its bimodal age–incidence curve that is characteristically seen in economically advantaged populations such as in the United States (Fig. 2.1),[20] where the majority of patients are young adults. With relatively few cases occurring among children, there is a rapid increase of incidence rates among teenagers, which peaks at about age 25. Thereafter, incidence rates decline to a plateau through middle age, after which they increase again with advancing age. There is a male excess of cases, especially in children and in the middle and later decades of life.

In interpreting this unusual variation with age, MacMahon[21] proposed in 1957 that the bimodality results from the overlap of distributions of two diseases with differing age peaks. He further suggested that among young adults, Hodgkin lymphoma is caused by a biologic agent of low infectivity, while among the elderly the cause is similar to those of the other lymphomas.[6] As discussed below, the evolving epidemiology and molecular evidence of the Epstein-Barr virus in many cases has supported his hypothesis for the origin of young-adult Hodgkin lymphoma, although it appears that more than one virus is involved. The Epstein-Barr virus is also implicated in the etiology of Hodgkin lymphoma in many elderly patients, but other risk factors for this age group are largely undefined.

Currently, about 7,370 new cases and about 1,410 deaths occur in the United States annually.[20] The age-adjusted incidence rate from 2000 to 2003 was 2.7 per 100,000 person-years, and the mortality rate was 0.5 per 100,000 person-years.[20] For patients diagnosed with Hodgkin lymphoma between 1998 and 2003, the 5-year relative survival rate was 84.2%. The incidence rates for American males and females from 2000 to 2003 were 3.0 and 2.3 per 100,000 person-years, respectively. The 5-year

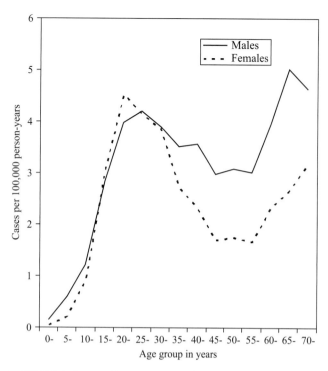

FIGURE 2.1. Age-specific average annual incidence rates of Hodgkin lymphoma, for all races by gender per 100,000 population, 2000-2003, in the United States SEER program.[20]

relative survival was higher for females (86.3%, non-Hispanic white; 85.7%, non-Hispanic black) than for males (83.8%, non-Hispanic white; 79.3%, non-Hispanic black).[20]

American whites have somewhat higher incidence rates of Hodgkin lymphoma than do other racial and ethnic subgroups, as shown in Table 2.1.[20] This observation reflects the role of socioeconomic status in modifying the risk of the disease in young adulthood, as well as the generally low rates in Asian populations. The current lifetime risk of developing Hodgkin lymphoma for American whites is 0.26% (1 in 385) and 0.21% (1 in 476) for males and females, respectively. That for American blacks is 0.19% (1 in 526) and 0.15% (1 in 667) for males and females, respectively. These estimates are conditional on surviving to age 95 years.[22]

TABLE 2.1

AGE-ADJUSTED AVERAGE ANNUAL INCIDENCE RATES OF HODGKIN LYMPHOMA, 2000-2003, IN MAJOR RACIAL/ETHNIC GROUPS IN THE UNITED STATES SEER PROGRAM[20]

Group	Incidence per 100,000 Person-Years	
	Males	Females
White (non-Hispanic)	3.5	2.9
Black (non-Hispanic)	2.8	2.1
Hispanic	2.9	1.6
Asian or Pacific Islander (non-Hispanic)	1.4	1.0
American Indian or Alaska Native (non-Hispanic)	1.1	0.7

Secular Trends

Between 1973 and 1994, the incidence of Hodgkin lymphoma decreased for both American blacks (−2.9%) and whites (−13.1%). Most of this decrease occurred in people aged 65 years and above—a total of 37.2%.[23] Glaser and Swartz[24] analyzed national data collected by the National Cancer Institute for 1969 to 1980 with correction for diagnostic error, based on time, age, and histology-specific confirmation rates from the Repository Center for Lymphoma Clinical Studies. Upon adjustment, they found that the incidence rates for older adults were lower than previously observed and showed no secular trend. Further, they found a slight increase for the nodular sclerosis subtype of Hodgkin lymphoma among young adults. An analysis of time trends and age-period-cohort patterns for the incidence in Hodgkin lymphoma in Connecticut between 1935 and 1992 concluded that the incidence increased among young adults aged 20 to 44 years. This increase was greater for women and primarily seen in the nodular sclerosis subtype of Hodgkin lymphoma.[25] More recently, between 1993 and 2003, the incidence rate did not change significantly among American non-Hispanic whites or blacks or Hispanics, whereas it increased by 5.2% per year among Asians and Pacific Islanders. The latter increase occurred primarily among young adults aged 15 to 39 years, with an annual percentage change of 8.3%.[20]

International Variation

The bimodality in the age-specific incidence rates of Hodgkin lymphoma, first noted in the late 1950s, continues to characterize populations living in economically advantaged, Westernized populations. Since that time, the peak incidence in the first (young-adult) mode has increased from about three to six cases per 100,000 person-years. In 1971, Correa and O'Conor[26] reported that a different age pattern was evident among economically disadvantaged populations. In these populations, there was an initial peak in childhood, but only for boys; relatively low rates among young-adults; followed by the late peak among those of advanced age. They further described an intermediate pattern, contrasting data from rural and urban Norwegians in the 1960s. The shift from the developing to an intermediate pattern in parallel with economic development has been noted by others.[27,28]

Currently, essentially all majority populations in Europe and North America have a well-defined, developed pattern of Hodgkin lymphoma incidence. The height of peak occurrence in young adulthood varies within this set of countries, being high in Canada, Switzerland, and Sweden, for example. The pattern within Eastern Europe is quickly evolving, which is also true for black Americans. In contrast, the pattern in Asia and Africa is generally intermediate or developing. Figure 2.2 shows characteristic age-incidence curves for females and males from various populations.[29] The malleability of the shape and age peaks within the first half of life in diverse populations in relation to economic and social environment underscores the importance of the generally protective effect of early childhood infections.

Variation with Socioeconomic Status

The association between the incidence of Hodgkin lymphoma in young adults and socioeconomic status has been found within populations based on the analysis of small-area socioeconomic status indices.[10,30] This association appears to be specific for the nodular sclerosis subtype of Hodgkin lymphoma.

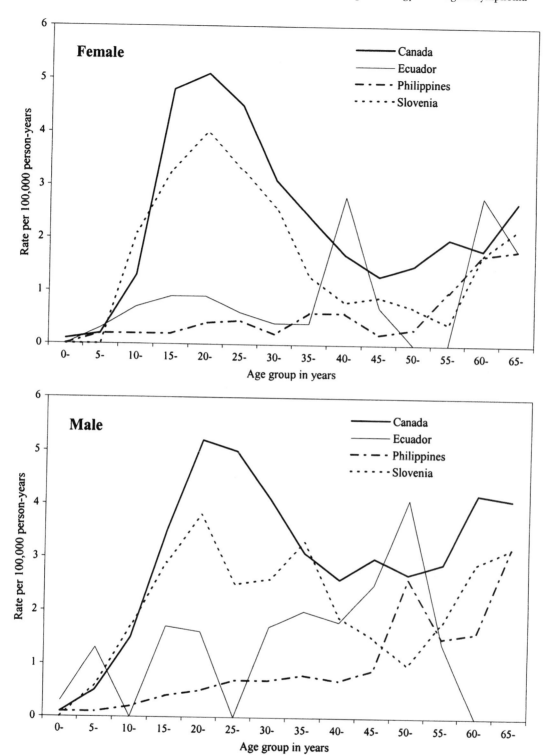

FIGURE 2.2. Female and male age-specific incidence rates of Hodgkin lymphoma in four countries per 100,000 population. (Reprinted with permission from Parkin DM, Whelan SL, Ferlay J, et al., eds. *Cancer incidence in five continents*, VIII, updated. IARC CancerBase No. 7. Lyon, France: International Agency for Research on Cancer, 2005.)

Henderson and associates[31] computed histology-specific incidence rates for Hodgkin lymphoma in Los Angeles County from 1972 to 1975 by socioeconomic status. They found that the incidence of the nodular sclerosis type was directly related to socioeconomic status, but there was no consistent association for the other histologic types. These data were confirmed and extended through 1985 by Cozen and co-workers,[32] who also found that the increase in incidence between 1972 and 1985 occurred only among cases of the nodular sclerosis subtype. They further reported that the risk pattern for mixed-cellularity Hodgkin lymphoma was quite distinct and negatively associated with socioeconomic status. More recently, Clarke and associates[33] evaluated the incidence of Hodgkin lymphoma in California from 1988 to 1992 in relation to an index of neighborhood socioeconomic status based on a set of census-based factors. As seen in Figure 2.3, the age-specific

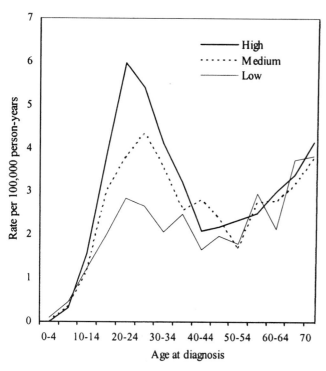

FIGURE 2.3. Age-specific incidence rates of Hodgkin lymphoma by tertile of neighborhood socioeconomic status (SES), California 1988–1992. (Reprinted with permission from Clarke CA, Glaser SL, Keegan TH, et al. Neighborhood socioeconomic status and Hodgkin's lymphoma incidence in California. *Cancer Epidemiol Biomarkers Prev* 2005;14:1441–1447.)

incidence rates varied directly with socioeconomic index tertiles for young adults, but not among older persons. This association was most apparent for the nodular sclerosis subtype in this age group.

These findings are consistent with national data. Using the United States Surveillance, Epidemiology, and End Results Registry (SEER) incidence data from 1969 to 1980, Glaser[34] reported that incidence rates for young adults were positively correlated with community-level socioeconomic status indicators, and that the incidence of the nodular sclerosis subtype increased in parallel with regional socioeconomic status indices. In general, the Hodgkin lymphoma cases occurring in economically developing populations and among lower socioeconomic status groups in developed populations are predominantly of the mixed cellularity and lymphocyte depletion subtypes,[35] and are more frequently Epstein-Barr virus–positive, as discussed below.

CLUSTERING

Given the long-standing notion of an infectious etiology for Hodgkin lymphoma, reports of clustering of cases have generated great interest. Clustering, which can be defined as the occurrence of cases close together in time and place at the time of their diagnosis, is a characteristic of infectious diseases. This is particularly the case for infectious diseases transmitted by direct person-to-person contact. It must be recognized that clusters of cases could also be due to common source exposure to noninfectious environmental agents. It should also be noted that many apparent clusters of cases are chance occurrences that become highlighted because of concerns about possibly causal environmental hazards.

In 1971, Vianna and colleagues[13,36] reported an extraordinary cluster of Hodgkin lymphoma cases centered around a single graduating class (1954) of a high school in Albany, New York. This reported cluster was noteworthy in several ways. First, the cluster was much larger than most previously reported cancer clusters, involving 31 cases of Hodgkin lymphoma. Second, the analysis of the cluster used epidemiologic methods more typical of infectious disease investigations. Third, cases were linked to one another both directly and indirectly through intermediate personal healthy contacts. This report generated a great deal of interest in the scientific community and in the lay media as evidence that an etiologic agent for Hodgkin lymphoma might be transmitted from person to person. Unfortunately, the Albany report did not employ appropriate control groups, and thus the significance of the findings remains undefined.

Since the Albany report was criticized for lack of a valid comparison group, Vianna and Polan[14] conducted another study on Long Island, near New York City. Here they used several infectious disease methods to assess whether students attending high schools in which diagnosed patients had been in attendance had an increased risk of developing Hodgkin lymphoma themselves. The first approach they used was a two–time period method. In this approach, schools were classified as positive or negative based on whether or not a student with Hodgkin lymphoma had been in attendance during an initial 5-year period. Students at high schools with cases (positive schools) and without cases (negative schools) during the first 5-year period were observed for a subsequent 5-year period. Comparisons were then made between the occurrence of Hodgkin lymphoma in positive schools and negative schools during the second period. Five of eight positive schools and none of 16 matched negative schools had cases diagnosed during the second period, a truly remarkable finding. The second approach they used was an index–secondary case method. The risk of Hodgkin lymphoma was assessed in those students and teachers who had overlapped in attendance with a diagnosed case for a period of a year. Comparison was then made between the expected occurrence of Hodgkin lymphoma in those subjects exposed to cases and that observed. There were 21 Hodgkin lymphoma cases observed in students versus 9.3 cases expected. For teachers, 7 Hodgkin lymphoma cases were observed versus 0.9 expected secondary cases. Both approaches yielded strong evidence of an increased risk of Hodgkin lymphoma in children and, to a lesser extent, in teachers, exposed to cases in the high school setting.

Several studies attempted to replicate the Long Island findings. Smith and co-workers[16] conducted a case-control study of Hodgkin lymphoma in Oxford, England, in which links between subjects were assessed. They found no evidence of person-to-person transmission. We performed a close replication of the Long Island study in the greater Boston area. Using two–time period approaches with varying time intervals and index–secondary case approaches, no increased risk of Hodgkin lymphoma was observed in students who had contact with Hodgkin lymphoma cases or attended positive schools in the Boston area.[17] Thus, the Long Island study findings could not be confirmed in other settings.

It is possible that the Long Island study findings are an artifact of cancer treatment referral patterns, because cases were identified via hospital and other treatment facility records.[17] Long Island is in close proximity to New York City, where there are several major cancer treatment centers. In contrast, Long Island at the time did not have any major cancer treatment centers. Attempts were made by the researchers to identify Long Island Hodgkin lymphoma cases in a search of selected hospitals in New York City. However, the hospitals surveyed were not the major cancer treatment centers. If patients living in close proximity to New York City were frequently referred to hospitals in the city and not entered into the study, and those patients residing further from

New York City received their treatment locally, then this could produce an artifact of clustering. Support for this interpretation is provided by the observation that the annual incidence rate of Hodgkin lymphoma on Long Island reported by Vianna and Polan was lower than the mortality rate for Hodgkin lymphoma reported by the National Cancer Institute for the same area at the same time.[17]

Newer statistical methods have been developed for assessing time-space clustering. Earlier methods were available for statistically assessing whether cases were closer together in time and space at diagnosis than would be expected by chance.[37–39] Simpler new methods have been developed that rely on closeness at time of diagnosis without need to consider the geographic frame. Although the earlier statistical methods of assessing time-space clustering essentially proved negative, some of the newer approaches suggest that there might be weak clustering of cases.[40]

In summary, at present there is little strong or persuasive evidence of clustering of Hodgkin lymphoma. This is important for clinical management in that patients can be reassured that there is no risk of their transmitting the disease to others. Relatives and friends may recall media reports of transmissibility of the disease and unnecessarily alarm patients about their possible contagiousness. Patients should be informed that this is definitely not the case.

GENETIC FACTORS

Familial Aggregation

Familial aggregation and genetic susceptibility play important roles in the causation of Hodgkin lymphoma. It is now well established that first-degree relatives of patients with Hodgkin lymphoma have about a threefold increased risk of developing the disease. As will be discussed below, this risk is greatest in identical twins, younger relatives, and siblings, particularly gender-concordant siblings of patients, and lowest in older relatives and parents of patients. Thus, the threefold increased risk is not uniform for all close relatives of patients. Several studies have also found an increased risk of other lymphoreticular malignancies (non-Hodgkin lymphoma and leukemia) in first-degree relatives of patients with Hodgkin lymphoma and vice versa. However, the increased risk of other lymphomas and leukemia is only slight, and on the order of about 1.2 to 2 times the expected population rates; and similarly weak results are found for the occurrence of Hodgkin lymphoma in relatives of patients with non-Hodgkin lymphoma.[41–43] In a recent, large Scandinavian we found a 3.3-fold, significantly increased risk of Hodgkin lymphoma in relatives of patients with non-Hodgkin lymphoma; however, we found no excess of non-Hodgkin lymphoma in relatives of patients with Hodgkin lymphoma.[44]

In an early population-based study in the greater Boston area, we found an increased Hodgkin lymphoma risk in siblings of young-adult patients but no increased risk in siblings of older adults with the disease.[45] Siblings of young-adult patients appeared to have a sevenfold increased risk of the disease. Curiously, siblings of the same gender as the patient were at higher risk of the disease (ninefold) than were opposite-gender siblings (fivefold). We hypothesized that this might be due to gender-concordant sibling pairs having more shared environmental exposures (for example, shared bedrooms or friends) than did gender-discordant sibling pairs. We reviewed the world literature on reported sibling pairs with Hodgkin lymphoma and found confirmation of our findings. A second, later review of the literature also found an excess of reported same-gender sibling pairs.[46]

More recently, excess gender-concordance of sibling pairs has been observed for non-Hodgkin lymphoma and for chronic lymphocytic leukemia, now considered to be a lymphoma.[41,47] Excess gender concordance of affected sibling pairs has also been reported for Behçet disease, multiple sclerosis, and sarcoidosis.[46] As pointed out by Sellick and associates, these are all diseases characterized by immunologic dysfunction and observed human leukocyte antigen (HLA) associations and most are also suspected of having an infectious etiology.[46,47] Such observations have led to the hypothesis that the gender concordance is due to interplay of genetic susceptibility and shared environmental exposures.[45,47] An alternative explanation for the gender concordance observations, proposed by Horwitz and Wiernik,[48] suggests that some of this excess might be related to genes located in the pseudoautosomal region of the sex chromosomes. Although this hypothesis needs further testing, it seems more likely that the unusual pattern of sibling occurrence of Hodgkin lymphoma is due to the interplay of both environmental and genetic factors.

Mack and co-workers[49] reported a remarkably increased risk in monozygotic twins of Hodgkin lymphoma cases. They found that among 179 monozygotic twin pairs with at least one twin affected with Hodgkin lymphoma, there were 10 pairs who became concordant for Hodgkin lymphoma, relative risk = 99(48–182). None of 187 pairs of dizygotic twins with one affected member became concordant for Hodgkin lymphoma. The authors indicated that the absence of an increased risk of Hodgkin lymphoma in the dizygotic twins of cases was probably due to a much lower genetic predisposition and to a very low risk of Hodgkin lymphoma in their small population of twins. Nevertheless, it is curious that a remarkably increased risk was observed for monozygotic twins, with no increased risk for the heterozygotic twins. This is an unusual study in that the subjects were identified via advertisements in newspapers and other media soliciting participation in the study of twins with cancer. The question arises as to whether the use of advertising to identify twin pairs might not have led to selective reporting of doubly affected pairs or of monozygotic twin pairs. Nevertheless, it is hard to imagine that such bias would lead to the extremely high relative risk observed. The earlier Boston study of sibling pairs with the disease suggested an interaction between genetic susceptibility and shared childhood exposures. The observation by Mack and associates of a remarkably increased risk of Hodgkin lymphoma in monozygotic twins, but not in heterozygotic twins, would argue in favor of a purely genetic basis for this susceptibility to this disease.

Other researchers have also concerned themselves with genetic issues relating to Hodgkin lymphoma. Chakravarti and colleagues[50] identified 41 pedigrees from a variety of sources and performed linkage analyses on these pedigrees. They found strong evidence of a recessive susceptibility gene tightly linked to the (HLA) complex and responsible for 60% of cases in multiplex families. The residual 40% was suggested to be due to other familial and/or environmental factors. They found no increase in gender concordance, but an increased concordance for histologic type. He concluded that there is etiologic heterogeneity in Hodgkin lymphoma with at least three independent determinants: an HLA-linked gene, an HLA-unlinked factor, and an environmental/genetic factor determining concordance in histologic type.

Attention was directed to observations of genetic anticipation in Hodgkin lymphoma and in other lymphoproliferative malignancies. Genetic anticipation is the phenomenon in which there is earlier age of onset or increased severity of a familial disease in successive generations. However, a recent, well-designed and analyzed, population-based study failed to find support for genetic anticipation in Hodgkin lymphoma, chronic lymphocytic leukemia, or non-Hodgkin lymphoma.[51]

Thus, it seems likely that previous observations of anticipation were the result of failing to account for confounders such as incidence changes over time or ascertainment bias.

No specific Hodgkin lymphoma gene has yet been identified. A recent study performed genome-wide linkage screening in 44 high-risk Hodgkin lymphoma families with 254 individuals.[52] The strongest linkage was found on chromosome 4p near the marker D4S394, and weaker linkage was found on chromosomes 2 and 11. Their results were also consistent with recessive inheritance for Hodgkin lymphoma. These promising results were for highly selected, high-risk families and thus may have limited generalizability to all patients with Hodgkin lymphoma.

Preliminary results from a large case-control study of childhood Hodgkin lymphoma currently in progress suggest that first-degree relatives of patients younger than 15 years of age at diagnosis had a 2.7-fold increased risk of *all* cancers. In a series of 464 patients with Hodgkin lymphoma and 699 individual-matched controls, 29 patients and 17 controls had a first-degree relative with a diagnosis of cancer. Four patients had parents with Hodgkin lymphoma but none of the controls did, and there appeared to be an increased occurrence of all lymphoreticular malignancies, melanoma, and testicular cancer in patient families.[53] A previous study by Olsen and associates[54] examined the risks of cancer in parents of childhood cancer cases from Denmark. Overall, they found no increased occurrence of cancer in parents of patients, and they specifically observed no increased risk of cancer in parents of children with Hodgkin lymphoma. This discrepancy may be accounted for by the fact that the case-control study from the United States and Canada obtained data by direct interview of parents of patients, whereas the Scandinavian study relied upon linkage of registry records, which are not subject to reporting bias.

Human Leukocyte Antigen

There have been many investigations of associations between human leukocyte antigen HLA types and risk of Hodgkin lymphoma. Early case-control studies from Scandinavia identified a slightly increased risk of Hodgkin lymphoma associated with the class I HLA antigens A1, B5, B8, and B18. It was found that persons with these HLA types had relative risks of Hodgkin lymphoma ranging from 1.3 to 1.5.[55,56] Subsequent studies of HLA and Hodgkin lymphoma risk have led to a good deal of confusion, some of which relates to the fact that some studies found HLA associations with only certain histologic subtypes of the disease and others did not. Nevertheless, there appears to be consistency in the findings of an association between Hodgkin lymphoma and HLA-A1 and, to a lesser degree, HLA-B5, -B8, and -B18.[56] More recently, Oza and co-workers[56] pooled data from 17 centers to obtain HLA data for 741 patients with Hodgkin lymphoma and 686 controls. Using more modern approaches defining specific alleles, they found a RR of 1.95 ($p <0.01$) for HLA-DPB1*0301 in white patients. There were significant reductions in the frequency of HLA-DPB1*0401 in patients from Japan and Taiwan, with a RR of 0.15 ($p <0.01$). They also found decreased duration of remission in patients with HLA-DPB1*0901 overall ($p <0.05$) and particularly in Japan and Taiwan ($p = 0.02$), where this type is most prevalent.

There have also been attempts to relate Epstein-Barr virus positivity of tumors from Hodgkin lymphoma patients with HLA types. This was done because HLA-A*0201 in healthy seropositive individuals is known to be associated with the cytotoxic T-cell response to the LMP-2 protein of the virus.[57] However, no associations could be found between Epstein-Barr virus status and HLA-A2 in two studies.[57,58] Subsequent studies of the relationship between HLA alleles and presence or absence of Epstein-Barr virus in Hodgkin lymphoma tumor tissues have yielded mixed results. A study from Scotland found that a higher proportion of EBV-positive cases typed positively for HLA-DPB1*0301 than did EBV-negative cases (43% versus 31%), but the difference was not statistically significant. This study also showed a strong association of this HLA allele with history of infectious mononucleosis in EBV-positive cases versus EBV-negative cases, odds ratio (OR) = 17.1(1.1–11.8), but this finding was based on very small numbers of cases.[59] A recent Dutch study performed very comprehensive analyses of HLA classes and polymorphisms in Epstein-Barr virus positive and negative Hodgkin lymphoma tumor specimens.[60] They found a significant association between EBV-positive tumors and the HLA class I region markers, D6S65 and D6S510. They also reported a significant difference in mean haplotype sharing between patients and controls surrounding the HLA class III marker D6S273. The authors conclude that areas within the HLA class I and class III regions are associated with susceptibility to Hodgkin lymphoma and the class I finding was specific for EBV-positive disease.

To summarize, the relationships between HLA types and Hodgkin lymphoma are generally weak and many findings have been inconsistent. Recent studies of the relationships between tumor Epstein-Barr virus status and HLA have not shed great light on susceptibility factors for the development of Epstein-Barr virus-positive disease. It appears that HLA type is a weak risk factor for Hodgkin lymphoma at best.

Increased Risk among Jews

It has been noted (but often overlooked) that Jews are at somewhat higher risk of Hodgkin lymphoma. In an early population-based case-control study conducted in Brooklyn, New York in the 1940s and 1950s, MacMahon found that older—but not younger—Jews were at increased risk.[21] However, in our population-based case-control study conducted in eastern Massachusetts in the 1970s, both young-adult and older Jews had notably higher rates of the disease than non-Jews.[12] As observed in our more recent study in eastern Massachusetts and Connecticut, the excess risk among young-adult and middle-aged Jews persisted through the late 1990s.[42] The level of affluence among American Jews increased substantially across these three generations. It is likely that in the earliest study, most subjects were infected with Epstein-Barr virus and other common infections in childhood due to more crowded living conditions and larger families, which reduced their risk for young-adult Hodgkin lymphoma. In our 1970s study, the risk related to being Jewish was still two to three times higher for all age groups after controlling for indices of socioeconomic status.[61] The finding of increased risk among Jews was confirmed by later population-based studies in Great Britain,[62,63] Los Angeles,[32] and Israel.[64] In our recent study there was an 80% excess risk among Jews between ages 15 and 54 years[42]; however, this finding was not evident among those subjects aged 55 years or more.

ENVIRONMENTAL/LIFESTYLE RISK FACTORS

Risk Factors Related to Age at Infection

There is a consistent body of evidence that risk of Hodgkin lymphoma is associated with factors in the childhood social environment that influence age at infection with the Epstein-Barr virus or very similar viruses. These associations pertain

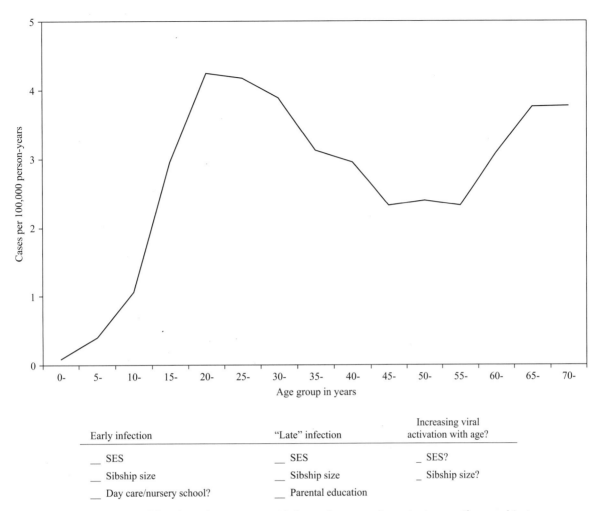

Early infection	"Late" infection	Increasing viral activation with age?
__ SES	__ SES	_ SES?
__ Sibship size	__ Sibship size	_ Sibship size?
__ Day care/nursery school?	__ Parental education	

FIGURE 2.4. Childhood social environment risk factors by age at diagnosis. Age-specific annual incidence rate of Hodgkin lymphoma for all races and both genders combined per 100,000 population, 2000-2003, in the United States SEER program.[20] SES, socioeconomic status.

to risk of the disease occurring from early childhood through middle age, that is, within the first incidence peak. Among patients who are diagnosed in their 50s or later, there is no apparent or consistent association with indicators of childhood socioeconomic status (Fig. 2.4).[20]

Children

Although a great deal is known about environmental risk factors for adult-onset Hodgkin lymphoma, relatively little is known about such factors for childhood Hodgkin lymphoma. This is not surprising, given the extreme rarity of this lymphoma diagnosed in children younger than 15 years of age. We conducted a population-based case-control study of Hodgkin lymphoma in the greater Boston area in which limited demographic data were collected from the annual town registers.[65] We found that the 14 very young children (less than age 10) with Hodgkin lymphoma came from lower socioeconomic status backgrounds than did the population controls. However, no socioeconomic status differences were observed for the 52 children who were 10 to 14 years of age at diagnosis. This finding suggests a transition in socioeconomic status of patients with Hodgkin lymphoma from early to later

childhood, in parallel with their probable age at infection with the Epstein-Barr virus.

We are currently conducting a large multi-institutional case-control study of childhood Hodgkin lymphoma in the United States and Canada at the University of New Mexico. Over 570 cases of Hodgkin lymphoma in children under age 15 years and matched controls are being compared for differences in environment and lifestyle factors. In an analysis of 506 cases and 763 community controls, we found inverse associations with risk of Hodgkin lymphoma with family income at birth (a 2.6 gradient in RR from lowest to highest category, p for trend ≤ 0.0001); similarly, a 1.6 gradient for income at time of interview ($p = 0.01$). In parallel, there was a nearly threefold inverse gradient for mothers' educational level ($p \leq 0.0001$). Sibship size was positively associated with Hodgkin lymphoma risk by a 2.4-fold direct gradient, ($p = 0.13$) (S. Grufferman, unpublished). As shown in Table 2.2, Westergaard and colleagues[66] conducted a population-based cohort study involving over two million Danes whose mothers were born in Denmark since 1935. They compared the sibship size and birth order among the 72 children (and 306 young adults) in Denmark who developed Hodgkin lymphoma to the rest of the cohort. For the children, they found there was a significant gradient of 1.28-fold in RR from children in the

TABLE 2.2

RELATIVE RISK (RR) AND 95% CONFIDENCE INTERVAL (CI) OF DEVELOPING HODGKIN LYMPHOMA IN A DANISH COHORT OF CHILDREN BY SIBSHIP SIZE AND BIRTH ORDER FOR DIAGNOSIS IN CHILDHOOD AND YOUNG ADULTHOOD

| | Age at diagnosis | | | |
| | <15 years | | ≥15 years | |
	RR (95% CI)	Trend[a](95% CI)	RR (95% CI)	Trend (95% CI)
Sibship Size[b]				
1	0.71(0.31–1.61)		0.80(0.50–1.28)	
2	1.00 ref.	1.28(1.00–1.63)	1.00 ref.	0.91(0.81–1.03)
3	0.94(0.53–1.68)	$p = 0.06$	0.94(0.73–1.22)	$p = 0.12$
4	1.11(0.46–2.66)		0.74(0.50–1.09)	
5+	3.31(1.36–8.02)		0.57(0.30–1.08)	
Birth Order[c]				
1	1.00 ref.		1.00 ref.	
2	0.93(0.50–1.70)	1.26(0.92–1.73)	0.98(0.74–1.28)	0.85(0.71–1.01)
3	2.04(0.97–4.26)	$p = 0.17$	0.78(0.50–1.22)	$p = 0.07$
4	1.50(0.42–5.33)		0.30(0.10–0.97)	

[a]Trend is the relative increase in risk of Hodgkin lymphoma per increase in sibship size or birth order.
[b]Adjusted for age, gender, year of diagnosis, and maternal age at birth of children.
[c]Adjusted for age, gender, year of diagnosis, maternal age at birth of child, and number of younger siblings.
Reprinted with permisssion from Westergaard T, Melbye M, Pedersen JB, et al. Birth order, sibship size and risk of Hodgkin's disease in children and young adults: a population-based study of 31 million person-years. *Int J Cancer* 1997;72:977–981.

smallest sibship size to those in the largest. Taken together, these findings regarding social environmental factors that influence age at infection for children with Hodgkin lymphoma are the mirror image of what is generally seen in young adults. In addition, in the American case-control study of childhood Hodgkin lymphoma, a statistically significant 40% protective effect of breast-feeding was found in this study. This finding confirms an earlier finding by Davis and associates[67] and by Schwartzbaum and co-workers.[68] Whether it is due to exposure of the child to viruses or other infectious agents transmitted in mother's milk, or due to a protective effect of antibodies, cytokines, or other substances in the milk that protects the child against Hodgkin lymphoma risk, is unknown. This association between breast-feeding status and Hodgkin lymphoma is not modified by Epstein-Barr virus status of the tumor specimens. Of interest, there is the report of Kusuhara and associates[69] that no differences were observed in the acquisition of Epstein-Barr virus infection between breast-fed and non–breast-fed Japanese infants.

In summary, little is known about environmental or lifestyle factors associated with the risk of Hodgkin lymphoma in children. This is an intriguing area for investigation, because the poliomyelitis hypothesis of Hodgkin lymphoma etiology would suggest that these cases, should they be due to infection by a common virus, would be analogous to the widespread unapparent infections or perhaps to the sporadic paralytic cases of the disease observed in countries with poor hygiene. The limited data that are available are consistent in suggesting that the youngest children who develop Hodgkin lymphoma are those at increased risk of early infections.

A very interesting feature of Hodgkin lymphoma in childhood is the marked male preponderance in very young cases. This observation was first made by MacMahon[6] and later confirmed by other investigators. Fraumeni and Li[70] found a 3:1 male excess in children with Hodgkin lymphoma. In children diagnosed before the age of 4, there is a 19-fold excess of affected males over females.[71] In another series examining

children diagnosed before the age of 7, a high gender ratio of 4.6:1 was also observed.[72] This finding is consistent with the notion of an infectious etiology of the disease. It is well known that males are far more susceptible to infections during childhood than are females.[73-76] This is true for bacterial, viral, and even parasitic diseases. This extreme male excess appears to diminish in Hodgkin lymphoma patients after age 10,[70] and suggests that the early childhood form of the disease might be quite different epidemiologically from other forms of the disease.

This notion of the childhood disease being different from young-adult disease received impetus from an early paper by Correa and O'Conor,[26] who, while using international registry data, observed that there was an inverse relationship in the relative frequencies of childhood- and young-adult–onset Hodgkin lymphoma. In less developed countries such as Colombia, there was a relatively high incidence of Hodgkin lymphoma in children, and, reciprocally, there was a relatively low incidence rate for young-adult Hodgkin lymphoma. Conversely, in developed countries like Denmark, the authors observed high incidence rates for young-adult disease and reciprocally low rates for childhood-onset Hodgkin lymphoma. This intriguing finding was reassessed in 1995 by Macfarlane and colleagues.[77] Using later data from the same source, they found that this inverse relationship no longer was present. Incidence rates for young-adult Hodgkin lymphoma had risen in developing countries while remaining fairly constant in more developed countries. These new findings suggest that environmental risk factors might be changing in Third World countries to more closely approximate those in the rest of the world.

Adults

Among young adults (mid-teens through the 30s), the occurrence of Hodgkin lymphoma is consistently associated with factors fostering escape from Epstein-Barr virus infection and other similar viruses in childhood.[8] In this age group, we and others have found a twofold or greater increased risk in persons with a higher socioeconomic status and educational level.[8,12,63,78–81] More relevantly, studies have demonstrated an inverse association of risk with sibship size, with the risk among persons from larger families only half that of persons from the smallest.[8,63,82] In addition, those persons in the later birth-order positions of large families are at lower risk than those born earlier.[8,12]

The sibship size and birth-order findings were replicated in a population-based cohort study involving over two million Danes whose mothers were born in Denmark since 1935, as shown in Table 2.2.[66] For young adults in the largest families (five or more children), the RR of Hodgkin lymphoma was 0.57(0.30–1.1) compared to those with only one sibling. There was a parallel graded relationship with birth order. In contrast, these associations were reversed for Hodgkin lymphoma among children, for whom being from a large family carried an RR of 3.3(1.4–8.0). Similarly, in a registry-based study in Sweden including 188 childhood, 1,708 young-adult, and 244 middle-aged and older Hodgkin lymphoma cases diagnosed between 1958 and 1998, we found that risk of Hodgkin lymphoma was significantly lower among young adults with three or more siblings.[83] There was no parallel decrease in risk with increasing sibship size among children under 15 years or adults 40 years and above. A case-control study in northern Italy involving cases of Hodgkin lymphoma diagnosed between 1983 and 1992 found a significant protective effect with increasing numbers of older siblings (that is, later birth order).[84]

In a population-based case-control study conducted in eastern Massachusetts in the 1970s, we evaluated whether the inverse sibship size association was explainable by its mixture with other risk factors including higher maternal education and parental socioeconomic status, lower housing density, Jewish religion, smaller number of playmates, and self-reported history of infectious mononucleosis.[12] However, adjustment for these correlated factors had little effect on the significant association with sibship size, indicating that reduced exposure to infectious agents within the family was associated with increased risk of Hodgkin lymphoma as a young adult. Similarly, living in a single-family house during childhood, as opposed to multiple-family housing, was a primary risk factor for the malignancy.

However, more recently in a population-based case-control study by Glaser and co-workers including young-adult women in the San Francisco area in the early 1990s,[81] and in our population-based case-control study in eastern Massachusetts and Connecticut in the late 1990s,[42] there was no apparent association between sibship size, birth order, maternal education, housing density, or number of childhood playmates and risk of Hodgkin lymphoma in young adults. Glaser and colleagues lacked information on preschool attendance, but reported marginally significant protective associations with having lived in a rented rather than a family-owned childhood home, and having had a shared rather than a single bedroom at age 11 years, and they suggested that the increased use of daycare and nursery school may explain the lack of association with sibship size.[81] We found that the only determinant of childhood social environment significantly associated with risk of young-adult Hodgkin lymphoma was having attended nursery school or daycare for at least one year before kindergarten, which carried a reduced RR of 0.64 (0.45–0.92).

The lack of association with childhood social class characteristics that predicted risk of Hodgkin lymphoma in earlier studies suggests that demographic changes in the United States over recent decades may have altered the childhood exposures that are most relevant to risk of Hodgkin lymphoma. The enrollment of young children in nursery school rose from 5% in 1964 to 50% between 1995 and 1999,[85] likely elevating the relative importance of preschool enrollment in shaping childhood infectious exposure. Similarly, general increases in standard of living may have increased the prevalence of homeownership and having one's own childhood bedroom. Nevertheless, the significant associations detected in these two most recent studies still indicate that reduced exposure to infectious agents in childhood, whether through not attending preschool, living in a family-owned home, or having a single bedroom, increases the risk of Hodgkin lymphoma in young adulthood.

A large number of studies have evaluated the risk of Hodgkin lymphoma among young adults with a history of infectious mononucleosis, which occurs most commonly when primarily infection with the Epstein-Barr virus is delayed until adolescence. These include seven cohort studies that evaluated the risk of Hodgkin lymphoma following the diagnosis of infectious mononucleosis.[86–92] Combined, these studies involved a total of approximately 80,000 young adults with serologically confirmed infectious mononucleosis, with the expected number of cases based on population data. Overall, there was about a threefold increased risk of Hodgkin lymphoma following a diagnosis of infectious mononucleosis. In the largest cohort study of this subject, with over 38,000 participants from Denmark and Sweden,[92] the relative risk of Hodgkin lymphoma remained elevated for up to 20 years after the onset of infectious mononucleosis (Fig. 2.5).[93] The excess risk diminished with increasing time since diagnosis and with younger age at diagnosis of infectious mononucleosis. The finding of a positive association between infectious mononucleosis and risk of young-adult Hodgkin lymphoma has been replicated in multiple case-control studies,[94] but not all.[95–97] A question that can be raised is whether this positive association simply reflects confounding by other risk factors related to susceptibility to late infection. However, in our earlier study conducted in eastern Massachusetts, where we controlled for the effects of other related risk factors (sibship size, birth order, density of childhood housing), history of infectious mononucleosis was still significantly associated with Hodgkin lymphoma, RR = 1.8.[12] Most convincingly, in a study by Hjalgrim and co-workers based on the large Scandinavian cohort study of infectious mononucleosis patients,[98] there was no excess risk of Hodgkin lymphoma in first-degree relatives, including parents, siblings, and offspring of these patients, indicating that confounding by socioeconomic status and living environment is unlikely to

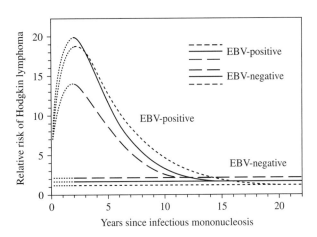

FIGURE 2.5. Relative risk of Epstein-Barr virus (EBV)-positive and EBV-negative Hodgkin lymphoma after infectious mononucleosis. (Reprinted with permission from Hjalgrim H, Askling J, Rostgaard, et al. Characteristics of Hogkin's lymphoma after infectious mononucleosis. N Engl J Med 2003;349:1324–1332.)

explain the positive association between infectious mononucleosis and risk of Hodgkin lymphoma.

Among middle-aged persons (40 to 54 years) in our 1970s Massachusetts study, increased risk of Hodgkin lymphoma was found to be associated with factors that reflect susceptibility to late infections (Fig. 2.4),[20] although the mix of these factors differed somewhat from that seen among the young adults. In the middle-aged group there was a threefold inverse gradient of risk associated with family size, a somewhat greater range than that among young adults. However, the gradient of risk was lost when the confounding effects of other factors were controlled. In contrast to the young adults, neither birth order nor number of playmates was a risk factor for the middle-aged subjects, and housing density was a weaker risk factor than among young adults. However, whether the subject had shared his or her bedroom with other children was of some importance: 57% of the Hodgkin lymphoma patients had their own bedrooms when they were 11 years old, as compared to 33% of controls. When controlled for sibship size, the association of risk with having one's own bedroom was evident only among subjects in families with three to five children, with an RR of 5.2 (1.9–14.3). Few subjects in this age group reported a history of infectious mononucleosis, with the adjusted RR being 1.3. The most important independent risk factor in this middle-age group was maternal education, with a fivefold increased risk among persons whose mothers had more than a high school education, compared to those whose mothers had not attended high school. Higher paternal socioeconomic status was also associated with Hodgkin lymphoma risk, but had no independent effect once maternal education was taken into account.

Our findings in the more recent Massachusetts and Connecticut-based study were in line with those of the earlier study, indicating an association between delayed childhood infection and increased risk of Hodgkin lymphoma.[42] Whereas we found the same lack of association with sibship size, birth order, maternal education, housing density, or number of childhood playmates as in young adults, having attended nursery school or daycare was associated with a reduced risk of Hodgkin lymphoma in middle-aged adults. The findings from a similar study in Israel[79] that provided data for this age group were consistent with the observation that middle-aged cases appear to be individuals whose childhood provided some protection from early infection. However, there was no clear association between childhood social class and risk of Hodgkin lymphoma among middle-aged women in the San Francisco area.[99] Overall, the combined evidence suggests that patients in this age group may be susceptible individuals who were infected as adults, perhaps by their children.

Among the oldest persons (55+ years) in both the Massachusetts study and the recent Massachusetts-Connecticut study, risk was not directly associated with socioeconomic status. If anything, patients came from a somewhat lower socioeconomic status than did controls. In the more recent study, higher parental education was associated with a reduced risk of Hodgkin lymphoma in older adults, whereas larger sibship size was associated with an increased risk.[42] There was no association between preschool attendance and risk of older-adult Hodgkin lymphoma, although only 3% of cases and controls reported having attended nursery school or daycare for at least one year before kindergarten. In the northern California study, there were inconsistent associations of both higher and lower childhood socioeconomic status with risk of Hodgkin lymphoma in older women.[99] However, within the Israeli population,[79] older cases appeared to come from somewhat higher socioeconomic status. Whether this latter observation is confounded by the apparent general increased risk of Hodgkin lymphoma among adult Jews (see above) is unknown.

In summary, children living under relatively poor conditions are at risk of Hodgkin lymphoma (Fig. 2.4).[20] For both young-adult and middle-aged persons, there is evidence that Hodgkin lymphoma may be a rare consequence of Epstein-Barr virus infection or other similar agents, which are strongly influenced by age at infection. The role of age at infection is not apparent for risk in the oldest ages, but the data are too sparse to reach a firm conclusion. The variation in known risk factors related to age of infection for the three epidemiologic types of Hodgkin lymphoma—childhood, young-adult, and older-adult—is somewhat unique in cancer epidemiology and suggests an important role for immune-related factors in the etiology of the disease. In particular, the apparent protective effect of exposure to other siblings and to other children in daycare in early childhood may be due to their effect on the maturation of the immune system, according to the "hygiene" hypothesis.[100] Of note, there is some evidence that Epstein-Barr virus infection before age 2 is protective against immunoglobulin (Ig)E sensitization, which is a marker of a "type 2" immune predominance.[101]

Epstein-Barr Virus

Multiple case-control studies conducted in the 1970s and 1980s evaluated whether patients with Hodgkin lymphoma had a different profile of antibodies to the major Epstein-Barr virus antigens compared to healthy controls, as had been documented in Burkitt lymphoma and nasopharyngeal carcinoma, two other malignancies strongly associated with Epstein-Barr virus infection. In interpreting antibody profiles, it is important to note that host control of latent Epstein-Barr virus infection is primarily accomplished by virus-specific cytotoxic T-cells, not antibodies. Rather, the relative level of specific antibodies appears to reflect the level of viral antigen. Seroepidemiologic studies have documented that patients with Hodgkin lymphoma as a group differ from controls in having elevated titers against the viral capsid antigen (VCA) and the early antigen (EA)—indicative of viral activation.[102] Studies that also tested for antibodies against the Epstein-Barr nuclear antigen (EBNA) complex had mixed findings.[19] We and a group from Finland have reported cohort studies on Epstein-Barr virus serology *preceding* Hodgkin lymphoma diagnosis[103,104]; these studies involved 43 cases[103] and 6 cases[104] that were diagnosed within the cohort years following blood collection. In the two early published studies, the elevated antibodies to the VCA and EA were confirmed. In addition, both studies found that elevated titers to the EBNA complex predicted subsequent Hodgkin lymphoma. In our study, multivariate analysis controlling for all antibodies measured, as well as histology, age, and gender, found that the strongest predictors were the prevalence of high titers against EBNA, RR = 6.7(90% CI, 1.8–24.5), and an inverse association with IgM antibodies against the VCA, RR = 0.07 (90% CI, 0.01–0.53).[103] This antibody profile is in itself paradoxical, as it suggests an enhanced level of Epstein-Barr virus replication *and* a vigorous immune response to the latent cycle antigens. These findings point to a protracted interaction between the host and the latent Epstein-Barr virus infection.

As detailed in Chapter 3, there is now overwhelming evidence that the Epstein-Barr virus plays a central role in the etiology of many, but by no means all, Hodgkin lymphoma cases.[19] This conclusion is based on the molecular analysis of multiple case series by numerous laboratories on patients from a range of populations throughout the world.[94] These studies document that in about one-third to one-half of Hodgkin lymphoma patients, Epstein-Barr virus genome is detectable in the Reed-Sternberg cells in affected lymph nodes, and that the genome itself is monoclonal. Further, the virus consistently expresses a restricted latent phenotype signature. The current standard of evidence for Epstein-Barr virus involvement in Hodgkin lymphoma requires detection of Epstein-Barr virus encoded RNA (EBER) by in situ hybridization and/or latent membrane protein 1 (LMP1) by immunohistochemical analysis.[105] The EBER and/or LMP1 signals must be unequivocally located to the malignant Reed-Sternberg cells, although in some cases only a subset of the malignant cells will be positive for technical or biological reasons.

Glaser and colleagues[106] recently reported a combined analysis of data from 14 international studies involving a total of 1,546 Hodgkin lymphoma patients, of whom 40% tested positive for the Epstein-Barr virus genome in tumor specimens. Using multivariate analysis, they found that Epstein-Barr virus positivity was more common among childhood and older-adult cases. Patients with Epstein-Barr virus–positive Hodgkin lymphoma were significantly more likely to have mixed cellularity than nodular sclerosis histology; the RR varied by age group: 7.3 (3.8–14.2) for children; 13.4 (9.0–19.9) for ages 15 to 49 years; and 4.9 (2.8–8.7) for those older. Young-adult cases with Epstein-Barr virus–positive disease were more likely to be male, RR = 2.5 (1.7–3.3); and childhood cases were more likely to be from less economically developed areas, RR = 6.0 (2.0–18.0). In addition, patients of Hispanic background were more likely to have Epstein-Barr virus–positive disease, RR = 4.1 (1.8–9.6), an association first reported by Gulley and associates.[107]

We found in Massachusetts and Connecticut that preschool attendance was inversely associated with risk of both Epstein-Barr virus–positive and negative Hodgkin lymphoma in young and middle-aged adults, and other indicators of childhood social environment did not distinguish between virus-positive and negative disease.[95] Alexander and co-workers studied the reported infectious disease history from 103 young adults with Hodgkin lymphoma, of whom 19 had Epstein-Barr virus–positive tumors. They found that for both virus-positive cases (OR = 0.18 [0.03-0.95]) and virus-negative cases (OR = 0.43 [0.21-0.86]), the greater number of reported infections for ages 2 years and above was protective.[108] However, Glaser and colleagues did not observe coherent patterns of childhood infection–related risk factors for either Epstein-Barr virus–positive or negative disease, although they observed some evidence that delayed childhood infections were positively associated only with risk of virus-positive disease in young adults.[96]

Because essentially all adult Hodgkin lymphoma cases have antibodies against the Epstein-Barr virus, these risk factors relate not to whether a patient has been infected with the virus, but how. The finding that children with Hodgkin lymphoma who come from economically underdeveloped areas were six times more likely to have Epstein-Barr virus–positive disease[106] would suggest that their risk was related to earlier age at infection. In contrast, Hjalgrim and associates found that among young adults—where susceptibility to delayed childhood infection is a consistent risk factor for Hodgkin lymphoma itself—those with serologically confirmed infectious mononucleosis were at a significantly increased risk of Epstein-Barr virus–positive Hodgkin lymphoma, RR = 4.0 (3.4–4.5), but not of virus-negative disease, RR = 1.5 (0.9–2.5).[93] The estimated median latency period between infectious mononucleosis and onset of Epstein-Barr virus–positive Hodgkin lymphoma was 4.1 years (1.8–8.3) (Fig. 2.5).[93] The specific association between infectious mononucleosis and Epstein-Barr virus–positive Hodgkin lymphoma was corroborated by Alexander and co-workers,[109] although not by three other case-control studies.[95–97] However, none of these four studies had information on serologically confirmed infectious mononucleosis. Thus, given that a patient has Hodgkin lymphoma, the likelihood that the tumor itself tests positive for Epstein-Barr virus genes or gene products appears to be related to factors indicative of somewhat poorer host response—namely, older age, male sex, living under somewhat poorer conditions, and having mixed cellularity histology. Whereas children, and possibly older adults, with Epstein-Barr virus–positive Hodgkin lymphoma appear to be prone to earlier childhood infection, young adults with virus-positive disease are more likely to have had postponed infection with Epstein-Barr virus.

Jarrett and associates[110] have proposed that infection with another oncogenic virus is responsible for Epstein-Barr virus–negative Hodgkin lymphoma, but no other known oncogenic DNA viruses have been convincingly detected in tumor specimens.[111] An alternative hypothesis to reconcile these paradoxical findings is that the Epstein-Barr virus is involved in the etiology of essentially every case a of Hodgkin lymphoma but the viral genome episome itself is somehow shed from the Reed-Sternberg cells in patients with a stronger host response.[112] However, the finding of Gallagher and colleagues that some patients with Epstein-Barr virus–negative Hodgkin lymphoma had no serologic evidence of ever having been infected with the virus indicates that Hodgkin lymphoma can arise in the absence of Epstein-Barr virus infection.[113] Furthermore, in the same study, the detection of virus genome fragments at equimolar proportions in tumor samples suggests that parts of the genome are not selectively deleted or retained, arguing against the "hit-and-run" hypothesis for Epstein-Barr virus–negative Hodgkin lymphoma.

A handful of studies, most based on small sample sizes, have evaluated the relationship between tumor Epstein-Barr virus status and Epstein-Barr virus antibody profiles in Hodgkin lymphoma. In an overlapping series of 107 cases, Brousset and associates[114] and Delsol and co-workers[115] concluded that there was no association between tumor Epstein-Barr virus positivity and a serologic pattern of reactivation, which they defined as anti-VCA >1:640, anti-EA >1:40, anti-EBNA >1:160. However, only one of 35 Epstein-Barr virus–negative and none of 16 virus-positive cases had this rather extreme pattern. Similarly, Levine and colleagues[116] found no differences in either anti-VCA or anti-EA between Epstein-Barr virus–positive and negative cases in a series of 39 patients. Enblad and co-workers[117] compared detailed Epstein-Barr virus serology between 27 Epstein-Barr virus–positive Hodgkin lymphoma cases and 80 virus-negative cases, and found only one significant difference: Epstein-Barr virus–positive cases were more likely to have IgG antibodies against the restricted component of EA. Comparing 19 Epstein-Barr virus–positive cases and 84 virus-negative cases, Alexander and colleagues[59] found that anti-VCA, but not anti-EA, titers were significantly higher in virus-positive cases than in virus-negative cases. In our study of 95 Epstein-Barr virus–positive cases and 303 virus-negative cases,[95] we found that virus-positive cases were significantly more likely to have detectable or elevated anti-VCA IgG and IgA, anti-EA IgG, and anti-EA-diffuse IgA, with elevated antibody titer defined as the upper 15% of the overall distribution; and to have a ratio of anti-EBNA-1 to anti-EBNA-2 less than or equal to 1.0, an indicator of defective immunity against the Epstein-Barr virus.[118] After mutually controlling for all independently associated antibodies, the RR for having elevated anti-VCA IgG was 3.6 (1.4–8.7), and that for having a low anti-EBNA-1/anti-EBNA-2 ratio was 3.2 (1.8–9.0), comparing Epstein-Barr virus–positive cases to negative cases. The latter finding was replicated in our companion study involving pre-diagnosis serum sampling of 139 Hodgkin lymphoma cases, of whom 40 had Epstein-Barr virus–positive tumor with control for the other antibodies against the Epstein-Barr virus; the relative risk associated with Epstein-Barr virus–positive Hodgkin lymphoma versus negative cases for a low anti-EBNA-1/anti-EBNA-2 ratio was significantly elevated

(L. Levin, Personal Communication). In addition, the presence of Epstein-Barr virus DNA has been reported in blood specimens in patients with Epstein-Barr virus–positive Hodgkin lymphoma.[119]

There is some evidence that risk of Hodgkin lymphoma is increased among patients with certain primary immunodeficiencies. Although there is a substantial risk of non-Hodgkin lymphoma primarily associated with loss of immunologic control of Epstein-Barr virus among such patients,[120] the number diagnosed with Hodgkin lymphoma is relatively small, about 9% of all malignancies (and 15% of all lymphomas).[121] These include children with ataxia telangiectasia (16 of 150 malignancies), Wiskott-Aldrich syndrome, (3 of 78 malignancies), or common variable immunodeficiency (8 of 120 malignancies).[122] Hodgkin lymphoma is even less common among the malignancies occurring in renal transplant patients, in whom it comprises about 2% of all lymphomas.[123–125] Whether this is greater than expected is not clear, as generally the number of patients and length of follow-up are not stated. In one report that did calculate the expected value, no Hodgkin lymphoma cases occurred, with 0.2 case expected[126]; in another cohort of organ transplant recipients, 2 Hodgkin lymphoma cases occurred with 2.2 cases expected.[127] One cohort study of stem-cell transplant recipients observed 4 Hodgkin lymphoma cases, with 0.27 expected, RR = 14.8 (3.8–32.9).[128] Post-transplant Hodgkin lymphomas are almost uniformly Epstein-Barr virus positive.[129] In addition, Hodgkin lymphoma has become recognized as part of the spectrum of opportunistic malignancies occurring in the natural history of human immunodeficiency virus-1 (HIV-1) infection.[130] In general, these HIV-1-infected patients present with advanced Hodgkin lymphoma with poor prognosis; the great majority have Epstein-Barr virus–positive tumors. In many, Hodgkin lymphoma appears to spread noncontiguously without mediastinal or splenic involvement.[131] This alteration in the natural history of Hodgkin lymphoma has been attributed to the loss of T-helper cells in HIV-1 infection.

Thus, overall, there is a substantial amount of evidence that age at infection, immune function, and the Epstein-Barr virus are central to the etiology of Hodgkin lymphoma. However, the enigma of Epstein-Barr virus–negative Hodgkin lymphoma remains.

Nonviral Factors

Occupation

Numerous cohort studies and fewer case-control studies have examined possible associations between occupational exposures and Hodgkin lymphoma risk. These results have been summarized in two earlier reviews.[94,132] The study of the possible etiologic role of occupational and environmental exposures in a relatively uncommon disease like Hodgkin lymphoma poses several basic methodological problems. In case-control approaches to the study of occupation, it is usually difficult to identify sufficient numbers of subjects with a particular job title or occupational exposure, especially if the exposure of interest is uncommon, to perform robust statistical analyses. On the other hand, cohort studies are efficient for the study of rare occupational exposures but inefficient for assessing Hodgkin lymphoma as an end-point, and very large cohorts would be necessary to generate sufficient numbers of Hodgkin lymphoma cases for conducting informative analyses. Furthermore, because most cohort studies can assess associations between occupational exposures and many different outcomes, some of the associations observed for Hodgkin lymphoma might be due to chance. This is the basic dilemma faced in studying occupational risk factors for Hodgkin lymphoma.

Several occupational exposures have been associated with Hodgkin lymphoma. Many reports center on occupational exposure to wood, herbicides, and other chemicals.[94,132,133] Unfortunately, the results of most studies have been inconsistent and few findings are statistically significant, let alone support a causal association. As a result, there are not well-established occupational risk factors for Hodgkin lymphoma. On the suspected, but not proven, list would be woodworking, herbicides, and other chemical exposures. However, the general lack of consistency of findings in occupational cohort studies of Hodgkin lymphoma risk suggests that chance may account for most of these positive findings. Recently, Kogevinas and co-workers[134] took an alternative approach based on the premise that Hodgkin lymphoma patients have a predisposing type 2 immune imbalance, which is associated with allergy and asthma. In a case-control study in Spain that included 41 Hodgkin lymphoma cases, they evaluated whether occupational exposure to high molecular weight agents that are associated with asthma predominately via an IgE hypersensitivity mechanism was associated with Hodgkin lymphoma. They found an OR of 2.3 (0.93–5.5). To study occupational risk factors for Hodgkin lymphoma would necessarily involve very expensive and very large studies. It is perhaps for that reason, as well as the weak associations previously observed, that we are left in a quandary of not knowing what role, if any, occupational exposures might play in the causation of Hodgkin lymphoma.

Medical History

Besides primary and acquired immunodeficiency, other immune-related disorders, including some autoimmune or chronic inflammatory diseases, may be associated with increased risk of Hodgkin lymphoma. In particular, patients hospitalized with rheumatoid arthritis in four very large cohorts in Finland, Denmark, Scotland, and Sweden[135–138] were found to have an elevated risk of subsequent Hodgkin lymphoma. Overall, the estimated relative risks ranged from twofold to fivefold for both men and women. In the largest Swedish study of 76,527 patients hospitalized with rheumatoid arthritis between 1964 and 1999,[138] 77 cases of Hodgkin lymphoma were observed, with 25.1 expected, RR = 3.1 (2.4–3.8).

An Italian cohort study of patients with inflammatory bowel disease found a significantly increased risk of Hodgkin lymphoma in 689 patients with ulcerative colitis, among whom 5 Hodgkin lymphoma cases arose, with 0.58 expected, RR = 8.6 (2.8–20.1). However, no excess risk was observed in 231 patients with Crohn disease. Studies of other autoimmune or chronic inflammatory disorders, such as multiple sclerosis[139–141] and psoriasis,[142] have also found no association with risk of developing of Hodgkin lymphoma. Landgren and associates reported a *negative* association between young-adult Hodgkin lymphoma and a personal history of diabetes mellitus, OR = 0.5 (0.2–1.1) in a Swedish cohort of 2,581 cases with matched population controls.[143] These findings, although mixed, support the notion that underlying immune dysregulation contributes to the development of Hodgkin lymphoma.

An Italian case-control study examined a wide range of infectious and noninfectious medical disorders, including chronic inflammatory conditions, and risk of Hodgkin lymphoma. They found that only infectious mononucleosis and tuberculosis were associated with an increased risk of Hodgkin lymphoma.[144]

Tonsillectomy

A considerable number of early epidemiologic studies addressed the question of whether tonsillectomy is a risk factor for Hodgkin lymphoma. Tonsillectomy is a risk factor for two diseases that share epidemiologic characteristics with Hodgkin lymphoma, paralytic poliomyelitis[145] and multiple sclerosis.[146] The relative risk of Hodgkin lymphoma among persons with prior tonsillectomy relative to those without has ranged from 0.46 to 3.6 in published studies.[147–149] Of note, there is great variation in the prevalence of tonsillectomy among the populations studied, from 9% in Denmark to 74% among Boston-area cases,[150] which does not correlate with Hodgkin lymphoma incidence rates. In those studies that used siblings as controls, thereby adjusting for childhood social environment, the association varied by sibship size.[151,152]

In all four of the published studies using sibling controls, a positive association was found. However, in two of the three of these that involved adult cases, the association was not uniformly present within all family-size groups.[151] This lack of a uniform association suggests either that tonsillectomy is not a causal factor or, if it is, its effect is complex, and modified by factors related to family size. The former explanation is favored by our findings from two companion population-based case-control studies on this question.[152] These studies involved 556 cases and 1,499 siblings from the metropolitan areas of Boston and Worcester, Massachusetts, and Detroit, Michigan. There was no evidence among young adults that prior tonsillectomy was a risk factor, RR = 1.0. Among middle-aged persons, the RR was 1.5 and not significant. Among older persons, the RR, 3.0, was significantly elevated, but the data were sparse. Taken together, the variability of findings, the variability of the practice of tonsillectomy, and the potential confounding with known risk factors for Hodgkin lymphoma argue against a causal association.

Other Factors

As Glaser[153] has pointed out, there appears to be a deficit of Hodgkin lymphoma cases among women in their late 30s and 40s in recent data from the United States and elsewhere. She proposes that this may represent a protective effect from childbearing, perhaps mediated by estrogen exposure. However, among women in this age group, Glaser and colleagues found that having had three or more children, compared to none, was positively associated with risk of Hodgkin lymphoma among women who had not breastfed their children; there was no association between parity and disease risk among women who had nursed.[154] Parity was also unassociated with risk of Hodgkin lymphoma among younger women (19 to 34 years) and older women (55 to 79 years), whereas long-term hormone use was marginally associated with lower risk overall. Kravdal and Hansen[155] found a protective effect of increasing number of births among mostly young-adult women in Norway, with an RR of 0.46 among women with three or more births, but no association in women aged 40 to 80 years or in men.[156] Other studies investigating parity and Hodgkin lymphoma risk[79,157–159] have generally found a slight or moderate, often statistically nonsignificant, inverse association that is sometimes stronger among women of reproductive age. One population-based case-control study in Slovenia found no association.[160] Taken together, there is limited evidence supporting a role of childbearing in women with Hodgkin lymphoma.

Several studies have evaluated the association between cigarette smoking and risk of Hodgkin lymphoma, with inconsistent results. Several studies found that current and/or former smoking increases the risk of Hodgkin lymphoma,[11,161–164] and Glaser and associates detected a positive association between exposure to environmental tobacco smoke and risk of young-adult Hodgkin lymphoma.[165] Nevertheless, just as many studies found no association between smoking and risk of Hodgkin lymphoma,[79,166–170] and Bernard and colleagues

reported an inverse association in a British case-control study.[63] However, we found an overall positive association between cigarette smoking and risk of Hodgkin lymphoma among young adults in Massachusetts and Connecticut,[42] with a twofold increase in risk limited to Epstein-Barr virus–positive disease.[95] Similarly, Glaser and co-workers reported a positive association between current smoking and Epstein-Barr virus–positive, but not negative, Hodgkin lymphoma in young-adult women.[165]

Likewise, studies of body mass index are inconclusive. In a Swedish cohort of individuals with a hospital discharge diagnosis of obesity,[171] the relative risk of Hodgkin lymphoma among men was 3.3 (1.4–6.5), whereas that among women was 0.9 (0.3–2.4). An early study of cancer mortality using college entrance health data from 50,000 male former students[11] also found an increased risk of death from Hodgkin lymphoma among "somewhat" obese men. However, in a large Scandinavian case-control study with 413 cases under 45 years and 205 cases age 45 or more years[172] we found no association between obesity and risk of Hodgkin lymphoma among males or females.

Recently, two novel findings were reported that call for confirmation in future studies. In our Massachusetts and Connecticut case-control study,[173] we found that regular use of aspirin, defined as consumption of at least two tablets per week on average over the preceding 5 years, was associated with a significantly reduced risk of Hodgkin lymphoma, RR = 0.60 (0.42–0.85); and use of acetaminophen was associated with increased risk, RR = 1.7 (1.3–2.3). These estimates were controlled for other analgesic use. This apparent protective effect of regular aspirin use is consistent with aspirin's unique ability to down-regulate the NFKB pathway, which is constitutively activated in Hodgkin lymphoma.

In a Scandinavian case-control study,[174] Smedby and associates found that greater exposure to ultraviolet radiation was associated with a significantly *lower* risk of Hodgkin lymphoma. For example, the relative risk among those who sunbathed four or more times per week 5 to 10 years ago, compared to those who never sunbathed, was 0.7 (0.5–1.0); and that for individuals sunburned at least two times per year 5 to 10 years ago, compared to those who were never sunburned, was also 0.7 (0.4–1.0). In addition, Hakansson and associates reported that among Swedish construction workers, those with the highest level of occupational sunlight had a significantly lower incidence of Hodgkin lymphoma, RR = 0.3 (0.1–0.9).[175] The inverse association between sun exposure and Hodgkin lymphoma risk could be mediated through an anticarcinogenic effect of vitamin D synthesized in the skin in response to ultraviolet radiation.[176] Smedby and colleagues[174] also reported that a history of skin cancer was associated with a twofold increase in risk of Hodgkin lymphoma. Their finding is consistent with several other reports.[177–179] These paradoxical findings of an apparent protective effect of sunlight and a positive association with history of skin cancer have also been reported for non-Hodgkin lymphoma,[174,177–179] but were not evident in the study of occupational exposure by Hakansson and associates.[175]

There are few other oncogenic exposures that appear to be related to risk of Hodgkin lymphoma. It is one of a handful of cancers that is clearly *not* associated with radiation exposure.[180,181] The roles of diet, physical activity, and alcohol use have received little attention.

SUMMARY

Hodgkin lymphoma continues to be an exceptional malignancy in its epidemiology and its biology. Few risk factors—other than those related to viral exposure and immune function—have been

TABLE 2.3

SUMMARY OF RISK FACTORS FOR HODGKIN LYMPHOMA

Factor	Strength of association	Consistency of association	Variation of subgroup
Epstein-Barr virus in Reed-Sternberg cells	Strong	Consistent	Mixed celluarity; males; children/older adults; Hispanics
Family history of Hodgkin lymphoma	Moderate to strong	Consistent	
Demographic characteristics	Moderate to strong	Consistent	Males; adults in Westernized populations; children in economically disadvantaged populations
Childhood social environment	Moderate	Consistent	Favors early infection in children; favors late infection in young adults (and middle-aged adults?)
History of infectious mononucleosis	Moderate	Consistent	Young adults (may be stronger in EBV genome-positive cases)
Jewish religion	Moderate	Consistent	(May be conditional on age of infection)
Family history of other hematopoietic disorders	Moderate to weak	Consistent	
Immunodeficiency syndromes	Weak to moderate	Fairly consistent	
HLA genotypes	Weak	Fairly consistent	
Occupation	Weak	Inconsistent	Possible association with wood-related occupations or herbicide exposure
Autoimmune or chronic inflammatory disorders	Weak	Inconsistent	
Tobacco smoking	Weak	Inconsistent	(May be restricted to EBV genome-positive cases)

HLA, human leukocyte antigen.

identified (Table 2.3). The major areas concern genetic risk, the validity of the apparent protective effects of aspirin, and of ultraviolet radiation exposure. The molecular breakthrough of the detection of the Epstein-Barr virus genes and gene products within the Reed-Sternberg cells has opened new avenues for inquiry. The question of how the virus plays a role in pathogenesis and why it is less frequently found in those cases most suggestive of an infectious etiology—young women with nodular sclerosis disease—is a challenge for epidemiologists, virologists, clinicians, and pathologists alike. Where these new clues will lead us remains to be seen. Thomas Hodgkin indeed started us all on a merry chase.

References

1. Hoster HA, Dratman MB. Hodgkin's disease (part I) 1832-1947. *Cancer Res* 1948;8:1–48.
2. Hoster HA, Dratman MB. Hodgkin's disease (part II) 1832-1947. *Cancer Res* 1948;8:49–78.
3. Cunningham WF. The status of diphtheroids with special reference to Hodgkin's disease. *Am J Med Sci* 1917;153:406–412.
4. Yates JL, Bunting CH. The rational treatment of Hodgkin's disease. *JAMA* 1915;64:1953–1961.
5. Bureau of the Census, United States Department of Commerce. *Manual of the International List of Causes of Death*, 4th edition, 1939. Washington, D.C.: U.S. Government Printing Office, 1940.
6. MacMahon B. Epidemiology of Hodgkin's disease. *Cancer Res* 1966;26:1189–1201.
7. Newell GR. Etiology of multiple sclerosis and Hodgkin's disease. *Am J Epidemiol* 1970;91:119–122.
8. Gutensohn (Mueller) N, Cole P. Epidemiology of Hodgkin's disease in the young. *Int J Cancer* 1977;19:595–604.
9. Gutensohn (Mueller) N, Cole P. Epidemiology of Hodgkin's disease. *Semin Oncol* 1980;7:92–102.
10. Alexander FE, McKinney PA, Williams J, et al. Epidemiological evidence for the two-disease hypothesis in Hodgkin's disease. *Int J Epidemiol* 1991;20:354–361.
11. Paffenbarger RS Jr, Wing AL, Hyde RT. Characteristics in youth indicative of adult onset Hodgkin's disease. *J Natl Cancer Inst* 1977;58:1489–1491.
12. Gutensohn (Mueller) N, Cole P. Childhood social environment and Hodgkin's disease. *N Engl J Med* 1981;304:135–140.
13. Vianna NJ, Greenwald P, Davies JNP. Extended epidemic of Hodgkin's disease in high school students. *Lancet* 1971;1:1209–1211.
14. Vianna NJ, Polan AK. Epidemiologic evidence for transmission of Hodgkin's disease. *N Engl J Med* 1973;289:499–502.
15. Grufferman S. Clustering and aggregation of exposures in Hodgkin's disease. *Cancer* 1977;39:1829–1833.
16. Smith PG, Pike MC, Kinlen LJ, et al. Contacts between young patients with Hodgkin's disease. A case-control study. *Lancet* 1977;2:59–62.
17. Grufferman S, Cole P, Levitan TR. Evidence against transmission of Hodgkin's disease in high schools. *N Engl J Med* 1979;300:1006–1011.
18. Weiss LM, Strickler JG, Warnke RA, et al. Epstein-Barr viral DNA in tissues of Hodgkin's disease. *Am J Pathol* 1987;129:86–91.
19. IARC. Epstein-Barr virus and Kaposi's sarcoma herpesvirus/human herpesvirus 8. In: *Monographs on the Evaluation of Carcinogenic Risks to Humans*. Volume 70. Lyon, France: International Agency for Research on Cancer, 1997;157.

20. Surveillance, Epidemiology, and End Results (SEER) Program (www.seer.cancer.gov) SEER*Stat Database. National Cancer Institute, DCCPS, Surveillance Research Program, Cancer Statistics Branch, released April 2006, based on the November 2005 SEER data submission.

21. MacMahon B. Epidemiological evidence on the nature of Hodgkin's disease. *Cancer* 1957;10:1045–1054.

22. Ries LAG, Harkins D, Krapcho M, et al., eds. *SEER Cancer Statistics Review, 1975-2003*. National Cancer Institute. Bethesda, MD. http://seer.cancer.gov/csr/1975_2003/, based on November 2005 SEER data submission, posted to the SEER website, 2006.

23. Ries LA G, Kosary CL, Hankey BF, et al., eds. SEER *Cancer Statistics Review, 1973–1994*. NIH publ. no. 97-2789. Bethesda: National Cancer Institute, 1997.

24. Glaser SL, Swartz WG. Time trends in Hodgkin's disease incidence: the role of diagnostic accuracy. *Cancer* 1990;66:2196–2204.

25. Chen YT, Zheng T, Chou MC, et al. The increase of Hodgkin's disease incidence among young adults. Experience in Connecticut, 1935–1992. *Cancer* 1997;79:2209–2218.

26. Correa P, O'Conor GT. Epidemiologic patterns of Hodgkin's disease. *Int J Cancer* 1971;8:192–201.

27. Hartge P, Devesa SS, Fraumeni JF, Jr. Hodgkin's disease and non-Hodgkin's lymphomas. *Cancer Surv* 1994;19/20:423–453.

28. Glaser SL. Hodgkin's disease in black populations: a review of the epidemiologic literature. *Semin Oncol* 1990;17:643–659.

29. Parkin DM, Whelan SL, Ferlay J, et al., eds. *Cancer incidence in five continents*, VIII (updated). IARC Cancer Base No. 7. Lyon, France: International Agency for Research on Cancer, 2005.

30. Alexander FE, Ricketts TJ, McKinney PA, et al. Community lifestyle characteristics and incidence of Hodgkin's disease in young people. *Int J Cancer* 1991;48:10–14.

31. Henderson BE, Dworsky R, Pike MC, et al. Risk factors for nodular sclerosis and other types of Hodgkin's disease. *Cancer Res* 1979;39:4507–4511.

32. Cozen W, Katz J, Mack T. Risk patterns of Hodgkin's disease in Los Angeles vary by cell type. *Cancer Epidemiol Biomarkers Prev* 1992;1:261–268.

33. Clarke CA, Glaser SL, Keegan TH, et al. Neighborhood socioeconomic status and Hodgkin's lymphoma incidence in California. *Cancer Epidemiol Biomarkers* Prev 2005;14:1441–1447.

34. Glaser SL. Regional variation in Hodgkin's disease incidence by histologic subtype in the US. *Cancer* 1987;60:2841–2847.

35. Hu E, Hufford S, Lukes R, et al. Third-world Hodgkin's disease at Los Angeles County-University of Southern California Medical Center. *J Clin Oncol* 1988;6:1285–1292.

36. Vianna NJ, Greenwald P, Brady J, et al. Hodgkin's disease: cases with features of a community outbreak. *Ann Intern Med* 1972;77:169–180.

37. Greenberg RS, Grufferman S, Cole P. An evaluation of space-time clustering in Hodgkin's disease. *J Chronic Dis* 1983;36:257–262.

38. Knox G. Detection of low intensity epidemics: application to cleft lip and palate. *Br J Prev Soc Med* 1963;17:121–127.

39. Ederer F, Myers MH, Mantel N. A statistical problem in space and time: do leukemia cases come in clusters? *Biometrics* 1964;20:626.

40. Alexander FE, Daniel CP, Armstrong AA, et al. Case clustering, Epstein-Barr virus Reed-Sternberg cell status and herpes virus serology in Hodgkin's disease: results of a case-control study. *Eur J Cancer* 1995;31A:1479–1486.

41. Goldin LR, Pfeiffer RM, Gridley G, et al. Familial aggregation of Hodgkin lymphoma and related tumors. *Cancer* 2004;100:1902–1908.

42. Chang ET, Zheng T, Weir EG, et al. Childhood social environment and Hodgkin's lymphoma: new findings from a population-based case-control study. *Cancer Epidemiol Biomarkers Prev* 2004;13:1361–1370.

43. Goldin LR, Landgren O, McMaster ML, et al. Familial aggregation and heterogeneity of non-Hodgkin lymphoma in population-based samples. *Cancer Epidemiol Biomarkers Prev* 2005;14:2402–2406.

44. Chang ET, Smedby KE, Hjalgrim H, et al. Family history of hematopoietic malignancy and risk of lymphoma. *J Natl Cancer Inst* 2005;97:1466–1474.

45. Grufferman S, Cole P, Smith PG, et al. Hodgkin's disease in siblings. *N Engl J Med* 1977;296:248–250.

46. Grufferman S, Barton JW, Eby NL. Increased sex concordance of sibling pairs with Behcet's disease, Hodgkin's disease, multiple sclerosis and sarcoidosis. *Am J Epidemiol* 1987;126:365–369.

47. Sellick GS, Allinson R, Matutes E, et al. Increased sex concordance of sibling pairs with chronic lymphocytic leukemia. *Leukemia* 2004;18:1162–1163.

48. Horwitz M, Wiernik PH. Pseudoautosomal linkage of Hodgkin disease. *Am J Hum Genet* 1999;65:1413–1422.

49. Mack TM, Cozen W, Shibata DK, et al. Concordance for Hodgkin's disease in identical twins suggesting genetic susceptibility to the young adult form of the disease. *N Engl J Med* 1995;332:413–418.

50. Chakravarti A, Halloran SL, Bale SJ, et al. Etiological heterogenicity in Hodgkin's disease: HLA linked and unlinked determinants of susceptibility independent of histological concordance. *Genet Epidemiol* 1986;3:407–415.

51. Daugherty SE, Pfeiffer RM, Mellenkjaer L, et al. No evidence for anticipation in lymphoproliferative tumors in population-based samples. *Cancer Epidemiol Biomarkers Prev* 2005;14:1245–1250.

52. Goldin LR, McMaster ML, Ter-Minassian M, et al. A genome screen of families at high risk for Hodgkin lymphoma: evidence for a susceptibility gene on chromosomes 4. *J Med Genet* 2005;42:595–601.

53. Grufferman S, Ambinder RF, Shugart YY, et al. Increased cancer risk in families of children with Hodgkin's disease. *Am J Epidemiol* 1998;147:S8. Abstract.

54. Olsen JH, Boice JD, Seersholm N, et al. Cancer in the parents of children with cancer. *N Engl J Med* 1995;333:1594–1599.

55. Hors J, Dausset J. HLA and susceptibility to Hodgkin's disease. *Immun Rev* 1983;70:167–192.

56. Oza AM, Tonks S, Lim J, et al. A clinical epidemiological study of human leukocyte antigen-DPB alleles in Hodgkin's disease. *Cancer Res* 1994;54:5101–5105.

57. Bryden H, MacKenzie J, Andrew L, et al. Determination of HLA-A*02 antigen status in Hodgkin's disease and analysis of an HLA-A*02-restricted epitope of the Epstein-Barr virus LMP-2 protein. *Int J Cancer* 1997;72:614–618.

58. Poppema S, Visser L. Epstein-Barr virus positivity in Hodgkin's disease does not correlate with an HLA A2-negative phenotype. *Cancer* 1994;73:3059–3063.

59. Alexander FE, Jarrett RF, Cartwright RA, et al. Epstein-Barr virus and HLA-DPB1-*0301 in young adult Hodgkin's disease: evidence for inherited susceptibility to Epstein-Barr virus in cases that are EBV+ve. *Cancer Epidemiol Biomarkers Prev* 2001;10:705–709.

60. Diepstra A, Niens M, Vellenga E, et al. Association with HLA class I in Epstein-Barr-virus-positive and with HLA class III in Epstein-Barr-virus negative Hodgkin's lymphoma. *Lancet* 2005;365:2216–2224.

61. Gutensohn (Mueller) N. Social class and age at diagnosis of Hodgkin's disease: new epidemiologic evidence on the two-disease hypothesis. *Cancer Treat Rep* 1982;66:689–695.

62. Bernard SM, Cartwright RA, Bird CC, et al. Aetiologic factors in lymphoid malignancies: a case-control epidemiological study. *Leuk Res* 1984;8:681–689.

63. Bernard SM, Cartwright RA, Darwin CM, et al. Hodgkin's disease: case-control epidemiological study in Yorkshire. *Br J Cancer* 1987;55:85–90.

64. Freedman LS, Barchana M, Al-Kayed S, et al. A comparison of population-based cancer incidence rates in Israel and Jordan. *Eur J Cancer* 2003;12:359–365.

65. Gutensohn (Mueller) N, Shapiro D. Social class risk factors among children with Hodgkin's disease. *Int J Cancer* 1982;30:433–435.

66. Westergaard T, Melbye M, Pedersen JB, et al. Birth order, sibship size and risk of Hodgkin's disease in children and young adults: a population-based study of 31 million person-years. *Int J Cancer* 1997;72:977–981.

67. Davis MK, Savitz DA, Graubard BI. Infant feeding and childhood cancer. *Lancet* 1988;2:365–368.

68. Schwartzbaum JA, George SL, Pratt CB, et al. An exploratory study of environmental medical factors potentially related to childhood cancer. *Med Pediatr Oncol* 1991;19:115–121.

69. Kusuhara K, Takabayashi A, Ueda K, et al. Breast milk is not a significant source for early Epstein-Barr virus or human herpesvirus 6 infection in infants: a seroepidemiologic study in two endemic areas of human T-cell lymphotropic virus type 1 in Japan. *Microbiol Immunol* 1997;41:309–312.

70. Fraumeni JF Jr, Li FP. Hodgkin's disease in childhood: an epidemiologic study. *J Natl Cancer Inst* 1969;42:681–691.

71. Kung FH. Hodgkin's disease in children four years of age or younger. *Cancer* 1991;67:1428–1430.

72. White L, McCourt BA, Isaacs H, et al. Patterns of Hodgkin's disease at diagnosis in young children. *Am J Pediatr Hematol Oncol* 1983;5:251–257.

73. Green MS. The male predominance in the incidence of infectious diseases in children: a postulated explanation for disparities in the literature. *Int J Epidemiol* 1992;21:381–386.

74. Melnick H. Enteroviruses. In: Evans AS, ed. *Viral infections of humans: epidemiology and control*, 3rd ed. New York: Plenum, 1989:214.

75. Washburn TC, Medearis DN, Childs B. Sex differences in susceptibility to infections. *Pediatrics* 1965;35:57–64.

76. Schlegel RJ, Bellanti JA. Increased susceptibility of males to infection. *Lancet* 1969;2:826–827.

77. Macfarlane GJ, Evstifeeva TV, Boyle P, et al. International patterns in the occurrence of Hodgkin's disease in children and young adult males. *Int J Cancer* 1995;61:165–167.

78. Cohen BM, Smetana HF, Miller RW. Hodgkin's disease: long survival in a study of 388 World War II Army cases. *Cancer* 1964;17:856–866.

79. Abramson JH, Pridan H, Sacks MI, et al. A case-control study of Hodgkin's disease in Israel. *J Natl Cancer Inst* 1978;61:307–314.

80. Serraino D, Franceschi S, Talamini R, et al. Socio-economic indicators, infectious diseases and Hodgkin's disease. *Int J Cancer* 1991;47:352–357.

81. Glaser SL, Clarke CA, Nugent RA, et al. Social class and risk of Hodgkin's disease in young-adult women in 1988–94. *Int J Cancer* 2002;98:110–107.

82. Bonelli L, Vitale V, Bistolfi F, et al. Hodgkin's disease in adults: association with social factors and age at tonsillectomy: a case-control study. *Int J Cancer* 1990;45:423–427.

83. Chang ET, Montgomery SM, Richiardi L, et al. Number of siblings and risk of Hodgkin's lymphoma. *Cancer Epidemiol Biomarkers Prev* 2004;13:1236–1243.

84. Charenoud L, Gallus S, Atieri A, et al. Numbers of siblings and risk of Hodgkin's and other lymphoid neoplasms. *Cancer Epidemiol Biomarkers Prev* 2005;14:552.

85. Jamieson A, Curry A, Martinez G. School enrollment in the United States—social and economic characteristics of students: October 1999. Washington, D.C.: U.S. Census Bureau, 2001.

86. Miller RW, Beebe GW. Infectious mononucleosis and the empirical risk of cancer. *J Natl Cancer Inst* 1973;50:315–321.

87. Rosdahl N, Larsen SO, Clemmesen J. Hodgkin's disease in patients with previous infectious mononucleosis: 30 years' experience. *Br Med J* 1974;2:253–256.

88. Connelly RR, Christine BW. A cohort study of cancer following infectious mononucleosis. *Cancer Res* 1974;34:1172–1178.

89. Carter CD, Brown Jr TM, Herbert JT, et al. Cancer incidence following infectious mononucleosis. *Am J Epidemiol* 1977;105:30–36.

90. Munoz N, Davidson RJ, Witthoff B, et al. Infectious mononucleosis and Hodgkin's disease. *Int J Cancer* 1978;22:10–13.

91. Kvale G, Hoiby EA, Pedersen E. Hodgkin's disease in patients with previous infectious mononucleosis. *Int J Cancer* 1979;23:593–597.

92. Hjalgrim H, Askling J, Sorenson P, et al. Risk of Hodgkin's disease and other cancers after infectious mononucleosis. *J Natl Cancer Inst* 2000;92:1522–1528.

93. Hjalgrim H, Askling J, Rostgaard, et al. Characteristics of Hogkin's lymphoma after infectious mononucleosis. *N Engl J Med* 2003;349: 1324–1332.

94. Mueller NE, Grufferman S. Hodgkin's disease. In: Schottenfeld D, Fraumeni JF Jr, eds. *Cancer epidemiology and prevention*, 2nd ed. New York: Oxford University Press, 1996;893–919.

95. Chang ET, Zheng T, Lennette ET, et al. Heterogeneity of risk factors and antibody profiles in Epstein-Barr virus genome-positive and –negative Hodgkin lymphoma. *J Infect Dis* 2004;189:2271–2281.

96. Glaser SL, Keegan TH, Clarke CA, et al. Exposure to childhood infections and risk of Epstein-Barr virus-defined Hodgkin's lymphoma in women. *Int J Cancer* 2005;115:599–605.

97. Sleckman BG, Mauch PM, Ambinder RF, et al. Epstein-Barr virus in Hodgkin's disease: correlation of risk factors and disease characteristics with molecular evidence of viral infection. *Cancer Epidemiol Biomarkers Prev* 1998;7:1117–1121.

98. Hjalgrim H, Rostgaard K, Askling J, et al. Hematopoietic and lymphatic cancers in relatives of patients with infectious mononucleosis. *J Natl Cancer Inst* 2002;94:678–681.

99. Glaser SL, Clarke CA, Stearns CB, et al. Age variation in Hodgkin's disease risk factors in older women: evidence from a population-based case-control study. *Leuk Lymphoma* 2001;42:997–1004.

100. Bain JF. The effect of infections on susceptibility to autoimmune and allergic diseases. *N Engl J Med* 2002;347:911–920.

101. Nilsson C, Linde A, Montgomery SM, et al. Does early EBV infection protect against IgE sensitization? *J Allergy Clin Immunol* 2005;116: 438–444.

102. Evans AS, Gutensohn (Mueller) N. A population-based case-control study of EBV and other viral antibodies among persons with Hodgkin's disease and their siblings. *Int J Cancer* 1984;34:149–157.

103. Mueller N, Evans, Harris NL, et al. Hodgkin's disease and Epstein-Barr virus. Altered antibody pattern before diagnosis. *N Engl J Med* 1989;320:689–695.

104. Lehtinen T, Lumio J, Dilner J, et al. Increased risk of malignant lymphoma indicated by elevated Epstein-Barr virus antibodies – a prospective study. *Cancer Causes Control* 1993;4:187–193.

105. Gulley ML, Glaser SL, Craig FE, et al. Guidelines for interpreting EBER in situ hybridization and LMP1 immunohistochemical tests for detecting Epstein-Barr virus in Hodgkin lymphoma. *Am J Clin Pathol* 2002;117:259–267.

106. Glaser SL, Lin RJ, Stewart SL, et al. Epstein-Barr virus-associated Hodgkin's disease: epidemiologic characteristics in international data. *Int J Cancer* 1997;70:375–382.

107. Gulley ML, Eagan PA, Quintanilla-Martinez L, et al. Epstein-Barr virus DNA is abundant and monoclonal in the Reed-Sternberg cells of Hodgkin's disease: association with mixed cellularity subtype and Hispanic American ethnicity. *Blood* 1994;83:1595–1602.

108. Alexander FE, Jarrett RF, Lawrence D, et al. Risk factors for Hodgkin's disease by Epstein-Barr virus (EBV) status: prior infection by EBV and other agents. *Br J Cancer* 2000;82:1117–1121.

109. Alexander FE, Lawrence DJ, Freeland J, et al. An epidemiologic study of index and family infectious mononucleosis and adult Hodgkin's disease (HD): evidence for a specific association with EBV+ve HD in young adults. *Int J Cancer* 2003;107:298–302.

110. Jarrett RF, MacKenzie J. Epstein-Barr virus and other candidate viruses in the pathogenesis of Hodgkin's disease. *Seminars in Hematology* 1999;36:260–269.

111. Armstrong AA, Shield L, Gallagher A, et al. Lack of involvement of known oncogenic DNA viruses in Epstein-Barr virus-negative Hodgkin's disease. *Br J Cancer* 1998;77:1045–1047.

112. Mueller NE. Epstein-Barr virus and Hodgkin's disease: an epidemiological paradox. *Epstein-Barr Virus Rep* 1997;4:1.

113. Gallagher A, Perry J, Freeland J, et al. Hodgkin lymphoma and Epstein-Barr virus (EBV): no evidence to support hit-and-run mechanism in cases classified as non-EBV-associated. *Int J Cancer* 2003;104:624–630.

114. Brousset P, Chittal S, Schlaifer D, et al. Detection of Epstein-Barr virus messenger RNA in Reed-Sternberg cells of Hodgkin's disease by in situ hybridization with biotinylated probes on specially processed modified acetone methyl benzoate xylene (ModAMeX) sections. *Blood* 1991;77:1781–1786.

115. Delsol G, Brousset P, Chittal S, et al. Correlation of the expression of Epstein-Barr virus latent membrane protein and in situ hybridization with biotinylated BamHI-W probes in Hodgkin's disease. *Am J Pathol* 1992;140:247–253.

116. Levine PH, Pallesen G, Ebbesen P, et al. Evaluation of Epstein-Barr virus antibody patterns and detection of viral markers in the biopsies of patients with Hodgkin's disease. *Int J Cancer* 1994;59:48–50.

117. Enblad G, Sandvej K, Lennette E, et al. Lack of correlation between EBV serology and presence of EBV in the Hodgkin and Reed-Sternberg cells of patients with Hodgkin's disease. *Int J Cancer* 1997;72:394–397.

118. Henle W, Henle G, Andersson J, et al. Antibody responses to Epstein-Barr virus-determined nuclear antigen EBNA-1 and EBNA-2 in acute and chronic Epstein-Barr virus infection. *Proc Natl Acad Sci USA* 1987;84:570–574.

119. Jarrett RF. Risk factors for Hodgkin's lymphoma by EBV status and sifnificance of detection of EBV genomes in serum of patients with EBV-associated Hodgkin's lymphoma. *Leuk Lymphoma* 2003;44(suppl 3):S27–S32.

120. List AF, Greco FA, Volger LB. Lymphoproliferative diseases in immunocompromised hosts: the role of Epstein-Barr virus. *J Clin Oncol* 1987;5:1673–1689.

121. Mueller N. Overview of the epidemiology of malignancy in immune deficiency. *JAIDS* 1999;21:S5–S10.

122. Filipovich AH, Mathur A, Kamat D, et al. Primary immunodeficiencies: genetic risk factors for lymphoma. *Cancer Res* 1992;52(suppl 19):5465s–5467s.

123. Sheil AG. Cancer in organ transplant recipients: part of an induced immune deficiency syndrome. *Br Med J (Clin Res Ed)* 1984;288:659–661.

124. Doyle TJ, Venkatachalam KK, Maeda K, et al. Hodgkin's disease in renal transplant recipients. *Cancer* 1983;51:245–247.

125. Bates WD, Gray DW, Dada MA, et al. Lymphoproliferative disorders in Oxford renal transplant recipients. *J Clin pathol* 2003;56:439–446.

126. Kinlen LJ, Sheil AG, Peto J, et al. Collaborative United Kingdom-Australasian study of cancer in patients treated with immunosuppressive drugs. *Br Med J* 1979;2:1461–1466.

127. Adami J, Gabel H, Lindelof B, et al. Cancer risk following organ transplantation: a nationwide cohort study in Sweden. *Br J Cancer* 2003;89:1221–1227.

128. Baker KS, Defor TE, Burns LJ, et al. New malignancies after blood or marrow stem-cell transplantation in children and adults: incidence and risk factors. *J Clin Oncol* 2003;21:1352–1358.

129. Ambinder RF. Posttransplant lymphoproliferative disease: pathogenesis, monitoring, and therapy. *Curr Oncol Rep* 2003;5:359–363.

130. Schulz TF, Boshoff CH, Weiss RA. HIV infection and neoplasia. *Lancet* 1996;348:587–591.

131. Knowles Dm, Chamulak GA, Subar M, et al. Lymphoid neoplasia associated with the acquired immunodeficiency syndrome (AIDS). The New York University Medical Center experience with 105 patients (1981-1986). *Ann Intern Med* 1988;108:744–753.

132. Grufferman S, Delzell E. Epidemiology of Hodgkin's disease. *Epidemiol Rev* 1984;6:76–106.

133. IARC Working Group on the Evaluation of Carcinogenic Risks to Humans, Wood Dust and Formaldehyde. *IARC Monographs on the Evaluation of Carcinogenic Risks to Humans*, vol. 62. Lyon, France: IARC Press, 1995; 404.

134. Kogevinas M, Zock J-P, Alvaro T, et al. Occupational exposure to immunologically active agents and risk for lymphoma. *Cancer Epidemiol Biomarkers Prev* 2004;13:1814–1818.

135. Hakulinen T, Isomaki H, Knekt P. Rheumatoid arthritis and cancer studies based on linking nationwide registries in Finland. *Am J Med* 1985;78:29–32.

136. Mellemkjaer L, Linet MS, Gridley G, et al. Rheumatoid arthritis and cancer risk. *Eur J Cancer* 1996;32A:1753–1757.

137. Thomas E, Brewster DH, Black RJ, et al. Risk of malignancy among patients with rheumatic conditions. *Int J Cancer* 2000;88:497–502.

138. Ekstrom K, Hjalgrim H, Brandt L, et al. Risk of malignant lymphomas in patients with rheumatoid arthritis and in their first-degree relatives. *Arthritis Rheum* 2003;48:963–970.

139. Vineis P, Crosignani P, Vigano C, et al. Lymphomas and multiple sclerosis in a multicenter case-control study. *Epidemiology* 2001;12:134–135.

140. Hjalgrim H, Rasmussen S, Rostgaard K, et al. Familial clustering of Hodgkin lymphomas and multiple sclerosis. *J Natl Cancer Inst* 2004;96:780–784.

141. Landgren O, Kerstann KF, Gridley G, et al. Re: Familial clustering of Hodgkin lymphoma and multiple sclerosis. *J Natl Cancer Inst* 2005;97:543–544; author reply 544-545.

142. Boffetta P, Gridley G, Lindelof B. Cancer risk in a population-based cohort of patients hospitalized for psoriasis in Sweden. *J Invest Dermatol* 2001;117:1531–1537.

143. Landgren O, Bjorkholm M, Montgomery SM, et al. Personal and family history of autoimmune diabetes mellitus and susceptibility to young-adult-onset Hodgkin lymphoma. *Int J Cancer* 2005;

144. Vineis P, Crosignani P, Sacerdote C, et al. Haematopoietic cancer and medical history: a multicentre case control study. *J Epidemiol Community Health* 2000;9:59–64.

145. Paffenbarger RS Jr, Wilson VO. Previous tonsillectomy and current pregnancy as they affect risk of poliomyelitis attack. *Ann NY Acad Sci* 1955;61:856–868.

146. Poskanzer DC. Tonsillectomy and multiple sclerosis. *Lancet* 1965;2:1264–1266.
147. Mueller NE. Hodgkin's disease. In: Schottenfeld D, Fraumeni JF Jr, eds. *Cancer epidemiology and prevention*, 2nd ed. New York: Oxford University Press, 1996:893–919.
148. Zwitter M, Primic-Zakelj M, Kosmelj K. A case-control study of Hodgkin's disease and pregnancy. *Br J Cancer* 1996;73:246–251.
149. Liaw KL, Adami J, Gridley G, et al. Risk of Hodgkin's disease subsequent to tonsillectomy: a population-based cohort study in Sweden. *Int J Cancer* 1997;72:711–713.
150. Mueller NE. The epidemiology of Hodgkin's disease. In: Selby D, McElwain TJ, eds. *Hodgkin's disease*. Oxford: Blackwell Scientific, 1987:68–93.
151. Gutensohn (Mueller) N, Li FP, Johnson RE, et al. Hodgkin's disease, tonsillectomy and family size. *N Engl J Med* 1975;292:22–25.
152. Mueller N, Swanson GM, Hsieh C-C, et al. Tonsillectomy and Hodgkin's disease: results from companion population-based studies. *J Natl Cancer Inst* 1987;78:1–5.
153. Glaser SL. Reproductive factors in Hodgkin's disease in women: a review. *Am J Epidemiol* 1994;139:237–246.
154. Glaser SL, Clarke CA, Nugent RA, et al. Reproductive factors in Hodgkin's disease in women. *Am J Epidemiol* 2003;158:553–563.
155. Kravdal O, Hansen S. Hodgkin's disease: the protective effect of childbearing. *Int J Cancer* 1993;55:909–914.
156. Kravdal O, Hansen S. The importance of childbearing for Hodgkin's disease: new evidence from incidence and mortality models. *Int J Epidemiol* 1996;25:737–743.
157. Franceschi S, Bidoli E, La Vecchia C. Pregnancy and Hodgkin's disease. *Int J Cancer* 1994;58:465–466.
158. Tavani A, Pregnolato A, La Vecchia C, et al. A case-control study of reproductive factors and risk of lymphomas and myelomas. *Leuk Res* 1997;21:885–888.
159. Lambe M, Hsieh CC, Tsaih SW, et al. Childbearing and the risk of Hodgkin's disease. *Cancer Epidemiol Biomarkers Prev* 1998; 7:831–834.
160. Zwitter M, Zakelj MP, Kosmelj K. A case-control study of Hodgkin's disease and pregnancy. *Br J Cancer* 1996;73:246–251.
161. Hammond EC, Horn D. Smoking and death rates—report on forty-four months of follow-up of 187,783 men. *JAMA* 1958;166:1294–1308.
162. Matthews ML, Dougan LE, Thomas DC, et al. Interpersonal linkage among Hodgkin's disease patients and controls in Western Australia. *Cancer* 1984;54:2571–2579.
163. Adami J, Nyren O, Bergstrom R, et al. Smoking and the risk of leukemia, lymphoma, and multiple myeloma (Sweden). *Cancer Causes Control* 1998;9:49–56.
164. Briggs NC, Hall HI, Brann EA, et al. Cigarette smoking and risk of Hodgkin's disease: a population-based case-control study. *Am J Epidemiol* 2002;156:1011–1020.
165. Glaser SL, Keegan TH, Clarke CA, et al. Smoking and Hodgkin lymphoma risk in women United States. *Cancer Causes Control* 2004; 15:387–397.
166. Siemiatycki J, Krewski D, Franco E, et al. Associations between cigarette smoking and each of 21 types of cancer: a multi-site case-control study. *Int J Epidemiol* 1995;24:504–514.
167. Stagnaro E, Ramazzotti V, Crosignani P, et al. Smoking and hematolymphopoietic malignancies. *Cancer Causes Control* 2001;12:325–334.
168. Gallus S, Giordano L, Altieri A, et al. Cigarette smoking and risk of Hodgkin's disease. *Eur J Cancer Prev* 2004;13:143–144.
169. Miligi L, Seniori-Costantini A, Crosignani P, et al. Occupational, environmental, and life-style factors associated with the risk of hematolymphopoietic malignancies in women. *Am J Ind Med* 1999;36:60–69.
170. Newell GR, Rawlings W. Evidence for environmental factors in the etiology of Hodgkin's disease. *J Chronic Dis* 1972;25:261–267.
171. Wolk A, Gridley G, Svensson M, et al. A prospective study of obesity and cancer risk (Sweden). *Cancer Causes Control* 2001;12:13–21.
172. Chang ET, Hjalgrim H, Smedby KE, et al. Body mass index and risk of malignant lymphoma in Scandinavian men and women. *J Natl Cancer Inst* 2005;97:210–218.
173. Chang ET, Zheng T, Weir EG, et al. Aspirin and the risk of Hodgkin's lymphoma in a population-based case-control study. *J Natl Cancer Inst* 2004;96:305–315.
174. Smedby KE, Hjalgrim H, Melbye M, et al. Ultraviolet radiation exposure and risk of malignant lymphomas. *J Natl Cancer Inst* 2005;97:199–209.
175. Hakansson N, Floderus B, Gustavsson P, et al. Occupation sunlight exposure and cancer incidence among Swedish construction workers. *Epidemiol* 2001;12:552–557.
176. Egan KM, Sosman JA, Blot WJ. Sunlight and reduced risk of cancer: is the real story vitamin D? *J Natl Cancer Inst* 2005;97:161–163.
177. Frisch M, Melby M. New primary cancers after squamous cell skin cancer. *Am J Epidemiol* 1995;141:916–922.
178. Levi F, Randimbison L, La Vecchia C, et al. Incidence of invasive cancers following squamous cell skin cancer. *Am J Epidemiol* 1997;146:734–739.
179. Kahn HS, Tatham LM, Patel AV, et al. Increased cancer mortality following a history of nonmelanoma skin cancer. *JAMA* 1998;260:910–912.
180 Boice Jr JD, Land CE, Preston DL. Ionizing radiation. In: Schottenfeld D, Fraulmeni JR JF, ed. *Cancer Epidemiology and Prevention*. 2nd ed. New York: Oxford University Press, 1996:319–354.
181. Halnanl KE. Failure to substantiate two cases of alleged occupation radiation carcinogenesis. *Lancet* 1988;1:639.

CHAPTER 3 ■ ASSOCIATION OF EPSTEIN-BARR VIRUS WITH HODGKIN LYMPHOMA

RICHARD F. AMBINDER AND LAWRENCE M. WEISS

The discovery of Epstein-Barr virus (EBV) DNA, RNA, and protein in Reed-Sternberg cells and their variants in cases of Hodgkin lymphoma fits neatly with epidemiologic observations that suggested that the tumor might be a rare consequence of a common infection.[1,2] The relationship was confirmed in a study that showed that serologically confirmed infectious mononucleosis increased the risk of EBV-associated Hodgkin lymphoma.[3] However, although EBV infection is nearly ubiquitous, viral infection of tumor cells is present in only some cases of Hodgkin lymphoma, and the frequency of the association varies among populations.[4] The young adult population, in which infectious mononucleosis is most common, is the population of patients with Hodgkin lymphoma where the association with EBV is least common. This chapter is focused on the association of the virus with the tumor. The chapter begins with an overview of relevant aspects of the epidemiology and biology of the virus and its association with other tumors, and concludes with consideration of the pathology, epidemiology, and clinical implications regarding prognosis and targeted therapy.

ASPECTS OF VIRUS BIOLOGY AND EPIDEMIOLOGY

EBV, like most of the other human herpesviruses, is nearly ubiquitous.[5] Serologic studies suggest that more than 90% of the adult population worldwide is infected by the virus. The virus is transmitted in saliva.[6,7] Replication of virus in the oropharynx may account for the pharyngitis that accompanies infectious mononucleosis.[8–10] Primary infection is usually asymptomatic in childhood, but in adolescence or young adulthood, it is associated with the syndrome of infectious mononucleosis in approximately one-third of cases.[11–13]

Structurally, the virion is an icosahedral capsid that contains a large genome (171 kb) of linear, double-stranded DNA, as shown in Figure 3.1.[14,15] It has a tropism for B-lymphocytes. Virion attachment to B-cells involves an interaction between CD21 and the viral envelope glycoprotein gp350/220, while viral entry requires a complex of three additional viral glycoproteins: gH, gL, and gp42 and an interaction with HLA class II acting as a coreceptor.[16,17] Other cell types can also be infected, and it is clear that there are other pathways for viral entry.

Latency and Lytic Infection

The life-cycle of all of the herpesviruses involves alternative states of infection.[5] During lytic (or productive) infection, the genetic program is active that selectively replicates virion components, including linear double-stranded viral DNA genomes and proteins. During latent infection, genetic programs that enable the viral genome to persist in host cells and to evade immune surveillance are active. It is lytic or productive infection that is associated with disease in herpes simplex infection (fever blisters, encephalitis), varicella-zoster infection (chickenpox, shingles), or cytomegalovirus infection (retinitis, pneumonia). Latent infection is not known to be associated with any pathologic manifestations with these latter viruses. In contrast, lytic EBV infection plays a role in oral hairy leukoplakia and perhaps in infectious mononucleosis, but it is latent infection that is associated with the most serious pathology: neoplasia.[18]

In vitro, EBV infection of resting B-cells leads to proliferation (Fig. 3.1).[19–21] In vivo, a similar process may expand the pool of latently infected cells even in the absence of new virion production and further cycles of infection. Studies of deletion mutants have shown that six viral genes are required for immortalization (Table 3.1).[22] EBNA1 activates the viral origin of replication used in latency and through chromatin interactions tethers viral episomes to chromosomes.[23] EBNA2 is a transcriptional transactivator that regulates viral and cellular gene expression. In these effects, EBNA2 mimics activated Notch, a receptor that mediates cell-to-cell signaling and influences cell fate and tissue development.[24] The viral protein competes away a corepressor complex and interacts with coactivator proteins to bring about transcriptional activation. Members of the EBNA3 family (EBNA3A, 3B, 3C) function in part by modulating the same signaling pathway. LMP1 is a member of the tumor necrosis factor receptor (TNFR) superfamily and resembles a constitutively activated CD40 molecule.[18,25] LMP1 expression is associated with transformation in model systems.[26] In transgenic mice, expression under the control of an immunoglobulin heavy-chain regulatory locus leads to lymphomagenesis. LMP1 expression leads to activation of NFκB; induction of activation markers including CD23, CD30, and CD40; and induction of cell adhesion molecules and anti-apoptotic genes. LMP1 recruits signaling adapter molecules, including tumor necrosis factor receptor associated-factors (TRAFs) 1, 2, and 3 and TNF receptor-associated death domain (TRADD).

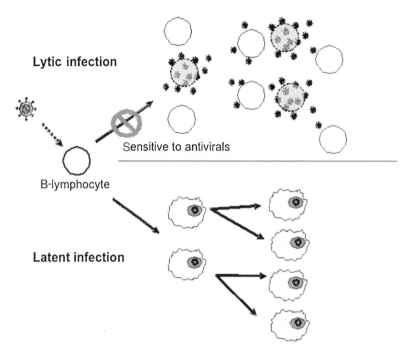

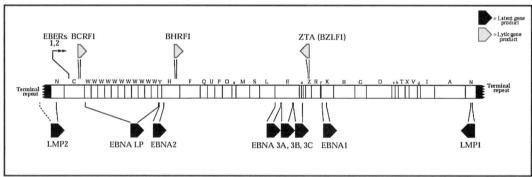

FIGURE 3.1. EBV infection of a B-lymphocyte. **Top:** When a virion harboring double-stranded linear DNA infects a B-lymphocyte, the lymphocyte may support the production of new virions, leading to the infection of other cells (lytic infection); or the viral genome may form an episome, express viral latency proteins that drive cell proliferation, and be passed on from mother to daughter cell without production of new virions. Replication of the viral genome and production of new virions can be inhibited by antivirals such as acyclovir and ganciclovir, but these agents have no effect on proliferation of infected cells. **Bottom:** Schematic map of the linear viral genome. Proteins discussed in the text are indicated. Vertical lines indicate Bam HI restriction sites. Restriction fragments are designated by letters. A variable number of terminal repeats are present at either end of the genome. See color insert. (Artwork courtesy of M. Victor Lemas.)

Other viral transcripts are expressed in immortalized lymphocytes but are not absolutely required for immortalization. LMP2A is an intrinsic membrane protein that includes an immunoreceptor tyrosine-based activation motif (ITAM) and provides a tonic signal that mimics the signal associated with Ig receptor engagement.[27] LMP2A expression appears to allow the survival of B-lymphocytes lacking Ig expression both in a transgenic murine model and in human lymphocytes in vitro.[28–30] As detailed later in the chapter, LMP2A may play a key role in Hodgkin lymphoma pathogenesis. EBER1 and EBER2 are polymerase III transcripts. These RNAs do not code for proteins. Suggested functions include modulation of pathways important in interferon response.[31,32] In addition to their biologic importance, their abundant expression has made them important tools for research and for the clinical detection of virus in tumor. The BamHI-A region of the genome encodes transcripts with open reading frames, although the predicted proteins have not been unambiguously

demonstrated in natural infection or in tumors.[33–35] Putative microRNAs have also been recognized in this region.

The latently infected B-cells in EBV-seropositive people differ markedly from lymphoblastoid B-cell lines. They are resting rather than proliferating and have very limited expression of viral genes.[36–39] Transcripts detected by reverse-transcriptase PCR in peripheral blood mononuclear cells include the EBERs, and sometimes LMP2A and EBNA1. However, analysis of individual cells at limiting dilution raises question as to whether any viral genes but the EBERs are expressed in most of the cells that harbor viral DNA.[21,40–43] The infected cells display a memory B-cell phenotype (CD20+CD27+IgD⁻CD5⁻), and carry somatically hypermutated immunoglobulin genes.[21,39] The genesis of the infected pool of resting cells is uncertain. The transition of EBV-infected naive B-cells expressing many viral latency genes to EBV-infected memory B-cells expressing few viral latency genes may involve a germinal center or germinal center-like reaction in which naive B-cells

TABLE 3.1

EBV LATENCY GENE PRODUCTS

Gene product	Function	Lymphocyte immortalization	CTL recognition	Hodgkin lymphoma expression
EBNA1	Latency replication, chromosome tethering of the viral episome	Yes	+/−	Yes
EBNA2	Transcriptional activator (mimics activated notch)	Yes	+	No
EBNA3A	Transcriptional modulation	Yes	++	No
EBNA3B	Transcriptional modulation	No	++	No
EBNA3C	Transcriptional modulation	Yes	++	No
LMP1	Transmembrane constitutively activated signaling molecule (TNFR superfamily)	Yes	+	Yes
LMP2A/2B	Transmembrane signaling molecule (ITAM motif)	No	+	Yes
EBERs 1/2	Unknown, do not code for protein	No	No	Yes

become memory cells.[39] The viral membrane proteins LMP1 and LMP2 may provide surrogate germinal center-like signals. Finally, immune surveillance may eliminate cycling cells expressing immunodominant viral antigens that drive cellular proliferation. Thus the virus may persist indefinitely in a sanctuary of long-lived resting memory cells with very limited viral gene expression.

Latency predominates in most EBV tissue culture systems and in lymphocytes in vivo. A small minority of EBV-immortalized B-lymphocytes will express lytic cycle viral antigens, and an even smaller number will produce virions.[44] Phorbol esters, butyrate, and other agents will increase the fraction of lytically infected cells.[45] Two immediate early sequence-specific DNA-binding proteins that act as transcriptional transactivators initiate the lytic cycle (Table 3.2).[46,47] Their expression initiates a cascade of events that leads to expression of delayed early genes, late genes, and ultimately packaging and release of infectious virus. ZTA expression blocks cell cycle progression through interactions with CCAAT/enhancer-binding protein alpha (CEBPα), leading to p21 accumulation and G1 cell cycle arrest, and thus refocusing cellular replication machinery on the viral genome.[48,49] The final steps of the viral lytic gene expression cascade, the synthesis of viral DNA and of the late proteins, can be blocked with antiviral agents such as acyclovir and ganciclovir that block the viral DNA polymerase (Fig. 3.1). These nucleoside analogues are selectively phosphorylated by the viral thymidine kinase (TK) and protein kinase (PK), and in turn are further phosphorylated by cellular kinases to triphosphates that inhibit the viral DNA polymerase.[50–52] However, the growth of the latently infected cells and maintenance of the viral genome are not inhibited by these agents.[53]

Viral Infection and the Immune Response

Primary infection with EBV in teenage or adult years is sometimes associated with the syndrome of infectious mononucleosis.[13] What cofactors are important in determining this association with symptoms (the dose of the viral innoculum in a kiss, the age of the host, host genetic factors, viral strain) are largely unknown. The typical manifestations of infectious mononucleosis include pharyngitis, fever, lymphadenopathy, splenomegaly, and lymphocytosis.[54,55] These are all thought to reflect an active cellular immune response. The peripheral lymphocytosis consists mainly of activated CD8+ T-lymphocytes that are largely EBV specific.[55–58] Activated CD4+ T-cells and NK cells are also present. All of these activated cell types directly lyse EBV-infected B-cell lines and natural killer (NK) targets in vitro.[59] Symptomatic infectious mononucleosis but not asymptomatic seroconversion may be associated with the long-term disappearance of T-cells expressing the α subunit of the IL15 receptor.

Primary infection is associated with the appearance of immunoglobulin M (IgM) titers to viral capsid antigen (VCA) and rising IgG titers to VCA and early antigen (EA). Over

TABLE 3.2

EBV LYTIC GENE PRODUCTS

Gene products	Function
Zta, Rta	Immediate early transcriptional transactivators that initiate lytic viral replication and mediate G(1) cell cycle arrest
BHRF1,BALF1	Anti-apoptotic proteins with homology to BCL2
Viral IL10 (BCRF1)	Immune modulatory with homology to IL10
Thymidine kinase (BXLF1)	Phosphorylates nucleosides (also antiviral analogues acyclovir and ganciclovir)
Protein kinase (BGLF1)	Phosphorylates a viral protein (also antiviral analogues including ganciclovir)
Viral DNA polymerase	Replicates viral DNA in lytic cycle (inhibited by phosphorylated nucleotide analogues such as acyclovir-triphosphate)

several months, IgM titers to VCA disappear, whereas IgG titers rise and then persist indefinitely. Titers to EBNA appear late but also persist indefinitely. For the diagnosis of primary EBV infection in the clinical setting, the most commonly used diagnostic assays detect heterophil antibodies that agglutinate sheep and horse erythrocytes. Their appearance coincides with the early phase of infectious mononucleosis, when polyclonal activation of B-cells leads to a general elevation of total IgM, IgG, and IgA.[13] Within weeks or months after the resolution of acute symptoms, these heterophil antibodies cease to be detectable. The explanation for their appearance and peculiar specificity remains elusive, and diagnostic use is entirely empiric.

Animal Models

Infection of cottontop marmosets and some other new world primates with EBV leads to polyclonal B-cell lymphoprolifera-tive disease.[60] In mice with severe combined immunodeficiency (SCID), EBV-associated B-cell tumors develop following transfer of peripheral blood mononuclear cells from EBV-seropositive donors, transfer of peripheral blood mononuclear cells from EBV-seronegative donors followed by inoculation with EBV, or simply transfer of EBV-immortalized B-cell lines.[61,62] Transgenic murine models have yielded conflicting results, with the EBNA1 transgene associated with lymphomagenesis in some reports but not others.[63,64]

EPSTEIN-BARR VIRUS IN NEOPLASIA

Characterization of EBV in Tumor Specimens

Before discussing the association of EBV with tumors, it is useful to consider the distinctive aspects of the application of Southern blot hybridization and in situ hybridization to the detection and characterization of EBV in tumor specimens. In both retroviral and papillomavirus-associated tumorigenesis, viral integration serves to mark clonal expansions of tumor cells. Integration of the EBV genome does not occur in lymphocyte immortalization, and integrated viral genomes are not commonly detected in tumors, although they have often been recognized in several tumor-derived cell lines.[65] Nonetheless, the state of the viral genome has allowed insights into clonality. Indeed, some of the evidence that Reed-Sternberg cells are clonal is inferred from analysis of the state of the EBV genome in tumor tissue. EBV episomes (closed, circular DNA molecules) are formed from the linear viral genomes present in virions (Fig. 3.2). Genomes in virions are bounded at either end by tandem direct repeats of approximately 0.5 kb. A viral genome may carry as many as 20 such repeats. These linear genomes circularize to form episomes. These episomes in turn serve as templates for the generation of multigenome-length con-catamers that are cleaved to form linear viral genomes.[66] Cleavage occurs semirandomly within the terminal repeat sequences, such that linear genomes generated from the same parental template differ in their numbers of terminal repeats. When these linear genomes circularize, the resultant episomes also differ from one another in terms of the number of terminal repeats. Episomal replication in latent infection generally pre-serves the number of terminal repeats of the parent episomes. Thus, numbers of terminal repeats in an episome are stable in latently infected cells. Linear and episomal viral genomes, and

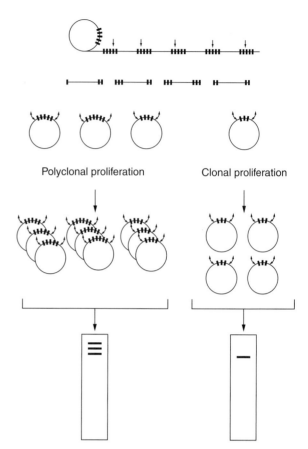

FIGURE 3.2. Analysis of clonality by Southern blot hybridization. Characterization of the state of the terminal repeats of the viral genome distinguishes polyclonal from monoclonal infected cell expansions. Rolling circle replication (**top**) leads to the generation of multiple-genome-length concatameric intermediates. These are cleaved semirandomly to yield single-genome-length linear DNA molecules with variable numbers of terminal repeats at the left and right ends of the viral genome. On infection, these linear genomes fuse to form episomes. The fusion joints carry variable numbers of terminal repeats. The size of the fusion joint reflecting the number of terminal repeats can be assessed by digestion with a restriction enzyme such as Bam HI followed by Southern blot hybridization with a terminal repeat probe. Bam HI restriction sites are shown. Because each infectious event leads to the circularization of a linear viral genome with a particular number of terminal repeats, and because the number of repeats is preserved in latently infected daugh-ter cells, the occurrence of one or many infectious events may be distinguished by the presence of one or more bands corresponding to the fused terminal repeats. Thus, in a polyclonal proliferation of cells, several bands will be detected (**bottom left**), whereas in a monoclonal proliferation of cells, only a single band will be detected. See color insert. (Artwork courtesy of M. Victor Lemas.)

number of terminal repeats incorporated in episomes, can be recognized by analysis of the terminal repeat fragments by Southern blot hybridization. The fused terminal repeats of epi-somes are readily distinguished from the shorter left and right terminal repeat fragments associated with linear genomes. Separate infectious events (i.e., different virions infecting dif-ferent cells) give rise to latent episomes with varying numbers of terminal repeats. On the other hand, when only a single infectious event gives rise to the latent episomes in a tissue (through proliferation of the infected cell), then all the episomes in the tissue will carry a fixed number of terminal repeats. With appropriate restriction enzymes and probe, separate infectious events can be distinguished from a single infectious event by the appearance of multiple versus single bands corresponding to the fused terminal repeats of viral genomes in an infected tissue.[67] Although the presence of clonality as assessed by study of the viral terminal repeats has often been interpreted as evidence that the viral infection preceded clonal expansion of tumor cells, data have been presented suggesting that fewer terminal repeats may be associated with higher levels of LMP2A expression and a selective advantage on infected cells.[68] Thus it is entirely possible that viral infection of a clonally expanded population of cells, while initially leading to apparent polyclonality with respect to EBV episomal terminal repeat number, might rapidly yield an apparently monoclonal population with respect to EBV.

The presence of the highly abundant EBER transcripts in most latently infected cells has provided an important marker of EBV latent infection by in situ hybridization.[69–72] Whereas most of the viral genes transcribed in latency including those required for immortalization are expressed at low copy numbers, the EBERs are expressed at copy numbers estimated at greater than 106 copies per cell.[73–75] Immunohistochemistry with monoclonal antibodies has helped define patterns of viral gene expression, although cross-reactivities of some monoclonal antibodies with cellular proteins has been problematic.[76]

Tumor Associations

EBV is associated with a number of human neoplasms, including malignant lymphoma, carcinoma, and even mesenchymal neoplasms. Specifically, EBV is associated with almost 100% of cases of nasopharyngeal carcinoma, regardless of the geographic location.[77] In addition, EBV can be identified in a subset of cases of gastric carcinoma, probably representing 5% to 10% of cases overall, with a particular predilection for cases of gastric carcinoma with a high content of lymphoid cells (so-called lymphoepithelioma).[78,79] EBV is associated with lymphoepitheliomas occurring at other sites, particularly foregut sites such as the salivary gland (especially in Eskimos), thymus, and nasal region.[77] Mesenchymal neoplasms that have been associated with EBV include smooth-muscle neoplasms occurring in immunocompromised patients, particularly children with AIDS;[80] and inflammatory pseudotumors of the liver and spleen, tumors that may represent a peculiar subset of follicular dendritic neoplasm.[81]

Both B-cell and T-cell lymphomas are associated with EBV (Table 3.3). B-cell lymphomas that are associated with EBV include Burkitt lymphoma, lymphoproliferations arising in cases of acquired or congenital immunodeficiencies, pulmonary

TABLE 3.3

EBV-ASSOCIATED LYMPHOID MALIGNANCIES

B lineage	
Non-Hodgkin lymphoma	
No immunodeficiency	
Burkitt lymphoma	Varies 20–100% (see text)
Diffuse large-cell lymphoma	<5%
Pyothorax lymphoma	>95%
Immunodeficiency	
Congenital	>90%
Post-transplant lymphoma	>90%
HIV	
Primary effusion lymphoma	>90%
Primary CNS lymphoma	>95%
Diffuse large-cell lymphoma	40–60%
Plasma cell tumors	>90%
Lymphomatoid granulomatosis	>90%
Hodgkin lymphoma	
No immunodeficiency	Varies 20–100% (see text)
Immunodeficiency	
Congenital	>90%
Post-transplant	>90%
HIV	>90%
T and NK cell lineage	
Nasal lymphoma	>95%
NK cell leukemia (aggressive)	>95%
Other peripheral T-cell l	Varies 5–70% (see text)

TABLE 3.4

PATTERNS OF VIRAL GENE EXPRESSIONS

B lineage	EBNA1	EBNA2, 3A, 3B, 3C	LMP1	LMP2	EBERs
Burkitt lymphoma	+	–	–	–	+
Pyothorax lymphoma	+	Variable	+	ND	+
Post-transplant lymphoma	+	Variable	+	+	+
Primary effusion lymphoma	+	–	–	–	+
Primary CNS lymphoma	+	Variable	+	ND	+
Hodgkin lymphoma	+	–	+++	+++	+

lymphomatoid granulomatosis, and pyothorax-associated pleural lymphoma (Table 3.4). Burkitt lymphoma was the first neoplasm found to have an association with EBV, as EBV viral particles were first identified in cell lines derived from African Burkitt lymphoma.[82] Burkitt lymphoma is endemic in malarial Africa but occurs only rarely in the United States and Europe and has an intermediate rate of occurrence in northern Africa and South America. The association of Burkitt lymphoma with EBV varies similarly, from a nearly 100% association in endemic areas, to less than 20% association in low-incidence areas, and an intermediate association in northern Africa and South America.[83–87] In the large majority of EBV-associated cases, a restricted latency pattern is seen (Fig. 3.3).[88,89]

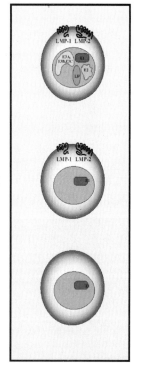

Post-Transplant Lymphoma

Hodgkin Lymphoma

Burkitt Lymphoma

FIGURE 3.3. Epstein-Barr virus (EBV) in three types of lymphoma. Post-transplant lymphoproliferative disease is associated with expression of the full range of viral latency antigens in immortalized B-cells (latency I). Hodgkin lymphoma is associated with a more restricted pattern (latency II). Burkitt lymphoma is associated with the most restricted pattern (latency III). In Burkitt lymphoma, MHC class I molecules are often downregulated, and antigens are not processed for presentation. (Artwork courtesy of M. Victor Lemas.)

However, cultured Burkitt lymphoma cells may drift to less restricted patterns of latency.[90]

Pyothorax-associated lymphoma is a rare tumor that has been described principally in Japan. It is of special interest because its existence points up the importance of poorly understood inflammatory cofactors that are part of EBV lymphomagenesis. These patients have a B-cell malignancy arising in the pleural space and presenting as a solid mass (in contrast to primary effusion lymphoma that may present in the pleural space as a malignant effusion). Patients had previously been treated for tuberculosis in the pre-antibiotic era with therapeutic pneumothorax maintained by placement of ping pong balls in the pleural space. Typically, these would become infected and chronic pyothorax would develop. Tumors are diagnosed with a latency more than 20 years from the time of the pneumothorax.

Lymphoproliferative disorders in patients with congenital immunodeficiencies, with iatrogenically induced immunodeficiencies (such as lymphoproliferative disorders following transplantation), and HIV infection are associated with EBV. Many congenital immunodeficiencies, including all varieties of severe combined immunodeficiency, are associated with EBV B-cell lymphoma.

X-linked immunodeficiency (XLP) is of particular interest in this regard. Approximately half of the boys with this infection die during the acute phase of primary EBV infection.[91] Many of the survivors succumb to EBV lymphoma or aplastic anemia. The signaling lymphocytic activation molecule (SLAM)-associated protein (SAP) is mutated or deleted in XLP.[92–94] This is a short adaptor molecule that is expressed in activated T and NK cells. It has been hypothesized that the clinical features of XLP are caused by dysregulated cellular immune response as a consequence of the absence of functional SAP, and that rapid elimination of EBV-infected B-cells might ameliorate the clinical syndrome. With this in mind, treatment with anti-CD20 (rituximab) at the time of primary EBV infection with rapid resolution of clinical symptoms and no progression of disease has been reported.[95]

Lymphoproliferative disorders develop in organ transplant recipients in part as a function of the organ transplanted, the immunosuppressive regimen, the occurrence of graft rejection, and patient characteristics (age and whether the recipient is EBV-seronegative).[96,97] Histologic features from benign hyperplasia, to polymorphic proliferations, to histologies that are indistinguishable from de novo malignant lymphoma are recognized.[98] The EBV-infected cells often show broad expression of viral latency antigens.

In AIDS, T-cell surveillance is also defective, leading to abnormally high numbers of EBV-infected B-cells in the peripheral blood and nonneoplastic lymphoid tissue.[99] Approximately 40% to 67% of AIDS-associated lymphomas are EBV-associated. The association is higher in systemic and central nervous system immunoblastic lymphomas, neoplasms that tend to occur in persons with long-standing AIDS who have extremely low T-cell counts; the association is lower in small noncleaved or large-cell lymphomas, which tend to occur in nodal sites in people with earlier-stage AIDS.[100,101] Dual viral infection with EBV and KSHV (also known as HHV8) is characteristic of primary effusion lymphoma in which tumor cells are found in serosal cavities without the formation of tumor masses.[102,103]

T-cell immunodeficiency, particularly in regard to the number of EBV-specific cytotoxic cells, may be a critical factor in the development of post-transplantation lymphoproliferations.[104] For example, in bone marrow transplantation, the period when the patient is at greatest risk for lymphoproliferations coincides with the nadir for EBV-specific cytotoxic T-cells.[105] Post-transplantation lymphoproliferative disorders in human marrow allograft recipients have been treated with small populations of donor-derived lymphocytes, with impressive success.[106] Others have used virus-specific T-cell lines to treat or prevent EBV-associated lymphoproliferative disease.[107,108] The results provide evidence that virus-specific T-cells are of critical importance in the pathogenesis of these lymphoproliferations.

EPSTEIN-BARR VIRUS IN HODGKIN LYMPHOMA

EBV Detection, Patterns of Gene Expression, Strain, and Immune Response

The presence of EBV genomic DNA in Hodgkin lymphoma was first reported by dot blot and Southern blot hybridization studies in 1987[1] and soon confirmed by others.[109–111] By means of DNA detection techniques, about 20% to 40% of cases of Hodgkin lymphoma were shown to harbor viral DNA. With a probe directed against DNA sequences adjacent to the EBV terminus, the viral DNA was shown to be present in a monoclonal population of cells in most cases, implying that the EBV was present in tumor lineage cells before clonal expansion or that particular clones of infected cells outgrow others.[1,109–112]

In situ hybridization studies localized the virus to Reed-Sternberg cells and their variants (Hodgkin cells) (Fig. 3.4).[70,109,111,113–115] EBV is also detected in rare small lymphocytes in tumor tissue by EBER in situ hybrization, both in cases of Hodgkin lymphoma in which EBER transcripts were detected, and were not detected, in the Reed-Sternberg cells.[116–121] Double-labeling showed that these EBER-expressing small lymphocytes are predominantly B-lineage (CD20+) lymphocytes, although some are T-lymphocytes (CD3+ and CD43+) and a small percentage did not mark with B-cell or T-cell antibodies.[120] Single-cell PCR has confirmed the presence of EBV DNA in individual Reed-Sternberg cells.[122,123] DNA amplification techniques applied to tumor extracts detects viral DNA more frequently insofar as they will detect virus in the occasional infiltrating lymphocyte.

Immunohistochemical studies also demonstrate viral gene expression in Hodgkin lymphoma (Fig. 3.4). In an early case report, EB nuclear antigen staining was reported in "Reed-Sternberg like" cells.[124] LMP1, LMP2, and EBNA1 are detected in series of patients with Hodgkin lymphoma.[125–130] In contrast to EBER detection, LMP1 antibodies do not stain small infiltrating lymphocytes.

EBV detection techniques in Hodgkin lymphoma have been studied to determine their sensitivity and reproducibility, and specific guidelines for interpretation have been elaborated.[71,72] In contrast to nasopharyngeal carcinoma, serologic analyses to date have shown no correlation between the presence or absence of EBV and patient serology, or stage of disease.[131–134]

PCR studies have been useful in determining that type 1 EBV is detected in most cases occurring in immunocompetent persons.[112,135] Partial deletions of the LMP1 gene were found in approximately 10% of cases, particularly those associated with numerous Reed-Sternberg cells, necrosis, and/or anaplasia, in at least one series.[136,137] These deletions are consistently found in a region near the 3' end of the LMP1 gene, identical to deletions seen in cases of nasopharyngeal carcinoma that behave aggressively when transplanted into nude mice.[138] These gene deletions lead to a loss of ten amino acids near the carboxyl terminus of the protein, extending the half-life of the protein. Our studies show a high prevalence of LMP1 gene deletions in cases from the United States and Brazil (33% and 46%, respectively).[139] However, we found no correlation between LMP1 gene deletions and numbers or anaplasia of Reed-Sternberg cells, and we found an even higher frequency of LMP1 gene deletions in reactive lymphoid tissues, which suggests that LMP1 gene deletions may not be relevant to the pathogenesis of Hodgkin lymphoma outside the setting of HIV infection.

When multiple sites of disease have been studied, EBV-associated cases harbor the viral genome in Reed-Sternberg cells at all sites; similarly, recurrences of EBV-associated cases usually harbor EBV as well.[114,140,141] However, exceptions have been noted.[142] Southern blotting studies in which a probe is directed against DNA near the EBV terminus have demonstrated EBV in the same clonal population at all involved sites.[140,143] Analysis of the EBV LMP1 gene has often, but not always, revealed deletions in diagnosis at different sites of Hodgkin lymphoma and at relapse, suggesting that some LMP1 gene deletions may be acquired after neoplastic transformation.[141,143]

Serology at the time of Hodgkin lymphoma diagnosis has not disntinguished between patients with virus-infected and other Hodgkin tumors.[131,144,145]

Other Viruses

A variety of other viruses have attracted the attention of investigators. Serologic and PCR studies of all of the human herpesviruses have occasionally detected cytomegalovirus, HHV6, and HHV7 viral DNA, but these are ubiquitous viruses and there is no evidence for localization to malignant cells.[146–148] Investigators have also failed to find evidence of adenovirus types 5 or 12, simian virus 40 (SV40), JC virus, or BK virus DNA in tumor.[149–151] Evidence of measles virus antigens and measles virus RNA sequences in some tumor biopsies has been presented but the findings have yet to be confirmed.[152,153] TT viruses are ubiquitous and have been detected at increased levels in the blood of patients with a variety of malignanices.[154] However, attempts to link TT viruses directly to lymphoma or Hodgkin lymphoma have thus far been unrewarding.[155,156]

Correlates of the EBV Association with Hodgkin Lymphoma

Histologic type, age, sex, ethnicity, and the physiologic effects of poverty all affect the association of EBV with Hodgkin lymphoma. A logistic regression analysis was used to examine EBV-associated Hodgkin lymphoma in a compilation of data from 1,546 patients in 14 studies.[4] The odds ratios for EBV-associated Hodgkin lymphoma were significantly elevated for mixed-cellularity versus nodular sclerosis histologic subtypes,

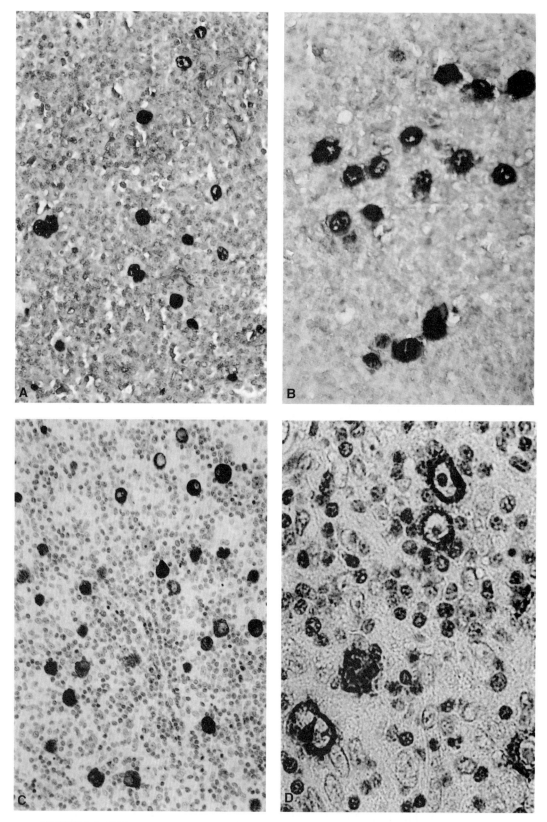

FIGURE 3.4. EBV gene expression in Reed-Sternberg cells. **A:** Polymerase III transcript (EBER) in situ hybridization. **B:** EBER in situ hybridization with CD15 labeling of Hodgkin cells. **C:** Latent membrane protein 1 (LMP1) immunohistochemistry. **D:** LMP2 immunohistochemistry. See color insert.

male versus female young adults, Hispanics versus whites, and children from economically underdeveloped versus better-developed regions. EBV is most commonly associated with the mixed-cellularity and lymphocyte-depletion subtypes of Hodgkin lymphoma[113,117,120,157–160] and less frequently with the nodular sclerosis subtype of Hodgkin lymphoma. Nodular lymphocyte predominant cases rarely contain EBV in the lymphocytic and histiocytic (L&H) cells,[113,120,128,160] although rare cases with EBV have been reported.[161]

Age is also associated with EBV positivity in Hodgkin lymphoma. Several studies have found an increased incidence in children (defined as younger than 16 years) in both developed and developing countries.[162–164] Some studies suggest an increased incidence of EBV positivity in cases in adults more than 50 years of age as opposed to cases in patients between the ages of 15 and 50 years.[163]

EBV positivity appears to correlate with geographic, cultural, genetic, and/or socioeconomic influences, all of which are difficult to separate. Among patients from the United States, most parts of Europe, and Israel, approximately 40% to 50% of cases of Hodgkin lymphoma have Reed-Sternberg cells that harbor virus.[4,119,120,165,166] In contrast, among populations from less developed regions, particularly those with large numbers of pediatric cases of Hodgkin lymphoma (e.g., populations from Central and South America), a very high EBV association has been found. In Hodgkin lymphoma among an indigenous Indian population in an underdeveloped area of Peru, an association of 94% was found.[167] Demographic features of the patient population were typical of those described for "third world" patients with Hodgkin lymphoma: a young median age (9 years), male predominance (male-female ratio of 3.5:1), and a predominance of the mixed-cellularity subtype. EBV RNA was identified in all or nearly all the Reed-Sternberg cells and variants in 30 of the 32 cases. This high rate of EBV positivity was statistically significantly higher than that found in typical Western cases, even after control for age and histologic subtype. Another study found a 100% incidence of EBV positivity in a series of pediatric cases of Hodgkin lymphoma from Honduras.[157] High rates of EBV positivity have also been reported in Brazilian,[162] Mexican,[168] and Argentine[169,170] series. The stronger association of EBV with Hodgkin lymphoma in Hispanics versus whites holds true even in U.S. series.[157,158] Series from various parts of Africa, Iran, Saudi Arabia, Greece, and China show a high incidence of EBV association.[121,164,171–173]

Infectious mononucleosis itself—that is, symptomatic primary infection—is a risk factor for the development of EBV-associated Hodgkin lymphoma. In a Scandinavian study of 38,555 patients tested for acute infectious mononucleosis, the acute disease was confirmed in 17,045 serologically.[3] Among the latter, the relative risk of developing EBV-associated Hodgkin lymphoma was increased 3.4- to 4.5-fold, whereas there was no increased risk of Hodgkin lymphoma without EBV. The median time from diagnosis of infectious mononucleosis to the diagnosis of Hodgkin lymphoma was 4.1 years (95% confidence interval, 1.8 to 8.3).

The incidence of EBV positivity in Hodgkin lymphoma occurring in HIV-infected patients is nearly 100%, which is higher than the rate of EBV positivity in HIV-associated non-Hodgkin lymphomas.[160,174,175] In contrast to Hodgkin lymphoma in immunocompetent persons, HIV-associated Hodgkin lymphoma is associated with both type 1 and type 2 EBV.[176,177]

Hodgkin lymphoma is in some cases familial. Cases of familial Hodgkin lymphoma are less likely to be EBV-associated than are sporadic cases.[178–180] In one large series of 60 patients from 27 families with familial Hodgkin lymphoma, the EBV association was 28%, with no excess of positive concordance.[178] There was no correlation between EBV serology and EBV positivity in the series. Genotyping of patients with Hodgkin lymphoma from the Netherlands and their first-degree relatives using microsatellite markers spanning the HLA region in combination with in situ hybridization studies to detect the presence or absence of virus in tumor showed an association of markers in the HLA class I region with EBV-positive tumors. These results are consistent with the possibility that antigenic presentation of viral peptides is important in the pathogenesis of Hodgkin lymphoma, although the result might also be explained by a neighboring gene or several that work in concert.[181]

EBV is infrequently identified in non-Hodgkin lymphomas that precede, develop simultaneously with, or follow the development of Hodgkin lymphoma. However, several cases of composite Hodgkin/non-Hodgkin lymphoma have been reported in which both the Reed-Sternberg cells and B-cell lymphoma cells contained EBV.[182] In addition, when chronic lymphocytic leukemia evolves into Hodgkin lymphoma, EBV is frequently detected in the RS cells or their variants and the histology is frequently mixed cellularity.[183–185] Hodgkin lymphoma in this setting is sometimes, but not always, clonally related to the preceeding chronic lymphocytic lymphoma as assessed by Ig gene rearrangements. Several authors have implicated fludarabine treatment in the development of EBV-associated Hodgkin lymphoma in chronic lymphocytic leukemia, and in at least some of these cases a distinct clonal origin of the tumor and the subsequent Hodgkin lymphoma have been clearly demonstrated.[186]

EBV in the Pathogenesis of Hodgkin Lymphoma

Many roles for EBV have been postulated in the pathogenesis of EBV-associated tumors. As reviewed above, several of the viral gene products are known to alter signaling pathways and transcription so as to modify cell growth and programmed cell death.[26,187–189] LMP1 and LMP2 are consistently expressed in EBV-associated Hodgkin lymphoma. The level of expression of these viral proteins as assessed by immunohistochemistry is as high as or higher than in other EBV-associated tumors. EBNA1 is expressed, and some investigators have suggested that EBNA1 may alter growth and apoptosis pathways, although there is no consensus in this regard. Finally, the EBERs and some of the BamHI-A transcripts are also expressed in Hodgkin lymphoma, and these have been suggested to be important in pathogenesis.

EBV may play a distinct role in the pathogenesis of Hodgkin lymphoma in comparison with other EBV-associated tumors.[190] One of the characteristics of Reed-Sternberg cells in classic Hodgkin lymphoma is the lack immunoglobulin gene expression, despite immunoglobulin gene rearrangement and somatic hypermutation. Crippling mutations that destroy the coding capacity of functional immunoglobulin rearrangements have been recognized in a subset of cases and these.[191] Literature review suggested a correlation with such crippling mutations and EBV association with EBV detected in 11 of 12 Hodgkin lymphoma cases with crippling mutations but only 19 of 43 cases lacking crippling mutations. The observation that in transgenic mice, LMP2A expression protects B-lineage cells from apoptosis normally associated with lack of immunoglobulin gene expression, led to the suggestion that LMP2A might play a key role in protecting tumor cells from apoptosis. Support for the hypothesis has come from the observation that destructive somatic hypermutation that precludes immunoglobulin expression appears to be highly associated with the presence of EBV in tumor cells, and EBV appears to be able to rescue and immortalize B-cells with stop codons in vitro.[30,192] Thus EBV may play a critical role in salvaging B-lineage cells with immunoglobulin stop codons from apoptosis.

The possibility that EBV might also play a role in the pathogenesis of Hodgkin lymphoma, even in patients where the commonly used tools for viral detection (immunohistochemistry for LMP1 or in situ hybridization for EBER expression) show no evidence of virus in tumor cells, has attracted interest but investigations to date do not favor the hypothesis. In particular, the idea that EBV-negative cases of Hodgkin lymphoma had previously been EBV positive but that tumor cells had lost the viral episome (the hit-and-run hypothesis) has some biologic plausibility in that the episome is readily lost from some tumor cell lines in culture, and it is not difficult to imagine that the viral genome might play a role early but after a series of genetic hits that it might no longer be required and the episome would be lost. If this were the case, it might be anticipated that the increase in Hodgkin lymphoma that follows infectious mononucleosis would include EBV-negative and EBV-positive cases, but an analysis from Scandinavia suggests that following serologically confirmed mononucleosis, the increased risk of Hodgkin lymphoma is accounted for by EBV-associated Hodgkin lymphoma.[3]

Similarly, the argument has been made that a defective EBV genome integrated in the chromosomal DNA of EBV-negative tumor cells might be missed by conventional EBV detection procedures including EBER in situ hybridization and LMP1 immunohistochemistry. Investigations using fluorescence in situ hybridization with large cosmid clones spanning the viral genome, PCR in situ hybridization, and PCR have yielded mixed results.[193–196]

Prognostic and Therapeutic Aspects

Investigators have variously reported no association, a more favorable prognosis for EBV-associated tumors, or a less favorable prognosis for EBV-associated tumors, as summarized in Table 3.5. Two large population-based studies, however, suggest explanations for discrepancies in previous reports.[197,198] Both studies were population based (in the United Kingdom and in northern California), and both teams of investigators reported an impact of age on the prognostic importance of the EBV association. Older patients' EBV-associated tumors had poorer survival even after adjusting for the effects of sex, stage, and B symptoms. Both groups also reported the inverse trend (better survival with EBV-associated tumors) in the youngest groups of patients with Hodgkin lymphoma.

Evidence that Reed-Sternberg cells express viral antigens and process these antigens for presentation has implications not only for the pathogenesis of Hodgkin lymphoma but also possibly for its treatment (Table 3.6). Adoptive cellular immunotherapy has proved effective in the prevention and treatment of lymphoproliferative disease in the setting of bone marrow transplantation.[106–108] Similar strategies for the treatment of Hodgkin lymphoma that specifically target tumor cells by virtue of their expression of viral antigens are presently

TABLE 3.5

EBV ASSOCIATION AND CLINICAL OUTCOME IN HODGKIN LYMPHOMA

	Reference	No. of patients	% EBV-associated	Prognostic significance of EBV association on overall survival
Population based	Jarrett et al[197]	437	35	Unfavorable in those ≥50 y
	Keegan et al[198]	922	27	Unfavorable in those >45 y
	Enblad et al[131]	117	27	None
	Stark et al[202]	102	34	Unfavorable
	Clarke et al[203]	311	17	Unfavorable in those >45 y
Clinical series	Armstrong et al[204]	59	36	None
	Claviez et al[205]	842	31	Unfavorable (age <21 y)
	Axdorph et al[206]	95	33	None
	Flavell et al[207]	273	29	None
	Murray et al[208]	190	27	None
	Vestlev et al[209]	66	41	None
	Kwon et al[210]	56	41	Positive impact on PFS in those <25 y
	Krugmann et al[211]	119	26	None
	Herling et al[212]	575	126	Favorable, but adjusted for stage and age
	Vassallo et al[213]	78	64	Favorable
	Glavina-Durdov et al[214]	100	26	None. Positive impact on DFS in those <30y
	Engel et al[215]	47	68	Favorable
	Morente et al[216]	140	51	Favorable
	Naresh et al[217]	110	78	Favorable

TABLE 3.6

POSSIBLE IMMUNOTHERAPY STRATEGIES FOR EBV RELATED HODGKIN LYMPHOMA

Intervention	Questions
VACCINE	
Prevent EBV infection	Can primary infection be prevented? If it were only delayed, might the consequences be more serious than natural infection?
Modify EBV infection	Can an immune response to a vaccine blunt the symptomatology associated with primary infection, even if primary infection is not prevented? Might this alter the risk of developing EBV-associated Hodgkin lymphoma?
Treat tumor/ prevent relapse	Can an immune response to viral antigens expressed by tumor cells kill tumor cells or prevent relapse?
ADOPTIVE IMMUNOTHERAPY	
Treat tumor/ prevent relapse	Can an immune response to viral antigens expressed by tumor cells kill tumor? Are there ex-vivo modifications of immune cells that might improve targeting or facilitate tumor-specific killing?

being explored with promising results.[199] Studies in 14 patients showed that infused effector cells could further expand in vivo, contribute to the memory pool, and traffic to tumor sites. Clinically, treatment was well tolerated and appeared to have antitumor activity. Two patients with measurable tumor at the time of treatment achieved complete remission, and in other cases remissions were maintained or disease appeared to have stabilized. New approaches to the selective expansion of antigen-specific T-cells that are particularly focused on antigens expressed in Hodgkin lymphoma, or strategies to overcome resistance to T-cell killing, promise to make treatment of Hodgkin lymphoma more effective.[200,201] Therapeutic vaccine trials with vaccines that express antigens or epitopes of EBV antigens expressed in Hodgkin lymphoma are underway at several centers. The goal of these vaccines is to boost cytotoxic responses to latency viral antigens expressed in tumor. Whereas adoptive immunotherapy approaches offer the possibility of specifically engineering effector cells, vaccines, if effective, may be more broadly applicable.

CONCLUSION

Epidemiologic, serologic, and direct-detection studies all independently point to EBV as a cofactor in the development of Hodgkin lymphoma. Clonality studies show that viral infection precedes clonal expansion of tumor cells. The ability of the virus to immortalize lymphocytes in tissue culture and other properties of the viral genome lend biologic plausibility to the theory of the virus as cofactor, as does the viral association with many other tumor types. However, as with other human tumor viruses, the relationship between infection and tumorigenesis remains complex and poorly understood.

Observations that crippling immunoglobulin gene mutations are commonly associated with Hodgkin lymphoma that harbors EBV suggests that the role that the virus plays in the pathogenesis of Hodgkin lymphoma may be intimately linked with the role that the B-cell plays in the viral life-cycle. Further investigation of the association promises not only to provide insights into pathogenesis but perhaps to open the way for new therapeutic strategies.

References

1. Weiss LM, Strickler JG, Warnke RA, et al. Epstein-Barr viral DNA in tissues of Hodgkin's disease. *Am J Pathol* 1987;129:86–91.
2. Macmahon B. Epidemiological evidence of the nature of Hodgkin's disease. *Cancer* 1957;10:1045–1054.
3. Hjalgrim H, Askling J, Rostgaard K, et al. Characteristics of Hodgkin's lymphoma after infectious mononucleosis. *N Engl J Med* 2003;349:1324–1332.
4. Glaser SL, Lin RJ, Stewart SL, et al. Epstein-Barr virus-associated Hodgkin's disease: epidemiologic characteristics in international data. *Int J Cancer* 1997;70:375–382.
5. Cohen JI. Epstein-Barr virus infection. *N Engl J Med* 2000;343:481–492.
6. Hoagland RJ. The transmission of infectious mononucleosis. *Am J Med Sci* 1955;229:262–272.
7. Yao QY, Rickinson AB, Epstein MA. Oropharyngeal shedding of infectious Epstein-Barr virus in healthy virus-immune donors. A prospective study. *Chin Med J (Engl)* 1985;98:191–196.
8. Lemon SM, Hutt LM, Shaw JE, et al. Replication of EBV in epithelial cells during infectious mononucleosis. *Nature* 1977;268:268–270.
9. Sixbey JW, Nedrud JG, Raab-Traub N, et al. Epstein-Barr virus replication in oropharyngeal epithelial cells. *N Engl J Med* 1984;310:1225–1230.
10. Pegtel DM, Middeldorp J, Thorley-Lawson DA. Epstein-Barr virus infection in ex vivo tonsil epithelial cell cultures of asymptomatic carriers. *J Virol* 2004;78:12613–12624.
11. Evans AS, Niederman JC, McCollum RW. Seroepidemiologic studies of infectious mononucleosis with EB virus. *N Engl J Med* 1968;279:1121–1127.
12. Henle G, Henle W, Diehl V. Relation of Burkitt's tumor-associated herpesytpe virus to infectious mononucleosis. *Proc Natl Acad Sci USA* 1968;59:94–101.
13. Williams H, Crawford DH. Epstein-Barr virus: the impact of scientific advances on clinical practice. *Blood* 2006;107:862–869.
14. Baer R, Bankier AT, Biggin MD, et al. DNA sequence and expression of the B95-8 Epstein-Barr virus genome. *Nature* 1984;310:207–211.
15. Farrell PJ. Epstein-Barr virus. The B95-8 strain map. *Methods Mol Biol* 2001;174:3–12.
16. Borza CM, Hutt-Fletcher LM. Alternate replication in B cells and epithelial cells switches tropism of Epstein-Barr virus. *Nat Med* 2002;8:594–599.
17. Speck P, Haan KM, Longnecker R. Epstein-Barr virus entry into cells. *Virology* 2000;277:1–5.
18. Young LS, Rickinson AB. Epstein-Barr virus: 40 years on. *Nat Rev Cancer* 2004;4:757–768.
19. Diehl V, Henle G, Henle W, et al. Demonstration of a herpes group virus in cultures of peripheral leukocytes from patients with infectious mononucleosis. *J Virol* 1968;2:663–669.
20. Moss DJ, Pope JH. Assay of the infectivity of Epstein-Barr virus by transformation of human leucocytes in vitro. *J Gen Virol* 1972;17:233–236.
21. Thorley-Lawson DA. Epstein-Barr virus: exploiting the immune system. *Nat Rev Immunol* 2001;1:75–82.
22. Kieff E. RAB. Epstein-Barr virus and its replication. In: Fields BN, Knipe DM, Howley PM, et al., eds. *Fields virology*, 4th ed. Philadelphia: Lippincott Williams & Wilkins; 2001:2511–2573.
23. Hung SC, Kang MS, Kieff E. Maintenance of Epstein-Barr virus (EBV) oriP-based episomes requires EBV-encoded nuclear antigen-1 chromosome-binding domains, which can be replaced by high-mobility group-I or histone H1. *Proc Natl Acad Sci USA* 2001;98:1865–1870.
24. Hayward SD. Viral interactions with the Notch pathway. *Semin Cancer Biol* 2004;14:387–396.
25. Wu S, Xie P, Welsh K, et al. LMP1 protein from the Epstein-Barr virus is a structural CD40 decoy in B lymphocytes for binding to TRAF3. *J Biol Chem* 2005;280:33620–33626.
26. Dirmeier U, Hoffmann R, Kilger E, et al. Latent membrane protein 1 of Epstein-Barr virus coordinately regulates proliferation with control of apoptosis. *Oncogene* 2005;24:1711–1717.
27. Portis T, Longnecker R. Epstein-Barr virus (EBV) LMP2A alters normal transcriptional regulation following B-cell receptor activation. *Virology* 2004;318:524–533.
28. Merchant M, Caldwell RG, Longnecker R. The LMP2A ITAM is essential for providing B cells with development and survival signals in vivo. *J Virol* 2000;74:9115–9124.
29. Chaganti S, Bell AI, Pastor NB, et al. Epstein-Barr virus infection in vitro can rescue germinal center B cells with inactivated immunoglobulin genes. *Blood* 2005;106:4249–4252.

30. Mancao C, Altmann M, Jungnickel B, et al. Rescue of "crippled" germinal center B cells from apoptosis by Epstein-Barr virus. *Blood* 2005;106: 4339–4344.

31. Ruf IK, Lackey KA, Warudkar S. Sample JT. Protection from interferon-induced apoptosis by Epstein-Barr virus small RNAs is not mediated by inhibition of PKR. *J Virol* 2005;79:14562–14569.

32. Wong HL, Wang X, Chang RC, et al. Stable expression of EBERs in immortalized nasopharyngeal epithelial cells confers resistance to apoptotic stress. *Mol Carcinog* 2005;44:92–101.

33. Chen H, Smith P, Ambinder RF, et al. Expression of Epstein-Barr virus BamHI-A rightward transcripts in latently infected B cells from peripheral blood. *Blood* 1999;93:3026–3032.

34. Thornburg NJ, Kusano S, Raab-Traub N. Identification of Epstein-Barr virus RK-BARF0-interacting proteins and characterization of expression pattern. *J Virol* 2004;78:12848–12856.

35. Pfeffer S, Sewer A, Lagos-Quintana M, et al. Identification of microRNAs of the herpesvirus family. *Nat Methods* 2005;2:269–276.

36. Miyashita EM, Yang B, Babcock GJ, et al. Identification of the site of Epstein-Barr virus persistence in vivo as a resting B cell. *J Virol* 1997;71: 4882–4891.

37. Miyashita EM, Yang B, Lam KM, et al. A novel form of Epstein-Barr virus latency in normal B cells in vivo. *Cell* 1995;80:593–601.

38. Hochberg D, Middeldorp JM, Catalina M, et al. Demonstration of the Burkitt's lymphoma Epstein-Barr virus phenotype in dividing latently infected memory cells in vivo. *Proc Natl Acad Sci USA* 2004;101:239–244.

39. Souza TA, Stollar BD, Sullivan JL, et al. Peripheral B cells latently infected with Epstein-Barr virus display molecular hallmarks of classical antigen-selected memory B cells. *Proc Natl Acad Sci USA* 2005;102:18093–18098.

40. Chen F, Zou JZ, di Renzo L, et al. A subpopulation of normal B cells latently infected with Epstein-Barr virus resembles Burkitt lymphoma cells in expressing EBNA-2 or LMP1. *J Virol* 1995;69:3752–3758.

41. Qu L, Rowe DT. Epstein-Barr virus latent gene expression in uncultured peripheral blood lymphocytes. *J Virol* 1992;66:3715–3724.

42. Tierney RJ, Steven N, Young LS, et al. Epstein-Barr virus latency in blood mononuclear cells: analysis of viral gene transcription during primary infection and in the carrier state. *J Virol* 1994;68:7374–7385.

43. Yang J, Tao Q, Flinn IW, et al. Characterization of Epstein-Barr virus-infected B cells in patients with posttransplantation lymphoproliferative disease: disappearance after rituximab therapy does not predict clinical response. *Blood* 2000;96:4055–4063.

44. Ryon JJ, Hayward SD, MacMahon EM, et al. In situ detection of lytic Epstein-Barr virus infection: expression of the NotI early gene and viral interleukin-10 late gene in clinical specimens. *J Infect Dis* 1993;168: 345–351.

45. Amon W, Farrell PJ. Reactivation of Epstein-Barr virus from latency. *Rev Med Virol* 2005;15:149–156.

46. Countryman J, Miller G. Activation of expression of latent Epstein-Barr herpesvirus after gene transfer with a small cloned subfragment of heterogeneous viral DNA. *Proc Natl Acad Sci USA* 1985;82:4085–4089.

47. Sarisky RT, Gao Z, Lieberman PM, et al. A replication function associated with the activation domain of the Epstein-Barr virus Zta transactivator. *J Virol* 1996;70:8340–8347.

48. Wu FY, Wang SE, Chen H, et al. CCAAT/enhancer binding protein alpha binds to the Epstein-Barr virus (EBV) ZTA protein through oligomeric interactions and contributes to cooperative transcriptional activation of the ZTA promoter through direct binding to the ZII and ZIIIB motifs during induction of the EBV lytic cycle. *J Virol* 2004;78:4847–4865.

49. Wu FY, Chen H, Wang SE, et al. CCAAT/enhancer binding protein alpha interacts with ZTA and mediates ZTA-induced p21(CIP-1) accumulation and G(1) cell cycle arrest during the Epstein-Barr virus lytic cycle. *J Virol* 2003;77:1481–1500.

50. Moore SM, Cannon JS, Tanhehco YC, et al. Induction of Epstein-Barr virus kinases to sensitize tumor cells to nucleoside analogues. *Antimicrob Agents Chemother* 2001;45:2082–2091.

51. Cannon JS, Hamzeh F, Moore S, et al. Human herpesvirus 8-encoded thymidine kinase and phosphotransferase homologues confer sensitivity to ganciclovir. *J Virol* 1999;73:4786–4793.

52. Wang JT, Yang PW, Lee CP, et al. Detection of Epstein-Barr virus BGLF4 protein kinase in virus replication compartments and virus particles. *J Gen Virol* 2005;86:3215–3225.

53. Gershburg E, Pagano JS. Epstein-Barr virus infections: prospects for treatment. *J Antimicrob Chemother* 2005;56:277–281.

54. Reynolds DJ, Banks PM, Gulley ML. New characterization of infectious mononucleosis and a phenotypic comparison with Hodgkin's disease. *Am J Pathol* 1995;146:379–388.

55. Woodberry T, Suscovich TJ, Henry LM, et al. Differential targeting and shifts in the immunodominance of Epstein-Barr virus—specific CD8 and CD4 T cell responses during acute and persistent infection. *J Infect Dis* 2005; 192:1513–1524.

56. Khanna R, Burrows SR, Kurilla MG, et al. Localization of Epstein-Barr virus cytotoxic T cell epitopes using recombinant vaccinia: implications for vaccine development. *J Exp Med* 1992;176:169–176.

57. Murray RJ, Kurilla MG, Brooks JM, et al. Identification of target antigens for the human cytotoxic T cell response to Epstein-Barr virus (EBV): implications for the immune control of EBV-positive malignancies. *J Exp Med* 1992;176:157–168.

58. Hislop AD, Annels NE, Gudgeon NH, et al. Epitope-specific evolution of human CD8(+) T cell responses from primary to persistent phases of Epstein-Barr virus infection. *J Exp Med* 2002;195:893–905.

59. Tomkinson BE, Maziarz R, Sullivan JL. Characterization of the T cell-mediated cellular cytotoxicity during acute infectious mononucleosis. *J Immunol* 1989;143:660–670.

60. Shope T, Dechairo D, Miller G. Malignant lymphoma in cottontop marmosets after inoculation with Epstein-Barr virus. *Proc Natl Acad Sci USA* 1973;70:2487–2491.

61. Mosier DE, Baird SM, Kirven MB, et al. EBV-associated B-cell lymphomas following transfer of human peripheral blood lymphocytes to mice with severe combined immune deficiency. *Curr Top Microbiol Immunol* 1990;166:317–323.

62. Rowe M, Young LS, Crocker J, et al. Epstein-Barr virus (EBV)-associated lymphoproliferative disease in the SCID mouse model: implications for the pathogenesis of EBV-positive lymphomas in man. *J Exp Med* 1991;173: 147–158.

63. Kang MS, Lu H, Yasui T, et al. Epstein-Barr virus nuclear antigen 1 does not induce lymphoma in transgenic FVB mice. *Proc Natl Acad Sci USA* 2005;102:820–825.

64. Wilson JB, Bell JL, Levine AJ. Expression of Epstein-Barr virus nuclear antigen-1 induces B cell neoplasia in transgenic mice. *EMBO J* 1996; 15:3117–3126.

65. Gulley ML, Raphael M, Lutz CT, et al. Epstein-Barr virus integration in human lymphomas and lymphoid cell lines. *Cancer* 1992;70:185–191.

66. Sato H, Takimoto T, Tanaka S, et al. Concatameric replication of Epstein-Barr virus: structure of the termini in virus-producer and newly transformed cell lines. *J Virol* 1990;64:5295–5300.

67. Gulley ML. Molecular diagnosis of Epstein-Barr virus-related diseases. *J Mol Diagn* 2001;3:1–10.

68. Moody CA, Scott RS, Su T, et al. Length of Epstein-Barr virus termini as a determinant of epithelial cell clonal emergence. *J Virol* 2003;77:8555–8561.

69. Wu TC, Mann RB, Epstein JI, et al. Abundant expression of EBER1 small nuclear RNA in nasopharyngeal carcinoma. A morphologically distinctive target for detection of Epstein-Barr virus in formalin-fixed paraffin-embedded carcinoma specimens. *Am J Pathol* 1991;138:1461–1469.

70. Wu TC, Mann RB, Charache P, et al. Detection of EBV gene expression in Reed-Sternberg cells of Hodgkin's disease. *Int J Cancer* 1990;46:801–804.

71. Glaser SL, Gulley ML, Borowitz MJ, et al. Inter- and intra-observer reliability of Epstein-Barr virus detection in Hodgkin lymphoma using histochemical procedures. *Leuk Lymphoma* 2004;45:489–497.

72. Gulley ML, Glaser SL, Craig FE, et al. Guidelines for interpreting EBER in situ hybridization and LMP1 immunohistochemical tests for detecting Epstein-Barr virus in Hodgkin lymphoma. *Am J Clin Pathol* 2002;117: 259–267.

73. Arrand JR, Rymo L. Characterization of the major Epstein-Barr virus-specific RNA in Burkitt lymphoma-derived cells. *J Virol* 1982;41:376–389.

74. Howe JG, Shu MD. Epstein-Barr virus small RNA (EBER) genes: unique transcription units that combine RNA polymerase II and III promoter elements. *Cell* 1989;57:825–834.

75. Howe JG, Steitz JA. Localization of Epstein-Barr virus-encoded small RNAs by in situ hybridization. *Proc Natl Acad Sci USA* 1986;83:9006–9010.

76. Murray PG, Lissauer D, Junying J, et al. Reactivity with a monoclonal antibody to Epstein-Barr virus (EBV) nuclear antigen 1 defines a subset of aggressive breast cancers in the absence of the EBV genome. *Cancer Res* 2003;63:2338–2343.

77. Iezzoni JC, Gaffey MJ, Weiss LM. The role of Epstein-Barr virus in lymphoepithelioma-like carcinomas. *Am J Clin Pathol* 1995;103:308–315.

78. Shibata D, Tokunaga M, Uemura Y, et al. Association of Epstein-Barr virus with undifferentiated gastric carcinomas with intense lymphoid infiltration. Lymphoepithelioma-like carcinoma. *Am J Pathol* 1991;139:469–474.

79. Shibata D, Weiss LM. Epstein-Barr virus-associated gastric adenocarcinoma. *Am J Pathol* 1992;140:769–774.

80. Lee ES, Locker J, Nalesnik M, et al. The association of Epstein-Barr virus with smooth-muscle tumors occurring after organ transplantation. *N Engl J Med* 1995;332:19–25.

81. Arber DA, Kamel OW, van de Rijn M, et al. Frequent presence of the Epstein-Barr virus in inflammatory pseudotumor. *Hum Pathol* 1995;26: 1093–1098.

82. Epstein MA, Achong BG, Barr YM. Virus particles in cultured lymphoblasts from Burkitt's lymphoma. *Lancet* 1964;15:702–703.

83. Bacchi MM, Bacchi CE, Alvarenga M, et al. Burkitt's lymphoma in Brazil: strong association with Epstein-Barr virus. *Mod Pathol* 1996;9:63–67.

84. Chan JK, Tsang WY, Ng CS, et al. A study of the association of Epstein-Barr virus with Burkitt's lymphoma occurring in a Chinese population. *Histopathology* 1995;26:239–245.

85. Gutierrez MI, Bhatia K, Barriga F, et al. Molecular epidemiology of Burkitt's lymphoma from South America: differences in breakpoint location and Epstein-Barr virus association from tumors in other world regions. *Blood* 1992;79:3261–3266.

86. Hummel M, Anagnostopoulos I, Korbjuhn P, et al. Epstein-Barr virus in B-cell non-Hodgkin's lymphomas: unexpected infection patterns and different infection incidence in low- and high-grade types. *J Pathol* 1995;175:263–271.

87. Shiramizu B, Barriga F, Neequaye J, et al. Patterns of chromosomal breakpoint locations in Burkitt's lymphoma: relevance to geography and Epstein-Barr virus association. *Blood* 1991;77:1516–1526.

88. Niedobitek G, Agathanggelou A, Rowe M, et al. Heterogeneous expression of Epstein-Barr virus latent proteins in endemic Burkitt's lymphoma. *Blood* 1995;86:659–665.

89. Tao Q, Robertson KD, Manns A, et al. Epstein-Barr virus (EBV) in endemic Burkitt's lymphoma: molecular analysis of primary tumor tissue. *Blood* 1998;91:1373–1381.

90. Rowe M, Rowe DT, Gregory CD, et al. Differences in B cell growth phenotype reflect novel patterns of Epstein-Barr virus latent gene expression in Burkitt's lymphoma cells. *EMBO J* 1987;6:2743–2751.

91. Morra M, Howie D, Grande MS, et al. X-linked lymphoproliferative disease: a progressive immunodeficiency. *Annu Rev Immunol* 2001;19:657–682.

92. Coffey AJ, Brooksbank RA, Brandau O, et al. Host response to EBV infection in X-linked lymphoproliferative disease results from mutations in an SH2-domain encoding gene. *Nat Genet* 1998;20:129–135.

93. Sayos J, Wu C, Morra M, et al. The X-linked lymphoproliferative-disease gene product SAP regulates signals induced through the co-receptor SLAM. *Nature* 1998;395:462–469.

94. Nichols KE, Harkin DP, Levitz S, et al. Inactivating mutations in an SH2 domain-encoding gene in X-linked lymphoproliferative syndrome. *Proc Natl Acad Sci USA* 1998;95:13765–13770.

95. Milone MC, Tsai DE, Hodinka RL, et al. Treatment of primary Epstein-Barr virus infection in patients with X-linked lymphoproliferative disease using B-cell-directed therapy. *Blood* 2005;105:994–996.

96. Swinnen LJ. Organ transplant-related lymphoma. *Curr Treat Options Oncol* 2001;2:301–308.

97. Gottschalk S, Rooney CM, Heslop HE. Post-transplant lymphoproliferative disorders. *Annu Rev Med* 2005;56:29–44.

98. Knowles DM, Cesarman E, Chadburn A, et al. Correlative morphologic and molecular genetic analysis demonstrates three distinct categories of post-transplantation lymphoproliferative disorders. *Blood* 1995;85:552–565.

99. Arber DA, Shibata D, Chen YY, et al. Characterization of the topography of Epstein-Barr virus infection in human immunodeficiency virus-associated lymphoid tissues. *Mod Pathol* 1992;5:559–566.

100. Hamilton-Dutoit SJ, Pallesen G, Franzmann MB, et al. AIDS-related lymphoma. Histopathology, immunophenotype, and association with Epstein-Barr virus as demonstrated by in situ nucleic acid hybridization. *Am J Pathol* 1991;138:149–163.

101. Raphael MM, Audouin J, Lamine M, et al. Immunophenotypic and genotypic analysis of acquired immunodeficiency syndrome-related non-Hodgkin's lymphomas. Correlation with histologic features in 36 cases. French study group of pathology for HIV-associated tumors. *Am J Clin Pathol* 1994;101:773–782.

102. Cesarman E, Chang Y, Moore PS, et al. Kaposi's sarcoma-associated herpesvirus-like DNA sequences in AIDS-related body-cavity-based lymphomas. *N Engl J Med* 1995;332:1186–1191.

103. Nador RG, Cesarman E, Chadburn A, et al. Primary effusion lymphoma: a distinct clinicopathologic entity associated with the Kaposi's sarcoma-associated herpes virus. *Blood* 1996;88:645–656.

104. O'Reilly RJ, Small TN, Papadopoulos E, et al. Biology and adoptive cell therapy of Epstein-Barr virus-associated lymphoproliferative disorders in recipients of marrow allograft. *Immunol Rev* 1997;157:195–216.

105. Lucas KG, Small TN, Heller G, et al. The development of cellular immunity to Epstein-Barr virus after allogeneic bone marrow transplantation. *Blood* 1996;87:2594–2603.

106. Papadopoulos EB, Ladanyi M, Emanuel D, et al. Infusions of donor leukocytes to treat Epstein-Barr virus-associated lymphoproliferative disorders after allogeneic bone marrow transplantation. *N Engl J Med* 1994;330:1185–1191.

107. Heslop HE, Ng CY, Li C, et al. Long-term restoration of immunity against Epstein-Barr virus infection by adoptive transfer of gene-modified virus-specific T lymphocytes. *Nat Med* 1996;2:551–555.

108. Rooney CM, Smith CA, Ng CY, et al. Use of gene-modified virus-specific T lymphocytes to control Epstein-Barr-virus-related lymphoproliferation. *Lancet* 1995;345:9–13.

109. Anagnostopoulos I, Herbst H, Niedobitek G, et al. Demonstration of monoclonal EBV genomes in Hodgkin's disease and Ki-1-positive anaplastic large cell lymphoma by combined Southern blot and in situ hybridization. *Blood* 1989;74:810–816.

110. Staal SP, Ambinder R, Beschorner WE, et al. A survey of Epstein-Barr virus DNA in lymphoid tissue. Frequent detection in Hodgkin's disease. *Am J Clin Pathol* 1989;91:1–5.

111. Weiss LM, Movahed LA, Warnke RA, et al. Detection of Epstein-Barr viral genomes in Reed-Sternberg cells of Hodgkin's disease. *N Engl J Med* 1989;320:502–506.

112. Gledhill S, Gallagher A, Jones DB, et al. Viral involvement in Hodgkin's disease: detection of clonal type A Epstein-Barr virus genomes in tumour samples. *Br J Cancer* 1991;64:227–232.

113. Brousset P, Chittal S, Schlaifer D, et al. Detection of Epstein-Barr virus messenger RNA in Reed-Sternberg cells of Hodgkin's disease by in situ hybridization with biotinylated probes on specially processed modified acetone methyl benzoate xylene (ModAMeX) sections. *Blood* 1991;77:1781–1786.

114. Coates PJ, Slavin G, D'Ardenne AJ. Persistence of Epstein-Barr virus in Reed-Sternberg cells throughout the course of Hodgkin's disease. *J Pathol* 1991;164:291–297.

115. Uhara H, Sato Y, Mukai K, et al. Detection of Epstein-Barr virus DNA in Reed-Sternberg cells of Hodgkin's disease using the polymerase chain reaction and in situ hybridization. *Jpn J Cancer Res* 1990;81:272–278.

116. Bellas C, Mampaso F, Fraile G, et al. Detection of Epstein-Barr genome in the lymph nodes of Hodgkin's disease. *Postgrad Med J* 1993;69:916–919.

117. Herbst H, Steinbrecher E, Niedobitek G, et al. Distribution and phenotype of Epstein-Barr virus-harboring cells in Hodgkin's disease. *Blood* 1992;80:484–491.

118. Hummel M, Anagnostopoulos I, Dallenbach F, et al. EBV infection patterns in Hodgkin's disease and normal lymphoid tissue: expression and cellular localization of EBV gene products. *Br J Haematol* 1992;82:689–694.

119. Jiwa NM, Kanavaros P, De Bruin PC, et al. Presence of Epstein-Barr virus harbouring small and intermediate-sized cells in Hodgkin's disease. Is there a relationship with Reed-Sternberg cells? *J Pathol* 1993;170:129–136.

120. Weiss LM, Chen YY, Liu XF, et al. Epstein-Barr virus and Hodgkin's disease. A correlative in situ hybridization and polymerase chain reaction study. *Am J Pathol* 1991;139:1259–1265.

121. Zhou XG, Hamilton-Dutoit SJ, Yan QH, et al. The association between Epstein-Barr virus and Chinese Hodgkin's disease. *Int J Cancer* 1993;55:359–363.

122. Roth J, Daus H, Gause A, et al. Detection of Epstein-Barr virus DNA in Hodgkin- and Reed-Sternberg-cells by single cell PCR. *Leuk Lymphoma* 1994;13:137–142.

123. Teramoto N, Akagi T, Yoshino T, et al. Direct detection of Epstein-Barr virus DNA from a single Reed-Sternberg cell of Hodgkin's disease by polymerase chain reaction. *Jpn J Cancer Res* 1992;83:329–333.

124. Poppema S, van Imhoff G, Torensma R, et al. Lymphadenopathy morphologically consistent with Hodgkin's disease associated with Epstein-Barr virus infection. *Am J Clin Pathol* 1985;84:385–390.

125. Pallesen G, Hamilton-Dutoit SJ, Rowe M, et al. Expression of Epstein-Barr virus latent gene products in tumour cells of Hodgkin's disease. *Lancet* 1991;337:320–322.

126. Herbst H, Dallenbach F, Hummel M, et al. Epstein-Barr virus latent membrane protein expression in Hodgkin and Reed-Sternberg cells. *Proc Natl Acad Sci USA* 1991;88:4766–4770.

127. Murray PG, Constandinou CM, Crocker J, et al. Analysis of major histocompatibility complex class I, TAP expression, and LMP2 epitope sequence in Epstein-Barr virus-positive Hodgkin's disease. *Blood* 1998;92:2477–2483.

128. Grasser FA, Murray PG, Kremmer E, et al. Monoclonal antibodies directed against the Epstein-Barr virus-encoded nuclear antigen 1 (EBNA1): immunohistologic detection of EBNA1 in the malignant cells of Hodgkin's disease. *Blood* 1994;84:3792–3798.

129. Deacon EM, Pallesen G, Niedobitek G, et al. Epstein-Barr virus and Hodgkin's disease: transcriptional analysis of virus latency in the malignant cells. *J Exp Med* 1993;177:339–349.

130. Niedobitek G, Kremmer E, Herbst H, et al. Immunohistochemical detection of the Epstein-Barr virus-encoded latent membrane protein 2A in Hodgkin's disease and infectious mononucleosis. *Blood* 1997;90:1664–1672.

131. Enblad G, Sandvej K, Lennette E, et al. Lack of correlation between EBV serology and presence of EBV in the Hodgkin and Reed-Sternberg cells of patients with Hodgkin's disease. *Int J Cancer* 1997;72:394–397.

132. Lennette ET, Rymo L, Yadav M, et al. Disease-related differences in antibody patterns against EBV-encoded nuclear antigens EBNA 1, EBNA 2 and EBNA 6. *Eur J Cancer* 1993;29A:1584–1589.

133. Levine PH, Pallesen G, Ebbesen P, et al. Evaluation of Epstein-Barr virus antibody patterns and detection of viral markers in the biopsies of patients with Hodgkin's disease. *Int J Cancer* 1994;59:48–50.

134. Fellbaum C, Hansmann ML, Niedermeyer H, et al. Influence of Epstein-Barr virus genomes on patient survival in Hodgkin's disease. *Am J Clin Pathol* 1992;98:319–323.

135. Lin JC, Lin SC, De BK, et al. Precision of genotyping of Epstein-Barr virus by polymerase chain reaction using three gene loci (EBNA-2, EBNA-3C, and EBER): predominance of type A virus associated with Hodgkin's disease. *Blood* 1993;81:3372–3381.

136. Knecht H, Bachmann E, Brousset P, et al. Deletions within the LMP1 oncogene of Epstein-Barr virus are clustered in Hodgkin's disease and identical to those observed in nasopharyngeal carcinoma. *Blood* 1993;82:2937–2942.

137. Knecht H, Bachmann E, Joske DJ, et al. Molecular analysis of the LMP (latent membrane protein) oncogene in Hodgkin's disease. *Leukemia* 1993;7:580–585.

138. Chen ML, Tsai CN, Liang CL, et al. Cloning and characterization of the latent membrane protein (LMP) of a specific Epstein-Barr virus variant derived from the nasopharyngeal carcinoma in the Taiwanese population. *Oncogene* 1992;7:2131–2140.

139. Hayashi K, Chen WG, Chen YY, et al. Deletion of Epstein-Barr virus latent membrane protein 1 gene in United States and Brazilian Hodgkin's disease and reactive lymphoid tissue: high frequency of a 30-bp deletion. *Hum Pathol* 1997;28:1408–1414.

140. Boiocchi M, Dolcetti R, De Re V, et al. Demonstration of a unique Epstein-Barr virus-positive cellular clone in metachronous multiple localizations of Hodgkin's disease. *Am J Pathol* 1993;142:33–38.

141. Vasef MA, Kamel OW, Chen YY, et al. Detection of Epstein-Barr virus in multiple sites involved by Hodgkin's disease. *Am J Pathol* 1995;147:1408–1415.

142. Delecluse HJ, Marafioti T, Hummel M, et al. Disappearance of the Epstein-Barr virus in a relapse of Hodgkin's disease. *J Pathol* 1997;182:475–479.

143. Brousset P, Schlaifer D, Meggetto F, et al. Persistence of the same viral strain in early and late relapses of Epstein-Barr virus-associated Hodgkin's disease. *Blood* 1994;84:2447–2451.

144. Meij P, Vervoort MB, Bloemena E, et al. Antibody responses to Epstein-Barr virus-encoded latent membrane protein-1 (LMP1) and expression of LMP1 in juvenile Hodgkin's disease. *J Med Virol* 2002;68:370–377.

145. Chang ET, Zheng T, Lennette ET, et al. Heterogeneity of risk factors and antibody profiles in epstein-barr virus genome-positive and -negative Hodgkin lymphoma. *J Infect Dis* 2004;189:2271–2281.

146. Evans AS, Gutensohn NM. A population-based case-control study of EBV and other viral antibodies among persons with Hodgkin's disease and their siblings. *Int J Cancer* 1984;34:149–157.

147. Clark DA, Alexander FE, McKinney PA, et al. The seroepidemiology of human herpesvirus-6 (HHV-6) from a case-control study of leukaemia and lymphoma. *Int J Cancer* 1990;45:829–833.

148. Torelli G, Marasca R, Luppi M, et al. Human herpesvirus-6 in human lymphomas: identification of specific sequences in Hodgkin's lymphomas by polymerase chain reaction. *Blood* 1991;77:2251–2258.

149. Armstrong AA, Shield L, Gallagher A, et al. Lack of involvement of known oncogenic DNA viruses in Epstein-Barr virus-negative Hodgkin's disease. *Br J Cancer* 1998;77:1045–1047.

150. Gallagher A, Perry J, Shield L, et al. Viruses and Hodgkin disease: no evidence of novel herpesviruses in non-EBV-associated lesions. *Int J Cancer* 2002;101:259–264.

151. Schmidt CA, Oettle H, Peng R, et al. Presence of human beta- and gamma-herpes virus DNA in Hodgkin's disease. *Leuk Res* 2000;24:865–870.

152. Benharroch D, Shemer-Avni Y, Myint YY, et al. Measles virus: evidence of an association with Hodgkin's disease. *Br J Cancer* 2004;91:572–579.

153. Glaser SL, Keegan TH, Clarke CA, et al. Exposure to childhood infections and risk of Epstein-Barr virus–defined Hodgkin's lymphoma in women. *Int J Cancer* 2005;115:599–605.

154. Jelcic I, Hotz-Wagenblatt A, Hunziker A, et al. Isolation of multiple TT virus genotypes from spleen biopsy tissue from a Hodgkin's disease patient: genome reorganization and diversity in the hypervariable region. *J Virol* 2004;78:7498–7507.

155. Garbuglia AR, Iezzi T, Capobianchi MR, et al. Detection of TT virus in lymph node biopsies of B-cell lymphoma and Hodgkin's disease, and its association with EBV infection. *Int J Immunopathol Pharmacol* 2003;16:109–118.

156. Zhong S, Yeo W, Tang MW, et al. Gross elevation of TT virus genome load in the peripheral blood mononuclear cells of cancer patients. *Ann NY Acad Sci* 2001;945:84–92.

157. Ambinder RF, Browning PJ, Lorenzana I, et al. Epstein-Barr virus and childhood Hodgkin's disease in Honduras and the United States. *Blood* 1993;81:462–467.

158. Gulley ML, Eagan PA, Quintanilla-Martinez L, et al. Epstein-Barr virus DNA is abundant and monoclonal in the Reed-Sternberg cells of Hodgkin's disease: association with mixed cellularity subtype and Hispanic American ethnicity. *Blood* 1994;83:1595–1602.

159. Pallesen G, Sandvej K, Hamilton-Dutoit SJ, et al. Activation of Epstein-Barr virus replication in Hodgkin and Reed-Sternberg cells. *Blood* 1991;78:1162–1165.

160. Uccini S, Monardo F, Stoppacciaro A, et al. High frequency of Epstein-Barr virus genome detection in Hodgkin's disease of HIV-positive patients. *Int J Cancer* 1990;46:581–585.

161. Khalidi HS, Lones MA, Zhou Y, et al. Detection of Epstein-Barr virus in the L & H cells of nodular lymphocyte predominance Hodgkin's disease: report of a case documented by immunohistochemical, in situ hybridization, and polymerase chain reaction methods. *Am J Clin Pathol* 1997;108:687–692.

162. Armstrong AA, Alexander FE, Paes RP, et al. Association of Epstein-Barr virus with pediatric Hodgkin's disease. *Am J Pathol* 1993; 142:1683–1688.

163. Jarrett RF, Gallagher A, Jones DB, et al. Detection of Epstein-Barr virus genomes in Hodgkin's disease: relation to age. *J Clin Pathol* 1991;44:844–848.

164. Weinreb M, Day PJ, Niggli F, et al. The consistent association between Epstein-Barr virus and Hodgkin's disease in children in Kenya. *Blood* 1996;87:3828–3836.

165. Benharroch D, Brousset P, Goldstein J, et al. Association of the Epstein-Barr virus with Hodgkin's disease in southern Israel. *Int J Cancer* 1997;71:138–141.

166. Lauritzen AF, Hording U, Nielsen HW. Epstein-Barr virus and Hodgkin's disease: a comparative immunological, in situ hybridization, and polymerase chain reaction study. *APMIS* 1994;102:495–500.

167. Chang KL, Albujar PF, Chen YY, et al. High prevalence of Epstein-Barr virus in the Reed-Sternberg cells of Hodgkin's disease occurring in Peru. *Blood* 1993;81:496–501.

168. Quintanilla-Martinez L, Gamboa-Domnquez A, Gamez-Ledesma I, et al. Association of Epstein-Barr virus latent membrane protein and Hodgkin's disease in Mexico. *Mod Pathol* 1995;8:675–679.

169. Preciado MV, De Matteo E, Diez B, et al. Presence of Epstein-Barr virus and strain type assignment in Argentine childhood Hodgkin's disease. *Blood* 1995;86:3922–3929.

170. Preciado MV, Diez B, Grinstein S. Epstein Barr virus in Argentine pediatric Hodgkin's disease. *Leuk Lymphoma* 1997;24:283–290.

171. Leoncini L, Spina D, Nyong'o A, et al. Neoplastic cells of Hodgkin's disease show differences in EBV expression between Kenya and Italy. *Int J Cancer* 1996;65:781–784.

172. Chan JK, Yip TT, Tsang WY, et al. Detection of Epstein-Barr virus in Hodgkin's disease occurring in an Oriental population. *Hum Pathol.* 1995;26:314–318.

173. Peh SC, Looi LM, Pallesen G. Epstein-Barr virus (EBV) and Hodgkin's disease in a multi-ethnic population in Malaysia. *Histopathology* 1997; 30:227–233.

174. Herndier BG, Sanchez HC, Chang KL, et al. High prevalence of Epstein-Barr virus in the Reed-Sternberg cells of HIV-associated Hodgkin's disease. *Am J Pathol* 1993;142:1073–1079.

175. Siebert JD, Ambinder RF, Napoli VM, et al. Human immunodeficiency virus-associated Hodgkin's disease contains latent, not replicative, Epstein-Barr virus. *Hum Pathol* 1995;26:1191–1195.

176. Boyle MJ, Vasak E, Tschuchnigg M, et al. Subtypes of Epstein-Barr virus (EBV) in Hodgkin's disease: association between B-type EBV and immuno-compromise. *Blood* 1993;81:468–474.

177. De Re V, Boiocchi M, De Vita S, et al. Subtypes of Epstein-Barr virus in HIV-1-associated and HIV-1-unrelated Hodgkin's disease cases. *Int J Cancer* 1993;54:895–898.

178. Lin AY, Kingma DW, Lennette ET, et al. Epstein-Barr virus and familial Hodgkin's disease. *Blood* 1996;88:3160–3165.

179. Mack TM, Cozen W, Shibata DK, et al. Concordance for Hodgkin's disease in identical twins suggesting genetic susceptibility to the young-adult form of the disease. *N Engl J Med* 1995;332:413–418.

180. Schlaifer D, Rigal-Huguet F, Robert A, et al. Epstein-Barr virus in familial Hodgkin's disease. *Br J Haematol* 1994;88:636–638.

181. Diepstra A, Niens M, Vellenga E, et al. Association with HLA class I in Epstein-Barr-virus-positive and with HLA class III in Epstein-Barr-virus-negative Hodgkin's lymphoma. *Lancet* 2005;365:2216–2224.

182. Kingma DW, Medeiros LJ, Barletta J, et al. Epstein-Barr virus is infrequently identified in non-Hodgkin's lymphomas associated with Hodgkin's disease. *Am J Surg Pathol* 1994;18:48–61.

183. Fong D, Kaiser A, Spizzo G, et al. Hodgkin's disease variant of Richter's syndrome in chronic lymphocytic leukaemia patients previously treated with fludarabine. *Br J Haematol* 2005;129:199–205.

184. Momose H, Jaffe ES, Shin SS, et al. Chronic lymphocytic leukemia/small lymphocytic lymphoma with Reed-Sternberg-like cells and possible transformation to Hodgkin's disease. Mediation by Epstein-Barr virus. *Am J Surg Pathol* 1992;16:859–867.

185. Rubin D, Hudnall SD, Aisenberg A, et al. Richter's transformation of chronic lymphocytic leukemia with Hodgkin's-like cells is associated with Epstein-Barr virus infection. *Mod Pathol* 1994;7:91–98.

186. De Leval L, Vivario M, De Prijck B, et al. Distinct clonal origin in two cases of Hodgkin's lymphoma variant of Richter's syndrome associated With EBV infection. *Am J Surg Pathol* 2004;28:679–686.

187. Hammerschmidt W, Sugden B. Epstein-Barr virus sustains Burkitt's lymphomas and Hodgkin's disease. *Trends Mol Med* 2004;10:331–336.

188. Ikeda M, Longnecker R. Pre-B-cell colony formation assay. *Methods Mol Biol* 2005;292:279–284.

189. Portis T, Ikeda M, Longnecker R. Epstein-Barr virus LMP2A: regulating cellular ubiquitination processes for maintenance of viral latency? *Trends Immunol* 2004;25:422–426.

190. Re D, Kuppers R, Diehl V. Molecular pathogenesis of Hodgkin's lymphoma. *J Clin Oncol* 2005;23:6379–6386.

191. Brauninger A, Schmitz R, Bechtel D, et al. Molecular biology of Hodgkin's and Reed/Sternberg cells in Hodgkin's lymphoma. *Int J Cancer* 2006;118:1853–1861.

192. Bechtel D, Kurth J, Unkel C, et al. Transformation of BCR-deficient germinal-center B cells by EBV supports a major role of the virus in the pathogenesis of Hodgkin and posttransplantation lymphomas. *Blood* 2005;106:4345–4350.

193. Ambinder RF. Gammaherpesviruses and "Hit-and-Run" oncogenesis. *Am J Pathol* 2000;156:1–3.

194. Gallagher A, Perry J, Freeland J, et al. Hodgkin lymphoma and Epstein-Barr virus (EBV): no evidence to support hit-and-run mechanism in cases classified as non-EBV-associated. *Int J Cancer* 2003;104:624–630.

195. Staratschek-Jox A, Kotkowski S, Belge G, et al. Detection of Epstein-Barr virus in Hodgkin-Reed-Sternberg cells: no evidence for the persistence of integrated viral fragments inLatent membrane protein-1 (LMP-1)-negative classical Hodgkin's disease. *Am J Pathol* 2000;156:209–216.

196. Gan YJ, Razzouk BI, Su T, et al. A defective, rearranged Epstein-Barr virus genome in EBER-negative and EBER-positive Hodgkin's disease. *Am J Pathol* 2002;160:781–786.

197. Jarrett RF, Stark GL, White J, et al. Impact of tumor Epstein-Barr virus status on presenting features and outcome in age-defined subgroups of patients with classic Hodgkin lymphoma: a population-based study. *Blood* 2005;106:2444–2451.

198. Keegan TH, Glaser SL, Clarke CA, et al. Epstein-Barr virus as a marker of survival after Hodgkin's lymphoma: a population-based study. *J Clin Oncol* 2005;23:7604–7613.

199. Bollard CM, Aguilar L, Straathof KC, et al. Cytotoxic T lymphocyte therapy for Epstein-Barr virus+ Hodgkin's disease. *J Exp Med* 2004; 200:1623–1633.

200. Wagner HJ, Bollard CM, Vigouroux S, et al. A strategy for treatment of Epstein-Barr virus-positive Hodgkin's disease by targeting interleukin 12 to the tumor environment using tumor antigen-specific T cells. *Cancer Gene Ther* 2004;11:81–91.

201. Bollard CM, Straathof KC, Huls MH, et al. The generation and characterization of LMP2-specific CTLs for use as adoptive transfer from patients with relapsed EBV-positive Hodgkin disease. *J Immunother* 2004;27:317–327.

202. Stark GL, Wood KM, Jack F, et al. Hodgkin's disease in the elderly: a population-based study. *Br J Haematol* 2002;119:432–440.

203. Clarke CA, Glaser SL, Dorfman RF, et al. Epstein-Barr virus and survival after Hodgkin disease in a population-based series of women. *Cancer* 2001;91:1579–1587.

204. Armstrong AA, Lennard A, Alexander FE, et al. Prognostic significance of Epstein-Barr virus association in Hodgkin's disease. *Eur J Cancer* 1994;30A: 1045–1046.

205. Claviez A, Tiemann M, Luders H, et al. Impact of latent Epstein-Barr virus infection on outcome in children and adolescents with Hodgkin's lymphoma. *J Clin Oncol* 2005;23:4048–4056.

206. Axdorph U, Porwit-MacDonald A, Sjoberg J, et al. Epstein-Barr virus expression in Hodgkin's disease in relation to patient characteristics, serum factors and blood lymphocyte function. *Br J Cancer* 1999;81:1182–1187.

207. Flavell KJ, Billingham LJ, Biddulph JP, et al. The effect of Epstein-Barr virus status on outcome in age- and sex-defined subgroups of patients with advanced Hodgkin's disease. *Ann Oncol* 2003;14:282–290.

208. Murray PG, Billingham LJ, Hassan HT, et al. Effect of Epstein-Barr virus infection on response to chemotherapy and survival in Hodgkin's disease. *Blood* 1999;94:442–447.

209. Vestlev PM, Pallesen G, Sandvej K, et al. Prognosis of Hodgkin's disease is not influenced by Epstein-Barr virus latent membrane protein. *Int J Cancer* 1992;50:670–671.

210. Kwon JM, Park YH, Kang JH, et al. The effect of Epstein-Barr virus status on clinical outcome in Hodgkin's lymphoma. *Ann Hematol* 2006.

211. Krugmann J, Tzankov A, Gschwendtner A, et al. Longer failure-free survival interval of Epstein-Barr virus-associated classical Hodgkin's lymphoma: a single-institution study. *Mod Pathol* 2003;16:566–573.

212. Herling M, Rassidakis GZ, Vassilakopoulos TP, et al. Impact of LMP-1 expression on clinical outcome in age-defined subgroups of patients with classical Hodgkin lymphoma. *Blood* 2006;107:1240; author reply 1241.

213. Vassallo J, Metze K, Traina F, et al. Expression of Epstein-Barr virus in classical Hodgkin's lymphomas in Brazilian adult patients. *Haematologica* 2001;86:1227–1228.

214. Glavina-Durdov M, Jakic-Razumovic J, Capkun V, et al. Assessment of the prognostic impact of the Epstein-Barr virus-encoded latent membrane protein-1 expression in Hodgkin's disease. *Br J Cancer* 2001;84:1227–1234.

215. Engel M, Essop MF, Close P, et al. Improved prognosis of Epstein-Barr virus associated childhood Hodgkin's lymphoma: study of 47 South African cases. *J Clin Pathol* 2000;53:182–186.

216. Morente MM, Piris MA, Abraira V, et al. Adverse clinical outcome in Hodgkin's disease is associated with loss of retinoblastoma protein expression, high Ki67 proliferation index, and absence of Epstein-Barr virus-latent membrane protein 1 expression. *Blood* 1997;90:2429–2436.

217. Naresh KN, Johnson J, Srinivas V, et al. Epstein-Barr virus association in classical Hodgkin's disease provides survival advantage to patients and correlates with higher expression of proliferation markers in Reed-Sternberg cells. *Ann Oncol* 2000;11:91–96.

BIOLOGY AND PATHOLOGY

CHAPTER 4 ▪ PATHOLOGY OF HODGKIN LYMPHOMA

LAWRENCE M. WEISS, ROGER A. WARNKE, MARTIN-LEO HANSMANN, JOHN K.C. CHAN, HANS KONRAD MUELLER-HERMELINK, NANCY LEE HARRIS, HARALD STEIN, AND ELAINE S. JAFFE

In recent years, it has been recognized that Hodgkin lymphoma subsumes two clinical, pathologic, and biologic disease entities: classical Hodgkin lymphoma and nodular lymphocyte predominant Hodgkin lymphoma. This realization is reflected in the most recent World Health Organization classification (Table 4.1), which is the classification system used in this chapter as well as throughout this book. Please see the previous edition of this book for a complete history of the pathology of Hodgkin lymphoma, including the description of previous classification systems.

CONSIDERATIONS IN TISSUE HANDLING

Optimally, the largest abnormal lymph node should be excised intact. It should be submitted fresh, preferably sterile, to allow the pathologist as many options as possible in pursuing special studies. It is best to place the node inside a capped empty container, and not on a dry towel or sponge, for these may introduce artifacts at the edge of the tissue. If there is a chance that the tissue will dry before the pathologist receives it, then the tissue may be placed in some sterile saline solution, although even this may make the subsequent preparation of frozen sections suboptimal. The pathologist may prepare touch preparations or, as we prefer, scrape preparations, which permit subsequent cytochemical studies and provide excellent preservation of cytologic characteristics. The differential diagnosis generally guides the allocation of tissue by the pathologist. The pathologist will always fix a generous aliquot in one or more fixatives, generally formalin and possibly a metal-based fixative such as B5. This provides for excellent morphology and allows virtually all immunohistochemical studies useful in the diagnosis of Hodgkin lymphoma to be performed. If non-Hodgkin lymphoma is in the differential diagnosis, then some tissue should be frozen and/or submitted for flow cytometric studies. The frozen tissue may be used for either immunohistochemical or molecular studies. Fresh tissue is required for conventional cytogenetic studies, which may be useful if these are readily available, and tissue may also be sent for microbiologic studies if an infectious process is a possibility.

Sometimes, a formal lymph node excisional biopsy specimen cannot be obtained, particularly from sites not easily accessible to the surgeon, such as the mediastinum. Hodgkin lymphoma may be diagnosed in small biopsy specimens, although immunohistochemical studies are often required to confirm the diagnosis. Fine-needle aspiration biopsy is being increasingly used for the diagnosis of lymphoid lesions.[1] Although a primary diagnosis of Hodgkin lymphoma can be rendered on fine-needle aspiration specimens by experts,[2] usually with the aid of immunohistochemistry, it is generally prudent for most pathologists without extensive experience to defer the diagnosis. However, fine-needle aspiration may still play a role in the diagnosis of a non-Hodgkin lymphoma or a specific type of reactive lymphadenopathy, particularly an infectious lymphadenopathy. Fine-needle aspiration biopsy is more reliable in the diagnosis of recurrent Hodgkin lymphoma and in staging cases of known Hodgkin lymphoma, although even in these circumstances, it must be used with great caution and by those experienced in using the technique.[3]

Frozen sections are usually not very reliable in the primary diagnosis of Hodgkin lymphoma, except when used by those with extensive experience. The diagnosis of Hodgkin lymphoma by frozen section is most accurate when frozen section is combined with a cytologic preparation, such as a touch or scrape preparation. Frozen sections are excellent for assessing lymph node architecture but are poor in revealing cytologic characteristics, whereas the opposite is true of touch or scrape preparations. Frozen section may still have an important role in the workup apart from determination of a specific diagnosis—it is most useful in determining the adequacy of a biopsy specimen and may prompt the pathologist to request additional tissue specimens from the surgeon.

CLASSICAL HODGKIN LYMPHOMA

Gross Appearance

Excised lymph nodes involved by classical Hodgkin lymphoma generally range in diameter from 2 to 5 cm. In cases of mixed cellularity (MC) or lymphocyte depletion (LD), the lymph nodes generally do not adhere to adjacent tissues and are soft to moderately firm. The cut section usually reveals a vague nodularity with a tan color. In cases of nodular sclerosis, the lymph node often adheres to adjacent tissues and is generally firm. The cut section usually reveals a distinct nodularity, gray-white to tan in color; foci of necrosis may be apparent.

TABLE 4.1

**WORLD HEALTH ORGANIZATION
CLASSIFICATION (1999)**

Nodular lymphocyte-predominant Hodgkin lymphoma

Classical Hodgkin lymphoma

    Nodular sclerosis

    Mixed cellularity

    Lymphocyte rich

    Lymphocyte depleted

Histopathology

The diagnosis of classical Hodgkin lymphoma is established with the identification of Hodgkin cells in the appropriate cellular milieu. Hodgkin cells encompass either diagnostic Reed-Sternberg cells or their variants (Figs. 4.1 to 4.3). For many years, the identification of so-called diagnostic Reed-Sternberg cells was required for the definitive diagnosis of classical Hodgkin lymphoma, and this was probably a prudent policy. However, it might have led to underdiagnosis of Hodgkin lymphoma—for example, when the tissue sampling was suboptimal. This policy might have also led to overdiagnosis of Hodgkin lymphoma, if the pathologist concentrated only on

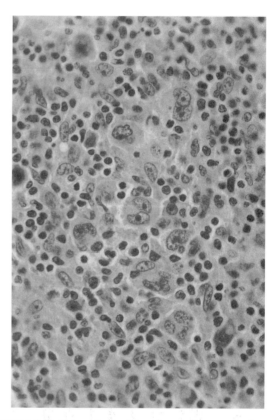

FIGURE 4.2. A diagnostic Reed-Sternberg cell is seen in the center, and many mononucleated and multinucleated Reed-Sternberg variants are seen throughout the field. See color insert.

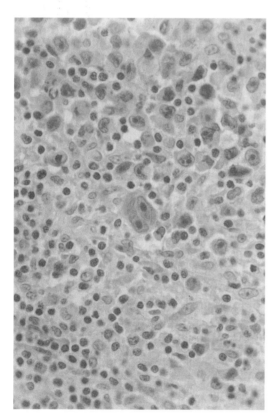

FIGURE 4.1. A diagnostic Reed-Sternberg cell with two nuclei is seen in the center, with a prominent eosinophilic nucleolus present in each nucleus. There is some chromatin clearing around each nucleolus. Several mononuclear Reed-Sternberg variants are also present in the upper half of the field. See color insert.

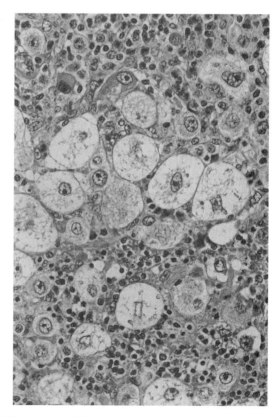

FIGURE 4.3. Several lacunar cells are present. A "mummified" Reed-Sternberg cell is in the upper left corner. See color insert.

the identification of diagnostic Reed-Sternberg cells to the exclusion of the cellular milieu, as cells closely resembling diagnostic Reed-Sternberg cells can be found in a wide variety of reactive and neoplastic diseases. At the current time, the definitive diagnosis of Hodgkin lymphoma can be made either by morphologic assessment alone, or by morphologic assessment combined with immunohistochemical studies, thus diminishing the importance of the definitive identification of diagnostic Reed-Sternberg cells.

Diagnostic Reed-Sternberg cells are large cells, either with a large polyploid nucleus or multinucleated (Figs. 4.1 and 4.2). Each lobe or nucleus contains one large inclusion-like eosinophilic nucleolus, ranging in size up to about 10 μm, the diameter of a small lymphocyte nucleus. The chromatin immediately surrounding the nucleolus often shows a clear zone. The remaining chromatin is generally vesicular but usually shows some degree of coarse clumping. The nuclear membrane is usually thick, and often chromatin is clumped against it. The nuclear outlines are usually rounded, but highly irregular nuclear outlines can be seen in some cases. Mitotic figures can be identified but are usually not as frequently encountered as in large-cell non-Hodgkin lymphoma. The cytoplasm is usually relatively abundant, so that an overall diameter of about 20 to 50 μm yields an area ranging from 4 to 25 times that of adjacent small lymphocytes. In sections stained with hematoxylin and eosin, the cytoplasm may be acidophilic, amphophilic, or basophilic, but it lacks the deep basophilia or paranuclear hof characteristic of immunoblasts. Most mononuclear Reed-Sternberg cell variants are similar to diagnostic Reed-Sternberg cells, but they are not multilobated or multinucleated. Lacunar cells are mononuclear or multinucleated (appearance of "pennies on a plate") Reed-Sternberg cell variants with abundant amphophilic cytoplasm (at least in metal-based fixatives) that is usually retracted to the nuclei in formalin-fixed sections (Fig. 4.3). Often, their nuclei have smaller lobes with more irregularities, and the eosinophilic nucleoli may be less prominent. Occasionally, apoptotic Hodgkin cells, sometimes termed mummified or zombie cells, are present. These cells contain pyknotic chromatin, often with barely recognizable nucleoli having fuzzy outlines, and deeply eosinophilic retracted cytoplasm.

The background infiltrate in Hodgkin lymphoma consists of a mixture of cell types (Fig. 4.4). Small lymphocytes usually predominate numerically, but scattered eosinophils, neutrophils, histiocytes, plasma cells, and fibroblasts are usually also present in variable numbers.

Eosinophils vary from rare to extremely numerous, even to the extent of forming eosinophilic abscesses, although they are most often moderate in number. In most cases, there are far fewer neutrophils than eosinophils, but neutrophils may predominate in rare cases, often associated with severe B symptoms (fever, weight loss, and night sweats). Histiocytes may have the appearance of tissue histiocytes or epithelioid histiocytes, or they may rarely be foamy. They most often occur singly but occasionally form well-defined granulomas, and multinucleated giant cells may also be seen. In rare cases, histiocytes may be so numerous as to give an appearance reminiscent of Lennert lymphoma (non-Hodgkin lymphoma with a high content of epithelioid cells), xanthogranulomatous inflammation, or lipid storage disease.[4] Plasma cells are usually present in scattered numbers, and if they are present in very large numbers or sheets, the diagnosis of Hodgkin lymphoma should be doubted. One rare manifestation is the appearance of Hodgkin cells in the midst of a reactive monocytoid B-cell proliferation.[5,6] Fibroblasts vary from isolated spindle cells, seen in typical cases, to widespread proliferation with areas resembling fibrous histiocytoma.[7,8] Rarely, small foci of Langerhans cell histiocytosis may be found in tissues involved by Hodgkin lymphoma.[9]

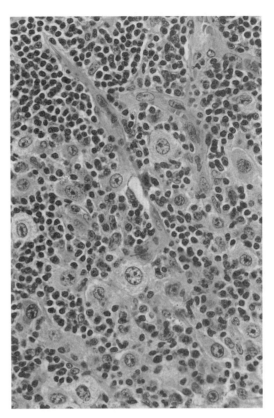

FIGURE 4.4. The background cells consist predominantly of small lymphocytes, along with scattered eosinophils, histiocytes, and plasma cells. See color insert.

Histologic Subtyping

Nodular Sclerosis

The nodular sclerosis subtype is characterized by collagenous bands and lacunar cells (Fig. 4.5). However, in practice, the presence of one or more sclerotic bands is the defining feature. These bands usually radiate from a thickened lymph node capsule, often following the course of a penetrating artery. The bands are composed of mature, laminated, relatively acellular collagen. They are described in textbooks as showing birefringence in polarized light, but in practice polarization is rarely carried out. In most cases, several broad collagenous bands can be identified, but a single band may be present, or fibrosis can be so extensive that only isolated nodules of lymphoid tissue remain. Can one recognize cases of nodular sclerosis in which bands are not yet present? This situation has been described by some as the cellular phase of nodular sclerosis, although in Lukes' original description of the cellular phase of nodular sclerosis, at least one intranodal collagen band was required for the diagnosis.[10] Some of these cases probably fit the recent description of "follicular" Hodgkin lymphoma,[11] and others may represent the follicular variant of lymphocyte-rich classical Hodgkin lymphoma. Clinical studies of small numbers of cases of the cellular phase of nodular sclerosis have demonstrated some clinical features and an overall survival rate similar to those of MC, but a relapse-free survival rate similar to that of nodular sclerosis.[12]

The collagenous bands of nodular sclerosis enclose nodules of lymphoid tissue containing variable numbers of Hodgkin cells and reactive infiltrate. Lacunar cells are the most common type of Hodgkin cell present, and may be found in large

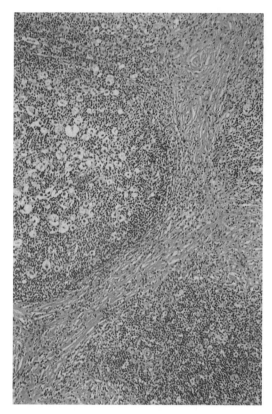

FIGURE 4.5. Nodular sclerosis Hodgkin lymphoma. Broad bands of fibrosis separate several nodules. See color insert.

intermediate subtype falls between lymphocyte-rich classical Hodgkin lymphoma and lymphocyte depletion. The capsule is usually intact and of normal thickness. A vague nodularity may be present at low magnification, but the presence of any definite fibrous bands would warrant classification as nodular sclerosis rather than mixed cellularity. At high magnification, a heterogeneous mixture of Hodgkin cells, small lymphocytes, eosinophils, neutrophils, epithelioid and nonepithelioid histiocytes, plasma cells, and fibroblasts is present (Fig. 4.6). Diagnostic Reed-Sternberg cells and mononuclear variants are usually easy to find. Small foci of necrosis may be present, but the extent is much less than that seen in nodular sclerosis.

Lymphocyte-Depleted Hodgkin Lymphoma

Lymphocyte-depleted Hodgkin lymphoma encompasses two types of Hodgkin lymphoma in the Lukes and Butler classification: diffuse fibrosis and reticular. In diffuse fibrosis, the most characteristic features are a marked degree of reticulin fibrosis surrounding single cells along with lymphocyte depletion (Fig. 4.7). In contrast to nodular sclerosis, this subtype is not characterized by the presence of thick fibrous bands, and the fibrosis envelops individual cells, not nodules of cells. Hodgkin cells are usually easily identified, but increased numbers of Hodgkin cells are not essential to the diagnosis. In the reticular variant, sheets of Hodgkin cells, often showing pleomorphic features, are found. Obviously, distinction from a large-cell non-Hodgkin lymphoma, particularly immunoblastic lymphoma, can be difficult, and immunohistochemical studies are essential to confirm the diagnosis of the reticular subtype. In some cases of lymphocyte depletion, features of both diffuse fibrosis and the reticular subtype may be present in different areas of the biopsy specimen.

numbers or in sheets. They tend to aggregate at the center of nodules, sometimes forming a rim around central areas of necrosis. Diagnostic Reed-Sternberg cells are usually not easily identified and may not be found in small biopsy specimens. Eosinophils and neutrophils are often numerous, but histiocytes and plasma cells are usually less conspicuous in nodular sclerosis. Fibrohistiocytic foci are sometimes found in the centers of nodules or extensively replacing the tissue.

In the practice of most Western centers, nodular sclerosis is by far the most common type of Hodgkin lymphoma, accounting for greater than two-thirds of all cases.[12] Therefore, various investigators have attempted to subclassify nodular sclerosis into prognostic groups.[13] The most successful effort has come from the British National Lymphoma Investigation.[14–17] These investigators have proposed the subclassification of nodular sclerosis into two grades. Cases are classified as grade 2 if (a) more than 25% of the cellular nodules show reticular or pleomorphic lymphocyte depletion, (b) more than 80% of the cellular nodules show the fibrohistiocytic variant of lymphocyte depletion, or (c) more than 25% of the nodules contain numerous bizarre and highly anaplastic-appearing Hodgkin cells without depletion of lymphocytes. All cases of nodular sclerosis not meeting these criteria are considered to be grade 1. Although this system appears to be somewhat hard to learn, some additional studies have demonstrated that cases classified as grade 2 have a significantly worse prognosis than those classified as grade 1[18,19]; other studies have failed to demonstrate a difference between these grades of nodular sclerosis.[20,21]

Mixed Cellularity

The subtype of MC comprises approximately 30% of cases of Hodgkin lymphoma in Western populations, but it may comprise 50% or more of cases in developing countries.[22] This

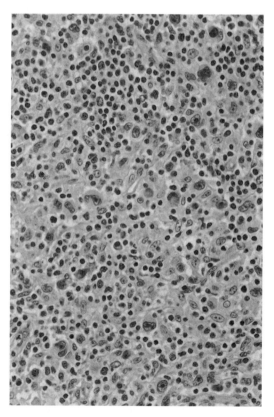

FIGURE 4.6. Mixed-cellularity Hodgkin lymphoma. There is an absence of fibrous bands. See color insert.

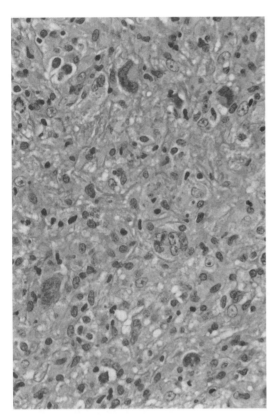

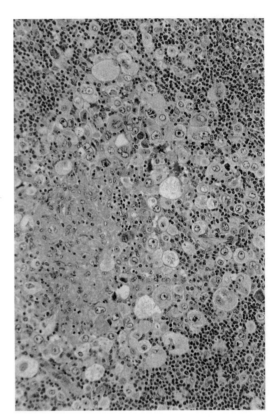

FIGURE 4.7. Lymphocyte depletion, diffuse fibrosis type. There is a reticulin collagen fibrosis around single cells. Although the Hodgkin cells appear atypical, results of immunophenotyping studies were characteristic of Hodgkin lymphoma in this case. See color insert.

FIGURE 4.8. Syncytial form of nodular sclerosis Hodgkin lymphoma; sheets of lacunar cells are clustered around a central area of necrosis. See color insert.

Lymphocyte-Rich Classical Hodgkin Lymphoma

Cases of lymphocyte-rich classical Hodgkin lymphoma may resemble either mixed cellularity, nodular sclerosis, or nodular lymphocyte-predominant Hodgkin lymphoma and may be either nodular or diffuse. Many cases of lymphocyte-rich classical Hodgkin lymphoma have a close resemblance to mixed-cellularity Hodgkin lymphoma, with a diffuse or vaguely nodular low-magnification appearance. Hodgkin and Reed-Sternberg cells are relatively rare, and the background is dominated by small mature lymphocytes. Eosinophils and neutrophils are usually restricted to blood vessels. Reed-Sternberg cells and variants are not easy to find but, when encountered, have identical features to the Hodgkin cells of mixed cellularity. Some cases of lymphocyte-rich classical Hodgkin lymphoma may show a distinctly nodular appearance that may closely mimic nodular lymphocyte-predominant Hodgkin lymphoma. The nodules of lymphocyte-rich classical Hodgkin lymphoma often contain small reactive germinal centers, with Hodgkin and Reed-Sternberg cells present in and near the mantle zones, a pattern that has been called follicular Hodgkin lymphoma.[23]

Other Histologic Types

Strickler and colleagues[24] described the syncytial variant of nodular sclerosis, in which cohesive aggregates of lacunar cells and other variants are seen, closely resembling non-Hodgkin lymphoma, carcinoma, or malignant melanoma (Fig. 4.8). Often, the centers of the aggregates are necrotic, rimmed by sheets of lacunar cells. Immunohistochemical studies are often necessary for accurate diagnosis. These cases probably represent a subset of the grade 2 nodular sclerosis cases according to the British National Lymphoma Investigation; therefore, this histologic appearance may be associated with an adverse prognosis.

Doggett and colleagues[25] described interfollicular Hodgkin lymphoma, in which Hodgkin cells are present in interfollicular regions between reactive follicles (Fig. 4.9). This variant of Hodgkin lymphoma can be easily dismissed as reactive hyperplasia, such as can be seen in a viral infection. This variant probably represents focal nodal involvement by Hodgkin lymphoma rather than a specific subtype, as other lymph nodes from the same patient, or even other foci in the same biopsy specimen, often show classic features of either nodular sclerosis or mixed-cellularity Hodgkin lymphoma.

In a large study of cases of Hodgkin lymphoma, a fibroblastic variant was recognized.[12] In this variant, increased numbers of fibroblasts are present, without significant collagen deposition. Many of these cases probably correspond to the fibrohistiocytic areas described by the British National Lymphoma Investigation in some cases of grade 2 nodular sclerosis. In the original description, the fibroblastic variant was associated with a shorter relapse-free survival period than were other types of Hodgkin lymphoma.

Finally, a small number of cases of Hodgkin lymphoma with a purely follicular pattern have been described; these have been termed follicular Hodgkin lymphoma.[11] In these cases, the Hodgkin cells had the phenotype of classical Hodgkin lymphoma but also expressed B-lineage antigens. In each case, the Hodgkin cells were confined to the follicles, which consisted mainly of mantle zone B-cells. The follicle centers were atrophic and usually eccentrically placed, and did not contain Hodgkin cells. Some or all of these cases may correspond to the follicular variant of lymphocyte-rich classical Hodgkin lymphoma.

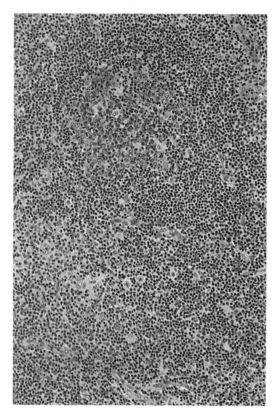

FIGURE 4.9. Interfollicular Hodgkin lymphoma. At the top is a reactive follicle. Several Hodgkin cells are seen in the interfollicular region in the bottom half of the field. See color insert.

Fine-Needle Aspiration Biopsy Studies

Fine-needle aspiration smears of Hodgkin lymphoma show a dispersed population of lymphoid and other cells in which scattered large cells are evident.[1,2] As expected, the lymphocytes are small with a mature chromatin pattern. The Hodgkin cells are recognizable as large cells with bilobed or multilobated nuclei and prominent nucleoli. Often, these cells appear to have more abundant cytoplasm than is generally appreciated in tissue sections. Immunohistochemical studies, particularly those employing an alkaline phosphatase detection (to circumvent interpretive problems associated with the pseudoperoxidase in red cells), may be very useful in confirming a presumptive fine-needle aspiration diagnosis of Hodgkin lymphoma.

Extranodal Disease and Staging Specimens

The same modern principles used to diagnose Hodgkin lymphoma in the lymph nodes should be applied to diagnosing it in extranodal sites. The diagnosis rests on the definitive identification of Hodgkin cells, either by histopathology or histopathology combined with immunohistochemical studies, in the appropriate cellular milieu.[26] Primary extranodal Hodgkin lymphoma is very uncommon outside the setting of HIV infection, but involvement of extranodal tissue is relatively common as a secondary phenomenon. Once a diagnosis of Hodgkin lymphoma has been established in a primary site, it is probably best not to provide a typing on staging biopsies of extranodal sites, where sclerosis may not be a type-specific feature.

Hodgkin lymphoma usually manifests in bone marrow as scattered foci of fibrosis in which Hodgkin cells can be identified.[27,28] Therefore, the aspirated specimen is rarely helpful in establishing a diagnosis, even in cases with extensive involvement. In the biopsy specimen, the patchy areas of fibrosis can usually be appreciated at low magnification. It is in these areas that a search for the Hodgkin cells should be made at high magnification; a search made in areas of normal marrow can lead to misidentification of hematopoietic precursors or megakaryocytes as Hodgkin cells. If Hodgkin cells are not seen in the areas of patchy fibrosis, serial levels should be obtained; immunohistochemical stains may be helpful in identifying Hodgkin cells. If Hodgkin cells cannot be demonstrated after serial levels have been obtained in a focal area of fibrosis in a random bone marrow biopsy specimen from patient with known Hodgkin lymphoma, these areas should still be suspected of harboring Hodgkin lymphoma, provided that another cause for the fibrosis cannot be discovered. The uninvolved marrow may show myeloid hyperplasia, eosinophilia, or increased numbers of plasma cells.[29]

Splenic involvement by Hodgkin lymphoma begins in the periarteriolar lymphoid sheath and the marginal B-cell zone and progresses to involve all the malpighian bodies of the white pulp.[30] In time, adjacent involved malpighian bodies may coalesce. Grossly, splenic involvement takes the form of discrete nodules ranging in size from 1 to 2 mm up to several centimeters; thus, splenic involvement may easily be missed by conventional radiologic studies. The pathologist who examines a spleen needs to section the organ very thinly and make a special effort to identify splenic hilar lymph nodes. Splenic hilar fat may yield small, grossly inapparent lymph nodes. The number of gross nodules should be recorded, and at least five, if present, should be documented histologically. Random sections of grossly normal spleen essentially never reveal evidence of Hodgkin lymphoma. Histologically, the splenic nodules of Hodgkin lymphoma usually resemble the nodules at other sites, although it is best not to try to type the disease, as nonspecific areas of fibrosis may be seen even in cases of mixed cellularity.

Liver involvement by Hodgkin lymphoma is almost never seen in the absence of splenic involvement outside the setting of HIV infection. The portal areas are affected at first, showing microscopic involvement, but in advanced cases, gross nodules can be seen in a portal distribution.[31,32] It is usually prudent to obtain immunohistochemical confirmation to distinguish Hodgkin lymphoma from nonspecific periportal lymphocytic infiltration in cases of early involvement.

The thymus is a common site of primary Hodgkin lymphoma and probably is the site of origin in a significant percentage of cases of Hodgkin lymphoma presenting in the mediastinum, particularly the nodular sclerosis type. At one time, involvement of the thymus by Hodgkin lymphoma was mistakenly labeled as granulomatous thymoma.[33] Thymic involvement by Hodgkin lymphoma often leads to cystic formations; these may persist as a residual mass following therapy, as may areas of sclerosis.

The lung is a relatively common site of secondary involvement and only rarely is the site of primary disease.[34] Secondary involvement manifests in two ways. Most commonly, it results from contiguous involvement by mediastinal disease, but it also may manifest as miliary involvement, reflective of vascular dissemination. Both primary and secondary involvement of the gastrointestinal tract and tonsillar tissue are very rare but have been reported.[35–38] Similarly, both primary and secondary involvement of the skin are unusual, except by contiguous spread from an underlying lesion. A diagnosis of primary Hodgkin lymphoma in the skin should be made with great caution and with confirmation by immunohistochemical studies, as CD30+ lymphoproliferative disease (including lymphomatoid papulosis), a much more common skin lymphoma, can closely mimic the histologic appearance of Hodgkin lymphoma.[39–41] Virtually every extranodal site, including the central nervous system, has been described as a primary or secondary site of Hodgkin lymphoma, but such cases are fortunately extremely rare.[42–44]

In addition, or more commonly, instead of disclosing evidence of Hodgkin lymphoma, staging biopsies may show sarcoidlike non-caseating epithelioid granulomas.[45] On rare occasions, these granulomas may coalesce to form gross nodules. Unless definite evidence of concurrent Hodgkin lymphoma is demonstrated, the finding of non-caseating granulomas should not be considered evidence of involvement by Hodgkin lymphoma. In the past, the presence of epithelioid granulomas in the liver or spleen of patients with Hodgkin lymphoma had been reported to be associated with a better 5-year overall and relapse-free survival;[46,47] however, this survival advantage may not be seen with long-term follow-up or with modern therapies.[48]

Post-Treatment, Relapse, and Autopsy Findings

Sites of successful treatment for Hodgkin lymphoma usually show dense collagenous scars, with only a few lymphocytes and fibroblasts and no identifiable Hodgkin cells; foamy macrophages may also be present.[49] Occasionally, the centers contain an amorphous eosinophilic necrotic debris surrounded by a poorly cellular fibrous rim, resembling an old infectious granuloma. These scars are most often found in lymph nodes, but they may also be encountered in liver, lung, bone marrow, and spleen. Large scars up to 4 cm in size may be evident on gross examination, and occasionally they may cause a clinically apparent mass—for example, in the mediastinum following successful treatment.

The histology of recurrent Hodgkin lymphoma is different, depending on whether the site of recurrence falls within or outside the treatment area. When the site of relapse is outside the treatment area, there is an impressive maintenance of the histologic appearance in the relapse biopsy specimens, with a change in histology seen in only a small percentage of cases.[50,51] When an unusual histologic pattern of Hodgkin lymphoma, such as extensive necrosis or large numbers of epithelioid histiocytes, has been present in the initial biopsy, it is often also present in the relapse specimen. The same histologic type is usually present in the initial and relapse specimens, although progression from one type to another occasionally occurs, most commonly lymphocyte-rich classical Hodgkin lymphoma to mixed cellularity, or mixed cellularity to lymphocyte depletion. Cases of nodular sclerosis tend to remain nodular sclerosis, although even this type can manifest as another type, usually mixed cellularity. However, there is a tendency for the number of eosinophils, histiocytes, and Hodgkin cells to increase in the relapse specimens. The increase in eosinophils is more marked in those patients who relapse 2 years or more after the initial diagnosis, whereas an increase in the number of Hodgkin cells is more often seen in patients who relapse early. Lymphocytes and reactive follicles appear to decrease in number between initial and relapse biopsy specimens. Those patients with a relapse-free interval longer than 1 year more often have a granulomatous reaction, in contrast to those who relapse in a shorter period of time.

When Hodgkin lymphoma recurs in irradiated sites, the tendency toward retention of the same histologic appearance is much smaller.[52] Recurrences may have an unusual appearance, often with a marked decrease in the number of lymphocytes, a decrease in the number of eosinophils, and increased numbers of Hodgkin cells with a greater range of cytologic

atypia. Recurrent cases of nodular sclerosis frequently exhibit fewer nodules and less sclerosis than formerly, and they are often difficult to subclassify. Nonetheless, histologic features of recurrence specimens cannot be used to identify those patients who will later die of Hodgkin lymphoma versus those who can be successfully retreated. The histologic appearance of Hodgkin lymphoma at autopsy is somewhat similar to that in treated sites but is often even more exaggerated.[53,54] Although in some patients the pretherapy histologic appearance is maintained, in many cases a marked increase in the number and atypia of Hodgkin cells is noted. Occasionally, sheets of Hodgkin cells may be present at autopsy. Most cases of nodular sclerosis lose their nodularity and sclerosis by the time of autopsy. Evidence of vascular dissemination of disease, to noncontiguous sites and to multiple extranodal sites, is common.

Patients successfully and unsuccessfully treated for Hodgkin lymphoma may show a wide range of other changes at autopsy, undoubtedly reflective of treatment effects.[53,54] Fibrosis and atrophy are common findings in multiple organs, including the lungs, gastrointestinal tract, liver, kidneys, endocrine organs (particularly the thyroid gland and gonads), and bone marrow. In addition, patients treated for Hodgkin lymphoma may show evidence of second neoplasms, most commonly acute nonlymphocytic leukemia and non-Hodgkin lymphoma, but also other neoplasms such as breast carcinoma and malignant melanoma (see Chapter 24).[55,56]

Ultrastructural Findings

Electron microscopic study is generally not useful in the diagnosis of Hodgkin lymphoma. The ultrastructural appearance of Hodgkin cells is similar to that of transformed lymphocytes.[57] As expected from the light microscopic findings, the nuclei of Hodgkin cells are large and multilobated, with uniformly dispersed chromatin. Nucleoli are very prominent and have well-developed nucleolonemata. The cytoplasm is abundant and shows evidence of synthetic activity, usually with numerous polyribosomes and prominent Golgi regions composed of numerous vesicles. Variable numbers of mitochondria are present, and lysosomes (a prominent constituent of macrophages) are usually few in number.

Immunophenotypic Findings

Immunophenotyping studies with frozen sections are of limited utility in the immunodiagnosis of Hodgkin lymphoma. With the suboptimal cytologic features of frozen sections and the relative rarity of Hodgkin cells, it is often difficult to ascertain staining results on Hodgkin cells with certainty. Similarly, flow cytometric studies, although useful in ruling out the presence of a non-Hodgkin lymphoma, particularly a B-cell lymphoma, are also of limited usefulness in making a positive diagnosis of Hodgkin lymphoma. Conventional flow cytometric studies are unable to gate easily on such an infrequent cell type as the Hodgkin cell in Hodgkin lymphoma, so that the results generally reflect the background cell population and not the Hodgkin cells. In fact, flow cytometric studies may even be misleading, as the profile usually seen—polyclonal B-cells with numerous immunophenotypically normal T-cells—is identical to that seen in a reactive lymph node.

Fortunately, immunohistochemical studies with paraffin sections are of great use in the diagnosis of Hodgkin lymphoma.[58–66] Rather than any one marker being both highly sensitive and specific for Hodgkin cells, a relatively limited panel of monoclonal antibodies, when analyzed in the aggregate, can provide very useful information. The phenotype of

TABLE 4.2

IMMUNOPHENOTYPE OF REED-STERNBERG CELLS IN PARAFFIN SECTIONS

	CD45 (%)	CD15 (%)	CD30 (%)	CD20 (%)
Classical Hodgkin lymphoma	7	87	89	24
Nodular lymphocyte predominant	65[a]	37[b]	38[c]	92
B-cell lymphoma	97	4	18	94
T-cell lymphoma	89	21	42	0

[a]Results are skewed by the inclusion of one large study in which all the cases were said to be CD45-negative.
[b]Results given may include cases of lymphocyte-rich classical Hodgkin lymphoma.
[c]Positive cells may be immunoblasts rather than lymphocytes and histiocytes (L&H cells).
Data adapted from Arber et al.[67], Chang et al.[69], Weiss et al.[70], and Chang et al.[77].

Hodgkin cells is summarized in Table 4.2. The percentages given are derived from compiled reviews of the literature[67–70] and therefore may differ from laboratory to laboratory. The data suggest, however, that CD45 may be one of the most useful markers in the immunodiagnosis of Hodgkin lymphoma. CD45 (or CD45RB, which is commonly assessed in paraffin sections) represents a group of antibodies directed against a family of related molecules present on virtually all hematolymphoid cells, with the exception of maturing erythroid cells and megakaryocytes; therefore, the antigen has been called leukocyte common antigen.[70] Its utility as a negative marker for Hodgkin cells (expressed in only 7% of cases) is enhanced by the finding that about 97% of B-cell lymphomas and 89% of T-cell lymphomas express CD45.[62,65,66,70–76] The category of non-Hodgkin lymphoma that is most likely to be confused histologically with Hodgkin lymphoma and that may lack CD45 expression is anaplastic large-cell lymphoma (negative for CD45 in about 33% of cases). Diffuse large B-cell lymphomas with immunoblastic features may on occasion also be nonreactive for CD45. The interpretation of CD45 staining may be difficult because it is important not to mistake membranous reactivity on adjacent cells as positivity of Hodgkin cells—not a trivial task, as Hodgkin cells are typically surrounded by T-cells. Staining results should be regarded as positive only if a clear, strong rim is observed entirely circling the cell (best assessed when two Hodgkin cells are adjacent to each other).

The CD30 cluster of antibodies is directed against the Ki-1 antigen.[77] In reactive tissues, these antibodies stain scattered large activated B- and T-lymphoid cells. Staining of the Reed-Sternberg cells and variants is seen in virtually all cases of classical Hodgkin lymphoma, if the quality of immunostaining is adequate.[62,77–83] The staining pattern for CD30 in Hodgkin lymphoma is usually strong and membranous and/or paranuclear in distribution, often associated with a weaker diffuse cytoplasmic positivity (Fig. 4.10). In addition to labeling Hodgkin cells, CD30 antibodies will also stain virtually all cases of anaplastic large-cell lymphoma and CD30+ cutaneous lymphoproliferative disease (including lymphomatoid papulosis), about 15% of B-lineage large-cell lymphomas, and about 40% of peripheral T-cell lymphomas. In most non-anaplastic non-Hodgkin lymphomas that show reactivity for CD30, the CD30 staining is usually seen on a subset of the neoplastic cells.

The CD15 cluster of antibodies is directed against the carbohydrate X hapten.[67] CD15 antibodies generally stain mature neutrophils, many macrophages, and a subset of T-cells, particularly after activation. Staining of the Reed-Sternberg cells and variants is seen in about 87% of cases of classical Hodgkin lymphoma (Fig. 4.11).[65–67,73,79,83,85–91] The staining pattern on Hodgkin cells is similar to that seen for CD30, but the labeling is often more heterogeneous with labeling of only a subset of cells. Patients whose Hodgkin cells are CD15− are older and predominantly male, and their clinical stage at diagnosis is more advanced than that of patients whose Hodgkin cells are CD15+; mixed cellularity is more common than nodular sclerosis among CD15− cases.[83] Cases that are CD30+, CD20−, and CD15− have significantly less freedom from treatment failure and poorer overall survival in comparison with cases that are CD30+, CD20−, and CD15+.

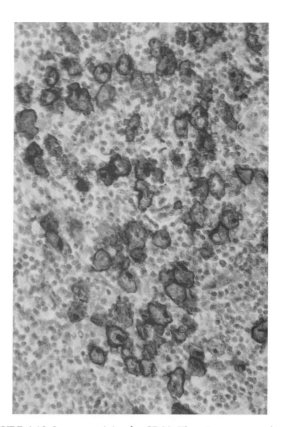

FIGURE 4.10. Immunostaining for CD30. There is strong membrane and paranuclear staining, and weaker cytoplasmic staining, of the Hodgkin cells. See color insert.

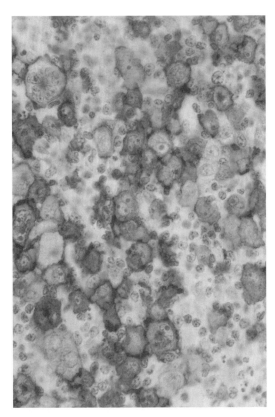

FIGURE 4.11. Immunostaining for CD15. There is strong membrane and paranuclear staining of the Hodgkin cells. See color insert.

CD20. Thus, one study found a small proportion of the neoplastic cells staining for CD79a in 20% of cases, in contrast to a small proportion of cells staining for CD20 in 30% of these cases.[100] Labeling of more than 50% of cells for CD79a was seen less frequently than for CD20 (1% versus 7% of cases). Similarly, CD45RA represents another B-lineage marker for which Hodgkin cells are usually negative.[70] In contrast, the B-cell associated transcription factor PAX-5 is expressed in a majority of cases. However, there is down-regulation of the B-cell transcription factors BOB.1/OBF.1, Oct-2, and PU.1, possibly explaining the absence of immunoglobulin expression seen.[101,102] In addition, there is down-regulation of the B-cell associated intracellular signaling molecules Syk, BLNK, and PLC-gamma2, and variable expression of the intracellular signaling molecules Lyn and Fyn.[103]

CD3, CD45RO, and CD43 are T-cell–related markers of varying specificity, with CD3 the most specific and CD43 the least specific. Hodgkin cells are rarely reported to stain for these markers in paraffin sections.[70,104] However, some expression of T-cell antigens, including the T-cell receptor beta chain antigen, has been reported in frozen sections as well as in plastic-embedded sections, in up to 40% of cases in one series.[60,61,105–108] CD4 is also commonly expressed.

Some laboratories perform additional paraffin section immunohistochemical studies to aid in the diagnosis of Hodgkin lymphoma, particularly in difficult cases in which the results derived from more commonly used markers are ambiguous. Antibodies against Epstein-Barr virus–latent membrane protein (EBV LMP) consistently stain Hodgkin cells in the subset of cases of Hodgkin lymphoma that are EBV related (Fig. 4.12).[109–111] Because cases of mixed cellularity

Multivariate analysis has shown that lack of CD15 staining is an independent adverse prognostic indicator.[83] In addition to staining most cases of classical Hodgkin lymphoma, CD15 antibodies also stain about two-thirds of cases of acute myeloid leukemia, 5% of B-cell lymphomas, and 20% of T-cell lymphomas. Often, the staining pattern in non-Hodgkin lymphoma is different from that seen in Hodgkin lymphoma, being cytoplasmic and granular, although staining patterns indistinguishable from those of Hodgkin cells may also be seen. In addition, CD15 antibodies label many carcinomas, particularly adenocarcinomas of the lung.[67,92]

The CD20 cluster of antibodies detects a mature B-cell antigen.[69] CD20 antibodies stain the vast majority of B-cell neoplasms, except the most immature cases of B-lineage acute lymphoblastic leukemia and plasma cell neoplasms. CD20 may rarely show reactivity with nonhematolymphoid cells, such as the epithelial cells in a subset of thymomas. There is a wide range of reported reactivity for CD20 in Hodgkin lymphoma, ranging from fewer than 5% to a majority of cases; the overall average is about 25%.[63,69,83,86,93–95] Typically, when a case of Hodgkin lymphoma is CD20+, only a subset of the Hodgkin cells stain, and these in a heterogeneous pattern (some cells strongly positive, some weakly positive, and some negative). This pattern contrasts with the consistently strong staining typically seen in B-cell non-Hodgkin lymphomas. Despite the positivity for CD20 in some cases, Hodgkin cells lack functional transcripts of immunoglobulin light and heavy chains.[96–98] Therefore, Hodgkin cells either lack detectable immunoglobulin light and heavy chain or, more commonly, stain for both κ and λ light chains as a consequence of passive absorption of immunoglobulin from tissue fluid.[99] The immunoglobulin-associated molecule CD79a may be expressed by Hodgkin cells in a manner similar to

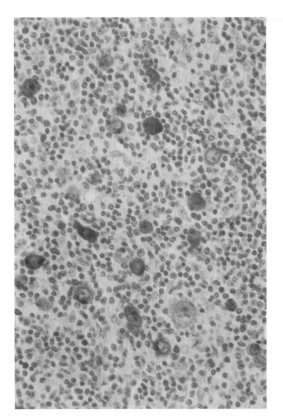

FIGURE 4.12. Immunostaining for Epstein-Barr virus (EBV) latent membrane protein (LMP) in a case of EBV-associated Hodgkin lymphoma. There is strong cytoplasmic staining, with paranuclear accentuation in the Hodgkin cells. EBV-positive small lymphocytes do not stain for LMP in Hodgkin lymphoma. See color insert.

and lymphocyte depletion as well as cases seen in the setting of HIV infection are most likely to be EBV associated, this stain is most useful when the differential diagnosis includes these types. Antibodies against CD40 recognize an antigen that, like CD30, is a member of the tumor necrosis/nerve growth receptor family. CD40 is expressed in 70% to 100% of cases of Hodgkin lymphoma, but in only 20% of cases of anaplastic large-cell lymphoma.[112] In addition, the pattern of staining in Hodgkin cells is somewhat different than in anaplastic large-cell lymphoma, resembling that of CD30 in Hodgkin lymphoma. Fascin is a 55-kd actin-bundling protein that is highly selective for dendritic cells in non-neoplastic tissues, although viral induction of fascin expression has been reported in EBV-infected B-cells.[113] Among neoplasms, fascin is a consistent marker for the Hodgkin cells of classical Hodgkin lymphoma, showing a strong diffuse cytoplasmic staining that frequently highlights dendritic shapes.[114] In contrast, no staining for fascin is seen in the L&H cells of nodular lymphocyte-predominant Hodgkin lymphoma, and only about 15% of non-Hodgkin lymphomas are positive for fascin. Hodgkin cells also stain with the lectins peanut agglutinin and Bauhinia purpurea in a majority of cases.[88,115]

We recommend the use of a panel of CD45RB, CD30, CD15, CD20, and CD3 in the routine immunodiagnosis of Hodgkin lymphoma. Additional, second-line markers that may be utilized in particularly difficult or immunohistochemically confusing cases may include EBV LMP, PAX-5, fascin, and other B- and T-cell markers.

One study has reported expression of the follicular dendritic cell marker CD21 in a significant percentage of cases,[116] but others have not confirmed this observation; differences in fixation and processing may explain the discrepancy. Other markers of dendritic cells, including fascin and CD83, have been identified in Hodgkin cells in a high percentage of cases.[114,117] Other markers reactive in Hodgkin cells include CD74 (most cases); the intermediate filament-associated protein restin (most cases), HLA-DR (Ia), class I antigens (variable expression, associated with EBV expression), CD25 (the interleukin-2 receptor), and CD71 (the transferrin receptor).[60,82,105,118–121] Most Hodgkin cells are positive for Ki-67, a nuclear proliferation marker expressed in cycling cells, as well as proliferating cell nuclear antigen (PCNA), p34, the protein product of the cell cycle control cdc2 gene, and cyclin D2.[122–129] Hodgkin cells are positive for p53 by immunohistochemistry, indicating the presence of higher-than-normal levels of the protein.[130–133] There is also variable expression of bcl2 and the p53-complexing protein mdm2, although there are no strong correlations between levels of the three proteins.[124,130,132] Hodgkin cells show increased expressed expression of several proteins indicative of activation of the NF-kB pathway, including c-Rel, TRAF1, and c-FLIP.[134,135]

Immunohistochemical studies have shown that most of the background lymphoid cells in Hodgkin lymphoma represent T-cells, with CD4+ helper cells predominating over CD8+ cytotoxic/suppressor cells.[116,119,136–140] In fact, low infiltration of FOXP3-positive (a marker for regulatory T-cells) cells in conjunction with high infiltration of TIA-1-positive cells may represent biological markers predicting an unfavorable outcome.[140] In addition, numerous macrophages can be identified. In many cases of Hodgkin lymphoma, expanded and disrupted networks of follicular dendritic cells can be identified, with Hodgkin cells often found embedded within them. This pattern is particularly well developed in cases of follicular Hodgkin lymphoma. One study has found that cases of Hodgkin lymphoma with prominent numbers of follicular dendritic cells have a better prognosis than other cases.[141]

Many cases of lymphocyte-rich classical Hodgkin lymphoma, particularly those with a nodular architecture, have a B-cell–rich infiltrate, in contrast to the marked T-cell predominance usually found in other types of classical Hodgkin lymphoma. Networks of follicular dendritic cells can be found in the nodules, representing the framework of follicles.

Diagnostic Molecular Findings

The molecular biology of Hodgkin cells is covered in Chapter 5, and the cytogenetics of Hodgkin lymphoma is covered in Chapter 8. From a diagnostic standpoint, the most important use of molecular studies is to rule out a non-Hodgkin lymphoma. Results of Southern blot studies for the detection of antigen receptor gene rearrangements are generally negative unless extremely large numbers of Hodgkin cells are present.[142–152] In the latter situation, light-rearranged bands of immunoglobulin light and/or heavy chains may be present; however, they can usually be distinguished from the more sizable bands observed in typical cases of non-Hodgkin lymphoma. Similarly, results of Southern blot studies to detect chromosomal translocations usually associated with subsets of non-Hodgkin lymphomas, such as t(14;18) and t(2;5), are also usually negative.[153–162] Caution needs to be exercised in the interpretation of the results of polymerase chain reaction (PCR) studies in Hodgkin lymphoma, as some of these translocations can rarely be detected by this methodology, and clonal immunoglobulin gene rearrangements may also be found in some cases, particularly those with large numbers of Hodgkin cells.[163–170]

Differential Diagnosis

The differential diagnosis of classical Hodgkin lymphoma is extremely broad, including carcinoma, malignant melanoma, sarcoma, reactive lymphoid lesions, non-Hodgkin lymphoma, and nodular lymphocyte-predominant Hodgkin lymphoma[171]; the differential diagnosis of classical Hodgkin lymphoma and the latter is covered below. Cases of the syncytial variant of nodular sclerosis Hodgkin lymphoma in particular may simulate carcinoma, melanoma, or a germ-cell tumor, whereas cases of undifferentiated nasopharyngeal carcinoma presenting in a cervical lymph node may closely simulate mixed-cellularity or nodular sclerosis Hodgkin lymphoma. When carcinoma is in the differential diagnosis, a keratin stain should either confirm or rule out that possibility (Table 4.3). Although embryonal carcinomas may be CD30+, they are also strongly positive for keratin and OCT-4. Germinomas (seminoma or dysgerminoma) are commonly negative for keratin, but they lack CD30 and CD15 and are also positive for OCT-4. Similarly, if malignant melanoma is in the differential diagnosis, an S-100 protein stain and possibly also an HMB-45 stain should be performed. Virtually all cases of malignant melanoma (as well as a wide variety of other neoplasms) are S-100+, but Hodgkin cells are consistently negative, although large numbers of S100+ dendritic cells may be seen in some cases. HMB-45 is a much more specific marker for malignant melanoma, but about 10% of cases may be negative. Rarely, fibroblastic areas in Hodgkin lymphoma can be confused with a spindle cell sarcoma. Attention to the cytologic features of the most spindled cells is important; they are bland in Hodgkin lymphoma, but atypical in sarcoma.

Two main patterns of reactive lymphoid proliferation can be easily confused with Hodgkin lymphoma. Cases of nodular sclerosis Hodgkin lymphoma in which necrosis is present in the center of one or more nodules may be misdiagnosed as a necrotizing or suppurative granulomatous lymphadenitis (the prototype being cat scratch disease). Attention should be given to the cells immediately rimming the areas of coagulative or suppurative necrosis. In necrotizing granulomatous

TABLE 4.3

IMMUNOHISTOLOGIC DIFFERENTIAL OF HODGKIN LYMPHOMA VERSUS NONHEMATOLYMPHOID NEOPLASMS

	Keratin	S-100	Alkaline phosphatase/OCT4	CD30
Hodgkin lymphoma	−	−	−	+
Carcinoma	+	−/+	−	−
Embryonal carcinoma	+	−	+	+
Germinoma	−/+	−	+	−
Malignant melanoma	−	+	−	−

CD, cluster of differentiation.

lymphadenitis, the cells lining the areas of necrosis are epithelioid histiocytes. In suppurative granulomatous lymphadenitis, the rimming cells are monocytoid cells and histiocytes with or without epithelioid features. In contrast, in Hodgkin lymphoma, at least some Hodgkin cells, usually lacunar cells, will be present. Hodgkin cells can be distinguished from histiocytes and monocytoid cells by the presence of at least some prominent nucleoli, and by the frequently multilobated nuclei. In cases of difficulty, immunohistochemical studies are of great help. Although histiocytes may occasionally show a granular cytoplasmic staining with CD15, they do not show membrane staining with CD15, they are always CD30−, and they are CD45+.

The second pattern of reactive lymphoid proliferation that can be easily confused with Hodgkin lymphoma is a reactive immunoblastic proliferation, including so-called interfollicular Hodgkinoid lymphadenitis.[172] In this setting, scattered immunoblasts or sheets of immunoblasts are present in the paracortical regions, either with or without hyperplastic follicles. When follicles are absent, the appearance can be easily confused with mixed-cellularity Hodgkin lymphoma; when follicles are present, the appearance can be easily confused with interfollicular Hodgkin lymphoma. Immunoblasts can closely resemble Hodgkin cells, as they have large nuclei, a vesicular chromatin pattern, and prominent nucleoli. Occasionally, they may be multilobated or multinucleated; cells resembling diagnostic Reed-Sternberg cells are well known to occur in virally induced reactive immunoblastic proliferations such as EBV-associated acute infectious mononucleosis. However, in contrast to Hodgkin cells, reactive immunoblasts usually have a basophilic cytoplasm, often with a distinct paranuclear hof (clear zone). They are usually associated with marked plasmacytosis, and transitional forms between frank plasma cells and immunoblasts are usually present. In addition, the immunoblasts are usually more evenly dispersed throughout the lymphoid proliferation; in contrast, Hodgkin cells in Hodgkin lymphoma are more irregularly clustered. Immunohistochemical studies are again of great help. Like Hodgkin cells, immunoblasts are often CD30+, but the intensity of staining is often variable from cell to cell. In contrast to Hodgkin cells, they are usually CD45+ and stain with either B- or T-cell markers. In addition, immunoblasts are usually CD15−, although the immunoblasts found in cytomegalovirus-associated lymphadenitis have been reported to be CD15+.

Many types of non-Hodgkin lymphoma can be easily confused with Hodgkin lymphoma. Lymphocyte-rich classical Hodgkin lymphoma must be distinguished from lymph node involvement by B-cell chronic lymphocytic leukemia/small-lymphocyte lymphoma. The latter often contains scattered cells with large nuclei, termed prolymphocytes and paraimmunoblasts, but does not usually contain eosinophils. Rarely, the phenomenon of chronic lymphocytic leukemia with Reed-Sternberg–like cells has been described (see below).[173,174] Histologically, lymph nodes involved by chronic lymphocytic leukemia/small-lymphocytic lymphoma usually show pale staining areas at low magnification (termed pseudofollicular growth centers), which is a highly characteristic feature of this neoplasm. The prolymphocytes and paraimmunoblasts do not possess nucleoli as large as those of Hodgkin cells. The differential diagnosis may be easily resolved by immunohistochemical studies, as the dominant small-lymphocytic cell type in chronic lymphocytic leukemia/small-lymphocyte lymphoma is a B-lymphocyte that shows aberrant coexpression of CD43 and CD5 and is usually also CD23+, whereas the dominant small-lymphocytic cell type is usually a T-lymphocyte in classical Hodgkin lymphoma.

T-cell–rich or histiocyte-rich B-cell lymphoma may be quite difficult to distinguish from MC Hodgkin lymphoma.[175,176] In the first case, the predominant cell type is a small lymphocyte that is a reactive T-cell component, whereas in the second case, large numbers of both reactive histiocytes and T-cells are present. In both lymphomas, which may represent variants of the same entity, a minority population of large cells represents the neoplastic B-cell component. The large-cell population can have nuclear features virtually indistinguishable from those of Hodgkin cells. Many cases of T-cell–rich B-cell lymphoma have other areas more consistent with a diffuse large B-cell lymphoma, but this is by no means always the case. In interpreting the results of immunohistochemical studies, one must remember that Hodgkin cells may express the B-lineage marker CD20 (albeit often in a heterogeneous pattern), but they usually lack expression of CD45RA, another B-lineage marker. The large cells in T-cell–rich B-cell lymphoma are CD45+, CD20+ (with all large cells showing the same intensity of staining), usually CD45RA+, and usually CD15− and CD30−. In addition, they are often positive for epithelial membrane antigen (a marker rarely present in Hodgkin lymphoma), and restriction of light chains can sometimes be demonstrated. Distinction between diffuse large-cell lymphoma of the mediastinum and the syncytial variant of nodular-sclerosis Hodgkin lymphoma can also be extremely difficult. The sclerosis in mediastinal large B-cell lymphoma usually consists of thin rather than the thick fibrous bands of nodular sclerosis Hodgkin lymphoma, and it usually compartmentalizes small groups of cells; however, this distinction may be very difficult to appreciate in the small biopsy specimens often obtained at this site. Immunohistochemical studies are often necessary for the distinction to be made (Table 4.2).

Peripheral T-cell lymphomas, particularly polymorphic examples, may also be difficult to distinguish from mixed-cellularity Hodgkin lymphoma.[177] Both neoplasms can demonstrate a mixed reactive infiltrate sometimes containing many eosinophils, and Hodgkin-like cells are not uncommonly seen in peripheral T-cell lymphoma. Cytologically, one tries to identify a range of cellular atypia in peripheral T-cell lymphoma, from atypical small to atypical medium to atypical large-sized lymphoid cells. The mitotic rate in peripheral T-cell lymphoma is also generally higher than that seen in Hodgkin lymphoma.[178] Immunohistochemical studies are of great use, as the large cells in peripheral T-cell lymphoma should stain with CD45 as well as one or more T-lineage markers, a rare phenomenon in Hodgkin cells. If necessary, immunophenotyping studies of frozen sections often can demonstrate an aberrant T-cell phenotype in peripheral T-cell lymphoma.[179–181] Molecular studies, with the demonstration of a sizable rearrangement of the β or γ T-cell receptor genes, would obviously favor a diagnosis of peripheral T-cell lymphoma. Anaplastic large-cell lymphoma may be extremely difficult to distinguish from Hodgkin lymphoma—so much so that terms such as anaplastic large-cell–like Hodgkin lymphoma and Hodgkin lymphoma-like anaplastic large-cell lymphoma have been introduced into the literature; PAX-5 staining can be very useful, as it is negative in anaplastic large-cell lymphoma but frequently positive in Hodgkin lymphoma. Cases of lymphocyte-depletion Hodgkin lymphoma are virtually always difficult to distinguish from non-Hodgkin lymphoma. Immunohistochemical studies should be performed to confirm the diagnosis of this rare type of Hodgkin lymphoma. In addition to the other immunohistochemical studies already mentioned to be helpful in the differential diagnosis of Hodgkin lymphoma versus non-Hodgkin lymphoma, EBV LMP may be of use, as cases of lymphocyte-depletion Hodgkin lymphoma are often associated with EBV (see Chapter 3), whereas fewer than 5% of cases of non-Hodgkin lymphoma occurring outside the setting of HIV infection are EBV+.[182]

NODULAR LYMPHOCYTE-PREDOMINANT HODGKIN LYMPHOMA

Gross Appearance

In nodular lymphocyte-predominant Hodgkin lymphoma, involved lymph nodes tend to be larger than those seen in classical Hodgkin lymphoma, typically ranging in size from 2 to 8 cm. The cut section usually reveals a vague or distinct nodular architecture, often with a rim of uninvolved lymphoid tissue.

Histopathology

At low magnification, the lymph node shows complete or subtotal effacement of the architecture. The capsule is usually intact without pericapsular infiltration, and there may be a rim of uneffaced lymphoid tissue, which may be normal or hyperplastic or may show progressive transformation of germinal centers. Fibrosis is uncommon but may be present and may be band-like, mimicking nodular sclerosis. In most cases, a nodular or a nodular and partly diffuse infiltration pattern is found in the effaced areas (Fig. 4.13). The nodules are typically large and relatively numerous, sometimes resembling progressively transformed germinal centers (Fig. 4.14); they are typically

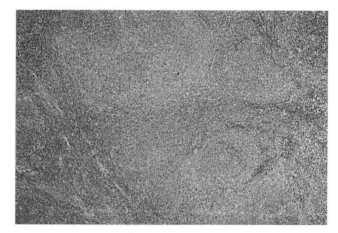

FIGURE 4.13. Nodular lymphocyte-predominant Hodgkin lymphoma showing large irregular nodules, which are closely packed (hematoxylin and eosin). See color insert.

closely packed, but in some cases the nodules are poorly demarcated and difficult to discern, and a diffuse architecture may be focally present. The existence of a purely diffuse form of nodular lymphocyte predominance is debated because typically some degree of nodularity is found when the entire lymph node is carefully examined. If a large number of well-prepared sections show no evidence of nodularity, the possibility of either lymphocyte-rich classical Hodgkin lymphoma or T-cell–rich large B-cell lymphoma should be seriously considered.

A mixture of lymphocytes and histiocytes, particularly epithelioid histiocytes, is characteristic of nodular lymphocyte-predominant Hodgkin lymphoma. Epithelioid histiocytes are preferentially found in the outer rim of nodular infiltrates. They are arranged in small groups or clusters, and well-formed granulomas may be present in rare cases. Eosinophils and neutrophils are rare. Plasma cells are not common and are seen only between follicles.

The neoplastic cells of nodular lymphocyte predominance are the L&H cells (popcorn cells), usually found in and around the nodules (Fig. 4.15). In diffuse areas, the L&H cells are still often arranged in a vaguely nodular pattern. Characteristically, L&H cells resemble centroblasts but are larger and have lobulated nuclei and small to moderate-sized basophilic nucleoli, often present adjacent to the nuclear membrane. The cytoplasm is broad and only slightly

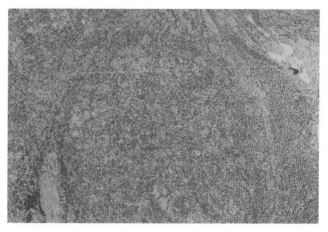

FIGURE 4.14. A nodule of nodular lymphocyte-predominant Hodgkin lymphoma is shown, composed mostly of small lymphocytes with scattered epithelioid histiocytes (hematoxylin and eosin). See color insert.

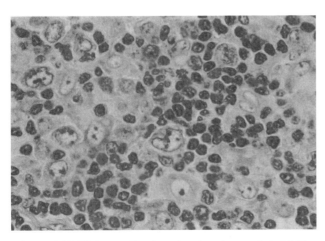

FIGURE 4.15. High magnification, showing characteristic L&H or "popcorn" cells (Giemsa stain). See color insert.

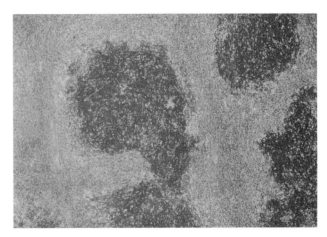

FIGURE 4.16. Follicular dendritic cells form large networks in nodular lymphocyte-predominant Hodgkin lymphoma (immuno-alkaline phosphatase, CD21). See color insert.

basophilic. Ultrastructural studies demonstrate that L&H cells have the appearance of centroblasts of germinal centers. In addition, follicular dendritic cells characteristic of the B-cell follicle can be found in the vicinity of the L&H cells.[183,184] Classical Hodgkin cells and Reed-Sternberg cells are few in number or completely lacking. If classic Hodgkin cells and Reed-Sternberg cells are easily detected, a diagnosis of lymphocyte-rich classical Hodgkin lymphoma should be suspected. In some cases, L&H cells may resemble lacunar cells because both cell types show irregularly shaped or lobulated nuclei, small nucleoli, and broad pale to slightly basophilic cytoplasm. Although in rare cases it may be difficult to distinguish between L&H cells and lacunar cells by routine histology, lacunar cells are usually larger, with more abundant cytoplasm than L&H cells.

The number of L&H cells varies considerably from case to case. When they are numerous, the distinction between nodular lymphocyte-predominant Hodgkin lymphoma and nodular lymphocyte-predominant Hodgkin lymphoma with transition to large B-cell lymphoma may be difficult to make. However, large-cell lymphoma should be diagnosed only when large areas of lymph nodes contain confluent L&H cells or centroblasts, particularly when they form sheets outside the nodules.

Immunophenotypic Findings

In typical cases, the nodules of nodular lymphocyte-predominant Hodgkin lymphoma demonstrate large numbers of small polyclonal B-lymphocytes in addition to L&H cells when stained with CD20 or CD79a.[184,185] The interfollicular areas are dominated by T-lymphocytes that are CD3-positive, and there may be only rare B-cells.[186] However, there is a wide variation in the number of T-cells in the nodules; T-cells tend to increase in numbers over time, and in some cases, the T-cells may outnumber B-cells, either in the entire section or in selected nodules. In all cases, individual L&H cells tend to be surrounded by T-cells. Often one or more of the T-cells forming rings around L&H cells are CD57 positive.[187] T-cells expressing CD57 are usually numerous in the nodules and are found to a lesser extent in the diffuse parts of nodular lymphocyte-predominant Hodgkin lymphoma.[185,188,189] The nodules are associated with large nodular meshworks of follicular dendritic cells staining positively with anti-CD21 (Fig. 4.16); follicular dendritic cells are absent in diffuse areas.[186,190,191]

The neoplastic cells in nodular lymphocyte-predominant Hodgkin lymphoma show a characteristic immunohistochemical

profile (Table 4.4).[192–195] The L&H cells are positive for leukocyte common antigen (CD45) and for B-cell antigens (CD20, PAX-5, CD45RA, CD79a) (Fig. 4.17), usually negative for CD30, and almost always negative for CD15. CD15 will become positive with a neuraminidase predigestion.[196] This marker profile has proved to be a consistent finding in nearly all cases.[197] Occasionally, a few CD30-positive blasts can be found. However, a careful evaluation of the morphology of these cells reveals that they lie either outside the nodules or in their outer rim, are smaller than L&H cells, show round to oval nuclei, and are most probably reactive immunoblasts, frequently found in the parafollicular regions of normal lymph nodes. The L&H cells are usually positive for J chain, a feature of B-cells,[198,199] as well as the B-cell transcription factors BOB.1/OBF.1 and Oct2.[101] In addition, there is consistent expression of the B-cell–associated intracellular signaling molecules Fyn, Syk, BLNK, and PLC-gamma2, although Lyn staining is only seen in a minority of cases.[103] In about 25% to 50% of cases, the L&H cells express epithelial membrane antigen[199]; this antigen is more easily detected in Bouin's-fixed sections. They are also usually positive for BCL6 but are negative for BCL2.[200,201] The L&H cells always lack positivity for T-cell markers such as CD3 and CD45RO and are virtually always negative for Epstein-Barr virus (EBV) latent membrane protein.[202]

The detection of immunoglobulins in L&H cells by immunohistochemistry is variable. Using conventional immunohistochemical techniques, most observers have found no good evidence of immunoglobulin expression in L&H cells.[192,203,204] Others have found L&H cells to express one or the other light chain in the same case.[183,187,199] However, there have been cases reported in which light-chain restriction could be demonstrated.[205,206] Notably, nearly all such cases have expressed κ light chains.

When proliferation markers such as Ki-67 are used, most L&H cells show positivity, whereas only a few bystander lymphocytes are in cycle.[207,208] If immunohistochemical double-staining techniques are used, the proliferating background lymphocytes are mainly T-cells, with infrequent B-cells showing evidence of proliferative activity.[207]

Diagnostic Molecular Studies

Considering the various technical problems and possibilities of misinterpretation of immunohistochemical staining for immunoglobulin in L&H, Hodgkin, and Reed-Sternberg cells, in situ hybridization studies have been used to visualize light-chain

TABLE 4.4

MORPHOLOGIC, IMMUNOPHENOTYPIC, AND GENETIC FEATURES
OF L&H CELLS VERSUS CLASSICAL HODGKIN CELLS

	L&H cells	Hodgkin cells
Nuclei	Polylobated	Mono- or binucleate
Nucleoli	Small to medium	Large
Classic Reed-Sternberg	Rare	Common
CD20	>95%	24% (97)
CD45	>95%	7% (98)
CD30	<5%	89% (99)
CD15	<5%	87% (100)
Epithelial membrane antigen	25–50%	5%
EBV-LMP	<1%	40–50%
In situ hybridization for light chains	Monotypic	–
Immunoglobulin genes rearranged	Clonal	Clonal
V-region mutations	+	+
Productive rearrangements	+	–

mRNA in neoplastic cells.[203,209–211] However, in situ hybridization techniques are limited by the sensitivity of the probes and the limitation in the identification of cells showing a positive signal. Probably as a consequence of the low copy numbers of mRNA and the relative low sensitivity of the method applied, the earliest studies could not identify mRNA for immunoglobulin light chains in L&H cells.[203,209] In subsequent studies, which enhanced the sensitivity by using special cocktails of digoxigenin-labeled probes or using radioactively labeled ribonucleic probes, it was possible to demonstrate monotypic light-chain mRNA expression in L&H cells; these studies detected nearly exclusively mRNA for kappa light chain.[210,211] In one of the studies, there was also evidence for light-chain restriction in a subset of the small B-cells in some cases.[211] EBV is rarely detectable in the L&H cells of nodular lymphocyte-predominant Hodgkin lymphoma[211–215]; however, a few well-documented cases of EBV-

positive nodular lymphocyte predominance have recently been reported.[216,216a] Using Southern blot hybridization techniques clonal rearrangements of the immunoglobulin gene locus, T-cell receptor genes, or the rearrangement of the *bcl-2* gene cannot be detected.[217,218]

Differential Diagnosis

Progressive Transformation of Germinal Centers

Progressively transformed germinal centers are enlarged germinal centers composed of increased numbers of mantle cells and decreased numbers of germinal center cells.[219–221] Single or clustered epithelioid histiocytes may occasionally be found but are less common than in nodular lymphocyte-predominant Hodgkin lymphoma. The progressively transformed germinal centers are typically round and widely spaced, and normal reactive lymphoid follicles are seen between them. Low magnification can provide important information for the differential diagnostic decision between progressive transformation of germinal centers and nodular lymphocyte-predominant Hodgkin lymphoma. In cases of reactive hyperplasia showing progressive transformation of germinal centers, germinal centers are characteristically numerous, and only a few progressively transformed germinal centers are found (Fig. 4.18).[221] In contrast, in nodular lymphocyte-predominant Hodgkin lymphoma, the nodules are closely packed, and germinal centers are almost never seen in involved areas of the lymph node. However, a peripheral rim of reactive lymphoid tissue may show well-preserved germinal centers.

In comparison with the centroblasts observed in progressive transformation of germinal centers, L&H cells are usually larger and show more lobulated nuclei. Moreover, L&H cells are often found at the periphery of or outside the nodules, in contrast to centroblasts, which are confined to follicles. The immunophenotype of progressively transformed

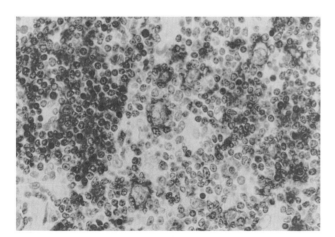

FIGURE 4.17. In addition to small lymphocytes, several L&H cells show a membrane-bound immunoreaction for CD20 (immuno-alkaline phosphatase). See color insert.

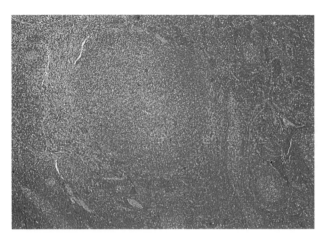

FIGURE 4.18. A large progressively transformed germinal center is surrounded by several small germinal centers (Giemsa stain). See color insert.

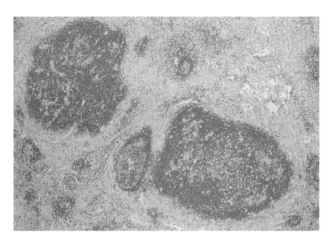

FIGURE 4.19. The progressively transformed germinal centers are composed mainly of B-cells, similar to the surrounding reactive follicles (immuno-alkaline phosphatase, CD20). See color insert.

germinal centers and nodular lymphocyte-predominant Hodgkin lymphoma are similar. However, some features are useful for differential diagnosis.[222] In progressive transformation of germinal centers, staining for CD20 reveals well-circumscribed nodules of B-cells, predominantly small, that occupy the entire nodule (Fig. 4.19). In contrast, in nodular lymphocyte-predominant Hodgkin lymphoma, staining for CD20 reveals irregular nodules showing a moth-eaten appearance, with frequent unstained T-cells surrounding large CD20-positive tumor cells. Staining for T-cell antigens may show many T-cells in both conditions; however, their distribution is distinctive. In progressive transformation of germinal centers, as in normal germinal centers, T-cells are scattered singly and are only rarely found rosetting around large B-cells or histiocytes. In contrast, in nodular lymphocyte predominance, the T-cells form irregular aggregates and clumps, with rosettes formed around the large B-cells. Staining for follicular dendritic cells or CD57 is not particularly helpful because the patterns may be similar unless there is distinct rosetting of CD57-positive cells around the large B-cells. In Bouin's-fixed tissue, most cases of nodular lymphocyte predominance express epithelial membrane antigen on

large cells; this reaction pattern is absent in progressive transformation of germinal centers.

Follicular Lymphoma

The differentiation between nodular lymphocyte-predominant Hodgkin lymphoma and follicular lymphoma is usually not difficult. The follicles of follicular lymphoma are usually smaller than the nodules of nodular lymphocyte-predominant Hodgkin lymphoma and often show extension outside of the capsule, a phenomenon that never occurs in nodular lymphocyte-predominant Hodgkin lymphoma. The follicles of follicular lymphomas are composed of centrocytes intermingled with a few up to moderate or large numbers of centroblasts. The latter may be large and can show features of L&H cells. In cases in which the centrocytes are relatively small and resemble lymphocytes, the differential diagnosis between follicular lymphoma and nodular lymphocyte-predominant Hodgkin lymphoma may become difficult. In these cases, immunostaining for CD20, CD3, CD57, J-chain, kappa/lambda-immunoglobulin light chain, and IgM heavy chain may help in establishing the diagnosis (Table 4.5).[223] The CD20-positive L&H cells in

TABLE 4.5

IMMUNOHISTOCHEMICAL AND MOLECULAR BIOLOGICAL STUDIES IN DIFFERENTIAL DIAGNOSIS BETWEEN NODULAR LYMPHOCYTE-PREDOMINANT HODGKIN LYMPHOMA AND FOLLICULAR LYMPHOMA

	Nodular lymphocyte-predominant Hodgkin lymphoma	Follicular lymphoma
CD20	L&H cells in nodules and interfollicular areas	Centroblasts/centrocytes within follicular structures
CD3, CD4, CD57	Aggregates of T-cells; T-cell rosettes around L&H cells	Scattered T-cells; no T-cell rosettes
Igκ/λ IgM	Polyclonal lymphocytes; L&H cells negative or rarely κ-positive	Clonal in centroblasts/centrocytes
Bcl-2 protein	L&H cells negative	Centroblasts/centrocytes usually positive
Immunoglobulin heavy-chain gene	No clonal band detected by Southern blot	Rearranged by Southern blot
t(14;18)	Absent	85%

nodular lymphocyte-predominant Hodgkin lymphoma are easily detected not only in the nodular but also in the interfollicular areas of the involved tissue. If T-cell antibodies (CD3, CD57) are used, in many cases of nodular-lymphocyte predominant Hodgkin lymphoma complete or incomplete rosettes around the L&H cells are detected, whereas in follicular lymphoma, rosetting T-cells are never found. The expression of one immunoglobulin light chain in small lymphoid cells and centroblasts can be found by immunohistochemistry in most cases of follicular lymphomas in frozen sections and in some cases in paraffin sections but not in nodular lymphocyte-predominant Hodgkin lymphoma. In contrast to follicular lymphoma, nodular lymphocyte-predominant Hodgkin lymphoma does not have detectable immunoglobulin heavy-chain gene rearrangements by Southern blotting and does not show the t(14;18).[217,218]

Nodular Lymphocyte-Predominant Hodgkin Lymphoma Versus Lymphocyte-Rich Classical Hodgkin Lymphoma

As in nodular lymphocyte-predominant Hodgkin lymphoma, small lymphocytes comprise the majority of the cells in lymphocyte-rich classical Hodgkin lymphoma. Eosinophils and plasma cells may or may not be admixed. This type of Hodgkin lymphoma may also show a nodular or follicular growth pattern, further mimicking nodular lymphocyte predominant Hodgkin lymphoma, as described by Ashton-Key and associates.[23] However, in contrast to nodular lymphocyte-predominant Hodgkin lymphoma, the nodules, when present, appear to represent expanded mantle zones. In typical cases, the neoplastic cells of lymphocyte-rich classical Hodgkin lymphoma have the characteristic features of classical Hodgkin and Reed-Sternberg cells. When a nodular architecture is present, the Hodgkin and Reed-Sternberg cells are typically found in the outer areas of the nodules, which seem to be expanded mantle zones, interfollicular areas, or adjacent monocytoid B-cell proliferations. Residual intact germinal centers are also frequently identified within the nodules, in contrast with nodular lymphocyte-predominant Hodgkin lymphoma. In cases with many classical Hodgkin and Reed-Sternberg cells, the diagnosis of lymphocyte-rich classical Hodgkin lymphoma may not be difficult. However, there are cases in which cells resembling L&H cells with occasional Hodgkin and Reed-Sternberg cells occur in a nodular lymphocytic background. These cases may be impossible to distinguish from nodular lymphocyte-predominant Hodgkin lymphoma on morphologic grounds and may require immunohistochemical studies. Some cases of lymphocyte-rich classical Hodgkin lymphoma may show a diffuse growth pattern. In such cases, the differential diagnosis with nodular lymphocyte-predominant Hodgkin lymphoma is less problematic. The presence of admixed eosinophils or plasma cells also argues against nodular lymphocyte-predominant Hodgkin lymphoma.

The immunohistochemical staining pattern of lymphocytes and follicular dendritic cells of lymphocyte-rich classical Hodgkin lymphoma is similar to that of nodular lymphocyte-predominant Hodgkin lymphoma in that the nodules are composed predominantly of B-cells with nodular meshworks of follicular dendritic cells. However, in lymphocyte-rich classical Hodgkin lymphoma, the B-cell–rich nodules sometimes show concentric rings of follicular dendritic cells with a central accumulation of follicular dendritic cells, similar to the pattern seen in Castleman's disease (Fig. 4.20). The Hodgkin and Reed-Sternberg cells of classical Hodgkin lymphoma are positive for CD30 and CD15 and negative for CD45 and may or may not express B-cell markers, whereas those of nodular lymphocyte-predominant Hodgkin lymphoma are CD20 positive and lack

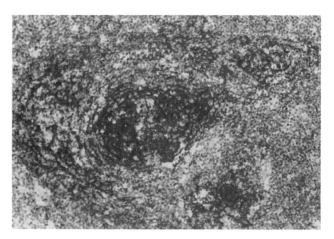

FIGURE 4.20. Nodular infiltrate of lymphocyte-rich classical Hodgkin lymphoma. Eccentrically localized remnants of germinal centers are visualized by immunostaining for follicular dendritic cells (immuno-alkaline phosphatase, CD21). See color insert.

CD15 and CD30 (Table 4.4). In situ hybridization for EBV or immunohistochemical studies for EBV latent membrane protein may show positivity in the tumor cells of lymphocyte-rich classical Hodgkin lymphoma but not in nodular lymphocyte-predominant Hodgkin lymphoma.

T-Cell–Rich Large B-Cell Lymphoma

The distinction between the diffuse variants of lymphocyte-predominant and lymphocyte-rich classical Hodgkin lymphoma and T-cell–rich large B-cell lymphoma may be extremely difficult and in some cases even impossible on morphologic and immunohistochemical grounds. The term T-cell–rich B-cell lymphoma was introduced by Ramsay and associates; it has been used to refer to B-cell lymphomas in which an unusually prominent reactive T-cell infiltrate is found.[224] The term has been used heterogeneously for cases with over 50% T-cells and for cases with over 90% T-cells.[225–227] Many reported cases probably represent "usual" diffuse large B-cell lymphomas or even low-grade lymphomas with many T-cells. However, Delabie and co-workers and Chittal and colleagues have described an unusual form of large B-cell lymphoma with a background of T-cells and histiocytes resembling diffuse lymphocyte-predominant Hodgkin lymphoma.[228,229] McBride and associates reported similar cases misdiagnosed as mixed-cellularity Hodgkin lymphoma; in that study, the atypical cells very closely resembled classical Reed-Sternberg cells and variants.[230] These cases appear to represent a distinct entity with an aggressive clinical course, often involving liver, spleen, and bone marrow. T-cell/histiocyte–rich large B-cell lymphoma is characterized by a diffuse infiltrate consisting mainly of T-lymphocytes and histiocytes that are not neoplastic and a minority of medium-sized to large neoplastic B-cells comprising 5% or less of the total cellular population.[224,228,229,231] The large B-cells may resemble L&H cells of nodular lymphocyte predominance or may resemble centroblasts or immunoblasts. This histologic picture may be extremely difficult to differentiate from nodular lymphocyte-predominant Hodgkin lymphoma with a diffuse pattern. Indeed, it has been debated whether T-cell–rich large B-cell lymphoma is a distinct entity or is rather an aggressive variant of nodular lymphocyte-predominant Hodgkin lymphoma.[232,233] In the REAL and WHO classifications, T-cell–rich large B-cell lymphoma is included as a variant of diffuse large cell B-cell lymphoma.

Criteria for the differential diagnosis between T-cell–rich large B-cell lymphoma and nodular lymphocyte predominance

TABLE 4.6

CRITERIA FOR DIFFERENTIAL DIAGNOSIS BETWEEN NODULAR LYMPHOCYTE-PREDOMINANT HODGKIN LYMPHOMA, INCLUDING ITS DIFFUSE VARIANT, AND T-CELL–RICH LARGE B-CELL LYMPHOMA

	Nodular lymphocyte predominant	T-cell–rich large B-cell lymphoma
Architecture	Nodular pattern (nearly always), sometimes bands of fibrosis	Diffuse pattern (occasional nodularity), sometimes diffuse fibrosis
Neoplastic component distribution	Found in "nodules"	Scattered
Popcorn appearance	+/–	–/+
Centroblast-like	–/+	+/–
RS/RS-like cells	–/+	–/+
CD45	+	+
CD20	+	+
CD30	–	–
CD15	–	–
EMA	–/+	–/+
J-chain	+	–
Monotypic Ig	–/+	+/–
MIB-1/Ki-67 index	High	High
EBV	–	–
Ig gene rearrangement studies on whole-tissue sections	–	+/–
Reactive component		
T-cells	++(CD4+)	++++(CD4,CD8+)
B or mixed B&T	+	–
T-cell rosettes	+	–
CD57+ cells	Varying, occasional rosettes	Rare
Histiocytes	Few to many (epitheloid)	Few to many
FDC meshworks	+	–
Clinical findings		
Stage	I or II	III or IV
Bone marrow involvement	–	Frequently +

Table modified from the E.A.H.P. Workshop, Toledo, October 1994.

are listed in Table 4.6. The immunophenotype of the neoplastic cells in T-cell/histiocyte–rich large B-cell lymphoma may be identical to that of lymphocyte-predominant Hodgkin lymphoma. The neoplastic cells of T-cell/histiocyte–rich large B-cell lymphoma express CD45, CD20, and CD79a and are often epithelial membrane antigen positive.[234] They may have cytoplasmic immunoglobulin and are CD15 and CD30 negative. Thus, the differential diagnosis rests on the background infiltrate. The presence of nodular meshworks of follicular dendritic cells, numerous small B-lymphocytes, and CD57-positive cells favors lymphocyte-predominant Hodgkin lymphoma, whereas their absence favors T-cell/histiocyte–rich large B-cell lymphoma. The presence of clear-cut immunoglobulin light-chain restriction by immunohistochemistry or clonal

immunoglobulin gene rearrangements by Southern blot would favor T-cell/histiocyte–rich large B-cell lymphoma. Finally, clinical features may provide a clue to the diagnosis, because lymphocyte-predominant Hodgkin lymphoma only rarely presents with disease involving the liver, spleen, and bone marrow, although these organs are commonly involved in T-cell/histiocyte–rich large B-cell lymphoma.

Some cases of T-cell–rich large B-cell lymphoma may contain neoplastic cells resembling classic Hodgkin or Reed-Sternberg cells, making the differential diagnosis with classical Hodgkin lymphoma even more problematic.[230,234,235] Distinction between classical Hodgkin lymphoma and T-cell/histiocyte–rich large B-cell lymphoma rests on the detection of CD15 and CD30 and the absence of CD45 on the neoplastic cells in classical Hodgkin lymphoma, as a significant subset of cases of classical Hodgkin lymphoma may express CD20. The identification of EBV in the Hodgkin and Reed-Sternberg cells of classical Hodgkin lymphoma may also be of benefit, as cases of T-cell/histiocyte–rich large B-cell lymphoma are rarely EBV positive.

The analysis of the rearranged V genes in the neoplastic cells of T-cell–rich large B-cell lymphoma reveals mutations indicating a germinal center cell origin of these lymphomas.[236] The evaluation of the mutation pattern speaks in favor of the involvement of the tumor cells of an antigen-driven selection process.

Transformation of Nodular Lymphocyte-Predominant Hodgkin Lymphoma to a Diffuse Large B-Cell Lymphoma

About 2% to 3% of patients with nodular lymphocyte predominance develop large-cell lymphoma of the B type.[237–239] Large-cell lymphoma may be found in the same lymph node that is involved by nodular lymphocyte predominance, in another lymph node at a distant site, or rarely at an extranodal localization. The occurrence of large-cell lymphoma in patients with nodular lymphocyte-predominant Hodgkin lymphoma may be simultaneous or subsequent, or in rare cases large-cell lymphoma may be seen before nodular lymphocyte-predominant Hodgkin lymphoma.[204,237,238,240–242] Patients with diffuse large B-cell lymphoma arising in nodular lymphocyte-predominant Hodgkin lymphoma have a prognosis similar to those with de novo diffuse large B-cell lymphoma and should be treated aggressively.[239]

The large-cell lymphomas are morphologically variable. Some are composed of cells resembling L&H cells. Others may span the spectrum of all subtypes of diffuse large-cell lymphomas of B type—centroblastic (monomorphic, polymorphic, or multilobated), immunoblastic, or anaplastic. Burkitt-like lymphomas may rarely develop. The large-cell lymphomas arising in nodular lymphocyte-predominant Hodgkin lymphoma characteristically express a B-cell phenotype (CD19- and CD20-positive) as well as immunoglobulin light-chain restriction. In lymph nodes containing both nodular lymphocyte-predominant Hodgkin lymphoma and large-cell lymphoma, the large-cell lymphoma is typically demarcated from the nodular lymphocyte-predominant Hodgkin lymphoma. However, in some cases, transitional areas containing numerous L&H cells may exist between the large-cell lymphoma and nodular lymphocyte-predominant Hodgkin lymphoma. It may occasionally be difficult to differentiate between nodular lymphocyte-predominant Hodgkin lymphoma with clusters of L&H cells and nodular lymphocyte-predominant Hodgkin lymphoma with transition to large-cell lymphoma. However, transformation to typical large-cell lymphoma should be diagnosed only when large areas of the lymph node are effaced by L&H cells.[194,237] Rare cases of nodular lymphocyte-predominant Hodgkin lymphoma may also relapse as T-cell–rich B-cell lymphoma.

In situ hybridization studies have shown the same immunoglobulin light-chain mRNA in the L&H cells of nodular lymphocyte-predominant Hodgkin lymphoma and in large-cell lymphoma in some of the cases investigated, indicating the presence of the same tumor clone.[243] In several studies, polymerase chain reaction techniques using tissue sections have been applied to examine cases of nodular lymphocyte predominance associated with large-cell lymphoma.[244–246] In these studies, consensus primers to the VH and JH regions were used to identify clonal B-cell populations. In the vast majority of cases of large-cell lymphoma associated with nodular lymphocyte-predominant Hodgkin lymphoma, clonal rearrangements could be found in the large-cell component.

However, clonal B-cell proliferations in nodular lymphocyte-predominant Hodgkin lymphoma were found in only a few cases. Identical sequences of rearranged V genes in two cases, both in the nodular lymphocyte-predominant Hodgkin lymphoma infiltrate and the large-cell lymphoma, were detected by Greiner and associates.[244]

Use of clonospecific oligonucleotides to detect rearranged V-gene sequences in large-cell lymphoma allowed Wickert and colleagues to identify a corresponding clonal B-cell proliferation in the associated nodular lymphocyte-predominant Hodgkin lymphoma in only a few cases.[246] No clonal immunoglobulin gene rearrangement was identified in any case of nodular lymphocyte-predominant Hodgkin lymphoma using polymerase chain reaction on whole sections or on enriched L&H cells by microdissection in another study.[245] In this study, clone-specific primers designed for the recognition of V-gene rearrangements of nodular lymphocyte-predominant Hodgkin lymphoma–associated large-cell lymphoma were not successful in detecting the corresponding clone in nodular lymphocyte-predominant Hodgkin lymphoma. In the above studies, the failure to detect clonal populations in nodular lymphocyte-predominant Hodgkin lymphoma may be related to the sensitivity of the methods used, as whole-section polymerase chain reaction usually does not detect monoclonality in nodular lymphocyte- predominant Hodgkin lymphoma.

RELATIONSHIP BETWEEN HODGKIN LYMPHOMA AND NON-HODGKIN LYMPHOMAS

Hodgkin lymphoma and non-Hodgkin lymphomas have long been regarded as distinct disease entities based on differences in pathology, immunophenotype, clinical features, and response to therapy. However, recent observations suggest that these disorders may be more closely related than previously thought. Considerable progress has been made regarding the origin of the neoplastic cell in Hodgkin lymphoma (see Chapter 5). Data suggest that the malignant cell of Hodgkin lymphoma is a B-cell in all, or nearly all, cases.[247–250] The existence of a T-cell form of Hodgkin lymphoma is not totally excluded, but if it exists, it is rare. If Hodgkin lymphoma is derived from an altered B-lymphocyte, it is not surprising that areas of overlap with B-cell non-Hodgkin lymphomas should occur both biologically and clinically (Table 4.7).[251] If the Reed-Sternberg cell is viewed as a crippled B-cell, the biological and molecular events leading to this state are complex. These events may occur in the context of a normal immune system, in the setting of non-Hodgkin lymphoma, or in the setting of immunodeficiency, such as the acquired immune deficiency syndrome or iatrogenic immune suppression following solid organ transplantation. Cells resembling Reed-Sternberg cells and variants may be observed in these diverse clinical settings and may represent early steps in the transformation to Hodgkin lymphoma. Studies of these cases at the interface of Hodgkin lymphoma and non-Hodgkin lymphoma may also provide insight into the pathogenesis of de novo Hodgkin lymphoma.

Composite Lymphoma: Hodgkin Lymphoma and B-Cell Non-Hodgkin Lymphoma

Composite lymphoma may be defined as the simultaneous occurrence of Hodgkin lymphoma and non-Hodgkin lymphoma in the same anatomic site or biopsy specimen.[252,253] Composite Hodgkin lymphoma and non-Hodgkin lymphoma

TABLE 4.7

INTERRELATIONSHIP BETWEEN CLASSICAL HODGKIN LYMPHOMA
AND NON-HODGKIN LYMPHOMAS

	NHL subtypes (%)[a]	Association with EBV
NHL following cHD	Large B-cell (45%)	14% of all B-cell subtypes: (mainly in high-grade subtypes)
	Burkitt/Burkitt-like (45%)	
	Other B-cell (10%)	
Composite cHD/NHL	Follicular (45%)	No
	Large B-cell (45%)	50% (in both HD and NHL)
	Other B-cell (10%)	No
cHD following NHL[b]	CLL	90% in (HD)
	Follicular lymphoma	No
	Large B-cell	No
	Mycosis fungoides	ND
	Other PTL (rare)	Yes

NHL, non-Hodgkin lymphoma; cHD, classical Hodgkin lymphoma; CLL, chronic lymphocytic leukemia;
EBV, Epstein-Barr virus; ND, not determined; PTL, peripheral T-cell lymphomas.
[a]Approximate distribution of associated lymphomas and lymphocytic leukemias based on published data.
[b]Accurate relative incidence figures for cHD following NHL are not available; only most common
associations are shown.

most often represents a B-cell non-Hodgkin lymphoma in association with classical Hodgkin lymphoma. The type of B-cell non-Hodgkin lymphoma involved reflects the incidence of B-cell lymphoma subtypes in the population. Therefore, most composite lymphomas involve follicular lymphomas and diffuse large B-cell lymphomas.[254–257] Uncommonly, other types of B-cell lymphoma may be seen in association with classical Hodgkin lymphoma, including marginal zone B-cell lymphomas and mantle-cell lymphomas.[258] The association of chronic lymphocytic leukemia with Hodgkin lymphoma has some distinctive features and is discussed separately.

Biopsy specimens usually show a segregation of the two histologic patterns within the lymph node. However, in some instances, the Hodgkin lymphoma and non-Hodgkin lymphoma may be more intertwined. For example, in some cases of follicular lymphoma with coexistent Hodgkin lymphoma, the Hodgkin lymphoma may be found in the interfollicular paracortical regions.

Immunohistochemical studies are usually required for the diagnosis of a composite lymphoma. The neoplastic cells of the Hodgkin lymphoma component should retain the classical phenotype of Hodgkin lymphoma.

The status of the Epstein-Barr virus has also been investigated in composite lymphomas. In most cases studied, the expression of Epstein-Barr virus was concordant in both components; that is, the neoplastic cells of both the Hodgkin lymphoma and the non-Hodgkin lymphoma were either both positive or both negative.[259] Approximately 33% of composite lymphomas were positive for Epstein-Barr virus sequences in the neoplastic cells. In all positive cases, the non-Hodgkin lymphoma component was an aggressive B-cell lymphoma, either large B-cell or Burkitt-like. Cases of composite follicular lymphoma and Hodgkin lymphoma were negative for Epstein-Barr virus in both components.

Only very limited molecular studies have been applied to composite lymphomas. In a few cases studied molecularly, the composite Hodgkin lymphoma showed the same translocation as the non-Hodgkin lymphoma—bcl-2/IgH in two cases of follicular lymphoma and CCND1/IgH in one case of

mantle-cell lymphoma.[260] No mutations were found in the FAS, NFKBIA, and ATM tumor-suppressor genes, and one case of Hodgkin lymphoma composite with diffuse large B-cell lymphoma showed mutations in the TP53 gene exclusively in the non-Hodgkin lymphoma component, suggesting a late transforming event.

Clinically, composite lymphoma presents in an older age group. In one series the median age at presentation was 62 years.[254] This clinical presentation is more typical of the underlying non-Hodgkin lymphoma and coincides with the second peak seen in epidemiologic studies of Hodgkin lymphoma, in which a bimodal age distribution is seen. The prognosis for patients with composite Hodgkin lymphoma and non-Hodgkin lymphoma is most dependent on the histologic subtype of the non-Hodgkin lymphoma identified. Patients with diffuse large B-cell lymphoma and Hodgkin lymphoma should be treated for the most "aggressive histology," in this instance the non-Hodgkin lymphoma. The clinical course of patients with composite follicular lymphoma and Hodgkin lymphoma is more indolent. Relapses of non-Hodgkin lymphoma, Hodgkin lymphoma, or composite lymphoma may be seen following therapy.

A situation closely related to composite lymphoma is the simultaneous presentation of Hodgkin lymphoma and non-Hodgkin lymphoma in different anatomic sites.[261] Only a small number of cases have been identified, perhaps because in a patient undergoing diagnostic biopsy, if a biopsy does lead to a definitive diagnosis, a second biopsy of another anatomic site is rarely performed. Although the true frequency of simultaneous Hodgkin lymphoma and non-Hodgkin lymphoma is difficult to assess, it seems to be a rare phenomenon. The distribution of the non-Hodgkin lymphoma subtypes encountered is similar to that of composite lymphoma, with follicular lymphomas and diffuse large B-cell lymphomas being the most frequent.

The coexistence of classical Hodgkin lymphoma with nodular lymphocyte-predominant Hodgkin lymphoma can be considered a type of composite lymphoma. Just as classical Hodgkin lymphoma may occur in the setting of a non-Hodgkin lymphoma of B-cell phenotype, classical Hodgkin lymphoma has also been reported in association with rare cases of nodular lymphocyte-predominant Hodgkin lymphoma.[262–264] This association has been reported as composite lymphoma as well as metachronous events involving biopsy specimens at different points in time.

Non-Hodgkin Lymphomas Following Hodgkin Lymphoma

An increased risk of non-Hodgkin lymphoma in patients successfully treated for Hodgkin lymphoma was first reported by Krikorian and associates.[265] All patients had been treated with both radiation and chemotherapy and had been in complete remission for 4 to 10 years. The actuarial risk of developing non-Hodgkin lymphoma was estimated at 4.4%, and it was postulated that the non-Hodgkin lymphomas represented a complication from a persistent immunologic deficit. It is known that patients with Hodgkin lymphoma have underlying defects in cell-mediated immunity and that these defects persist following therapy.[266,267] The most common subtypes of non-Hodgkin lymphoma have been diffuse large B-cell lymphoma or other high-grade B-cell lymphomas classified as Burkitt-like or small noncleaved, non-Burkitt in the Working Formulation.[268,269] However, rare cases of low-grade non-Hodgkin lymphoma also have been reported.[270]

Subsequent series have confirmed the previous findings. The time to non-Hodgkin lymphoma following a diagnosis of Hodgkin lymphoma has ranged from 1 to 26 years. The risk of secondary non-Hodgkin lymphoma is approximately 5%. The risk of non-Hodgkin lymphoma appears greater in patients showing evidence of underlying immunodeficiency or immune suppression, such as low peripheral blood lymphocyte counts, advanced clinical stage, or systemic symptoms.[269]

The histologic subtype of non-Hodgkin lymphoma does not appear related to the subtype of Hodgkin lymphoma or the treatment received. All of the non-Hodgkin lymphomas have been of B-cell phenotype, and most patients have presented with intra-abdominal disease. The pathologic and clinical features are similar to those of the aggressive B-cell non-Hodgkin lymphomas reported in association with other immunodeficiency states, such as acquired immune deficiency syndrome. Thus, although these findings are of interest, they do not necessarily shed light on the nature of the malignant cell in Hodgkin lymphoma or point to a clonal relationship between the two tumors. One recent study of a single case provided evidence for distinct B-cell clones in the two tumors using a single-cell microdissection assay and PCR amplification.[271] A "small noncleaved" Burkitt-like lymphoma presented as an abdominal mass involving the cecum 41 months after the initial presentation with nodular sclerosis Hodgkin lymphoma. As has been the case in previous reports, the patient was in remission for Hodgkin lymphoma at the time of presentation with the non-Hodgkin lymphoma. Epstein-Barr viral sequences were not studied in this case.

Based on the similarities of these lymphomas to those seen in immunodeficiency states, and the underlying immunologic deficits in patients with Hodgkin lymphoma, one might expect these lymphomas to be positive for Epstein-Barr virus. However, Epstein-Barr virus was identified uncommonly in non-Hodgkin lymphoma associated with Hodgkin lymphoma. Only 2 of 14 (14%) non-Hodgkin lymphomas that followed Hodgkin lymphoma contained Epstein-Barr virus.[259] Additionally, 2 cases of simultaneous Hodgkin lymphoma and large-cell lymphoma of B-cell type were also Epstein-Barr virus-negative.

Although the pathogenesis of most non-Hodgkin lymphomas following Hodgkin lymphoma remains uncertain, it still may be related to the underlying immunodeficiency of Hodgkin lymphoma. Parallels may be drawn with many of the non-Hodgkin lymphomas associated with human immunodeficiency virus infection (HIV). Most such Epstein-Barr virus-negative non-Hodgkin lymphomas are Burkitt lymphomas with rearrangements of the *c-myc* oncogene.[272] A common pathogenesis may be operative in non-Hodgkin lymphoma following Hodgkin lymphoma and HIV-associated non-Hodgkin lymphoma. In support of this possibility, a number of the non-Hodgkin lymphomas following Hodgkin lymphoma have been small noncleaved or Burkitt-like. In addition, patients with Hodgkin lymphoma often exhibit evidence of polyclonal B-cell hyperplasia and plasmacytosis, as is commonly seen in HIV-positive patients, perhaps suggesting that similar immunologic stimuli may be involved in both groups of patients.

Mediastinal Large B-Cell Lymphoma and Nodular Sclerosis Hodgkin Lymphoma

One of the more common occurrences in patients with composite lymphoma, or non-Hodgkin lymphoma following Hodgkin lymphoma, is the association of mediastinal or thymic B-cell lymphoma with nodular sclerosis Hodgkin lymphoma.[254,268,273,273a] Mediastinal large B-cell lymphomas have been reported following treatment for Hodgkin lymphoma, but in contrast to most non-Hodgkin lymphomas, which usually present more than 10 years after primary diagnosis and treatment, the mediastinal lymphomas have presented early in the course of disease, frequently within 1 year of diagnosis. Similarly, Hodgkin lymphoma has been reported following mediastinal large B-cell lymphoma, and composite cases containing distinct components of each lymphoma have also been well described. In addition, a number of cases have been described in which it has been extremely difficult to impossible to distinguish these two entities, raising consideration of a transitional or intermediate entity, tentatively designated mediastinal gray-zone lymphoma.[273a,274–276] These patients present with a large mediastinal mass; unexpectedly, mostly men are affected. About one-half of the cases resemble classical Hodgkin lymphoma, albeit with a large number of mononuclear variants and diminished inflammatory background. Others most closely resemble a large B-cell lymphoma, but have admixed Hodgkin cells. Fibrous bands are either absent or focal. Necrosis, which is usually a prominent feature in histologically aggressive nodular sclerosis Hodgkin lymphoma (grade II), is either absent or focal. However, most of the cases do show some vague nodularity, reminiscent of that seen in nodular sclerosis Hodgkin lymphoma. The immunohistochemical phenotype of these cases is also "transitional." Cases resembling Hodgkin lymphoma often have strong consistent reactivity for CD20, while cases resembling large B-cell lymphoma often have absent or weak CD20 expression, and are often CD15 positive. B-cell transcription factor expression in the gray zone cases more closely resembles large B-cell lymphoma than Hodgkin lymphoma. All cases are negative for Epstein-Barr virus, arguing against a role for Epstein-Barr virus in the process. Clinically, it is recommended that patients with features of both Hodgkin lymphoma and mediastinal B-cell lymphoma should be treated for an aggressive non-Hodgkin lymphoma. The clinical course in these patients is generally aggressive, and many have relapsed following conventional treatment for Hodgkin lymphoma with either radiation or chemotherapy. In addition, relapse often occurs at distant sites, such as kidneys or central nervous system, common sites of spread for mediastinal large B-cell lymphoma.

Nodular sclerosis Hodgkin lymphoma and mediastinal large B-cell lymphoma share a number of common features.

Clinically, they both show a female predominance and present in young adults, with the median age of presentation for thymic B-cell lymphoma being slightly older than that of nodular sclerosis Hodgkin lymphoma.[277–279] Both lymphomas present with an anterior mediastinal mass with involvement of the thymus gland and frequent involvement of supraclavicular lymph nodes. In addition to the clinical similarities, both lymphomas share a similar cell of origin, a B-cell situated between the germinal center and the plasma cell. They also share a number of other biological characteristics, including similar gene expression profiles,[280,281] a lack of immunoglobulin expression, low levels of B-cell receptor-signaling molecules, secretion of the chemokine TARC, and high expression of the IL-13 receptor and downstream effectors of IL-13 signaling.[272] Finally, these two neoplasms have karyotypic abnormalities at common sites, including 2p15, site of the REL oncogene, and 9p24, site of the tyrosine kinase gene JAK2.[272]

Hodgkin Lymphoma Following Non-Hodgkin Lymphoma

Although a risk for non-Hodgkin lymphoma following Hodgkin lymphoma has been known for some time, Hodgkin lymphoma following non-Hodgkin lymphoma has been considered rare. Carrato and colleagues reported five cases occurring 5 to 23 years after a primary diagnosis of non-Hodgkin lymphoma.[282] Travis and colleagues reviewed the experience of the national SEER Cancer Registry.[283] They found that Hodgkin lymphoma was the most common cancer occurring after treatment for non-Hodgkin lymphoma, with an observed-to-expected risk ratio of 4.16:1. Hodgkin lymphoma was more common than acute leukemia, a malignancy often associated with the carcinogenic effects of alkylating agent chemotherapy.

In a study expanding on Hodgkin lymphoma following non-Hodgkin lymphoma, all of the non-Hodgkin lymphomas were of B-cell origin, with a median age at presentation of the non-Hodgkin lymphoma of 54 years.[284] The most common histologic subtypes of the underlying non-Hodgkin lymphoma were follicular lymphoma or diffuse large B-cell lymphoma. The median interval between non-Hodgkin lymphoma and Hodgkin lymphoma was 5 years. The patients had generally received chemotherapy, either alone or in combination with radiation therapy. Lymph nodes represented the site of presentation of Hodgkin lymphoma in all cases. Although it is difficult to draw firm conclusions in a heterogeneously treated patient population, most of the patients did respond to therapy for Hodgkin lymphoma. The most common histologic subtype of Hodgkin lymphoma was nodular sclerosis. Hodgkin lymphoma has also been reported in association with certain T-cell malignancies, most commonly mycosis fungoides as well as B-cell chronic lymphocytic leukemia (see below).

As expected, the immunologic phenotypes of the Hodgkin lymphoma and non-Hodgkin lymphoma were discordant. In one study in which bcl-2 rearrangements were investigated by polymerase chain reaction (PCR) in an unselected series of 32 cases of Hodgkin lymphoma, bcl-2 rearrangements were found in only two cases, both of which arose in the setting of prior follicular lymphoma.[285] In one case, identical chromosomal breakpoints were identified in the Hodgkin lymphoma and the follicular lymphoma. This finding would suggest a clonal relationship between the two tumors. However, given the sensitivity of the PCR technique, it is difficult to rule out the presence of small numbers of follicular lymphoma B-cells in the lymph node involved by Hodgkin lymphoma, even if they were not detected by conventional histologic or immunohistochemical means.

In a separate study in which the role of Epstein-Barr virus was investigated in cases of Hodgkin lymphoma following non-Hodgkin lymphoma, in none of the cases was Epstein-Barr virus positive in the Reed-Sternberg cells.[261] This finding is perhaps unexpected because Epstein-Barr virus has been shown to play a role in the occurrence of Hodgkin lymphoma following chronic lymphocytic leukemia.

Chronic Lymphocytic Leukemia and Classical Hodgkin Lymphoma

The development of classical Hodgkin lymphoma in a patient with chronic lymphocytic leukemia has been recognized for some time and has been considered a form of Richter transformation.[286,287] Early reports had described Reed-Sternberg–like cells in the setting of chronic lymphocytic leukemia or in Richter syndrome.[288] However, it was often assumed that these cases represented pleomorphic non-Hodgkin lymphomas resembling Hodgkin lymphoma rather than true occurrences of Hodgkin lymphoma.[289–291] More recently, several groups have documented both histologically and immunophenotypically the association of Hodgkin lymphoma and chronic lymphocytic leukemia, suggesting that the association is real.[292–297]

Two histologic patterns are observed. In one, the Hodgkin lymphoma is histologically segregated from the chronic lymphocytic leukemia, either involving a different lymph node or anatomic site or within a single lymph node.[293,298] In these cases, Reed-Sternberg cells and variants are found in the usual cellular milieu of Hodgkin lymphoma, with numerous T-lymphocytes, plasma cells, eosinophils, and other inflammatory cells. The Reed-Sternberg cells display the usual phenotype of classical Hodgkin lymphoma and are typically positive for Epstein-Barr virus sequences by in situ hybridization. Expression of CD20 by at least some of the Reed-Sternberg cells is commonly observed.

A second pattern is more frequently encountered. In this instance, Reed-Sternberg cells and variants are seen in a background of otherwise typical chronic lymphocytic leukemia, without the apparent cellular background of Hodgkin lymphoma.[255,292,299] However, on closer inspection, although the Reed-Sternberg cells are surrounded by small lymphocytes, with immunohistochemical studies they are found to be rosetted by T-cells, as is typical of Hodgkin lymphoma.[292] The surrounding B-cells have the usual phenotype of chronic lymphocytic leukemia and are monoclonal with coexpression of CD5. This process can be considered a form of composite lymphoma because both diseases are present in the same anatomic site.

By immunohistochemical studies, the Reed-Sternberg cells display the usual phenotype of Hodgkin lymphoma: CD30 positive and CD15 positive. Expression of some B-cell–associated antigens is variable. Epstein-Barr virus appears to play a major role in the development of Hodgkin lymphoma in this setting.[300] The Reed-Sternberg cells have been positive for Epstein-Barr virus by in situ hybridization or staining for latent membrane protein (LMP-1) in more than 80% of the cases studied. Although most of the background chronic lymphocytic leukemia cells are negative for Epstein-Barr virus, a small number of Epstein-Barr virus–positive cells are often found. In one study, Epstein-Barr virus positivity was identified in a small population of the lymphocytes in the underlying chronic lymphocytic leukemia several years before the development of Hodgkin lymphoma. This observation suggests that a first step in this transformation may be Epstein-Barr virus infection of chronic lymphocytic leukemia B-lymphocytes.[295] Rare cases in which the Reed-Sternberg cells are negative for Epstein-Barr virus have been described, indicating that there may be other mechanisms involved in this transformation.[301]

Recent studies have attempted to examine the clonal relationship between chronic lymphocytic leukemia and Hodgkin lymphoma using microdissection techniques and PCR amplification of immunoglobulin heavy-chain genes (IgH).[296,297,302] In cases associated with EBV, separate clones have been identified in the two neoplasms. However, in cases in which the Hodgkin cells are EBV negative, the same B-cell clone has been identified in both the Hodgkin cells and the chronic lymphocytic leukemia cells, suggesting a different pathogenesis in the EBV-positive and EBV-negative cases.

Clinically, the development of Hodgkin lymphoma in a patient with chronic lymphocytic leukemia usually portends an aggressive clinical course.[294,300] Most of the patients have developed progressive dissemination of Hodgkin lymphoma, usually with a poor response to therapy. The median survival is under 2 years following the diagnosis of Hodgkin lymphoma. It is interesting to speculate on the role of immune deficiency in the development of Hodgkin lymphoma following chronic lymphocytic leukemia. Patients with chronic lymphocytic leukemia typically display defects in both cellular and humoral immunity, with an increased risk of viral infections. Perhaps an increased viral load of Epstein-Barr virus is associated with the secondary development of Hodgkin lymphoma. In this regard, it has been suggested that treatment with fludarabine, which leads to profound lymphocytopenia, may increase the risk of secondary Hodgkin lymphoma.[303]

Hodgkin Lymphoma and T-Cell Lymphoma

In general, T-cell lymphomas are less often reported in association with Hodgkin lymphoma than B-cell lymphomas.[261] This observation may reflect the lower frequency of T-cell malignancies, with the risk of coincidence with Hodgkin lymphoma being equal to that for B-cell disease. Alternatively, it might indicate that patients with T-cell lymphomas are not at risk to develop Hodgkin lymphoma. Finally, the coincidence may be underreported because of the difficulty in distinguishing Hodgkin lymphoma from peripheral T-cell lymphoma. However, if the association of Hodgkin lymphoma with non-Hodgkin lymphoma is an indication of the clonal relationship of the two disorders, as a B-cell origin is likely for most cases of Hodgkin lymphoma, it is not surprising that Hodgkin lymphoma is rarely found with T-cell lymphomas. In one well-documented case, cytogenetic studies were performed on both the Hodgkin lymphoma and the associated peripheral T-cell lymphoma.[304] Evidence of two distinct clones was obtained.

Cells resembling Reed-Sternberg cells both morphologically and immunophenotypically have been reported in a number of T-cell malignancies including mycosis fungoides, adult T-cell leukemia/lymphoma, and peripheral T-cell lymphomas, unspecified.[305–307] The most common association is that of Hodgkin lymphoma and mycosis fungoides. Since 1979, more than 20 well-documented reports of Hodgkin lymphoma in association with mycosis fungoides have appeared in the literature.[308–312] In one case studied with molecular techniques, a common clonal T-cell gene rearrangement was found in tissues involved by lymphomatoid papulosis, mycosis fungoides, and Hodgkin lymphoma.[313] However, a second report provided evidence for distinct clonal origins of mycosis fungoides and Hodgkin lymphoma in two patients studied with molecular techniques.[312] The confirmation of an association between mycosis fungoides, lymphomatoid papulosis, and Hodgkin lymphoma is complicated by the existence of common morphological and even phenotypical characteristics of the neoplastic cells.[305] Expression of both CD15 and

CD30 has been reported in the pleomorphic tumor cells of both mycosis fungoides and lymphomatoid papulosis.[314,315] Therefore, do cases of Hodgkin lymphoma in the setting of mycosis fungoides and lymphomatoid papulosis represent instances of true Hodgkin lymphoma, or are these pleomorphic T-cell malignancies simulating Hodgkin lymphoma?[316]

In instances of mycosis fungoides and Hodgkin lymphoma occurring in the same patient, the diagnosis of mycosis fungoides usually precedes that of Hodgkin lymphoma by months to years. This observation would further support the view that some of these cases might represent pleomorphic T-cell lymphomas simulating Hodgkin lymphoma. However, in some cases the diagnosis of Hodgkin lymphoma may precede the appearance of mycosis fungoides, or the two disorders may present simultaneously.[308,317–319] An association of mycosis fungoides and Hodgkin lymphoma is further supported by the diagnosis of Hodgkin lymphoma in the relatives of patients with mycosis fungoides.[320] In a large epidemiologic study, Hodgkin lymphoma was the most common lymphoproliferative or hematopoietic malignancy occurring in family members. Of 526 consecutive patients with mycosis fungoides or Sézary syndrome, 21 had first-degree relatives with some form of lymphoma or leukemia. Hodgkin lymphoma accounted for one-third of the total cases reported. These observations further support an association between mycosis fungoides and Hodgkin lymphoma and suggest that genetically determined immunoregulatory pathways may represent shared pathways of oncogenesis in these disorders.

A relationship between Hodgkin lymphoma and mycosis fungoides is further complicated by controversy as to whether a T-cell form of Hodgkin lymphoma exists (see Chapter 5). It is generally agreed that the vast majority of cases of Hodgkin lymphoma are of B-cell origin. However, cases of Hodgkin lymphoma expressing T-cell–associated antigens, including the relatively specific marker CD3, have been described,[320] and rare cases have been reported to have clonal T-cell receptor rearrangements.[320a–320c] Whether such cases represent true T-cell forms of Hodgkin lymphoma is not yet resolved.

The existence of a T-cell form of Hodgkin lymphoma is complicated by cases of anaplastic large-cell lymphoma, which may contain Reed-Sternberg–like cells and may closely simulate nodular sclerosing Hodgkin lymphoma histologically. Both anaplastic large-cell lymphoma and Hodgkin lymphoma are CD30 positive. However, studies for the expression of cytotoxic-associated molecules have confirmed the distinction of anaplastic large-cell lymphoma from Hodgkin lymphoma. Although most cases of anaplastic large-cell lymphoma express cytotoxic molecules such as TIA-1, granzyme B, and perforin, the neoplastic cells of Hodgkin lymphoma are negative for these antigens in most cases.[322,323] In addition, many cases of anaplastic large-cell lymphoma are also positive for ALK-1, which detects the anaplastic large-cell lymphoma kinase.[324–326] Furthermore, cases of Hodgkin lymphoma usually express the B-cell transcription factor PAX-5, a marker that is negative in anaplastic large-cell lymphoma.[327]

Reed-Sternberg–like cells have been observed in a number of other peripheral T-cell lymphomas, including angioimmunoblastic T-cell lymphoma. A Hodgkin-like morphology has also been reported in adult T-cell leukemia/lymphoma.[306,307] This histologic pattern appears to precede the development of acute adult T-cell leukemia/lymphoma in the few published cases. One report suggested that the Reed-Sternberg–like cells were Epstein-Barr virus-positive transformed B-cells and not part of the neoplastic T-cell process.[328] In contrast to the neoplastic T-cells, the Reed-Sternberg–like cells lacked HTLV-I–associated sequences. We too have observed such Reed-Sternberg–like cells in peripheral T-cell lymphomas (unpublished observations). The Reed-Sternberg–like cells contained Epstein-Barr virus sequences and expressed the CD20 antigen, as distinct from the expression of T-cell antigens on the neoplastic T-cells. Notably, both adult T-cell leukemia/lymphoma and angioimmunoblastic T-cell lymphoma are malignancies associated with immune suppression and an increased risk of opportunistic infections. The presence of Epstein-Barr virus-transformed B-cell blasts may represent a manifestation of the underlying immunodeficiency in these conditions.

Hodgkin Lymphoma and Epstein-Barr Virus–Positive Lymphoproliferative Disorders

It has been shown that patients with rheumatologic disorders receiving long-term immunosuppressive therapy with methotrexate are at increased risk to develop Epstein-Barr virus–positive lymphoproliferative disorders, which may either resemble Hodgkin lymphoma or represent true cases of Hodgkin lymphoma.[329–331] In most cases the patients have been receiving immunosuppressive therapy for at least 1 year. Cases of lymphoproliferative disorder resembling Hodgkin lymphoma often occur in soft tissue or other non-nodal sites, whereas cases with features of more typical Hodgkin lymphoma tend to present in lymph nodes.

Immunohistochemical studies may be of value in distinguishing typical Hodgkin lymphoma from other lymphoproliferative disorders because the lymphoproliferative disorders are usually negative for CD15 in the atypical cells. The clinical management of these cases is complex. Often, the immunosuppression is withdrawn, and the patient observed for spontaneous regression. The same approach may be followed even in lymph nodes resembling more typical Hodgkin lymphoma, because some cases will spontaneously regress. However, if the lesions persist, conventional therapy for Hodgkin lymphoma is recommended.

It is of interest that classical Hodgkin lymphoma is relatively uncommon following solid organ transplantation. However, an increased risk of Hodgkin lymphoma following allogeneic bone marrow transplantation has been observed[332]. Such cases are virtually always positive for Epstein-Barr virus. In addition, Hodgkin lymphoma-like post-transplant lymphoproliferative disorders may occur.[333] Despite their histologic appearance resembling Hodgkin lymphoma, these cases usually have clinical, immunophenotypic, and molecular genetic differences from Hodgkin lymphoma and are more similar to monomorphic B-cell post-transplant lymphoproliferative disorders.

Hodgkin Lymphoma and T-Cell–Rich B-Cell Lymphoma

In recent years several groups have reported the existence of cases histologically resembling Hodgkin lymphoma but having the immunophenotype of T-cell–rich B-cell lymphoma.[334–336] The cases may resemble either classical Hodgkin lymphoma or, more often, lymphocyte- predominant Hodgkin lymphoma. The differential diagnosis of such cases is discussed in detail above. We comment only briefly on the biological significance of T-cell–rich B-cell lymphomas resembling classical Hodgkin lymphoma.

Modern studies of the biology of Hodgkin lymphoma have suggested that classical Hodgkin lymphoma may in fact be a T-cell–rich B-cell lymphoma.[247] A B-cell origin for the malignant cells of Hodgkin lymphoma is apparent in nearly all cases. Reed-Sternberg cells elaborate numerous cytokines, which lead to the prominent inflammatory background that is an essential component of the histologic diagnosis.[337] T-cells comprise the majority of the non-neoplastic lymphocytes in most cases of classical Hodgkin lymphoma.

The events that lead to the development of a Reed-Sternberg cell are as yet unknown. However, it is likely that this process involves multiple steps. Moreover, cases of Hodgkin lymphoma show significant variation from case to case in the expression of B-cell–associated antigens.[338,339] By definition, if all of the neoplastic cells are CD20 positive, the diagnosis of T-cell–rich B-cell lymphoma over Hodgkin lymphoma is favored. However, cases of T-cell–rich B-cell lymphoma resembling classical Hodgkin lymphoma may be related to Hodgkin lymphoma. Interestingly, T-cell–rich B-cell lymphoma has a more aggressive course than Hodgkin lymphoma, with these patients frequently failing to respond to conventional therapy for Hodgkin lymphoma.[334–336] Moreover, the expression of B-cell antigens by a high proportion of the malignant cells (>20%) was shown to be an adverse prognostic factor in a large series from the German Hodgkin Study Group.[340]

References

1. Pitts WC, Weiss LM. The role of fine needle aspiration biopsy in diagnosis and management of hematopoietic neoplasms. In: Knowles DM, ed. *Neoplastic hematopathology*. Baltimore: Williams & Wilkins, 1992:385.
2. Das DK, Gupta SK, Datta BM, et al. Fine needle aspiration cytodiagnosis of Hodgkin's disease and its subtypes. I. Scope and limitations. *Acta Cytol* 1989;34:329.
3. Friedman M, Kim U, Shimaoka K, et al. Appraisal of aspiration cytology in management of Hodgkin's disease. *Cancer* 1980;45:1653–1663.
4. Variakojis D, Strum SB, Rappaport H. The foamy macrophages in Hodgkin's disease. *Arch Pathol* 1972;93:453.
5. Mohrmann RL, Nathwani BN, Brynes RK, et al. Hodgkin's disease occurring in monocytoid B-cell clusters. *Am J Clin Pathol* 1991;95:802.
6. Plank L, Hansmann ML, Fisher R. Monocytoid B-cells occurring in Hodgkin's disease. *Virchows Arch* 1994;424:321.
7. Khalidi HS, Singleton TP, Weiss SW. Inflammatory malignant fibrous histiocytoma: distinction from Hodgkin's disease and non-Hodgkin's lymphoma by a panel of leukocyte markers. *Mod Pathol* 1997;10:438.
8. Suster S. Transformation of Hodgkin's disease into malignant fibrous histiocytoma. *Cancer* 1986;57:264.
9. Burns BF, Colby TV, Dorfman RF. Langerhans' cell granulomatosis (histiocytosis X) associated with malignant lymphomas. *Am J Surg Pathol* 1983;7:529.
10. Lukes RJ. Criteria for involvement of lymph node, bone marrow, spleen, and liver in Hodgkin's disease. *Cancer Res* 1971;31:1755.
11. Ashton-Key M, Thorpe PA, Allen JP, et al. Follicular Hodgkin's disease. *Am J Surg Pathol* 1995;19:1294.
12. Colby TV, Hoppe RT, Warnke RA. Hodgkin's disease: a clinicopathologic study of 659 cases. *Cancer* 1981;49:1848.
13. Mann RB, Jaffe ES, Berard CW. Malignant lymphomas—a conceptual understanding of morphologic diversity. A review. *Am J Pathol* 1979;94:105.
14. Bennett MH, MacLennan KA, Easterling MJ, et al. The prognostic significance of cellular subtypes in nodular sclerosing Hodgkin's disease: an analysis of 271 non-laparotomised cases (BNLI report no. 22). *Clin Radiol* 1983;34:497.
15. MacLennan KA, Bennett MH, Vaughan HB, et al. Diagnosis and grading of nodular sclerosing Hodgkin's disease: a study of 2190 patients. *Int Rev Exp Pathol* 1992;33:27.
16. MacLennan KA, Bennett MH, Tu A, et al. Relationship of histopathologic features to survival and relapse in nodular sclerosing Hodgkin's disease: a study of 1,659 patients. *Cancer* 1989;64:1686.
17. Haybittle JL, Hayhoe FGJ, Easterling MJ, et al. Review of British National Lymphoma Investigation studies of Hodgkin's disease and development of prognostic index. *Lancet* 1985;1:967.
18. Ferry JA, Linggood RM, Convery KM, et al. Hodgkin's disease, nodular sclerosis type: implications of histologic subclassification. *Cancer* 1993;71:457.
19. Wijlhuizen TJ, Vrints LW, Jairam R, et al. Grades of nodular sclerosis (NSI–NSII) in Hodgkin's disease: are they of independent prognostic value? *Cancer* 1989;63:1150.
20. Masih AS, Weisenburger DD, Vose JM, et al. Histologic grade does not predict prognosis in optimally treated, advanced-stage nodular sclerosing Hodgkin's disease. *Cancer* 1992;69:228.
21. Hess JL, Bodis S, Pinkus G, et al. Histopathologic grading of nodular sclerosis Hodgkin's disease. Lack of prognostic significance in 254 surgically staged patients. *Cancer* 1994;74:708.

22. Correa P, O'Conor GT. Epidemiologic patterns of Hodgkin's disease. *Int J Cancer* 1971;8:192.
23. Ashton-Key M, Thorpe PA, Allen JP, et al. Follicular Hodgkin's disease. *Am J Surg Pathol* 1995;19:1294.
24. Strickler JG, Michie SA, Warnke RA, et al. The "syncytial variant" of nodular sclerosing Hodgkin's disease. *Am J Surg Pathol* 1986;10:470.
25. Doggett RS, Colby TV, Dorfman RF. Interfollicular Hodgkin's disease. *Am J Med* 1983;78:22.
26. Rappaport H, Berard CW, Butler JJ, et al. Report of the committee on histopathological criteria contributing to staging of Hodgkin's disease. *Cancer Res* 1971;31:1864.
27. O'Carroll DI, McKenna RW, Brunning RD. Bone marrow manifestations of Hodgkin's disease. *Cancer* 1976;38:1717.
28. Bartl R, Frisch B, Burkhardt R, et al. Assessment of bone marrow histology in Hodgkin's disease: correlation with clinical factors. *Br J Haematol* 1982;51:345.
29. Te Velde J, Den Ottolander GJ, Spaander PJ, et al. The bone marrow in Hodgkin's disease: the non-involved marrow. *Histopathology* 1978;2:31.
30. Dorfman RF, Colby TV. The pathologist's role in management of patients with Hodgkin's disease. *Cancer Treat Rep* 1982;66:675.
31. Dich NH, Goodman ZD, Klein MA. Hepatic involvement in Hodgkin's disease: clues to histologic diagnosis. *Cancer* 1989;64:2121.
32. Bagley CM Jr, Roth JA, Thomas LB, et al. Liver biopsy in Hodgkin's disease: clinicopathologic correlations in 127 patients. *Ann Intern Med* 1972;76:219.
33. Katz A, Lattes R. Granulomatous thymoma or Hodgkin's disease of the thymus? A clinical and histological study and a re-evaluation. *Cancer* 1969;23:1.
34. Kern WH, Crepeau A, Jones JC. Primary Hodgkin's disease of the lung: report of four cases and review of the literature. *Cancer* 1961;14:1151.
35. Söderström K-O, Joensuu H. Primary Hodgkin's disease of the stomach. *Am J Clin Pathol* 1988;89:806.
36. Todd GB, Michaels L. Hodgkin's disease involving Waldeyer's lymphoid ring. *Cancer* 1974;34:1769.
37. Devaney K, Jaffe ES. The surgical pathology of gastrointestinal Hodgkin's disease. *Am J Clin Pathol* 1991;95:794.
38. Quinones-Avila MP, Gonzalez-Longoria AA, Admirand JH, et al. Hodgkin lymphoma involving Waldeyer ring: a clinicopathologic study of 22 cases. *Am J Clin Pathol* 2005;123:651.
39. Kaudewitz P, Stein H, Dallenbach F. Primary and secondary Ki-1+ (CD30+) anaplastic large cell lymphomas. *Am J Pathol* 1989;135:359.
40. Sioutos N, Kerl H, Murphy SB, et al. Primary cutaneous Hodgkin's disease. Unique clinical, morphologic, and immunophenotypic findings. *Am J Dermatopathol* 1994;16:2.
41. Smith JLJ, Butler JJ. Skin involvement in Hodgkin's disease. *Cancer* 1980;45:345.
42. Ashby MA, Barber PC, Holmes AE, et al. Primary intracranial Hodgkin's disease: a case report and discussion. *Am J Surg Pathol* 1988;12:294.
43. Meis JM, Butler JJ, Osborne BM. Hodgkin's disease involving the breast and chest wall. *Cancer* 1986;57:1859.
44. Saponzink MD, Kaplan HS. Intracranial Hodgkin's disease: a report of 12 cases and review of the literature. *Cancer* 1983;14:1151.
45. Kadin ME, Donaldson S, Dorfman RF. Isolated granulomas in Hodgkin's disease. *N Engl J Med* 1970;283:859.
46. O'Connell MJ, Schimpff SC, Kirschner RH, et al. Epithelioid granulomas in Hodgkin's disease. A favorable prognostic sign? *JAMA* 1975;233:886.
47. Sacks EL, Donaldson SS, Gordon J, et al. Epithelioid granulomas associated with Hodgkin's disease: clinical correlations in 55 previously untreated patients. *Cancer* 1978;41:562.
48. Abrams J, Pearl P, Moody M, et al. Epithelioid grnaulomas revisited: long-term follow-up in Hodgkin's disease. *Am J Clin Oncol* 1988;11:456.
49. Chen JL, Osborne BM, Butler JJ. Residual fibrous masses in treated Hodgkin's disease. *Cancer* 1982;60:407.
50. Colby TV, Warnke RA. The histology of the initial relapse of Hodgkin's disease. *Cancer* 1980;45:289.
51. Strum SB, Rappaport H. Consistency of histologic subtypes in Hodgkin's disease in simultaneous and sequential biopsy specimens. *Natl Cancer Inst Monogr* 1973;36:253.
52. Dolginow D, Colby TV. Recurrent Hodgkin's disease in treated sites. *Cancer* 1981;48:1124.
53. Colby TV, Hoppe RT, Warnke RA. Hodgkin's disease at autopsy: 1972–1977. *Cancer* 1981;47:1852.
54. Grogan TM, Berard CW, Steinhorn SC, et al. Changing patterns of Hodgkin's disease at autopsy: a 25-year experience at the National Cancer Institute, 1953–1978. *Cancer Treat Rep* 1982;66:653.
55. Krikorian JG, Burke JS, Rosenberg SA, et al. Occurrence of non-Hodgkin's lymphoma after therapy for Hodgkin's disease. *N Engl J Med* 1979;300:452.
56. Bookman MA, Longo DL. Concomitant illness in patients treated for Hodgkin's disease. *Cancer Treat Rev* 1986;13:77.
57. Glick AD, Leech JH, Flexner JM, et al. Ultrastructural study of Reed-Sternberg cells. Comparison with transformed lymphocytes and histiocytes. *Am J Pathol* 1976;85:195.
58. Giffler RF, Gillespie JJ, Ayala AG, et al. Lymphoepithelioma in cervical lymph nodes of children and young adults. *Am J Surg Pathol* 1977;1:293.
59. Angel C, Warford A, Campbell A, et al. The immunohistology of Hodgkin's disease—Reed-Sternberg cells and their variants. *J Pathol* 1987;153:21.
60. Agnarsson BA, Kadin ME. The immunophenotype of Reed-Sternberg cells. A study of 50 cases of Hodgkin's disease using fixed frozen tissues. *Cancer* 1989;63:2083.
61. Casey TT, Olson SJ, Cousar JB, et al. Immunophenotypes of Reed-Sternberg cells: a study of 19 cases of Hodgkin's disease in plastic-embedded sections. *Blood* 1989;74:2624.
62. Chittal SM, Caveriviere P, Schwarting R, et al. Monoclonal antibodies in the diagnosis of Hodgkin's disease: the search for a rational panel. *Am J Surg Pathol* 1988;12:9.
63. Chu W-S, Abbondanzo SL, Frizzera G. Inconsistency of the immunophenotype of Reed-Sternberg cells in simultaneous and consecutive specimens from the same patients. A paraffin section evaluation in 56 patients. *Am J Pathol* 1992;141:11.
64. Strauchen JA, Dimitriu-Bona A. Immunopathology of Hodgkin's disease. Characterization of Reed-Sternberg cells with monoclonal antibodies. *Am J Pathol* 1989;123:293.
65. Vasef MA, Alsabeh R, Medeiros LJ, et al. Immunophenotype of Reed-Sternberg and Hodgkin's cells in sequential biopsy specimens of Hodgkin's disease. A HIER-based study. *Am J Clin Pathol* 1997;108:54.
66. Hall PA, D'Ardenne AJ, Stansfeld AG. Paraffin section immunohistochemistry. II. Hodgkin's disease and large cell anaplastic (Ki1) lymphoma. *Histopathology* 1988;13:161.
67. Arber DA, Weiss LM. CD15: a review. *Appl Immunohistochem* 1993;1:17.
68. Chang K-L, Chen Y-Y, Shibata D, et al. In situ hybridization methodology for the detection of EBV EBER-1 RNA in paraffin-embedded tissues, as applied to normal and neoplastic tissues. *Diagn Mol Pathol* 1992;1:246.
69. Chang KL, Arber DA, Weiss LM. CD20: a review. *Appl Immunohistochem* 1996;4:1.
70. Weiss LM, Arber DA, Chang KL. CD45: a review. *Appl Immunohistochem* 1993;1:166.
71. Pinkus GS, Said JW. Hodgkin's disease, lymphocyte predominance type, nodular—a distinct entity? Unique staining profile of L&H variants of Reed-Sternberg cells defined by monoclonal antibodies to leukocyte common antigen, granulocyte specific antigen, and B-cell specific antigen. *Am J Pathol* 1985;116:1.
72. Warnke RA, Gatter KC, Falini B, et al. Diagnosis of human lymphoma with monoclonal antileukocyte antibodies. *N Engl J Med* 1983;309:1275.
73. Dorfman RF, Gatter KC, Pulford KAF, et al. An evaluation of the utility of anti-granulocyte and anti-leukocyte monoclonal antibodies in the diagnosis of Hodgkin's disease. *Am J Pathol* 1986;123:508.
74. Medeiros LJ, Weiss LM, Warnke RA, et al. Utility of combining antigranulocyte with antileukocyte antibodies in differentiating Hodgkin's disease from non-Hodgkin's lymphoma. *Cancer* 1988;62:2475.
75. Strickler J, Weiss L, Copenhaver C, et al. Monoclonal antibodes reactive in routinely processed tissue sections of malignant lymphoma, with emphasis on T-cell lymphomas. *Hum Pathol* 1987;18:808.
76. Wieczorek R, Burke JS, Knowles DM. Leu-M1 antigen expression in T-cell neoplasia. *Am J Pathol* 1985;121:374.
77. Chang KL, Arber DA, Weiss LM. CD30: a review. *Appl Immunohistochem* 1993;1:244.
78. Miettinen M. Immunohistochemical study on formaldehyde-fixed, paraffin-embedded Hodgkin's and non-Hodgkin's lymphomas. *Arch Pathol Lab Med* 1992;116:1197.
79. De Mascarel I, Trojani M, Eghbali H, et al. Prognostic value of phenotyping by Ber-H2, Leu-M1, EMA in Hodgkin's disease. *Arch Pathol Lab Med* 1990;114:953.
80. Ree HJ, Neiman RS, Martin AW, et al. Paraffin section markers for Reed-Sternberg cells. A comparative study of peanut agglutinin, Leu-M1, LN-2, and Ber H2. *Cancer* 1989;63:2030.
81. Schwarting R, Gerdes J, Durkop H, et al. BER-H2: a new anti-Ki-1 (CD30) monoclonal antibody directed at a formol-resistant epitope. *Blood* 1989;74:1678.
82. Stein H, Mason DY, Gerdes J, et al. The expression of the Hodgkin's disease associated antigen Ki-1 in reactive and neoplastic lymphoid tissue: evidence that Reed-Sternberg cells and histiocytic malignancies are derived from activated lymphoid cells. *Blood* 1985;66:848.
83. von Wasielewski R, Mengel M, Fischer R, et al. Classical Hodgkin's disease: clinical impact of the immunophenotype. *Am J Pathol* 1997;151:1123.
84. Pallesen G, Hamilton DS. Ki-1 (CD30) antigen is regularly expressed by tumor cells of embryonal carcinoma. *Am J Pathol* 1988;133:446.
85. Stein H, Hansmann ML, Lennert K, et al. Reed-Sternberg and Hodgkin cells in lymphocyte-predominant Hodgkin's disease of nodular subtype contain J chain. *Am J Clin Pathol* 1986;86:292.
86. Pinkus GS, Said JW. Hodgkin's disease, lymphocyte predominance type, nodular—further evidence for a B cell derivation: L&H variants of Reed-Sternberg cells express L26, a pan B cell marker. *Am J Pathol* 1988;133:211.
87. Frierson HF, Innes DJ. Sensitivity of anti-Leu-M1 as a marker in Hodgkin's disease. *Arch Pathol Lab Med* 1985;109:1024.
88. Hsu SM, Jaffe ES. Leu-M1 and peanut agglutinin stain the neoplastic cells of Hodgkin's disease. *Am J Clin Pathol* 1984;82:29.
89. Fellbaum C, Hansmann ML, Parwaresch MR, et al. Monoclonal antibodies Ki-B3 and Leu M1 discriminate giant cells of infectious mononucleosis and of Hodgkin's disease. *Hum Pathol* 1988;19:1168.
90. Hyder DM, Schnitzer B. Utility of Leu M1 monoclonal antibody in the differential diagnosis of Hodgkin's disease. *Arch Pathol Lab Med* 1986;110:416.

91. Hall PA, D'Ardenne AJ. Value of CD15 immunostaining in diagnosing Hodgkin's disease: a review of published literature. *J Clin Pathol* 1987;40:1298.

92. Sheibani K, Battifora H, Burke JS, et al. Leu-M1 antigen in human neoplasms: an immunohistologic study of 400 cases. *Am J Surg Pathol* 1986;10:227.

93. Zukerberg L, Collins A, Ferry J, et al. Coexpression of CD15 and CD20 by Reed-Sternberg cells in Hodgkin's disease. *Am J Pathol* 1991;139:475.

94. Enblad G, Sundstrom C, Glimerius B. Immunohistochemical characteristics of Hodgkin and Reed-Sternberg cells in relation to age and clinical outcome. *Histopathology* 1993;22:535.

95. Bai MC, Jiwa NM, Horstman A, et al. Decreased expression of cellular markers in Epstein-Barr virus-positive Hodgkin's disease. *J Pathol* 1994;174:49.

96. Hummel M, Ziemann K, Lammert H, et al. Hodgkin's disease with monoclonal and polyclonal populations of Reed-Sternberg cells. *N Engl J Med* 1995;333:901.

97. Küppers R, Rajewsky K, Zhao M, et al. Hodgkin disease: Hodgkin and Reed-Sternberg cells picked from histological sections show clonal immunoglobulin gene rearrangements and appear to be derived from B cells at various stages of development. *Proc Natl Acad Sci USA* 1994;91:10962.

98. Ruprai AK, Pringle JH, Angel CA, et al. Localization of immunoglobulin light chain mRNA expression in Hodgkin's disease by in situ hybridization. *J Pathol* 1991;164:37.

99. Kadin ME, Stites DP, Levy R, et al. Exogenous immunoglobulin and the macrophage origin of Reed-Sternberg cells in Hodgkin's disease. *N Engl J Med* 1978;299:1208.

100. Korkolopoulou P, Cordell J, Jones M, et al. The expression of the B-cell marker mb-1 (CD79a) in Hodgkin's disease. *Histopathology* 1994;24:511.

101. Jundt F, Kley K, Anagnostopoulos I, et al. Loss of PU .1 expression is associated with defective immunoglobulin transcription in Hodgkin and Reed-Sternberg cells of classical Hodgkin disease. *Blood* 2002;99:3060.

102. Stein H, Marafioti T, Foss HD, et al. Down-regulation of BOB.1/OBF.1 and Oct2 in classical Hodgkin disease but not in lymphocyte predominant Hodgkin disease correlates with immunoglobulin transcription. *Blood* 2001:97;496.

103. Marafioti T, Pozzobon M, Hansmann ML, et al. Expression of intracellular signaling molecules in classical and lymphocyte predominance Hodgkin disease. *Blood* 2004:103;188.

104. Arber DA, Weiss LM. CD43: a review. *Appl Immunohistochem* 1993;1:88.

105. Kadin M, Muramoto L, Said J. Expression of T cell antigens on Reed-Sternberg cells in a subset of patients with nodular sclerosis and mixed cellularity Hodgkin's disease. *Am J Pathol* 1988;130:345.

106. Falini B, Stein H, Pileri S, et al. Expression of T-cell antigens on Hodgkin's and Sternberg-Reed cells of Hodgkin's disease. A combined immunocytochemical and immunohistological study using monoclonal antibodies. *Histopathology* 1987;12:129.

107. Falini B, Stein H, Pileri S, et al. Expression of lymphoid-associated antigens on Hodgkin's and Reed-Sternberg cells of Hodgkin's disease. An immunocytochemical study on lymph node cytospins using monoclonal antibodies. *Histopathology* 1987;11:1229.

108. Dallenbach FE, Stein H. Expression of T-cell-receptor beta chain in Reed-Sternberg cells. *Lancet* 1989;2:828.

109. Chang KL, Albujar PF, Chen Y-Y, et al. High prevalence of Epstein-Barr virus in the Reed-Sternberg cells of Hodgkin's disease occurring in Peru. *Blood* 1993;81:496.

110. Pallesen G, Hamilton-Dutoit SJ, Rowe M, et al. Expression of Epstein-Barr virus latent gene products in tumour cells of Hodgkin's disease. *Lancet* 1991;337:320.

111. Herbst H, Dallenbach F, Hummel M, et al. Epstein-Barr virus latent membrane protein expression in Hodgkin and Reed-Sternberg cells. *Proc Natl Acad Sci U S A* 1991;88:4766.

112. O'Grady JT, Stewart S, Lowrey J, et al. CD40 expression in Hodgkin's disease. *Am J Pathol* 1994;144:21.

113. Mosialos G, Yamashiro S, Baughman RW, et al. Epstein-Barr virus infection induces expression in B lymphocytes of a novel gene encoding an evolutionarily conserved 55-kilodalton actin-bundling protein. *J Virol* 1994;68:7320.

114. Pinkus GS, Pinkus JL, Langhoff E, et al. Fascin, a sensitive new marker for Reed-Sternberg cells of Hodgkin's disease. Evidence for a dendritic or B cell derivation? *Am J Pathol* 1997;150:543.

115. Chang KL, Curtis CM, Momose H, et al. Sensitivity and specificity of Bauhinia purpurea as a paraffin section marker for the Reed-Sternberg cells of Hodgkin's disease. *Appl Immunohistochem* 1993;1:208.

116. Delsol G, Meggetto F, Brousset P, et al. Relation of follicular dendritic reticulum cells to Reed-Sternberg cells of Hodgkin's disease with emphasis on the expression of CD21 antigen. *Am J Pathol* 1993;142:1729.

117. Sorg UR, Morse TM, Patton WN, et al. Hodgkin's cells express CD83, a dendritic cell lineage associated antigen. *Pathology* 1997;29:294.

118. Sherrod AE, Felder B, Levy JN, et al. Immunohistologic identification of phenotypic antigens associated with Hodgkin and Reed-Sternberg cells. A paraffin section study. *Cancer* 1986;57:2135.

119. Poppema S, Visser L. Absence of HLC class I expression by Reed-Sternberg cells. *Am J Pathol* 1994;145:37.

120. Delabie J, Shipman R, Bruggen J, et al. Expression of the novel intermediate filament-associated protein restin in Hodgkin's disease and anaplastic large-cell lymphoma. *Blood* 1992;80:2891.

121. Hsu S, Yang K, Jaffe E. Phenotypic expression of Hodgkin's and Reed-Sternberg cells in Hodgkin's disease. *Am J Pathol* 1985;118:209.

122. Gerdes J, van Baarlen J, Pileri S, et al. Tumor cell growth fraction in Hodgkin's disease. *Am J Pathol* 1987;128:390.

123. Sabattini E, Gerdes J, Gherlinzoni F, et al. Comparison between the monoclonal antibodies Ki-67 and PC10 in 125 malignant lymphomas. *J Pathol* 1993;169:397.

124. LeBrun DP, Ngan BY, Weiss LM, et al. Involvement of the bcl-2 oncogene in the origin of Hodgkin's disease from follicular non-Hodgkin's lymphoma. *Blood* 1994;83:223.

125. Freeman J, Kellock DB, Yu CCW, et al. Proliferating cell nuclear nuclear antigen (PCNA) and nucleolar organiser regions in Hodgkin's disease: correlation with morphology. *J Clin Pathol* 1993;46:446.

126. Hell K, Lorenzen J, Hansmann ML, et al. Expression of the proliferating cell nuclear antigen in the different types of Hodgkin's disease. *Am J Clin Pathol* 1993;99:598.

127. Schmid C, Sweeney E, Isaacson PG. Proliferating cell nuclear antigen (PCNA) expression in Hodgkin's disease. *J Pathol* 1992;168:1.

128. Gupta RK, Lister TA, Bodmer JG. Proliferation of Reed-Sternberg cells and variants in Hodgkin's disease. *Ann Oncol* 1994;5(suppl 1):S117.

129. Bai M, Tsanou E, Agnantis NJ, et al. Proliferation profile of classical Hodgkin's lymphomas. Increased expression of the protein cyclin D2 in Hodgkin's and Reed-Sternberg cells. *Mod Pathol* 2004:17;1338.

130. Chen W-G, Chen Y-Y, Kamel OW, et al. p53 mutations in Hodgkin's disease. *Lab Invest* 1996;75:519.

131. Gupta RK, Norton AJ, Thompson IW, et al. p53 expression in Reed-Sternberg cells in Hodgkin's disease. *Br J Cancer* 1992;66:649.

132. Doussis IA, Pezzella F, Lane DP, et al. An immunocytochemical study of p53 and bcl-2 protein expression in Hodgkin's disease. *Am J Clin Pathol* 1993;99:663.

133. Doglioni C, Pelosio P, Mombello A, et al. Immunohistochemical evidence of abnormal expression of the antioncogene-encoded p53 phosphoprotein in Hodgkin's disease and CD30+ anaplastic lymphomas. *Hematol Pathol* 1991;5:67.

134. Rodig SJ, Savage KJ, Nguyen V, et al. TRAF1 expression and c-Rel activation anre useful adjuncts in distinguishing classical Hodgkin lymphoma from a subset of morphologically or immunophenotypically similar lymphomas. *Am J Surg Pathol* 2005:29;196.

135. Uherova P, Olson S, Thompson MA, et al. Expression of c-FLIP in classic and nodular lymphocyte-predominant Hodgkin lymphoma. *Appl Immunohistochem Mol Morphol* 2004;12;105.

136. Pinkus GS, Barbuto D, Said J, et al. Lymphocyte subpopulations of lymph nodes and spleens in Hodgkin's disease. *Cancer* 1978;42:1270.

137. Abdulaziz Z, Mason D, Stein H, et al. An immunohistological study of the cellular constituents of Hodgkin's disease using a monoclonal antibody panel. *Histopathology* 1984;8:1.

138. Valente G, Ferrara P, Stramignoni A. Lymphocyte populations of non-scleronodular Hodgkin's disease subtypes in different stages of lymphocyte depletion. An immunophenotypic and quantitative study. *Virchows Arch B* 1990;58:289.

139. Alavaikko JF, Hansmann ML, Nebendahl C, et al. Follicular dendritic cells in Hodgkin's disease. *Am J Clin Pathol* 1991;95:194.

140. Alvaro T, Lejeune M, Salvado MT, et al. Outcome in Hodgkin's lymphoma can be predicted from the presence of accompanying cytotoxic and regulatory T cells. *Clin Cancer Res* 2005:11;1467.

141. Alavaikko MJ, Blanco G, Aine R. Follicular dendritic cells have prognostic relevance in Hodgkin's disease. *Am J Clin Pathol* 1994;101:761.

142. Jacobson JO, Wilkes BM, Harris NL. Polyclonal rearrangement of the T-cell antigen receptor genes in Hodgkin's disease: implications for diagnosis. *Mod Pathol* 1991;4:172.

143. Roth MS, Schnitzer B, Bingham EL, et al. Rearrangement of immunoglobulin and T-cell receptor genes in Hodgkin's disease. *Am J Clin Pathol* 1988;131:331.

144. Brinker MGL, Poppema S, Buys CHCM, et al. Clonal immunoglobulin gene rearrangements in tissues involved by Hodgkin's disease. *Blood* 1987;70:186.

145. Griesser H, Feller AC, Mak TW, et al. Clonal rearrangements of T-cell receptor and immunoglobulin genes and immunophenotypic antigen expression in different subclasses of Hodgkin's disease. *Int J Cancer* 1987;40:157.

146. Herbst H, Tippelmann G, Anagnostopoulos I, et al. Immunoglobulin and T cell receptor gene rearrangements in Hodgkin's disease and Ki-1-positive anaplastic large cell lymphoma: dissociation between phenotype and genotype. *Leuk Res* 1989;13:103.

147. Hu EHL, Ellison D, Zovich D, et al. Molecular analysis of Hodgkin's disease with abundant Reed-Sternberg cells. *Hematol Pathol* 1990;4:27.

148. O'Connor N, Crick J, Gatter K, et al. Cell lineage in Hodgkin's disease. *Lancet* 1987;1:158.

149. Weiss LM, Strickler JG, Hu E, et al. Immunoglobulin gene rearrangements in tissues involved by Hodgkin's disease. *Hum Pathol* 1986;17:1006.

150. Weiss LM, Warnke RA, Sklar J. Clonal antigen receptor gene rearrangements and Epstein-Barr viral DNA in tissues in Hodgkin's disease. *Hematol Oncol* 1988;6:233.

151. Knowles D, Neri A, Pelicci P, et al. Immunoglobulin and T-cell receptor beta-chain gene rearrangement analysis of Hodgkin's disease: implications for lineage determination and differential diagnosis. *Proc Natl Acad Sci USA* 1986;83:7942.

152. Sundeen J, Lipford E, Uppenkamp J, et al. Rearranged antigen receptor genes in Hodgkin's disease. *Blood* 1987;70:96.

153. Chan WC, Elmberger G, Lozano MD, et al. Large-cell anaplastic lymphoma-specific translocation in Hodgkin's disease. *Lancet* 1994;345:920.

154. Weiss LM, Lopategui JR, Sun L-H, et al. Absence of the t(2;5) in Hodgkin's disease. *Blood* 1995;85:2845.

155. Weiss LM, Warnke RA, Sklar J, et al. Molecular analysis of the t(14;18) chromosomal translocation in malignant lymphomas. *N Engl J Med* 1987;317:1185.

156. Wellmann A, Otsuki T, Vogelbruch M, et al. Analysis of the t(2;5)(p23;q35) by RT-PCR in CD30+ anaplastic large cell lymphomas, in other non-Hodgkin's lymphomas of T-cell phenotype, and in Hodgkin's disease. *Blood* 1995;86:2321.

157. Ladanyi M, Cavalchire G, Morris SW, et al. Reverse transcriptase polymerase chain reaction for the Ki-1 anaplastic large cell lymphoma-associated t(2;5) translocation in Hodgkin's disease. *Am J Pathol* 1994; 145:1296.

158. Lamant L, Meggetto F, Al Saati T, et al. High incidence of the t(2;5)(p23;q35) translocation in anaplastic large cell lymphoma and its lack of detection in Hodgkin's disease. Comparison of cytogenetic analysis, RT-PCR and P-80 immunostaining. *Blood* 1996;87:284.

159. Koduru PRK, Susin M, Schulman P, et al. Phenotypic and genotypic characterization of Hodgkin's disease. *Am J Hematol* 1993;44:117.

160. Shibata D, Hu E, Weiss LM, et al. Detection of specific t(14;18) chromosomal translocations in fixed tissues. *Hum Pathol* 1990;21:199.

161. Athan E, Chadburn A, Knowles DM. The bcl-2 gene translocation is undetectable in Hodgkin's disease by Southern blot hybridization and polymerase chain reaction. *Am J Pathol* 1992;141:193.

162. Louie DC, Kant JA, Brooks JJ, et al. Absence of t(14;18) major and minor breakpoints and of bcl-2 protein overproduction in Reed-Sternberg cells of Hodgkin's disease. *Am J Pathol* 1991;139:1231.

163. Orscheschek K, Mere H, Hell J, et al. Large-cell anaplastic lymphoma-specific translocation (t[2;5][p23;q35]) in Hodgkin's disease—indication of a common pathogenesis? *Lancet* 1995;345:87.

164. Stetler-Stevenson M, Crush-Stanton S, Cossman J. Involvement of the bcl-2 gene in Hodgkin's disease. *J Natl Cancer Inst* 1990;82:855.

165. Gupta RK, Whelan JS, Lister TA, et al. Direct sequence analysis of the t(14;18) chromosomal translocation in Hodgkin's disease. *Blood* 1992; 79:2084.

166. Reid AH, Cunningham RE, Frizzera G, et al. bcl-2 rearrangement in Hodgkin's disease. Results of polymerase chain reaction, flow cytometry, and sequencing on formalin-fixed, paraffin-embedded tissue. *Am J Pathol* 1993;142:395.

167. LeBrun DP, Ngan BY, Weiss LM, et al. The bcl-2 oncogene in Hodgkin's disease arising in the setting of follicular non-Hodgkin's lymphoma. *Blood* 1994;83:223.

168. Tamaru J, Hummel M, Zemlin M, et al. Hodgkin's disease with a B-cell phenotype often shows a VDJ rearrangement and somatic mutations in the VH genes. *Blood* 1994;84:708.

169. Orazi A, Jiang B, Lee CH, et al. Correlation between presence of clonal rearrangements of immunogloublin heavy chain genes and B-cell antigen expression in Hodgkin's disease. *Am J Clin Pathol* 1995;104:413.

170. Kamel OW, Chang PP, Hsu FS, et al. Clonal VDJ recombination of the immunoglobulin heavy chain gene by PCR in classical Hodgkin's disease. *Am J Clin Pathol* 1995;104:419.

171. Warnke RA, Weiss LM, Chan JKC, et al. Tumors of the lymph nodes and spleen. In: Rosai J, ed. *Atlas of tumor pathology,* vol 14. Washington, DC: Armed Forces Institute of Pathology, 1995.

172. Fellbaum CH, Hansmann M-L, Lennert K. Lymphadenitis mimicking Hodgkin's disease. *Histopathology* 1988;12:253.

173. Williams J, Schned A, Cotelingam JD, et al. Chronic lymphocytic leukemia with coexistent Hodgkin's disease. Implications for the origin of the Reed-Sternberg cell. *Am J Surg Pathol* 1991;15:33.

174. Momose H, Jaffe ES, Shin SS, et al. Chronic lymphocytic leukemia/small lymphocytic lymphoma with Reed-Sternberg–like cells and possible transformation to Hodgkin's disease. Mediation by Epstein-Barr virus. *Am J Surg Pathol* 1992;16:859.

175. Macon WR, Williams ME, Greer JP, et al. T-cell-rich B-cell lymphomas. A clinicopathologic study of 19 cases. *Am J Surg Pathol* 1992;16:351.

176. Delabie J, Vandenberghe E, Kennes C, et al. Histiocyte-rich B-cell lymphoma. A distinct clinicopathologic entity possibly related to lymphocyte predominant Hodgkin's disease, paragranuloma subtype. *Am J Surg Pathol* 1992;16:37.

177. Banks PM. The distinction of Hodgkin's disease from T-cell lymphoma. *Semin Diag Pathol* 1992;9:279.

178. Osborne BM, Uthman MO, Butler JJ, et al. Differentiation of T-cell lymphoma from Hodgkin's disease: mitotic rate and S-phase analysis. *Am J Clin Pathol* 1990;93:227.

179. Picker LJ, Weiss LM, Medeiros LJ, et al. Immunophenotypic criteria for the diagnosis of non-Hodgkin's lymphma. *Am J Pathol* 1987;128:181.

180. Weiss LM, Crabtree GS, Rouse RV, et al. Morphologic and immunologic characterization of 50 peripheral T-cell lymphomas. *Am J Pathol* 1985;118:316.

181. Borowitz M, Reichert TA, Brynes RK, et al. The phenotypic diversity of peripheral T-cell lymphomas. The Southeastern Cancer Study Group experience. *Hum Pathol* 1986;17:567.

182. Weiss LM, Chang KL. Association of the Epstein-Barr virus with hematolymphoid neoplasia. *Adv Anat Pathol* 1996;3:1.

183. Poppema S, Kaiserling E, Lennert K. Nodular paragranuloma and progressively transformed germinal centers. Ultrastructural and immunohistologic findings. *Virchows Arch [Cell Pathol]* 1979;31:211.

184. Hansmann ML, Wacker HH, Radzun HJ. Paragranuloma is a variant of Hodgkin's disease with predominance of B-cells. *Virchows Arch [Pathol Anat Histopathol]* 1986;409:171.

185. Poppema S. The nature of the lymphocytes surrounding Reed-Sternberg cells in nodular lymphocyte predominance and in other types of Hodgkin's disease. *Am J Pathol* 1989;135:351.

186. Hansmann ML, Stein H, Dallenbach F, et al. Diffuse lymphocyte-predominant Hodgkin's disease (diffuse paragranuloma): a variant of the B-cell-derived nodular type. *Am J Pathol* 1991;138:29.

187. Timens W, Visser L, Poppema S. Nodular lymphocyte predominance type of Hodgkin's disease is a germinal center lymphoma. *Lab Invest* 1986; 54:457.

188. Hansmann ML, Fellbaum C, Hui PK, et al. Correlation of content of B cells and Leu 7-positive cells with sybtype and stage in lymphocyte predominance type Hodgkin's disease. *Cancer Res Clin Oncol* 1988;114:405.

189. Kamel OW, Gelb AB, Shibuya RB, et al. Leu7 (CD57) reactivity distinguishes nodular lymphocyte predominance Hodgkin's disease, T cell rich B cell lymphoma and follicular lymphoma. *Am J Pathol* 1993;142:541.

190. Alavaikko JF, Hansmann ML, Nebendahl C, et al. Follicular dendritic cells in Hodgkin's disease. *Am J Clin Pathol* 1991; 95:194.

191. Alavaikko MJ, Blanco G, Aine R. Follicular dendritic cells have prognostic relevance in Hodgkin's disease. *Am J Clin Pathol* 1994;101:761.

192. Pinkus GS, Said JW. Hodgkin's disease, lymphocyte predominance type, nodular—a distinct entity? Unique staining profile of L&H variants of Reed-Sternberg cells defined by monoclonal antibodies to leukocyte common antigen, granulocyte specific antigen, and B-cell specific antigen. *Am J Pathol* 1985;116:1.

193. Pinkus GS, Said JW. Hodgkin's disease, lymphocyte predominance type, nodular—further evidence for a B cell derivation. L & H variants of Reed-Sternberg cells express L26, a pan B cell marker. *Am J Pathol* 1988;133:211.

194. Chittal SM, Alard C, Rossi JF, et al. Further phenotypic evidence that nodular, lymphocyte-predominant Hodgkin's disease is a large B-cell lymphoma in evolution. *Am J Surg Pathol* 1990;14:1024.

195. Chittal SM, Caveriviere P, Schwarting R, et al. Monoclonal antibodies in the diagnosis of Hodgkin's disease: the search for a rational panel. *Am J Surg Pathol* 1988;12:9.

196. Hsu SM, Ho YS, Li PJ, et al. L&H variants of Reed-Sternberg cells express sialylated Leu M1 antigen. *Am J Pathol* 1986;122:199.

197. Anagnostopoulos I, Hansmann ML, Franssila K, et al. European task force on lymphoma project on lymphocyte predominance Hodgkin disease: histologic and immunohistologic analysis of submitted cases reveals 2 types of Hodgkin disease with a nodular growth pattern and abundant lymphocytes. *Blood* 2000;96; 1889.

198. Stein H, Hansmann ML, Lennert K, et al. Reed-Sternberg and Hodgkin's cells in lymphocyte-predominant Hodgkin's disease of nodular subtype contain J chain. *Am J Clin Pathol* 1986;86:292.

199. Poppema S. The diversity of the immunohistological staining pattern of Sternberg-Reed cells. *J Histochem Cytochem* 1980;28:788.

200. Falini B, Bigerna B, Pasqualucci L, et al. Distinctive expression pattern of the BCL-6 protein in nodular lymphocyte prodominance Hodgkin's disease. *Blood* 1996;87:465.

201. Algara P, Martinez P, Sanchez L, et al. Lymphocyte predominance Hodgkin's disease (nodular paragranuloma)-A bcl-2 negative germinal centre lymphoma. *Histopathology* 1991;19:69.

202. Weiss LM, Chang KL. Association of the Epstein-Barr virus with hematolymphoid neoplasia. *Adv Anat Pathol* 1996;3:1.

203. Momose H, Chen Y-Y, Ben-Ezra J, et al. Nodular, lymphocyte predominant Hodgkin's disease: study of immunoglobulin light chain protein and mRNA expression. *Hum Pathol* 1992;23:1115.

204. Sundeen JT, Cossman J, Jaffe ES. Lymphocyte predominant Hodgkin's disease nodular subtype with coexistent "large cell lymphoma." Histological progression or composite malignancy? [See comments.] *Am J Surg Pathol* 1988;12:599.

205. Li G, Hansmann M. Lymphocyte predominant Hodgkin's disease of nodular subtype combined with pulmonary lymphoid infiltration and hypogammaglobulinemia. *Virchows Arch [Pathol Anat Histopathol]* 1989;145:481.

206. Schmid C, Pan L, Diss T, et al. Expression of B-cell antigens by Hodgkin's and Reed-Sternberg cells. *Am J Pathol* 1991;139:701.

207. Hell K, Lorenzen J, Hansmann ML, et al. Expression of the proliferating cell nuclear antigen in the different types of Hodgkin's disease. *Am J Clin Pathol* 1993;99:598.

208. Gerdes J, van Baarlen J, Pileri S, et al. Tumor cell growth fraction in Hodgkin's disease. *Am J Pathol* 1987;128:390.

209. Ruprai AK, Pringle JH, Angel CA, et al. Localization of immunoglobulin light chain mRNA expression in Hodgkin's disease by in situ hybridization. *J Pathol* 1991;164:37.

210. Hell K, Pringle JH, Hansmann ML, et al. Demonstration of light chain mRNA in Hodgkin's disease. *J Pathol* 1993;171:137.

211. Stoler MH, Nichols GE, Symbula M, et al. Nodular L&H lymphocyte predominance Hodgkin's disease: evidence for a kappa light chain-restricted monotypic B cell neoplasm. *Am J Pathol* 1995;146:812.

212. Weiss LM, Chen YY, Liu X, et al. A correlative in situ hybridization and polymerase chain reaction study. *Am J Pathol* 1991;139:1259.

213. Brousset P, Chittal S, Schlaifer D, et al. Detection of Epstein-Barr virus messenger RNA in Reed-Sternberg cells of Hodgkin's disease by in situ hybridization with biotinylated probes on specially processed modified acetone methyl benzoate xylene (ModAMeX) sections. *Blood* 1991;77:1781.

214. Shibata D, Hansmann ML, Weiss LM, et al. Epstein-Barr virus infection and Hodgkin's disease: a study of fixed tissues using the polymerase chain reaction. *Hum Pathol* 1991;22:1262.

215. Hansmann ML, Shibata D, Lorenzen J, et al. Incidence of Epstein-Barr virus, bcl-2 expression and chromosomal translocation t(14;18) in large cell lymphoma associated with paragranuloma (lymphocyte-predominant Hodgkin's disease). *Hum Pathol* 1994;25:240.

216. Khalidi H, Lones MA, Zhou Y, et al. Detection of Epstein-Barr virus in the L&H cells of nodular lymphocytic predominance Hodgkin's disease. Report of a case documented by immunohistochemical, in situ hybridization, and polymerase chain reaction methods. *Am J Clin Pathol* 1997;108:687.

216a. Chang K-C, Khen NT, Jones D, et al. Epstain Barr virus is associated with all histological subtypes of Hodgkin lymphoma in Vietnamese children with special emphasis on the entity of lymphocyte predominance subtype. *Hum Pathol* 2005;36:747.

217. Lorenzen J, Hansmann ML, Pezzella F, et al. Expression of the bcl-2 oncogene product and chromosomal translocation t(14;18) in Hodgkin's disease. *Hum Pathol* 1992;23:1205.

218. Said JW, Sassoon AF, Shintaku IP, et al. Absence of bcl-2 major breakpoint region and J_H gene rearrangement in lymphocyte predominance Hodgkin's disease: results of Southern blot analysis and polymerase chain reaction. *Am J Pathol* 1991;138:261.

219. Burns BF, Colby TV, Dorfman RF. Differential diagnostic features of nodular L&H Hodgkin's disease, including progressive transformation of germinal centers. *Am J Surg Pathol* 1984;8:253.

220. Osborne BM, Butler JJ. Clinical implications of progressive transformation of germinal centers. *Am J Surg Pathol* 1984;8:725.

221. Hansmann ML, Fellbaum C, Hui PK, et al. Progressive transformation of germinal centers with and without association to Hodgkin's disease. *Am J Clin Pathol* 1990;93:219.

222. Nguyen P, Ferry J, Harris NL. Progressive transformation of germinal centers and nodular lymphocyte predominance Hodgkin's disease: a comparative immunohistochemical study. *Am J Surg Pathol* 1999;23:27–33.

223. Hansmann ML, Küppers R. Pathology and "molecular histology" of Hodgkin's disease and the border to non-Hodgkin's lymphomas. *Baillieres Clin Haematol* 1996;9:459.

224. Ramsay AP, Smith WJ, Isaacson PG. T-cell-rich B-cell lymphoma. *Am J Surg Pathol* 1988;12:433.

225. Macon WR, Williams ME, Greer JP, et al. T-Cell-rich B-cell lymphomas. A clinicopathologic study of 19 cases. *Am J Surg Pathol* 1992;16:351.

226. Ng C, Chan J, Hui P, et al. Large B-cell lymphomas with a high content of reactive T-cells. *Hum Pathol* 1989;20:1145.

227. Scarpa A, Bonetti F, Zamboni G, et al. T-cell-rich B-cell lymphoma. *Am J Surg Pathol* 1989;13:335. Letter.

228. Chittal SM, Brousset P, Voigt JJ, et al. Large B-cell lymphoma rich in T-cells and simulating Hodgkin's disease. *Histopathology* 1991;19:211.

229. Delabie J, Vandenberghe E, Kennes C, et al. Histiocyte-rich B-cell lymphoma. A distinct clinicopathologic entity possibly related to lymphocyte predominant Hodgkin's disease, paragranuloma subtype. *Am J Surg Pathol* 1992;16:37.

230. McBride JA, Rodriguez J, Luthra R, et al. T-cell-rich B large cell lymphoma simulating lymphocyte-rich Hodgkin's disease. *Am J Surg Pathol* 1996;20:193.

231. Chan A. T-cell-Rich B-Cell Lymphoma. What is new? What is cool? *Am J Clin Pathol* 1997;108:489.

232. De Jong D, Van Gorp J, Sie-Go D, et al. T-cell-rich B-cell non-Hodgkin's lymphoma: a progressed form of follicle center cell lymphoma and lymphocyte predominance Hodgkin's disease. *Histopathology* 1996;28:15.

233. Skinnider B, Connors J, Gascoyne R. Bone marrow involvement in T-cell-rich-B-cell lymphoma. *Am J Clin Pathol* 1997;108:570.

234. Osborne BM, Buttler JJ, Pugh WC. The value of immunophenotyping on paraffin sections in the identification of T-cell rich B-cell large cell lymphomas. *Am J Surg Pathol* 1990;14:933.

235. Osborne BM, Butler JJ, Pugh WC. The value of immunophenotyping on paraffin sections in the identification of T-cell rich B-cell large cell lymphoma: lineage confirmed by JH rearrangement. *Am J Surg Pathol* 1990;14:933.

236. Küppers R, Rajewsky K, Hansmann ML. Diffuse large cell lymphomas are derived from mature B-cells carrying V region genes with a high load of somatic mutations and evidence of selection for antibody expression. *Eur J Immunol* 1997;27:1398.

237. Hansmann ML, Stein H, Fellbaum C, et al. Nodular paragranuloma can transform into high-grade malignant lymphoma of B type. *Hum Pathol* 1989;20:1169.

238. Miettinen M, Franssila KO, Saxen E. Hodgkin's disease, lymphocyte predominance nodular: increased risk for subsequent non-Hodgkin's lymphomas. *Cancer* 1983;51:2293.

239. Huang JZ, Weisenburger DD, Vosey JM, et al. Diffuse large B-cell lymphoma arising in nodular lymphocyte predominant Hodgkin lymphoma: a report of 21 cases from the Nebraska Lymphoma Study Group. *Leuk Lymph* 2004;45; 1551.

240. Gonzalez CL, Medeiros LJ, Jaffe ES. Composite lymphoma. A clinicopathologic analysis of nine patients with Hodgkin's disease and B-cell non-Hodgkin's lymphoma. *Am J Clin Pathol* 1991;96:81.

241. Grossman DM, Hanson CA, Schnitzer B. Simultaneous lymphocyte predominant Hodgkin's disease and large cell lymphoma. *Am J Surg Pathol* 1991;15:668.

242. Jaffe ES, Zarate-Osorno A, Kingma DW, et al. The interrelationship between Hodgkin's disease and non-Hodgkin's lymphoma. *Ann Oncol* 1994;5(suppl 1):S7.

243. Hell K, Hansmann ML, Pringle JH, et al. Combination of Hodgkin's disease and diffuse large cell lymphoma: an in situ hybridization study for immunoglobulin light chain messenger RNA. *Histopathology* 1995;27:491.

244. Greiner TC, Gascoyne RD, Anderson ME, et al. Nodular lymphocyte-predominant Hodgkin's disease associated with large cell lymphoma: Analysis of Ig gene rearrangements by V-J polymerase chain reaction. *Blood* 1996;88:657.

245. Pan LX, Diss TC, Peng HZ, et al. Nodular lymphocyte predominance Hodgkin's disease: a monoclonal or polyclonal B-cell disorder? *Blood* 1996;87:2428.

246. Wickert RS, Weisenburger DD, Tierens A, et al. Clonal relationship between lymphocyte predominance Hodgkin's disease and concurrent or subsequent large cell lymphoma of B lineage. *Blood* 1995;86:2312.

247. Stewards RS. Hodgkin's disease—time for a change. *N Engl J Med* 1997;337:495. Editorial, comment.

248. Kanzler H, Kuppers R, Hansmann ML, et al. Hodgkin and Reed-Sternberg cells in Hodgkin's disease represent the outgrowth of a dominant tumor clone derived from (crippled) germinal center B cells. *J Exp Med* 1996;184:1495.

249. Tamaru J, Hummel M, Zemlin M, et al. Hodgkin's disease with a B-cell phenotype often shows a VDJ rearrangement and somatic mutations in the VH genes. *Blood* 1994;84:708.

250. Küppers R, Rajewsky K, Zhao M, et al. Hodgkin's disease: Hodgkin and Reed Sternberg cells picked from histological sections show clonal immunoglobulin gene rearrangements and appear to be derived from B cells at various stages of development. *Proc Natl Acad Sci USA* 1994;91:1092.

251. Jaffe ES, Zarate-Osorno A, Medeiros LJ. The interrelationship of Hodgkin's disease and non-Hodgkin's lymphomas—lessons learned from composite and sequential malignancies. *Semin Diagn Pathol* 1992;9:297.

252. Custer R, Bernard W. The interrelationship of Hodgkin's disease and other lymphatic tumors. *Am J Med Sci* 1948;216:625.

253. Kim H, Hendrickson M, Dorfman R. Composite lymphoma. *Cancer* 1977;40:959.

254. Gonzalez CL, Medeiros LJ, Jaffe ES. Composite lymphoma. A clinicopathologic analysis of nine patients with Hodgkin's disease and B-cell non-Hodgkin's lymphoma. *Am J Clin Pathol* 1991;96:81.

255. Hansmann ML, Fellbaum C, Hui PK, et al. Morphological and immunohistochemical investigation of non-Hodgkin's lymphoma combined with Hodgkin's disease. *Histopathology* 1989;15:35.

256. Paulli M, Rosso R, Kindl S, et al. Nodular sclerosing Hodgkin's disease and large cell lymphoma. Immunophenotypic characterization of a composite case. *Virchows Arch Pathol Anat Histopathol* 1992;421:271.

257. Guarner J, del Rio C, Hendrix L, et al. Composite Hodgkin's and non-Hodgkin's lymphoma in a patient with acquired immune deficiency syndrome. In-situ demonstration of Epstein-Barr virus. *Cancer* 1990;66:796.

258. Aguilera NS, Howard LN, Brissette MD, et al. Hodgkin's disease and an extranodal marginal zone B-cell lymphoma in the small intestine: an unusual composite lymphoma. *Mod Pathol* 1996;9:1020.

259. Kingma DW, Medeiros LJ, Barletta J, et al. Epstein-Barr virus is infrequently identified in non-Hodgkin's lymphomas associated with Hodgkin's disease. *Am J Surg Pathol* 1994;18:48.

260. Schmitz R, Renne C, Rosenquist R, et al. Insights into the multistep transformation of lymphomas: IgH-associated translocations and tumor suppressor gene mutations in clonally related composite Hodgkin's and non-Hodgkin's lymphoma. *Leukemia* 2005;19:1452.

261. Jaffe ES, Zarate-Osorno A, Kingma DW, et al. The interrelationship between Hodgkin's disease and non-Hodgkin's lymphomas. *Ann Oncol* 1994;5(suppl 1):s7.

262. Gelb AB, Dorfman RF, Warnke RA. Coexistence of nodular lymphocyte predominance Hodgkin's disease and Hodgkin's disease of the usual type. *Am J Surg Pathol* 1993;17:364.

263. Hansmann M, Stein H, Fellbaum C, et al. Nodular paragranuloma can transform into high-grade malignant lymphoma of B type. *Hum Pathol* 1989;20:1169.

264. Miettinen M, Franssila KO, Saxen E. Hodgkin's disease, lymphocytic predominance nodular. Increased risk for subsequent non-Hodgkin's lymphomas. *Cancer* 1983;51:2293.

265. Krikorian JG, Burke JS, Rosenberg SA, et al. Occurrence of non-Hodgkin's lymphoma after therapy for Hodgkin's disease. *N Engl J Med* 1979;300:452.

266. Levy R, Kaplan HS. Impaired lymphocyte function in untreated Hodgkin's disease. *N Engl J Med* 1974;290:181.

267. Fisher RI, DeVita VT Jr, Bostick F, et al. Persistent immunologic abnormalities in long-term survivors of advanced Hodgkin's disease. *Ann Intern Med* 1980;92:595.

268. Zarate-Osorno A, Medeiros LJ, Longo DL, et al. Non-Hodgkin's lymphomas arising in patients successfully treated for Hodgkin's disease. A clinical, histologic, and immunophenotypic study of 14 cases. *Am J Surg Pathol* 1992;16:885.

269. Bennett M, MacLennan K, Hudson G, et al. Non-Hodgkin's lymphoma arising in patients treated for Hodgkin's disease in the BNLI: a 20-year experience. *Ann Oncol* 1991;2(suppl 2):83.

270. Shimizu K, Hara K, Kunii A. Non-Hodgkin's lymphoma following Hodgkin's disease. A case report and immunohistochemical corroboration. *Am J Clin Pathol* 1986;86:370.

271. Ohno T, Trenn G, Wu G, et al. The clonal relationship between nodular sclerosis Hodgkin's disease with a clonal Reed-Sternberg cell population and a subsequent B-cell small non-cleaved cell lymphoma. *Mod Pathol* 1998;11:485.

272. Gaidano G, Carbone A, Dalla-Favera R. Pathogenesis of AIDS-related lymphomas: molecular and histogenetic heterogeneity. *Am J Pathol* 1998;152:623.

273. Perrone T, Frizzera G, Rosai J. Mediastinal diffuse large-cell lymphoma with sclerosis. A clinicopathologic study of 60 cases. *Am J Surg Pathol* 1986;10:176.

273a. Traverse-Glehen A, Pittaluga S, Gaulard P, et al. Mediastinal gray zone lymphoma: the missing link between classic Hodgkin's lymphoma and mediastinal large B-cell lymphoma. *Am J Surg Pathol* 2005;29:2005.

274. Poppema S, Kluiver JL, Atayar C, et al. Report: workshop on mediastinal grey zone lymphoma. *Eur J Haematol* 2005;75;45.

275. Rudiger T, Jaffe ES, Delsol G, et al. Workshop report on Hodgkin's disease and related diseases ('grey zone' lymphoma). *Ann Oncol* 1998:9;S31.

276. Calvo KR, Traverse-Glehen A, Pittaluga S, et al. Molecular profiling provides evidence of primary mediastinal large B-cell lymphoma as a distinct entity related to classic Hodgkin lymphoma: implications for mediastinal gray zone lymphomas as an intermediate form of B-cell lymphoma. *Adv Anat Pathol* 2004:11; 227.

277. The Non-Hodgkin's Lymphoma Classification Project. A clinical evaluation of the International Lymphoma Study Group classification of non-Hodgkin's lymphoma. *Blood* 1997;89:3909.

278. Moller P, Moldenhauer G, Momburg F, et al. Mediastinal lymphoma of clear cell type is a tumor corresponding to terminal steps of B cell differentiation. *Blood* 1987;69:1087.

279. Lamarre L, Jacobson J, Aisenberg A, et al. Primary large cell lymphoma of the mediastinum. *Am J Surg Pathol* 1989;13:730.

280. Savage K, Monti S, Kutok JL, et al. The molecular signature of mediastinal large B-cell lymphoma differs from that of other didfuse large B-cell lymphomas and shares features with classical Hodgkin's lymphoma. *Blood* 2003:102; 3871.

281. Rosenwald A, Wright G, Leroy K, et al. Molecular diagnosis of primary mediastinal B-cell lymphoma identifies a clinically favorable subgroup of diffuse large B-cell lymphoma related to Hodgkin lymphoma. *J Exp Med* 2003:198;851.

282. Carrato A, Filippa D, Koziner B. Hodgkin's disease after treatment of non-Hodgkin's lymphoma. *Cancer* 1987;60:887.

283. Travis LB, Gonzalez CL, Hankey BF, et al. Hodgkin's disease following non-Hodgkin's lymphoma. *Cancer* 1992;69:2337.

284. Zarate-Osorno A, Medeiros J, Jaffe ES. Hodgkin's disease coexistent with plasma cell dyscrasia. *Arch Pathol Lab Med* 1992;116:969.

285. LeBrun DP, Ngan BY, Weiss LM, et al. The bcl-2 oncogene in Hodgkin's disease arising in the setting of follicular non-Hodgkin's lymphoma. *Blood* 1994;83:223.

286. Richter M. Generalized reticular cell sarcoma of lymph nodes associated with lymphatic leukemia. *Am J Pathol* 1928;4:285.

287. Choi H, Keller RH. Coexistence of chronic lymphocytic leukemia and Hodgkin's disease. *Cancer* 1981;48:48.

288. Han T. Chronic lymphocytic leukemia in Hodgkin's disease. Report of a case and review of the literature. *Cancer* 1971;28:300.

289. Dick F, Maca R. The lymph node in chronic lymphocytic leukemia. *Cancer* 1978;41:283.

290. Foucar K, Rydell RE. Richter's syndrome in chronic lymphocytic leukemia. *Cancer* 1980;46:118.

291. Caveriviere P, Mallem O, Al Saati T, et al. Reed-Sternberg-like cells in Richter's syndrome express granulocytic- associated-antigen (Leu-M1). *Am J Clin Pathol* 1986;85:755. Letter.

292. Williams J, Schned A, Cotelingam JD, et al. Chronic lymphocytic leukemia with coexistent Hodgkin's disease: Implications for the origin of the Reed-Sternberg cell. *Am J Surg Pathol* 1991;15:33.

293. Brecher M, Banks P. Hodgkin's disease variant of Richter's syndrome: report of eight cases. *Am J Clin Pathol* 1990;93:333.

294. Fayad L, Robertson LE, O'Brien S, et al. Hodgkin's disease variant of Richter's syndrome: experience at a single institution. *Leuk Lymphoma* 1996;23:333.

295. Rubin D, Hudnall SD, Aisenberg A, et al. Richter's transformation of chronic lymphocytic leukemia with Hodgkin's-like cells is associated with Epstein-Barr virus infection. *Mod Pathol* 1994;7:91.

296. Pescarona E, Pignoloni P, Mauro FR, et al. Hodgkin/Reed-Sternberg cells and Hodgkin's disease in patients with B-cell chronic lymphocytic leukaemia: an immunohistological, molecular and clinical study of four cases suggesting a heterogenous pathogenetic background. *Virchows Arch* 2000:437;129.

297. de Leval L, Vivario M, De Prijck B, et al. Distinct clonal origin in two cases of Hodgkin's lymphoma variant of Richter's syndrome associated with EBV infection. *Am J Surg Pathol* 2004;8:679.

298. Weisenberg E, Anastasi J, Adeyanju M, et al. Hodgkin's disease associated with chronic lymphocytic leukemia. Eight additional cases, including two of the nodular lymphocyte predominant type. *Am J Clin Pathol* 1995;103:479.

299. Chittal S, Caveriviere P, Schwarting R, et al. Monoclonal antibodies in the diagnosis of Hodgkin's disease. The search for a rational panel. *Am J Surg Pathol* 1988;12:9.

300. Momose H, Jaffe ES, Shin SS, et al. Chronic lymphocytic leukemia/small lymphocytic lymphoma with Reed-Sternberg-like cells and possible transformation to Hodgkin's disease. Mediation by Epstein-Barr virus. *Am J Surg Pathol* 1992;16:859.

301. Cha I, Herndier BG, Glassberg AB, et al. A case of composite Hodgkin's disease and chronic lymphocytic leukemia in bone marrow. Lack of Epstein-Barr virus. *Arch Pathol Lab Med* 1996;120:386.

302. Ohno T, Smir BN, Weisenburger DD, et al. Origin of the Hodgkin/Reed-Sternberg cells in chronic lymphocytic leukemia with "Hodgkin's transformation." *Blood* 1998;91:1757.

303. Giles FJ, O'Brien SM, Keating MJ. Chronic lymphocytic leukemia in (Richter's) transformation. *Semin Oncol* 1998;25:117.

304. Wlodarska I, Delabie J, De Wolf-Peeters C, et al. T-cell lymphoma developing in Hodgkin's disease: evidence for two clones. *J Pathol* 1993;170:239.

305. van der Putte SC, Toonstra J, Go DM, et al. Mycosis fungoides. Demonstration of a variant simulating Hodgkin's disease. A report of a case with a cytomorphological analysis. *Virchows Arch B Cell Pathol Incl Mol Pathol* 1982;40:231.

306. Picard F, Dreyfus F, Le Guern M, et al. Acute T-cell leukemia/lymphoma mimicking Hodgkin's disease with secondary HTLV I seroconversion. *Cancer* 1990;66:1524.

307. Ohshima K, Kikuchi M, Yoshida T, et al. Lymph nodes in incipient adult T-cell leukemia-lymphoma with Hodgkin's disease-like histologic features. *Cancer* 1991;67:1622.

308. Simrell CR, Boccia RV, Longo DL, et al. Coexisting Hodgkin's disease and mycosis fungoides. Immunohistochemical proof of its existence. *Arch Pathol Lab Med* 1986;110:1029.

309. Hawkins KA, Schinella R, Schwartz M, et al. Simultaneous occurrence of mycosis fungoides and Hodgkin disease: clinical and histologic correlations in three cases with ultrastructural studies in two. *Am J Hematol* 1983;14:355.

310. Clement M, Bhakri H, Monk B, et al. Mycosis fungoides and Hodgkin's disease. *J R Soc Med* 1984;77:1037.

311. Kaufman D, Gordon LI, Variakojis D, et al. Successfully treated Hodgkin's disease followed by mycosis fungoides: case report and review of the literature. *Cutis* 1987;39:291.

312. Brousset P, Lamant L, Viraben R, et al. Hodgkin's disease following mycosis fungoides: phenotypic and molecular evidence for different tumour cell clones. *J Clin Pathol* 1996;49:504.

313. Davis T, Morton C, Miller-Cassman R, et al. Hodgkin's disease, lymphomatoid papulosis, and cutaneous T-cell lymphoma derived from a common T-cell clone. *N Engl J Med* 1992;326:1115.

314. Ralfkiaer E, Bosq J, Gatter KC, et al. Expression of a Hodgkin and Reed-Sternberg cell associated antigen (Ki-1) in cutaneous lymphoid infiltrates. *Arch Dermatol Res* 1987;279:285.

315. Wieczorek R, Suhrland M, Ramsay D, et al. Leu-M1 antigen expression in advanced (tumor) stage mycosis fungoides. *Am J Clin Pathol* 1986;86:25.

316. Scheen SR3rd Banks PM, Winkelmann RK. Morphologic heterogeneity of malignant lymphomas developing in mycosis fungoides. *Mayo Clin Proc* 1984;59:95.

317. Caya JG, Choi H, Tieu TM, et al. Hodgkin's disease followed by mycosis fungoides in the same patient. Case report and literature review. *Cancer* 1984;53:463.

318. Park CS, Chung HC, Lim HY, et al. Coexisting mycosis fungoides and Hodgkin's disease as a composite lymphoma: a case report. *Yonsei Med J* 1991;32:362.

319. Lipa M, Kunynetz R, Pawlowski D, et al. The occurrence of mycosis fungoides in two patients with preexisting Hodgkin's disease. *Arch Dermatol* 1982;118:563.

320. Greene MH, Pinto HA, Kant JA, et al. Lymphomas and leukemias in the relatives of patients with mycosis fungoides. *Cancer* 1982;49:737.

320a. Seitz V, Hummel M, Marafioti T, et al. Detection of clonal T-cell receptor gamma-chain gene rearrangements in Reed-Sternberg cells of classic Hodgkin disease. *Blood* 2000;10:3020.

320b. Muschen M, Rajewsky K, Brauninger A, et al. Rare occurrence of classical Hodgkin's disease as a T cell lymphoma. *J Exp Med* 2000;2:387.

320c. Willenbrock K, Ichinohasama R, Kadin ME, et al. T-cell variant of classical Hodgkin's lymphoma with nodal and cutaneous manifestations demonstrated by single-cell polymerase chain reaction. *Lab Invest* 2002;9:1103.

321. Kadin ME, Muramoto L, Said J. Expression of T-cell antigens on Reed-Sternberg cells in a subset of patients with nodular sclerosing and mixed cellularity Hodgkin's disease. *Am J Pathol* 1988;130:345.

322. Foss HD, Anagnostopoulos I, Araujo I, et al. Anaplastic large-cell lymphomas of T-cell and null-cell phenotype express cytotoxic molecules. *Blood* 1996;88:4005.

323. Krenacs L, Wellmann A, Sorbara L, et al. Cytotoxic cell antigen expression in anaplastic large cell lymphomas of T- and null-cell type and Hodgkin's disease: evidence for distinct cellular origin. *Blood* 1997;89:980.

324. Benharroch D, Meguerian-Bedoyan Z, Lamant L, et al. ALK-positive lymphoma: a single disease with a broad spectrum of morphology. *Blood* 1998;91:2076.

325. Chittal SM, Delsol G. The interface of Hodgkin's disease and anaplastic large cell lymphoma. *Cancer Surv* 1997;30:87.

326. Pittaluga S, Wiodarska I, Pulford K, et al. The monoclonal antibody ALK1 identifies a distinct morphological subtype of anaplastic large cell lymphoma associated with 2p23/ALK rearrangements. *Am J Pathol* 1997; 151:343.

327. Falini B, Mason DY. Proteins encoded by genes involved in chromosomal alterations in lymphoma and leukemia: clinical value of their detection by immunocytochemistry. *Blood* 2002;99:409.

328. Ohshima K, Suzumiya J, Kato A, et al. Clonal HTLV-I-infected CD4-T-lymphocytes and non-clonal non-HTLV-I- infected giant cells in incipient ATLL with Hodgkin-like histologic features. *Int J Cancer* 1997; 72:592.

329. Georgescu L, Quinn GC, Schwartzman S, et al. Lymphoma in patients with rheumatoid arthritis: association with the disease state or methotrexate treatment. *Semin Arthritis Rheum* 1997;26:794. See comments.

330. Kamel OW, van de Rijn M, Weiss, LM, et al. Brief report: reversible lymphomas associated with Epstein-Barr virus occurring during methotrexate therapy for rheumatoid arthritis and dermatomyositis. *N Engl J Med* 1993;328:1317.

331. Kamel OW, Weiss LM, van de Rijn M, et al. Hodgkin's disease and lymphoproliferations resembling Hodgkin's disease in patients receiving long-term low-dose methotrexate therapy. *Am J Surg Pathol* 1996; 20:1279.

332. Rowlings PA, Curtis RE, Kingma DW, et al. Hodgkin disease following allogeneic bone marrow transplantation: Long latency and association with Epstein-Barr virus. *Blood* 1997;90(suppl 1):379a. Abstract.

333. Pitman S, Huang Q, Zuppan CW, et al. Hodgkin lymphoma–like post transplant lymphoproliferative disorder (HL-like PTLD) simulates monomorphic B-cell PTLD both clinically and pathologically. *Am J Surg Pathol* 2006;30:470.

334. Chittal S, Brousset P, Voigt J, et al. Large B-cell lymphoma rich in T-cells and simulating Hodgkin's disease. *Histopathology* 1991;19:211.

335. Delabie J, Vandenberghe E, Kennes C, et al. Histiocyte-rich B-cell lymphoma. A distinct clinicopathologic entity possibly related to lymphocyte predominant Hodgkin's disease, paragranuloma subtype. *Am J Surg Pathol* 1992;16:37.

336. McBride JA, Rodriguez J, Luthra R, et al. T-cell–rich B large-cell lymphoma simulating lymphocyte rich Hodgkin's disease. *Am J Surg Pathol* 1996; 20:193.

337. Gruss HJ, Pinto A, Duyster J, et al. Hodgkin's disease: a tumor with disturbed immunological pathways. *Immunol Today* 1997;18:156.

338. Schmid C, Pan L, Diss T, et al. Expression of B-cell antigens by Hodgkin's and Reed-Sternberg cells. *Am J Pathol* 1991;139:701.

339. Zukerberg L, Collins A, Ferry J, et al. Coexpression of CD15 and CD20 by Reed-Sternberg cells in Hodgkin's disease. *Am J Pathol* 1991;139:475.

340. von Wasielewski R, Mengel M, Fischer R, et al. Classical Hodgkin's disease. Clinical impact of the immunophenotype. *Am J Pathol* 1997;151:1123.

CHAPTER 5 ■ NATURE OF REED-STERNBERG AND L & H CELLS, AND THEIR MOLECULAR BIOLOGY IN HODGKIN LYMPHOMA

RALF KÜPPERS AND DANIEL RE

DISCOVERY OF THE REED-STERNBERG CELLS AND LYMPHOCYTIC AND/OR HISTIOCYTIC (L & H) CELLS

In 1832, Thomas Hodgkin described the anatomic findings of seven patients with enormous lymph node swellings.[1] Independently, Samuel Wilks published an article in 1856 summarizing ten cases (including four of the seven cases already investigated by Hodgkin) having the same anatomic features.[2] As soon as he became aware of his mistake, he appended an appropriate comment to his article. In the following years, Wilks collected additional cases and interpreted them as pathognomonic for a new disease entity.[3] Although it was Wilks who separated Hodgkin's disease from other diseases associated with lymph node swellings, he was sufficiently magnanimous to name the disease after Hodgkin in acknowledgment of Hodgkin's first report of some cases. The histopathologic features of this disease were initially described by Langhans in 1872[4] and Greenfield in 1878.[5] However, Carl Sternberg in 1898[6] and Dorothy Reed in 1902[7] published independently of each other a more detailed description of the cytologic features of the multinucleated giant cells, which have since been known as Reed-Sternberg cells. The mononucleated blasts were later designated Hodgkin cells. In 1966, Lukes and Butler[8] described a multilobated variant of the Hodgkin and Reed-Sternberg (HRS) cells that occurs mainly in the nodular lymphocyte-predominance type of Hodgkin's disease. These multilobated blasts were called L & H cells because in lymphocyte-predominant Hodgkin's disease the cellular background consists of lymphocytes and histiocytes. Because of the multilobated nuclear morphology of these cells, Neiman[9] suggested the name "popcorn cells." HRS and L & H cells are only a minor population of cells in tissues affected by Hodgkin's disease, usually accounting for less than 1% of the cellular infiltrate.

Immunohistological studies of the last 20 years have shown that the classical HRS cells and the L & H cells show strikingly distinct immunophenotypes.[10,11] L & H cells are characterized by the consistent expression of CD20 and J chain, and the constant absence of CD30 and CD15, whereas typical HRS cells are characterized by the constant expression of CD30, frequent expression of CD15, and absence of J chain. These findings demonstrate that L & H cells and HRS cells represent different types of cells and that Hodgkin's disease therefore comprises two distinct diseases: lymphocyte-predominant Hodgkin's disease and non-lymphocyte-predominant Hodgkin's disease. This distinction correlates well with the clinical findings that the early stages of lymphocyte-predominant Hodgkin's disease may be quite indolent, and that all other forms of Hodgkin's disease progress steadily without treatment and therefore require immediate treatment.[12] In view of these findings, the International Lymphoma Study Group proposed to subsume all Hodgkin's disease histotypes with classical HRS cells, which include nodular-sclerosis, mixed-cellularity, and lymphocyte-depleted Hodgkin's disease, under the term classical Hodgkin's disease, to emphasise their relationship to each other and their distinctness from lymphocyte-predominant Hodgkin's disease.[13] As it has been revealed that both HRS and L & H cells derive from B-lymphocytes (or very rarely T-cells in classical Hodgkin's disease, discussed later), Hodgkin lymphoma is the term used in the new World Health Organization (WHO) classification of malignant lymphomas.[14]

In the past, the clear difference between lymphocyte-predominant Hodgkin lymphoma and classical Hodgkin lymphoma was often not recognized. A recent study of lymphocyte-predominant Hodgkin lymphoma clarified the reason for this confusion by finding a Hodgkin lymphoma form that closely resembles, in growth pattern and cellular composition, nodular lymphocyte-predominant Hodgkin lymphoma but that resembles, in the immunophenotype of its atypical blasts, classical Hodgkin lymphoma.[10] In the WHO classification of malignant lymphomas,[14] this form is designated as nodular lymphocyte-rich classical Hodgkin lymphoma, a new histologic subtype of classical Hodgkin lymphoma (Table 5.1).

ANTIGENS ASSOCIATED WITH HRS AND L & H CELLS

CD15

The first antigen found to be commonly associated with HRS cells was CD15. This association was first recognized by use of the antibodies Tü9[15] and 3C4,[16] and later of Leu-M1[17] and C3D1.[18] The CD15 antibodies are directed at the trisaccharide antigen lacto-N-fucipentaose III, also termed X-hapten.[19] The

TABLE 5.1

WORLD HEALTH ORGANIZATION CLASSIFICATION
OF HODGKIN LYMPHOMA

Nodular lymphocyte-predominant Hodgkin lymphoma
+/− Diffuse areas
Classic Hodgkin lymphoma
Lymphocyte rich
Nodular sclerosis (grades I and II)
Mixed cellularity
Lymphocyte depleted

detection of the CD15 moiety has achieved diagnostic significance because it is present in HRS cells in most cases of classical Hodgkin lymphoma but is constantly absent from L & H cells of lymphocyte-predominant Hodgkin lymphoma. However, CD15 has no value as a marker of cell lineage because in normal subjects it is expressed on a variety of cells, including late cells of granulopoiesis, epithelioid-type macrophages, various epithelial cells, and a subset of B-cells and T-cells following activation and/or transformation by Epstein-Barr virus (EBV). It may also be found on some HRS-like cells in infectious mononucleosis, and on the neoplastic cells of some non-Hodgkin lymphomas (NHL).[17,19–21]

CD30

In search of viral antigens in HRS cells, the research team of Stein in 1981 generated polyclonal antibodies,[22] and one year later monoclonal antibodies,[23,24] against the Hodgkin lymphoma cell line L428. These studies led to the discovery of the Ki-1 molecule,[23,24] which was clustered as CD30 in 1987.[25] By molecular cloning, the CD30 antigen was identified as a cytokine receptor of the tumor necrosis factor receptor family.[26] Gene disruption and functional studies revealed that CD30 is involved in the negative selection of thymocytes and in the regulation of apoptosis and proliferation of activated lymphoid cells.[27–29] The CD30 antigen proved to be an ideal marker for HRS cells because it selectively labels HRS cells in tissues affected by classical Hodgkin lymphoma.[23,24,30] The detection of the CD30 molecule on some large perifollicular and intrafollicular blasts in normal lymphoid tissue, and the finding that expression of this molecule can be induced on normal peripheral blood B-cells and T-cells by mitogens and viruses such as EBV and human T-cell leukemia virus (HTLV) I and II,[30] indicate that the CD30 antigen does not represent a viral antigen but rather a differentiation antigen whose expression is associated with activation of lymphoid cells. The restriction of the occurrence of the CD30 antigen in normal subjects to occasional activated lymphoid cells favors a lymphocytic origin of HRS cells.[30]

B-Cell and T-Cell Marker Molecules

B-cell antigens (e.g., CD19, CD20, CD22, CD79a) or T-cell antigens (e.g., CD3, CD4, CD8, T-cell receptor (TCR) β-chain) are detected on variable proportions of HRS cells in approximately 10% to 20% of cases of classical Hodgkin lymphoma.[31–38] Although these findings were in harmony with the cell lineage characteristics of Hodgkin lymphoma cell lines (discussed later), they evoked much skepticism. Because

the B- and T-cell markers were not demonstrable in most cases of classical Hodgkin lymphoma, and when they were demonstrable it was only on varying proportions of HRS cells, it was widely believed that the detectability of B- and T-cell antigens on HRS cells represents an aberrant antigen expression phenomenon that does not permit any conclusions to be drawn concerning the cellular origin of HRS cells. Fortunately, the situation is clearer for L & H cells. These cells were shown to express constantly the B cell-associated molecules J chain,[18,39] CD20,[34,40] and CD79a,[37] and to lack CD30, CD15, and T-cell antigens,[10] indicating their distinctness from HRS cells and their derivation from B-cells.

Molecules Associated with Dendritic Cells

An interesting but not yet fully understood finding is the expression of restin,[41,42] fascin,[43] and thymus and activation regulated chemokine (TARC) by HRS cells.[44] All three molecules are expressed in normal tissues on dendritic cells.[43,45] These properties prompted some authors to believe that HRS cells are related to dendritic cells rather than to lymphoid cells. Beyond that, the expression of TARC could possibly explain the mechanism by which CD4-positive T-cells form rosettes around the HRS cells. TARC is a chemokine that attracts CD4-positive T-cells by binding to chemokine receptor 4 (CCR4).[44]

Conclusions of the Immunophenotypic Studies

In summary, the immunophenotypic studies agree that the L & H cells of lymphocyte-predominant Hodgkin lymphoma consistently carry B-cell antigens, so that their derivation from B-cells was generally suspected. For the HRS cells of classical Hodgkin lymphoma, the situation was less clear because these cells in most instances lack lineage-specific antigens and express some unusual molecules, including those characteristic of dendritic antigen-presenting cells. However, the antigen profile of the HRS cells pointed toward a derivation from activated lymphoid cells.

IN VITRO MODELS OF HODGKIN LYMPHOMA

Most attempts to establish permanently growing cell lines derived from a pure HRS cell population failed up until the late 1970s, mainly due to outgrowth of EBV-positive lymphoblastoid cell lines derived from short-term cultures of normal EBV-infected B-cells,[46] or contamination with nonhuman monkey kidney cells.[47] The first two permanent cell lines (designated L428 and L540) that were highly likely to be derived from HRS cells were established in Volker Diehl's laboratory in 1979.[48] Both cell lines were established from patients with advanced-stage Hodgkin lymphoma (CS IVB). The L428 line grew out from pleural effusion and the L540 cell line from bone marrow. With few exceptions, all other cell lines were also established from body fluids (pleural effusion, bone marrow, peripheral blood) of patients with advanced-stage lymphoma. Possibly, this observation reflects an in vivo adaption of the cells to the conditions of suspension culture as a prerequisite for in vitro outgrowth. These cell lines resembled in situ HRS cells in morphology, ability to bind T-cells to form rosettes, expression of certain cell surface markers such as major histocompatibility complex class II molecules, and absence of immunoglobulin and macrophage characteristics.[49]

More than ten bona fide Hodgkin lymphoma cell lines have been established (summarized in Table 5.2). Despite the close resemblance in immunophenotype, these cell lines are not generally accepted as being truly derived from HRS or L & H cells in all instances. Although two-thirds display a B-cell and one-third displays a T-cell phenotype and genotype, this ratio does not reflect the in vivo situation where B-cell cases far outnumber T-cell cases (>95%; see below). Furthermore, HRS cells are EBV-infected in 40% to 50% of classical Hodgkin lymphoma cases, whereas only one of the Hodgkin lymphoma cell lines (the L591 cell line) is EBV-positive. One of the cell lines (the HD-Myz cell line) differs strikingly from in situ HRS cells as it expresses the macrophage-associated CD68 antigen and lacks expression of CD30 and CD15 as well as rearrangement of immunoglobulin or TCR genes.[50]

It must be stressed in this context that for only one of the above-mentioned Hodgkin lymphoma cell lines (the L1236 cell line) a direct derivation from the in situ HRS cells was proven. L1236 cells harbor the same CDR3 sequences in the rearranged immunoglobulin genes as the in situ HRS cells of the patient from whom the cell line was established.[51,52] With the exception of the DEV cell line, all Hodgkin lymphoma cell lines established to date are derived from cases of classical Hodgkin lymphoma. DEV is a cell line that was established in Sibrand Poppema's laboratory from a case that originally was thought to be nodular-sclerosis Hodgkin lymphoma, but which subsequently was retyped as nodular lymphocyte-predominant

Hodgkin lymphoma.[53] This is in line with the observation that these cells are CD20-positive and express immunoglobulin, which is uncharacteristic of classical Hodgkin lymphoma but typical for lymphocyte-predominant Hodgkin lymphoma.

The establishment of Hodgkin lymphoma cell lines represents a very important step in the progress of Hodgkin lymphoma research, as these cells were used for the successful discovery of HRS cell-associated antigens such as CD30[23,24] or CD70,[54] as well as for the analysis of multiple signaling pathways in HRS cells. Lately, these cell lines are used together with animal models as preclinical models for targeted therapeutic approaches for Hodgkin lymphoma.

Analysis of primary tumor material fron patients with Hodgkin lymphoma is hampered by the fact that HRS cells represent only a minority of cells in the affected lymph nodes and that these cells rarely grow in vitro. Therefore, one has to consider animal models for Hodgkin lymphoma in order to study HRS cell biology in vivo. After subcutaneous transplantation in athymic T-cell deficient nude mice, neither primary HRS cells nor the Hodgkin lymphoma cell lines described above were tumorigenic.[55] Only after intracranial transplantation into nude mice was growth of Hodgkin lymphoma cell lines observed.[56] Severe combined immunodeficient (SCID) or nonobese diabetic (NOD)/SCID mice lacking functional B- and T-lymphocytes seem to be a better alternative to nude mice, as xenotransplanted Hodgkin lymphoma cell lines (L428, L540, L591, HDLM2, KMH2) did grow progressively after subcutaneous inoculation into SCID mice without prior

TABLE 5.2

IMMUNOPHENOTYPE AND GENOTYPE OF CELL LINES ESTABLISHED FROM CASES OF HODGKIN LYMPHOMA

Cell line[a]	CD30	CD15	B-AG	T-AG	Rearranged Ig or TCR gene	BCR or TCR expression	EBV	Reference
L428	+	+	−	−	IgH,L	−	−	48
L591	+	+/−	CD19, CD20	CD2	IgH,L	IgAλ	+	190
KM-H2	+	+	−	−	IgH,L	−	−	191
L540	+	(+)	−	−	TCRα,β,δ	−	−	190, 192
HO	+	−	−	CD3,5,7	TCRβ,δ	TCRβ?	−	193
HDLM2	+	+	−	CD2	TCRα,β,δ	−	−	194, 195
DEV[b]	+	+	CD20, CD22	−	IgH,L	cyIgA	−	196, 197
HD-70[c]	+	+	−	−	IgH,L	cyIgAκ	−	198
ZO[c]	+	+	−	−	IgH,L	nd	−	197
SUP-HD1[c]	−	+	−	−	IgH,L, TCRβ	κ	−	199
HD-MyZ[d]	−	−	−	−	−	−	−	50
L1236	+	+	−	−	IgH,L	−	−	52
HKB-1	+	+	CD19, CD20	−	IgH	nd	−	200

CD, cluster of differentiation; AG, antigen; Ig, immunoglobulin; BCR, B-cell receptor; EBV, Epstein-Barr virus; cy, cytoplasmic; TCR, T-cell receptor; +, constantly positive; (+) faintly positive; +/− variably positive; −, constantly negative; nd, not done

[a]One further cell line originally considered as Hodgkin lymphoma-derived, the CO line, was later identified as a cell culture contamination [201].

[b]This cell line was originally reported to derive from a case of classical Hodgkin lymphoma. However, the case was later reclassified as nodular lymphocyte-predominant Hodgkin lymphoma, so that DEV is presumably the first line derived from nodular lymphocyte-predominant Hodgkin lymphoma.

[c]It is not known whether these cell lines are still alive or whether the diagnosis of the primary material was correct; most of these cell lines have not been made available.

[d]This line has been established from a patient with nodular-sclerosis Hodgkin lymphoma. However, it is unlikely that the cell line is derived from the HRS cells because the HRS cells in the tissue biopsy specimen proved to be CD30+, CD15+, and CD68−, whereas the cell lines cells are CD30−, CD15−, and CD68+. Moreover, all informative Hodgkin lymphoma cases analyzed so far showed a B-cell or, rarely, a T-cell origin, whereas HD-Myz lacks immunoglobulin and TCR gene rearrangements and is hence of a nonlymphoid origin.

treatment of animals.[55] Based on these observations, Hodgkin lymphoma cell lines were also inoculated intravenously into the tail veins of SCID mice to achieve disseminated growth resembling the growth pattern of HRS cell in humans. When this approach was used, of three cell lines tested (L540, L428, and KMH2), only the L540 cell line gave rise to tumors.[57] After intravenous inoculation, L540 cells showed progressive disseminated growth and preferentially localized to lymph nodes, particularly the cervical, iliac, and inguinal nodes. The spleen was found to be involved only rarely. The disseminated SCID mouse model for the growth of Hodgkin lymphoma cells was used for preclinical testing of novel immunotherapeutic modalities, such as monoclonal CD30 antibodies. Although mice were cured in up to 100% of instances, clinical responses in humans were only modest, which might be attributed to the fact that patients with Hodgkin lymphoma are heavily pretreated due to multiple relapses before qualifying for clinical trials using experimental strategies.

Lymph node or spleen tissue affected by Hodgkin lymphoma was also transplanted into the subrenal capsule of SCID mice. From the material of 3 patients (from a total of 13), tumors of human origin deveoped and spread predominantly into the lymph nodes.[58] These tumors, however, did not consist of HRS cells. Rather, an outgrowth of EBV-positive B-lymphocytes was observed.[58] Of note, B-cells growing out from xenografted Hodgkin lymphoma tissue displayed a high number of numeric as well as structural chromosomal aberrations compared with EBV-positive B-cells growing out in SCID mice after transplantation of B cells from healthy donors.

In summary, the use of Hodgkin cell lines for in vitro studies provided invaluable insights into the pathogenesis of HRS cells in Hodgkin lymphoma. Furthermore, in vivo growth of these cell lines in SCID mice serves as a model for preclinical testing of novel treatment modalities such as immunotherapy or small molecules. Nevertheless, results obtained with these models are of limited use to predict efficacy of novel treatment strategies in patients with Hodgkin lymphoma. Therefore, new preclinical models are needed to validate more accurately the therapeutic potential of biologically based translational treatment strategies for patients with Hodgkin lymphoma in the future.

CLONALITY AND ORIGIN OF HRS AND L & H CELLS

HRS Cells in Classical Hodgkin Lymphoma

The origin of the HRS cells was much debated for a long time. This was mainly due to the rarity of these cells in the tumor tissue, which hampered their molecular analysis; and to their unusual immunophenotype, which does not resemble any normal cell in the hematopoietic system (discussed earlier). Moreover, as discussed, only a few cell lines could be established

TABLE 5.3

GENETIC AND PHENOTYPIC CHARACTERISTICS OF HRS AND L & H CELLS IN RELATION TO THEIR B-CELL ORIGIN

Feature	HRS cells in classical Hodgkin lymphoma	L & H cells in lymphocyte-predominant Hodgkin lymphoma
Somatically mutated Ig V genes	Yes	Yes
Destructive somatic mutations[a]	Yes (25%)	No
Ongoing somatic mutation	No	Yes
Proposed cellular origin	Pre-apoptotic germinal-center B-cell	Antigen-selected, mutating germinal-center B-cell
Expression of a BCR	No	Yes
Expression of B-cell–specific transcription factors (Oct-2, Bob1, Pu1)	Very rarely	Yes
Expression of B-lineage commitment factor Pax-5	Yes (low level)	Yes
Expression of B-cell surface molecules (CD20, CD79)	No or rarely	Yes
Expression of germinal center B-cell markers (bcl-6, AID)	Rarely	Yes
Expression of plasma cell markers (Mum1, CD138)	Often	No
Expression of molecules involved in antigen presentation (MHC class II, CD40, CD80, CD86)	Yes	Yes
Expression of markers for non–B-cells (e.g., TARC, granzyme B, CD15, CD3)	Occasionally/frequently	No
Rare cases with a T-cell origin	Yes (<2%)	No

[a]This refers to obviously crippling mutations that can be easily identified (e.g., nonsene mutations).

from Hodgkin lymphoma tissues. The origin of the HRS cells was finally clarified when microdissection and single-cell PCR methods were applied to single HRS cells to analyze them for immunoglobulin or TCR gene rearrangements. Immunoglobulin and TCR gene rearrangements are highly diverse and specific for B- and T-cells, respectively, thus representing ideal markers for clonality and a B- or T-cell origin of the cells carrying such rearrangements.[59] The single-cell studies showed that HRS cells of classical Hodgkin lymphoma in nearly all cases carry clonal immunoglobulin gene rearrangements, thereby establishing their clonality and B-cell lineage origin.[60–64] Nearly all cases carried somatically mutated immunoglobulin variable (V) gene rearrangements. Such mutations happen in antigen-activated B-cells participating in immune responses in germinal centers through the process of somatic hypermutation.[65] Thus, the detection of somatic mutations in the rearranged V-genes of HRS cells suggested that these cells were derived from germinal-center or postgerminal-center B-cells (Table 5.3). The V-gene sequences of the HRS cells obtained from a given case did not carry intraclonal sequence variations, showing that the somatic hypermutation process was silenced in the HRS cells. Surprisingly, 25% of cases of classical Hodgkin lymphoma carried somatic mutations that rendered originally functional V-gene rearrangements nonfunctional.[60–64,66,67] Such "crippling" somatic mutations included nonsense mutations and deletions. Germinal-center B-cells acquiring destructive somatic mutations normally very efficiently undergo apoptosis within

the germinal-center microenvironment and are removed by macrophages. Therefore, HRS cells carrying destructive V-gene mutations likely derive from pre-apoptotic germinal-center B-cells that escaped apoptosis (Fig. 5.1).[61,67,68] Importantly, nonsense mutations and deletions or duplications represent only a small fraction of disadvantageous mutations that cause apoptotic death of germinal-center B-cells. Many germinal-center B cells will undergo apoptosis because of unfavorable replacement mutations that impair proper folding of the antibody variable domain or heavy- and light-chain pairing, or that reduce the affinity of the antibody to the cognate antigen. As such mutations can usually not be easily identified, it is likely that HRS cells as a rule derive from crippled germinal-center B-cells (Table 5.3).

A few cases of classical Hodgkin lymphoma lack somatic mutations in their rearranged V-genes.[69,70] These cases may principally derive from pre-germinal-center, naive B-cells. However, as germinal-center founder cells start to proliferate and become sensitive for apoptosis even before the onset of somatic hypermutation,[71] the unmutated Hodgkin lymphoma cases may well derive from germinal-center founder cells, and it is indeed to be expected that among the pool of pre-apoptotic germinal-center B cells, there are cells that are driven into apoptosis even before the hypermutation machinery is activated.

As lymphocyte-rich classical Hodgkin lymphoma was only recently recognized as a distinct subtype of Hodgkin lymphoma and grouped together with the other types of classical

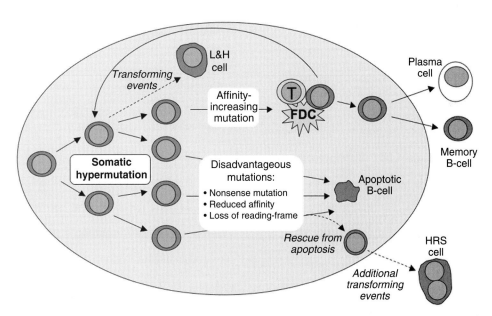

FIGURE 5.1. B-cell differentiation processes in the germinal center and scenario for the generation of HRS and L & H cells. Antigen-activated B cells migrate into B-cell follicles of secondary lymphoid organs and establish germinal centers[189]. Germinal-center B-cells undergo clonal expansion and activate the process of somatic hypermutation that introduces mutations at a high rate into rearranged immunoglobulin variable genes. Germinal-center B-cells acquiring affinity-increasing mutations are positively selected by interaction with T-helper cells and follicular dendritic cells. Presumably after repeated rounds of proliferation, mutation, and selection, positively selected B-cells differentiate into memory B-cells or plasma cells and leave the germinal center. Most somatic mutations are disadvantageous for germinal-center B-cells, such as amino acid replacement mutations resulting in reduced affinity to the immunizing antigen or deletions that result in loss of the correct reading-frame. Germinal-center B-cells with such unfavorable mutations are functionally crippled and undergo programmed cell death (apoptosis). The pattern of somatic mutations in rearranged immunoglobulin genes of HRS cells from classical Hodgkin lymphoma indicates that these cells are derived from the pool of pre-apoptotic, crippled germinal-center B-cells. The reason for the apoptosis resistance of the HRS cell precursors is largely unclear, but may involve several distinct transforming events, such as EBV infection in a fraction of the cases. The L & H cells of lymphocyte-predominant Hodgkin lymphoma lack crippling mutations, express a BCR, and often show intraclonal V-gene diversity, indicating hypermutation activity during clonal expansion. L & H cells hence appear to derive from selected, mutating germinal-center B-cells.

Hodgkin lymphoma (discussed earlier),[10] this prompted a molecular V-gene analysis of several such cases. That study supported the assignment of lymphocyte-rich classical Hodgkin lymphoma to classical Hodgkin lymphoma, because the HRS cells lacked intraclonal V-gene diversity like the HRS cells of the other types of classical Hodgkin lymphoma and cases with crippled B-cell receptor (BCR) were identified.[72]

Rare T-Cell Origin of HRS Cells in Classical Hodgkin Lymphoma

Since HRS cells in about 5% to 15% of cases of classical Hodgkin lymphoma express one or more molecules normally expressed by T-cells (e.g., granzyme B, perforin, CD3), such cases were analyzed for a potential T-cell derivation. In three studies of a total of 27 cases, clonal TCR gene rearrangements were identified in 5 of the lymphomas.[73–75] Thus, in very rare cases (likely less than 2%), HRS cells may derive from T-cells. The differentiation stage of the respective T-cell precursors of the HRS cells, and whether these were pre-apoptotic T-lymphocytes, is unclear. Importantly, most of the Hodgkin lymphoma cases with partial T-cell phenotype of the HRS cells lack TCR gene rearrangements and carry rearranged immunoglobulin V-genes, showing that T-cell markers can be aberrantly expressed by B- lineage-derived HRS cells.[73,74]

HRS Cells as Cell Fusions?

The unusual immunophenotype of the HRS cells, often showing coexpression of markers typical for distinct hematopoietic cell types, and the frequent detection of additional chromosomal copies even in the mononucleated Hodgkin cells, prompted speculations that the HRS cell clones may derive from cell fusion.[76,77] In light of the consistent detection of clonal immunoglobulin gene rearrangements in HRS cells, it was principally possible that the HRS cell clones may stem from fusion between a B-cell and a non-B-cell. Because non-B-cells have their IgH alleles in germline configuration, while most B-cells carry two rearranged IgH alleles, several cases of classical Hodgkin lymphoma with B-cell origin were analyzed for the presence of immunoglobulin loci in germline configuration in addition to two rearranged immunoglobulin loci. However, in none of the cases were additional germline IgH alleles observed.[78] Similarly, in a case of T-cell–derived Hodgkin lymphoma, no TCRβ alleles in germline configuration were found in addition to two clonal TCRβ gene rearrangements.[78] Therefore, these results argue against a role of cell fusion in HRS cell generation.

Regarding the relationship between the mononucleated Hodgkin and the multinucleated Reed-Sternberg cells, there is evidence that Reed-Sternberg cells develop from Hodgkin cells by endomitosis.[79,80]

L & H Cells in Lymphocyte-Predominant Hodgkin Lymphoma

The expression of multiple B-cell markers by the L & H cells in lymphocyte-predominant Hodgkin lymphoma already suggested their B-cell origin (discussed earlier). This was molecularly proven by the demonstration of clonal immunoglobulin gene rearrangements in the L & H cells.[62,81–83] All cases analyzed so far carried somatically mutated V-genes.[62,81,82] In many of the cases, intraclonal V-gene diversification was observed, indicating ongoing hypermutation activity during clonal expansion.[62,81,82] As active hypermutation is a

hallmark of germinal-center B-cells,[65] this indicates a germinal-center B-cell origin of the L & H cells (Table 5.3). This is supported by the expression of the germinal-center B-cell–specific transcription factor Bcl-6 by these cells and their positivity for activation-induced cytidine deaminase (AID), an enzyme that plays a key role in somatic hypermutation and immunoglobulin class switching, and that is mainly expressed by germinal center B-cells.[84,85] At variance to the situation in classical Hodgkin lymphoma, no lymphocyte-predominant Hodgkin lymphoma cases with crippling mutations have been found. Thus, L & H cells appear to represent transformed selected, mutating germinal-center B-cells.

COMPOSITE LYMPHOMAS

In very rare instances, Hodgkin and non-Hodgkin lymphoma occur in the same patient, either concurrently or sequentially. A key issue regarding the pathogenesis of composite lymphomas is whether they represent a chance occurrence of two independent lymphomas in the same patient, or whether the two malignancies are clonally related and hence have a common derivation. This question has been addressed by performing immunoglobulin V-gene studies in microdissected HRS cells of classical Hodgkin lymphoma and B-NHL cells.[86–88] In a few cases, distinct clonal origins of the lymphomas were reported,[89–91] but in the majority of cases, the HRS and B-NHL cells were found to harbour the same V-gene rearrangements, proving the clonal relationship of the two lymphomas.[70,86–88,92–95] The identification of a common origin of HRS cells of classical Hodgkin lymphoma and B-NHL derived from mature B-cells in these composite lymphomas is a further strong argument for the B-cell derivation of HRS cells.

The clonally related V-gene rearrangements carried by the HRS and B-NHL cells in most composite lymphomas showed both identical, shared somatic mutations as well as mutations that were present only in the HRS or the B-NHL cells. Because immunoglobulin V-gene diversification by somatic hypermutation happens in germinal-center B-cells in the course of their clonal expansion, this finding indicates that the common precursor of the two lymphomas was a germinal-center B-cell that had already acquired some somatic V-gene mutations, and that the lymphomas developed from distinct descendents of that common precursor (Fig. 5.2). Therefore, the somatic mutation pattern reveals that such lymphomas usually do not develop as the transformation of one malignant clone into another, but as a parallel transformation of two members of a (pre-malignant) B-cell clone.

The association between B-cell chronic lymphocytic leukemia (B-CLL) and HRS cells not only includes concurrent composite lymphomas of B-CLL and Hodgkin lymphoma and "transformation" of B-CLL into Hodgkin lymphoma (Hodgkin lymphoma variant of Richter syndrome), but also cases of B-CLL in which HRS-like cells are detectable intermingled with B-CLL cells without the typical cellular infiltrate of Hodgkin lymphoma.[96,97] These scattered HRS-like cells represent monoclonal populations and are often infected by EBV.[95,96,98] Notably, although EBV-negative Hodgkin lymphoma or HRS-like cells combined with B-CLL are mostly clonally related and hence share a common origin, EBV-positive HRS-like clones are mostly unrelated to the B-CLL.[87,95,96,98] This suggests that an EBV-infected B-cell with the morphology of HRS cells may sometimes clonally expand in the setting of a B-CLL and perhaps represents a precursor for an EBV-positive case of Hodgkin lymphoma developing on the background of the B-CLL.

Classical Hodgkin lymphoma not only can be combined with B-NHL but also with T-cell lymphomas. In three instances,

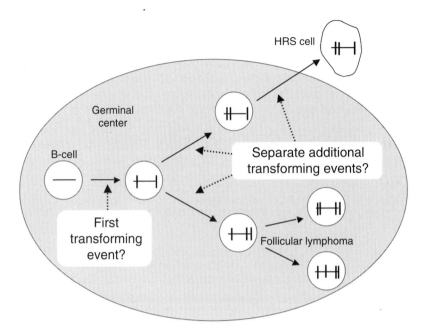

FIGURE 5.2. Scenario for the development of composite lymphomas. The horizontal lines within the cells indicate a V-gene rearrangement; vertical lines within the cells indicate somatic mutations. The somatic mutation patterns in most clonally related composite lymphomas analyzed indicates that the two lymphomas do not represent a transformation of one lymphoma into the other, but the parallel transformation of two "sister" cells into the two distinct lymphomas. The shared, premalignant precursor of both lymphomas was likely a germinal-center B-cell. This scenario for the development of composite lymphomas indicates that there are both shared transforming events, present already in the common tumor precursor, and distinct transforming events that are restricted to one or the other of the two lymphomas. First examples supporting this scenario have recently been described.[108]

combinations of classical Hodgkin and T-cell lymphomas have been molecularly analyzed.[99–101] Also in these cases, indication or proof for a common origin was obtained, further confirming that in rare instances HRS cells derive from T-cells.

About 3% to 5% of patients with lymphocyte-predominant Hodgkin lymphoma develop diffuse large B-cell lymphomas. It has been speculated that the B-NHL developing after lymphocyte-predominant Hodgkin lymphoma represents transformations of the L & H cells, but only a few of these cases have indeed shown a clonal relationship at the molecular level.[102–107] However, one has to take into consideration that whole-tissue DNA was analyzed in some of the studies, so that the clonal rearrangement of the L & H cells might have been missed due to their rarity in the tissue. In addition, even in studies using sensitive diffuse large B-cell lymphoma-specific primers to search for the same rearrangement in the lymphocyte-predominant Hodgkin lymphoma biopsies, it may well be that amplification of a clonally related rearrangement in the L & H cells failed due to distinct somatic mutation patterns, as they were frequently seen in combinations of classical Hodgkin lymphoma and B-NHL, as described earlier.

In cases of clonally related composite lymphomas, the multistep transformation process of lymphomagenesis and the development of two distinct tumors from a shared precursor can be studied. So far, six clonally related composite lymphomas were analyzed for shared and distinct transforming events.[108] In two combinations of Hodgkin lymphoma and follicular lymphoma, bcl-2/IgH translocations, which are a hallmark of follicular lymphomas, were identified not only in the follicular lymphomas but also in the HRS cells. Similarly, in a composite mantle cell and Hodgkin lymphoma the same bcl-1/IgH translocation (the hallmark of mantle-cell lymphomas) was detected in both lymphoma clones. Thus, this shows at the DNA sequence level that HRS cells can harbor IgH-associated translocations and such translocations involving bcl-2 or bcl-1 can represent an early step in the pathogenesis of composite lymphomas.[108] In a composite Hodgkin lymphoma and diffuse large B-cell lymphoma, clonal replacement mutations of the p53 gene on both alleles were found exclusively in the diffuse large B-cell lymphoma, exemplifying a late-transforming event, and suggesting that the p53 mutations happened in a germinal-center B-cell that was the precursor of the diffuse large B-cell lymphoma.

LOSS OF THE B-CELL PHENOTYPE OF HRS CELLS

Immunohistochemical studies showed down-regulation of numerous B-cell markers, such as CD20, CD79, Oct-2, Bo, and Pu.1 in the HRS cells of classical Hodgkin lymphoma.[109–112] The lack of expression of transcription factors regulating immunoglobulin gene transcription (Oct-2, Bob1, und Pu.1) most likely also explains the absence or very low level of immunoglobulin gene transcription observed in HRS cells.[110] However, there is now an indication that the immunoglobulin loci are also silenced by epigenetic mechanisms, in particular DNA methylation.[113] This epigenetic silencing by promoter methylation not only affects the immunoglobulin genes but also other B-cell–specific genes, such as Pu.1, CD19, CD79b, and Bob1.[114,115]

Gene expression profiling studies of Hodgkin lymphoma cell lines (L428, L1236, KMH2, HDLM2) and normal mature B-cells as well as the main types of B-cell NHL revealed that the down-regulation of B-cell–specific genes is much more general than indicated from earlier studies.[116] Decreased mRNA levels of the vast majority of known B-lineage–specific genes in the HRS cells were identified.[116] The down-regulated genes include components of the BCR signaling pathway (e.g., Blk, Syk, SLP-65), transcription factors (e.g., Pu.B, A-myb, Spi-B), and surface markers (e.g., CD37, CD53). Thus, there appears to be a global loss of the B-cell phenotype of HRS cells in classical Hodgkin lymphoma.

Because normal B-cells are stringently selected for expression of a BCR throughout their life, one may speculate that there is a connection between the proposed origin of HRS cells from crippled germinal-center B-cells and their global loss of the B-cell phenotype. Perhaps a germinal-center B-cell that, because of unfavorable immunoglobulin V-gene mutations, fails to express a high-affinity BCR and normally would undergo apoptosis, can escape the selection for expression of a (high-affinity) BCR by losing its B-cell identity, and hence also expression of the signaling machinery that induces apoptosis upon loss of (high-affinity) BCR expression. However, although not mutually exclusive, the lost B-cell identity of HRS cells could also reflect an involvement of transforming events in the pathogenesis of classical Hodgkin lymphoma that renders the cells independent from the normal survival signals of B-cells, enabling these cells to adopt another phenotype.

Because down-regulation of many B-cell markers is also a feature of plasma cells, and because it was reported that HRS cells in a large fraction of cases express the plasma cell marker CD138, it has been proposed that HRS cells may derive from postgerminal-center (plasma) cells.[84,117] However, the CD138-positivity of HRS cells could not be confirmed in other studies,[118] and the lack of expression of immunoglobulin and the plasma cell marker BLIMP-1,[110,119] and the retained expression of Pax-5 and MHC class II, are not compatible with a plasma cell phenotype. Thus, although some aspects of the HRS cell phenotype resemble plasma cells, there are major differences in key features of their gene-expression patterns.

The down-regulation of B-cell–specific molecules does not include factors important for antigen presentation (CD40, CD80, CD86, MHC class II), implying that it is essential for HRS cells to retain antigen-presenting capacities.[120] Moreover, as already described earlier, also the transcription factor Pax-5, a key B-cell lineage commitment and maintenance factor, is still expressed by HRS cells, although several of its direct target genes are not expressed.[121]

SIGNALING PATHWAYS ACTIVE IN HRS AND L & H CELLS

The heterodimeric NFκB is a key transcription factor involved in many inflammatory and immunologic processes. Activation of several cell-surface receptors (e.g., CD40) leads to degradation of the NFκB inhibitor IκBα or other members of the IκB family, that normally bind to NFκB and prevent its translocation into the cell nucleus. Inactivation of IκB is mediated by IκB kinases (IKK), which phosphorylate IκB and cause its ubiquitination and degradation. Upon degradation of IκB, NFκB can move into the nucleus and activate expression of multiple genes. NFκB (p65/RelA) was first described in 1996 to be constitutively active in Hodgkin lymphoma cell lines[122] and to be critical for HRS cell survival in vivo in SCID mice.[123] NFκB has been shown to mediate both proliferative and anti-apoptotic gene expression programmes in HRS cells.[124] Inhibition of NFκB activity and induction of spontaneous cell death in Hodgkin lymphoma cell line cells by overexpression of an IκBα super-repressor has provided further evidence that NFκB is critical for HRS cell suriival.[124] NFκB therefore might be regarded as a transforming master switch for HRS cells in Hodgkin lymphoma, although constitutive NFκB activation is not a specific feature of HRS cells but is also characteristic for inflammatory disease and other lymphomas, such as a subset of diffuse large B-cell lymphomas.

There are various explanations for NFκB up-regulation in HRS cells: gene amplification of c-rel[125,126]; activation of cell-surface receptors such as CD30,[127] CD40,[128] RANK,[129] or Notch1[130]; expression of viral latent membrane proteins 1 (LMP1) and LMP2a in EBV-positive cases; or loss-of-function mutations of the NFκB suppressor IκBα or IκBε (see below).

Upon TNFR ligation, NFκB activation is induced via TRAF signaling[127,131] and the mitogen-activated protein kinase (MAPK) pathway.[132] It has been shown that activation of the MEK kinase leads to phosphorylation of downstream ERK in HRS cells, thus promoting cell survival.[132] Inhibition of ERK phosphorylation was efficient in inhibiting ligand-induced cell survival in HRS cell lines. Of note, CD30 signaling has recently been linked to the non-canonical NFκB activation pathway involving RelB/p52 in HRS cells.[133]

Analysis of the PI3K/AKT signaling cascade revealed constitutive activity of this pathway in HRS cell lines, which has been linked to IL6 secretion and expression of EHG homeobox gene HLXB9 of HRS cells in vitro.[134] It has been demonstrated that targeting of the PI3K/AKT pathway with small molecule inhibitors might be of potential use for future treatment strategies in patients with Hodgkin lymphoma.[135]

The activator protein 1 (AP-1) complex is formed by hetero- or homodimers of jun, Fos, and ATF family proteins. In Hodgkin lymphoma and also in anaplastic large-cell lymphoma (ALCL) but not in other lymphoma entities, c-jun and junB have been decribed to be aberrantly expressed in the malignant cell population.[136] C-jun seems to be the major transactivating force of the constitutive AP-1 complex. Its activity in HRS cells is independent of JNK but relies on an unknown autoregulatory mechanism, whereas junB activity is NFκB dependent.[136] Both c-jun and junB support proliferation of HRS cells, possibly via induction of cyclin D2 and c-MET expression.[136]

Notch1 is a cell transmembrane receptor that upon ligand binding is cleaved, so that the intracellular domain can translocate into the nucleus and function as a transcription factor.[137] Notch1 signaling plays an important role in various cell fate decisions, including B- and T-cell development: In Notch1 expressing lymphoid precursors B-cell development is suppressed and T-cell differentiation is promoted.[137] With this background, it was surprising that strong Notch1 expression was detected in B-cell–derived HRS cells.[130] The Notch1 ligand Jagged1 is expressed in HRS cells and also in other cells in the tumor tissue, suggesting that Notch1 is activated and functioning in HRS cells.[130] This is supported by studies with Hodgkin lymphoma cell lines, which showed that activation of Notch1 promotes cell proliferation and survival,[130] although another study could not verify the growth-promoting effect of Notch1 activation in a Hodgkin lymphoma line.[138] The aberrant expression of Notch1 in HRS cells may also contribute to the lost B-cell phenotype of HRS cells discussed above, although the B- cell–specific target genes inhibited by Notch1 are still largely unknown.

Many cytokines signal through the Jak/STAT pathway. Upon cytokine receptor activation, Jak kinases become activated, and these can then phosphorylate members of the STAT family of transcription factors. Posphorylated STATs can enter the cell nucleus and activate transcription of target genes. In HRS cells, STAT3, STAT5a, and STAT6 are expressed and constitutively activated.[139,140] The activation of STAT6 is likely mediated by an autocrine stimulation loop, because this factor is activated by Il-13R signaling, and HRS cells express both Il-13 and the Il-13R.[140,141] For STAT5a, it has been shown that both its expression as well as its activation is positively regulated by NFκB activitiy in HRS cells.[139] STAT signaling is presumably important for HRS cell proliferation, because inhibition of Il-13 signaling or STAT3 activity in Hodgkin lymphoma cell lines inhibits cell proliferation.[142–144]

Based on gene expression profiling studies, aberrant expression of multiple receptor tyrosine kinases, which are not normally expressed by B-cells, was recently identified in Hodgkin lymphoma.[145] The coexpression of several receptor tyrosine kinases, including PDGFRA, DDR2, EPHB1, RON, TRKA, and TRKB, was most pronounced in classical Hodgkin lymphoma, but was also identified in lymphocyte-predominant Hodgkin lymphoma. Activation of these tyrosine kinases was implicated by the phosphorylation of several kinases themselves and by an elevated phospho-tyrosine content of the HRS cells in a considerable fraction of cases.[145] The receptor tyrosine kinase activity seems not to be due to somatic mutations, but to ligand-induced activation, as the ligands for several of the tyrosine kinases were detected in the cells surrounding the HRS cells or in the HRS cells themselves, indicating both paracrine and autocrine activation mechanisms.[145] A coexpression and activation of multiple receptor tyrosine kinases appears to be unique to Hodgkin lymphoma among lymphoid malignancies and suggests that this activation may play a central role in Hodgkin lymphoma pathogenesis. However, the critical downstream targets of the kinase activities remain to be identified.

In summary, multiple signaling pathways are aberrantly activated in HRS cells in vitro and in vivo and critically contribute to the proliferation and survival of the HRS cells. For some of the signaling pathways mechanisms for their aberrant and constitutive activation were elucidated in recent years. Future functional studies using knockdown experiments such as RNA interference technology might help to clarify the relative contribution of each of the mentioned pathways for the pathogenesis of Hodgkin lymphoma.

ROLE OF EBV IN HODGKIN LYMPHOMA PATHOGENESIS

In about 40% of cases of classical Hodgkin lymphoma in the western world, the HRS cells are infected by EBV.[146] EBV persists throughout the course of the disease and shows a monoclonal pattern of infection, suggesting an involvement of the virus in the pathogenesis of such cases of Hodgkin lymphoma.[147] In EBV-positive cases of Hodgkin lymphoma, three viral proteins are expressed, the EBV nuclear antigen 1 (EBNA1) and the latent membrane proteins LMP1 and LMP2a.[146] EBNA1 is essential for replication of the viral genome, but may have some additional functions.[146] LMP1 mimics an activated CD40 receptor that has a central role in B-cell differentiation and the survival of germinal-center B-cells.[148] LMP2a harbors a cytoplasmatic motif that is also found in the coreceptors of the BCR and that mediates signal transduction of cross-linked BCR.[149] Through this motif, LMP2a recruits cytoplasmic kinases that normally bind to the BCR and thereby mimic an immunoglobulin receptor. The capability of LMP2a to replace the function of the BCR as an essential survival signal for B-cells was recently shown in transgenic mice expressing LMP2a already in B-cell precursors. In these mice, Ig-negative B-cells lacking productive immunoglobulin heavy-chain rearrangements can bypass normal developmental checkpoints and colonize peripheral lymphoid organs.[150,151] If LMP2a has a similar function in germinal-center B-cells that acquired unfavorable somatic mutations in their BCR, so that they fail to receive appropriate survival signals through their BCR, LMP2a may rescue such germinal-center B-cells from apoptosis. Hence, LMP2a may play an important role in the pathogenesis of EBV-positive Hodgkin lymphoma.

The capability of EBV to rescue BCR-deficient human germinal-center B-cells from apoptosis was recently directly tested in three studies.[152–154] In these studies tonsillar germinal-center B-cells were isolated and infected in vitro with EBV to establish lymphoblastoid cell lines. Among the monoclonal cell lines, several lines were identified that carried destructive mutations rendering originally functional immunoglobulin V-gene rearrangements nonfunctional. These destructive mutations were most likely introduced by somatic hypermutation in the germinal center and normally would have caused rapid cell death. Thus, EBV is principally capable of rescuing BCR-deficient germinal-center B-cells from apoptosis, further supporting a role of EBV in the pathogenesis of Hodgkin lymphoma.

The role of EBV in the rescue of crippled germinal-center B-cells that lost the capacity to express a BCR is additionally substantiated by an analysis of somatic mutation patterns in V-genes of HRS cells from classical Hodgkin lymphoma and the EBV status of the cases. This analysis revealed a striking correlation between the detection of crippling mutations preventing BCR expression (e.g., nonsense mutations generating stop codons) and the presence of EBV in the HRS cells.[155] Of 12 cases of classical Hodgkin lymphoma with such crippling mutations, 11 were EBV-infected, and the only EBV-negative case typed as crippled is perhaps not entirely impaired to express a BCR, as it carries a point mutation in the heavy-chain promoter octamer motif and has a Vκ leader peptide with two additional amino acids, so that it cannot be ruled out that these mutations would still allow BCR expression.[66] Among 43 cases lacking evidence for crippling mutations, 19 were EBV-positive, a fraction close to the overall frequency of EBV-positive Hodgkin lymphoma cases. Thus, (nearly) all cases of Hodgkin lymphoma with crippling mutations that prevent BCR expression are EBV-positive. As discussed in more detail elsewhere,[155] this finding indicates that a germinal-center B-cell that had acquired BCR-destructive mutations can survive and become a precursor of an HRS tumor clone only if it is EBV-infected. Presumably, the BCR-substituting function of LMP2a is needed to replace the tonic BCR survival signal. In HRS cell precursors that acquired disadvantageous somatic mutations still allowing BCR expression (e.g., replacement mutations reducing affinity to the respective antigen), lymphoma development can occur by other mechanisms, because such cells are apparently not dependent on the LMP2a gene as a substitute for the BCR.

The association between crippling mutations and presence of EBV also implies that EBV infection is an early event in Hodgkin lymphoma pathogenesis, before or at the time when the crippling mutations happened and when the HRS cell precursors still had a B-cell phenotype and were dependent on BCR expression. In the established HRS cell clone LMP2a may be less important, because HRS cells have lost their B-cell phenotype and expression of the key signaling molecules for BCR (or LMP2a) signaling,[156] so that HRS cells presumably no longer depend on the BCR or its substitute LMP2a. Indeed, LMP2a expression is detected by immunohistochemistry only in about half of EBV-positive cases of Hodgkin lymphoma.[157]

TRANSFORMING MECHANISMS IN HRS AND L & H CELLS

Numerical and structural chromosome abnormalities are detected in most cases of classical Hodgkin lymphoma in the HRS cell population.[158] Although it is known from classical cytogenetic studies that several breakpoints such as 3q27, 6q15, 7q22, 11q23, and 14q32 are detected nonrandomly at a higher frequency in HRS cells,[159] known translocation partners such as BCL6, MYC, and MALT1 were identified only in a minority of cases.[160] Similarly, translocations typically found in follicular lymphoma and anaplastic large-cell lymphoma, that is, t(14;18)(q32;q21) and t(2;5)(p23;q35), which involve the bcl-2 gene and the alk gene, respectively, are not or only very rarely found in HRS cells (Table 5.4).[161–163] Similar to most other B-cell lymphomas, HRS cells do not display a mutator phenotype.[164]

Applying whole-genome approaches such as comparative genomic hybridization (CGH), recurrent genomic imbalances were detected in most cases of classical Hodgkin lymphoma. Among these imbalances, 2p13-p16, 9p23-p24, and 12q14 were involved most frequently affecting the c-rel, Jak2, and MDM2 gene loci, respectively.[125,126,165,166] The observed gene amplifications have been shown to have functional consequences in that a higher Jak2 gene copy number might account for constitutively phosphorylated STAT proteins observed in HRS cells. MDM2 gene amplifications possibly result in increased amounts of MDM2 protein that is known

TABLE 5.4

ONCOGENE AND TUMOR SUPPRESSOR GENE ALTERATIONS IN HRS CELLS
OF CLASSICAL HODGKIN LYMPHOMA[a]

Gene name	Material studied	Total no. cases	No. mutated cases[b]	Reference
Bcl-2	Single cells	115	0	161
	Single cells	2[c]	2	108
N-Ras	Single cells	12	0	173
P53	Single cells	4	0	166
	Single cells	8	0	168
	Enriched cells	26	3	167
IκBα	Enriched cells	8	2	179
	Single cells	10	1	180
	Single cells	5	2	181
IκBε	Single cells	6	1	182
CD95[d]	Single cells	10	1	171
	Enriched cells	20	1	170
SOCS-1	Single cells	19	8	178

[a]Several mutations were also identified in Hodgkin lymphoma cell lines: p53 in HDLM2[169], IκBα in L428, and KMH2[179–181], IκBε in L428[182], and CD95 in L1236.[170]
[b]Translocations in the case of bcl-2
[c]Composite follicular lymphoma and Hodgkin lymphoma.
[d]Only one of the mutations affects the death domain, although the functional importance of the other mutations remains unclear.

to bind and block the transactivation domain of p53. This could explain the well-documented overexpression of wild-type p53 in Hodgkin lymphoma-affected tissue. Mutations in the p53 gene itself occur only rarely in HRS cells.[166–169] Similar to p53, other tumor-suppressor genes such as CD95[170–172] and oncogenes such as n-ras[173] were also shown to lack genetic mutations in most cases (Table 5.4). Caspase 8, caspase 10, or the FADD genes, which are additional members of the CD95 signaling pathway, were analyzed for inactivating mutations, as HRS cells were shown to be apoptosis resistant despite wild-type CD95 expression, but no mutations were identified in these genes.[174] There is now strong evidence that the resistance of HRS cells against CD95-mediated apoptosis induction is indeed due to strong expression of cFLIP, a negative regulator of CD95 signaling.[170,175–177]

Recently, frequent mutations in the SOCS1 gene, an inhibitor of STAT signaling, were detected in HRS cells of classical Hodgkin lymphoma, suggesting that SOCS1 inactivation acts as a tumor suppressor in Hodgkin lymphoma, contributing to constitutive STAT activity.[178]

Constitutive NFκB activity might be considered a transforming event for Hodgkin lymphoma as its activity has been shown to be crucial for HRS cell survival.[123] Genetic mechanisms that are likely involved in NFκB upregulation include c-rel gene amplifications,[125,126] somatic IκBα mutations in approximately 30% of cases,[179–181] and, rarely, IκBε mutations.[182] Notably, IκBα mutations are not found in the ABC type of diffuse large B-cell lymphoma that is also characterized by high activity of the NFκB transcription factor.[183]

Little is known about the transforming events involved in the pathogenesis of lymphocyte-predominant Hodgkin lymphoma. L & H cells have been described to harbor bcl-6 gene translocations in a considerable fraction of cases.[184,185] A recent study also found recurrent gains of 2q, 4q, 5q, 6, and 11q in L & H cells using CGH. It was speculated that these regions might be more specifically associated with the pathogenesis of lymphocyte-predominant Hodgkin lymphoma.[186] Finally, aberrant somatic hypermutation of several protooncogenes (Pax5, c-myc, RhoH/TTF, Pim1), as is seen at high frequency specifically in diffuse large B-cell lymphomas but not other B-NHL,[187] was recently reported to occur frequently also in L & H cells.[188] The pathogenetic relevance of these mutations remains to be clarified.

References

1. Hodgkin T. On some morbid appearances of the absorbent glands and spleen. *Med Chir Trans* 1832;17:68–114.
2. Wilks S. Cases of lardaceous disease and some allied affections, with remarks. *Guy's Hosp Rep* 1856;17:103–132.
3. Wilks S. Enlargement of the lymphatic glands and spleen (or, Hodgkin's disease), with remarks. *Guy's Hosp Rep* 1865;11:56–57.
4. Langhans T. Das maligne Lymphosarkom (Pdeudoleukämie). *Virchows Arch Pathol Anat* 1872;54:509–536.
5. Greenfield WS. Specimens illustrative of the pathology of lymphadenoma and leucocythemia. *Trans Pathol Soc London* 1878;29:272–304.
6. Sternberg C. Über eine eigenartige unter dem Bilde der Pseudoleukämie verlaufende Tuberkolose des lymphatischen Apparates. *Z Heilkunde* 1898;19:21–90.
7. Reed D. On the pathological changes in Hodgkin's disease with special reference to its relation to tuberculosis. *John Hopkins Hosp Rep* 1902;10:133–193.
8. Lukes RJ, Butler JJ. The pathology and nomenclature of Hodgkin's disease. *Cancer Res* 1966;26:1063–1083.
9. Neiman RS. Current problems in the histopathologic diagnosis and classification of Hodgkin's disease. *Pathol Annu* 1978;13Pt 2:289–328.
10. Anagnostopoulos I, Hansmann ML, Franssila K, et al. European Task Force on Lymphoma project on lymphocyte predominance Hodgkin disease: histologic and immunohistologic analysis of submitted cases reveals 2 types of Hodgkin disease with a nodular growth pattern and abundant lymphocytes. *Blood* 2000;96:1889–1899.
11. Mason DY, Banks PM, Chan J, et al. Nodular lymphocyte predominance Hodgkin's disease. A distinct clinicopathological entity. *Am J Surg Pathol* 1994;18:526–530.

12. Hansmann ML, Zwingers T, Boske A, et al. Clinical features of nodular paragranuloma (Hodgkin's disease, lymphocyte predominance type, nodular). *J Cancer Res Clin Oncol* 1984;108:321–330.

13. Harris NL, Jaffe ES, Stein H, et al. A revised European-American classification of lymphoid neoplasms: a proposal from the International Lymphoma Study Group. *Blood* 1994;84:1361–1392.

14. Jaffe ES, Harris NL, Stein H, et al. *WHO classification of tumors: pathology and genetics of tumors of haematopoietic and lymphoid tissues.* Lyon: IARC Press; 2001.

15. Stein H, Uchanska-Ziegler B, Gerdes J, et al. Hodgkin and Sternberg-Reed cells contain antigens specific to late cells of granulopoiesis. *Int J Cancer* 1982;29:283–290.

16. Schienle HW, Stein N, Muller-Ruchholtz W. Neutrophil granulocytic cell antigen defined by a monoclonal antibody—its distribution within normal haemic and non-haemic tissue. *J Clin Pathol* 1982;35:959–966.

17. Pinkus GS, Thomas P, Said JW. Leu-M1—a marker for Reed-Sternberg cells in Hodgkin's disease. An immunoperoxidase study of paraffin-embedded tissues. *Am J Pathol* 1985;119:244–252.

18. Stein H, Hansmann ML, Lennert K, et al. Reed-Sternberg and Hodgkin cells in lymphocyte-predominant Hodgkin's disease of nodular subtype contain J chain. *Am J Clin Pathol* 1986;86:292–297.

19. Knapp W, Dörken B, Gilks WR, et al. 1989. Appendix A: CD guide. In: Knapp W, Dörken B, Gilks WR, eds. *Leucocyte typing IV—activation antigens.* New York: Oxford University Press; 1074.

20. Sheibani K, Battifora H, Burke JS, et al. Leu-M1 antigen in human neoplasms. An immunohistologic study of 400 cases. *Am J Surg Pathol* 1986;10:227–236.

21. Wieczorek R, Burke JS, Knowles DM II. Leu-M1 antigen expression in T-cell neoplasia. *Am J Pathol* 1985;121:374–380.

22. Stein H, Gerdes J, Kirchner H, et al. Hodgkin and Sternberg-Reed cell antigen(s) detected by an antiserum to a cell line (L428) derived from Hodgkin's disease. *Int J Cancer* 1981;28:425–429.

23. Schwab U, Stein H, Gerdes J, et al. Production of a monoclonal antibody specific for Hodgkin and Sternberg-Reed cells of Hodgkin's disease and a subset of normal lymphoid cells. *Nature* 1982;299:65–67.

24. Stein H, Gerdes J, Schwab U, et al. Identification of Hodgkin and Sternberg-Reed cells as a unique cell type derived from a newly-detected small-cell population. *Int J Cancer* 1982;30:445–459.

25. Schwarting R, Gerdes J, Stein H. Ber-H2: a new monoclonal antibody of the Ki-1 family for the detection of Hodgkin's disease in formaldehyde-fixed tissue sections. In: McMichael AJ, ed. *Leucocyte typing III—white blood cell antigens.* New York: Oxford University Press;1987:74.

26. Dürkop H, Latza U, Hummel M, et al. Molecular cloning and expression of a new member of the nerve growth factor receptor family that is characteristic for Hodgkin's disease. *Cell* 1992;68:421–427.

27. Amakawa R, Hakem A, Kundig TM, et al. Impaired negative selection of T cells in Hodgkin's disease antigen CD30-deficient mice. *Cell* 1996; 84:551–562.

28. Shanebeck KD, Maliszewski CR, Kennedy MK, et al. Regulation of murine B cell growth and differentiation by CD30 ligand. *Eur J Immunol* 1995;25:2147–2153.

29. Smith CA, Gruss HJ, Davis T, et al. CD30 antigen, a marker for Hodgkin's lymphoma, is a receptor whose ligand defines an emerging family of cytokines with homology to TNF. *Cell* 1993;73:1349–1360.

30. Stein H, Mason DY, Gerdes J, et al. The expression of the Hodgkin's disease associated antigen Ki-1 in reactive and neoplastic lymphoid tissue: evidence that Reed-Sternberg cells and histiocytic malignancies are derived from activated lymphoid cells. *Blood* 1985;66: 848–858.

31. Agnarsson BA, Kadin ME. The immunophenotype of Reed-Sternberg cells. A study of 50 cases of Hodgkin's disease using fixed frozen tissues. *Cancer* 1989;63:2083–2087.

32. Angel CA, Warford A, Campbell AC, et al. The immunohistology of Hodgkin's disease–Reed-Sternberg cells and their variants. *J Pathol* 1987;153:21–30.

33. Casey TT, Olson SJ, Cousar JB, et al. Immunophenotypes of Reed-Sternberg cells: a study of 19 cases of Hodgkin's disease in plastic-embedded sections. *Blood* 1989;74:2624–2628.

34. Chittal SM, Caveriviere P, Schwarting R, et al. Monoclonal antibodies in the diagnosis of Hodgkin's disease. The search for a rational panel. *Am J Surg Pathol* 1988;12:9–21.

35. Dallenbach FE, Stein H. Expression of T-cell-receptor beta chain in Reed-Sternberg cells. *Lancet* 1989;2:828–830.

36. Drexler HG. Recent results on the biology of Hodgkin and Reed-Sternberg cells. I. Biopsy material. *Leuk Lymphoma* 1992;8:283–313.

37. Korkolopoulou P, Cordell J, Jones M, et al. The expression of the B-cell marker mb-1 (CD79a) in Hodgkin's disease. *Histopathology* 1994; 24:511–515.

38. Stein H, Herbst H, Anagnostopoulos I, et al. The nature of Hodgkin and Reed-Sternberg cells, their association with EBV, and their relationship to anaplastic large-cell lymphoma. *Ann Oncol* 1991;2(suppl 2): 33–38.

39. Poppema S. The diversity of the immunohistological staining pattern of Sternberg-Reed cells. *J Histochem Cytochem* 1980;28:788–791.

40. Said JW. The immunohistochemistry of Hodgkin's disease. *Semin Diagn Pathol* 1992;9:265–271.

41. Bilbe G, Delabie J, Bruggen J, et al. Restin: a novel intermediate filament-associated protein highly expressed in the Reed-Sternberg cells of Hodgkin's disease. *EMBO J* 1992;11:2103–2113.

42. Delabie J, Shipman R, Bruggen J, et al. Expression of the novel intermediate filament-associated protein restin in Hodgkin's disease and anaplastic large-cell lymphoma. *Blood* 1992;80:2891–2896.

43. Pinkus GS, Pinkus JL, Langhoff E, et al. Fascin, a sensitive new marker for Reed-Sternberg cells of hodgkin's disease. Evidence for a dendritic or B cell derivation? *Am J Pathol* 1997;150:543–562.

44. van den Berg A, Visser L, Poppema S. High expression of the CC chemokine TARC in Reed-Sternberg cells. A possible explanation for the characteristic T-cell infiltration Hodgkin's lymphoma. *Am J Pathol* 1999;154:1685–1691.

45. Said JW, Pinkus JL, Shintaku IP, et al. Alterations in fascin-expressing germinal center dendritic cells in neoplastic follicles of B-cell lymphomas. *Mod Pathol* 1998;11:1–5.

46. Kaplan HS, Gartner S. "Sternberg-Reed" giant cells of Hodgkin's disease: cultivation in vitro, heterotransplantation, and characterization as neoplastic macrophages. *Int J Cancer* 1977;19:511–525.

47. Harris NL, Gang DL, Quay SC, et al. Contamination of Hodgkin's disease cell cultures. *Nature* 1981;289:228–230.

48. Schaadt M, Fonatsch C, Kirchner H, et al. Establishment of a malignant, Epstein-Barr-virus (EBV)-negative cell-line from the pleura effusion of a patient with Hodgkin's disease. *Blood* 1979;38:185–190.

49. Schaadt M, Diehl V, Stein H, et al. Two neoplastic cell lines with unique features derived from Hodgkin's disease. *Int J Cancer* 1980;26:723–731.

50. Bargou RC, Mapara MY, Zugck C, et al. Characterization of a novel Hodgkin cell line, HD-MyZ, with myelomonocytic features mimicking Hodgkin's disease in severe combined immunodeficient mice. *J Exp Med* 1993;177:1257–1268.

51. Kanzler H, Hansmann ML, Kapp U, et al. Molecular single cell analysis demonstrates the derivation of a peripheral blood-derived cell line (L1236) from the Hodgkin/Reed-Sternberg cells of a Hodgkin's lymphoma patient. *Blood* 1996;87:3429–3436.

52. Wolf J, Kapp U, Bohlen H, et al. Peripheral blood mononuclear cells of a patient with advanced Hodgkin's lymphoma give rise to permanently growing Hodgkin-Reed Sternberg cells. *Blood* 1996;87:3418–3428.

53. van den Berg A, Kroesen BJ, Kooistra K, et al. High expression of B-cell receptor inducible gene BIC in all subtypes of Hodgkin lymphoma. *Genes Chromosomes Cancer* 2003;37:20–28.

54. Stein H, Gerdes J, Schwab U, et al. Evidence for the detection of the normal counterpart of Hodgkin and Sternberg-Reed cells. *Hematol Oncol* 1983;1:21–29.

55. von Kalle C, Wolf J, Becker A, et al. Growth of Hodgkin cell lines in severely combined immunodeficient mice. *Int J Cancer* 1992;52:887–891.

56. Diehl V, Kirchner HH, Schaadt M, et al. Lymphoproliferation and heterotransplantation in nude mice: tumor cells in Hodgkin's disease. *Haematol Blood Transfus* 1981;26:229–234.

57. Kapp U, Dux A, Schell-Frederick E, et al. Disseminated growth of Hodgkin's-derived cell lines L540 and L540cy in immune-deficient SCID mice. *Ann Oncol* 1994;5(suppl 1):121–126.

58. Kapp U, Wolf J, Hummel M, et al. Hodgkin's lymphoma-derived tissue serially transplanted into severe combined immunodeficient mice. *Blood* 1993;82:1247–1256.

59. Rajewsky K. Clonal selection and learning in the antibody system. *Nature* 1996;381:751–758.

60. Irsch J, Nitsch S, Hansmann ML, et al. Isolation of viable Hodgkin and Reed-Sternberg cells from Hodgkin disease tissues. *Proc Natl Acad Sci USA* 1998;95:10117–10122.

61. Kanzler H, Küppers R, Hansmann ML, et al. Hodgkin and Reed-Sternberg cells in Hodgkin's disease represent the outgrowth of a dominant tumor clone derived from (crippled) germinal center B cells. *J Exp Med* 1996; 184:1495–1505.

62. Küppers R, Rajewsky K, Zhao M, et al. Hodgkin disease: Hodgkin and Reed-Sternberg cells picked from histological sections show clonal immunoglobulin gene rearrangements and appear to be derived from B cells at various stages of development. *Proc Natl Acad Sci USA* 1994; 91: 10962–10966.

63. Marafioti T, Hummel M, Foss H-D, et al. Hodgkin and Reed-Sternberg cells represent an expansion of a single clone originating from a germinal center B-cell with functional immunoglobulin gene rearrangements but defective immunoglobulin transcription. *Blood* 2000;95:1443–1450.

64. Spieker T, Kurth J, Küppers R, et al. Molecular single-cell analysis of the clonal relationship of small Epstein-Barr virus-infected cells and Epstein-Barr virus-harboring Hodgkin and Reed/Sternberg cells in Hodgkin disease. *Blood* 2000;96:3133–3138.

65. Küppers R, Zhao M, Hansmann ML, et al. Tracing B cell development in human germinal centres by molecular analysis of single cells picked from histological sections. *EMBO J* 1993;12:4955–4967.

66. Jox A, Zander T, Küppers R, et al. Somatic mutations within the untranslated regions of rearranged Ig genes in a case of classical Hodgkin's disease as a potential cause for the absence of Ig in the lymphoma cells. *Blood* 1999;93:3964–3972.

67. Küppers R. Molecular biology of Hodgkin's lymphoma. *Adv Cancer Res* 2002;84:277–312.

68. Küppers R, Rajewsky K. The origin of Hodgkin and Reed/Sternberg cells in Hodgkin's disease. *Annu Rev Immunol* 1998;16:471–493.

69. Müschen M, Küppers R, Spieker T, et al. Molecular single-cell analysis of Hodgkin- and Reed-Sternberg cells harboring unmutated immunoglobulin variable region genes. *Lab Invest* 2001;81:289–295.

70. Rosenquist R, Roos G, Erlanson M, et al. Clonally related splenic marginal zone lymphoma and Hodgkin lymphoma with unmutated V gene rearrangements and a 15-yr time gap between diagnoses. *Eur J Haematol* 2004;73:210–214.

71. Lebecque S, de Bouteiller O, Arpin C, et al. Germinal center founder cells display propensity for apoptosis before onset of somatic mutation. *J Exp Med* 1997;185:563–571.

72. Bräuninger A, Wacker HH, Rajewsky K, et al. Typing the histogenetic origin of the tumor cells of lymphocyte-rich classical Hodgkin's lymphoma in relation to tumor cells of classical and lymphocyte-predominance Hodgkin's lymphoma. *Cancer Res* 2003;63:1644–1651.

73. Müschen M, Rajewsky K, Bräuninger A, et al. Rare occurrence of classical Hodgkin's disease as a T cell lymphoma. *J Exp Med* 2000;191:387–394.

74. Seitz V, Hummel M, Marafioti T, et al. Detection of clonal T-cell receptor gamma-chain gene rearrangements in Reed-Sternberg cells of classic Hodgkin disease. *Blood* 2000;95:3020–3024.

75. Tzankov A, Bourgau C, Kaiser A, et al. Rare expression of T-cell markers in classical Hodgkin's lymphoma. *Mod Pathol* 2005;18:1542–1549.

76. Bucsky P. Hodgkin's disease: the Sternberg-Reed cell. *Blood* 1987;55:413–420.

77. Michels KB. The origins of Hodgkin's disease. *Eur J Cancer Prev* 1995;4:379–388.

78. Küppers R, Bräuninger A, Müschen M, et al. Evidence that Hodgkin and Reed-Sternberg cells in Hodgkin disease do not represent cell fusions. *Blood* 2001;97:818–821.

79. Drexler HG, Gignac SM, Hoffbrand AV, et al. Formation of multinucleated cells in a Hodgkin's-disease-derived cell line. *Int J Cancer* 1989;43:1083–1090.

80. Re D, Benenson E, Beyer M, et al. Cell fusion is not involved in the generation of giant cells in the Hodgkin-Reed Sternberg cell line L1236. *Am J Hematol* 2001;67:6–9.

81. Braeuninger A, Küppers R, Strickler JG, et al. Hodgkin and Reed-Sternberg cells in lymphocyte predominant Hodgkin disease represent clonal populations of germinal center-derived tumor B cells. *Proc Natl Acad Sci USA* 1997;94:9337–9342.

82. Marafioti T, Hummel M, Anagnostopoulos I, et al. Origin of nodular lymphocyte-predominant Hodgkin's disease from a clonal expansion of highly mutated germinal-center B cells. *N Engl J Med* 1997;337:453–458.

83. Ohno T, Stribley JA, Wu G, et al. Clonality in nodular lymphocyte-predominant Hodgkin's disease. *N Engl J Med* 1997;337:459–465.

84. Carbone A, Gloghini A, Gaidano G, et al. Expression status of BCL-6 and syndecan-1 identifies distinct histogenetic subtypes of Hodgkin's disease. *Blood* 1998;92:2220–2228.

85. Greiner A, Tobollik S, Buettner M, et al. Differential expression of activation-induced cytidine deaminase (AID) in nodular lymphocyte-predominant and classical Hodgkin lymphoma. *J Pathol* 2005;205:541–547.

86. Bräuninger A, Hansmann ML, Strickler JG, et al. Identification of common germinal-center B-cell precursors in two patients with both Hodgkin's disease and Non-Hodgkin's lymphoma. *N Engl J Med* 1999;340:1239–1247.

87. Küppers R, Sousa AB, Baur AS, et al. Common germinal-center B-cell origin of the malignant cells in two composite lymphomas, involving classical Hodgkin's disease and either follicular lymphoma or B-CLL. *Mol Med* 2001;7:285–292.

88. Marafioti T, Hummel M, Anagnostopoulos I, et al. Classical Hodgkin's disease and follicular lymphoma originating from the same germinal center B cell. *J Clin Oncol* 1999;17:3804–3809.

89. Caleo A, Sanchez-Aguilera A, Rodriguez S, et al. Composite Hodgkin lymphoma and mantle cell lymphoma: two clonally unrelated tumors. *Am J Surg Pathol* 2003;27:1577–1580.

90. Ohno T, Trenn G, Wu G, et al. The clonal relationship between nodular sclerosis Hodgkin's disease with a clonal Reed-Sternberg cell population and a subsequent B-cell small noncleaved cell lymphoma. *Mod Pathol* 1998;11:485–490.

91. Thomas RK, Wickenhauser C, Kube D, et al. Repeated clonal relapses in classical Hodgkin's lymphoma and the occurrence of a clonally unrelated diffuse large B cell non-Hodgkin lymphoma in the same patient. *Leuk Lymphoma* 2004;45:1065–1069.

92. Bellan C, Lazzi S, Zazzi M, et al. Immunoglobulin gene rearrangement analysis in composite Hodgkin disease and large B-cell lymphoma: evidence for receptor revision of immunoglobulin heavy chain variable region genes in Hodgkin-Reed-Sternberg cells? *Diagn Mol Pathol* 2002;11:2–8.

93. Rosenquist R, Menestrina F, Lestani M, et al. Indications for peripheral light-chain revision and somatic hypermutation without a functional B-cell receptor in precursors of a composite diffuse large B-cell and Hodgkin's lymphoma. *Lab Invest* 2004;84:253–262.

94. Tinguely M, Rosenquist R, Sundstrom C, et al. Analysis of a clonally related mantle cell and Hodgkin lymphoma indicates Epstein-Barr virus infection of a Hodgkin/Reed-Sternberg cell precursor in a germinal center. *Am J Surg Pathol* 2003;27:1483–1488.

95. van den Berg A, Maggio E, Rust R, et al. Clonal relation in a case of CLL, ALCL, and Hodgkin composite lymphoma. *Blood* 2002;100:1425–1429.

96. Kanzler H, Küppers R, Helmes S, et al. Hodgkin and Reed-Sternberg-like cells in B-cell chronic lymphocytic leukemia represent the outgrowth of single germinal-center B-cell-derived clones: potential precursors of Hodgkin and Reed-Sternberg cells in Hodgkin's disease. *Blood* 2000;95:1023–1031.

97. Ohno T, Smir BN, Weisenburger DD, et al. Origin of the Hodgkin/Reed-Sternberg cells in chronic lymphocytic leukemia with "Hodgkin's transformation." *Blood* 1998;91:1757–1761.

98. de Leval L, Vivario M, De Prijck B, et al. Distinct clonal origin in two cases of Hodgkin's lymphoma variant of Richter's syndrome associated with EBV infection. *Am J Surg Pathol* 2004;28:679–686.

99. Davis TH, Morton CC, Miller-Cassman R, et al. Hodgkin's disease, lymphomatoid papulosis, and cutaneous T-cell lymphoma derived from a common T-cell clone. *N Engl J Med* 1992;326:1115–1122.

100. Kadin ME, Drews R, Samel A, et al. Hodgkin's lymphoma of T-cell type: clonal association with a CD30+ cutaneous lymphoma. *Hum Pathol* 2001;32:1269–1272.

101. Willenbrock K, Ichinohasama R, Kadin ME, et al. T-cell variant of classical Hodgkin's lymphoma with nodal and cutaneous manifestations demonstrated by single-cell polymerase chain reaction. *Lab Invest* 2002;82:1103–1109.

102. Greiner TC, Gascoyne RD, Anderson ME, et al. Nodular lymphocyte-predominant Hodgkin's disease associated with large-cell lymphoma: analysis of Ig gene rearrangements by V-J polymerase chain reaction. *Blood* 1996;88:657–666.

103. Ohno T, Huang JZ, Wu G, et al. The tumor cells in nodular lymphocyte-predominant Hodgkin disease are clonally related to the large cell lymphoma occurring in the same individual. Direct demonstration by single cell analysis. *Am J Clin Pathol* 2001;116:506–511.

104. Pan LX, Diss TC, Peng HZ, et al. Nodular lymphocyte predominance Hodgkin's disease: a monoclonal or polyclonal B-cell disorder? *Blood* 1996;87:2428–2434.

105. Shimodaira S, Hidaka E, Katsuyama T. Clonal identity of nodular lymphocyte-predominant Hodgkin's disease and T-cell-rich B-cell lymphoma. *N Engl J Med* 2000;343:1124–1125.

106. Wickert RS, Weisenburger DD, Tierens A, et al. Clonal relationship between lymphocytic predominance Hodgkin's disease and concurrent or subsequent large-cell lymphoma of B lineage. *Blood* 1995;86:2312–2320.

107. Yoshinaga H, Ohashi K, Yamamoto K, et al. Clonal identification of Burkitt's lymphoma arising from lymphocyte-predominant Hodgkin's disease. *Br J Haematol* 1996;95:380–382.

108. Schmitz R, Renné; C, Rosenquist R, et al. Insight into the multistep transformation process of lymphomas: IgH-associated translocations and tumor suppressor gene mutations in clonally related composite Hodgkin's and non-Hodgkin's lymphomas. *Leukemia* 2005;19:1452–1458.

109. Re D, Müschen M, Ahmadi T, et al. Oct-2 and Bob-1 deficiency in Hodgkin and Reed Sternberg cells. *Cancer Res* 2001;61:2080–2084.

110. Stein H, Marafioti T, Foss HD, et al. Down-regulation of BOB.1/OBF.1 and Oct2 in classical Hodgkin disease but not in lymphocyte predominant Hodgkin disease correlates with immunoglobulin transcription. *Blood* 2001;97:496–501.

111. Watanabe K, Yamashita Y, Nakayama A, et al. Varied B-cell immunophenotypes of Hodgkin/Reed-Sternberg cells in classic Hodgkin's disease. *Histopathology* 2000;36:353–361.

112. Torlakovic E, Tierens A, Dang HD, et al. The transcription factor PU.1, necessary for B-cell development is expressed in lymphocyte predominance, but not classical Hodgkin's disease. *Am J Pathol* 2001;159:1807–1814.

113. Ushmorov A, Ritz O, Hummel M, et al. Epigenetic silencing of the immunoglobulin heavy-chain gene in classical Hodgkin lymphoma-derived cell lines contributes to the loss of immunoglobulin expression. *Blood* 2004;104:3326–3334.

114. Doerr JR, Malone CS, Fike FM, et al. Patterned CpG methylation of silenced B cell gene promoters in classical Hodgkin lymphoma-derived and primary effusion lymphoma cell lines. *J Mol Biol* 2005;350:631–640.

115. Ushmorov A, Leithäuser F, Sakk O, et al. Epigenetic processes play a major role in B-cell-specific gene silencing in classical Hodgkin lymphoma. *Blood* 2005;107:2493–2500.

116. Schwering I, Bräuninger A, Klein U, et al. Loss of the B-lineage-specific gene expression program in Hodgkin and Reed-Sternberg cells of Hodgkin lymphoma. *Blood* 2003;101:1505–1512.

117. Carbone A, Gloghini A, Larocca LM, et al. Human immunodeficiency virus-associated Hodgkin's disease derives from post-germinal center B cells. *Blood* 1999;93:2319–2326.

118. O'Connell FP, Pinkus JL, Pinkus GS. CD138 (syndecan-1), a plasma cell marker immunohistochemical profile in hematopoietic and nonhematopoietic neoplasms. *Am J Clin Pathol* 2004;121:254–263.

119. Cattoretti G, Angelin-Duclos C, Shaknovich R, et al. PRDM1/Blimp-1 is expressed in human B-lymphocytes committed to the plasma cell lineage. *J Pathol* 2005;206:76–86.

120. Poppema S. Immunology of Hodgkin's disease. *Baillieres Clin Haematol* 1996;9:447–457.

121. Foss HD, Reusch R, Demel G, et al. Frequent expression of the B-cell-specific activator protein in Reed-Sternberg cells of classical Hodgkin's disease provides further evidence for its B-cell origin. *Blood* 1999;94:3108–3113.

122. Bargou RC, Leng C, Krappmann D, et al. High-level nuclear NF-kappa B and Oct-2 is a common feature of cultured Hodgkin/Reed-Sternberg cells. *Blood* 1996;87:4340–4347.

123. Bargou RC, Emmerich F, Krappmann D, et al. Constitutive nuclear factor-kappaB-RelA activation is required for proliferation and survival of Hodgkin's disease tumor cells. *J Clin Invest* 1997;100:2961–2969.

124. Hinz M, Loser P, Mathas S, et al. Constitutive NF-kappaB maintains high expression of a characteristic gene network, including CD40, CD86, and a set of antiapoptotic genes in Hodgkin/Reed-Sternberg cells. *Blood* 2001;97:2798–2807.

125. Joos S, Menz CK, Wrobel G, et al. Classical Hodgkin lymphoma is characterized by recurrent copy number gains of the short arm of chromosome 2. *Blood* 2002;99:1381–1387.

126. Martin-Subero JI, Gesk S, Harder L, et al. Recurrent involvement of the REL and BCL11A loci in classical Hodgkin lymphoma. *Blood* 2002; 99:1474–1477.

127. Horie R, Watanabe T, Morishita Y, et al. Ligand-independent signaling by overexpressed CD30 drives NF-kappaB activation in Hodgkin-Reed-Sternberg cells. *Oncogene* 2002;21:2493–2503.

128. Annunziata CM, Safiran YJ, Irving SG, et al. Hodgkin disease: pharmacologic intervention of the CD40-NF kappa B pathway by a protease inhibitor. *Blood* 2000;96:2841–2848.

129. Fiumara P, Snell V, Li Y, et al. Functional expression of receptor activator of nuclear factor kappaB in Hodgkin disease cell lines. *Blood* 2001;98:2784–2790.

130. Jundt F, Anagnostopoulos I, Förster R, et al. Activated Notch 1 signaling promotes tumor cell proliferation and survival in Hodgkin and anaplastic large cell lymphoma. *Blood* 2001;99:3398–3403.

131. Rodig SJ, Savage KJ, Nguyen V, et al. TRAF1 expression and c-Rel activation are useful adjuncts in distinguishing classical Hodgkin lymphoma from a subset of morphologically or immunophenotypically similar lymphomas. *Am J Surg Pathol* 2005;29:196–203.

132. Zheng B, Fiumara P, Li YV, et al. MEK/ERK pathway is aberrantly active in Hodgkin disease: a signaling pathway shared by CD30, CD40, and RANK that regulates cell proliferation and survival. *Blood* 2003;102:1019–1027.

133. Nonaka M, Horie R, Itoh K, et al. Aberrant NF-kappaB2/p52 expression in Hodgkin/Reed-Sternberg cells and CD30-transformed rat fibroblasts. *Oncogene* 2005;24:3976–3986.

134. Nagel S, Scherr M, Quentmeier H, et al. HLXB9 activates IL6 in Hodgkin lymphoma cell lines and is regulated by PI3K signalling involving E2F3. *Leukemia* 2005;19:841–846.

135. Georgakis GV, Li Y, Rassidakis GZ, et al. Differential effects of three small molecules blocking phosphatidylinositol-3 kinase or AKT in Hodgkin disease cell lines: Induction of apoptosis and cell cycle arrest. *Blood* 2004;104(suppl):125a. Abstract.

136. Mathas S, Hinz M, Anagnostopoulos I, et al. Aberrantly expressed c-Jun and JunB are a hallmark of Hodgkin lymphoma cells, stimulate proliferation and synergize with NF-kappa B. *EMBO J* 2002;21:4104–4113.

137. Radtke F, Wilson A, Mancini SJ, et al. Notch regulation of lymphocyte development and function. *Nat Immunol* 2004;5:247–253.

138. Zweidler-McKay PA, He Y, Xu L, et al. Notch signaling is a potent inducer of growth arrest and apoptosis in a wide range of B-cell malignancies. *Blood* 2005;106:3898–3906.

139. Hinz M, Lemke P, Anagnostopoulos I, et al. Nuclear factor kappaB-dependent gene expression profiling of Hodgkin's disease tumor cells, pathogenetic significance, and link to constitutive signal transducer and activator of transcription 5a activity. *J Exp Med* 2002;196:605–617.

140. Skinnider BF, Elia AJ, Gascoyne RD, et al. Signal transducer and activator of transcription 6 is frequently activated in Hodgkin and Reed-Sternberg cells of Hodgkin lymphoma. *Blood* 2002;99:618–626.

141. Skinnider BF, Elia AJ, Gascoyne RD, et al. Interleukin 13 and interleukin 13 receptor are frequently expressed by Hodgkin and Reed-Sternberg cells of Hodgkin lymphoma. *Blood* 2001;97:250–255.

142. Holtick U, Vockerodt M, Pinkert D, et al. STAT3 is essential for Hodgkin lymphoma cell proliferation and is a target of tyrphostin AG17 which confers sensitization for apoptosis. *Leukemia* 2005;19:936–944.

143. Kapp U, Yeh WC, Patterson B, et al. Interleukin 13 is secreted by and stimulates the growth of Hodgkin and Reed-Sternberg cells. *J Exp Med* 1999;189:1939–1946.

144. Baus D, Pfitzner E. Specific function of STAT3, SOCS1, and SOCS3 in the regulation of proliferation and survival of classical Hodgkin lymphoma cells. *Int J Cancer* 2006;118:1404–1413.

145. Renné C, Willenbrock K, Küppers R, et al. Autocrine and paracrine activated receptor tyrosine kinases in classical Hodgkin lymphoma. *Blood* 2005;105:4051–4059.

146. Rickinson AB, Kieff E. Epstein-Barr virus. In: Knipe DM, Howley PM, eds. *Fields virology*. Philadelphia: Lippincott-Raven; 2001: 2575–2627.

147. Brousset P, Schlaifer D, Meggetto F, et al. Persistence of the same viral strain in early and late relapses of Epstein-Barr virus-associated Hodgkin's disease. *Blood* 1994;84:2447–2451.

148. Kilger E, Kieser A, Baumann M, et al. Epstein-Barr virus-mediated B-cell proliferation is dependent upon latent membrane protein 1, which simulates an activated CD40 receptor. *EMBO J.* 1998;17:1700–1709.

149. Alber G, Kim KM, Weiser P, et al. Molecular mimicry of the antigen receptor signalling motif by transmembrane proteins of the Epstein-Barr virus and the bovine leukemia virus. *Curr Biol* 1993;3:333–339.

150. Caldwell RG, Wilson JB, Anderson SJ, et al. Epstein-Barr virus LMP2A drives B cell development and survival in the absence of normal B cell receptor signals. *Immunity* 1998;9:405–411.

151. Casola S, Otipoby KL, Alimzhanov M, et al. B cell receptor signal strength determines B cell fate. *Nat Immunol* 2004;5:317–327.

152. Bechtel D, Kurth J, Unkel C, et al. Transformation of BCR-deficient germinal-center B cells by EBV supports a major role of the virus in the pathogenesis of Hodgkin and posttransplantation lymphomas. *Blood* 2005; 106:4345–4350.

153. Chaganti S, Bell AI, Begue-Pastor N, et al. Epstein-Barr virus infection in vitro can resue germinal centre B cells with inactivated immunoglobulin genes. *Blood* 2005; 106:4249–4252.

154. Mancao C, Altmann M, Jungnickel B, et al. Rescue of "crippled" germinal center B cells from apoptosis by Epstein-Barr virus. *Blood* 2005; 106:4339–4344.

155. Bräuninger A, Schmitz R, Bechtel D, et al. Molecular biology of Hodgkin and Reed/Sternberg cells in Hodgkin's lymphoma. *Int J Cancer* 2006;118:1853–1861.

156. Schwering I, Bräuninger A, Klein U, et al. Loss of the B-lineage-specific gene expression program in Hodgkin and Reed-Sternberg cells of Hodgkin lymphoma. *Blood* 2003;101:1505–1512.

157. Niedobitek G, Kremmer E, Herbst H, et al. Immunohistochemical detection of the Epstein-Barr virus-encoded latent membrane protein 2A in Hodgkin's disease and infectious mononucleosis. *Blood* 1997;90:1664–1672.

158. Weber-Matthiesen K, Deerberg J, Poetsch M, et al. Numerical chromosome aberrations are present within the CD30+ Hodgkin and Reed-Sternberg cells in 100% of analyzed cases of Hodgkin's disease. *Blood* 1995; 86:1464–1468.

159. Falzetti D, Crescenzi B, Matteuci C, et al. Genomic instability and recurrent breakpoints are main cytogenetic findings in Hodgkin's disease. *Haematologica* 1999;84:298–305.

160. Martin-Subero JI, Renné C, Grohmann S, et al. Chromosomal rearrangements affecting the BCL6, MYC and MALT1 loci are rare events in classical Hodgkin lymphoma. *Eur J Hematol* 2004;73(suppl. 65):B23. Abstract.

161. Gravel S, Delsol G, Al Saati T. Single-cell analysis of the t(14;18)(q32;p21) chromosomal translocation in Hodgkin's disease demonstrates the absence of this transformation in neoplastic Hodgkin and Reed-Sternberg cells. *Blood* 1998;91:2866–2874.

162. Weber-Matthiesen K, Deerberg-Wittram J, Rosenwald A, et al. Translocation t(2;5) is not a primary event in Hodgkin's disease. Simultaneous immunophenotyping and interphase cytogenetics. *Am J Pathol* 1996;149:463–468.

163. Weiss LM, Lopategui JR, Sun LH, et al. Absence of the t(2;5) in Hodgkin's disease. *Blood* 1995;85:2845–2847.

164. Re D, Benenson L, Wickenhauser C, et al. Proficient mismatch repair protein expression in Hodgkin and Reed Sternberg cells. *Int J Cancer* 2002;97:205–210.

165. Joos S, Küpper M, Ohl S, et al. Genomic imbalances including amplification of the tyrosine kinase gene JAK2 in CD30+ Hodgkin cells. *Cancer Res* 2000;60:549–552.

166. Küpper M, Joos S, Von Bonin F, et al. MDM2 gene amplification and lack of p53 point mutations in Hodgkin and Reed-Sternberg cells: results from single-cell polymerase chain reaction and molecular cytogenetic studies. *Br J Haematol* 2001;112:768–775.

167. Maggio EM, Stekelenburg E, Van den Berg A, et al. TP53 gene mutations in Hodgkin lymphoma are infrequent and not associated with absence of Epstein-Barr virus. *Int J Cancer* 2001;94:60–66.

168. Montesinos-Rongen M, Roers A, Küppers R, et al. Mutation of the p53 gene is not a typical feature of Hodgkin and Reed-Sternberg cells in Hodgkin's disease. *Blood* 1999;94:1755–1760.

169. Garcia JF, Villuendas R, Sanchez-Beato M, et al. Nucleolar p14(ARF) overexpression in Reed-Sternberg cells in Hodgkin's lymphoma: absence of p14(ARF)/Hdm2 complexes is associated with expression of alternatively spliced Hdm2 transcripts. *Am J Pathol* 2002;160:569–578.

170. Maggio EM, van den Berg A, de Jong D, et al. Low frequency of FAS mutations in Reed-Sternberg cells of Hodgkin's lymphoma. *Am J Pathol* 2003;162:29–35.

171. Müschen M, Re D, Bräuninger A, et al. Somatic mutations of the CD95 gene in Hodgkin and Reed-Sternberg cells. *Cancer Res* 2000;60:5640–5643.

172. Re D, Hofmann A, Wolf J, et al. Cultivated H-RS cells are resistant to CD95L-mediated apoptosis despite expression of wild-type CD95. *Exp Hematol* 2000;28:31–35.

173. Trümper L, Pfreundschuh M, Jacobs G, et al. N-ras genes are not mutated in Hodgkin and Reed-Sternberg cells: results from single cell polymerase chain-reaction examinations. *Leukemia* 1996;10:727–730.

174. Thomas RK, Schmitz R, Harttrampf AC, et al. Apoptosis-resistant phenotype of classical Hodgkin's lymphoma is not mediated by somatic mutations within genes encoding members of the death-inducing signaling complex (DISC). *Leukemia* 2005;19:1079–1082.

175. Dutton A, O'Neil JD, Milner AE, et al. Expression of the cellular FLICE-inhibitory protein (c-FLIP) protects Hodgkin's lymphoma cells from autonomous Fas-mediated death. *Proc Natl Acad Sci USA* 2004; 101:6611–6616.

176. Mathas S, Lietz A, Anagnostopoulos I, et al. c-FLIP Mediates Resistance of Hodgkin/Reed-Sternberg Cells to Death Receptor-induced Apoptosis. *J Exp Med* 2004;199:1041–1052.

177. Thomas RK, Kallenborn A, Wickenhauser C, et al. Constitutive expression of c-FLIP in Hodgkin and Reed-Sternberg cells. *Am J Pathol* 2002; 160:1521–1528.

178. Weniger MA, Melzner I, Menz CK, et al. Mutations of the tumor suppressor gene SOCS-1 in classical Hodgkin lymphoma are frequent and associated with nuclear phospho-STAT5 accumulation. *Blood* 2005;106. Abstract.

179. Cabannes E, Khan G, Aillet F, et al. Mutations in the IkBa gene in Hodgkin's disease suggest a tumour suppressor role for IkBa. *Oncogene* 1999; 18:3063–3070.

180. Emmerich F, Meiser M, Hummel M, et al. Overexpression of I kappa B alpha without inhibition of NF-kappaB activity and mutations in the I kappa B alpha gene in Reed-Sternberg cells. *Blood* 1999;94:3129–3134.

181. Jungnickel B, Staratschek-Jox A, Bräuninger A, et al. Clonal deleterious mutations in the ikBa gene in the malignant cells in Hodgkin's disease. *J Exp Med* 2000;191:395–401.

182. Emmerich F, Theurich S, Hummel M, et al. Inactivating I kappa B epsilon mutations in Hodgkin/Reed-Sternberg cells. *J Pathol* 2003;201: 413–420.

183. Thomas RK, Wickenhauser C, Tawadros S, et al. Mutational analysis of the IkappaBalpha gene in activated B cell-like diffuse large B-cell lymphoma. *Br J Haematol* 2004;126:50–54.

184. Wlodarska I, Nooyen P, Maes B, et al. Frequent occurrence of BCL6 rearrangements in nodular lymphocyte predominance Hodgkin lymphoma but not in classical Hodgkin lymphoma. *Blood* 2003;101:706–710.

185. Renné C, Martin-Subero JI, Hansmann ML, et al. Molecular cytogenetic analyses of immunoglobulin loci in nodular lymphocyte predominant Hodgkin's lymphoma reveal a recurrent IGH-BCL6 juxtaposition. *J Mol Diagn* 2005;7:352–356.

186. Franke S, Wlodarska I, Maes B, et al. Lymphocyte predominance Hodgkin disease is characterized by recurrent genomic imbalances. *Blood* 2001;97:1845–1853.

187. Pasqualucci L, Neumeister P, Goossens T, et al. Hypermutation of multiple proto-oncogenes in B-cell diffuse large-cell lymphomas. *Nature* 2001;412:341–346.

188. Liso A, Capello D, Marafioti T, et al. Aberrant somatic hypermutation in tumor cells of nodular-lymphocyte-predominant and classic Hodgkin lymphoma. *Blood* 2006;108:1013–1020.

189. MacLennan IC. Germinal centers. *Annu Rev Immunol* 1994;12:117–139.

190. Diehl V, Kirchner HH, Burrichter H, et al. Characteristics of Hodgkin's disease-derived cell lines. *Cancer Treat Rep* 1982;66:615–632.

191. Kamesaki H, Fukuhara S, Tatsumi E, et al. Cytochemical, immunologic, chromosomal, and molecular genetic analysis of a novel cell line derived from Hodgkin's disease. *Blood* 1986;68:285–292.

192. Diehl V, Kirchner HH, Schaadt M, et al. Hodgkin's disease: establishment and characterization of four in vitro cell lines. *J Cancer Res Clin Oncol* 1981;101:111–124.

193. Jones D, Furley AWJ, Gerdes J, et al. Phenotypic and genotypic analysis of two cell lines derived from Hodgkin's disease tissue biopsies. In: Diehl V, Pfreundschuh M, Loeffler M, eds. *New aspects in the diagnosis and treatment of Hodgkin's disease.* Berlin: Springer-Verlag; 1989:62–66.

194. Drexler HG, Gaedicke G, Lok MS, et al. Hodgkin's disease derived cell lines HDLM-2 and L-428: comparison of morphology, immunological and isoenzyme profiles. *Leuk Res* 1986;10:487–500.

195. Drexler HG, Gignac SM, Hoffbrand AV, et al. Characterisation of Hodgkin's disease derived cell line HDLM-2. In: Diehl V, Pfreundschuh M, Loeffler M, eds. *New aspects in the diagnosis and treatment of Hodgkin's disease.* Berlin: Springer-Verlag; 1989:75–82.

196. Poppema S, De Jong B, Atmosoerodjo J, et al. Morphologic, immunologic, enzymehistochemical and chromosomal analysis of a cell line derived from Hodgkin's disease. Evidence for a B-cell origin of Sternberg-Reed cells. *Cancer* 1985;55:683–690.

197. Poppema S, Visser L, De Jong B, et al. The typical Reed-Sternberg phenotype and Ig gene rearrangement of Hodgkin's disease derived cell line ZO indicating a B cell origin. In: Diehl V, Pfreundschuh M, Loeffler M, eds. *New aspects in the diagnosis and treatment of Hodgkin's disease.* Berlin: Springer-Verlag; 1989.

198. Kanzaki T, Kubonishi I, Eguchi T, et al. Establishment of a new Hodgkin's cell line (HD-70) of B-cell origin. *Cancer* 1992;69:1034–1041.

199. Naumovski L, Utz PJ, Bergstrom SK, et al. SUP-HD1: a new Hodgkin's disease-derived cell line with lymphoid features produces interferon-g. *Blood* 1989;74:2733–2742.

200. Wagner HJ, Klintworth F, Jabs W, et al. Characterization of the novel, pediatric Hodgkin disease-derived cell line HKB-1. *Med Pediatr Oncol* 1998;31:138–143.

201. Drexler HG, Dirks WG, MacLeod RA. False human hematopoietic cell lines: cross-contaminations and misinterpretations. *Leukemia* 1999; 13:1601–1607.

CHAPTER 6 ■ CYTOKINES, CYTOKINE RECEPTORS, AND CHEMOKINES IN HODGKIN LYMPHOMA

YUE MA, ANKE VAN DEN BERG, CIGDEM ATAYAR, LYDIA VISSER, AND SIBRAND POPPEMA

Hodgkin lymphomas are characterized by a small minority of generally less than 1% neoplastic cells, the so called Hodgkin and Reed-Sternberg cells, and a large majority of inflammatory cells, including lymphocytes, histiocytes, plasma cells, eosinophils, mast cells, neutrophils, fibroblasts, and other stroma cells. Several lines of evidence suggest that the reactive tissue elements are attracted by cytokines and chemokines secreted by the Hodgkin and Reed-Sternberg cells (Tables 6.1 and 6.2).[1] The inflammatory cells also produce a range of factors that recruit additional inflammatory cells, support the growth of the Hodgkin and Reed-Sternberg cells, and stimulate collagen synthesis. Hodgkin lymphoma almost appears like a lexicon of cytokines, chemokines, and their receptors in which almost all cytokines are represented in the Hodgkin and Reed-Sternberg cells, the inflammatory cells, or both.

Presence of constitutive activated transcription factor NF-κB is one of the hallmarks of Hodgkin lymphoma and is believed to play a major role in the pathogenesis. Most of the cytokines and chemokines expressed in Hodgkin and Reed-Sternberg cells are thought to be indeed regulated by NF-κB. Several mechanisms, including CD30, CD40, LMP-1, and defective IκBα, have been shown to play a role in the induction of the constitutively activated NF-κB. In recent decades, many studies have been published on the expression of cytokines and chemokines. An overview of the cytokines and chemokines expressed in the malignant cells of Hodgkin lymphomas and Hodgkin cell lines and in serum samples of patients with Hodgkin lymphoma is given below.

CYTOKINES IN HODGKIN AND REED-STERNBERG CELLS IN HODGKIN LYMPHOMA TISSUE AND CELL LINES

IFN-γ

IFN-γ is a TH1-cell–associated cytokine that supports cell-mediated immunity primarily through its effects on the monocyte/macrophage population and inhibits TH2 cells. IFN-γ was reported to be present in 14 out of 30 cases of Hodgkin lymphoma in a quite variable percentage of Hodgkin and Reed-Sternberg cells, ranging from 1% to 90%.[2] These results were largely confirmed in another study that demonstrated IFN-γ expression in all cases, ranging from 3% to 52% of Hodgkin and Reed-Sternberg cells.[3] Comparison of nodular-sclerosis and mixed-cellularity subtypes revealed higher expression levels in the mixed-cellularity cases[4] In Hodgkin lymphoma-derived cell lines, IFN-γ mRNA expression has been reported in HDLM2, L591 and DEV[5] and IFN-γ protein production by ELISA in L1236[6] and by immunohistochemistry in L540.[2] Incubation of the cell lines HDLM2 and KMH2 with recombinant IFN-γ had no effect on proliferation.[7]

Interleukin-1α and -1β

IL-1 is a proinflammatory cytokine that plays pleiotropic roles in host defense mechanisms. Several studies analyzed expression of IL-1α and IL-1β by immunohistochemistry and frequently found expression of IL-1α in the Hodgkin and Reed-Sternberg cells. In addition, these studies also demonstrated that several other cell types, including small to medium-sized cells of uncertain origin, granulocytes, macrophages, interdigitating reticulum cells, and endothelial cells also produce IL-1α and IL-1β.[8–10] Cells positive for IL-1β were much lower in number and consisted mainly of macrophages.[10] High IL-1 mRNA levels were reported in several studies, but this type of analysis does not allow identification of the specific cell types that actually produce this cytokine.[11] In Hodgkin cell lines, high IL-1α secretion was found in HDLM2 and high IL-1β secretion in was found in KMH2.[12]

Interleukin-2

IL-2 is an important growth factor for T-cells, and it augments the NK cytolytic activity. Expression studies for IL-2 revealed positive Hodgkin and Reed-Sternberg cells varying from less than 5%[3] to more than 30%.[13] However, no IL-2 expression has been observed in several Hodgkin cell lines[5,6,13–15] confirming the lack of IL-2 expression in Hodgkin and Reed-Sternberg cells.[13] Highly variable results have also been reported for IL-2R.[16–19] Adding IL-2 to the culture medium of Hodgkin cell lines had no effects, indicating that IL-2 and IL-2R do not play an important role in the growth and survival of Hodgkin and Reed-Sternberg cells. However, the IL-2R on these cells may play a role as decoy receptors, depleting IL-2 from the T-cells.

Interleukin-3

IL-3 acts as a growth factor for B-cells, activates monocytes, and enhances survival and proliferation of mast cells, eosinophils, and stromal cells. IL-3 expression has been demonstrated in Hodgkin cell lines,[20] but to date no studies

TABLE 6.1

CYTOKINE EXPRESSION IN TUMOR CELLS OF HODGKIN LYMPHOMA

| Cytokine | % Positive HL cases | Produced by | | Relevance for HL | References |
		HRS	Lines		
IFN γ	50–100	+	+	Stimulation of macrophages/ induction of CXCL10	3, 120, 121
IL-1a	75	+	+	Fibrosis and sclerosis	8–10
IL-1b	<5	−	+	Fibrosis and sclerosis	8–10
IL-2	?	+	−	?	3,6,13,14
IL-3	0	−	+	Growth factor for HRS cells	20–22
IL-4	0	−	+	Induction CCL17 and CCL22	3,6,14,23,25
IL-5	?	+	+	Induction of eosinophils	14,27,28
IL-6	65–100	+	+	Stimulation of B-cells and plasma cells	6,14,23,24, 31,33,41
IL-7	77	+	+	Growth factor for T-cells	36
IL-9	50	+	−	Autocrine growth factor/ positive effect on mast cells	37,38
IL-10	21–36	+	+	Immune suppression of TH1 cells	3,5,40,41
IL-12	0	−	+	n.a.	42,43
IL-13	86	+	+	Fibrosis and sclerosis/ autocrine growth factor/ induction of CCL17 and CCL22	25,28,35,44
IL-15	?	?	+	?	11
TNFα	100	+	+	Enhance CCL11 production by fibroblasts/collagen synthesis	10,13,31
LT-a	100	+	+	B-cell growth factor/ collagen synthesis	31
TGFβ	70–80	+	+	Immunesuppressive/ induction of fibrosis	5,48,49
bFGF	90	+	+	Fibrosis and sclerosis	52,53

?, not known; −, negative; +, positive.

are available about IL-3 expression in Hodgkin and Reed-Sternberg cells of tissue samples. More than 90% of Hodgkin and Reed-Sternberg cells express the alpha chain of the IL-3R (IL-3Rα).[21] Hodgkin cell lines also express the α and β chains that form IL-3R, both at the mRNA and protein level. Exogenous IL-3 promotes the growth of cultured Hodgkin cells, and this effect can be potentiated by IL-9 and stem cell factor (SCF) co-stimulation. IL-3 is able to partially rescue tumor cells from apoptosis induced by serum deprivation. Cultured Hodgkin cells also increase the production of IL-3 by preactivated T- cells, suggesting an involvement of IL-3/IL-3R interactions in the cellular growth of Hodgkin lymphoma through paracrine mechanisms.[21,22]

Interleukin-4

IL-4 is a pleiotropic factor that affects different steps of antigen-dependent maturation of human B-cells and acts as a positive factor for survival of T-cells. Expression of IL-4 in cases of Hodgkin lymphoma could not be demonstrated in the tumor cells.[3,23] In Hodgkin cell lines the results for production of IL-4 protein were not consistent.[5,14,23,25] Stimulation of L428 with IL-4 revealed enhanced growth, but incubation with anti-IL-4 antibodies had no effect on their growth.[26] Based on these results it is unlikely that IL-4 acts as an autocrine growth factor for Hodgkin and Reed-Sternberg cells.

Interleukin-5

IL-5 mRNA transcripts are present in the cytoplasm of Hodgkin and Reed-Sternberg cells in a proportion of cases of classical Hodgkin lymphoma[27] and in some of the cell lines.[5,14,28] Proliferation of IL-5 positive Hodgkin cell lines is not affected by neutralizing antibodies[28] indicating that IL-5 probably does not act as an autocrine growth factor. Because IL-5 is responsible for the growth and differentiation of

TABLE 6.2

CHEMOKINE EXPRESSION IN TUMOR CELLS OF HODGKIN LYMPHOMA

Chemokine	% Positive Cases		Produced by		Relevance for HL	References
	CHL	NLP	HRS	Lines		
CCL1 (I-309)	?	?	?	+	?	54, 55
CCL5 (Rantes)	0–70	0–70	+	+	Recruitment reactive cells and mast cells	54,56–58
CCL11 (Eotaxin)	0		−	+	TNF-α induced enhanced production by fibroblasts	4,59,69
CCL13 (MCP-4)	40	70	+	+	?	54
CCL17 (TARC)	80–93	0	+	+	Induction of TH2 and regulatory T-cells	42,54,55,58,60–62
CCL19 (MIP-3β/ELC)			?	+	Induction of T-cells	54,63
CCL20 (MIP-3α)			?	+	?	54
CCL22 (MDC)	90–100	17–100	+	+	Induction of TH2 and regulatory T-cells	54,55,58,64,69
CCL28 (MEC)	75		+	+	Recruitment of Eosinophils and plasma cells	55
CXCL8 (IL-8)	0–10	0	−	−	Density of neutrophils	54,67,68
CXCL9 (MIG)	70	0	+	+	Reactive infiltrate EBV+ HL	4,58,62,69
CXCL10 (IP-10)	25–70	0–85	+	+	Reactive infiltrate EBV+ HL	4,54,55,58,62,69,70
CXCL12 (SDF1)	0	0	−	−	?	63
CXCL13 (BLC)			+	+	?	54,63
CXCL16	?	?	?	+	Attraction of plasma Cells	55

?, not known; −, negative; +, positive.

Interleukin-6

IL-6 was first identified as a T-cell–derived cytokine that induces maturation of B-cells into antibody-producing plasma cells and stimulates plasma cells. Several studies report on the expression of IL-6 in Hodgkin and Reed-Sternberg cells. Overall, expression was observed in 65% to 100% of cases of classical Hodgkin lymphoma,[23,24,31–33] with a significantly higher expression level in EBV-positive (84%) than EBV-negative cases (51%).[32] Besides the Hodgkin and Reed-Sternberg cells, reactive histiocytes and endothelial cells also stained positive for IL-6.[23] High expression levels have been confirmed in most Hodgkin cell lines.[6,14,23,33]

IL-6R has been detected on Hodgkin and Reed-Sternberg cells in some cases and cell lines in some studies but not in others.[23] Tesch and associates[34] reported that IL-6R protein was expressed more commonly in mixed-cellularity than nodular-sclerosis cases. Incubation of six Hodgkin cell lines with neutralizing antibodies against IL-6 or IL-6R did not affect the proliferation, and these studies do not support a putative autocrine growth effect of IL-6 on Hodgkin and Reed-Sternberg cells.[14,23,35]

Interleukin-7

IL-7 can induce growth of mature T-cells but not mature B-cells and may act as an antitumor cytokine, involved in activation of the immune response. IL-7 expression was demonstrated in Hodgkin and Reed-Sternberg cells of 24 out of 31 cases by RNA in situ hybridization.[36] Moreover, IL-7 mRNA transcripts were also frequently observed in Hodgkin cell lines.[36]

Interleukin-9

IL-9 is a T-cell and mast cell growth factor that can also potentiate IL-4–induced IgG4 and IgE production. Hodgkin and Reed-Sternberg cells are positive for IL-9 by RNA in situ hybridization[37] and immunohistochemistry in approximately

eosinophils, it may be associated with the presence of eosinophils in tissues involved by Hodgkin lymphoma.[29,30]

50% of the cases. In 19% of the cases the cytoplasm of the tumor cells stains for IL-9R.[38] In L428 expression of IL-9 was observed only upon stimulation with PHA/PMA.[37] A moderate stimulatory effect on the proliferation was observed upon treatment of KMH2 with IL-9, suggesting that it acts as a growth factor for Hodgkin and Reed-Sternberg cells.[39]

Interleukin-10

IL-10 is a TH2 cytokine with strong anti-inflammatory properties. IL-10 inhibits T-cell growth, blocks IL-2 and IFN-γ production by TH1 cells, and down-regulates pro-inflammatory cytokine production. IL-10 is a growth and differentiation factor for B-cells. IL-10 mRNA and protein were detected in a variable percentage of Hodgkin and Reed-Sternberg cells in 21% to 36% of samples of primary classical Hodgkin lymphoma.[3,40,41] Much higher levels are observed in EBV-positive than in EBV-negative cases.[3,40] IL-10 mRNA and protein were detected in two of seven Hodgkin cell lines.[6,40] In a more recent study, high IL-10 levels were detected by RT-PCR in all cell lines.[5]

Interleukin-12

IL-12 is a cytokine with in vitro and in vivo immunomodulatory effects; it enhances TH1 responses and inhibits TH2 responses. In tissue samples of Hodgkin lymphoma, expression of the p35 and p40 subunits was reported mainly in small lymphoid cells and not in the Hodgkin and Reed-Sternberg cells.[42] By RNAse protection assay two Hodgkin cell lines showed high expression of IL-12 p35, but not of the p40 subunit.[43] EBI3 is an EBV-induced cytokine homologous to the IL-12 p40 subunit and was found to be strongly expressed in Hodgkin and Reed-Sternberg cells in 32 of 33 cases, independently of the EBV status of the tumour cells.[43] It has been suggested that EBI3 may function to antagonize IL-12 and to inhibit the development of a TH1 immune response.

Interleukin-13

IL-13 induces fibrosis and stimulates fibroblasts to produce CCL11 and is a positive factor for TH2 cells. IL-13 expression was identified by RNA in situ hybridization in Hodgkin and Reed-Sternberg cells in 86% of cases.[28,35] At the protein level, IL-13 was demonstrated in 93% of the cases.[44] Most Hodgkin cell lines express IL-13.[5,25,28] In contrast to various other cytokines, a dose-dependent inhibition of proliferation was observed in IL-13–positive cell lines HDLM2 and L1236 upon treatment with neutralizing antibodies against IL-13,[25,28,45] suggesting an autocrine effect for IL-13. However, treatment of the IL-13–positive cell lines L428 and KMH2 had no effect on proliferation.[25]

Interleukin-15

IL-15 is a T-cell growth factor. IL-15 mRNA expression has been identified in tissue samples from Hodgkin lymphoma but the responsible cells are not known.[11] All Hodgkin cell lines showed high expression of IL-15 mRNA by RT-PCR, which suggests that Hodgkin and Reed-Sternberg cells in involved tissues contribute to the IL-15 production.[11]

TNF-α

TNF-α is an important modulator of inflammation, tissue remodelling, and wound healing. RNA in situ hybridization revealed that expression of TNF-α is restricted predominantly to Hodgkin and Reed-Sternberg cells.[10] High expression levels were confirmed by two other studies in all cases of Hodgkin lymphoma.[14,31] Hodgkin cell lines were all positive for TNF-α mRNA but no protein expression could be detected.[31] The receptor for TNF-α has only been studied in a small number of primary cases and was found to be expressed in a proportion of the cases,[46] suggesting that TNF-α might have an autocrine effect on Hodgkin and Reed-Sternberg cells by stimulating activation of NF-κB.

Lymphotoxin-α

LT-α shares approximately 50% structural homology with TNF-α and shares the same receptors. Expression of LT-α was observed in Hodgkin and Reed-Sternberg cells of all cases, and this was supported by the high mRNA and protein expression levels in Hodgkin cell lines.[31] LT-α might also act as an autocrine factor for Hodgkin and Reed-Sternberg cells.

TGF-β

TGF-β is one of the main immunosuppressive cytokines that inhibit IL-2–dependent T-cell proliferation. In addition, it induces fibrosis and collagen synthesis. TGF-β expression has been observed in the majority of cases of classical Hodgkin lymphoma.[47–49] In situ hybridization indicated that TGF-β mRNA can be localized to Hodgkin and Reed-Sternberg cells[48] and eosinophils,[50] which are known to make TGF-β. In Hodgkin cell lines a very high level of TGF-β mRNA was detected by qRT-PCR.[5] High TGF-β levels have been found especially in cases of nodular sclerosis, and this is thought to be responsible for the formation of the collagen bands in that subtype.[47] TGF-β secreted by Hodgkin and Reed-Sternberg cells suppresses T-cell activation and in addition also induces enhanced TGF-β production by lymphocytes, resulting in an autocrine-suppressed state of these lymphocytes.[51]

bFGF (FGF2)

bFGF is responsible for collagen synthesis. Presence of bFGF was demonstrated by immunohistochemistry and RNA in situ hybridization in Hodgkin and Reed-Sternberg cells, histiocytes, and stromal cells in the vast majority of cases of nodular sclerosis and also in Hodgkin lymphoma cell lines.[52,53] bFGF might contribute to the induction of sclerosis in Hodgkin lymphoma.

CHEMOKINES IN HODGKIN AND REED-STERNBERG CELLS IN HODGKIN LYMPHOMA TISSUE AND CELL LINES

CCL1

CCL1 (I-309) reacts with CCR8, which is expressed on TH2 cells, activated NK cells, and monocytes. CCL1 expression has been detected in several Hodgkin cell lines.[54,55] In Hodgkin tissue, high CCL1 mRNA transcript levels have been demonstrated, but it is unclear whether this chemokine is produced by the tumor cells. Despite the lack of confirmation of CCL1 transcripts in Hodgkin and Reed-Sternberg cells, its expression seems to be specific for Hodgkin tissue because it is not observed in control lymphoid tissues and in other B-cell malignancies.[54]

CCL5

CCL5 (Rantes) is a so-called pro-inflammatory chemokine that attracts cells positive for CC-chemokine receptors CCR1, 3, 4, and 5. These receptors can be found on monocytes, eosinophils, mast cells, basophils, and T lymphocytes. All Hodgkin cell lines express significant levels of CCL5 mRNA.[54–56] Protein expression was found in the Hodgkin and Reed-Sternberg cells in Hodgkin tissue, independent of subtype, and also in many cells of the reactive background.[54] RNA in situ hybridization for CCL5 transcripts revealed that positive cells were confined largely to the infiltrating cells, which mainly were of T-cell origin.[57] More recently, CCL5 expression was found specifically in the lymphocytes surrounding the Hodgkin and Reed-Sternberg cells.[58]

High levels of CCL5 and the presence of high numbers of CCR3- and CCR5-positive eosinophils, monocytes, and T-cells[57] indicate that this chemokine contributes to the recruitment of the reactive cells in Hodgkin lymphoma.

CCL11

CCL11 (Eotaxin) attracts CCR2-, 3-, and 5-positive eosinophils, monocytes, and T-cells. Expression of CCL11 has been observed only in the L1236 cell line.[59] In Hodgkin tissue CCL11 is found predominantly in fibroblasts, some macrophages, and in the smooth muscle of blood vessels.[59] In one report limited expression of CCL11 was found in the Hodgkin and Reed-Sternberg cells with a higher expression level in the nodular-sclerosis subtype and a positive correlation with the presence of eosinophils.[4] Although Hodgkin and Reed-Sternberg cells usually do not produce CCL11 themselves, they do contribute to the high CCL11 levels by production of TNF-α, which has been shown to enhance CCL11 production by fibroblasts.[59]

CCL13

CCL13 (MCP-4) attracts cells with CCR1, 2, 3, or 5 expression, which can be observed on monocytes, eosinophils, and T-cells. Only the mixed-cellularity Hodgkin lymphoma–derived cell line L1236 expresses CCL13.[54] In tissue samples, low CCL13 protein expression was found in Hodgkin and Reed-Sternberg cells in 6 of 14 classical and in 5 of 7 cases of nodular lymphocyte-predominant Hodgkin lymphoma.[54]

CCL17

CCL17 (TARC) binds to CCR4 and 8 on TH2 cells, regulatory T-cells, basophils, and monocytes. All Hodgkin cell lines express TARC, albeit at variable levels.[54,55] Using serial analysis of gene expression (SAGE), RNA in situ hybridization, and immunohistochemistry, CCL17 was found to be highly expressed in the neoplastic cells of classical and not in nodular lymphocyte-predominant Hodgkin lymphomas or non-Hodgkin lymphomas.[60] Eighty-six percent of classical Hodgkin lymphoma cases were reported to stain for CCL17.[61] High expression levels of CCL17 might explain the influx of lymphocytes with a TH2-like phenotype, and CCL17-positive cases are indeed associated with a higher percentage of CCR4-positive cells.[60,62] In turn, TH2 type cytokines (IL-4, IL-13) can induce the production of CCL17 by Hodgkin and Reed-Sternberg cells.

CCL19

CCL19 (MIP3β/ELC) attracts CCR7 positive-dendritic cells, T-cells, and B-cells. In Hodgkin cell lines, expression of CCL19

has only been demonstrated in L591.[54] This is consistent with the results in tissues, which revealed expression only in endothelial and stromal cells and not in the Hodgkin and Reed-Sternberg cells. CCR7, the receptor for CCL19, is expressed by Hodgkin cell lines and Hodgkin and Reed-Sternberg cells of classical but not of nodular lymphocyte-predominant Hodgkin lymphomas.[63] This suggests that this chemokine may play an important role in the migration and dissemination of Hodgkin and Reed-Sternberg cells. Moreover, the expression levels of CCL19 might also contribute to the migration of CCR7-positive T-cells into the areas involved by Hodgkin lymphoma.

CCL20

CCL20 (MIP3α) attracts CCR6-positive cells; this receptor is expressed on a subset of immature dendritic cells and memory T-cells. Expression of CCL20 mRNA was found in Hodgkin cell lines L428 and L591.[54] In tissues, a low expression of CCL20 was found at mRNA levels, but it is not known whether CCL20 is produced by Hodgkin and Reed-Sternberg cells or by the infiltrating cells.

CCL22

CCL22 (MDC) binds CCR4 and CCR8 receptors that are expressed on dendritic cells, TH2 cells, regulatory T-cells, basophils, and monocytes. Most Hodgkin cell lines express high levels of CCL22 transcripts.[54,55] High protein expression levels were also found in the cytoplasm of Hodgkin and Reed-Sternberg cells of 90% to 100% of classical and also variably in cases of nodular lymphocyte-predominant Hodgkin lymphoma and non-Hodgkin lymphoma.[54,64,65,66] CCL22 production can also be stimulated by TH2 cytokines IL-4 and IL-13 and may serve to reinforce the attraction of TH2 and regulatory T-lymphocytes, initiated by CCL17.

CCL28

CCL28 (MEC) attracts CCR3- and CCR10-positive eosinophils and plasma cells. CCL28 is expressed only in Hodgkin cell line L428.[55] In tissue, expression was found in the Hodgkin and Reed-Sternberg cells of a large majority of cases. CCL28 expression correlated with the amount of infiltrating eosinophils and plasma cells.[55] The CCL28 receptor, CCR10, was found to be expressed in the cells of 7 out of 19 cases, suggesting also an autocrine mode of action.

CXCL8

CXCL8 (IL-8) attaches to CXCR1 and CXCR2, which are found on neutrophils. No CXCL8 expression was observed in any of the Hodgkin cell lines.[54] Lack of expression was confirmed in Hodgkin tissues, both at the RNA[54,67] and protein level.[68] CXCL8 expression was observed in Hodgkin and Reed-Sternberg cells of only 10% of cases of classical Hodgkin lymphoma, whereas positive reactive cells were observed in 60% of the cases.[68] The CXCL8-positive cells were more numerous in cases of nodular-sclerosis than mixed-cellularity subtype. The number of CXCL8-positive cells and the density of neutrophils were positively correlated. In nodular lymphocyte-predominant Hodgkin lymphoma cases CXCL8 expression was absent.[68]

CXCL9

CXCL9 (MIG) reacts with CXCR3, which is expressed on TH1 and NK cells. CXCL9 mRNA is found at low levels in Hodgkin cell lines. A homogeneous expression was found in all Hodgkin and control tissues with RT-PCR.[54] Teruya-Feldstein and colleagues[69] demonstrated presence of CXCL9 in Hodgkin and Reed-Sternberg cells that was most pronounced in EBV-positive cases. High expression levels were also observed in nodular lymphocyte-predominant Hodgkin lymphoma.[69] In a more recent study, all mixed-cellularity cases stained strongly positive for CXCL9, whereas only 40% of the nodular-sclerosis cases were positive including only one strongly positive case.[58] In addition to positive tumor cells, some of the histiocytes were also positive for CXCL9.

CXCL10

CXCL10 (IP-10) is a proinflammatory chemokine that can be induced by IFN-γ. Like CXCL9, it binds to CXCR3. CXCL10 is expressed in the majority of Hodgkin cell lines.[54,55] In tissue, the highest expression levels have been observed in EBV-positive cases and were produced mainly by the Hodgkin and Reed-Sternberg cells.[62,69] Expression was very high in all cases of mixed cellularity and in only some (40%) cases of nodular sclerosis, similar to the findings for CXCL9.[4,62] Some expression was also found in the reactive background cells.[54,70] CXCL10 was not detected in nodular lymphocyte-predominant Hodgkin lymphoma.[70] The receptor for CXCL10 (CXCR3) was also found to be expressed in Hodgkin cell lines,[63] whereas CXCR3-positive lymphocytes were observed directly surrounding Hodgkin and Reed-Sternberg cells. This suggests a direct effect of CXCL10 and CXCL9 on the reactive infiltrate in EBV-positive cases.

CXCL12

CXCL12 attracts CXCR4-positive cells, which is expressed on all T-cells. CXCL12 (SDF-1) was not found in Hodgkin cell lines and Hodgkin and Reed-Sternberg cells, but its receptor CXCR4 has been reported to be highly expressed in most cell lines and cases. This receptor could therefore be important for the migration and dissemination of Hodgkin and Reed-Sternberg cells.[63]

CXCL13

CXCL13 (BLC/BCA-1) attracts CXCR5-positive naive B-cells and CD4/CD57-positive TH cells. CXCL13 was found to be strongly expressed by cell line L428 and weakly by L591.[54] Hodgkin and Reed-Sternberg cells weakly expressed CXCL13, especially in cases of nodular sclerosis. Infiltrating cells in both classical and nodular lymphocyte-predominant Hodgkin lymphoma did express CXCL13.[63] CXCR5 was only expressed in Hodgkin cell line L591.

CXCL16

CXCL16 attracts CXCR6-positive plasma cells. Expression of this chemokine has only been studied in Hodgkin cell lines which were consistently positive.[55]

Role of Dipeptidyl-Peptidase IV (CD26)

Several chemokines including CCL22, CCL5, CXCR10, and CCL11 may be natural substrates of CD26. This glycoprotein has intrinsic dipeptidyl-peptidase IV activity and can truncate its substrates, resulting in products with reduced chemotactic activity. Because the T-lymphocytes surrounding the Hodgkin and Reed-Sternberg cells lack CD26 expression they are incapable of modulating the chemotaxis exerted by the Hodgkin and Reed-Sternberg cells, in contrast to CD26-positive cells,

such as TH1 cells and cytotoxic cells, which thus are less sensitive to these chemokines.[30]

CYTOKINE AND CHEMOKINE SERUM LEVELS IN PATIENTS WITH HODGKIN LYMPHOMA

Several studies have analyzed cytokine levels in sera of patients with Hodgkin lymphoma in comparison to levels observed in normal controls, whereas only a few studies have focused on the analysis of chemokine serum levels (Table 6.3). For most cytokines studied thus far (i.e., IL-1α, IL-1β, IL-2, IL-3, IL-4, IL-13, IFN-γ, TNFα, and LTα), the vast majority of patients with Hodgkin lymphoma had normal levels and increased levels were observed in less than 15% of the samples. For part of the cytokines (IL-7, IL-8, IL-10, G-CSF, and GM-CSF), a variable percentage of patients presenting with increased serum levels was observed, probably reflecting the variation in detection levels of the individual ELISA assays used in the various studies. Gene polymorphisms, especially those that are located in the promotor regions, might also influence the serum levels of the corresponding cytokines. An overview of the most prominently increased cytokines and chemokines and their possible clinical relevance is given next.

Increased IL-6 serum levels have been reported in variable percentages of patients with Hodgkin lymphoma.[71,72] No relation of increased IL-6 levels with various clinical factors and freedom from treatment failure was reported.[71] In another study a correlation was observed between high IL-6 levels and poor prognosis.[73] This was confirmed by Cozen et. al[74] who demonstrated higher IL-6 levels in a high risk-group according to international prognostic score status as compared to lower levels in the low-risk group. There was also an association between increased IL-6 serum levels with increased IL-3 and GM-CSF levels in the majority of cases.[75] Genotyping of the IL-6 gene region revealed a decreased risk to develop Hodgkin lymphoma for the C allele of the IL-6 174G>C promotor polymorphism.[76] However, these results could not be confirmed by another study[77] that analyzed DNA samples in 408 cases and 349 controls. In the latter study, a significant difference was only observed for G alleles in patients with nodular lymphocyte-predominant Hodgkin lymphoma.

Increased serum IL-9 levels were observed in 40% of the patients and this was most pronounced in the nodular sclerosis subtype. High IL-9 levels correlated with several negative prognostic factors.[78]

Many studies have been performed on serum IL-10 levels in patients with Hodgkin lymphoma, and increased IL-10 levels were found in from 10% to more than 50% of the cases.[79–84] Increased IL-10 levels were associated with older age[79] and emerged as an independent predictor of inferior failure-free survival. Progression-free survival was 50% in the group with high IL-10 levels versus 81% in patients with normal IL-10 levels for all patients with Hodgkin lymphoma and 43% versus 77% for the patients with classical Hodgkin lymphoma.[85] EBV-positive cases had higher IL-10 levels than EBV-negative cases.[85] This is consistent with the significantly worse prognosis for older patients with EBV-positive Hodgkin lymphoma.[86] Genotyping of two IL-10 promoter polymorphisms (-1082G>A and -592C>A) in 147 Hodgkin patients revealed no significant differences.[87]

IL-13 is a cytokine that has been suggested to be an autocrine growth factor for Hodgkin and Reed-Sternberg cells and was found to be elevated in serum samples of only 11% of newly diagnosed patients with Hodgkin lymphoma. No correlations were observed with clinical factors. In patients who relapsed, increased serum levels were found in 16%.[88]

TABLE 6.3

CYTOKINE AND CHEMOKINE SERUM LEVELS IN PATIENTS WITH HODGKIN LYMPHOMA

Cytokine	% Patients[a]	Related to/Proposed Relevance for HL	References
IFN-γ	<15	—	118
IL-1α	<15	—	97,122
IL-1β	<15	—	75,97,118
IL-2	<15	IPS	97,122
IL-3	<15	—	97
IL-4	<15	—	96,97,122
IL-6	>35	Poor prognosis/IPS/disease activity/ clinical symptoms/B-symptoms	71–73,75,118,122
IL-7	>29	Disease activity/clinical symptoms/ B-symptoms	96,97
IL-9	40	Autocrine growth factor	78
IL-10	10–50	Failure-free survival/EBV status	79–81,84,85,123
IL-13	<15	Relapse/autocrine growth factor	78,88
G-CSF	Variable	Disease activity/clinical symptoms	75
GM-CSF	<39	—	75,97
VEGF	?	Survival	126
HGF	?	—	126
TNF-α	<15	Clinical symptoms/B-symptoms	73,75,97,120,124,125,127
TNF-β	<15	—	97,127
CXCL8	<27	Disease activity/clinical symptoms/ B-symptoms	96,97
CCL17	90	Tumor load/poor survival	98

IPS, International Prognostic Score.

[a]In many studies the percentage of patients with increased levels is not given, due to comparison of only the group mean or median values.

Analysis of the TNF-α promotor polymorphism (-308G>A) in 36 patients with Hodgkin lymphoma demonstrated no significant difference compared to normal controls. The incidence of TNF-α4, a microsatellite allele associated with low TNF production, was significantly higher in responders than in nonresponders in a group of 61 patients.[89] Because this gene is located in the HLA class III region, which shows strong linkage disequilibrium over a large area, it is difficult to determine whether this indeed represents the causative variation.[90]

Analysis of a single nucleotide polymorphism in the IL-1Rα gene revealed no significant correlation with Hodgkin lymphoma compared to normal controls.[91] In 88 children presenting with Hodgkin lymphoma, increased IL-2R serum levels were observed. This effect was most pronounced in patients with stage III and IV disease and patients presenting with B-symptoms.[92] High IL-2R levels correlated with poor prognosis.[93–95]

Increased serum levels of CXCL8 were observed in 27% of patients with Hodgkin lymphoma,[96,97] were associated with B-symptoms, and occurred more often in patients with the nodular-sclerosis subtype.[96]

In a retrospective study, TARC serum levels were found to be elevated in 90% of a group of 62 patients with classical Hodgkin lymphoma.[98] So far, this is the most consistently up-regulated serum marker in Hodgkin lymphoma. At diagnosis, TARC serum levels correlated with stage, erythrocyte sedimentation rate, leukocyte counts, and lymphocyte counts. TARC serum levels also correlated with tumor load and levels dropped after therapy. A TARC serum level >2,000 pg/mL after completed treatment was found to correlate with a poor survival rate.

EFFECTS OF CYTOKINES AND CHEMOKINES ON THE HISTOPATHOLOGY OF HODGKIN LYMPHOMA

EOSINOPHILIA, PLASMA CELLS, AND MAST CELLS

Eosinophils are frequently present in the inflammatory infiltrate of classical Hodgkin lymphomas, and in some patients eosinophilia can be detected in the peripheral blood. Eosinophilia can also be found in some T-cell lymphomas, but is an infrequent finding in B-cell non-Hodgkin lymphomas. Eosinophilia was found to be associated with the presence of IL-5 mRNA in the cytoplasm of Hodgkin and Reed-Sternberg cells in some cases of mixed cellularity and nodular sclerosis.[27] IL-5 normally is produced by activated TH2 cells and stimulates the production of eosinophils. Some human B-cells have been shown to express IL-5 receptors, but it is not clear whether these cells can also respond to IL-5. Another cytokine highly produced by Hodgkin and Reed-Sternberg cells and promoting eosinophilia is IL-9.

A strong direct correlation was found between tissue eosinophilia and expression of CCL11 mRNA expression in Hodgkin tissues.[4,99] A high expression of CCL11 was found specifically in nodular sclerosis compared to other subtypes. In contrast, no CCL11 was found in B- or T-cell lymphomas with tissue eosinophilia, suggesting another pathway for eosinophilia in these disorders. Hodgkin and Reed-Sternberg cells did not secrete CCL11 themselves, but induced fibroblasts to produce eotaxin through TNF-α.[59]

Hodgkin and Reed-Sternberg cells were found to be positive for CCL28 in a majority of cases and CCL28 significantly correlated with the presence of eosinophils expressing CCR3, and plasma cells expressing CCR10. Thus, the production of CCL28 by Hodgkin and Reed-Sternberg cells may play a major role in tissue accumulation of eosinophils in classical Hodgkin lymphoma. In addition to eosinophils, CCL28 also attracts plasma cells.[55]

Interestingly, eosinophils strongly express the CD30 ligand, which can stimulate the CD30 molecule on the Hodgkin and Reed-Sternberg cells.[100] This may explain why tissue eosinophilia is a poor prognostic sign. Mast cells also strongly express CD30 ligand and may thus also stimulate Hodgkin and Reed-Sternberg cells via CD30.[101] IL-9 and CCL5 are two of the factors produced by Hodgkin and Reed-Sternberg cells cells that may attract mast cells,[38] and mast cells are indeed present in most cases of Hodgkin lymphoma, especially in the nodular-sclerosis subtype. Patients with a higher degree of mast cell infiltration have a worse failure-free survival rate.[102]

SCLEROSIS AND FIBROSIS

Bands of collagen surrounding and separating abnormal lymphoid nodules and surrounding blood vessels are characteristic of nodular sclerosis, the most common histologic type of Hodgkin lymphoma. There are at least two mechanisms that may explain fibroblast activation and fibrosis in Hodgkin lymphoma: unbalanced production of pro-fibrogenic cytokines like IL-1, IL-13, TNF-α, TGF-β, and bFGF[103] by the tumor cells and/or the reactive cells, and activation of fibroblasts by CD40L-expressing cells of the Hodgkin lymphoma microenvironment. Supernatants of cell cultures from nodular sclerosis were shown to potentiate the growth of fibroblasts in vitro.[104] Fibroblast-activating activity was also found in cell culture supernatants of Hodgkin lymphoma and at least part of this activity could be attributed to IL-1,[105,106] whereas TNF-α also contributed to fibroblast growth in Hodgkin lymphoma.[107,108] However, the growth factor most consistently associated with nodular sclerosis is TGF-β. TGF-β has been known for several years to stimulate fibroblast proliferation and collagen synthesis both in vitro and in vivo.[109,110] A high-molecular-weight TGF-β, active at physiologic pH, was demonstrated in supernants from the L428 cell line.[111] Activated TGF-β was found to be associated with the extracellular matrix mainly around blood vessels, zones of necrosis, at the margins of bands of collagen sclerosis, and in areas containing syncytia of Hodgkin and Reed-Sternberg cells in tissue sections of nodular-sclerosis cases.[47] The presence of activated TGF-β in situ on the cell membrane and within the cytoplasm of Hodgkin and Reed-Sternberg cells suggests that these cells are secreting activated TGF-β continuously. In situ hybridization showed that TGF-β mRNA was localized in the Hodgkin and Reed-Sternberg cells[48] and in eosinophils,[50] which are known to make TGF-β.[112]

TGF-β may interact with other cytokines, particularly bFGF in causing the fibrosis in Hodgkin lymphoma. In a murine model of cutaneous fibrosis, simultaneous application of TGF-β and bFGF causes persistent fibrosis.[113] Ohshima and co-workers demonstrated the presence of bFGF by immunohistochemistry and in situ hybridization in Hodgkin and Reed-Sternberg cells, histiocytes, and stromal cells in nodular-sclerosis cases.[52] Thus, both TGF-β and bFGF appear to contribute to the induction of collagen sclerosis in Hodgkin lymphoma. Another factor that may promote fibrosis is IL-13, which was found to be produced by the Hodgkin and Reed-Sternberg cells as well as the TH2 lymphocytes and acts as an autocrine stimulatory factor, but also can stimulate fibroblasts that have IL-13 receptors.[44]

EFFECTS OF CYTOKINES ON THE CLINICAL MANIFESTATIONS OF HODGKIN LYMPHOMA

Patients with Hodgkin lymphoma experience fever, weight loss, and night sweats, known as B-symptoms, much more frequently than patients with B-cell non-Hodgkin lymphomas.[114] Fever is not specifically associated with inflammation or necrosis, and most patients with the nodular-sclerosis subtype do not have fever.[115] The immediate cause of the B-symptoms is unknown, but there is good reason to suspect that certain cytokines are responsible.

Interleukin-1β, TNF-α, IFN-γ, and IL-6 are pro-inflammatory pyrogenic molecules that can also mediate inhibition of lipogenic enzymes and lead to development of anorexia and weight loss.[115–121] Administration of these molecules to animals or humans can cause B-symptoms. Thus, several investigators have attempted to correlate B-symptoms with presence of these molecules in tissues of Hodgkin lymphoma patients. Indeed, high levels of IL-1,[8] TNF-α,[10] and LT-α[115] have been detected in a variable proportion of tissues involved by Hodgkin lymphoma, but generally no clear association with B-symptoms could be identified. However, IL-1β was found to be increased about two to ten times in five of eight lymph nodes from patients with Hodgkin lymphoma and B-symptoms, whereas other cytokines (IL-1α, TNF-α, LT-α, and IL-6) were expressed heterogeneously in both symptomatic and asymptomatic patients.[121] Statistical analysis demonstrated that this difference in IL-1β expression between symptomatic and asymptomatic patients was significant.

Others have tried to correlate B-symptoms with serum cytokine levels of patients with Hodgkin lymphoma.[71,75,97,120] Increased levels of IL-2R, IL-6, IL-7, G-CSF, and CXCL8, were found in many patients with Hodgkin lymphoma as opposed to healthy individuals. Serum concentrations of IL-2R, IL-6, and IL-7 were significantly correlated with advanced-stage disease and, together with G-CSF levels, with the presence of B-symptoms. Patients with normal IL-6 levels also had better event-free survivals than patients with elevated IL-6 levels, but this difference did not reach significance. These findings indicate that enhanced levels of sIL-2R, IL-6, IL-7, G-CSF, and CXCL8 are correlated with disease activity and clinical symptoms in Hodgkin lymphoma.

SUMMARY AND CONCLUSIONS

Many studies have been performed to understand the complex crosstalk between Hodgkin and Reed-Sternberg cells and the much more abundant infiltrating cells. Although much remains unsolved, some clear relations and interactions have been observed (Fig. 6.1). Chemokines largely account for the attraction of various infiltrating cells. CCL17 and CCL22 are the most prominent and characteristic for Hodgkin lymphoma

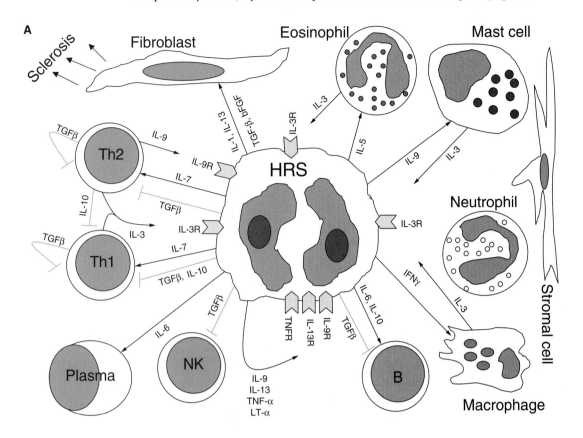

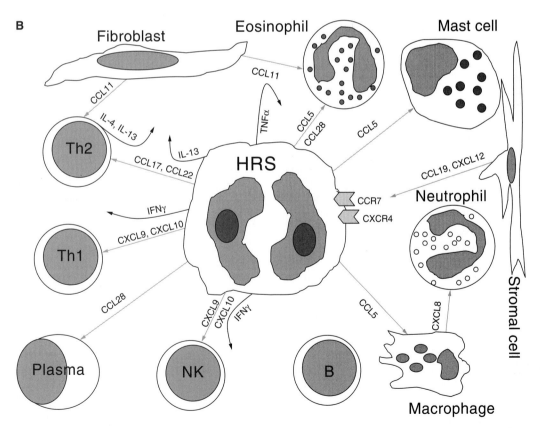

FIGURE 6.1. Schematic representation of effects of cytokines and chemokines on Hodgkin and Reed-Sternberg cells and infiltrating cells. **A:** Schematic presentation of the cytokine effects. Black arrows represent positive/stimulating effects of cytokines and gray arrows represent negative/blocking effects. **B:** Schematic presentation of chemokine effects. Gray arrows present the chemokine attracting effects. Black arrows present the stimulatory effects of cytokines on chemokine production. See color insert.

and may explain the presence of TH2-like lymphocytes that provide positive signals for the Hodgkin and Reed-Sternberg cells by producing IL-4, IL-10, and IL-13. IL-4 and IL-13 also reinforce the production of CCL17 and CCL22 by the Hodgkin and Reed-Sternberg cells. To escape an effective immune response, Hodgkin and Reed-Sternberg cells produce immunosuppressive cytokines like IL-10 and TGF-β.

Although several cytokines have been postulated to be autocrine growth factors, this has only been proven for IL-9 and IL-13 by treatment of Hodgkin cell lines with these cytokines or with blocking antibodies. Presence of eosinophilia in Hodgkin tissues can be explained by high levels of CCL11, IL-5, and CCL28, which are induced either indirectly by the fibroblasts through stimulation with TNF-α or produced by Hodgkin and Reed-Sternberg cells. Presence of sclerotic bands specifically in the nodular-sclerosis subtype is associated with high expression levels of various cytokines, including TGF-β, IL-13, bFGF, and IL-1.

Serum cytokine and chemokine levels in patients with Hodgkin lymphoma have been correlated with various clinical symptoms. The most convincing association is that between elevated IL-6 and presence of B-symptoms. Some of the other cytokines, including IL-7, TNF-α, and CXCL8, are also associated with B-symptoms. The most consistently elevated serum marker is CCL17, and this chemokine may indeed be useful to monitor disease activity of Hodgkin lymphoma.

References

1. Gruss HJ, Pinto A, Duyster J, et al. Hodgkin's disease: a tumor with disturbed immunological pathways. *Immunol Today*. 1997;18:156–163.
2. Gerdes J, Kretschmer C, Zahn G, et al. Immunoenzymatic assessment of interferon-gamma in Hodgkin and Sternberg- Reed cells. *Cytokine* 1990; 2:307–310.
3. Dukers DF, Jaspars LH, Vos W, et al. Quantitative immunohistochemical analysis of cytokine profiles in Epstein-Barr virus-positive and -negative cases of Hodgkin's disease. *J Pathol* 2000;190:143–149.
4. Teruya-Feldstein J, Jaffe ES, Burd PR, et al. Differential chemokine expression in tissues involved by Hodgkin's disease: direct correlation of eotaxin expression and tissue eosinophilia. *Blood* 1999;93:2463–2470.
5. Atayar C, Poppema S, Blokzijl T, et al. Expression of the T-cell transcription factors, GATA-3 and T-bet, in the neoplastic cells of Hodgkin lymphoma. *Am J Pathol* 2005;166:127–134.
6. Wolf J, Kapp U, Bohlen H, et al. Peripheral blood mononuclear cells of a patient with advanced Hodgkin's lymphoma give rise to permanently growing Hodgkin-Reed Sternberg cells. *Blood* 1996;87: 3418–3428.
7. Hsu SM, Hsu PL. Lack of effect of colony-stimulating factors, interleukins, interferons, and tumor necrosis factor on the growth and differentiation of cultured Reed-Sternberg cells. Comparison with effects of phorbol ester and retinoic acid. *Am J Pathol* 1990;136:181–189.
8. Ree HJ, Crowley JP, Dinarello CA. Anti-interleukin-1 reactive cells in Hodgkin's disease. *Cancer* 1987;59:1717–1720.
9. Ruco LP, Pomponi D, Pigott R, et al. Cytokine production (IL-1a, IL-1b, TNFa) and endothelial cell activation (ELAM-1 and HLA-DR) in reactive lymphadenitis, Hodgkin's disease, and in non-Hodgkin's lymphomas. An immunocytochemical study. *Am J Pathol* 1990;137:1163–1171.
10. Xerri L, Birg F, Guigou V, et al. In situ expression of the IL-1a and TNF-a genes by Reed-Sternberg cells in Hodgkin's disease. *Int J Cancer* 1992; 50:689–693.
11. Malec M, Soderqvist M, Sirsjo A, et al. Real-time polymerase chain reaction determination of cytokine mRNA expression profiles in Hodgkin's lymphoma. *Haematologica* 2004;89:679–685.
12. Hsu S-M, Krupen K, Lachman LB. Heterogeneity of interleukin 1 production in cultured Reed-Sternberg cell lines HDLM-1, HDLM-1d and KM-H2. *Am J Pathol* 1989;135:33–38.
13. Hsu SM, Tseng CK, Hsu PL. Expression of p55 (Tac) interleukin-2 receptor (IL-2R), but not p75 IL-2R, in cultured H-RS cells and H-RS cells in tissues. *Am J Pathol* 1990;136:735–744.
14. Klein S, Jucker M, Diehl V, et al. Production of multiple cytokines by Hodgkin's disease derived cell lines. *Hematol Oncol* 1992;10:319–329.
15. Tesch H, Herrmann T, Abts H, et al. High affinity IL-2 receptors on a Hodgkin's derived cell line. *Leuk Res* 1990;14:953–960.
16. Strauchen JA, Breakstone BA. IL-2 receptor expression in human lymphoid lesions. Immunohistochemical study of 166 cases. *Am J Pathol* 1987; 126:506–512.
17. Sheibani K, Winberg CD, van de Velde S, et al. Distribution of lymphocytes with interleukin-2 receptors (TAC antigens) in reactive lymphoproliferative processes, Hodgkin's disease, and non-Hodgkin's lymphomas. An immunohistologic study of 300 cases. *Am J Pathol* 1987;127:27–37.
18. Agnarsson BA, Kadin ME. The immunophenotype of Reed-Sternberg cells. A study of 50 cases of Hodgkin's disease using fixed frozen tissues. *Cancer* 1989;63:2083–2087.
19. Levi E, Butmarc J, Kourea HP, et al. Detection of interleukin-2 receptors on tumor cells in formalin-fixed, paraffin-embedded tissues. *Appl Immunohistochem* 1997;5:234–238.
20. Gruss HJ, Brach MA, Drexler HG, et al. Expression of cytokine genes, cytokine receptor genes, and transcription factors in cultured Hodgkin and Reed-Sternberg cells. *Cancer Res* 1992;52:3353–3360.
21. Aldinucci D, Poletto D, Gloghini A, et al. Expression of functional interleukin-3 receptors on Hodgkin and Reed-Sternberg cells. *Am J Pathol* 2002;160:585–596.
22. Aldinucci D, Olivo K, Lorenzon D, et al. The role of interleukin-3 in classical Hodgkin's disease. *Leuk Lymphoma* 2005;46:303–311.
23. Hsu SM, Xie SS, Hsu PL, et al. Interleukin-6, but not interleukin-4, is expressed by Reed-Sternberg cells in Hodgkin's disease with or without histologic features of Castleman's disease. *Am J Pathol* 1992;141: 129–138.
24. Merz H, Fliedner A, Orscheschek K, et al. Cytokine expression in T-cell lymphomas and Hodgkin's disease. Its possible implication in autocrine or paracrine production as a potential basis for neoplastic growth. *Am J Pathol* 1991;139:1173–1180.
25. Skinnider BF, Elia AJ, Gascoyne RD, et al. Signal transducer and activator of transcription 6 is frequently activated in Hodgkin and Reed-Sternberg cells of Hodgkin lymphoma. *Blood*. 2002;99:618–626.
26. Newcom SR, Ansari AA, Gu L. Interleukin-4 is an autocrine growth factor secreted by the L-428 Reed-Sternberg cell. *Blood* 1992;79:191–197.
27. Samoszuk M, Nansen L. Detection of interleukin-5 messenger RNA in Reed-Sternberg cells of Hodgkin's disease with eosinophilia. *Blood* 1990;75:13–16.
28. Kapp U, Yeh WC, Patterson B, et al. Interleukin 13 is secreted by and stimulates the growth of Hodgkin and Reed-Sternberg cells. *J Exp Med* 1999;189:1939–1945.
29. Poppema S, van den Berg A. Interaction between host T cells and Reed-Sternberg cells in Hodgkin lymphomas. *Semin Cancer Biol* 2000;10:345–350.
30. Maggio E, van den Berg A, Diepstra A, et al. Chemokines, cytokines and their receptors in Hodgkin's lymphoma cell lines and tissues. *Ann Oncol* 2002;13(suppl 1):52–56.
31. Foss HD, Herbst H, Oelmann E, et al. Lymphotoxin, tumour necrosis factor and interleukin-6 gene transcripts are present in Hodgkin and Reed-Sternberg cells of most Hodgkin's disease cases. *Br J Haematol* 1993; 84:627–635.
32. Herbst H, Samol J, Foss HD, et al. Modulation of interleukin-6 expression in Hodgkin and Reed-Sternberg cells by Epstein-Barr virus. *J Pathol* 1997;182:299–306.
33. Jucker M, Abts H, Li W, et al. Expression of interleukin-6 and interleukin-6 receptor in Hodgkin's disease. *Blood* 1991;77:2413–2418.
34. Tesch H, Jucker M, Klein S, et al. Hodgkin and Reed-Sternberg cells express interleukin 6 and interleukin 6 receptors. *Leuk Lymphoma* 1992;7: 297–303.
35. Skinnider BF, Elia AJ, Gascoyne RD, et al. Interleukin 13 and interleukin 13 receptor are frequently expressed by Hodgkin and Reed-Sternberg cells of Hodgkin lymphoma. *Blood* 2001;97:250–255.
36. Foss HD, Hummel M, Gottstein S, et al. Frequent expression of IL-7 gene transcripts in tumor cells of classical Hodgkin's disease. *Am J Pathol* 1995;146:33–39.
37. Merz H, Houssiau FA, Orscheschek K, et al. Interleukin-9 expression in human malignant lymphomas: unique association with Hodgkin's disease and large cell anaplastic lymphoma. *Blood* 1991;78:1311–1317.
38. Glimelius I, Edström A, Amini RM, et al. IL-9 expression contributes to the cellular composition in Hodgkin lymphoma. *Eur J Haematol* 2006; 76:278–283.
39. Carbone A, Gloghini A, Gattei V, et al. Expression of functional CD40 antigen on Reed-Sternberg cells and Hodgkin's disease cell lines. *Blood* 1995;85:780–789.
40. Herbst H, Foss H-D, Samol J, et al. Frequent expression of interleukin-10 by Epstein-Barr virus-harboring tumor cells of Hodgkin's disease. *Blood* 1996;87:2918–2929.
41. Beck A, Pazolt D, Grabenbauer GG, et al. Expression of cytokine and chemokine genes in Epstein-Barr virus-associated nasopharyngeal carcinoma: comparison with Hodgkin's disease. *J Pathol* 2001;194:145–151.
42. Schwaller J, Tobler A, Niklaus G, et al. Interleukin-12 expression in human lymphomas and nonneoplastic lymphoid disorders. *Blood* 1995;85: 2182–2188.
43. Niedobitek G, Pazolt D, Teichmann M, et al. Frequent expression of the Epstein-Barr virus (EBV)-induced gene, EBI3, an IL-12 p40-related cytokine, in Hodgkin and Reed-Sternberg cells. *J Pathol* 2002;198:310–316.
44. Ohshima K, Akaiwa M, Umeshita R, et al. Interleukin-13 and interleukin-13 receptor in Hodgkin's disease: possible autocrine mechanism and involvement in fibrosis. *Histopathology* 2001;38:368–375.
45. Oshima Y, Puri RK. Suppression of an IL-13 autocrine growth loop in a human Hodgkin/Reed-Sternberg tumor cell line by a novel IL-13 antagonist. *Cell Immunol* 2001;211:37–42.

46. Ryffel B, Brockhaus M, Durmuller U, et al. Tumor necrosis factor receptors in lymphoid tissues and lymphomas. Source and site of action of tumor necrosis factor alpha. *Am J Pathol* 1991;139:7–15.
47. Kadin ME, Agnarsson BA, Ellingsworth LR, et al. Immunohistochemical evidence of a role for transforming growth factor beta in the pathogenesis of nodular sclerosing Hodgkin's disease. *Am J Pathol* 1990;136:1209–1214.
48. Newcom SR, Gu L. Transforming growth factor beta 1 messenger RNA in Reed-Sternberg cells in nodular sclerosing Hodgkin's disease. *J Clin Pathol* 1995;48:160–163.
49. Hsu SM, Lin J, Xie SS, et al. Abundant expression of transforming growth factor-beta 1 and -beta 2 by Hodgkin's Reed-Sternberg cells and reactive T lymphocytes in Hodgkin's disease. *Hum Pathol* 1993;24:249–255.
50. Kadin M, Butmarc J, Elovic A, et al. Eosinophils are the major source of transforming growth factor-beta 1 in nodular sclerosing Hodgkin's disease. *Am J Pathol* 1993;142:11–16.
51. Obberghen-Schilling E, Roche NS, Flanders KC, et al. Transforming growth factor beta 1 positively regulates its own expression in normal and trans-formed cells. *J Biol Chem* 1988;263:7741–7746.
52. Ohshima K, Sugihara M, Suzumiya J, et al. Basic fibroblast growth factor and fibrosis in Hodgkin's disease. *Pathol Res Pract* 1999;195:149–155.
53. Khnykin D, Troen G, Berner JM, et al. The expression of fibroblast growth factors and their receptors in Hodgkin's lymphoma. *J Pathol* 2006;208:431–438.
54. Maggio EM, Van Den Berg A, Visser L, et al. Common and differential chemokine expression patterns in rs cells of NLP, EBV positive and negative classical Hodgkin lymphomas. *Int J Cancer* 2002;99:665–672.
55. Hanamoto H, Nakayama T, Miyazato H, et al. Expression of CCL28 by Reed-Sternberg cells defines a major subtype of classical Hodgkin's disease with frequent infiltration of eosinophils and/or plasma cells. *Am J Pathol* 2004;164:997–1006.
56. Fischer M, Juremalm M, Olsson N, et al. Expression of CCL5/RANTES by Hodgkin and Reed-Sternberg cells and its possible role in the recruitment of mast cells into lymphomatous tissue. *Int J Cancer* 2003;107:197–201.
57. Buri C, Korner M, Scharli P, et al. CC chemokines and the receptors CCR3 and CCR5 are differentially expressed in the nonneoplastic leukocyte infil-trates of Hodgkin's disease. *Blood* 2001;97:1543–1548.
58. Ohshima K, Karube K, Hamasaki M, et al. Imbalances of chemokines, chemokine receptors and cytokines in Hodgkin lymphoma: classical Hodgkin lymphoma vs. Hodgkin-like ATLL. *Int J Cancer* 2003;106:706–712.
59. Jundt F, Anagnostopoulos I, Bommert K, et al. Hodgkin/Reed-Sternberg cells induce fibroblasts to secrete eotaxin, a potent chemoattractant for T cells and eosinophils. *Blood* 1999;94:2065–2071.
60. Van den Berg A, Visser L, Poppema S. High expression of the CC chemokine TARC in Reed-Sternberg cells. A possible explanation for the characteristic T-cell infiltrate in Hodgkin's lymphoma. *Am J Pathol* 1999;154:1685–1691.
61. Peh SC, Kim LH, Poppema S. TARC, a CC chemokin, is frequently expressed in classic Hodgkin's lymphoma but not in NLP Hodgkin's lym-phoma, T-cell-rich B-cell lymphoma, and most cases of anaplastic large cell lymphoma. *Am J Surg Pathol* 2001;25:925–929.
62. Ohshima K, Tutiya T, Yamaguchi T, et al. Infiltration of Th1 and Th2 lym-phocytes around Hodgkin and Reed-Sternberg (H&RS) cells in Hodgkin disease: relation with expression of CXC and CC chemokines on H&RS cells. *Int J Cancer* 2002;98:567–572.
63. Hopken UE, Foss HD, Meyer D, et al. Up-regulation of the chemokine receptor CCR7 in classical but not in lymphocyte-predominant Hodgkin disease correlates with distinct dissemination of neoplastic cells in lymphoid organs. *Blood* 2002;99:1109–1116.
64. Hedvat CV, Jaffe ES, Qin J, et al. Macrophage-derived chemokine expres-sion in classical Hodgkin's lymphoma: application of tissue microarrays. *Mod Pathol* 2001;14:1270–1276.
65. Andrew DP, Chang MS, McNinch J, et al. STCP-1 (MDC) CC chemokine acts specifically on chronically activated Th2 lymphocytes and is produced by monocytes on stimulation with Th2 cytokines IL-4 and IL-13. *J Immunol* 1998;16:5027–5038.
66. Imai T, Chantry D, Raport CJ, et al. Macrophage-derived chemokine is a functional ligand for the CC chemokine receptor 4. *J Biol Chem* 1998;273:1764–1768.
67. Luciani MG, Stoppacciaro A, Peri G, et al. The monocyte chemotactic pro-tein 1 (MCP-1) and interleukin 8 (IL-8) in Hodgkin's disease and in solid tumours. *J Clin Pathol* 1998;51:273–276.
68. Foss HD, Herbst H, Gottstein S, et al. Interleukin-8 in Hodgkin's disease. Preferential expression by reactive cells and association with neutrophil density. *Am J Pathol* 1996;148:1229–1236.
69. Teruya-Feldstein J, Tosato G, Jaffe ES. The role of chemokines in Hodgkin's disease. *Leuk Lymphoma* 2000;38:363–371.
70. Teichmann M, Meyer B, Beck A, et al. Expression of the interferon-inducible chemokine IP-10 (CXCL10), a chemokine with proposed anti-neoplastic functions, in Hodgkin lymphoma and nasopharyngeal carcinoma. *J Pathol* 2005;206:68–75.
71. Gause A, Scholz R, Klein S, et al. Increased levels of circulating interleukin-6 in patients with Hodgkin's disease. *Hematol Oncol* 1991;9:307–313.
72. Seymour JF, Talpaz M, Hagemeister FB, et al. Clinical correlates of elevated serum levels of interleukin 6 in patients with untreated Hodgkin's disease. *Am J Med* 1997;102:21–28.
73. Vener C, Guffanti A, Pomati M, et al. Soluble cytokine levels correlate with the activity and clinical stage of Hodgkin's disease at diagnosis. *Leuk Lymphoma* 2000;37:333–339.
74. Aydin F, Yilmaz M, Ozdemir F, et al. Correlation of serum IL-2, IL-6 and IL-10 levels with International Prognostic Index in patients with aggressive non-Hodgkin's lymphoma. *Am J Clin Oncol* 2002;25:570–572.
75. Gause A, Jung W, Keymis S, et al. The clinical significance of cytokines and soluble forms of membrane-derived activation antigens in the serum of patients with Hodgkin's disease. *Leuk Lymphoma* 1992;7:439–447.
76. Cozen W, Gill PS, Ingles SA, et al. IL-6 levels and genotype are associated with risk of young adult Hodgkin lymphoma. *Blood* 2004;103:3216–3221.
77. Cordano P, Lake A, Shield L, et al. Effect of IL-6 promoter polymorphism on incidence and outcome in Hodgkin's lymphoma. *Br J Haematol* 2005;128:493–495.
78. Fischer M, Bijman M, Molin D, et al. Increased serum levels of interleukin-9 correlate to negative prognostic factors in Hodgkin's lymphoma. *Leukemia* 2003;17:2513–2516.
79. Bohlen H, Kessler M, Sextro M, et al. Poor clinical outcome of patients with Hodgkin's disease and elevated interleukin-10 serum levels. Clinical significance of interleukin-10 serum levels for Hodgkin's disease. *Ann Hematol* 2000;79:110–113.
80. Viviani S, Notti P, Bonfante V, et al. Elevated pretreatment serum levels of Il-10 are associated with a poor prognosis in Hodgkin's disease, the Milan Cancer Institute experience. *Med Oncol* 2000;17:59–63.
81. Vassilakopoulos TP, Nadali G, Angelopoulou MK, et al. Serum interleukin-10 levels are an independent prognostic factor for patients with Hodgkin's lymphoma. *Haematologica* 2001;86:274–281.
82. Axdorph U, Sjoberg J, Grimfors G, et al. Biological markers may add to prediction of outcome achieved by the International Prognostic Score in Hodgkin's disease. *Ann Oncol* 2000;11:1405–1411.
83. Salgami EV, Efstathiou SP, Vlachakis V, et al. High pretreatment inter-leukin-10 is an independent predictor of poor failure-free survival in patients with Hodgkin's lymphoma. *Haematologia (Budap)* 2002;32:377–387.
84. Visco C, Vassilakopoulos TP, Kliche KO, et al. Elevated serum levels of IL-10 are associated with inferior progression-free survival in patients with Hodgkin's disease treated with radiotherapy. *Leuk Lymphoma* 2004;45:2085–2092.
85. Herling M, Rassidakis GZ, Medeiros LJ, et al. Expression of Epstein-Barr virus latent membrane protein-1 in Hodgkin and Reed-Sternberg cells of classical Hodgkin's lymphoma: associations with presenting features, serum interleukin 10 levels, and clinical outcome. *Clin Cancer Res* 2003;9:2114–2120.
86. Jarrett RF, Stark GL, White J, et al. Impact of tumor Epstein-Barr virus sta-tus on presenting features and outcome in age-defined subgroups of patients with classic Hodgkin lymphoma: a population-based study. *Blood* 2005;106:2444–2451.
87. Munro LR, Johnston PW, Marshall NA, et al. Polymorphisms in the inter-leukin-10 and interferon gamma genes in Hodgkin lymphoma. *Leuk Lymphoma* 2003;44:2083–2088.
88. Fiumara P, Cabanillas F, Younes A. Interleukin-13 levels in serum from patients with Hodgkin disease and healthy volunteers. *Blood* 2001;98:2877–2878.
89. Libura J, Bettens F, Radkowski A, et al. Polymorphic tumor necrosis factors microsatellite TNFa4 is associated with resistance of Hodgkin lymphoma to chemotherapy and with replapses after therapy. *Anticancer Res* 2002;22:921–926.
90. Diepstra A, Niens M, Vellenga E, et al. Association with Hodgkin lym-phoma class I in Epstein-Barr-virus-positive and with Hodgkin lymphoma class III in Epstein-Barr-virus-negative Hodgkin lymphoma. *Lancet* 2005;365:2216–2224.
91. Demeter J, Messer G, Ramisch S, et al. Polymorphism within the second intron of the IL-1 receptor antagonist gene in patients with hematopoietic malignancies. *Cytokines Mol Ther* 1996;2:239–242.
92. Pui CH, Ip SH, Thompson E, et al. High serum interleukin-2 receptor levels correlate with a poor prognosis in children with Hodgkin's disease. *Leukemia* 1989;3:481–484.
93. Ambrosetti A, Nadali G, Vinante F, et al. Serum levels of soluble inter-leukin-2 receptor in Hodgkin disease. Relationship with clinical stage, tumor burden, and treatment outcome. *Cancer* 1993;72:201–206.
94. Enblad G, Sundstrom C, Gronowitz S, et al. Serum levels of interleukin-2 receptor (CD 25) in patients with Hodgkin's disease, with special reference to age and prognosis. *Ann Oncol* 1995;6:65–70.
95. Viviani S, Camerini E, Bonfante V, et al. Soluble interleukin-2 receptors (sIL-2R) in Hodgkin's disease: outcome and clinical implications. *Br J Cancer* 1998;77:992–997.
96. Trumper L, Jung W, Dahl G, et al. Interleukin-7, interleukin-8, soluble TNF receptor, and p53 protein levels are elevated in the serum of patients with Hodgkin's disease. *Ann Oncol* 1994;5(suppl 1):93–96.
97. Gorschluter M, Bohlen Hasenclever D, et al. Serum cytokine levels corre-late with clinical parameters in Hodgkin's disease. *Ann Oncol* 1995;6:477–482.
98. Weihrauch MR, Manzke O, Beyer M, et al. Elevated serum levels of CC thymus and activation-related chemokine (TARC) in primary Hodgkin's disease: potential for a prognostic factor. *Cancer Res* 2005;65:5516–5519.
99. Teruya-Feldstein J, Jaffe ES, Berkowitz JR, et al. Eotaxin-1, a specific chemoattractant for eosinophils in Hodgkin's tissues. *Blood* 1997;90:388a.
100. Pinto A, Aldinucci D, Gloghini A, et al. Human eosinophils express func-tional CD30 ligand and stimulate proliferation of a Hodgkin's disease cell line. *Blood* 1996;88:3299–3305.

101. Molin D, Fischer M, Xiang Z, et al. Mast cells express functional CD30 ligand and are the predominant CD30L-positive cells in Hodgkin's disease. *Br J Haematol* 2001;114:616–623.
102. Molin D, Edstrom A, Glimelius I, et al. Mast cell infiltration correlates with poor prognosis in Hodgkin's lymphoma. *Br J Haematol* 2002;119:122–124.
103. Drexler HG. Recent results on the biology of Hodgkin and Reed-Sternberg cells. II. Continuous cell lines. *Leuk Lymphoma* 1993;9:1–25.
104. Newcom SR, O'Rourke L. Potentiation of fibroblast growth by nodular sclerosing Hodgkin's disease cell cultures. *Blood* 1982;60:228–237.
105. Ford RJ, Mehta S, Davis F, et al. Growth factors in Hodgkin's disease. *Cancer Treat Rep* 1982;66:633–638.
106. Kortmann C, Burrichter H, Monner D, et al. Interleukin-1-like activity constitutively generated by Hodgkin derived cell lines. I. Measurement in a human lymphocyte co-stimulator assay. *Immunobiology* 1984;166: 318–333.
107. Kretschmer C, Jones DB, Morrison K, et al. Tumor necrosis factor alpha and lymphotoxin production in Hodgkin's disease. *Am J Pathol* 1990; 137:341–351.
108. Sugarman BJ, Aggarwal BB, Hass PE, et al. Recombinant human tumor necrosis factor-alpha: effects on proliferation of normal and transformed cells in vitro. *Science* 1985;230:943–945.
109. Roberts AB, Sporn MB, Assoian RK, et al. Transforming growth factor type beta: rapid induction of fibrosis and angiogenesis in vivo and stimulation of collagen formation in vitro. *Proc Natl Acad Sci USA* 1986;83:4167–4171.
110. Mustoe TA, Pierce GF, Thomason A, et al. Accelerated healing of incisional wounds in rats induced by transforming growth factor-beta. *Science* 1987;237:1333–1336.
111. Newcom SR, Kadin ME, Ansari AA. Production of transforming growth factor-beta activity by Ki-1 positive lymphoma cells and analysis of its role in the regulation of Ki-1 positive lymphoma growth. *Am J Pathol* 1988;131:569–577.
112. Wong DT, Elovic A, Matossian K, et al. Eosinophils from patients with blood eosinophilia express transforming growth factor beta 1. *Blood* 1991;78:2702–2707.
113. Shinozaki M, Kawara HN, Kakinuma T, et al. Induction of subcutaneous tissue fibrosis in newborn mice by transforming growth factor-b—simultaneous application with basic fibroblast growth factor causes persistent fibrosis. *Biochem Biophys Res Commun* 1997;237:292–296.
114. Ree HJ, Pezzullo JC. Inflammation and/or necrosis of tumors cannot account for fever in most febrile patients with Hodgkin's disease. *Cancer* 1987;60:1787–1789.
115. Sappino AP, Seelentag W, Pelte MF, et al. Tumor necrosis factor/cachectin and lymphotoxin gene expression in lymph nodes from lymphoma patients. *Blood* 1990;75:958–962.
116. Quesada JR, Talpaz M, Rios A, et al. Clinical toxicity of interferons in cancer patients: a review. *J Clin Oncol* 1986;4:234–243.
117. Feinberg B, Kurzrock R, Talpaz M, et al. A phase I trial of intravenously-administered recombinant tumor necrosis factor-alpha in cancer patients. *J Clin Oncol* 1988;6:1328–1334.
118. Lahdevirta J, Maury CP, Teppo AM, et al. Elevated levels of circulating cachectin/tumor necrosis factor in patients with acquired immunodeficiency syndrome. *Am J Med* 1988;85:289–291.
119. Opp M, Obal F Jr, Cady AB, et al. Interleukin-6 is pyrogenic but not somnogenic. *Physiol Behav* 1989;45:1069–1072.
120. Kurzrock R, Redman J, Cabanillas F, et al. Serum interleukin 6 levels are elevated in lymphoma patients and correlate with survival in advanced Hodgkin's disease and with B symptoms. *Cancer Res* 1993;53:2118–2122.
121. Perfetti V, Dragani TA, Paulli M, et al. Gene expression of pyrogenic cytokines in Hodgkin's disease lymph nodes. *Haematologica* 1992;77: 221–225.
122. Pinto A, Aldinucci D, Gloghini A, et al. Human eosinophils express functional CD30 ligand and stimulate proliferation of a Hodgkin's disease cell line. *Blood* 1996;88:3299–3305.
123. Baker SJ, Reddy EP. Transducers of life and death: TNF receptor superfamily and associated proteins. *Oncogene* 1996;12:1–9.
124. Blay JY, Farcet JP, Lavaud A, et al. Serum concentrations of cytokines in patients with Hodgkin's disease. *Eur J Cancer* 1994;30A:321–324.
125. Sarris AH, Kliche KO, Pethambaram P, et al. Interleukin-10 levels are often elevated in serum of adults with Hodgkin's disease and are associated with inferior failure-free survival. *Ann Oncol* 1999;10:433–440.
126. Giles FJ, Vose JM, Do KA, et al. Clinical relevance of circulating angiogenic factors in patients with non-Hodgkin's lymphoma or Hodgkin's lymphoma. *Leuk Res* 2004;28:595–604.
127. Warzocha K, Bienvenu J, Ribeiro P, et al. Plasma levels of tumour necrosis factor and its soluble receptors correlate with clinical features and outcome of Hodgkin's disease patients. *Br J Cancer* 1998;77:2357–2362.

CHAPTER 7 ■ DYSREGULATED IMMUNE RESPONSE IN HODGKIN LYMPHOMA

SIBRAND POPPEMA

Hodgkin lymphoma is a malignant lymphoma characterized by the presence of multinucleated giant cells, the Reed-Sternberg cells, and their mononuclear variants, the Hodgkin cells. These are now generally believed to be a clonal neoplastic population that derives from transformed B-lymphocytes. The malignant cells usually comprise less than 1% of the total cell population and are surrounded by a prominent infiltrate of reactive cells. These are mostly T-lymphocytes with variable admixtures of eosinophils, histiocytes, plasma cells, and, in cases of nodular lymphocyte-predominant Hodgkin lymphoma, also considerable numbers of small B-lymphocytes.

IMPAIRED IMMUNE RESPONSE IN PATIENTS WITH HODGKIN LYMPHOMA

In the late 19th century, Hodgkin's disease, now termed Hodgkin lymphoma, was believed to be a granulomatous inflammatory lesion because Hodgkin lymphoma and tuberculosis were found to coexist in many autopsies. Sternberg even stated that it was simply an atypical form of tuberculosis.[1] Some years later, evidence emerged that the two diseases were different, and in this context the precise definition of the morphologic features of the Hodgkin and Reed-Sternberg cells was an important step.[2-6] The coexistence of the two diseases remained, however, and in 1947 Jackson and Parker reported a frequency of 20% tuberculosis in autopsies of patients with Hodgkin lymphoma.[7] Better treatment of tuberculosis led to a reduced incidence, and nowadays the combination of Hodgkin lymphoma and tuberculosis is extremely infrequent in North America and Western Europe, but can still be encountered in countries where tuberculosis is endemic.[8]

Dorothy Reed was the first to document that patients with Hodgkin lymphoma have an impaired immune response.[3] She demonstrated the absence of a reaction to tuberculin in patients with Hodgkin lymphoma. In the early 1930s, Parker and Steiner provided further evidence that an immunologic defect might be the cause of the increased susceptibility to tuberculosis because the tuberculin reaction was negative in a majority of patients with Hodgkin lymphoma even while some of these patients had active tuberculosis.[9,10] In 1947, Dubin found only one positive tuberculin reaction among 38 patients with Hodgkin lymphoma, while at that time the positivity rate in the general population was over 52%.[11] He also noted that the positivity of serologic reactions for syphilis was less than expected and that some patients with coexisting brucellosis were unable to produce anti-*Brucella* antibody titers. Based on this, Dubin postulated that the immunologic deficiency of Hodgkin lymphoma was not restricted to tuberculosis but was generalized.[11]

Schier and co-workers conducted systematic tests of the capacity of 43 patients with Hodgkin lymphoma to react to tuberculoprotein, *Trychophyton gypseum*, *Candida albicans*, and mumps skin test antigen, and found the delayed-type responses to be severely depressed as compared to control individuals.[12] From that moment on, numerous reports confirmed an impairment of the immune response in Hodgkin lymphoma (Table 7.1). This lack of response has also been described as "anergy." Lamb and colleagues reported that this anergy was also present in patients with Hodgkin lymphoma in good condition, in contrast to the anergy of other malignancies, which was virtually restricted to patients in poor condition.[13] In other words, it was concluded that the anergy of Hodgkin lymphoma is a primary attribute of the disease. However, in a carefully performed study, Brown and associates showed that patients in clinical stage I were comparable to those of normal controls and that the frequency of anergy increased with advancing stage.[14] This suggested that the disease needs to have a certain extent before it is reflected in a general reduction of delayed-type responses. Sokal and Primikirios observed that two patients who had a long remission from Hodgkin lymphoma recovered the ability to react to tuberculin.[15] This was confirmed in a later study that also suggested that the tuberculin test might serve as a prognostic index.[16]

The major clinical importance of these observations is that individuals with Hodgkin lymphoma have greater susceptibility to infections with bacteria, viruses, fungi, and parasites.[17] Before chemotherapy and radiotherapy were available, infectious diseases were a major cause of death in patients with Hodgkin lymphoma. Even now, infections account for a major cause of death in patients with treated Hodgkin lymphoma. The most commonly observed infections after treatment are pneumonia, bacteremia, skin infections, and meningitis.[18] *Streptococcus pneumoniae*, *Staphylococcus aureus*, and *Staphylococcus epidermidis* are the microorganisms most often isolated from patients with Hodgkin lymphoma. Herpes zoster infections, which are commonly observed in immune-comprised individuals, are also frequently seen in individuals with Hodgkin lymphoma. Infections with gram-negative bacteria are less frequently observed. The infections in treated patients are partly also the result of therapy-induced immune deficiency.

Skin testing with natural antigens such as tuberculin does not really distinguish between true anergy in a previously sensitized individual and the lack of response in individuals

TABLE 7.1

NATURE OF THE IMMUNE RESPONSE IN PATIENTS WITH HODGKIN LYMPHOMA

	In vitro	In vivo
T-cells	Increased spontaneous proliferation Decreased mitogen-induced proliferation Reduced response to recall antigens Reduced mixed leukocyte reaction Normal allogenic leukocyte reaction Increased spontaneous cytokine production Reduced mitogen/antigen induced cytokine production Decreased CD3 ζ-chain expression	Reduced response against tuberculin Reduced response against DNCB Increased shedding of CD25, CD8, CD95
B-cells	Increased mitogen-induced Ig production Reduced antigen-induced Ig production	Increased total Ig titer Increased antiviral Ig titer

DNCB, dinitrochlorobenzene; Ig, Immunoglobulin.

never previously exposed to the antigen. Certain chemicals, like the extremely potent contact allergen 2,4-dinitrochlorobenzene (DNCB), elicit a tuberculin-type reaction, the delayed-type hypersensitivity reaction. In the early 1960s it was shown that patients with Hodgkin lymphoma had a reduced response toward dinitrochlorobenzene and that on remission there was a transition toward a normal reaction (Table 7.1).[19] In this study, one of the patients relapsed, and this was accompanied by a transition toward unresponsiveness. It was concluded that the immunologic defect manifested by anergy for 2,4-dinitrochlorobenzene and other delayed-type hypersensitivity antigens is an early manifestation of Hodgkin lymphoma and is closely correlated with disease activity.[19]

Attempts to convert anergic patients with Hodgkin lymphoma by active immunization with the bacillus of Calmette-Guérin (BCG) were found to show a good correlation between the inability to respond and poor prognosis. This suggested that the test was a measure of the activity of the mechanism responsible for resistance to the disease. The question whether there is indeed an effective antitumor response in some cases is still unresolved.

IMPAIRED PERIPHERAL BLOOD CELL RESPONSES IN VITRO

Lymphocyte counts in patients with Hodgkin lymphoma were found to be only slightly lower than normal in early stages but significantly lower in the higher stages and severely depressed in late stages.[14] In vitro, a reduced proliferative response of lymphocytes from patients with Hodgkin lymphoma to phytohemagglutinin (PHA) was first demonstrated by Hersh and Oppenheim in 1965, and later Aisenberg used ^{14}C-labeled thymidine to quantify the blastoid transformation.[21,22] The response to other mitogens such as concanavalin A and pokeweed mitogen and to recall antigens such as dinitrochlorobenzene or tuberculin was also found to be reduced (Table 7.1).[23] The response in an autologous mixed leukocyte reaction (MLR) was depressed as well.[24] In contrast, the response in an allogeneic mixed leukocyte reaction was observed as normal.[25] There was a reduction in the production of cytokines and a decreased immunoglobulin production on stimulation with mitogens or antigens.[26,27] In contrast, increased spontaneous production of immunoglobulins[28] and

an increased proportion of peripheral T-cells that spontaneously synthesize DNA have been observed.[29] In particular, an increase of IgE has been noted in up to 50% of the patients.[30] These results indicate that there is a population of activated lymphocytes present in the peripheral blood of patients with Hodgkin lymphoma that do not have normal antigen responsiveness.

It has been demonstrated that peripheral blood T-cells from patients with untreated Hodgkin lymphoma have decreased T-cell receptor (TCR) ξ-chain expression (Table 7.1).[31] This defect resulted in an altered signal transduction, as was shown by an impaired Ca^{2+} mobilization. Adequate stimulation with anti-CD3 and anti-CD28 antibodies resulted in normal expression of the ξ-chain and in the restoration of IL-2 production and cytotoxicity to normal values. Surprisingly, in the lymphocytes in the involved tissues of Hodgkin lymphoma, this reduction in TCR ξ-chain expression is much less pronounced than in the peripheral blood cells (S. Poppema, unpublished observations, 1999). Sjoberget and associates recently compared patient PBLs with the corresponding tumor infiltrating lymphocytes, and also showed a significantly higher (CD3+/4+) or equal (CD3+/8+) ξ-chain expression in the latter.[32]

CD30, a member of the tumor necrosis factor receptor (TNFR) superfamily, is consistently detected on Hodgkin and Reed-Sternberg cells, and a soluble form of CD30 (sCD30) is found in the serum of Hodgkin patients.[33,34] The level of sCD30 correlates with the tumor burden, suggesting that the Hodgkin—Reed-Sternberg cells are the major source of sCD30. The sCD30 has been found to have prognostic value for the outcome of treatment in Hodgkin lymphoma.[34] CD30 can interact with its natural ligand CD30L, expressed on most hematopoietic cell types, and this interaction is associated with enhanced shedding of sCD30. In vitro CD30 indeed inhibits T-cell proliferation. Anti-CD3-stimulated T-cells in the presence of CD30 do not increase tritium uptake and fail to express CD25 and CD26 and to produce interleukin 2. This inability of the T-cells to express CD26 is in accordance with the results of immunohistochemistry on disease-involved tissues. Increased levels of sCD95, sCD8, and sCD25 are also observed in patients with Hodgkin lymphoma.[34,35] It is very likely that these and perhaps other soluble factors, including the so-called E-rosette—inhibiting factor, influence the immune response in patients with Hodgkin lymphoma by inhibiting interactions between antigen-presenting cells and T-cells or otherwise by interfering with T-cell activation.[36] Of particular interest is the finding that Hodgkin and

Reed-Sternberg cells produce large amounts of various chemokines, including the Th2-type chemokines TARC and MDC[37–39] and that high serum levels of these chemokines correlate with disease activity and prognosis.[40]

ABSENCE OF IMMUNE RESPONSE AGAINST EPSTEIN-BARR VIRUS— POSITIVE HODGKIN AND REED-STERNBERG CELLS

The presence of an extensive population of reactive lymphocytes and plasma cells in the lymph nodes from patients with Hodgkin lymphoma suggests that there is an immunologic reaction in progress. An impairment of the local immune response is suggested by the absence of an effective cytotoxic response against Epstein-Barr virus (EBV) antigens by lymphocytes derived from EBV-positive Hodgkin lymph nodes (Table 7.1). Most patients with Hodgkin lymphoma have overcome an EBV infection earlier in life, and specific cytotoxic T-cells can be found in the peripheral blood of these same patients.[41] The absence of a cytotoxic response in EBV-positive cases is probably relevant because there is a cytotoxic response against EBV antigens by lymphocytes derived from EBV-negative Hodgkin lymph nodes.[41,42] The EBV latent membrane proteins LMP-1 and LMP-2 in association with human leukocyte antigen (HLA) class I serve as potential targets for specific CD8+ T-cells.[43] The presentation of LMP-2 is restricted through the HLA class I antigen A2, and therefore it has been hypothesized that HLA-A2—positive individuals would be underrepresented among Caucasians with EBV-associated Hodgkin lymphoma. However, there was no significant difference between the frequency of HLA A2 positivity in Hodgkin lymphoma cases and controls and between EBV-associated and -nonassociated cases of Hodgkin lymphoma.[44,45] However, HLA class I was frequently found to be absent altogether from Hodgkin and Reed-Sternberg cells in the classical forms of Hodgkin lymphoma, although some cases of mixed-cellularity Hodgkin lymphoma and all cases of nodular lymphocyte-predominant Hodgkin lymphoma were positive.[46] Interestingly, others have reported HLA class I to be usually present in EBV-positive cases and absent in EBV-negative cases of Hodgkin lymphoma.[47] Absence of HLA class I presents a mechanism to escape the specific cytotoxic immune response. In EBV-positive Hodgkin lymphoma, normal expression of HLA class I and transporters associated with antigen processing can be found.[48] However, in a large genotyping study in Groningen, patients with EBV-positive Hodgkin lymphoma were found to have a polymorphism in HLA class I that was not present in patients with EBV-negative Hodgkin lymphoma. This polymorphism may have an effect on the recognition of antigen by CD8 cells and prevent a cytotoxic response or induce a regulatory response.[49] Absence of HLA class I on the Hodgkin and Reed-Sternberg cells generally should lead to recognition of antigens by NK cells. In human placenta this is prevented by HLA G; and indeed, Hodgkin and Reed-Sternberg cells that lack HLA class I frequently do express HLA G.[50]

Until recently it was assumed that only CD8-positive cytotoxic T-cells played a role in MHC class I-restricted immune surveillance, but now it is clear that also CD4-positive T-cells play an important role in anti EBNA-1 immune responses. Antigen presentation to CD4-positive T-cells requires MHC class II processing that is not dependent on proteasomal digestion. Whether antigen presentation by HLA class II-positive RS cells can induce an effective immune response in HL is not known. HLA class II is expressed on Hodgkin and Reed-Sternberg cells in approximately 70% cases of Hodgkin lymphoma, and it is of interest that HLA class II negative cases have a worse prognosis.[50] The various molecules involved in antigen recognition, co-stimulation and cell adhesion in Hodgkin lymphoma are summarized in Table 7.2 and Figure 7.1.

Whether the observed impaired systemic cellular immunity is the result of, or constitutes a predisposition for, Hodgkin lymphoma remains unclear. Some studies from Scandinavia found immunologic defects in unaffected siblings of patients with Hodgkin lymphoma, but this could not be confirmed in other studies.[52,53] Our recent finding on a polymorphism in HLA class I in EBV-positive patients and another polymorphism in HLA class III in EBV-negative patients suggests that there might be indeed be predisposing abnormalities. On the other hand, the data mentioned earlier on the presence or absence of a normal response to delayed-type antigens in early versus later stages of the disease suggest that most of the immunologic abnormalities are secondary phenomena. Obviously, currently available radiotherapy and chemotherapy also contribute to the short-term and long-term immunodeficiency in patients treated for Hodgkin lymphoma, but there are no exact data on the precise contributions of the disease and its therapy.

TABLE 7.2

POSSIBLE INTERACTIONS BETWEEN HODGKIN AND REED-STERNBERG (HRS) CELLS AND T-LYMPHOCYTES

	HRS cells	Interaction	T-cells	Other cell types
Antigen recognition	Antigen?	?	TCR/CD3	
	HLA class I (some)	±	CD8	
	HLA class II	+	CD4	
Costimulation	CD80	+	CD28, CTLA4	
	CD86	+	CD28, CTLA4	
	CD30	?	CD30L	Eosinophils
	CD40	+	CD40L	
Cell—cell contact	CD58	+	CD2	
	CD54	+	CD11a/CD18	

TCR, T-cell receptor; HLA, human leukocyte antigen.

Infectious Mononucleosis   **Hodgkin Lymphoma**

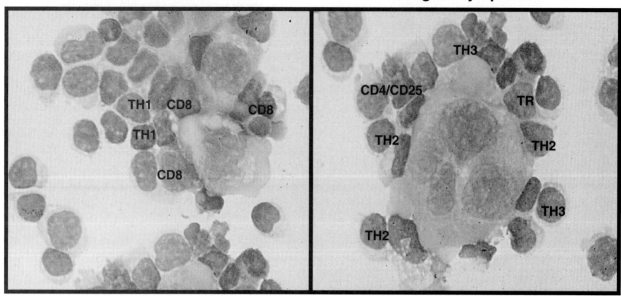

FIGURE 7.1. Immune response towards Epstein-Barr virus-infected cells in infectious mononucleosis and in Hodgkin lymphoma. In infectious mononucleosis, virus antigens are presented by HLA class I to CD8+ T-cells, which results in stimulation and co-stimulation, followed by proliferation and a cytotoxic response toward the virus-infected cells. The CD4+ T_H1-cells are activated by antigen-presenting cells and can give CD8+ T-cells help by producing IL-2 and several other T_H1-associated cytokines. In Hodgkin lymphoma there are only CD4+ T_H-cells present in the vicinity of the Hodgkin and Reed-Sternberg cells, and no CD8+ T-cells. This could be the result of a polymorphism or of absence of HLA class I molecules on the Hodgkin and Reed-Sternberg cells. Moreover, the CD4+ cells that surround the Hodgkin and Reed-Sternberg cells produce T_H2-associated cytokine IL-13, T_H3-associated cytokine TGF-β and T_R-associated cytokine IL-10. In addition, CD4/CD25 as well as Foxp3-positive regulatory T-cells are present. These cytokines (IL-13) may support the growth of the Hodgkin and Reed-Sternberg cells and further suppress a Th1-type cytotoxic response (IL-10, TGF-β). See color insert.

ACTIVATED CD4-POSITIVE T-CELLS SURROUNDING THE HODGKIN AND REED STERNBERG CELLS

The lymphocytes in close vicinity to Hodgkin and Reed-Sternberg cells are almost exclusively positive for CD4, whereas usually only very few CD8+ or natural killer (NK) cells are present in this area (Tables 7.3 and 7.4).[54] In patients who are HIV positive, however, CD8+ cells predominate, but it is not known whether these CD8+ cells are cytotoxic or regulatory CD8 cells. The generally observed increase of CD4+ cells in Hodgkin nodes is associated with a decrease in CD4+ cells in the circulation and predominantly reflects increased influx of mature CD4+ T-lymphocytes into the involved tissues.[54] Results of imaging with indium-111—labeled lymphocytes showing positivity in involved nodes support this concept.[55] Activated CD8+ T-cells, as determined by granzyme positivity, have been described in some cases but not immediately surrounding the Hodgkin and Reed-Sternberg cells. Surprisingly, the presence of these granzyme-positive lymphocytes was associated with an unfavorable prognosis.[56]

The CD4+ T-cells that surround the Hodgkin and Reed-Sternberg cells are in a state of activation, as indicated by the presence of several activation-associated surface markers, including CD38, CD69, CD71, and HLA class II (Tables 7.3 and 7.4).[57,58] A proportion of these CD4+ cells also stain for the cytotoxic granule-associated molecule TIA-1, but the significance of this staining is not known. There are no indications

TABLE 7.3

IMMUNOPHENOTYPE OF LYMPHOCYTES SURROUNDING THE HODGKIN—REED-STERNBERG CELLS IN HODGKIN LYMPHOMA

	Nodular lymphocyte-predominant	Classical
	Hodgkin lymphoma	Hodgkin lymphoma
CD3	+	+
TCRαβ	+	+
CD4	+	+
CD8	−	−
CD57	+	−
CD26	−	−
CD28	+	+
CTLA-4	+	+
CD40L	−	+
CD69	+	+
CD45RA	−	−
CD45R0	+	+
CD45RB	dim	dim

TCR, T-cell receptor; CTLA-4, cutaneous T-lymphocyte antigen.

TABLE 7.4

THE IMMUNE RESPONSE IN HODGKIN LYMPHOMA—INVOLVED LYMPH NODES

Lymphocyte subtypes	Predominance of activated CD4+ cells
	Few CD8+ cells
	Absence of NK cells
	Absence of CD26+ cells
Immune response characteristics	CD45 isotype expression indicative of Th2 cells
	Absence of IL-2 production by CD4+/CD26− cells
	Lymphocytes have characteristics of anergy
	No specific cytotoxic response against EBV in EBV+ cases

NK, natural killer; EBV, Epstein—Barr virus.

that the lymphocytes are of clonal origin or have a restricted TCR β-chain gene variable-region repertoire.[59,60] The lymphocytes lack expression of another activation marker, CD26 (dipeptidylpeptidase IV),[57] a surface molecule involved in co-stimulation of T-lymphocytes.[61,62]

Further characterization of CD4+ T-cells derived from lymph nodes of classical as well as the nodular lymphocyte-predominant subtype of Hodgkin lymphoma, by flow cytometry, has revealed that they are predominantly CD45RO+/ CD45RB^{dim}, suggesting an activated/memory T$_H$2 phenotype (Tables 7.3 and 7.4).[57,63] The T$_H$1/T$_H$2 paradigm was originally described by Mossman and associates in mice[64] and allowed the distinction of T$_H$1 cells that supported inflammatory responses by producing interleukin-2 (IL-2) and interferon-γ (IFN-γ) from T$_H$2 cells that support humoral responses by producing cytokines such as interleukin-4 (IL-4), IL-5, IL-6, and IL-10. When a single-cell suspension is prepared from lymph nodes involved by Hodgkin lymphoma, and these cells are optimally stimulated in vitro with phorbol ester and ionomycin, they produce IL-2, IFN-γ, and IL-4. When the CD4+/CD26− lymphocytes that immediately surround the Hodgkin and Reed-Sternberg cells are sorted from Hodgkin lymph nodes, these do not produce IL-2 but, when optimally stimulated in vitro, secrete increased amounts of IL-4. However, in a recent study we have shown that the lymphocytes in classical Hodgkin lymphoma, but not NLP Hodgkin lymphoma, spontaneously do produce IL-13 mRNA.[65] This cytokine profile suggests a T$_H$2 phenotype of at least a subset of these T-cells. The notion that the response in Hodgkin lymphoma is of T$_H$2 type is consistent with the finding that Hodgkin patients have elevated serum levels of T$_H$2-type cytokines IL-6 and IL-13 and frequently have elevated levels of IgG and also IgE.[30] For further discussion see also the section below on the potential anergy and/or regulatory nature of the surrounding T-cells.

CD57+ T-CELLS SURROUNDING HODGKIN AND REED-STERNBERG CELLS IN NLP HODGKIN LYMPHOMA: A SPECIAL T-CELL SUBSET

The CD4+ lymphocytes surrounding the so called lymphocytic and histiocytic (L&H)-type Reed-Sternberg cells in the nodular lymphocyte predominant subtype express CD57 on their surface, in contrast to those surrounding Hodgkin and Reed-Sternberg cells in the classical subtypes of Hodgkin lymphoma, which do not express CD57 (Table 7.3).[58] The CD57-positive cells do not express CD40L. CD4 and CD57

coexpression is normally almost exclusively seen on T-cells in the light zone of reactive germinal centers,[68] and these cells also lack CD40L expression. In germinal centers there are at least two CD4 T-cell subsets: CD4+/CD40L+ cells are located at the rim of germinal center light zone and mantle zone; and CD4+/CD57+ cells are distributed within the light zone. The CD4+/CD57+ cells are similar to murine CD4+/NK1.1+ cells in their tissue distribution and cytokine production, indicating a possible similar function for both lymphocyte subpopulations. The murine CD4+/NK1.1+ cells are known to produce IL-4 early in the immune response and direct it toward a T$_H$2-type response.[69] In human tonsillar germinal centers, the CD4+/CD57+ cells also express IL-4 mRNA.[70] We have recently confirmed this finding by quantitative pcr in sorted CD4+/CD57+ tonsillar T-cells and found that upon activation these cells produce IL2, IL4, and IL10 as well as TGF βmRNA's. However, the CD4/CD57-positive cells sorted from NLP HL and from progressively transformed germinal centers that are considered to be precursor lesions of NLP HL, could not produce IL4 mRNA.[65] The absence of IL4 and presence of IL10 mRNA would be consistent with a Tr1 cytokine profile. The relevance of this finding is not yet clear.

It has been suggested that CD57 expression is a marker of activation.[71] It has also been demonstrated that CD57+ T-cells have undergone more cell divisions than memory cells with other phenotypes, and can be considered senescent cells.[67] The lack of IL2 and IL4 transcripts in NLP HL may therefore simply reflect a history of more cell divisions in NLP HL than in reactive tonsils.[65]

ANERGY AND/OR REGULATORY NATURE OF SURROUNDING T-CELLS IN CLASSICAL HODGKIN LYMPHOMA AS A POSSIBLE CAUSE FOR IMPAIRED CYTOTOXICITY

As mentioned earlier, the T-cells surrounding the Hodgkin and Reed-Sternberg cells in the classical types of Hodgkin lymphoma do not express CD26 (Tables 7.3 and 7.4), although more than 60% of normal peripheral blood and lymph node T-cells are CD26+.[72,73] CD26 physically interacts with adenosine deaminase (ADA) and with CD45R0, both of which are important in the immune response.[74,75] CD26− T-cells become CD26+ by stimulation with antigens/mitogens under physiologic conditions,[74] but the CD26− cells from Hodgkin lesions remain negative after stimulation.[57] This indicates that the absence of CD26 is potentially relevant with respect to the impaired immune response observed in Hodgkin lymphoma. Inability to produce IL-2 and reduced proliferation are the hallmarks of anergic T-cells (Fig. 7.1). Marshall and colleagues reported that the lymphocytes in HL indeed do not produce cytokines, such as IL-2, IL-4, and interferon-γ (IFN-γ), with primary (keyhole limpet hemocyanin [KLH]) and recall (purified protein derivative [PPD]) antigens and the mitogen concanavalin A (ConA).[76] However, sorted CD26⁻ lymphocytes from cases of classical Hodgkin lymphoma can be stimulated in vitro to produce IFN-γ and IL-4, but not IL-2.[57]

Anergic T-cells can be obtained by several mechanisms: lack of co-stimulation,[77,78] activation by superantigens,[79] or the effect of certain cytokines (IL-10, TGF-β).[80,81] Thus, a possible way for Hodgkin and Reed-Sternberg cells to escape cytotoxic killing is by induction of anergy in T-cells. The anergic state of the lymphocytes is probably not the result of lack of co-stimulation by CD80 (B7.1), CD86 (B7.2), and other adhesion/co-stimulatory molecules such as CD58 (LFA-3) and CD54 (ICAM-1), because these are highly expressed on Hodgkin and Reed-Sternberg cells (Fig. 7.1, Table 7.2).[33,82]

Hodgkin and Reed-Sternberg cells are capable of producing a wide variety of cytokines, including IL-1, IL-5, IL-6, IL-9, IL-10, IL-13, and TGF-β,[83,84] and it is suspected that constitutive nuclear expression of NF-κB is responsible for this phenomenon.[85] Remarkably, Hodgkin and Reed-Sternberg cells generally express the T-cell transcription factors T-bet and GATA-3 that regulate the production of Th1 and Th2 cytokines in T-cell subsets.[86] The cytokines produced by Hodgkin and Reed-Sternberg cells also include IL-10 and TGF-β,[87–89] which are indeed known to be capable of anergy induction.[90] Supernatant from Hodgkin cell line L-428 was found to inhibit CD25 expression and IL-2 production when peripheral blood mononuclear cells were stimulated with anti-CD3, although the cells still became CD69 positive. This indicates that a soluble factor is responsible for the improper activation.[91] L-428 is known to produce TGF-β and IL-10.[92] Depletion of TGF-β from L-428 supernatant was found to completely prevent the inhibitory effect, while adding the removed TGF to RPMI resulted in a similar reduced CD25 and IL-2 expression pattern as with L-428 supernatant and IL-10 depletion did not affect the inhibitory effect of L-428 supernatant.[91] These findings strongly suggest that TGF-β is the T-cell inhibitory factor in the L-428 cell line. Marshall and colleagues confirmed that HL-infiltrating lymphocytes directly suppress peripheral blood mononuclear cell (PBMC) responses. They identified the presence of IL-10 secreting cells and CD4⁺CD25⁺ regulatory T-cells. The immunosuppressive effect of the infiltrating cells could be neutralized with anti—IL-10, by preventing cell-to-cell contact, and by anti—cytotoxic T-lymphocyte—associated antigen 4 (anti—CTLA-4).[76] FOXP3 is considered a marker for regulatory T-cells and TIA-1 as a cytotoxic cell marker. In a recent study it was found that, perhaps counterintuitively, a relatively low number of FOXP3-positive cells and a relatively high number of TIA-1 predict for unfavorable outcome.[93]

TGF-β is generally produced in a latent, inactive complex composed of the bioactive TGF-β homodimer (25 kd) and a noncovalently bonded precursor protein.[94] Often a latent TGF-β binding protein is associated with this complex. Bioactive TGF-β homodimer can be released from the complex after very strong acidification. The TGF-β produced by the L-428 cell line was found to be active at physiologic pH and had a much higher molecular weight than the usual active form.[95] By SDS-PAGE, the L-428 TGF-β was shown to contain a 25-kd molecule that cross-reacted with antibodies against TGF-β. High-molecular-weight TGF-β was also observed in the urine of patients with Hodgkin lymphoma, although it was absent from healthy controls, suggesting that it is also produced in vivo by the tumor.[95] Production of TGF-β that is already active at physiologic pH by Hodgkin and Reed-Sternberg cells might enable them to (de)regulate the immune response in their favor. TGF-β is also a potent growth factor for fibroblasts and is known to promote the formation of extracellular matrix and fibrosis.[89] The L-428 cell line was derived from a patient with the nodular-sclerosis subtype of Hodgkin lymphoma and is EBV negative. By in situ hybridization we have demonstrated the presence of TGF-β mRNA in the Hodgkin and Reed-Sternberg cells of nodular sclerosis cases.[91] Therefore, TGF-β may shape the environment for Hodgkin and Reed-Sternberg cells by suppressing the T-cell response and inducing the collagen formation in the nodular sclerosis subtype. There are indications that EBV-positive Hodgkin and Reed-Sternberg cells as frequently found in mixed cellularity relatively frequently produce IL-10, and less frequently produce TGF-β and this may result in the different inflammatory infiltrate and morphology in this subtype.

The findings indicate that there are variations in the populations involved in different cases. It can be concluded that, as an overall population, the infiltrating lymphocytes do not have Th1- or Th2-type functions, because they do not spontaneously produce IL-2 or IL-4 and may therefore be considered anergic. However, they include cells producing IL-10, despite not being fully activated, and therefore function as Tr1 cells. In addition, there are CD4/CD25-positive and also FOXP3-positive regulatory T-cells, and also TGF-β producing, so-called Th3 cells, present in the infiltrate.

POSSIBLE ROLE FOR MEMBERS OF THE TNFR/NGFR AND TNFL SUPERFAMILIES IN HODGKIN LYMPHOMA

CD30, now identified as a member of the tumor necrosis factor receptor (TNFR) family, was first discovered with a monoclonal antibody prepared against the cell line L-428 that shows a consistently high expression on Hodgkin and Reed-Sternberg cells.[96] Further investigations revealed that CD30 expression is not restricted to these cells alone but is also expressed on activated T- and B-lymphocytes. The abundant presence of CD30 on Hodgkin and Reed-Sternberg cells and its absence in most non-Hodgkin lymphomas suggest that it might play an important role in the development of Hodgkin lymphoma. However, it is not quite clear how CD30 might be involved because the CD30 ligand can not be demonstrated on the T-cells surrounding the Hodgkin and Reed-Sternberg cells, although it has been found on the eosinophils.[97] The known TNF receptor superfamily has gradually grown in recent years.[98] Their natural ligands form two superfamilies, the neutrophins [nerve growth factor (NGF) ligand superfamily] and the tumor necrosis factor (TNF) ligand superfamily. Several other members of both the TNF receptor and TNF ligand superfamily have also been observed in Hodgkin lymphoma: CD27L (CD70), CD40, and CD95 (Fas/Apo) are all highly expressed on Hodgkin and Reed-Sternberg cells.[99] Some of their ligands, notably CD40L, are expressed on the surrounding activated T-cells.[100] These T-cells also express Fas (CD95) but only minimal amounts of Fas ligand (CD95L). Somewhat surprisingly, CD40L is absent from the CD57⁺ lymphocytes in the nodular lymphocyte-predominant subtype of Hodgkin lymphoma.[100] Several members of these superfamilies have an important role in the regulation of proliferation and apoptosis, and CD40/CD40L interaction is extremely important in B-cell activation.[101]

CD95/CD95L interaction is capable of apoptosis induction and is involved in the maintenance of immune privilege and peripheral tolerance.[102] It is also one of the mechanisms used in the cytotoxic response by T-cells. It is therefore interesting that there is no adequate cytotoxic response toward Hodgkin and Hodgkin and Reed-Sternberg cells, although they express substantial amounts of CD95.

A possible mechanism for tumor cells to escape a cytotoxic response is deletion of the T_H1 cells, resulting in the absence of help to the effector cells. T_H1 cells, cytotoxic T-cells, and NK cells are more sensitive than T_H2 cells to CD95-mediated activation-induced cell death.[103] This difference in susceptibility is already present in T_H0 cells.[104] In Hodgkin lymphoma, the lymphocytes surrounding the tumor cells predominantly express a T_H2 phenotype. A polyclonal antibody reactive with membrane-bound as well as secreted CD95L and a monoclonal antibody reactive with a cytoplasmic determinant of CD95L both give strong staining of Hodgkin and Reed-Sternberg cells, whereas the surrounding lymphocytes have a very low expression of CD95L and relatively high expression of CD95 (S. Poppema, unpublished results). CD95L expression has also been detected on malignant cells in several other malignancies, giving these malignant cells yet another possible mechanism to escape the immune response.[105] It is therefore possible that Hodgkin and Reed-Sternberg cells escape a cytotoxic and T_H1 immune response through the induction of apoptosis in surrounding cytotoxic T and NK lymphocytes and T_H1 cells.

Traditionally, starting from the early observations that low numbers of lymphocytes were associated with a poor prognosis and normal numbers with a better prognosis, it has been accepted that the lymphocytes present a more or less effective immune response against the tumor cells or an associated etiologic agent.

Migration of T- as well as B-lymphocytes into normal as well as neoplastic lymphoid tissues requires the interaction between chemokines like CCL19 and CCL21 that are expressed on high endothelial venules and receptors like CCR7 that are expressed on subsets of T and B lymphocytes. Interestingly, not only the T-lymphocytes in Hodgkin lymphoma, but also the RS cells themselves express CCR7, perhaps explaining the predominant location in T-cell areas of lymph nodes.[105] On the other hand, the L&H cells of NLP HL, as well as the CD57-positive T-cells surrounding them, only express CXCR4, a receptor influencing migration to follicles.[106] An explanation for the specific phenotype of Hodgkin lymphoma is offered by the finding that the tumor cells of the classical subtypes of Hodgkin lymphoma produce high quantities of the CC chemokine TARC.[107] As mentioned before, constitutive nuclear NF-κB expression may induce the production of several chemokines by Hodgkin and Reed-Sternberg cells. NF-κB activation caused by the HTLV-1—encoded transactivator Tax can lead to the expression of several chemokines.[108] It is therefore possible that the up-regulation of TARC also results from NF-κB activation. It has also been demonstrated that inhibitors of NF-κB—like roxithromycin can suppress the production of TARC.[110]

TARC is normally produced in much smaller amounts by a subset of antigen-presenting cells and strongly attracts T-lymphocytes expressing the CCR4 receptor.[111] Activated T_H2 lymphocytes express the CCR4 receptor, whereas T_H1 lymphocytes express the CCR5 receptor.[112,113] A significant proportion of the lymphocytes of Hodgkin tissue indeed express CCR4 mRNA and have predominantly cytoplasmic protein expression of the CCR4 receptor,[37] probably indicating previous receptor ligand interaction. In addition, Hodgkin and Reed-Sternberg cells also produce large amounts of macrophage-derived chemokine (MDC) that also interacts with the CCR4 receptor.[38,39] The production of TARC by Hodgkin and Reed-Sternberg cells may therefore result in specific attraction of T_H2-type T-lymphocytes. The paradox of an extensive but apparently ineffective immune infiltrate may thus reflect chemotactic attraction of T_H2 cells by an aberrantly produced chemokine instead of an antitumor response.

SUMMARY

Hodgkin lymphoma is characterized by the presence of Hodgkin and Reed-Sternberg cells surrounded by predominantly CD4+ T-lymphocytes. These lymphocytes express a variety of activation markers but are incapable of mounting an effective immune response against the tumor cells. The lymphocytes typically are CD45RO+/CD45RB^{dim}/CD69+; lack the expression of CD26; can be stimulated in vitro with PMA/ionomycin, but not with recall antigens like KLH or PPD or with ConA, to produce IFN-γ and IL-4 but not IL-2; and spontaneously only produce suppressive cytokines like IL-10 and TGFβ. The CD45 isotype expression, the absence of CD26, and the potential for IL-4 production suggest that these lymphocytes have a T_H2 origin. The production of the CC chemokine TARC by the Hodgkin and Reed-Sternberg cells of the classical subtypes of Hodgkin lymphoma may contribute to the predominance of T_H2-like cells in the lesions because TARC strongly binds to CCR4, a chemokine receptor that is expressed on activated T_H2 cells. Lack of IL-2 production, the induction of a predominant T_H2 response, or the induction of anergy would each contribute to an ineffective immune response. Another factor involved in the lack of an effective immune response may be the cytokine TGF-β, which is produced in an active form by Hodgkin and Reed-Sternberg cells and has potent immunosuppressive effects on T-cells as well as a fibrosis-promoting effect. Interleukin-10, which is also produced by some Hodgkin and Reed-Sternberg cells, may also modulate the immune response toward a T_H2 type.

In this manner, Reed-Sternberg cells are able to create a T_H2-type environment that benefits their own survival because it supports the proliferation of (abnormal) B-cells and prevents the development of a cytotoxic immune response.

The TNF/TNFR superfamilies probably play an important role in Hodgkin lymphoma, as several members of these families, notably CD30, CD40, CD70, CD95, and also CD95L, are highly expressed on the Hodgkin and Reed-Sternberg cells. Moreover, their natural ligands are expressed on the surrounding lymphocytes. A general feature of members of the TNF/TNFR family is their involvement in cell activation and/or apoptosis, and therefore, they may play a crucial role in improper activation of the lymphocytes. Unequal susceptibility of lymphocyte subpopulations to Fas-mediated cell death could result in absence of effector cells such as CD8+ T-cells and NK cells, or appropriate helper cells such as T_H1 CD4+ cells.

In conclusion, there are a range of factors present in Hodgkin lymphoma that may contribute to the paradox of an extensive inflammatory infiltrate and concomitant ineffectiveness of the host antitumor response as well as the generalized cellular immune deficiency in patients with active Hodgkin lymphoma.

References

1. Sternberg C. Über einem eigenartige unter dem bilde der pseudoleukämie verlaufende tuberculose des lymphatischen apparates. *Z Heilkd* 1898;19: 21–90.
2. Clarke JM. Discussion on lymphadenoma. *Br Med J* 1901;2:701.
3. Reed DM. On the pathological changes in Hodgkin's disease; with especial reference to its relation to tuberculosis. *Johns Hopkins Hosp Rep* 1902;10:133–196.

4. Longcope WT. On the pathological histology of Hodgkin's disease, with a report of a series of cases. *Bull Ayer Clin Lab Penn Hosp* 1903;1:1.
5. Hoster HA, Dratman MV, Craver LF, et al. Hodgkin's disease 1832–1947. *Cancer Res* 1948;8:1,49–78.
6. Waldhauser A. Hodgkin's disease. *Arch Pathol* 1933;16:522–672.
7. Jackson H Jr, Parker F Jr. *Hodgkin's disease and allied disorders.* New York: Oxford University Press; 1947.
8. Centkowski P, Sawczuk-Chabin J, Prochorec M, et al. Hodgkin's lymphoma and tuberculosis coexistence in cervical lymph nodes. *Leuk Lymphoma* 2005;46:471–475.
9. Parker F, Jackson H, Green H, et al. Studies of diseases of the lymphoid and myeloid tissues. IV. Skin reaction to human and avian tuberculin. *J Immunol* 1932;22:277.
10. Steiner PE. Etiology of Hodgkin's disease. *Arch Intern Med* 1934;54:11.
11. Dubin IN. The poverty of the immunological mechanism in patients with Hodgkin's disease. *Ann Intern Med* 1947;27:898–911.
12. Schier WW, Roth A, Ostroff G, et al. Hodgkin's disease and immunity. *Am J Med* 1956;20:94–99.
13. Lamb D, Pilney F, Kelly WD, et al. A comparative study of the incidence of anergy in patients with carcinoma, leukemia, Hodgkin's disease and other lymphomas. *J Immunol* 1962;89:555–558.
14. Brown RS, Haynes HA, Foley HT, et al. Hodgkin's disease. Immunologic, clinical and histologic features of 50 untreated patients. *Ann Intern Med* 1967;67:291–302.
15. Sokal JE, Primikirios M. The delayed skin test response in Hodgkin's disease and lymphosarcoma. *Cancer* 1961;14:597–607.
16. Ciampelli E, Pelu G. Compartamento dello intradermoreazione alla tubercolina nei pazienti affetti da morbo di Hodgkin trattati radiologicamente. *Radiol Med* 1963;48:683–690.
17. Armstrong D, Minamoto GY. Infectious complications of infections of Hodgkin's disease. In: Lacher MJ, Redmann JR, eds. *Hodgkin's disease: the consequences of survival.* Philadelphia: Lea & Febiger; 1990:151.
18. Bookman MA, Longo DL. Concomitant illness in patients treated for Hodgkin's disease. *Cancer Treat Rev* 1986;13:77–111.
19. Aisenberg AC. Studies on the delayed hypersensitivity in Hodgkin's disease. *J Clin Invest* 1962;41:1964–1970.
20. Aisenberg AC. Manifestations of immunologic unresponsiveness in Hodgkin's disease. *Cancer Res* 1966;26:1152–1164.
21. Aisenberg AC. Quantitative estimation of the reactivity of normal and Hodgkin's disease lymphocytes with thymidine-2-C14. *Nature* 1965;205:1233.
22. Hersh EM, Oppenheim JJ. Impaired in vitro lymphocyte transformation in Hodgkin's disease. *N Engl J Med* 1965;273:1006–1012.
23. Clerici M, Ferrario E, Trabattoni D, et al. Multiple defects of T helper cell function in newly diagnosed patients with Hodgkin's disease. *Eur J Cancer* 1994;30A:1464–1470.
24. Gaines JD, Gilmer MA, Remington JS. Deficiency of lymphocyte antigen recognition in Hodgkin's disease. *Natl Cancer Inst Monogr* 1975;36:117–121.
25. Engleman EG, Benike CJ, Hoppe RT, et al. Autologous mixed lymphocyte reaction in patients with Hodgkin's disease. *J Clin Invest* 1980;66:149–158.
26. Bjorkholm M, Holm G, Mellstedt H, et al. Immunological capacity of lymphocytes with Hodgkin's disease evaluated in mixed lymphocyte culture. *Clin Exp Immunol* 1977;22:373–377.
27. Ford RJ, Tsao J, Kouttab NM, et al. Association of an interleukin abnormality with the T cell defect in Hodgkin's disease. *Blood* 1984;64:386–392.
28. Longmire RL, McMillan R, Yelenosky R, et al. In vitro splenic IgG synthesis in Hodgkin's disease. *N Engl J Med* 1973;289:763–767.
29. Huber C, Michlmayr G, Falkensamer M, et al. Increased proliferation of T lymphocytes in the blood of patients with Hodgkin's disease. *Clin Exp Immunol* 1973;21:47–53.
30. Amlot PL, Slaney J. Hypergammaglobulinaemia E in Hodgkin's disease and its relationship to atopy or a familial predisposition to atopy. *Int Arch Allergy Appl Immunol* 1981;64:138–145.
31. Renner C, Ohnesorge S, Held G, et al. T cells from patients with Hodgkin's disease have a defective T-cell receptor chain expression that is reversible by T-cell stimulation with CD3 and CD28. *Blood* 1996;88:236–241.
32. Sjoberg J, Andersson M, Garcia C, et al. Expression of the signal transduction molecule zeta in peripheral and tumour-associated lymphocytes in Hodgkin's disease in relation to the Epstein-Barr virus status of the tumour cells. *Br J Haematol* 2002;116:765–773.
33. Gruss H-J, Pinto A, Duyster J, et al. Hodgkin's disease: a tumor with disturbed immunological pathways. *Immunol Today* 1997;18:156–163.
34. Gause A, Jung W, Schmits R, et al. Soluble CD8, CD25 and CD30 antigens as prognostic markers in patients with untreated Hodgkin's lymphoma. *Ann Oncol* 1992;3:S49–S52.
35. Nadali G, Vinante F, Chilosi M, et al. Soluble molecules as biological markers in Hodgkin's disease. *Leuk Lymphoma* 1997;26(suppl 1):99–105.
36. Katay I, Wirnitzer U, Burrichter H, et al. L-428 cells derived from Hodgkin's disease produce E-rosette inhibiting factor. *Blood* 1990;76:791–796.
37. van den Berg A, Visser L, Poppema S. High expression of CC chemokine TARC in the Reed-Sternberg cells: A possible explanation for the characteristic lymphocytic infiltrate in Hodgkin's disease. *Am J Pathol* 1999;154:1685–1691.
38. Maggio EM, van den Berg A, Visser L, et al. Common and differential chemokine expression patterns in RS cells of NLP, EBV positive and negative classical Hodgkin lymphomas. *Int J Cancer* 2002;99:665–672.
39. Maggio E, van den Berg A, Diepstra A, et al. Chemokines, cytokines and their receptors in Hodgkin's lymphoma cell lines and tissues. *Ann Oncol* 2002;13s1:52–56.
40. Weihrauch MR, Manzke O, Beyer M, et al. Elevated serum levels of CC thymus and activation-related chemokine (TARC) in primary Hodgkin's disease: potential for a prognostic factor. *Cancer Res* 2005;65:5516–5519.
41. Frisan T, Sjoberg J, Dolcetti R, et al. Local suppression of Epstein-Barr (EBV)-specific cytotoxicity in biopsies of EBV-positive Hodgkin's disease. *Blood* 1995;86:1493–1501.
42. Dolcetti R, Frisan T, Sjoberg J, et al. Identification and characterization of an Epstein-Barr virus-specific T-cell response in the pathologic tissue of a patient with Hodgkin's disease. *Cancer Res* 1995;55:3675–3681.
43. Khanna R, Burrows SR, Nichols J, et al. Identification of cytotoxic T cell epitopes within Epstein-Barr virus (EBV) oncogene latent membrane protein 1 (LMP1): evidence for HLA A2 supertype-restricted immune recognition of EBV-infected cells by LMP-1 specific cytotoxic T lymphocytes. *Eur J Immunol* 1998;28:451–458.
44. Poppema S, Visser L. Epstein-Barr virus positivity in Hodgkin's disease does not correlate with HLA A2 negative phenotype. *Cancer* 1994;73:3059–3063.
45. Bryden H, MacKenzie J, Andrew L, et al. Determination of HLA-A*02 antigen status in Hodgkin's disease and analysis of an HLA-A*02 restricted epitope of the Epstein-Barr virus LMP-2 protein. *Int J Cancer* 1997;72:614–618.
46. Poppema S, Visser L. Absence of HLA class I expression by Reed-Sternberg cells. *Am J Pathol* 1994;145:37–41.
47. Oudejans JJ, Jiwa NM, Kummer JA, et al. Analysis of major histocompatibility complex class I expression on Reed-Sternberg cells in relation to the cytotoxic T-cell response in Epstein-Barr virus-positive and -negative Hodgkin's disease. *Blood* 1996;87:3844–3851.
48. Lee SP, Constandinou CM, Thomas WA, et al. Antigen presenting phenotype of Hodgkin Reed-Sternberg cells: analysis of the HLA class I processing pathway and the effects of interleukin-10 on Epstein-Barr virus-specific cytotoxic T-cell recognition. *Blood* 1998;92:1020–1030.
49. Diepstra A, Niens M, Vellenga E, et al. Association with HLA class I in Epstein-Barr-virus-positive and with HLA class III in Epstein-Barr-virus-negative Hodgkin's lymphoma. *Lancet* 2005;365:2216–2224.
50. Diepstra A, Poppema S, Boot M, et al. HLA-G expression as an immune escape mechanism in classical Hodgkin lymphoma and primary mediastinal B-cell lymphoma. *J Pathol* 2006.
51. Bjorkholm M, Holm G, De Faire U, et al. Immunological defects in healthy twin siblings to patients with Hodgkin's disease. *Scand J Haematol* 1977;19:396–404.
52. Ricci M, Romagnani S. Immune status in Hodgkin's disease. In: Doria G, Eskol A, eds. *The immune system: function and therapy of dysfunction.* New York: Academic Press; 1980:105–112.
53. Poppema S, Bhan AK, Reinherz EL, et al. In situ immunologic characterization of cellular constituents in lymph nodes and spleens involved by Hodgkins's disease. *Blood* 1982;59:226–232.
54. Romagnani S, Del Prete GF, Maggi E, et al. Displacement of T lymphocytes with the helper/inducer phenotype from peripheral blood to lymphoid organs in untreated patients with Hodgkin's disease. *Scand J Haematol* 1983;31:305–314.
55. Lavender P, Goldman JM, Arnot RN, et al. Kinetics of indium-111 labeled lymphocytes in normal subjects and patients with Hodgkin's disease. *Br Med J* 1977;2:797–799.
56. Oudejans JJ, Jiwa NM, Kummer JA, et al. Activated cytotoxic T cells as prognostic marker in Hodgkin's disease. *Blood* 1997;89:1376–1382.
57. Poppema S. Immunology of Hodgkin's disease. *Baillieres Clin Haematol* 1996;9:447–457.
58. Poppema S. The nature of the lymphocytes surrounding Reed-Sternberg cells in nodular lymphocyte predominance and in other types of Hodgkin's disease. *Am J Pathol* 1989;135:351–357.
59. Poppema S, Hepperle B. Restricted V gene usage in T-cell lymphomas as detected by anti-T-cell receptor variable region reagents. *Am J Pathol* 1991;138:1479–1484.
60. Rubin B, Martin EPG, Arnaud J, et al. Expression and signal transduction of T-cell antigen receptor (TCR)/CD3 complexes on fresh or in vitro expanded T lymphocytes from patients with Hodgkin's and non-Hodgkin's lymphomas. *Scand J Immunol* 1997;45:715–725.
61. Morimoto C, Schlossman SF. CD26 a key costimulatory molecule on CD4 memory T cells. *Immunologists* 1994;2:4–7.
62. Fleischer B. CD26: a surface protease involved in T-cell activation. *Immunol Today* 1997;15:180–184.
63. Poppema S, Lai R, Visser L, et al. CD45 (leucocyte common antigen) expression in T and B lymphocyte subsets. *Leuk Lymphoma* 1996;20:217–222.
64. Mosmann TR, Cherwinski H, Bond MW, et al. Two types of helper T cell clone. I. Definition according to profiles of lymphokine activities and secreted proteins. *J Immunol* 1986;136:2348–2357.
65. Atayar C, Poppema S, Visser L, et al. Cytokine gene expression profile distinguishes CD4+/CD57+ T-cells of nodular lymphocyte predominance type of Hodgkin lymphoma from their tonsillar counterparts. *J Pathol* 2006;208: in press.

66. Brenchley JM, Karandikar NJ, Betts MR, et al. Expression of CD57 defines replicative senescence and antigen-induced apoptotic death of CD8+ T cells. *Blood* 2003;101:2711–2720.

67. Gorschluter M, Bohlen H, Hasenclever D, et al. Serum cytokine levels correlate with clinical parameters in Hodgkin's disease. *Ann Oncol* 1995;6: 477–482.

68. Poppema S, Visser L, De Leij L. Reactivity of presumed anti–natural killer cell antibody Leu 7 with intrafollicular T lymphocytes. *Clin Exp Immunol* 1983;54:834–837.

69. Yoshimoto T, Bendelac A, Hu-Li J, et al. Defective IgE production by SJL mice is linked to the absence of CD4+, NK1.1+ T cells that promptly produce interleukin 4. *Proc Natl Acad Sci USA* 1995;92: 11931–11934.

70. Butch AW, Chung G, Hoffmann JW, et al. Cytokine expression by germinal center cells. *J Immunol* 1997;150:39–47.

71. Vollenweider L, Lazzarato M, Groscurth P. Proliferation of IL-2 activated lymphocytes preferably occurs in aggregates by cells expressing the CD57 antigen. *Scand J Immunol* 1995;42:381–386.

72. Fox DA, Hussey RE, Fitzgerald KA, et al. Ta₁, a novel 105 kD human T cell activation antigen defined by a monoclonal antibody. *J Immunol* 1984;133:1250–1256.

73. Mattern T, Scholz W, Feller AC, et al. Expression of CD26 (dipeptidyl peptidase IV) on resting and activated human T lymphocytes. *Scand J Immunol* 1991;33:737–748.

74. Kameoka J, Tanaka T, Nojima Y, et al. Direct association of adenosine deaminase with a T cell activation antigen, CD26. *Science* 1993;261:466–469.

75. Torimoto T, Dang NH, Vivier E, et al. Coassociation of CD26 (dipeptidyl peptidase IV) with CD45 on the surface of human T lymphocytes. *J Immunol* 1991;147:2514–2517.

76. Marshall NA, Christie LE, Munro LR, et al. Immunosuppressive regulatory T cells are abundant in the reactive lymphocytes of Hodgkin lymphoma. *Blood* 2004;103:1755–1762.

77. Sloan-Lancaster J, Evavold BD, Allen PM. Induction of T cell anergy by altered T-cell receptor ligand on live antigen-presenting cells. *Nature* 1993;363:156–159.

78. Schwarz RH. Models of T cell anergy: Is there a common molecular mechanism? *J Exp Med* 1996;184:1–8.

79. Tsiagbe VK, Yoshimoto T, Asakawa J, et al. Linkage of superantigen-like stimulation of syngeneic T cells in a mouse model of follicular center cell B cell lymphoma to transcription of endogenous mammary tumor virus. *EMBO J* 1993;12:2313–2320.

80. Groux H, Bigler M, de Vries JE, et al. Interleukin-10 induces a long-term antigen-specific anergic state in human CD4+ T cells. *J Exp Med* 1996; 184:19–29.

81. Kehrl JH, Wakefield LM, Roberts AB, et al. Production of transforming growth factor beta by human T lymphocytes and its potential role in the regulation of T cell growth. *J Exp Med* 1986;163:1037–1050.

82. Munro JM, Freedman AS, Aster JC, et al. In vivo expression of the B7 costimulatory molecule by subsets of antigen-presenting cells and the malignant cells of Hodgkin's disease. *Blood* 1994;83:793–798.

83. Hsu S, Waldron JW, Hsu P, et al. Cytokines in malignant lymphomas: Review and prospective evaluation. *Hum Pathol* 1993;24:1040–1057.

84. Kadin ME, Agnarsson BA, Ellingsworth LR, et al. Immunohistochemical evidence of a role for transforming growth factor beta in the pathogenesis of nodular sclerosing Hodgkin's disease. *Am J Pathol* 1990;136:1209–1214.

85. Bargou RC, Emmerich F, Krappmann D, et al. Constitutive nuclear factor-κB-RelA activation is required for proliferation and survival of Hodgkin's disease tumor cells. *J Clin Invest* 1997;100:2961–2969.

86. Atayar C, Poppema S, Blokzijl T, et al. Expression of the T-cell transcription factors, GATA-3 and T-bet, in the neoplastic cells of Hodgkin lymphomas. *Am J Pathol* 2005;166:127–134.

87. Ohshima K, Suzumiya J, Akamatu M, et al. Human and viral interleukin-10 in Hodgkin's disease, and its influence on CD4+ and CD8+ T lymphocytes. *Int J Cancer* 1995;62:5–10.

88. Hsu S-M, Lin J, Xie S-S, et al. Abundant expression of transforming growth factor-β1 and -β2 by Hodgkin's Reed-Sternberg cells and by reactive T lymphocytes in Hodgkin's disease. *Hum Pathol* 1993;24:249–255.

89. Newcom SR, Kadin ME, Ansari AA. Production of transforming growth factor-beta activity by Ki-1 positive lymphoma cells and analysis of its role in the regulation of Ki-1 positive lymphoma growth. *Am J Pathol* 1988;131:569–577.

90. Reinhold D, Bank U, B₁hling F, et al. Transforming growth factor-β1 (TGF- β1) inhibits DNA synthesis of PMW-stimulated PBMC via suppression of IL-2 and IL-6 production. *Cytokine* 1994;6:382–388.

91. Potters M, Diepstra A, Meulenaar R, et al. The absence of effective T-cell activation in Hodgkin's disease may be the result of TGF-β production by Reed-Sternberg cells. *Blood* 1997;10:265b. Abstract.

92. Newcom SR, Kadin ME, Ansari AA, et al. L-428 nodular sclerosing Hodgkin's cell secrete a unique transforming growth factor-beta active at physiologic pH. *J Clin Invest* 1988;82:1915–1921.

93. Alvaro T, Lejeune M, Salvado MT, et al. Outcome in Hodgkin's lymphoma can be predicted from the presence of accompanying cytotoxic and regulatory T cells. *Clin Cancer Res* 2005;11:1467–1473.

94. Lawrence DA. Transforming growth factor-β: a general review. *Eur Cytokine Netw* 1996;7:363–374.

95. Newcom SR, Tagra KK. High molecular weight transforming growth factor β is excreted in the urine in active nodular sclerosing Hodgkin's disease. *Cancer Res* 1992;52:6768–6773.

96. Schwab U, Stein H, Gerdes J, et al. Production of a monoclonal antibody specific for Hodgkin and Sternberg-Reed cells of Hodgkin's disease and a subset of normal lymphoid cells. *Nature* 1982;299:65–67.

97. Pinto A, Aldinucci D, Gloghini A, et al. The role of eosinophils in the pathobiology of Hodgkin's disease. *Ann Oncol* 1997;8(suppl 2):89–95.

98. Smith CA, Farrah T, Goodwin RG. The TNF receptor superfamily of cellular and viral proteins: activation, costimulation, and death. *Cell* 1994;76: 959–962.

99. Gruss H-J, Pinto A, Gloghini A, et al. CD30 ligand expression in nonmalignant and Hodgkin's disease-involved lymphoid tissues. *Am J Pathol* 1996; 149:469–481.

100. Carbone A, Gloghini A, Gruss H, et al. CD40 ligand is constitutively expressed in a subset of T cell lymphomas and on the microenvironmental reactive T cells of follicular lymphomas and Hodgkin's disease. *Am J Pathol* 1995;147:912–922.

101. Grewal I, Flavell RA. A central role of CD40 ligand in the regulation of CD4+ T-cell responses. *Immunol Today* 1996;17:410.

102. Abbas AK. Die and let live: eliminating dangerous lymphocytes. *Cell* 1996;84:655–657.

103. Zhang X, Brunner T, Carter L, et al. Unequal death in T helper cell (Th)1 and Th2 effectors: Th1, but not Th2, effectors undergo rapid Fas/FasL-mediated apoptosis. *J Exp Med* 1997;185:1837–1849.

104. Varadhachary AS, Perdow SN, Hu C, et al. Differential ability of T cell subsets to undergo activation-induced cell death. *Proc Natl Acad Sci USA* 1997;94:5778–5783.

105. Walker PS, Saas P, Dietrich PY. Role of Fas ligand (CD95L) in immune escape: the tumor cell strikes back. *J Immunol* 1997;158:4521–4524.

106. Hopken UE, Foss HD, Meyer D, et al. Up-regulation of the chemokine receptor CCR7 in classical but not in lymphocyte-predominant Hodgkin disease correlates with distinct dissemination of neoplastic cells in lymphoid organs. *Blood* 2002;99:1109–1116.

107. Poppema S, Potters M, Visser L, et al. Immune escape mechanisms in Hodgkin's disease. *Ann Oncol* 1998;9:S21–S24.

108. Komine M, Kakinuma T, Kagami S, et al. Mechanism of thymus- and activation-regulated chemokine (TARC)/CCL17 production and its modulation by roxithromycin. *J Invest Dermatol* 2005;125:491–498.

109. Baba M, Imai T, Yoshida T, et al. Constitutive expression of various chemokine genes in human T-cell lines infected with human T-cell leukemia virus type 1: role of the viral transactivator Tax. *Int J Cancer* 1996;66: 124–129.

110. Imai T, Yoshida T, Baba M, et al. Molecular cloning of a novel T-cell directed CC chemokine expressed in thymus by signal sequence trap using Epstein-Barr virus vector. *J Biol Chem* 1996;271:21514–21521.

111. Imai T, Baba M, Nishimura M, et al. The T-cell directed CC-chemokine TARC is a highly specific ligand for CC chemokine receptor 4. *J Biol Chem* 1997;272:15036–15042.

112. Bonecchi R, Bianchi G, Bordignon PP, et al. Differential expression of chemokine receptors and chemotactic responsiveness of type 1 T helper cells (Th1s) and Th2s. *J Exp Med* 1998;187:129–134.

113. Sallusto F, Lenig D,Mackay CR, et al. Flexible programs of chemokine receptor expression on human polarized T helper 1 and 2 lymphocytes. *J Exp Med* 1998;187:875–883.

114. Loetscher P, Uguccioni M, Bordoli L, et al. CCR5 is characteristic of TH1 lymphocytes. *Nature* 1998;391:344–345.

CHAPTER 8 ■ CYTOGENETICS OF CLASSICAL HODGKIN LYMPHOMA

STEFAN JOOS AND REINER SIEBERT

It is now widely accepted that the malignant Hodgkin and Reed-Sternberg cells (HRS cells) in classical Hodgkin lymphoma (HL) are derived from B-cells in the vast majority of cases. Evidence for this was provided by single-cell analyses demonstrating immunoglobulin variable (V) gene rearrangements as well as crippling mutations, which are highly specific for antigen-activated B-cells.[1-7] In case these rearrangements remain unproductive, B-cells within the germinal center normally undergo apoptosis. However, for as yet unknown reasons, HRS cells escape this mechanism, which is considered one of the key steps in the pathogenesis of this disease. Rearrangements of the *TCR* genes were also found in rare cases (~2%), indicating that HRS cells might also originate from T-cells.[8-10] Further support for the B- or T-cell origin of HRS cells came from analyses of composite lymphoma from Hodgkin lymphoma and non-Hodgkin lymphoma (NHL), in which clonal relationships between the tumor cells from the different tumor compartments were observed. This indicated that the malignant cells originated from a common ancestor but subsequently performed an independent development of cytogenetic and molecular changes.[11-18]

Although the B- or T-cell origin of HRS cells is now generally accepted and has, for example, resulted in a renaming "Hodgkin's disease" to "Hodgkin lymphoma,"[19] our knowledge about the molecular mechanisms leading to this malignancy is still poor. This is mainly due to the fact that HRS cells represent only a minority (~1%) of the cells within an affected lymph node, which makes cytogenetic and molecular analyses of these cells a highly challenging task. They have to be specifically distinguished and isolated from bystander cells, for example, by immunodetection and micromanipulation techniques, and generally there is only a minor amount of material available for detailed molecular studies. Therefore, cell lines derived from HRS cells became very important for the progression of classical HL research. However, the relevance of experiments with cell lines often remained limited, because only few classical HL-derived cell lines could be established. Furthermore, all were derived from patients at late stages of the disease.[20,21]

Analysis and identification of characteristic chromosomal aberrations in tumor cells are powerful tools to provide insights into the molecular mechanisms underlying the development of individual tumors. Here we summarize the major results obtained from cytogenetic analyses of classical HL as well as from classical HL-derived cell lines. Initial cytogenetic studies were started as long as 40 years ago, and particularly after chromosome banding techniques were established, there was hope to be able to identify specific structural chromosomal aberrations that would shed light on the genes and the molecular mechanisms involved in the pathogenesis of this disease. However, chromosome banding analysis of HRS cells turned out to be difficult, in particular because of the scarcity of abnormal metaphase cells as well as the high complexity of the chromosomal aberrations identified. With the advent of molecular cytogenetics in the 1980s, several of these difficulties could be overcome, for example, by applying fluorescence in situ hybridization (FISH) on interphase nuclei or by screening the entire genome for HRS cells using comparative genomic hybridization (CGH). Although no classical HL-specific chromosomal aberration similar to that known for several subtypes of non-Hodgkin lymphoma has yet been identified, these approaches allowed the localization of a number of chromosomal regions characteristically altered in HRS cells. Several of these aberrant regions were found to harbor genes coding for members of cellular signalling pathways, which become deregulated in this way. Prominent examples include the NF-κB and the JAK/STAT pathways, which were shown in further studies to be frequently deregulated in HRS cells.

ANALYSIS OF PRIMARY HODGKIN LYMPHOMA USING CLASSICAL CYTOGENETICS

The first reports on cytogenetic changes in classical HL were published in the early 1960s.[22] They showed that two different types of metaphase cells are distinguishable in Hodgkin cells: normal ones, most probably derived from nonmalignant cells; and highly aneuploid cells, most likely representing the malignant cells.

With the advent of chromosomal banding techniques, it became possible to analyze numerical and in particular structural cytogenetic aberrations in more detail. However, chromosomal banding analysis of HRS cells turned out to be rather difficult.[23,24] First, the culturing conditions are critical. HRS cells generally exhibit a low proliferation index and if the culturing period is too short, either no or very few metaphase cells are obtained. If the culturing period is too long, preferentially normal lymphoid cells begin to divide, resulting in a high frequency of unrearranged metaphases not representative of the malignant clone. Many studies were performed in which short-term conditions of less than 72 hours were applied. Another difficulty was that aneuploid clones often showed a highly complex rearrangement pattern, while the chromosome morphology was frequently poor.[23] For these reasons, abnormal chromosomes often could not be identified and had

TABLE 8.1

CYTOGENETIC ANALYSES IN HODGKIN LYMPHOMA

Author	Patients	Patients with analyzable metaphases	Patients with abnormal metaphases All	%[a]
Hossfeld et al.[103]	6	6	6	100
Kristoffersson et al.[104]	20	18	11	61
Cabanillas et al.[59]	49	29	18	62
Dennis et al.[105]	12	12	9	75
Koduru et al.[30]	51	39	5	13
Schouten et al.[106]	37	29	13	45
Reeves and Pickup[107]	5	5	4	80
Banks et al.[29]	7	5	3	60
Ladanyi et al.[31]	95	57	13	23
Tilly et al.[28]	60	49	33	67
Poppema et al.[108]	28	25	23	89
Döhner[27]	33	25	9	36
Schlegelberger et al.[26]	21	20	14	70
Pedersen et al.[109]	31	27	16	59
Falzetti et al.[33]	27	24	14	58
Total	482	370	191	52

Series are listed in chronological order with respect to publication date. Only series reporting banded chromosomes from Hodgkin lymphoma tissue are shown here.
[a]Percentage of those with analyzable metaphases.

to be listed as "marker chromosomes" with unknown composition.[25]

In Table 8.1, results are summarized from serial investigations performed between 1978 and 1999 on 482 patients with primary classical HL. Analyzable metaphases could be obtained from 370 patients. In about half of them (48%), only normal karyotypes were detected. This high incidence led to the hypothesis that HRS cells sometimes might lack cytogenetic changes, an issue that later could be disproved by applying the FICTION approach (see below). Abnormal metaphases, defined as those with either numerical or structural chromosomal abnormalities, were found in 191 of the 370 patients (52%). As shown in Table 8.1, there is a high variability with regard to the frequency of tumors showing abnormal metaphases. This ranged from 13% to 92%, and probably reflects methodologic differences, including the analysis of samples that have variable cellularity or contain different numbers of malignant cells. In addition, differences in elapsed time from biopsy to placing the cells in culture, the exact culture conditions used to generate metaphases, and the exact banding techniques can all affect the number of abnormal metaphases observed. Finally, a reporting bias cannot be excluded. In the authors' own unpublished series of 455 cases diagnosed or suspicious for HL ascertained over more than two decades, 43% showed a normal karyotype, 6% showed nonclonal or "simple" changes, and 10% carried a complex karyotype characteristic for HRS cells. In the remaining samples, no metaphases could be obtained (J.I. Martin-Subero, M. Giefing, L. Harder, and R. Siebert, unpublished data).

As can be further seen from Table 8.1, chromosome-banding analyses from HL are relatively scanty, as compared to the situation for non-Hodgkin lymphomas. However, some important findings were obtained. One major result was that the karyotypic changes observed in HRS cells were found to be clonal, which suggested for the first time that Hodgkin lymphoma represents a neoplastic (and not an inflammatory) condition.

In general, polyploidy was found to be very common amongst HRS cells. Early cytogenetic studies predominantly revealed near-diploid karyotypes with only minor chromosome anomalies,[23] while more recent publications present mostly near-triploid to near-tetraploid karyotypes with many numerical and structural chromosome aberrations.[26–28] A compilation of published cytogenetic data comprising 105 chromosomally aberrant classical HL cases revealed the presence of a karyotype in the near-triploid to near-tetraploid range in 57 of the cases (54%).[23,26–32] A near-diploid karyotype with complex numerical and structural aberrations was found in 30 of the cases (29%). In 18 cases (17%), a near-diploid chromosome number containing only minor numerical or structural chromosome abnormalities, such as gains or losses of single chromosomes or chromosome segments, was observed.

Considering numerical aberrations of individual chromosomes, gains exceed losses in most of the cases. Among the most frequent gains were those of chromosomes 2, 5, 9, and 12, while losses mostly involved chromosomes 6, 10, 13, 15, 17, 18, 21, 22, and Y.[20,27,28] With regard to structural abnormalities, translocations, inversions, deletions, or duplications

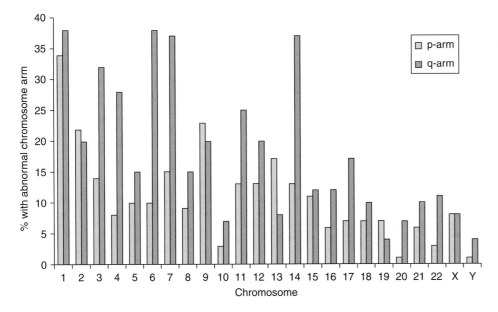

FIGURE 8.1. Alterations of specific chromosome arms in Hodgkin lymphoma as detected by chromosome-banding analysis. Compiled from the 167 abnormal karyotypes from the series of Table 8.1 that were reported in detail.[26–31,33,59,60,103–106,108,109]

were reported. Their distribution on the different arms of each chromosome is summarized in Figure 8.1. Taking into account the relative size of the different chromosomes and the short (p) and the long (q) arms, these data suggest that 2p, 3q, 4q, 6q, 7q, 9p, 11q, 13p, 14p, 14q, 15p, and 17q are altered more frequently than expected from their relative size. This is particularly striking, when chromosome 9p as well as the short arms of the acrocentric chromosomes 13, 14, and 15 are considered, because the p arms are much smaller than the q arms in these cases. In fact, aberrations on these chromosomes were also frequently detected later on by molecular cytogenetics.

A strategy to address candidate genes that might be involved in classical HL oncogenesis is to determine how often specific chromosomal bands are involved in aberrations. Falzetti and associates summarized the breakpoints of 177 classical HL cases[33] and found a nonrandom distribution of breakpoints, most frequently affecting chromosomal bands 1p13, 1q21, 1q22, 5p15, 12p13, and 19p13 in 5%; 1p36, 6q15, 6q21, and 8q24 in 6%; 7q22, 7q32, 12q24, 13p11, 14p11, and 15p11 in 7%; 11q23 in 10%; and 14q32 in 12% of the metaphases analyzed. Interestingly, several of the affected subbands correspond to well-known chromosomal breakpoints described in other lymphoid malignancies. Examples are rearrangements of bands 6q15-21, 7q22, 7q32, and 11q23.[34,35] The chromosomal band most frequently affected by rearrangements in this compilation is 14q32, which is consistent with the B-cell origin of classical HL. As could be demonstrated later by molecular cytogenetics, the IGH (immunoglobulin heavy chain) locus is frequently involved in these rearrangements.

Due the high number of affected subregions and the relatively low resolution of chromosome banding analysis (~5 Mb), there are a large number of possible genes that could be affected by these rearrangements. Which of these genes actually represent critical targets and contribute to classical HL pathogenesis remains speculative at this stage.

Overall, the results from classical chromosome banding analyses provided the first evidence that classical HL is a neoplastic condition. Furthermore, they showed the presence of nonrandom cytogenetic changes in HRS cells that could result in inactivation of tumor suppressor genes and/or activation of oncogenes. However, the number of cases analyzed by this approach remained relatively small. In addition, the resolution

of chromosome banding analysis is relatively low (about 5 Mb), and therefore the candidate genes that might be directly affected by these aberrations could not be narrowed down to reasonable numbers. This situation improved with the advent of molecular cytogenetic techniques, described in the following section.

ANALYSIS OF HODGKIN LYMPHOMA USING MOLECULAR CYTOGENETICS

With the advent of novel cytogenetic strategies like fluorescence in situ hybridization (FISH) or comparative genomic hybridization (CGH), a deeper insight into the characteristic genomic changes of HRS cells could be obtained. In the next section, the principles and major advantages of these methods for the analysis of HRS cells will be outlined. This is followed by a description of the most important findings in classical HL-derived cell lines and primary HL tumors.

Molecular Cytogenetic Techniques

Fluorescence In Situ Hybridization (FISH)

In FISH, delineation of specific chromosomal sequences is performed in morphologically preserved biological specimens using fluorochrome-labeled DNA-probes. A particular advantage of FISH is the potential to detect very small, submicroscopic chromosomal changes. Thus deletions or other structural rearrangements of only several kb can be detected by FISH, while the resolution of chromosomal banding analysis is in the range of 5 to 10 Mb. Furthermore, FISH can analyze chromosomal changes not only on metaphase chromosomes but also in interphase nuclei (interphase cytogenetics). This constitutes a decisive advantage over previous techniques for the analysis of HRS cells, because interphase nuclei are much more frequent in cellular preparations than metaphase spreads. A second advantage is that tumor cells do not have to be precultured and analyses can be performed on paraffin-embedded material.[36]

A special feature of FISH is that various DNA-probes can be used simultaneously by labelling them with different fluorochromes. Frequently, dual-color FISH is performed, in which in addition to the probe to be tested, a second, differentially labeled probe is used to serve as an internal standard. This approach was further improved and extended in order to facilitate the identification of chromosomal subregions of individual chromosomes. In principle, this is achieved by using a set of *painting* probes specific for all human chromosomes, each of which is labelled by a different combination of five fluorochromes. After hybridization of this probe set, the individual chromosomes exhibit different signal patterns, which are recognized and transformed in defined pseudocolors using suitable hardware and software packages.[37,38] The multicolor approach (M-FISH) is a powerful tool to analyze the composition of heavily rearranged chromosomes, which are typical for HRS cells, and has been used in particular for detailed cytogenetic analyses of HRS-derived cell lines (described later).

Fiction

A further development that became particularly important for cytogenetic analyses of classical HL is the FICTION technique (fluorescence-immunophenotyping and interphase cytogenetics as a tool for investigation of neoplasms), which combines the interphase FISH approach with immunohistochemistry.[39,40] FICTION takes advantage of the characteristic expression of antigens on certain cell types such as CD30 on the HRS cells. CD30 is rarely expressed by the reactive mononuclear cell infiltrate, and therefore its staining coupled with the size and number of nuclei allows a clear identification of HRS cells. Simultaneous FISH analysis then allows the detection of numerical or structural chromosomal aberrations specifically in HRS cells. In this way, it was possible to demonstrate that HRS cells, in contrast to the surrounding bystander cells, harbor the complex karyotypic rearrangements and therefore represent the malignant cell clone in classical HL.

By its design, FICTION allows the specific evaluation of Reed-Sternberg cells because they bear a selectable immunohistochemical marker. Nevertheless, FICTION cannot determine a global karyotype, because it can only probe for specific numerical or structural aberrations. Such analyses became possible with the advent of genome screening techniques, like chromosomal and array-based CGH.

Comparative Genomic Hybridization (CGH)

CGH allows a genome wide screening of chromosomal gains and losses without prior knowledge of genomic regions of interest and independent of the availability of metaphase cells from the specimens to be investigated.[41–44] The principles of this approach are shown in Figure 8.2. For CGH analysis, whole genomes of tumor cells and normal control cells are used as probes (Fig. 8.2B). Hybridization of this probe is directed against metaphase chromosomes prepared from normal individuals. This allows the comparison of the signal intensities of tumor DNA and normal DNA along every individual chromosome. The signal intensity ratios of both probes are measured and indicate relative copy number changes of chromosomal regions within the tumor genome.

In array CGH, which represents an extension of the chromosomal CGH approach, the genomic DNA probes are hybridized on DNA arrays instead of metaphase chromosomes (Fig. 8.2C).[45,46] The DNA arrays are composed primarily of BAC clones with an average length of 100 to 200 kb or of oligonucleotides of about 70 nucleotides in length. Array CGH as compared to conventional chromosomal CGH there-

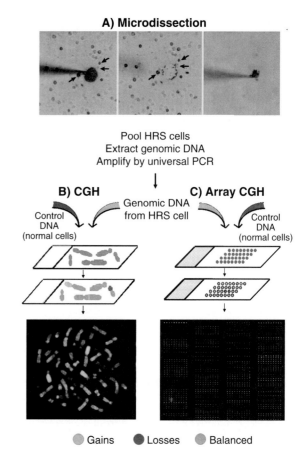

A) Microdissection

Pool HRS cells
Extract genomic DNA
Amplify by universal PCR

B) CGH   **C) Array CGH**

Control DNA (normal cells)   Genomic DNA from HRS cell   Control DNA (normal cells)

● Gains   ● Losses   ● Balanced

FIGURE 8.2. Genome-wide screening for chromosomal imbalances by CGH and array CGH. **A:** Before CGH-analysis, HRS cells have to be enriched, for example, by microdissection using glass needles. Subsequently, the genomic DNA is amplified by universal PCR and labeled with suitable fluorochromes. **B:** In chromosomal CGH, the labeled probe is hybridized together with a differentially labeled genomic DNA probe from normal cells against metaphase chromosomes prepared from normal peripheral blood cells. Gains *(green)* and losses *(red)* within the tumor genome are recognized by different signal intensity ratios on the corresponding chromosomal target sequences of the hybridized chromosomes. **C:** In array CGH, arrays of genomic sequences (oligonucleotides, BAC clones) are hybridized instead of metaphase chromosomes. This allows the detection of chromosomal imbalances with higher resolution ($\sim$ 50 kb) as compared to chromosomal CGH ($\sim$5 Mb). See color insert.

fore has a higher resolution (about 200-fold) and, in addition, can be fully automated.[47,48]

A major advantage of CGH and array CGH, as compared to other cytogenetic methods such as chromosome banding or FISH, is the fact that, instead of metaphase chromosomes or interphase nuclei, only genomic DNA is required from the tumor cells to be studied. With regard to classical HL this means, however, that the malignant HRS cells have to be physically enriched, for example, by cell sorting or micromanipulation devices, and the genomic DNA amplified (Fig. 8.2A). The latter has been performed by *universal* PCR methods, such as DOP-PCR (degenerate oligo-primed polymerase chain reaction), where primers with degenerate sequence cassettes are used.[49] Alternatively, linker-adapter strategies such as SCOMP (single-cell comparative genomic hybridization, described by Klein and associates), have been applied successfully.[50] With the latter approach it was possible to amplify genomic DNA from single cells, while pools of 10 to 20 cells are required for CGH analysis with DOP-PCR.[44,51,52]

CYTOGENETIC ANALYSIS OF HODGKIN LYMPHOMA CELL LINES BY COMBINED CLASSICAL AND MOLECULAR CYTOGENETICS

As indicated, the paucity of malignant cells in HL represents a general problem for molecular and cytogenetic studies of classical HL. It was therefore of high practical importance that cell lines derived from HRS cells could be established. However, an important question is how representative these cell lines are, because only about 10 have been established and all of them were isolated from patients at a time when the tumor had recurred.[20,21] To answer this question, cytogenetic aberrations in about half of these cell lines were analyzed in great detail. Because the pattern of chromosomal aberrations is highly complex, it was necessary to apply different cytogenetic approaches in order to unravel the numerous and often very subtle changes present in these cell lines.

A detailed combined chromosomal banding and FISH analysis of three HRS-derived cell lines (L428, L-1236, and L-540) was described by Fonatsch and co-workers.[32] One of the major results from this analysis was that despite the extreme genomic instability resulting in a sporadic occurrence of chromosomal abnormalities in only subsets of HRS cells from individual cases, several nearly identical chromosomal aberrations were found. In addition, several aberrations were observed in more than one cell line. For example, a deleted chromosome 11 with breakpoint in 11q14~q21 was seen in L-428 and L-1236, while two other marker chromosomes in these cell lines showed a duplication of the region 7q22-36. In addition, common breakpoints were detected in all three cell lines, involving, for example, chromosomal bands 1p22 (L428, L-1236), 2p23-25 (L428, L-1236), 2q37 (L-540, L-1236), 8q13~q21 (L-428, L-540), 8q24 (L-540, L-1236), and 14q24 (L-540, L1236).

Interestingly, rearrangements involving rDNA from the short arm of acrocentric chromosomes (13, 14, 15, 21, and 22) were found in two of the three cell lines. L-428 harbors a rearrangement of an unidentified chromosome segment with the short arm of chromosome 13 and parts of the long arm of an X chromosome are translocated to 21p. In L-540, a rearrangement of the short arm of chromosome 15 with 14q11 and 1p as well as a translocation of 7q22-qter to 21p12 is found. These results have led to the hypothesis that the genes encoding for ribosomal RNA play a critical role in the recombination process in these cell lines. As will be described below, this was further supported by M-FISH experiments, which were performed on these and further classical HL-derived cell lines.[53,54]

Chromosome 14 is involved in rearrangements in all three cell lines. In cell line L428, there is a translocation between chromosome 14q23 and chromosome 9 material; in L-540, 14q11 is intercalated between chromosome 15 and chromosome 1p material. In L-1236 a complex t(10;14) translocation involving the IGH locus (J.I. Martin-Subero and R.Siebert, unpublished data) and a deletion del(14)(q24) was detected.

Comparing these results with chromosome banding studies from primary classical HLs, the nonrandomness of numerical as well as structural aberrations of chromosome 14 has already been recognized in previous banding studies. In particular, Tilly,[28] Döhner,[27] Schlegelberger,[26] and their colleagues often found rearrangements of 14q11 and 14q32 in HRS cells from primary tumors. Other cytogenetic aberrations found in both primary classical HL as well as in cell lines included deletions, translocations, and duplications on the short arm of chromosome 1[23,26,27,55–58]; the short arm of chromosome 2 (2p23~p25)[26,28]; chromosome 7q22-35[26–28,58]; the long arm of chromosome 11, in particular 11q23[23,27,28,59,60]; as well as the long arm of chromosome 12 from 12q15-24.[26–28]

The same cell lines and one more line, HDLM-2, were also analyzed by multicolor FISH, which provided further important results, in particular concerning the composition of the numerous translocated chromosomes.[53,54] In general, this analysis again revealed a large number of numerical and structural aberrations, as shown in Figure 8.3 for KM-H2. Similar to observations in previous banding studies, individual cell

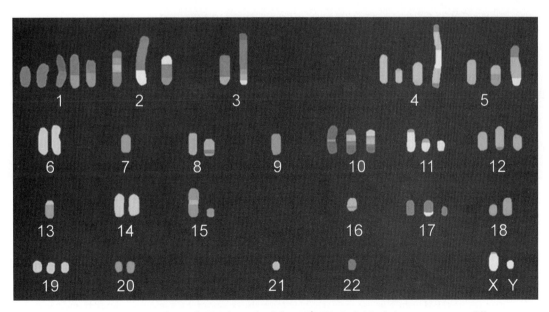

FIGURE 8.3. M-FISH analysis of HRS-derived cell line KM-H2. Individual chromosomes are differentially colored, making it possible to visualize the multiple rearrangements present in HRS cells. Note the complex composition of several translocated chromosomes and the frequently small size of translocated chromosomal bands, which are difficult to identify (e.g., by chromosomal banding analysis). See color insert. (Image was provided by Dr. Anna Jauch, Human Genetics Department, University of Heidelberg, Germany.)

lines exhibited a set of consistent chromosomal aberrations, which were found in all metaphases analyzed, but in addition a large number of abnormalities were observed sporadically in only a few metaphases.[54] In fact, there was not a single pair of metaphases that was completely identical in the four cell lines investigated, which underlines the high degree of chromosomal instability in these cells.

Concerning the structural aberrations, a large number of translocated chromosomes (22 to 57) were observed. Often, they were composed of material derived from multiple (up to 6) different chromosomes. Recurrent translocated chromosomes observed in more than one cell line included t(2;9) in KM-H2, HDLM-2, and L1236; t(7;11) in KM-H2, L428, and L1236; and t(12;13) and t(14;15) in KM-H2, HDLM-2, and L428. Similar data have also been obtained for HDLM-2 in a second M-FISH study.[53] Consistent translocations found in all HRS cells of individual cell lines were less frequent (4 in KM-H2, 7 in HDLM-2, 6 in L428, and 10 in L1236). Only one of them, a t(2;8), was detected in more than one cell line (HDLM-2 and in L428). The breakpoints were located on chromosome 2p12-15, which, among other genes, contains *REL* (see discussion below). *REL* was never found to be directly affected by these translocations.

However, for HDLM2, the breakpoint of the t(2;8) translocation could be mapped within a 1,7 Mb region of *REL*, while in other cell lines (KM-H2, L-428, and L-1236), intrachromosomal duplications of the 2p12-16 band including *REL* were detected.[54] As will be described below, copy number gains of the short arm of chromosome 2 were also recurrently found by CGH and FISH/FICTION in primary classical HL.

In contrast to chromosomal banding, the M-FISH approach made it possible to identify higher numbers of chromosomal translocations in the cell lines mentioned. This is most probably due to the potential of M-FISH to efficiently detect material of different origin in composite translocated chromosomes including only small chromosomal segments, each only a few megabases in size. Such segments were often found in classical HL cell lines (Fig. 8.4). They originated from different chromosomes and frequently represented distal parts containing subtelomeric sequences. Notably, in some instances they were present in multiple copies, which were translocated to different partner chromosomes, as has been demonstrated for the distal parts of chromosomal arms 4p, 5q, 8q, 9p, 12p, 17q, and Xp.[54] These structures could be termed *segmental chromosome aberrations* and resembled *segmental jumping translocations*, which were previously described in rare cases of treatment-related leukemias by Tanaka and associates.[61,62] It has been proposed that they might be generated by nonreciprocal, transchromosomal recombination of hyperreplicative or fragile sites or by the involvement of recombinogenic repetitive sequences, such as those occurring in centromeric/pericentromeric heterochromatin, telomeres, or subtelomeric regions. Further support for such a mechanism in HRS cells was provided by MacLeod and co-workers,[53] who could demonstrate, that a number of segmental chromosome aberrations in the cell line HDLM-2 was associated with subtelomeric microsatellite repeats or rDNA sequences (Fig. 8.4B). This could be confirmed in other cell lines as well as in primary tumors.[54,63] A prominent role of rDNA sequences had also been discussed in chromosome

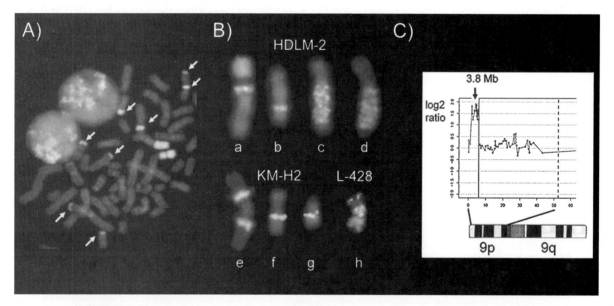

FIGURE 8.4. Segmental chromsome aberrations in HRS cell lines. **A:** Metaphase spread derived from cell line KM-H2 hybridized with a chromosome 7-specific painting probe. A number of segments inserted into different chromosomes *(arrows)* are visible, which are all derived from the distal part of chromosome 7q as demonstrated by the array CGH experiment (data not shown). **B:** Segmental chromosome aberrations of chromosomal region 9p24 in three different cHL cell lines. In *red*, the signal of a chromosome 9-specific painting probe is visible, while the *green* signal corresponds to a probe representing the *JAK2* locus on 9p24. **a–c:** Segmental chromosome aberrations of band 9p24 in three different chromosomes of cell line HDLM-2. In one chromosome, multiple insertions occurred. Segmental chromosome aberrations are flanked by r-DNA sequences, as shown in (**d**), where an r-DNA-specific probe *(blue)* has been used for FISH. **g–h:** Three segmental chromosome aberrations of 9p24 in cell line KM-H2 and one in cell line L-428. **C:** Array CGH analysis of chromosome 9 in cell line HDLM-2. The hybridization intensity ratios (log2 ratio) of HDLM-2 DNA and normal DNA are shown for BAC clones distributed from the telomere to the centromere of chromsome 9p. As expected from the M-FISH results, the distal 9p region is strongly amplified. The size of this segmental chromosome aberration is 3.8 Mb and harbors *JAK2* as well as a number of other candidate genes like *PD-L1* and *PD-L2*. See color insert. (From B. Radlwimmer, S. Ohl, P. Lichter, and S. Joos, unpublished data.)

banding studies due to the frequent finding of translocations involving acrocentric chromosomes in HRS cells.[26–28,32]

Due to the partial polysomy generated by segmental chromosome aberrations, oncogenes located within these regions become co-amplified in HRS cells, which has been shown, for example, for CCND2, MYC, MMSET and JAK2.[54] The janus kinase gene JAK2 was particularly interesting, because segmental chromosome aberrations including this gene were found in three different cell lines (Fig. 4). Moreover, as will be described below, this locus also is frequently amplified in HRS cells from primary tumors.[51,64]

The results of the cell lines described were complemented by CGH as well array CGH analyses, making it possible to generate a comprehensive genome-wide map of all numerical changes.[54] This revealed gains most frequently involving chromosomal bands 9p24 in all four cell lines, as well as 2p13-16 (KM-H2, L428, L1236), 5p15 (KM-H2, HDLM-2, L428), and 12p13 (HDLM-2, L428, L1236). Losses most frequently affected chromosome 18 (KM-H2, HDLM-2 and L428). Finally, distinct high-level amplifications, which had never been described before in HRS cells, were identified. They affected chromosomal bands 7q36, 9p24, 9q22, 11q24-25, 16q24, and 17q25; that is, they mostly involved distal chromosomal parts, which is in accordance with the identification of segmental chromosome aberrations from telomeric regions in the M-FISH experiments described above.

Array CGH analysis of the cell lines was initiated because chromosomal imbalances below the resolution of chromosomal CGH can be identified in this way. In fact, one such hidden amplification was detected, which, among others, included the STAT6 gene (signal transducer and activator 6) (S. Joos, B. Radlwimmer, P. Lichter, et al., personal communication; and R. Siebert, J.I. Martin-Subero, et al., personal communication). A further aim of the array-CGH studies was to measure the extension of amplified chromosomal subregions with high resolution in order to define potentially relevant oncogenes with higher precision. One example is the 9p24 amplicon in cell line HDLM-2, which could be shown to extend over 3.8 Mb (Fig. 8.4C) and, beside JAK2, additionally includes further potential oncogenes, including PD-L1 and PD-L2 coding for immunomodulating B-7 proteins.

Finally, recent array-based analyses of Hodgkin lymphoma cell lines using gene chips detecting single nucleotide polymorphisms (SNPs) provided evidence for partial uniparental disomy (pUPD) as another means of chromosomal complexity in classical HL (R. Siebert, J.I. Martin-Subero, et al., unpublished data). The term UPD refers to the fact that the two (or more) copies of a given chromosome or chromosomal segment derive only from the mother or the father. This is due to loss of one parental chromosome and duplication (or multiplication) of the other. For example, chromosome 6 in cell line L-1236 is derived only from one of the parents, which is in line with loss of heterozygosity (LOH) reported for this chromosome.[65] Remarkably, chromosome 6 contains so-called "imprinted" genes that are only expressed from one of the parental chromosomes.

FICTION ANALYSIS OF CHROMOSOMAL ABERRATIONS IN PRIMARY HODGKIN LYMPHOMA

FICTION has contributed significantly to our understanding of Hodgkin lymphoma. In early studies, HRS cells from classical Hodgkin lymphoma were analyzed for numerical chromosomal aberrations applying chromosome-specific centromere probes. Using this approach, Weber-Matthiesen and associates were able to show for the first time that only CD30-positive HRS cells harbored numerical chromosomal aberrations, while this was not the case in reactive cells.[66] Recurrent tri- or tetraploid HRS cells with often more than 70 chromosomes and up to 8 copies of individual chromosomes were detected.[66,67] Overall, the numerical alterations resembled those obtained by classical cytogenetics. Thus, chromosomes 1, 2, 4, 8, 12, 17, X, and Y were most frequently affected in 60% to 90% of HRS cells. Furthermore, in cases with complex and hyperdiploid karyotypes, the FICTION results agreed with those detected by conventional chromosome banding.

FICTION as well as FISH were also extensively used for the analysis of structural rearrangements in HRS cells from primary tumors. One focus was the analysis of chromosomal breakpoints affecting the immunoglobulin (IG) loci, because breakpoints at the respective chromosomal sites had been frequently observed. Therefore, Martin-Subero and co-workers have investigated a large series of classical HL for chromosomal breakpoints in the heavy and light immunoglobulin gene loci (IGH, IGL, and IGK) and found breakpoints in IGH in 17% of the cases. Though the IGH partners were heterogeneous and remain to be determined in most of the cases, individual tumors showed translocations of IG sequences to the REL locus on chromosomal band 2p16, the BCL6 gene on 3q27, the MYC gene on 8q24, and BCL3/RELB gene on 19q13. Other translocation partners involved chromosomal bands 14q23, 16p13, and 17q12. In addition to these results, HRS cells frequently showed evidence for a (partial) deletion of the IGH constant region, suggesting the presence of class switch recombination.

Given the role of the MYC, BCL6, and MALT1 oncogenes in lymphomagenesis, a series of classical HLs lacking an IG break was also evaluated by Martin-Subero and associates for chromosomal breakpoints affecting the corresponding gene loci. Only a single classical HL showed a chromosomal breakpoint in the BCL6 locus and none of these cases displayed breakpoints in MYC or MALT. However, genomic amplifications and gains of the MYC locus were observed in a subset of cases (R. Siebert, J.I. Martin-Subero, et al., unpublished data).

GENOMIC SCREENING OF PRIMARY HODGKIN LYMPHOMA

As shown in Figure 8.2, for CGH analysis whole-genomic DNA of HRS and control cells is used as a probe for FISH hybridization of chromosomes of normal metaphase cells. Therefore, pools of HRS cells have to be isolated and the genomic DNA amplified before CGH analysis can be performed.

The first CGH analysis of a series of 9 cases of HL (6 mixed cellularity and 3 nodular sclerosis) was described by Ohshima and colleagues.[68] Genomic DNA amplified from about 100 CD30-positive HRS cells that were isolated by FACS cell sorting was used as a probe for CGH. This analysis revealed a large number of chromosomal imbalances, mainly gains of 1p13 and 7q35-36, as well as losses of chromosomal arm 16q. Based on these results, further studies were initiated by the authors, which confirmed that deletions within the long arm are often present in HRS cells. One of the critical genes located within these deletions is E-catherin. In fact, the corresponding gene product representing a well-known adhesion molecule protein was found to be rarely expressed in classical HL.[69]

A large CGH analysis of 40 classical HL cases was described by Joos and associates.[51] About 20 to 30 HRS cells were isolated from each tumor by microdissection and amplified by DOP-PCR for subsequent CGH analysis. Again, this analysis revealed a high number of chromosomal imbalances in individual cases with gains occurring about three times more frequently than losses. Chromosomal losses most frequently affected chromosomal arms 13q (22%), Xp, and Xq (12% each); as well as 1p, 4q, and 17p (7% each). Gains were detected at higher frequencies than losses, most prominently on chromosomal arms 2p in 54%, as well as on 12q in 37% and 17p in 27%, of the cases. Lower frequencies (<25%) were detected for 9p and 16p (24% each), 17q and 20q (20% each), as well as 9q, 22q, and Xq (17% each). Notably, CGH identified various distinct high-level amplifications, which involved chromosomal bands 2p14-16, 3q21, 4p16, 4q23-24, 5p15, 5p11-13, and 12q13-14.

Table 8.2 summarizes the consensus regions of the recurrently imbalanced chromosomal regions as well as high-level amplifications together with various candidate genes located in the corresponding areas. As already indicated, the short arm of chromosome 2 was most frequently found imbalanced, and the consensus region, which is defined by a distinct amplification, again covers chromosomal bands 2p15-16 including, for example, REL (Fig. 8.5). As mentioned above, the same region has been found frequently rearranged in classical HL-derived cell lines. The REL protein is part of the NF-κB transcription factors associated with cell proliferation and tumor development.[70–73] Interestingly, a further high-level amplification affecting chromosomal band 4q23-24 also resulted in a co-amplification of a NF-κB encoding gene, namely NFKB1, which further underlines the critical role of these proteins in classical HL.

TABLE 8.2

CHROMOSOMAL REGIONS SHOWING NUMERICAL CHANGES IN HRS CELLS IN MORE THAN 20% AND DISTINCT HIGH-LEVEL AMPLIFICATIONS ACCORDING TO CGH ANALYSIS OF 40 HODGKIN LYMPHOMAS

Band	%	Genetic loci mapping in area
GAINS		
2p13-16	54	*REL* (oncogene REL, avian reticuloendotheliosis); *BCL11A* (B-cell CLL/lymphoma 11A); *TGFA* (transforming growth factor, alpha); *TLX2* (T-cell leukemia, homeobox 2) *RAB1* (member RAS oncogene family), *CDK7* (cyclin-dependent kinase 7)
9p24	23	*PD-L1, PD-L2* (programmed cell death 1 ligands 1 and 2); *NFIB* (nuclear factor I/B); *INSL4, INSL6* (Insulin-like protein 4 and 6); *JAK2* (janus kinase 2); *OVC* (ovarian adenocarcinoma oncogene)
12q23-24	37	*IGF1* (insulin-like growth factor-1); *NUP* (nucleoporin); *THRAP2* (thyroid hormone receptor-associated protein 2); *BCL7A* (B-cell CLL/lymphoma-7A); *CMKLR1* (chemokine-like receptor 1); *SHP2* (protein tyrosine phosphatase, nonreceptor-type, 11); *PRKAB1* (protein kinase, AMP-activated, noncatalytic, beta-1); *PPP1CC* (protein phosphatase-1, catalytic subunit, gamma isoform); *STK21* (serine/threonine protein kinase-21); *STK21* (serine/threonine protein kinase-21); *GPR81* (G-protein-coupled receptor 81); *GPR109A; GPR109B; RSN* (restin); *FZD10* (frizzled 10)
16p13	23	*CCNF* (cyclin F); *IL32* (interleukin 32); *RAB26* (RAS-associated protein RAB26); *TNFRSF12A* (tumor necrosis factor receptor superfamily, member 12A); *LITAF* (LPS-induced TNFA factor); *MHC2TA* (major histocompability complex, class II, transactivator)
17p	27	*CRK* (avian sarcoma virus CT10 (v-crk) oncogene homolog); *TNFSF12* (tumor necrosis factor ligand superfamily, member 12); TNFRSF13B (tumor necrosis factor receptor superfamily, member 13B); *BCL6B* (B-cell lymphoma 6B); *MAPK7* (mitogen-activated protein kinase 7); *JNKK1* (SAPK/ERK kinase-1)
HIGH-LEVEL AMPLIFICATIONS		
2p14-16		*REL* (oncogene REL, avian reticuloendotheliosis); *BCL11A* (B-cell CLL/lymphoma 11A); *TGFA* (transforming growth factor alpha); *TLX2* (T-cell leukemia, homeobox 2); *RAB1* (member RAS oncogene family); *CDK7* (cyclin-dependent kinase 7)
3q13		*CD80* (CD28 antigen ligand 1, B7-1 antigen); *CD86* (CD28 antigen ligand 2, B7-2 antigen); *RAB7* (Ras-associated protein RAB7)
4p16		*FGFR3* (fibroblast growth factor receptor-3); *JAMIP1* (janus kinase interacting protein gene)
4q23-24		*NFKB1* (nuclear factor of kappa light chain gene enhancer in B-cells 1 (p105); *LEF1* (lymphoid enhancer-binding factor-1)
5p15		*TRIO* (triple functional domain); *IRX* (Iroquois homeo box protein); *TERT* (telomerase reverse transcriptase); *NKD2* (naked 2)
5p11-13		*FGF10* (fibroblast growth factor-10); *IL7R* (interleukin-7 receptor); *LIFR* (inhibitory factor receptor); *SKP2* (S-phase kinase-associated protein 2 (p45).
12q13-14		*WNT1* (wingless-type MMTV integration site family, member 1, oncogene INT1); *WNT10B; LFG* (FAS apoptotic inhibitory molecule 2); *RAB5B* (Ras-associated protein RAB5B) *RAB13, STAT6* (signal transducer and activator of transcription-6); SHP2 (protein tyrosine phosphatase, nonreceptor-type); *MDM2*.

From Joos S, Menz CK, Wrobel G, et al. Classical Hodgkin lymphoma is characterized by recurrent copy number gains of the short arm of chromosome 2. *Blood* 2002;99:1381–1387. With permission.

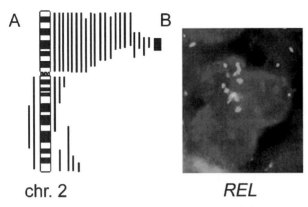

FIGURE 8.5. Copy number gains of the short arm of chromosome 2 in primary Hodgkin lymphoma. **A:** Results from CGH analysis performed on pools of HRS cells derived from 40 different cHLs.[51] Gain of 2p or parts of it occur in more than half of the cases, while losses were never observed. The consensus region of these aberrations was defined by a distinct high-level amplification, which affects subband 2p15-16, where, for example, the *REL* gene is located. **B:** FISH analysis of a single HRS cell showing multiple *REL* signals *(green)* but only two signals of the centromere of chromosome 2 *(red)*. See color insert.

The CGH results mentioned prompted a series of further interphase FISH/FICTION studies, which where performed on more than 100 primary classical HL cases. Among them, imbalances of the *REL* locus were found in 46% of cases (Martin-Subero and Siebert and associates, unpublished data). Furthermore, gains of the *REL* locus were found to be associated with nuclear accumulation of the REL protein,[74] which is indicative for the functionally active form of this protein. Finally, recurrent gains of the *BCL3/RELB* locus and losses of the *NFKBIA* locus were observed in HRS cells.[73]

In addition to the NF-κB system, CGH provided evidence for an involvement of the JAK/STAT signalling pathway in classical HL pathogenesis. As has been described above, the *JAK2* gene is involved in segmental chromosome aberrations in HRS-derived cell lines and becomes amplified in this way (Fig. 8.4). The same region (9p24) was also found overrepresented in 24% of primary tumors. Furthermore, high-level amplifications of chromosomal band 4p16 and 12q21 harboring the genes for janus kinase-interacting protein Jamip1 and for STAT6, respectively, were found involved in high-level amplifications[51] (S. Joos et al. and J.I. Martin-Subero et al., unpublished data). Further systematic FISH analyses finally revealed gains of *JAK2* and *STAT2/6* in roughly 40% and 30% of classical HL (R. Siebert, personal communication).

Other interesting candidates arising from CGH analysis are factors that modulate T-cell receptor signalling. An important family includes the B-7 proteins,[75,76] of which four were found in commonly amplified chromosomal regions: the genes for programmed cell death ligands 1 and 2 (*PDL1, PDL2*) on 9p24; and CD80 and CD86, which are located within chromosomal band 3q13. Remarkably, preliminary analyses suggest involvement of *PDL2* in chromosomal translocations in HL (R. Siebert et al., unpublished data). Certainly, this class of proteins deserves further investigation, for example, with regard to their impact on differentiation and down-regulation of T-cells and whether these proteins prevent T-cells surrounding the HRS cells from attacking them.

The frequent gains and high-level amplifications involving the long arm of chromosome 12, and in particular a high-level amplification on 12p13-14, suggested that the *MDM2* gene might frequently be increased in copy number. In fact, this could be demonstrated by FICTION analysis in HRS cells in four of six cases tested.[77] Gain of *MDM2* could account for

the frequent finding of accumulated p53 in HRS cells. Alternatively, this observation could also be due to p53 point mutations, but results from different laboratories concerning this matter are discrepant, most likely due to methodological differences.[78–80]

Other candidate genes depicted in this study point to the involvement of the WNT signalling pathway like *WNT1* and *WNT10B*, as well as *NKD2*, which interacts with the dishevelled protein DVL. Genes coding for G-proteins or their regulators include *RAB1*, *RAB5B*, *RAB7*, and *RAB13* as well as *TRIO*, an enhancing factor for Rho-like GTPases. Finally, genes encoding for *MMSET*, involved in t(4;14) translocations found in multiple myeloma; BCL7A, involved in translocations found in malignant lymphoma; fibroblast growth factor genes *FGF4* and *FGF10*; the telomerase subunit gene *TERT*, involved in different malignancies; as well the antiapoptotic genes *FAIM2* and *CTBP1* should be mentioned as potentially interesting candidates for further investigations in classical HL.

SUMMARY AND CONCLUSIONS

Molecular cytogenetic approaches like FISH, FICTION, and CGH have provided a number of new insights about characteristic chromosomal changes in HRS cells. As described above, there is a high degree of chromosomal instability, which is characterized by aneuploidy as well as large numbers of chromosomal translocations in HRS cells. Individual tumors and cell lines exhibit consistent cytogenetic changes found in all HRS cells as well as variable aberrations, which are observed only in HRS subpopulations. Repetitive sequences from subtelomeres as well as rDNA regions from the short arm of acrocentric chromosomes were frequently found adjacent to translocation breakpoints, confirming previous suggestions from chromosome-banding analyses that these sequences play an essential role in the formation of recombination events in HRS cells. This is also true for segmental chromosome aberrations, which appear to be a characteristic feature of HRS cells. As described, these structures very much resemble segmental jumping translocations previously described by Tanaka and co-workers in rare cases of hematologic diseases,[61] but up to now it remains unclear whether they share the same typical features. Segmental chromosome aberrations represent rather small chromosomal segments of 1 to 8 Mb in size from a particular chromosomal region, which are inserted or attached to other chromosomes. This can result in a co-amplification of oncogenes, as has been shown, for example, for *JAK2* and neighboring genes in three different cell lines. Furthermore, because segmental chromosome aberrations were frequently found to be derived from distal chromosomal parts, it is possible that they provide telomere sequences to chromosomes that have otherwise lost them, a mechanism termed *telomere capture*.[81]

One of the major technical breakthroughs in recent classical HL cytogenetics was the possibility of performing genome-wide screens for chromosomal imbalances. For the first time it was possible in this way to identify distinct high-level amplifications in HRS cells and to measure their extension with high resolution. In addition, CGH identified chromosomal imbalances that occurred at relatively high frequencies among classical HL tumors, such as gains of chromosomal arms 2p, 9p, and 12q in 20% to 50%. This is in contrast to the situation in chromosome-banding studies, where abnormal chromosomal subregions were usually detected in not more than 10%,[33] which often rendered their relevance questionable.

Aberrations of chromosomal band 2p25-16 as well as 9p24 belong to the most prominent cytogenetic changes identified up to now in HRS cells. A considerable amount of data have accumulated showing that this affects the NF-κB and JAK/STAT signalling pathways via the genes *REL* and *JAK2*. There is also cytogenetic evidence that other members of these pathways become deregulated by chromosomal aberrations.

Gain of chromosomal band 2p15-16 including the *REL* gene constitutes the most frequent aberration found in HRS cells by CGH and subsequent FISH analyses. It was found in every second tumor and was especially frequent among those of the nodular-sclerosis subtype (88%). *REL* codes for a subunit of NF-κB transcription factors associated with cell proliferation and tumor development,[82] as does *NFKB1*, the gene of which was also found amplified in HRS cells. It has been shown by several groups that the NF-κB pathway is constitutively activated in HRS cells.[83–85] For example, mutations in the IκB gene, a potent inhibitor of NF-κB, have been described, which might account for NF-κB activation at least in a subset of tumors.[86,87]

Gains of chromosomal arm 9p24 were detected in 24% of classical HLs. This subregion has attracted particular attention because, as described above, it was also involved in segmental chromosomal aberrations in three classical HL cell lines.[54,64] One of the candidate genes, *JAK2*, codes for a janus kinase, which is involved in the JAK/STAT signalling pathway of cytokines. Further aberrations that affected genes from this pathway included high-level amplifications of 4p16 and 12q13, including the genes coding for Jamip1, a janus kinase-binding protein, and STAT6, which acts downstream of JAK proteins.

The initial CGH findings prompted a number of further molecular analyses showing that *JAK2* as well as *STAT3*, *STAT5*, and *STAT6* acting downstream of janus kinases are overexpressed and constitutively phosphorylated in HRS-derived cell lines and primary tumors.[88–93] Furthermore, Melzner and associates recently demonstrated that *SOCS1*, an inhibitor of JAK2, is frequently mutated in Hodgkin cells.[94] Taken together, these results point to an important pathogenic role of this pathway in classical HL.

With respect to the frequent gains of chromosome 2p and 9p, including amplifications of *REL* and *JAK2*, the pattern of chromosomal aberrations was found strikingly similar to what has been observed in primary mediastinal large B-cell lymphoma.[71] Although *REL* amplifications have been observed frequently among other diffuse large B-cell lymphomas,[70] gains of 9p are often only found in these tumor entities, while they are rare (2%) among other lymphomas.[95] This has prompted discussions whether Hodgkin lymphoma and mediastinal large B-cell lymphoma are pathogenically related and/or share common deregulated molecular mechanisms.[74] This hypothesis is supported by rare cases of composite lymphomas with features of both lymphoma entities.[96] In addition, both tumor entities share a number of clinical and immunological features, including their frequent mediastinal origin and the lack of functional expression of HLA class I and Ig molecules.[97–99]

In conclusion, the introduction of new cytogenetic approaches and experimental strategies has provided significant new insights into the molecular mechanisms underlying classical HL. Less is known about the nonclassical Hodgkin subtype, nodular lymphocyte-predominant Hodgkin lymphoma (NLPHL), where only a few (less than a dozen) aberrant karyotypes have been characterized by chromosome banding. Basically, several chromosomal changes where detected similar to those found in highly malignant B-NHL. In addition, Franke and colleagues published a CGH study of 19 NLPHLs in which recurrent gains and losses as well as distinct high-level amplifications were identified.[112] Overall, the pattern of imbalances was significantly different from that of classical HL, suggesting a different pathogenic mechanism in this tumor type. Furthermore, various studies reported that the *BCL6* gene is more frequently involved in chromosomal translocations in NLPHL than in classical Hodgkin lymphoma.[100–102]

Acknowledgments

We wish to particularly thank C. Mecucci, A. Jauch, L. Harder, J.I. Martin-Subero, B. Radlwimmer, G. Toedt, S. Ohl, and P. Lichter for providing unpublished material and helpful discussions. We regret that not all of the colleagues who contributed to this field of research could be mentioned. Finally, we are very grateful to the Deutsche Krebshilfe and the Deutsche Forschungsgemeinschaft, which supported the research on Hodgkin lymphoma in the authors' laboratories.

References

1. Irsch J, Nitsch S, Hansmann ML, et al. Isolation of viable Hodgkin and Reed-Sternberg cells from Hodgkin disease tissues. *Proc Natl Acad Sci USA* 1998;95:10117–10122.
2. Kanzler H, Kuppers R, Hansmann ML, et al. Hodgkin and Reed-Sternberg cells in Hodgkin's disease represent the outgrowth of a dominant tumor clone derived from (crippled) germinal center B cells. *J Exp Med* 1996;184: 1495–1505.
3. Kuppers R, Rajewsky K, Zhao M, et al. Hodgkin disease:Hodgkin and Reed-Sternberg cells picked from histological sections show clonal immunoglobulin gene rearrangements and appear to be derived from B cells at various stages of development. *Proc Natl Acad Sci USA* 1994;91: 10962–10966.
4. Marafioti T, Hummel M, Foss HD, et al. Hodgkin and Reed-sternberg cells represent an expansion of a single clone originating from a germinal center B-cell with functional immunoglobulin gene rearrangements but defective immunoglobulin transcription. *Blood* 2000;95:1443–1450.
5. Spieker T, Kurth J, Küppers R, et al. Molecular single-cell analysis of the clonal relationship of small Epstein-Barr virus-infected cells and Epstein-Barr virus-harboring Hodgkin and Reed/Sternberg cells in Hodgkin disease. *Blood* 2000;96:3133–3138.
6. Jox A, Zander T, Kuppers R, et al. Somatic mutations within the untranslated regions of rearranged Ig genes in a case of classical Hodgkin's disease as a potential cause for the absence of Ig in the lymphoma cells. *Blood* 1999;93:3964–3972.
7. Küppers R. Molecular biology of Hodgkin's lymphoma. *Adv Cancer Res* 2002;84:277–312.
8. Muschen M, Rajewsky K, Brauninger A, et al. Rare occurrence of classical Hodgkin's disease as a T cell lymphoma. *J Exp Med* 2000;191:387–394.
9. Seitz V, Hummel M, Marafioti T, et al. Detection of clonal T-cell receptor gamma-chain gene rearrangements in Reed-Sternberg cells of classic Hodgkin disease. *Blood* 2000;95:3020–3024.
10. Tzankov A, Bourgau C, Kaiser A, et al. Rare expression of T-cell markers in classical Hodgkin's lymphoma. *Mod Pathol* 2005;18:1542–1549.
11. Rosenquist R, Roos G, Erlanson M, et al. Clonally related splenic marginal zone lymphoma and Hodgkin lymphoma with unmutated V gene rearrangements and a 15-yr time gap between diagnoses. *Eur J Haematol* 2004;73: 210–214.
12. Brauninger A, Hansmann ML, Strickler JG, et al. Identification of common germinal-center B-cell precursors in two patients with both Hodgkin's disease and non-Hodgkin's lymphoma. *N Engl J Med* 1999;340:1239–1247.
13. Kuppers R, Sousa AB, Baur AS, et al. Common germinal-center B-cell origin of the malignant cells in two composite lymphomas involving classical Hodgkin's disease and either follicular lymphoma or B-CLL. *Mol Med* 2001;7:285–292.
14. Marafioti T, Hummel M, Anagnostopoulos I, et al. Classical Hodgkin's disease and follicular lymphoma originating from the same germinal center B cell. *J Clin Oncol* 1999;17:3804–3809.
15. Bellan C, Lazzi S, Zazzi M, et al. Immunoglobulin gene rearrangement analysis in composite hodgkin disease and large B-cell lymphoma: evidence for receptor revision of immunoglobulin heavy chain variable region genes in Hodgkin-Reed-Sternberg cells? *Diagn Mol Pathol* 2002;11:2–8.
16. Rosenquist R, Menestrina F, Lestani M, et al. Indications for peripheral light-chain revision and somatic hypermutation without a functional B-cell receptor in precursors of a composite diffuse large B-cell and Hodgkin's lymphoma. *Lab Invest* 2004;84:253–262.
17. Tinguely M, Rosenquist R, Sundstrom C, et al. Analysis of a clonally related mantle cell and Hodgkin lymphoma indicates Epstein-Barr virus infection of a Hodgkin/Reed-Sternberg cell precursor in a germinal center. *Am J Surg Pathol* 2003;27:1483–1488.
18. van den Berg A, Maggio E, Rust R, et al. Clonal relation in a case of CLL ALCL and Hodgkin composite lymphoma. *Blood* 2002;100:1425–1429.

19. Stein H, Delsol G, Pileri S, et al. Classical Hodgkin's lymphoma. In: Jaffe E, Harris N, Stein H, et al., eds. *World Health Organization classification of tumours. Pathology and genetics of tumours of the hematopoietic and lymphoid tissue.* Lyon: IARC Press;2001:244–253.

20. Drexler HG. Recent results on the biology of Hodgkin and Reed-Sternberg cells. I. Biopsy material. *Leuk Lymphoma* 1993;8:1–25.

21. Kanzler H, Hansmann ML, Kapp U, et al. Molecular single cell analysis demonstrates the derivation of a peripheral blood-derived cell line (L1236) from the Hodgkin/Reed-Sternberg cells of a Hodgkin's lymphoma patient. *Blood* 1996;87:3429–3436.

22. Spriggs AI, Boddingtom MM. Chromosomes of Sternberg-Reed cells. *Lancet* 1962;2:153.

23. Thangavelu M, Le Beau MM. Chromosomal abnormalities in Hodgkin's disease. *Hematol Oncol Clin North Am* 1989;3:221–236.

24. Atkin NB. Cytogenetics of Hodgkin's disease. *Cytogenet Cell Genet* 1998;80:23–27.

25. Mitelman F, ed. Guidelines for cancer cytogenetics. Supplement to an International System for Human Cytogenetic Nomenclature. In: *ISCN 1995.* Basel: Karger;1995:1–54.

26. Schlegelberger B, Weber-Matthiesen K, Himmler A, et al. Cytogenetic findings and results of combined immunophenotyping and karyotyping in Hodgkin's disease. *Leukemia* 1994;8:72–80.

27. Döhner H, Bloomfield CD, Frizzera G, et al. Recurring chromosome abnormalities in Hodgkin's disease. *Genes Chromosom Cancer* 1992;5:392–398.

28. Tilly H, Bastard C, Delastre T, et al. Cytogenetic studies in untreated Hodgkin's disease. *Blood* 1991;77:1298–1304.

29. Banks RE, Gledhill S, Ross FM, et al. Karyotypic abnormalities and immunoglobulin gene rearrangements in Hodgkin's disease. *Cancer Genet Cytogenet* 1991;51:103–111.

30. Koduru PR, Offit K, Filippa D. A, Lieberman PH, et al. Cytogenetic and molecular genetic analysis of abnormal cells in Hodgkin's disease. *Cancer Genet Cytogenet* 1989;43:109–118.

31. Ladanyi M, Parsa NZ, Offit K, et al. Clonal cytogenetic abnormalities in Hodgkin's disease. *Genes Chromosomes Cancer* 1991;3:294–299.

32. Fonatsch C, Jox A, Streubel B, et al. Cytogenetic findings in Hodgkin's disease cell lines. In: Mauch PM, Armitage JO, Diehl V, et al. eds. *Hodgkin's disease.* Philadelphia: Lippincott Wiliams & Wilkins; 1999:213–219.

33. Falzetti D, Crescenzi B, Matteuci C, et al. Genomic instability and recurrent breakpoints are main cytogenetic findings in Hodgkin's disease. *Haematologica* 1999;84:298–305.

34. Offit K, Louie DC, Parsa NZ, et al. Del (7)(q32) is associated with a subset of small lymphocytic lymphoma with plasmacytoid features. *Blood* 1995;86:2365–2370.

35. Gaidano G, Hauptschein RS, Parsa NZ, et al. Deletions involving two distinct regions of 6q in B-cell non-Hodgkin lymphoma. *Blood* 1992;80:1781–1787.

36. Joos J, Fink TM, Rätsch A, et al. Mapping and chromosome analysis:the potential of fluorescence in situ hybridization. *J Biotech* 1994;35:135–153.

37. Schrock E, du Manoir S, Veldman T, et al. Multicolor spectral karyotyping of human chromosomes. *Science* 1996;273:494–497.

38. Speicher MR, Ballard GS, Ward DC. Karyotyping human chromosomes by combinatorial multi-fluor FISH. *Nat Genet* 1996;12:368–375.

39. Weber-Matthiesen K, Winkemann M, Müller-Hermelink A, et al. Simultaneous fluorescence immunophenotyping and interphase cytogenetics: a contribution to the characterization of tumour cells. *J Histochem Cytochem* 1992;40:171–175.

40. Weber-Matthiesen K, Deerberg J, Muller-Hermelink A, et al. Rapid immunophenotypic characterization of chromosomally aberrant cells by the new FICTION method. *Cytogenet Cell Genet* 1993;63:123–125.

41. Kallioniemi A, Kallioniemi OP, Sudar D, et al. Comparative genomic hybridization for molecular cytogenetic analysis of solid tumors. *Science* 1992;258:818–821.

42. Du Manoir S, Speicher MR, Joos S, et al. Detection of complete and partial chromosome gains and losses by comparative genomic in situ hybridization. *Hum Genet* 1993;90:590–610.

43. Joos S, Scherthan H, Speicher MR, et al. Detection of amplified genomic sequences by reverse chromosome painting using genomic tumor DNA as probe. *Hum Genet* 1993;90:584–589.

44. Joos S, Lichter P. Comparative genomic hybridization. In: Spector D, ed. *Cells—a Cold Spring Habor laboratory manual.* New York: Cold Spring Habor Laboratory Press;1997:112.1–112.11.

45. Solinas-Toldo S, Lampel S, Stilgenbauer S, et al. Matrix-based comparative genomic hybridization:Biochips to screen for genomic imbalances. *Genes Chromosom Cancer* 1997;20:399–407.

46. Pinkel D, Segraves R, Sudar D, et al. High resolution analysis of DNA copy number variation using comparative genomic hybridization to microarrays. *Nat Genet* 1998;20:207–211.

47. Wessendorf S, Lichter P, Schwänen C, et al. Potential of chromosomal and matrix-based comparative genomic hybridization for molecular diagnostics in lymphomas. *Ann Hematol* 2001;80(suppl 3):B35–37.

48. Wessendorf S, Fritz B, Wrobel G, et al. Automated screening for genomic imbalances using matrix-based comparative genomic hybridization. *Lab Invest* 2002;82:47–60.

49. Telenius H, Pelmear A, Tunnacliffe A, et al. Cytogenetic analysis by chromosome painting using DOP-PCR amplified flow-sorted chromosomes. *Genes Chromosom Cancer* 1992;4:257–263.

50. Klein CA, Schmidt-Kittler O, Schardt JA, et al. Comparative genomic hybridization loss of heterozygosity and DNA sequence analysis of single cells. *Proc Natl Acad Sci USA* 1999;96:4494–4499.

51. Joos S, Menz CK, Wrobel G, et al. Classical Hodgkin lymphoma is characterized by recurrent copy number gains of the short arm of chromosome 2. *Blood* 2002;99:1381–1387.

52. Joos S, Schwänen C, Lichter P. Comparative genomic hybridization on metaphase chromosomes and DNA-chips. In: Beatty B, Mai S, Squire JA, eds. *FISH: a practical approach.* Oxford: Oxford University Press; 2002: 159–182.

53. MacLeod RA, Spitzer D, Bar-Am I, et al. Karyotypic dissection of Hodgkin's disease cell lines reveals ectopic subtelomeres and ribosomal DNA at sites of multiple jumping translocations and genomic amplification. *Leukemia* 2000;14:1803–1814.

54. Joos S, Granzow M, Holtgreve-Grez H, et al. Hodgkin's lymphoma cell lines are characterized by frequent aberrations on chromosomes 2p and 9p including REL and JAK2. *Int J Cancer* 2003;103:489–495.

55. Fonatsch C, Diehl V, Schaadt M, et al. Cytogenetic investigations in Hodgkin's disease: I. Involvement of specific chromosomes in marker formation. *Cancer Genet Cytogenet* 1989;20:39–52.

56. Fonatsch C, Gradl G, Rademacher J. Genetics of Hodgkin's lymphoma. In: Diehl V, Pfreundschuh M, Löffler M, eds. *Recent results in cancer research. New aspects in the diagnosis and treatment of Hodgkin's disease.* Berlin:Springer Verlag; 1989:35.

57. Wolf J, Kapp U, Bohlen H, et al. Peripheral blood mononuclear cells of a patient with advanced Hodgkin's lymphoma give rise to permanently growing Hodgkin-Reed Sternberg cells. *Blood* 1996;8:3418–3428.

58. Heim S, Mitelman F, eds. *Cancer cytogenetics:chromosomal and molecular genetic aberrations of tumor cells.* New York:Wiley-Liss;1995.

59. Cabanillas F, Pathak S, Trujillo J, et al. Cytogenetic features of Hodgkin's disease suggest possible origin from a lymphocyte. *Blood* 1988;71:1615–1617.

60. Reeves BR, Pickup VL. The chromosome changes in non-Burkitt lymphomas. *Hum Genet* 1980;53:349–355.

61. Tanaka K, Arif M, Eguchi M, et al. Frequent jumping translocations of chromosomal segments involving the ABL Oncogene alone or in combination with CD3-MLL genes in secondary leukemias. *Blood* 1997;89:596–600.

62. Coleman AE, Kovalchuk AL, Janz S, et al. Jumping translocation breakpoint regions lead to amplification of rearranged Myc. *Blood* 1999;93:4442–4444.

63. Martin-Subero JI, Knippschild U, Harder L, et al. Segmental chromosomal aberrations and centrosome amplifications:pathogenetic mechanisms in Hodgkin and Reed-Sternberg cells of classical Hodgkin's lymphoma? *Leukemia* 2003;17:2214–2219.

64. Joos S, Küpper M, Ohl S, et al. Genomic imbalances including amplification of the tyrosine kinase gene JAK2 in CD30+ Hodgkin cells. *Cancer Res* 2000;60:549–552.

65. Staratschek-Jox A, Thomas RK, Zander T, et al. Loss of heterozygosity in the Hodgkin-Reed Sternberg cell line L1236. *Br J Cancer* 2001;84:381–387.

66. Weber-Matthiesen K, Deerberg J, Poetsch M, et al. Numerical chromosome aberrations are present within the CD30+ Hodgkin and Reed-Sternberg cells in 100% of analysed cases of Hodgkin's Disease. *Blood* 1995;86:1464–1468.

67. Weber-Matthiesen K, Deerberg J, Poetsch M, et al. Clarification of dubious kyryotypes in Hodgkin's disease by simultaneous fluorescence immunophenotyping and interphase cytogenetics (FICTION). *Cytogenet Cell Genet* 1995;70:243–245.

68. Ohshima K, Ishiguro M, Ohgami A, et al. Genetic analysis of sorted Hodgkin and Reed-Sternberg cells using comparative genomic hybridization. *Int J Cancer* 1999;82:250–255.

69. Ohshima K, Haraoka S, Yoshioka S, et al. Chromosome 16q deletion and loss of E-cadherin expression in Hodgkin and Reed-Sternberg cells. *Int J Cancer* 2001;92:678–682.

70. Houldsworth D, Mathew S, Rao PH, et al. Rel proto-oncogene is frequently amplified in extranodal diffuse large cell lymphoma. *Blood* 1996;87:25–29.

71. Joos S, Otaño-Joos MI, Ziegler S, et al. Primary mediastinal (thymic) B-cell lymphoma is characterized by gains of chromosomal material including 9p and amplification of the REL gene. *Blood* 1996;87:1571–1578.

72. Mathew S, Murty VS, Dalla-Favera R, et al. Chromosomal localization of genes encoding the transcription factors c-rel NF-kBp50 NF-kBp65 and lyt-10 by fluorescence in situ hybridization. *Oncogene* 1993;8:191–193.

73. Martin-Subero JI, Gesk S, Harder L, et al. Recurrent involvement of the REL and BCL11A loci in classical Hodgkin lymphoma. *Blood* 2002;99:1474–1477.

74. Barth TF, Martin-Subero JI, Joos S, et al. Gains of 2p involving the REL locus correlate with nuclear c-Rel protein accumulation in neoplastic cells of classical Hodgkin's lymphoma. *Blood* 2003;109:3681–3686.

75. Blank C, Gajewski TF, Mackensen A. Interaction of PD-L1 on tumor cells with PD-1 on tumor-specific T cells as a mechanism of immune evasion:implications for tumor immunotherapy. *Cancer Immunol Immunother* 2005;54:307–314.

76. Latchman Y, Wood CR, Chernova T, et al. PD-L2 is a second ligand for PD-1 and inhibits T cell activation. *Nat Immunol* 2001;2:261–268.

77. Kupper M, Joos S, von Bonin F, et al. MDM2 gene amplification and lack of p53 point mutations in Hodgkin and Reed-Sternberg cells: results from single-cell polymerase chain reaction and molecular cytogenetic studies. *Br J Haematol* 2001;112:768–775.

78. Gupta RK, Patel K, Bodmer WF, et al. Mutation of p53 in primary biopsy material and cell lines from Hodgkin disease. *Proc Natl Acad Sci USA* 1993;90:2817–2821.
79. Chen WG, Chen YY, Kamel OW, et al. p53 mutations in Hodgkin's disease. *Lab Invest* 1996;75:519–527.
80. Sanchez-Beato M, Piris MA, Martinez-Montero JC, et al. MDM2 and p21WAF1/CIP1 wild-type p53-induced proteins are regularly expressed by Sternberg-Reed cells in Hodgkin's disease. *J Pathol* 1996;180:58–64.
81. Meltzer P, Guan X, Trent G. Telomere capture stabilizes chromosome breakage. *Nat Genet* 1993;4:252–255.
82. Gilmore TD, Kalaitzidis D, Liang MC, et al. The c-Rel transcription factor and B-cell proliferation: a deal with the devil. *Oncogene* 2004;23:2275–2286.
83. Bargou R, Emmerich F, Krappmann D, et al. Constitutive nuclear factor-kappaB-RelA activation is required for proliferation and survival of Hodgkin's disease tumor cells. *J Clin Invest* 1997;100:2961–2969.
84. Hinz M, Loser P, Mathas S, et al. Constitutive NF-kappaB maintains high expression of a characteristic gene network including CD40 CD86 and a set of antiapoptotic genes in Hodgkin/Reed-Sternberg cells. *Blood* 2001;97:2798–2807.
85. Horie R, Watanabe T, Morishita Y, et al. Ligand-independent signaling by overexpressed CD30 drives NF-kappaB activation in Hodgkin-Reed-Sternberg cells. *Oncogene* 2002;21:2493–2503.
86. Emmerich F, Meiser M, Hummel M, et al. Overexpression of I kappa B alpha without inhibition of NF-kappaB activity and mutations in the I kappa B alpha gene in Reed-Sternberg cells. *Blood* 1999;94:3129–3134.
87. Emmerich F, Theurich S, Hummel M, et al. Inactivating I kappa B epsilon mutations in Hodgkin/Reed-Sternberg cells. *J Pathol* 2003;201:413–420.
88. Kube D, Holtick U, Vockerodt M, et al. STAT3 is constitutively activated in Hodgkin cell lines. *Blood* 2001;98:762–770.
89. Skinnider BF, Elia AJ, Gascoyne RD, et al. Signal transducer and activator of transcription 6 is frequently activated in Hodgkin and Reed-Sternberg cells of Hodgkin lymphoma. *Blood* 2002;99:618–626.
90. Holtick U, Vockerodt M, Pinkert D, et al. STAT3 is essential for Hodgkin lymphoma cell proliferation and is a target of tyrphostin AG17 which confers sensitization for apoptosis. *Leukemia* 2005;19:936–944.
91. Baus D, Pfitzner E. Specific function of STAT3 SOCS1 and SOCS3 in the regulation of proliferation and survival of classical Hodgkin lymphoma cells. *Int J Cancer* 2006;118:1404–1413.
92. Cochet O, Frelin C, Peyron JF, et al. Constitutive activation of STAT proteins in the HDLM-2 and L540 Hodgkin lymphoma-derived cell lines supports cell survival. *Cell Signal* 2006;18:449–465.
93. Weniger MA, Melzner I, Menz CK, et al. Mutations of the tumor suppressor gene SOCS-1 in classical Hodgkin lymphoma are frequent and associated with nuclear phospho-STAT5 accumulation. *Oncogene* 2006;25:2679–2684.
94. Melzner I, Bucur AJ, Bruderlein S, et al. Biallelic mutation of SOCS-1 impairs JAK2 degradation and sustains phospho-JAK2 action in the MedB-1 mediastinal lymphoma line. *Blood* 2005;105:2535–2542.
95. Bentz M, Barth TF, Brüderlein S, et al. Gain of chromosome arm 9p is characteristic of primary mediastinal B-cell lymphoma (MBL):Comprehensive molecular cytogenetic analysis and presentation of a novel MBL cell line. *Genes Chromosomes Cancer* 2001;30:393–401.
96. Rüdiger T, Jaffe E, Delsol G, et al. Workshop report on Hodgkin's disease and related diseases ("grey zone" lymphoma). *Ann Oncol* 1998;9(suppl 5):31–38.
97. Stein H, Gerdes J, Schwab U, et al. Identification of Hodgkin and Sternberg-reed cells as a unique cell type derived from a newly-detected small-cell population. *Int J Cancer* 1982;30:445–459.
98. Möller P, Herrmann B, Moldenhauer G, et al. Defective expression of MHC class I antigens is frequent in B-cell lymphomas of high-grade malignancy. *Int J Cancer* 1987;40:32–39.
99. Ruprai A, Pringle J, Angel C, et al. Localization of immunoglobulin light chain mRNA expression in Hodgkin's disease by in situ hybridization. *J Pathol* 1991;164:37–40.
100. Renne C, Martin-Subero JI, Hansmann ML, et al. Molecular cytogenetic analyses of immunoglobulin loci in nodular lymphocyte predominant Hodgkin's lymphoma reveal a recurrent IGH-BCL6 juxtaposition. *J Mol Diagn* 2005;7:352–356.
101. Wlodarska I, Stul M, De Wolf-Peeters C, et al. Heterogeneity of BCL6 rearrangements in nodular lymphocyte predominant Hodgkin's lymphoma. *Haematologica* 2004;89:965–972.
102. Atayar C, Kok K, Kluiver J, et al. BCL6 alternative breakpoint region break and homozygous deletion of 17q24 in the nodular lymphocyte predominance type of Hodgkin's lymphoma-derived cell line DEV. *Hum Pathol* 2006;37:675–683.
103. Hossfeld DK, Schmidt CG. Chromosome findings in effusions from patients with Hodgkin's disease. *Int J Cancer* 1978;21:147–156.
104. Kristoffersson U, Heim S, Mandahl N, et al. Cytogenetic studies in Hodgkin's disease. *Acta Pathol Microbiol Immunol Scand* 1987;95: 289–295.
105. Dennis TR, Stock AD, Winberg CD, et al. Cytogenetic studies of Hodgkin's disease. Analysis of involved lymph nodes from 12 patients. *Cancer Genet Cytogenet* 1989;37:201–208.
106. Schouten HC, Sanger WG, Duggan M, et al. Chromosomal abnormalities in Hodgkin's disease. *Blood* 1989;73:2149–2154.
107. Reeves BR, Nash R, Lawler SD, et al. Serial cytogenetic studies showing persistence of original clone in Hodgkin's disease. *Cancer Genet Cytogenet* 1990;50:1–8.
108. Poppema S, Kaleta J, Hepperle B. Chromosomal abnormalities in patients with Hodgkin's disease:evidence for frequent involvement of the 14q chromosomal region but infrequent bcl-2 gene rearrangement in Reed-Sternberg cells. *J Natl Cancer Inst* 1992;84:1789–1793.
109. Pedersen RK, Sorensen AG, Pedersen NT, et al. Chromosome aberrations in adult Hodgkin disease in a Danish population-based study. *Cancer Genet Cytogenet* 1999;110:128–132.
110. Koduru PR, Lichtman SM, Smilari TF, et al. Serial phenotypic cytogenetic and molecular genetic studies in Richter's syndrome:demonstration of lymphoma development from the chronic lymphocytic leukaemia cells. *Br J Haematol* 1993;85:613–616.
111. Kohno S, Van den Berghe H. Chromosomes and causation of human cancer and leukemia: XXXI. Dq- deletions and their significance in proliferative disorders. *Cancer* 1979;43:1350–1357.
112. Franke S, Wlodarska I, Maes B, et al. Lymphocyte predominance Hodgkin disease is characterized by recurrent genomic imbalances. *Blood* 2001;97;1845–1853.

STAGING AND INITIAL EVALUATION

CHAPTER 9 ■ CLINICAL EVALUATION AND STAGING OF HODGKIN LYMPHOMA

DAVID C. HODGSON AND MARY K. GOSPODAROWICZ

The initial clinical evaluation and staging of patients with Hodgkin lymphoma (HL) serves to (a) confirm the HL diagnosis, (b) determine the extent and distribution of disease, (c) evaluate fitness to receive standard treatments, and (d) provide prognostic information.

HISTORICAL PERSPECTIVE

The early staging classifications for Hodgkin's disease reflected the natural history of the disease, because no effective therapy was available. The first recorded classification, proposed in 1865, divided the disease into three stages: latent, progressive, and cachectic.[1] The latent stage was characterized by "enlarged nodes (glands), arising from some cause. . . . Blood shows no appreciable abnormality." The progressive stage was "initially localized but becomes generalized over a period of 18–24 months. . . . Anemia becomes apparent only in the second phase of the disease. . . . There is loss of appetite and digestive difficulty." The final stage of cachexia is "associated with an alteration in the blood picture. . . . The illness results in anemia and cachexia and is not accompanied by leucocytosis."

In 1879, Gowers[2] also proposed a three-stage classification: local growth only, local enlargement "preponderating," and general uniform infection.

In 1902 Dorothy Reed[3] described the features of what are now known as Reed-Sternberg cells, and also two functional stages of Hodgkin's disease, including an initial stage of increasing lymphadenopathy during which the individual was in apparently normal physical condition and a second stage of advancing disease with progressive cachexia and anemia. The clinical course was further defined in 1911 by Ziegler,[4] who described 11 distinct patterns; and was again recategorized, in 1920, by Longcope and McAlpin,[5] dividing Hodgkin's disease into seven distinct clinical forms: localized, mediastinal, generalized, acute, larval, splenomegalic, and osteoperiostitic.

The antecedents of contemporary anatomic staging were proposed by Jackson and Parker,[6,7] and later by Craver,[8] who created a classification based on the distribution of disease: class I, localized disease; class II, regional or intermediate disease; and class III, generalized disease. Peters proposed more specific definitions[9] with a three-stage classification: stage I involving a single lymph node region or a single lesion elsewhere in the body, stage II involving two or more proximal lymph node regions of either the upper or lower trunk, and stage III involving two or more lymph node regions of both upper and lower trunk. This system was further modified by Peters and Middlemiss[10] to take into account constitutional symptoms of generalized disease in stage II. In 1964, Kaplan and colleagues[11] proposed modification of Peters' stage III to distinguish nodal disease above and below the diaphragm as defined by lymphangiography (stage III) from disease that involved extralymphatic tissues (stage IV). They also proposed extending the concept of classification of constitutional symptoms from stage II to all four stages.

These changes were ratified at both the Paris meeting in February 1965[12] and at the Rye conference in New York in September 1965,[13] and lymph node chains were designated as regions for the purpose of staging (Fig. 9.1). At that time all stages were subclassified as A or B to indicate the absence or presence, respectively, of defined systemic symptoms. Those symptoms were otherwise explained as (a) fever, (b) night sweats, or (c) pruritus. Weight loss was not considered to be a B-symptom at that time.

Changes were proposed to the Rye classification by Peters,[14] Musshoff and associates,[15] and Rosenberg[16] to maximize the effectiveness of radiation therapy (RT). Two major modifications were adopted in the Ann Arbor staging classification in 1971.[17] The first addressed the ambiguity in defining extranodal stage I and stage IV disease. Musshoff and colleagues found that patients with nodal disease that extended to involve contiguous extranodal sites had a significantly better prognosis than those with disseminated extra-lymphatic involvement. Therefore, the designation "E" emerged to distinguish contiguous extranodal extension that could be encompassed within a tolerable radiation field and safely treated with radical dose.

The second modification introduced the concept of pathologic stage. This was made possible by performing staging laparotomy with splenectomy, and biopsies of the liver, bone marrow, and multiple lymph nodes in order to accurately describe the extent of disease. The designations of clinical stage (CS) and pathologic stage (PS) were suggested to clarify on which basis the anatomic stage was determined. Clinical stage referred to the extent of disease determined on the basis of diagnostic tests following a diagnostic biopsy. Pathologic stage was developed primarily to acknowledge the greater accuracy of disease extent determined by staging laparotomy, although a positive bone marrow biopsy, even in the absence of staging laparotomy, would permit the designation of stage IV disease. In practice, however, most clinicians used the designation PS to indicate stage determined after exploratory laparotomy with splenectomy. As this procedure is now rarely performed, most patients are considered clinically staged.[18,19]

The changes were agreed to at the Workshop on the Staging of Hodgkin's disease, held at Ann Arbor, Michigan, in 1971, and form the basis for the Ann Arbor Classification.[20,21] All cases of Hodgkin's disease continued to be subclassified as A or B to indicate the respective absence or presence of constitutional symptoms. These are defined as unexplained night

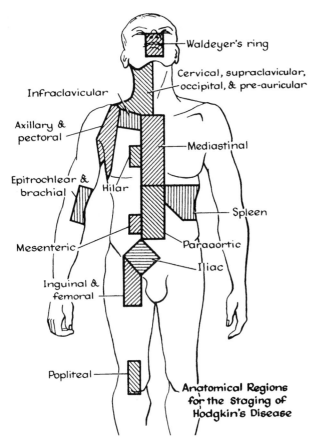

FIGURE 9.1. The anatomic definitions of separate lymph node regions adopted for staging purposes at the Rye symposium on Hodgkin lymphoma. (Reprinted with permission from Kaplan HS, Rosenberg SA. The treatment of Hodgkin's disease. *Med Clin North Am* 1966;50:1591–1610.)

TABLE 9.1

COTSWOLDS MODIFICATION TO ANN ARBOR STAGING SYSTEM

Stage	Definitions
I	Involvement of a single lymph node region or lymphoid structure (e.g., spleen, thymus, Waldeyer ring)
II	Involvement of two or more lymph node regions on the same side of the diaphragm (the mediastinum is a single site; hilar lymph nodes are lateralized); the number of anatomic sites should be indicated by a suffix (e.g., II3)
III	Involvement of lymph node regions or structures on both sides of the diaphragm
III$_1$	With or without splenic, hilar, celiac, or portal nodes
III$_2$	With paraaortic, iliac, mesenteric nodes
IV	Involvement of extranodal site(s) beyond that designated E

Annotation:
A, no B-symptoms.
B, fever, drenching sweats, or weight loss.
X, bulky disease, >1/3 widening of mediastinum at T5-6, or >10 cm maximum dimension of nodal mass.
E, involvement of a single extranodal site, contiguous or proximal to known nodal site.
CS, clinical stage.
PS, pathologic stage.
Reprinted with permission from Lister TA, Crowther D, Sutcliffe SB, et al. Report of a committee convened to discuss the evaluation and staging of patients with Hodgkin lymphoma: Cotswolds meeting. *J Clin Oncol* 1989;7:1630–1636.

sweats, persistent or recurrent fever with temperatures above 38°C during the month prior to diagnosis, and/or loss of 10% or more of body weight during the 6 months prior to diagnosis. Pruritus was excluded, having been shown to have little influence on prognosis.[19] The Cotswolds modification of the Ann Arbor staging system was introduced 1989 to recognize the use of CT scanning for the detection of intra-abdominal disease, to formalize a definition of bulk of disease, and to provide guidelines for evaluating response (Table 9.1).[20] This staging classification provides a basis for selecting initial treatment and has been widely adopted, with most clinical trial groups, the Union Internationale Centre le Cancer (UICC), and the American Joint Committee on Cancer (AJCC) following the guidelines laid down by the Committee on Hodgkin's Lymphoma Staging.[20–24] During the early 1970s, patients with stages I, II, and IIIA disease were usually treated with radiotherapy following laparotomy; the remainder were mostly treated with combination chemotherapy. Since the Ann Arbor meeting, several significant changes in the management of Hodgkin lymphoma have taken place. Additional factors have been recognized, (e.g., tumor bulk and number of sites of disease) that adversely affect the prognosis of patients treated with radiation alone. Such prognostic factors are utilized to define risk-adapted therapy, and combined modality treatment has become standard for patients with early-stage disease. Also, computed tomography (CT), and fluorine-18-deoxyglucose positron emission tomography (FDG-PET) are now routinely used for staging and evaluation of response.

SITES OF INVOLVEMENT AND PRESENTING FEATURES

It is thought that Hodgkin lymphoma typically originates at a single lymphatic site, and progresses to adjacent lymphoid tissues before disseminating to distant nonadjacent sites and organs.[9,23–27] This is particularly true for patients in the younger age groups with classic histologic subtypes of disease.

Although surgical staging is no longer part of initial evaluation, the results of surgical staging studies provided information that is relevant to contemporary management, because an understanding of the probable distribution of disease can facilitate the interpretation of clinical staging tests. Figure 9.2 illustrates the most common anatomic distribution of Hodgkin lymphoma in a series of 100 consecutive patients undergoing surgical staging at Stanford, and reveals the orderly progression of disease spread along adjacent nodal regions.[26] The pattern of disease at presentation also appears to be associated with the histologic subtype, as described by Mauch and colleagues[28] in a study of 719 patients with Hodgkin lymphoma who underwent staging laparotomy. For example, most patients with nodular lymphocyte-predominant Hodgkin lymphoma present with localized peripheral disease often in the upper neck, whereas the majority of patients with nodular sclerosis histology have disease above the diaphragm and mediastinal node involvement. Disease in the liver is most frequently seen in patients with mixed-cellularity or lymphocyte-depletion Hodgkin lymphoma and systemic symptoms.

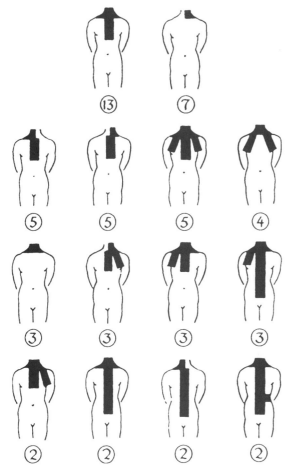

TABLE 9.2

INVOLVED SITES OF DISEASE IN UNTREATED PATHOLOGICALLY STAGED PATIENTS WITH HODGKIN LYMPHOMA

Site	Percentage involved
Waldeyer ring	1–2
Cervical nodes	
Right side	50–60
Left side	60–70
Axillary nodes	
Right side	25–35
Left side	30–35
Mediastinal nodes	50–60
Hilar nodes	15–35
Spleen	30–35
Liver	2–6
Paraaortic nodes	30–40
Iliac nodes	15–20
Mesenteric nodes	1–4
Inguinal nodes	8–15
Bone marrow	1–4
Other extranodal sites (lung, bone, etc.)	10–12
Total extranodal	10–15

FIGURE 9.2. Evidence of an orderly progression in the spread of Hodgkin lymphoma. Most common anatomic patterns of Hodgkin lymphoma in 100 consecutive patients who underwent staging laparotomy at Stanford. The number of patients is given in the *circles*. (Reprinted with permission from Rosenberg SA, Kaplan HS. Evidence for an orderly progression in the spread of Hodgkin's disease. *Cancer Res* 1966;26:1225.)

Evaluating the extent and distribution of disease has important therapeutic implications, because in many cases the intensity of chemotherapy and the decision to use or omit radiation therapy depends on the clinical stage. In circumstances in which a patient with nodular-sclerosis HL (NSHL) in the neck is found to have lymph nodes of borderline size on an abdominal CT, it is useful to know that it is uncommon to have NSHL in the neck and the lower abdomen without disease also present in the upper abdomen.[26] Similarly, many patients will have small CT-detected abnormalities found in the liver or lungs. However, it is uncommon to have pulmonary disease at presentation without involvement of intrathoracic lymph nodes, usually on the ipsilateral side.

SYMPTOMS AND PRESENTING FEATURES

For a discussion of unusual syndromes associated with Hodgkin lymphoma, the reader is referred to Chapter 28.

The most common clinical presentation of Hodgkin lymphoma is a young adult noticing an enlarged nontender lymph gland in the neck or supraclavicular fossa (60–80%), axilla (10–20%), or less often in the inguinal-femoral region (5–15%) (Table 9.2). Another common presentation is the discovery of a mediastinal mass on imaging, and approximately 60% of patients have mediastinal involvement at diagnosis. Mediastinal disease may be very bulky with minimal symptoms. Bulky mediastinal disease is often associated with pericardial or pleural effusions, which frequently do not harbor malignant cells; symptoms of superior vena cava obstruction are uncommon.

Systemic symptoms often precede the diagnosis. Typical symptoms of Hodgkin lymphoma are fever, night sweats, pruritus, fatigue, and weight loss, none of which is specific. B-symptoms are reported by approximately 25% to 30% of patients, and more commonly in those with other adverse risk factors.[29,30] Pel-Ebstein fever[31,32] is the characteristic intermittent fever: it is uncommon and recurs at variable intervals of several days or weeks lasting for 1 to 2 weeks before waning. More commonly, an HL-associated fever is more noticeable in the evening, and becomes more severe and continuous over time. Low-grade fever and drenching night sweats are usually found in the setting of advanced disease. Pruritus, if severe, may be a symptom of disease.[33] It may occur early in the course of Hodgkin lymphoma in 10% to 15% of all patients, often preceding the diagnosis, and it has been reported that 85% of patients may experience pruritus at some time during the course of the disease. Pain with alcohol ingestion is a rare but well-described symptom associated with HL. The pain is characteristically severe, occurring within a few minutes of the ingestion of even a small amount of alcohol, and localizing to areas involved by lymphoma.

Several paraneoplastic neurologic syndromes have been reported in association with the disease, but these are rare.

Symptomatic hypercalcemia is extremely uncommon in patients presenting with Hodgkin lymphoma and is usually associated with involvement of bone or, rarely, abnormalities in vitamin D metabolism. Skin lesions associated with Hodgkin lymphoma include ichthyosis, urticaria, erythema multiforme, erythema nodosum, necrotizing lesions, or hyperpigmentatio. Skin involvement with HL itself is very rare.

INITIAL EVALUATION

Pathologic Diagnosis

A full discussion of the pathologic diagnosis of HL is given in Chapter 4. The oncologist must be certain that the HL diagnosis was based on an adequate biopsy specimen that was examined utilizing appropriate morphologic and immunohistochemical criteria. In uncommon circumstances, a diagnosis can be made on a core or needle biopsy; however, a whole lymph node excision is preferred for pathologic examination. When the diagnosis of Hodgkin lymphoma is made from biopsy of an extranodal site, a node biopsy confirmation of diagnosis is desirable unless the diagnosis is considered unequivocal.

In some cases, drugs (e.g., phenytoin or antibiotics) may provoke histologic changes within lymph nodes that may mimic HL, particularly the mixed cellularity subtype. Other benign conditions, such as infectious mononucleosis, lymphoid hyperplasia with progressive transformation of germinal centers, or Castleman disease, may produce lymphadenopathy with histologic features similar to HL. Moreoever, certain forms of non-Hodgkin lymphoma (NHL) may have features that may be difficult to distinguish from HL. Most commonly, T-cell rich large B-cell lymphoma is in the differential diagnosis of both nodular lymphocyte-predominant HL and classical HL, while anaplastic CD30-positive NHL may have histology similar to classical HL. If the clinical presentation of disease is not typical for the given pathologic diagnosis (for example, if an elderly male with noncontiguous involvement of multiple nonbulky lymph nodes has a diagnosis of nodular-sclerosis HL), then a review of the pathology by an expert hematopathologist, or even a re-biopsy should be considered.

History and Physical Examination

Obtaining a detailed history facilitates several goals: to assess prognosis, to facilitate the appropriate performance and interpretation of staging tests, to identify co-morbid conditions that might influence selection of treatment, and to establish risk factors for late effects. A review of medications is warranted because, as noted above, certain drugs may produce lymphadenopathy with histologic features mimicking HL. Patient age, the presence of B-symptoms, and performance status directly affect treatment selection. Similarly, a history of active heart, lung, liver, or kidney disease, or HIV/AIDS, may influence the provision of chemotherapy, while the presence of scleroderma or similar autoimmune disorders is a relative contraindication to RT. Prior respiratory infections may cause lung nodules on CT imaging that could be mistaken for lymphoma. Smoking status may influence the decision to use mediastinal RT, as smokers are known to be at significant risk of secondary lung cancer following this treatment. Similarly, a strong family history of heart disease or breast cancer may influence the follow-up of patients treated for HL.

Physical examination of the palpable lymph node regions is crucial to document the distribution, number, and size of involved nodes. Explicit measurement of enlarged lymph nodes facilitates evaluation of response after treatment. The Waldeyer ring should be examined, especially in patients with high neck disease. The size of the liver and spleen in centimeters below the costal margin in the midclavicular line should be recorded.

Imaging Evaluation of Extent of Disease

The Cotswolds committee made modifications to the Ann Arbor staging system in part to recognize the use of CT scanning to evaluate the extent of disease (Table 9.3).[20] Radiologic

TABLE 9.3

RECOMMENDED STUDIES FOR INITIAL EVALUATION

Mandatory for the Cotswolds classification	Histology and immunophenotyping Past and familial history, clinical examination as per Cotswolds recommendations Blood counts and routine workup: ESR, LDH, alkaline phosphatase, albumin, liver function, virology Chest radiograms: CT of chest, abdomen, and pelvis; bone marrow aspiratation and biopsy if indicated
Recommended for disease assessment	FDG-PET or gallium scanning/gallium SPECT β2-microglobulin, interleukin-6, and interleukin-10 levels
Investigational noninvasive	MRI (bone/bone marrow), technetium bone scanning Immunoscintigram with antiferritin or anti-CD30 antibodies Histologic expression and/or serum levels of soluble CD8, CD25, CD30, IL-6, and other cytokines
Recommended for toxicity assessment	Heart: ECG, MUGA, or echocardiogram Pulmonary: lung function tests Thyroid and gonadal functions: FSH, LH, and TSH (semen analysis and sperm storage) Psychosocial adaptation

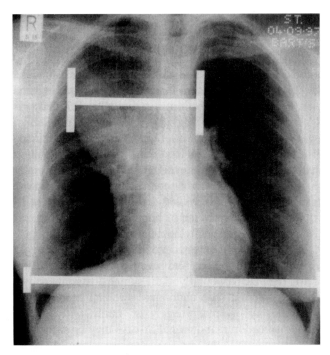

FIGURE 9.3. A chest radiograph of a female patient with mediastinal involvement of Hodgkin lymphoma at presentation. The maximum transverse diameter of the mass (11.5 cm) is divided by the maximal diameter of the chest (26.5 cm) to yield a ratio of 0.43. (Note that the internal thoracic diameter at the T5-6 interspace is 22.5 cm—a ratio of 0.51.)

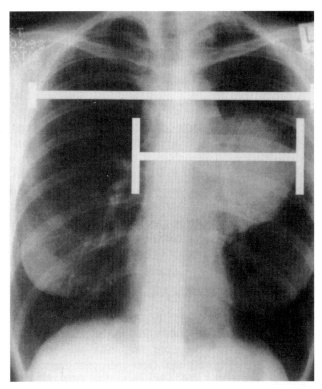

FIGURE 9.4. A chest radiograph of another female patient with mediastinal involvement of Hodgkin lymphoma at presentation. The maximum transverse diameter of the mass (14.0 cm) is divided by the internal thoracic diameter at the T5-6 interspace (26.0 cm) as described in the Cotswolds report (20), yielding a ratio of 0.54. (Note that the maximal diameter of the chest is 28.5 cm—a ratio of 0.49.)

investigation should include postero-anterior and lateral chest radiographs. Measurements of the mediastinal mass size (or ratio to chest dimensions) on chest x-ray have been correlated with prognosis and are used to assign treatment in some clinical trials (Fig. 9.3 and 9.4). A CT of the neck, thorax, abdomen, and pelvis should be performed. Intravenous contrast allows one to distinguish lymph nodes from vessels seen in cross-section. Until recently, imaging of the neck had been considered optional, as bilateral whole-neck RT was typically given to most stage I and II patients with supra-diaphragmatic disease, regardless of the degree of neck involvement. This is no longer the case, however, as the neck volume encompassed by modern involved-field RT will vary depending on the presence and location of enlarged neck nodes at diagnosis. Consequently, inadequate neck imaging can potentially lead to unnecessary over-treatment of the neck, if the radiation oncologist is unable to determine the extent of disease prior to treatment.

Gallium-67 citrate scanning was initially investigated in the 1960s and 1970s following the observation that uptake was most pronounced in viable tumor.[34] The major role of gallium imaging is to evaluate the response of disease before and after treatment, rather than to stage patients (see below).[35,36] Gallium imaging is not exceptionally sensitive in the detection of small-volume disease, particularly in the abdomen; where enlarged lymph nodes are seen on CT, the absence of corresponding uptake on gallium imaging should not be used to downstage patients. In such circumstances PET may reveal evidence of disease in the abdomen that is missed by gallium (see below).[37]

Occasionally CT imaging may reveal equivocal findings in the spleen or liver. Splenic cysts can usually be adequately characterized by CT, but ultrasound may occasionally be required to rule out solid lesions. Vascular malformations in the liver may at times have an appearance similar to lymphoma, and MRI may better characterize liver abnormalities where CT findings are ambiguous (see Chapter 10).

FDG-PET is a useful modality in the staging of HL patients when used in conjunction with CT imaging[38] (see also Chapter 11). It is more sensitive than gallium imaging, and compared to CT-based imaging alone, FDG-PET will change the stage in approximately 25% of HL patients.[38] Most, but not all, of these changes will result in upstaging and often in treatment modifications. Treatment modifications may be minor (Fig. 9.5) or major, such as an increased duration or intensity of chemotherapy. A major limitation of studies examining the value of FDG-PET in HL staging is the absence of biopsy findings to adjudicate discrepancies between CT and FDG-PET findings. In one study, 6/18 (33%) of discordant results occurred because FDG-PET did not detect areas of involvement seen on other imaging or proven by biopsy,[39] and false-positives may be even more likely to occur. In clinical practice, it is preferable to have two imaging modalities indicating the same stage of disease before proceeding with treatment. Selection of different treatment approaches based on stage makes it necessary to have as accurate clinical staging as possible.

Ideally, FDG-PET should be co-registered with CT scans to improve accuracy. It is important to recognize that modern treatment based on conventional staging with CT with or without gallium imaging produces excellent results, and decisions to intensify or reduce therapy based on discordant FDG-PET results should be undertaken cautiously, preferably as part of a clinical study.[38]

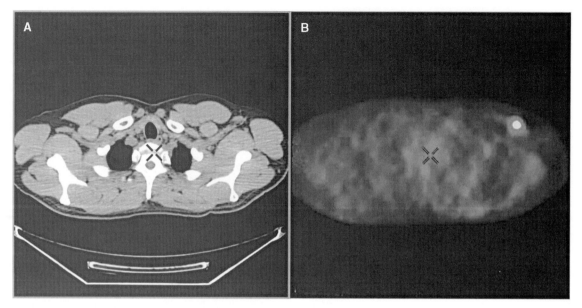

FIGURE 9.5. Patient with classical Hodgkin lymphoma with clinical involvement of left supraclavicular area. CT scan (**A**) showed small adenopathy in left axilla (did not meet size criteria), but the node was PET+ (**B**). Radiation field was extended to include the left axilla. See color insert.

Criteria for Nodal Involvement by Hodgkin Lymphoma

There is normal variation in the size of mediastinal and hilar nodes, but those measuring more than 10 mm in shortest cross-section can be considered abnormal. Retrocrural lymph nodes larger than 6 mm can be considered abnormal. In the remaining abdomen and pelvis, lymph nodes of more than 15 mm in shortest cross-section are typically considered to be involved, particularly in the paraaortic region. However, although unequivocal abnormal findings on CT scanning may represent Hodgkin lymphoma, there is a risk of false-positives, particularly within the abdomen, when using these criteria. Therefore, when lymph nodes in the 15- to 20-mm range are seen, further evaluation is warranted using FDG-PET or gallium imaging.

As discussed previously, it is important that equivocal imaging results be interpreted in the context of the known patterns of spread and other prognostic factors. In an asymptomatic young patient with nonbulky HL otherwise confined to the neck and no other adverse risk factors, it is unlikely that an equivocal paraaortic node actually contains lymphoma. However, in the context of multiple supradiaphragmatic sites of disease and B-symptoms, stage III disease is more likely.[40] Lymph nodes that are enlarged on CT but normal on FDG-PET should be biopsied whenever feasible before downstaging a patient, particularly if a change in treatment recommendation would result from the change in stage.[38]

Criteria For Extranodal Involvement

The 1989 Cotswolds modification to the Ann Arbor staging system explicitly indicated that involvement of extralymphatic tissue on one side of the diaphragm by direct extension of nodal disease should be staged according to the nodal extent, with an associated extranodal (E) designation.[20] This was determined on the basis of data indicating that patients with this presentation had a better prognosis than patients with stage IV disease, and it was implied that their prognosis was comparable to

patients with disease confined to the lymph nodes.[20] Studies examining the impact of extranodal involvement have differed in their findings, with some reporting that the location or number of extranodal sites involved influenced prognosis[41,42] while others found no impact on overall survival.[43,44]

Substantial variation in stage assignment has been demonstrated among patients with extranodal involvement, specifically in the distinction between stage IV and early-stage extranodal disease. Experienced oncologists vary in their stage assignment of patients with nearby, but discontinuous, extranodal involvement.[45] It is important to recognize that the original intent of the extranodal designation was to acknowledge that in some cases, involved lymph nodes could invade adjacent tissues, and that these patients had a better prognosis than stage IV patients. In rare cases, patients may present with a single extranodal site with enlarged adjacent lymph nodes (e.g., humeral involvement with axillary lymph nodes enlarged), and such cases might reasonably be categorized as early stage, extranodal. However, the involvement of 2 or more noncontiguous extranodal sites should typically be considered indicative of stage IV disease.

Criteria for Bulk

The definition of bulk has varied considerably in the literature. The definition that found greatest acceptance for the mediastinum involved measuring the greatest transverse diameter of the mediastinal mass on a standard postero-anterior chest radiograph and dividing by the maximal diameter of the chest wall at its pleural surfaces, usually at the level of the diaphragm[46] or alternatively at the T5-T6 interspace (the Cotswolds committee recommending the latter approach). A ratio exceeding one-third was considered bulky and an adverse feature among patients treated with RT alone or chemotherapy alone. There are no widely accepted criteria for the definition of bulk using measurements obtained from CT scans: the Cotswolds committee recommended that a nodal mass must be greater than 10 cm in diameter to be designated as bulky,[20] while recent and ongoing trials have defined bulk as confluent nodal masses greater than 7 cm[47] or greater than 5 cm.[48]

Identification of Other Prognostic Factors

The identification of adverse prognostic factors is a key feature of selecting the appropriate intensity of treatment and the modalities to be used (see Chapter 12). Clinical features used to indicate the necessity for more intensive treatment typically include older age, advanced stage, large tumor bulk, the presence of B-symptoms, elevated ESR, anemia, and elevated white cell count.[49,50] These factors are typically grouped together to create risk categories, and cooperative group clinical trials have assigned risk-adapted therapy according to these categories. Other factors that are important to document are the presence of hypoalbumineamia or lymphopenia.[50]

It is notable that many of the clinical factors included in current risk categorization systems were associated with an increased risk of relapse among patients treated with RT alone. When adequate treatment that includes modern chemotherapy is provided, some of these factors are no longer associated with the risk of relapse, largely because that risk is so low.[51] However, the provision of adequate treatment still relies on accurate ascertainment of these clinical factors.

CLINICAL EVALUATION DURING THERAPY

Clinical evaluation during treatment is an important component of individualizing treatment intensity. Re-evaluation should be made prior to each cycle of chemotherapy, to document resolution of lymphadenopathy and to identify acute toxicities that may require modification of treatment (e.g., bleomycin lung toxicity, congestive heart failure, persistent neutropenia). If palpable lymphadenopathy was not present at the initiation of treatment, imaging should be obtained after every 2 or 3 cycles of chemotherapy, and treatment should be changed if the patient fails to show objective evidence of response.

Rapid early response to initial therapy is increasingly recognized as a favorable prognostic factor among HL patients that may potentially be used to guide the overall intensity of a course of treatment. Response may be evaluated by CT, gallium, or FDG-PET, after 2 or 3 cycles of chemotherapy. Resolution of gallium[35,52] or FDG-PET[38,53] scan abnormities midway through chemotherapy is associated with a better prognosis.

Recent and ongoing clinical trials in children have assigned additional chemotherapy and/or RT to patients with a slow early response to the first 2 to 4 cycles of chemotherapy (measured by CT), while reducing treatment for those with rapid early responses.[54,55] Early results of these trials show excellent outcomes. Ongoing trials (e.g., GHSG HD15; UK Leukemia Research Fund FDG-PET study) will help determine the extent to which midtreatment evaluation with FDG-PET can contribute to the tailoring of treatment intensity.

CLINICAL EVALUATION AFTER THERAPY

Definition of Treatment Outcome

In patients with advanced-stage disease who are treated with chemotherapy alone, response should be documented one month following completion of treatment based on clinical findings and repetition of imaging investigations that were abnormal at presentation (typically CT and PET). As discussed below, false-positive PET scans may occur shortly after RT, so that repeat imaging should be delayed for patients treated with combined modality therapy if they are clinically well. Re-evaluation should occur if there is doubt about the response to treatment. After completion of treatment, regression of disease may be slow, and a residual fibrotic mass may still be visible on a chest radiograph or CT images.

The Cotswold criteria[20] for reporting response to therapy are described in the next sections.

Complete Remission

The patient has no clinical, radiologic, or other evidence of Hodgkin lymphoma. Changes consistent with the effects of previous therapy (i.e., radiation fibrosis) may be present.

Complete Remission (Unconfirmed/Uncertain)

This category, CR(u), of response has been included to denote patients in whom remission status is unclear, as the patient is otherwise in good health with no clinical evidence of Hodgkin lymphoma, but some radiologic abnormality, not absolutely consistent with the effects of therapy, persists at a site of previous disease. It is well recognized that imaging abnormalities may persist following treatment, and that these do not necessarily signify active disease.[56,57] Guidelines for criteria used to assign response category based on measurements of residual abnormalities on post-treatment CT scans have been published (Table 9.4).[58]

It is often appropriate to investigate residual abnormalities seen on post-treatment CT scans with MRI, gallium, or FDG-PET to help distinguish persistent disease versus residual scar tissue. Whole-body FDG-PET is a useful tool in evaluating disease regression.[59–61] However, it must be recognized that thymic rebound, reactive lymph node hyperplasia, or subclinical radiation pneumonitis may lead to abnormalities on FDG-PET following mediastinal RT.[38,62] To avoid "false-positive" interpretation, some authors recommend that FDG-PET re-evaluation should be delayed until 3 months following completion of mediastinal RT, although the characteristic appearance of post-RT lung changes occurring before 3 months can usually be distinguished from lymphoma by experienced nuclear radiographers.[38,63] The positive predictive value of an abnormal FDG-PET scan following treatment (i.e., the probability that a patient with an abnormal scan will relapse) is not as high for patients with HL as for those with non-Hodgkin lymphoma,[38,61,62] and confirmation of relapse with other tests or re-imaging is required before proceeding to salvage therapy. FDG-PET results should not be considered in

TABLE 9.4

CRITERIA USED TO ASSIGN CR, CR(U), AND PR CATEGORIES FROM POST-TREATMENT CT SCAN

Anatomic site	CR	CR(u)	PR[a]
Thorax (cm)	<1.0	1.1–2.0	>2.1
Retrocrural (cm)	<0.6	0.7–1.6	>1.7
Abdomen (cm)	<1.5	1.6–2.5	>2.6

[a]Less than 50% of original nodal mass.
CR, complete remission; CR(u), unconfirmed/uncertain complete remission; PR, partial remission.
Reprinted with permission from Radford JA, Crowther D, Rohatiner AZ, et al. Results of a randomized trial comparing MVPP chemotherapy with a hybrid regimen, ChlVPP/EVA, in the initial treatment of Hodgkin's disease. *J Clin Oncol* 1995;13:2379–2385.

isolation, but in the context of other imaging test results and the patient's clinical condition.

Re-biopsy may be warranted to evaluate persistent imaging abnormalities depending on the degree of suspicion, the morbidity of biopsy, and whether salvage treatment will vary significantly depending on the result. If re-biopsy is undertaken, the difficulties of sampling artifacts should be recognized. Persistent elevation of the ESR, while not diagnostic of active Hodgkin lymphoma, is an indication for very close surveillance.[64,65]

Partial Remission

Partial remission is defined as a decrease by at least 50% in the sum of the products of the largest perpendicular diameters of all measurable lesions. This would include patients with an abnormal but improved PET scan. Other manifestations of disease (e.g., B-symptoms) should also improve. As described above, re-imaging and/or re-biopsy to detect persistent active disease should be aggressively undertaken if the results would substantially influence treatment decisions (e.g., if the patient is a candidate for aggressive salvage therapy).

Progressive Disease

Progressive disease is defined as 25% or more increase in the size of a least one measurable lesion, or the appearance of a new lesion, or recurrence of B-symptoms that cannot otherwise be explained.

Follow-Up Management

Following completion of therapy, restaging, and documentation of response, follow-up guidelines vary, but most recommend that patients be seen at approximately 3-month intervals during the first and second year of therapy, 4-month intervals in the third year, 6-month intervals in the fourth and fifth years, and annually thereafter. The frequency and type of radiologic studies should reflect the initial sites of disease and the risk of relapse.

There are few data upon which to base recommendations for the routine performance of bloodwork or imaging. The Cotswolds committee recommended the follow-up schedule outlined above, with a full blood count, ESR, biochemical profile, and chest radiograph to be performed at each visit. The National Comprehensive Cancer Network (NCCN) and the European Society of Medical Oncology (ESMO) have independently defined and published recommended guidelines for follow-up care.[66]

Although some clinicians will perform routine CT re-imaging in asymptomatic patients, three studies suggest that the yield of routine tests in asymptomatic patients is low. A retrospective study of the follow-up of 210 patients with Hodgkin lymphoma treated with chemotherapy and in complete or partial remission following treatment was reported by Radford and associates.[67] In 2,512 outpatient visits, 37 relapses were detected. In only 4 cases (11%) was relapse detected as a result of routine physical examination or investigation of a patient who had no symptoms. The report concluded that relapse of Hodgkin lymphoma after treatment is usually detected as a result of the investigation of symptoms, rather than by routine screening of asymptomatic patients. It was proposed that the frequency of routine tests visits should be reduced, and greater emphasis placed on patient education. Patients should be informed about the importance of symptoms and encouraged to arrange an earlier appointment should these develop.

In another study from the UK,[68] routine surveillance CT scanning was responsible for the detection of only 2 of 22

relapses and the authors concluded that routine CT scanning during the follow-up period was expensive and inefficient.

A third retrospective study examined the cost and benefit of routine follow-up evaluation in 709 patients treated with radiotherapy for early-stage Hodgkin lymphoma.[69] Only 1 of 157 relapses was detected by routine bloodwork. The rate of relapse detection was highest for a combination of history and physical examination (78 of 10,000 examinations) followed by chest x-ray (26 of 10,000 examinations). Patients whose relapse was detected on imaging did not have significantly better survival than those whose relapse was detected by history and physical examination. The authors concluded that chest radiographs were useful during the first 3 years of follow-up, but routine abdominal x-rays, full blood counts, and other laboratory tests rarely led to the detection of recurrence.[69] In general, re-imaging is not indicated more than twice per year in the absence of clinical signs or symptoms of recurrence.

One limitation of these studies is that chest x-ray is less sensitive for the detection of relapse than modern CT imaging, which may increase the proportion of relapses detected prior to the development of symptoms.[70] A recent study employed decision analysis to evaluate CT-based follow-up strategies for patients with stage I to II, or stage III to IV, HD, treated with ABVD-based chemotherapy with or without radiation therapy. Three strategies for following patients after CR were compared: routine annual CT for 10 years, annual CT for 5 years, or follow-up with non-CT modalities only for asymptomatic patients. Annual CT follow-up was associated with minimal survival benefit. With adjustments for quality of life, a decrement in quality-adjusted life expectancy was found for early-stage patients followed with CT compared with non-CT modalities. The authors concluded that the cost-effectiveness ratio for annual routine follow-up CT was substantially higher than those of most well-accepted cancer interventions.[71]

FDG-PET is also emerging as a potential tool to detect relapse. A prospective study of 36 HL patients found that routine FDG-PET correctly identified all 5 relapses that occurred following treatment.[72] However, the false-positive rate was 55% (6/11 with abnormal FDG-PET did not have relapse confirmed) (see Fig. 9.6) and 2/5 of relapsed patients developed symptoms shortly after the detection by FDG-PET, so the marginal benefit of the test was unclear. The authors concluded that further studies, including cost-benefit analyses, are warranted before FDG PET can be recommended as a routine part of follow-up for HL patients.[72]

Detection of Late Effects

The likelihood of HL relapse more than 5 years following completion of treatment is small, but routine follow-up becomes important to reduce the morbidity of long-term complications of therapy (see Chapter 26). Thyroid function should be evaluated at least annually, with a total thyroxine (T_4) and thyroid-stimulating hormone (TSH) level, particularly for those patients who received neck or mediastinal RT. A full blood count may reveal bone marrow dysfunction. The elevated risk of breast cancer among females treated with mediastinal RT warrants screening 8 to 10 years after treatment.[35] Although mammography is the only test definitively shown to be an effective tool for breast cancer screening, its suboptimal performance in women with dense breast tissue has led some authors to recommend ultrasound or MRI screening for young high-risk women.[73] Clinical trials are needed to investigate the utility of MRI screening for breast cancer among young HL survivors. Women are also advised to undergo annual cervical smears. The risk of colon cancer is elevated among HL survivors, although the risk does not increase as rapidly as that for

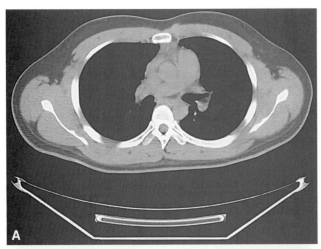

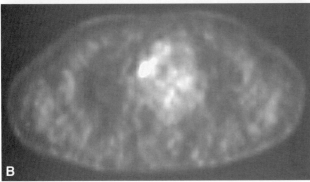

FIGURE 9.6. This patient was treated with combined modality therapy for CS IIA disease. PET scan was negative 2 months after completion of therapy. One year later, repeat CT showed small anterior mediastinal adenopathy (**A**) and PET scan was positive (**B**). Biopsy revealed only reactive changes.

breast cancer[74,75]; colonoscopic screening should be considered 10 to 15 years following treatment.

The risk of symptomatic or fatal heart disease has been shown to be significantly elevated among HL survivors[76,77] (see Chapter 25). Most clinically significant cardiac disease occurs in survivors with additional cardiac risk factors (abnormal blood pressure or serum lipids, smoking).[76,78] Patients should be educated about these risk factors, and these should be monitored and treated aggressively. Progressive fatigue or chest pain requires cardiac investigation and should not be attributed to noncardiac causes unless heart disease has been ruled out. Although survivors have been shown to have an increased risk of asymptomatic electrocardiographic or echocardiographic abnormalities, currently there is no clear evidence that routine screening with these tests leads to earlier intervention with useful treatment. Future studies may clarify the value of routine screening of cardiac function. Female survivors who become pregnant, however, should undergo a cardiac evaluation due to the significant cardiac stress associated with pregnancy and childbirth.

References

1. Hodgkin T. On some morbid appearances of the absorbent glands and spleen. *Med Chir Trans* 1832;17:68.
2. Gowers WR. Hodgkin's disease. In: Reynolds JR., ed. *A System of Medicine.* London: Macmillan; 1879:306.
3. Reed DM. *On the pathological changes in Hodgkin's disease, with especial reference to tuberculosis.* Baltimore: Johns Hopkins Hospital; 1902:10.
4. Ziegler K. *Die Hodgkinsche Krankheit.* Jena: Gustav Fischer; 1911.
5. Longcope WT, McAlpin KR. *Hodgkin's disease,* vol. 4. Oxford: Oxford Medical; 1920.
6. Jackson H Jr. PFJ. Hodgkin's disease. I. General considerations. *N Engl J Med* 1944;230:1.
7. Jackson H Jr., Parker F Jr. Hodgkin's disease. II. Pathology. *N Engl J Med* 1944;231:35.
8. Craver LF. Hodgkin's disease. In: Tice F., ed. *Practice of medicine,* vol. 5. Hagerstown, MD: WF Pryor; 1951:152.
9. Peters MV. A study of survivals in Hodgkin's disease treated radiologically. *Am J Roentegenol* 1950;63:299.
10. Peters MV, Middlemiss KCH. A Study of Hodgkin's disease treated by irradiation. *Am J Roentegenol* 1958;79:114.
11. Kaplan HS, Bagshaw MA, Rosenberg SA. Presentation de protocoles d'essai radiotherapuetiques des lymphomes malins de L'Universite de Stanford. *Nouv Rev Fr Hematol* 1964;4:95.
12. Tubiana M. Hodgkin's disease: historical perspective and clinical presentation. *Baillieres Clin Haematol* 1996;9:503.
13. Rosenberg SA. Report of the committee on the staging of Hodgkin's disease. *Cancer Res* 1966;26:1310.
14. Peters MV. The need for a new clinical classification in Hodgkin's disease. *Cancer Res* 1971;31:1713–1722.
15. Musshoff K, Renemann H, Boutis L, et al. Extranodular lymphogranulomatosis-diagnosis, therapy and prognosis in two different types of organ involvement. Contribution to the phase classification of Hodgkin's disease. *Fortschr Geb Rontgentstr Nuklearmed* 1968;109:776–786.
16. Rosenberg SA, Kaplan HS. Hodgkin's disease and other malignant lymphomas. *Calif Med* 1970;113:23.
17. Rosenberg SA, Boiron M, DeVita VTJ, et al. Report of the committee on Hodgkin's disease staging procedures. *Cancer Res* 1971;31:1862.
18. Carbone PP, Kaplan HS, Musshoff KAU. –KEA as initials for Musshoff?}. Report of the committee on Hodgkin's disease staging classification. *Cancer Res* 1971;31:1860.
19. Tubiana M, Attie R, Flamant R, et al. Prognostic factors in 454 cases of Hodkin's disease. *Cancer Res* 1971;31:1801.
20. Lister TA, Crowther D, Sutcliffe SB, et al. Report of a committee convened to discuss the evaluation and staging of patients with Hodgkin's disease: Cotswolds meeting. *J Clin Oncol* 1989;7:1630–1636.
21. UICC. *TNM Classification of malignant tumours,* 6th ed. New York: Wiley; 2002.
22. Greene FL PD, Morrow M, Balch C, et al. *AJCC cancer staging handbook,* 6th ed. New York: Springer; 2002.
23. Gilbert R. Radiotherapy in Hodgkin's disease (malignant granulomatosis): anatomic and clinical foundations, governing principles, results. *Am J. Roentgenol* 1939;41:198.
24. Peters MV, Alison RE, Bush RS. Natural history of Hodgkin's disease as related to staging. *Cancer* 1966;19:308.
25. Kaplan HS. The radical radiotherapy of regionally localized Hodgkin's disease. *Radiology* 1962;78:553.
26. Rosenberg SA. Evidence for an orderly progression in the spread of Hodgkin's disease. *Cancer Res* 1966;26:1225.
27. Kaplan HS. *On the natural history, treatment and prognosis of Hodgkin's disease. Harvey Lectures 1968–1969.* New York: Academic Press; 1970.
28. Mauch PM, Kadin M, Coleman CN, et al. Patterns of presentation of Hodgkin's Disease. *Cancer* 1993;71:2062.
29. Hoppe RT, Hanlon AL, Hanks GE, et al. Progress in the treatment of Hodgkin's disease in the United States, 1973 versus 1983. The Patterns of Care Study. *Cancer* 1994;74:3198–3203.
30. Kennedy BJ, Loeb V, Jr., Peterson VM, et al. National survey of patterns of care for Hodgkin's disease. *Cancer* 1985;56:2547–2556.
31. Pel PK. Pseudoleukamie oder chronisches ruckfallsfieber? *Zur Symptomatologie der sorgenannten Pseudoleukamie II* 1887:644.
32. Ebstein W. Von das chronische ruckfallsfieber, eine neu infections-krankheit. *Berl Klin Wochenschr* 1887;24:565.
33. Gobbi PG, Cavalli C, Gendarini A, et al. Reevaluation of prognostic significance of symptoms in Hodgkin's disease. *Cancer* 1985;56:2874–2880.
34. Edwards CL, Hayes RL. Tumor scanning with 67Ga citrate. *J Nucl Med* 1969;10:103–105.
35. Ng AK, Bernardo MV, Silver B, et al. Mid- and post-ABVD gallium scanning predicts for recurrence in early-stage Hodgkin's disease. *Int J Radiat Oncol Biol Phys* 2005;61:175–184.
36. Bogart JA, Chung CT, Mariados NF, et al. The value of gallium imaging after therapy for Hodgkin's disease. *Cancer* 1998;82:754–759.
37. Friedberg JW, Fischman A, Neuberg D, et al. FDG-PET is superior to gallium scintigraphy in staging and more sensitive in the follow-up of patients with de novo Hodgkin lymphoma: a blinded comparison. *Leuk Lymphoma* 2004;45:85–92.
38. Jerusalem G, Hustinx R, Beguin Y, et al. Positron emission tomography imaging for lymphoma. *Curr Opin Oncol* 2005;17:441–445.
39. Naumann R, Beuthien-Baumann B, Reiss A, et al. Substantial impact of FDG PET imaging on the therapy decision in patients with early-stage Hodgkin's lymphoma. *Br J Cancer* 2004;90:620–625.
40. Mauch P, Larson D, Osteen R, et al. Prognostic factors for positive surgical staging in patients with Hodgkin's disease. *J Clin Oncol* 1990;8:257–265.

41. Meis JM, Butler JJ, Osborne BM. Hodgkin's disease involving the breast and chest wall. *Cancer* 1986;57:1859–1865.

42. Hodgson DC, Tsang RW, Pintilie M, et al. Impact of chest wall and lung invasion on outcome of stage I-II Hodgkin's lymphoma after combined modality therapy. *Int J Radiat Oncol Biol Phys* 2003;57:1374–1381.

43. Gobbi PG, Comelli M, Grignani GE, et al. Estimate of expected survival at diagnosis in Hodgkin's disease: a means of weighting prognostic factors and a tool for treatment choice and clinical research. A report from the International Database on Hodgkin's Disease (IDHD). *Haematologica* 1994;79:241–255.

44. Longo DL, Glatstein E, Duffey PL, et al. Alternating MOPP and ABVD chemotherapy plus mantle-field radiation therapy in patients with massive mediastinal Hodgkin's disease. *J Clin Oncol* 1997;15:3338–3346.

45. Connors JM, Klimo P. Is it an E lesion or stage IV? An unsettled issue in Hodgkin's disease staging. *J Clin Oncol* 1984;2:1421–1423.

46. Mauch P, Goodman R, Hellman S. The significance of mediastinal involvement in early stage Hodgkin's disease. *Cancer* 1978;42:1039–1045.

47. Laskar S, Gupta T, Vimal S, et al. Consolidation radiation after complete remission in Hodgkin's disease following six cycles of doxorubicin, bleomycin, vinblastine, and dacarbazine chemotherapy: is there a need? *J Clin Oncol* 2004;22:62–68.

48. Ballova V, Ruffer JU, Haverkamp H, et al. A prospectively randomized trial carried out by the German Hodgkin Study Group (GHSG) for elderly patients with advanced Hodgkin's disease comparing BEACOPP baseline and COPP-ABVD (study HD9$_{elderly}$). *Ann Oncol* 2005;16:124–131.

49. Josting A, Wolf J, Diehl V. Hodgkin disease: prognostic factors and treatment strategies. *Curr Opin Oncol* 2000;12:403–411.

50. Hasenclever D, Diehl V. A prognostic score for advanced Hodgkin's disease. International Prognostic Factors Project on Advanced Hodgkin's Disease. *N Engl J Med* 1998;339:1506–1514.

51. Hasenclever D. The disappearance of prognostic factors in Hodgkin's disease. *Ann Oncol* 2002;13(suppl 1):75–78.

52. Tuli MM, Al-Shemmari SH, Ameen RM, et al. The use of gallium-67 scintigraphy to monitor tumor response rates and predict long-term clinical outcome in patients with lymphoma. *Clin Lymphoma* 2004;5:56–61.

53. Hutchings M, Loft A, Hansen MT, et al. FDG-PET after two cycles of chemotherapy predicts treatment failure and progression-free survival in Hodgkin lymphoma. *Blood* 2005;107:52–59.

54. Ruhl U, Albrecht M, Dieckmann K, et al. Response-adapted radiotherapy in the treatment of pediatric Hodgkin's disease: an interim report at 5 years of the German GPOH-HD 95 trial. *Int J Radiat Oncol Biol Phys* 2001;51:1209–1218.

55. Kelly KM, Hutchinson RJ, Sposto R, et al. Feasibility of upfront dose-intensive chemotherapy in children with advanced-stage Hodgkin's lymphoma: preliminary results from the Children's Cancer Group Study CCG-59704. *Ann Oncol* 2002;13(suppl 1):107–111.

56. Jochelson M, Mauch P, Balikian J, et al. The significance of the residual mediastinal mass in treated Hodgkin's disease. *J Clin Oncol* 1985;3:637–640.

57. Radford JA, Cowan RA, Flanagan M, et al. The significance of residual mediastinal abnormality on the chest radiograph following treatment for Hodgkin's disease. *J Clin Oncol* 1988;6:940–946.

58. Radford JA, Crowther D, Rohatiner AZ, et al. Results of a randomized trial comparing MVPP chemotherapy with a hybrid regimen, ChlVPP/EVA, in the initial treatment of Hodgkin's disease. *J Clin Oncol* 1995;13:2379–2385.

59. Reinhardt MJ, Herkel C, Altehoefer C, et al. Computed tomography and 18F-FDG positron emission tomography for therapy control of Hodgkin's and non-Hodgkin's lymphoma patients: when do we really need FDG-PET? *Ann Oncol* 2005;16:1524–1529.

60. Dittmann H, Sokler M, Kollmannsberger C, et al. Comparison of 18FDG-PET with CT scans in the evaluation of patients with residual and recurrent Hodgkin's lymphoma. *Oncol Rep* 2001;8:1393–1399.

61. Rigacci L, Castagnoli A, Dini C, et al. (18)FDG-positron emission tomography in post treatment evaluation of residual mass in Hodgkin's lymphoma: Long-term results. *Oncol Rep* 2005;14:1209–1214.

62. Kazama T, Faria SC, Varavithya V, et al. FDG PET in the evaluation of treatment for lymphoma: clinical usefulness and pitfalls. *Radiographics* 2005;25:191–207.

63. Castellucci P, Zinzani P, Nanni C, et al. 18F-FDG PET early after radiotherapy in lymphoma patients. *Cancer Biother Radiopharm* 2004;19:606–612.

64. Friedman S, Henry-Amar M, Cosset JM, et al. Evolution of erythrocyte sedimentation rate as predictor of early relapse in posttherapy early-stage Hodgkin's disease. *J Clin Oncol* 1988;6:596–602.

65. Henry-Amar M, Friedman S, Hayat M, et al. Erythrocyte sedimentation rate predicts early relapse and survival in early-stage Hodgkin disease. The EORTC Lymphoma Cooperative Group. *Ann Intern Med* 1991;114:361–365.

66. Hoppe RT, Advani RH, Bierman PJ, et al. Hodgkin disease/lymphoma. Clinical practice guidelines in oncology. *J Natl Compr Canc Netw* 2006;4:210–230.

67. Radford JA, Eardley A, Woodman C, et al. Follow up policy after treatment for Hodgkin's disease: too many clinic visits and routine tests? A review of hospital records. *BMJ* 1997;314:343–346.

68. Dryver ET, Jernstrom H, Tompkins K, et al. Follow-up of patients with Hodgkin's disease following curative treatment: the routine CT scan is of little value. *Br J Cancer* 2003;89:482–486.

69. Torrey MJ, Poen JC, Hoppe RT. Detection of relapse in early-stage Hodgkin's disease: role of routine follow-up studies. *Journal of Clinical Oncology* 1997;15:1123–1130.

70. Khan A, Herman PG, Jojas KA, et al. Comparison of CT and chest radiographs in the evaluation of post-therapy lymphoma patients. *Eur J Radiol* 1989;9:96–100.

71. Guadagnolo BA, Punglia RS, Kuntz KM, et al. Cost-effectiveness of routine computerized tomography in follow-up of patients with complete response after primary treatment for Hodgkin's disease. *Int J Radiat Oncol Biol Phys* 2005;63:S114–S115.

72. Jerusalem G, Beguin Y, Fassotte MF, et al. Early detection of relapse by whole-body positron emission tomography in the follow-up of patients with Hodgkin's disease. *Ann Oncol* 2003;14:123–130.

73. Elmore JG, Armstrong K, Lehman CD, et al. Screening for breast cancer. *JAMA* 2005;293:1245–1256.

74. Dores GM, Metayer C, Curtis RE, et al. Second malignant neoplasms among long-term survivors of Hodgkin's disease: a population-based evaluation over 25 years. *J Clin Oncol* 2002;20:3484–3494.

75. Swerdlow AJ, Barber JA, Hudson GV, et al. Risk of second malignancy after Hodgkin's disease in a collaborative British cohort: the relation to age at treatment. *J Clin Oncol* 2000;18:498–509.

76. Hull MC, Morris CG, Pepine CJ, et al. Valvular dysfunction and carotid, subclavian, and coronary artery disease in survivors of hodgkin lymphoma treated with radiation therapy. *JAMA* 2003;290:2831–2837.

77. Hancock SL, Tucker MA, Hoppe RT. Factors affecting late mortality from heart disease after treatment of Hodgkin's disease. *JAMA* 1993;270:1949–1955.

78. Strasser JF, Li S, Neuberg D, et al. Late cardiac toxicity after mediastinal radiation therapy for Hodgkin's disease. *Int J Radiat Oncol Biol Phys* 2004;60:S216–S217.

79. Kaplan HS, Rosenberg SA. The treatment of Hodgkin's disease. *Med Clin North Am* 1966;50:1591–1610.

CHAPTER 10 ■ ANATOMIC IMAGING

AXEL GOSSMANN

In Hodgkin lymphoma, initial staging is crucial to determine the location and extent of disease, to define manifestations and prognostic factors, and is the hallmark for the choice of treatment. Furthermore, staging allows comparison of treatment results between different study groups. Due to the availability of imaging techniques such as computed tomography (CT), magnetic resonance imaging (MRI), and ultrasonography (US), it has been possible to improve the accuracy of clinical staging, so that invasive pathologic staging is now seldom necessary. At present, the established radiological technique for the diagnosis of lymphoma is computed tomography, which might be supplemented by initial MRI and ultrasonography.[1,2] Beside these techniques, positron emission tomography (PET) using fluorine-18 (FDG) is increasingly used in the staging and follow-up of malignant lymphomas, although its precise role has not yet been determined.[3]

CONVENTIONAL IMAGING

Prior to the era of computed tomography, conventional imaging was the only way to perform accurate staging in Hodgkin lymphoma. A conventional x-ray of the chest was performed to detect mediastinal masses and involvement of the lung (Fig. 10.1A), and lymphangiography was used to detect enlarged abdominal or pelvic lymph nodes (Fig. 10.1B). However, the drawback of both techniques is the limited sensitivity and specificity for the detection of enlarged lymph nodes and, subsequently, the limited capability to perform precise staging. It is known that a conventional x-ray of the chest fails to detect enlarged lymph nodes of the mediastinum in many cases (Fig. 10.2). In addition, lymphangiography is a technically demanding procedure where small lymphatic vessels have to be cannulated on the dorsum of the foot for the injection of a lymphotropic contrast agent. Lymphangiography mainly detects enlarged lymph nodes of the retroperitoneum and fails to detect enlarged lymph nodes, for instance, of the mesentery or the porta hepatis. By contrast, computed tomography has an excellent sensitivity for the detection of enlarged lymph nodes in all anatomic regions of the body (Fig. 10.3) and has, therefore, now completely replaced conventional imaging as the method of choice for staging Hodgkin lymphoma.

Today, conventional x-ray of the chest is mainly used for the assessment of a large mediastinal involvement in advanced Hodgkin lymphoma. A large mediastinal involvement is considered when the ratio of the maximal mediastinal width to the thoracic dimension (mediastinum/thorax ratio) is larger than 0.33, and it is considered to be very large when the ratio is greater than 0.45.[4] The detection of a large mediastinal involvement in Hodgkin lymphoma is important because patients have a poorer prognosis and require different treatment strategies.[5,6]

COMPUTED TOMOGRAPHY

CT of the thorax and abdomen is an established procedure for the diagnosis and staging of tumors. The possibility of demonstrating pathologic enlargements of lymph nodes has led to the routine use of CT in the staging of malignant lymphomas.[1] Disadvantages that are considered with CT are the exposure to ionizing radiation and, in general, the need for oral and intravenous administration of contrast agents. Notwithstanding these limitations, a rapid development in the technology of CT has been seen during recent years. First, spiral CT was introduced, which made it possible to make the optimum use of contrast agent bolus. More recently, multidetector row CT has brought further advantages. This rapidly evolving technique allows a unique spatial resolution of below 1 mm by giving almost isotropic voxel sizes at the same time. As a result, high spatial resolution images can be generated; and by using multiplanar reconstruction (MPR) techniques, high-resolution images of the body can be reconstructed in all desired planes (Fig. 10.3). This multiplanar imaging technique allows the precise assessment of enlarged lymph nodes and tumor masses in the x-, y-, and z-planes. With the help of MPR, even small lymph nodes in complex anatomic areas such as the porta hepatis or the mesentery can be easily differentiated from surrounding tissues (Fig. 10.3). A multiplanar imaging technique is therefore no longer restricted to MRI and has improved the diagnostic confidence of CT. Modern multidetector row CT allows fast imaging of the whole body. With a spatial resolution of approximately 1 mm, the whole neck, thorax, and abdomen from the base of the skull to the groin can be imaged during a single breath hold with an approximate acquisition time of 25 seconds (Fig. 10.3). Thus, even in patients who are not able to lie on their back or to hold the breath for a longer time, CT can be performed for staging Hodgkin lymphoma.

When Hodgkin lymphoma is diagnosed, extensive staging must be performed to determine whether extranodal involvement represents a primary manifestation or dissemination of systemic disease. By using different reconstruction algorithms and different window presets (Fig. 10.4), CT is not solely limited to the detection of nodal involvement. Instead, CT is also a useful tool to detect extranodal disease. Especially for the detection of involvement of the lung parenchyma (Figs. 10.4B, and 10.8), the pleura and the chest wall, CT is considered to be the method of choice.[7]

MAGNETIC RESONANCE IMAGING

In addition to CT, MRI is another cross-sectional imaging modality for staging Hodgkin lymphoma. The excellent soft-tissue contrast and the lack of exposure to ionizing radiation

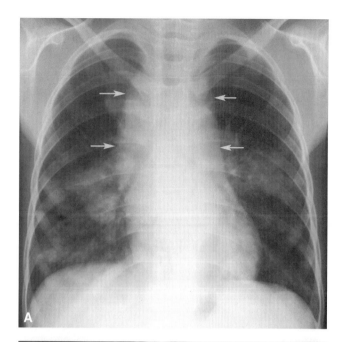

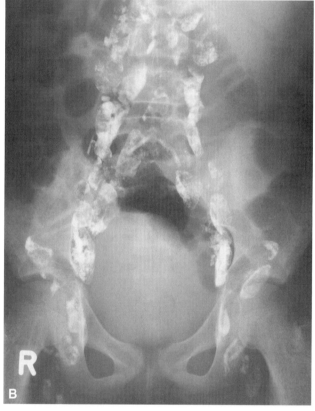

FIGURE 10.1. Conventional x-ray of the chest (**A**) and lymphogram (**B**) of a 9-year-old boy with advanced Hodgkin lymphoma. X-ray of the chest shows clearly the mediastinal mass *(arrows)* as well as the involvement of the lung parenchyma on both sides. Lymphogram shows multiple enlarged lymph nodes with an inhomogeneous contrast enhancement. Findings are indicative for involvement of Hodgkin lymphoma.

are the main advantages of MRI. Furthermore, the application of oral or intravenous contrast agents can frequently be avoided. On the other hand, longer acquisition times than those of CT and the relatively high costs are considered to be disadvantages of this technique. At present, MRI is therefore

mainly used to assess for lymphomatous involvement of the central nervous system and to evaluate suspected bone or bone marrow involvement.[8] However, during the past years, improvements of technology, especially the development of fast imaging techniques, have considerably reduced MRI time without compromising the quality of MR images. Moreover, faster imaging results in reduced artifacts of the MR images due to fewer movement artifacts (e.g. breathing, heart and bowel movements). As a consequence, the use of MRI is no longer limited to the detection of involvement of the central nervous system or the bone marrow. MRI is now considered to be as diagnostic as CT for staging Hodgkin lymphoma[9–11] (Figs. 10.5 and 10.6) and parenchymal organs.[9,12] Further technical improvements of MRI with specially designed fast spin-echo (FSE) short inversion time inversion recovery (STIR) sequences in combination with sliding table platforms have made it possible to perform whole-body MRI with short acquisition times (Fig. 10.5). The three-dimensional data sets are collected within a single breath hold with nearly isotropic resolution and provide image quality comparable to that of conventional fat-saturated two-dimensional gradient-echo images. The total acquisition time for the whole body can be achieved as fast as approximately 15 minutes.[13] This new technique has already shown its potential for staging lymphomas (Fig. 10.5)[13–16] and various cancers.[13,17–18] Although initial results of whole-body MRI are promising, there is certainly a need for evaluation in larger patient cohorts.[13,16]

NODAL INVOLVEMENT BY HODGKIN LYMPHOMA

Adequate staging of newly diagnosed patients with Hodgkin lymphoma is important to determine the best therapy regimen. In essence, the staging is based on the number of sites of lymph node involvement, whether lymph nodes are involved on both sides of the diaphragm, whether there is extranodal disease, and whether B-symptoms are present.[19] In clinical practice, a CT of the neck, thorax, abdomen, and pelvis is used as an established radiological technique for staging Hodgkin lymphoma.[1,2] It is considered to be the method of choice for staging of Hodgkin lymphoma and its use is recommended by the National Comprehensive Cancer Network (NCCN). Although US of the neck and the abdomen might be also used for the detection of enlarged lymph nodes, the high interobserver variability and the limited diagnostic value in cases of adiposity or gaseous distension make CT the method of choice for staging Hodgkin lymphoma.

Once Hodgkin lymphoma is diagnosed, the number of sites of lymph node involvement and the presence of extranodal disease have to be assessed. The diagnosis of nodal involvement of Hodgkin lymphoma relies mainly on size, number, and morphologic criteria that are insensitive. Despite technical improvements, the detection of Hodgkin lymphoma involvement in normal-sized lymph nodes and the differentiation between enlarged lymph nodes due to inflammatory reactions and Hodgkin lymphoma involvement are still major problems. Therefore, a biopsy has to be performed in some cases to test whether or not nodal involvement by Hodgkin lymphoma is present.

In clinical practice, a lymph node size of more than approximately 1.5 cm in its largest diameter is considered to be suspicious for the involvement of Hodgkin lymphoma. Usually, the size of enlarged lymph nodes is assessed in the plane with the maximum diameter of the tumor mass (Fig. 10.7A). In addition, the determination of additional axes, orthogonal to

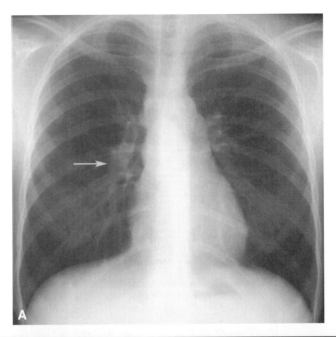

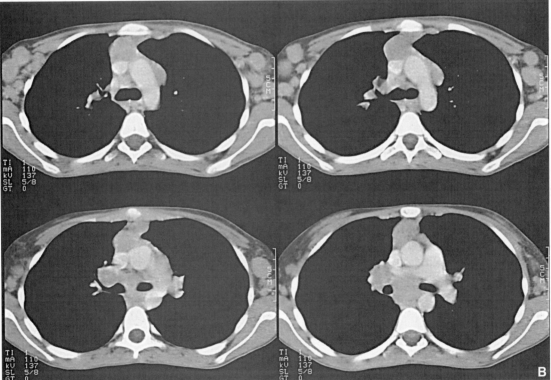

FIGURE 10.2. Conventional x-ray of the chest (**A**) and contrast-material–enhanced computed tomography of the thorax (**B**) in a 14-year-old girl with Hodgkin lymphoma. X-ray of the chest shows mild right hilar adenopathy *(arrow)*. By contrast, computed tomography of the thorax shows the full extent of the disease with multiple enlarged lymph nodes of the mediastinum, the hilum, and bilateral axillae. Due to the limited sensitivity of conventional x-rays in detecting enlarged lymph nodes, cross-sectional imaging techniques have replaced conventional x-rays in staging Hodgkin lymphoma.

the maximum diameter (Fig.10.7B) or according to the second largest diameter of the enlarged lymph node (Fig. 10.7C), might be helpful to appreciate treatment results more precisely. The best estimation of the total tumor amount, however, is given by a volumetric assessment of the total tumor mass (Fig. 10.7D to F). By the measurement and subsequent summation of all areas on all slices with tumor tissue (Fig. 10.7D to F), the closest estimation of the total tumor amount is yielded. Although this technique is time consuming, it is the only approach where the total tumor burden is estimated, and therefore allows an exact assessment of treatment benefit according to a reduction of tumor volume.

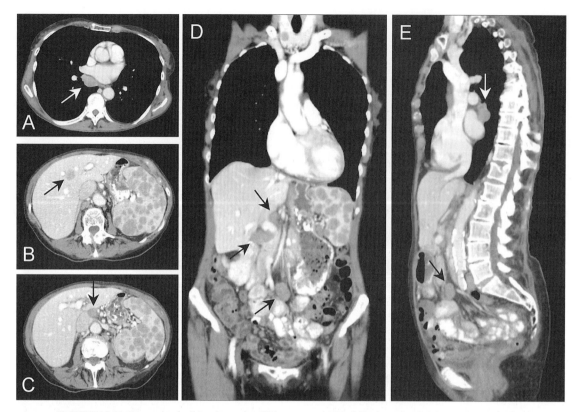

FIGURE 10.3. Contrast-material–enhanced multidetector row CT of the thorax and abdomen (**A** to **C**) with coronal (**D**) and sagittal (**E**) reconstructions of a patient with Hodgkin lymphoma. The excellent spatial resolution in combination with the coronal and sagittal reconstructions allows a precise detection of enlarged lymph nodes of the mediastinum (**A, E**), the porta hepatis (**C, D**) and the mesentery (**D, E**). In addition, a focal involvement of the spleen (**B to D**) and the liver (**B**) is also clearly demonstrated. The whole data set was acquired during one single breath hold. Due to the possibility of the detection of both nodal involvement and extranodal disease, CT is considered the method of choice for staging Hodgkin lymphoma.

EXTRANODAL INVOLVEMENT BY HODGKIN LYMPHOMA

In 80% to 90% of patients with Hodgkin lymphoma, the first manifestation is lymphadenopathy, most frequently located supradiaphragmatically. Hodgkin disease is usually almost entirely confined to the lymph nodes while extranodal involvement is much less common compared to non-Hodgkin lymphoma. Extranodal invasion of adjacent tissue is seen in up to 15% of cases and hematogenous spread in 5% to 10%. Even when dissemination occurs beyond the lymphoreticular system, certain patterns of associated spread are frequently evident.[7]

Lungs and Pericardium

Involvement of the lung parenchyma sometimes occurs in Hodgkin lymphoma. Pulmonary involvement is usually associated with hilar nodal disease at presentation. Mediastinal adenopathy has a usually predictable pattern involving anterior and middle mediastinal nodes with or without disease in the hila. Hilar adenopathy is uncommon without detectable mediastinal disease and the lung is virtually never involved alone. Lung manifestations include direct extension from involved nodes, nodules with or without cavitation, atelectasis secondary to endobronchial or nodal obstruction, and, rarely,

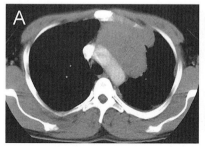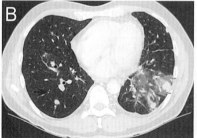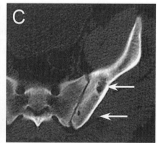

FIGURE 10.4. Based on the same raw data as in Figure 10.3, CT demonstrates Hodgkin involvement of lymph nodes of the mediastinum (**A**), lung parenchyma (**B**), and the skeletal system (**C**) by using different reconstruction algorithms and window presets.

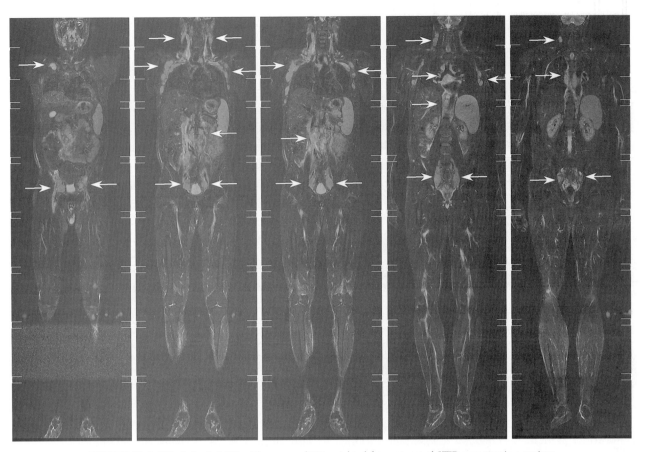

FIGURE 10.5. Whole-body MRI with a coronal T2-weighted fat-suppressed STIR sequence in a patient with Hodgkin lymphoma demonstrates clearly extensive nodal involvement of cervical, supra- and infra-clavicular, axillary, mediastinal, lung and liver hilum, celiac, retroperitoneal, mesenteric, iliac, and inguinal lymph nodes *(arrows)*. Note the normal signal of the bone marrow without evidence for Hodgkin lymphoma and the moderate reactive splenomegaly. Acquisition time for the whole sequence was 11 minutes. Although initial results of whole-body MRI are promising, evaluation of its clinical value needs to be assessed in larger patient cohorts.

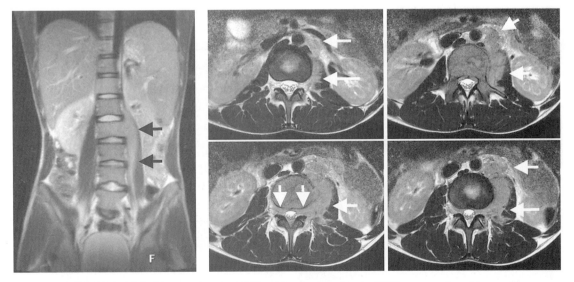

FIGURE 10.6. MRI with coronal and axial T2-weighted turbo spin echo (TSE) sequences in an 11-year-old boy with Hodgkin lymphoma shows a retroperitoneal and paravertebral tumor mass with infiltration of the psoas muscle and the adjacent vertebral body *(arrows)*. In addition, infiltration of the spinal canal along the posterior longitudinal ligament is demonstrated. In comparison to CT, MRI is superior for assessment of infiltration of the spinal canal.

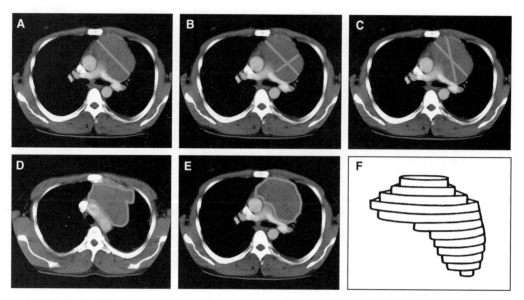

FIGURE 10.7. CT in a patient with Hodgkin lymphoma of the upper mediastinum with different approaches for the evaluation of the tumor burden. In clinical practice, the sizes of enlarged lymph nodes are assessed in only one plane according to the maximum diameter of enlarged lymph nodes or bulky tumor masses, respectively (**A**). The determination of additional axes, orthogonal to the maximum tumor diameter (**B**) or according to the second-largest diameter (**C**), are helpful to appreciate treatment results more precisely. A volumetric assessment of the total tumor mass (**D, E**) with the summation of different tumor areas for the determination of the tumor volume (**F**) represents the best estimation of the total tumor amount.

an interstitial pattern. Also nodular lesions that are often peripheral with poorly defined borders are present in Hodgkin lymphoma (Figs. 10.4B and 10.8). The nodules, with or without cavitation, tend to be single or few in number, with a predilection for the upper lobes. Pleural effusions are not uncommon, but solid pleural masses are less frequent. Invasion of the pericardium is not often seen, although masses are commonly seen along the pericardium. Invasion of the chest wall occurs particularly with involvement of internal mammary nodes.[19] The most common feature of primary pulmonary Hodgkin lymphoma is a direct extension from hilar nodes toward the lung. Especially for the detection of involve-

ment of the lung parenchyma, pleura, and chest wall, CT is considered to be the method of choice.[1,7]

Thymus

Although thymic enlargement is seen in 30% to 50% of patients with intrathoracic involvement, Hodgkin lymphoma involving only the thymus is rare.[19,20] Thymic involvement does not change the stage of the disease. Usually, the enlarged thymus shrinks with therapy and adopts a typical triangular thymic configuration. However, in about one-third of cases, the thymus

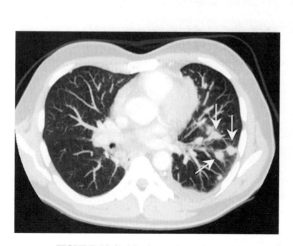
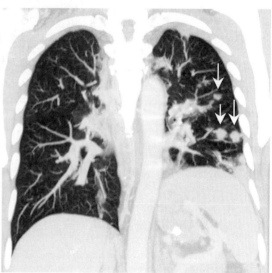

FIGURE 10.8. Maximum intensity projections of computed tomography of the lung in an axial plane and a coronal reconstruction show multiple nodular peripheral lesions with poorly defined borders in the left lung. The findings are indicative for involvement of Hodgkin lymphoma.

remains enlarged after therapy although a full clinical remission appears.[20] Such post-therapeutic enlargement is often caused by thymic rebound or the persistence of thymic cysts. In general, the timing of thymic enlargement relative to therapy in combination with therapeutic effects of Hodgkin lymphoma elsewhere, and the typical configuration of the thymus, allow the differentiation between Hodgkin involvement or thymic rebound. Thymic enlargement can be detected easily with CT as well as with MRI. In addition, parasternal US has been suggested as an alternative technique for the diagnosis of thymic involvement but is of limited value because it does not obviate CT.[20]

Spleen

Diagnostic laparotomy is no longer routinely performed in Hodgkin lymphoma and noninvasive diagnosis of spleen involvement remains uncertain. Thus, the problem in detecting splenic involvement is still largely unsolved. Staging laparotomy has shown that the spleen is involved in about 30% to 40% of patients at presentation.[21] Splenic involvement can appear diffuse or as multiple nodules of up to 1 cm in diameter (Fig. 10.3). The size of the spleen is not an exact marker for the assessment of involvement of Hodgkin lymphoma, because a diffuse infiltration may be present even in normal-sized spleens and mild to moderate reactive splenomegaly occurs in about 30% of patients without involvement (Fig. 10.5). Only a marked splenomegaly is highly suggestive for Hodgkin lymphoma of the spleen.[1] One approach to detect a diffuse splenic involvement might be the use of a spleen index. In a recent study[22] we could show that splenic weight is highly correlated with a spleen index defined as the product of length, width, and thickness measured by CT (correlation coefficient 0.93). By applying the identified risk factors in clinically staged patients, spleen involvement could be determined. The spleen weight could be estimated with the help of a spleen index. Above an index of 1,000 the probability of spleen involvement is higher than 90%.

Liver

Primary hepatic Hodgkin lymphoma is rare while secondary liver involvement in Hodgkin lymphoma occurs more often. It is usually associated with lymph node disease and is almost invariably associated with Hodgkin lymphoma of the spleen (Fig. 10.3). The more extensive the splenic disease is, the greater is the likelihood of hepatic involvement.[21] Hepatic involvement is usually diffuse with several nodular lesions (Fig. 10.3). The diffuse or infiltrative form of the disease results in patchy, irregular infiltrates originating primarily in the portal areas. Both CT and MRI are considered the methods of choice for the detection of liver involvement. However, the small number of positive findings with cross-sectional imaging techniques relative to the relatively large number of studies reviewed suggests that both methods do not reveal a high sensitivity in detecting hepatic involvement.

Bone and Bone Marrow

The diagnosis of neoplastic bone marrow infiltration is important to identify suitable treatment protocols. According to the Ann Arbor Classification, bone marrow infiltration by Hodgkin lymphoma indicates the most advanced stage (stage IV). Although bone marrow involvement is relatively uncommon in Hodgkin lymphoma, a bone marrow biopsy is recommended due to the high impact of positive bone marrow on treatment planning. Usually, bone marrow biopsy is performed by iliac crest biopsy, which may be false negative when the bone marrow infiltration is focal rather than diffuse (Fig. 10.9).[23,24]

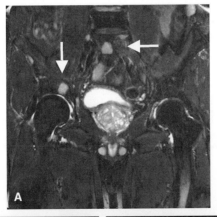

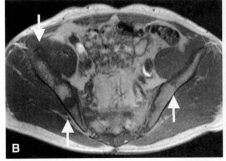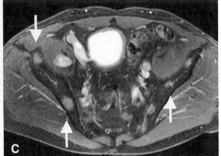

FIGURE 10.9. MRI with a coronal T2-weighted fat-suppressed STIR sequence (**A**), axial T1-weighted TSE sequences (**B**), and axial T1-weighted TSE sequences with fat suppression after intravenous contrast injection (**C**) in a patient with Hodgkin lymphoma shows several areas of focal bone marrow infiltration *(arrows)*. On the T1-weighted sequence (**B**) the normal bone marrow has a hyperintensive signal as compared to the adjacent muscle (see also Fig. 10.10).

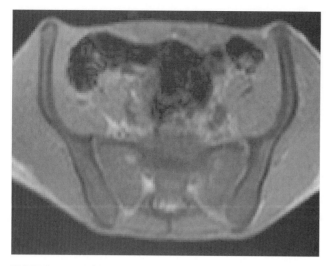

FIGURE 10.10. The same 11-year-old boy with Hodgkin lymphoma as shown in Fig. 10.6 demonstrates on MRI on the axial T1-weighted TSE sequence a hypointense signal of the bone marrow. The signal of the bone marrow appears darker than the surrounding muscle tissue, which is indicative for a diffuse infiltration of the bone marrow. Note the different appearance of a diffuse and a focal involvement (see Fig. 10.9) of the bone marrow.

By contrast, with modern whole-body MRI the evaluation of almost the entire bone marrow is possible (Fig. 10.5). Moreover, MRI is highly sensitive for both the detection of focal infiltration of the bone marrow (Fig. 10.9) as well as a diffuse infiltration (Fig. 10.10). Various studies have highlighted the importance of MRI in staging Hodgkin involvement of the bone marrow.[8,25,26] According to recent studies, patients with bone marrow infiltration at MRI but negative bone marrow biopsy have a worse prognosis than patients with both negative MRI and negative bone marrow biopsy.[25, 26] In addition to a primary involvement of the bone or the bone marrow, occasionally posterior nodes can invade the adjacent vertebrae and spinal canal (Fig. 10.6), which can be nicely seen with MRI. For the detection of bone marrow involvement and the infiltration of the spinal canal, MRI is superior to CT (Fig. 10.11) and is the method of choice.

RESIDUAL TUMOR MASSES

At present over 90% of patients with early-stage Hodgkin lymphoma will be cured.[28] Both radiotherapy and combination chemotherapy are effective treatment modalities. However, a common problem is residual tumor masses that are detected in follow up examinations after therapy. The HD12 protocol is a multicenter prospective randomized trial of the German Hodgkin Study Group (GHSG) for advanced stages of Hodgkin disease (IIB with risk factors: bulky mediastinal mass and/or extranodal disease; III; IV). In this trial, a multidisciplinary panel of radiologists, radiation oncologists, and medical oncologists reviews the diagnostic imaging from patients with advanced Hodgkin lymphoma.[29] Based on the results of this multidisciplinary panel, almost every second patient (214 out of 500 patients; 43%) had residual tumor masses (definition of residual tumor mass: reduction of the initial maximum tumor diameter of more than 50% and a remaining maximum tumor diameter of more than 2 cm after therapy). In patients with initially bulky tumor masses (maximum tumor diameter of more than 5 cm) nearly all patients (93%) had residual tumor masses (Fig. 10.12C and D). The upper mediastinum was the most common localization of residual tumor masses (178 out of 214 patients; 83%). Thus, residual tumor masses in patients with Hodgkin lymphoma are common findings that have to be expected at the end of therapy. In general, a reduction of the tumor volume of more than 50% is considered to be a good response to therapy. However, the question remains how scar tissue or granulomatous tissue can be differentiated from persistent tumor tissue. At present, neither CT nor MRI can answer this question. In the future, lymphotropic contrast agents and positron emission tomography might be helpful to differentiate scar tissue from persistent tumor tissue.

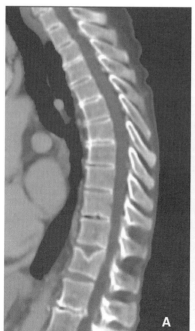
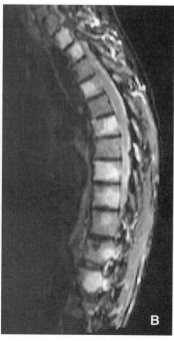

FIGURE 10.11. CT with sagittal reconstructions of the thoracic spine (**A**) and MRI with a sagittal T2-weighted fat suppressed STIR sequence (**B**) of the same patient with Hodgkin lymphoma as shown in Figure 10.3. MRI clearly demonstrates the severe involvement of the bone marrow in many vertebral bodies. CT is less sensitive for the detection of bone marrow involvement and only shows degenerative changes of the vertebral bodies.

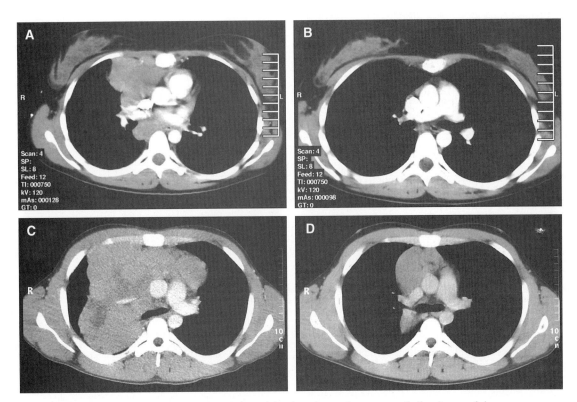

FIGURE 10.12. CT of two patients with Hodgkin lymphoma demonstrates bulky disease of the upper mediastinum before therapy in both patients (**A, C**). The first patient showed a complete response after eight cycles of BEACOPP (**B**), while in the other patient a large residual tumor mass persisted after therapy (**D**). Residual tumor masses after therapy are common findings that have to be expected. In general, a reduction of the tumor volume of more than 50% is considered to be a good response to therapy. However, neither CT nor MRI can differentiate scar or granulomatous tissue from persistent tumor tissue.

LYMPHOTROPIC CONTRAST AGENTS

All current cross-sectional imaging techniques (US, CT, and MRI) are limited in detecting nodal metastases primarily because detection relies mainly on insensitive size criteria.[30,31] Attempts to use the signal intensity with MRI for differentiating normal from metastatic or tumor-involved lymph nodes have also proved unreliable.[32] Lymphotropic contrast agents are a new promising approach to detect small tumor nodules in normal-sized lymph nodes. These newly developed compounds are reticuloendothelial system (RES)-targeted MRI contrast agents consisting of ultrasmall superparamagnetic iron oxide particles (USPIO), which were specifically developed for MR lymphangiography[33–35] and to improve the detection of minimal nodal metastases. Ferumoxides were investigated in phase I to III studies as RES-specific contrast agents. There are different compounds under clinical investigation at present, such as NC100150 (Clariscan) or ferumoxtran (Sinerem, Combidex). Ferumoxtran is a prototype colloid-based USPIO, also representing Fe_2O_3 and Fe_3O_4 particles with a dextran layer. These nanoparticles have a diameter of 20 to 50 nm (mean, 35 nm) and a blood half-life of about 24 hours in humans.[36] After intravenous injection, USPIO are transported into the interstitial space and subsequently via lymph vessels into the lymph nodes. Once within normally functioning nodes, the iron particles are phagocytosed by the macrophages, reducing the signal intensity of normal lymph nodes in which they accumulate due to the susceptibility effects of iron oxide reducing $T2^*$. In areas

of lymph nodes replaced by malignant cells, there is absence of macrophage activity and hence lack of USPIO uptake. Thus, normal lymph nodes turn black postcontrast, namely on $T2^*$-weighted images, while tumor-bearing lymph nodes remain unchanged in signal.[37] Therefore, post-USPIO MRI allows identification of tumor areas within lymph nodes independently of lymph node size. Several studies have demonstrated enhanced sensitivity and specificity for lymph node evaluation after ferumoxtran administration, for pelvic, head and neck, and chest malignancies.[33,37–40] Moreover, one recent study has shown that USPIO contrast-enhanced MRI allows the detection of small and otherwise undetectable lymph-node metastases in patients with prostate cancer.[41] Although there are no studies published yet regarding the usefulness of USPIO in Hodgkin lymphoma, this new group of contrast agents offers the possibility to identify tumor nodules within lymph nodes independent of size criteria. However, the results of the ongoing phase III studies have to be awaited to learn more about the capability of USPIO for staging Hodgkin lymphoma.

In addition to the improved detection of nodal involvement of Hodgkin lymphoma, USPIO might be also useful to differentiate normal, hypercellular, and neoplastic bone marrow. After chemotherapy or radiation therapy, the normal bone marrow might undergo a reconversion from fatty to cellular hematopoietic marrow. A common clinical problem is therefore the differentiation between reconverted hematopoietic marrow and recurrent tumor after therapy. Unfortunately, this important differentiation is not possible with conventional MR techniques, because relaxation rates and MR signal characteristics of highly cellular hematopoietic and highly cellular neoplastic bone marrow are similar.[42] Superparamagnetic iron oxides, however, might be able to answer this question. Because neoplastic bone marrow lesions do not contain intact RES, but normal and hypercellular reconverted bone marrow do, only the latter take up superparamagnetic iron oxides. Therefore, contrast-enhanced MRI using superparamagnetic iron oxides might be useful to differentiate normal from neoplastic bone marrow.[43]

CONCLUSION

CT and MRI are useful cross-sectional imaging techniques for staging Hodgkin lymphoma. By using modern CT and MRI scanners, both imaging modalities allow fast imaging of large parts of the body with an excellent spatial resolution. However, due to short acquisition times in combination with the possibility of the detection of both nodal involvement and extranodal disease, CT is considered as the method of choice for staging Hodgkin lymphoma. In clinical practice, MRI is mainly used as an adjunct to assess for lymphomatous involvement of the central nervous system and to evaluate suspected bone or bone marrow involvement. In the assessment of extranodal involvement, CT is superior to MRI for the evaluation of lung disease.

Major problems in staging Hodgkin lymphoma are still the detection of nodal involvement in normal-sized lymph nodes and residual tumor masses after therapy. In the future, newly developed lymphotropic contrast agents for MRI as well as positron emission tomography might be helpful to answer these questions.

References

1. Fishman EK, Kuhlman JE, Jones RJ. CT of lymphoma: spectrum of disease. *Radiographics* 1991;11:647–669.
2. Munker R, Stengel A, Stabler A, et al. Diagnostic accuracy of ultrasound and computed tomography in the staging of Hodgkin's disease. Verification by laparotomy in 100 cases. *Cancer* 1995; 76:1460–1466.
3. Burton C, Ell P, Linch D. The role of PET imaging in lymphoma. *Br J Haematol* 2004;126:772–784.
4. Schomberg PJ, Evans RG, O'Connell MJ, et al. Prognostic significance of mediastinal mass in adult Hodgkin's disease. *Cancer* 1984;53:324–328.
5. Hasenclever D, Diehl V. A prognostic score for advanced Hodgkin's disease. International Prognostic Factors Project on Advanced Hodgkin's Disease. *N Engl J Med* 1998;339:1506–1514.
6. Brice P, Colin P, Berger F, et al. Advanced Hodgkin disease with large mediastinal involvement can be treated with eight cycles of chemotherapy alone after a major response to six cycles of chemotherapy. *Cancer* 2001; 92:453–459.
7. Guermazi A, Brice P, de Kerviler EE, et al. Extranodal Hodgkin disease: spectrum of disease. *Radiographics* 2001;21:161–179.
8. Linden A, Zankovich R, Theissen P, et al. Malignant lymphoma: bone marrow imaging versus biopsy. *Radiology* 1989;173:335–339.
9. Jung G, Heindel W, von Bergwelt-Baildon M, et al. Abdominal lymphoma staging: is MR imaging with T2-weighted turbo-spin-echo sequence a diagnostic alternative to contrast-enhanced spiral CT? *J Comput Assist Tomogr* 2000;24:783–787.
10. Tesoro-Tess JD, Balzarini L, Ceglia E, et al. Magnetic resonance imaging in the initial staging of Hodgkin's disease and non-Hodgkin lymphoma. *Eur J Radiol* 1991;12:81–90.
11. Hanna SL, Fletcher BD, Boulden TF, et al. MR imaging of infradiaphragmatic lymphadenopathy in children and adolescents with Hodgkin disease: comparison with lymphography and CT. *J Magn Reson Imaging* 1993; 3:461–470.
12. Greco A, Jelliffe AM, Maher EJ, et al. MR imaging of lymphomas: impact on therapy. *J Comput Assist Tomogr* 1988;12:785–791.
13. Lauenstein TC, Goehde SC, Herborn CU, et al. Whole-body MR imaging: evaluation of patients for metastases. *Radiology* 2004;233:139–148.
14. Iizuka-Mikami M, Nagai K, Yoshida K, et al. Detection of bone marrow and extramedullary involvement in patients with non-Hodgkin's lymphoma by whole-body MRI: comparison with bone and 67Ga scintigraphies. *Eur Radiol* 2004;14:1074–1081.
15. Kellenberger CJ, Miller SF, Khan M, et al. Initial experience with FSE STIR whole-body MR imaging for staging lymphoma in children. *Eur Radiol* 2004;14:1829–1841.
16. Kellenberger CJ, Epelman M, Miller SF, et al. Fast STIR whole-body MR imaging in children. *Radiographics* 2004;24:1317–1330.
17. Steinborn MM, Heuck AF, Tiling R, et al. Whole-body bone marrow MRI in patients with metastatic disease to the skeletal system. *J Comput Assist Tomogr* 1999;23:123–129.
18. Walker R, Kessar P, Blanchard R, et al. Turbo STIR magnetic resonance imaging as a whole-body screening tool for metastases in patients with breast carcinoma: preliminary clinical experience. *J Magn Reson Imaging* 2000; 11:343–350.
19. North LB, Libshitz HI, Lorigan JG. Thoracic lymphoma. *Radiol Clin North Am* 1990;28:745–762.
20. Wernecke K, Vassallo P, Rutsch F, et al. Thymic involvement in Hodgkin disease: CT and sonographic findings. *Radiology* 1991;181:375–383.
21. Shirkhoda A, Ros PR, Farah J, et al. Lymphoma of the solid abdominal viscera. *Radiol Clin North Am* 1990;28:785–799.
22. Rueffer U, Sieber M, Stemberg M, et al. Spleen involvement in Hodgkin's lymphoma: assessment and risk profile. *Ann Hematol* 2003; 82:390–396.
23. Coller BS, Chabner BA, Gralnick HR. Frequencies and patterns of bone marrow involvement in non-Hodgkin lymphomas: observations on the value of bilateral biopsies. *Am J Hematol* 1977;3:105–119.
24. Brunning RD, Bloomfield CD, McKenna RW, et al. Bilateral trephine bone marrow biopsies in lymphoma and other neoplastic diseases. *Ann Intern Med* 1975;82:365–366.
25. Mariette X, Zagdanski AM, Guermazi A, et al. Prognostic value of vertebral lesions detected by magnetic resonance imaging in patients with stage I multiple myeloma. *Br J Haematol* 1999;104:723–729.
26. Vande Berg BC, Michaux L, Scheiff JM, et al. Sequential quantitative MR analysis of bone marrow: differences during treatment of lymphoid versus myeloid leukemia. *Radiology* 1996;201:519–523.
27. Urba WJ, Longo DL. Hodgkin's disease. *N Engl J Med* 1992;326:678–687.
28. Sieber M, Ruffer U, Josting A, et al. Treatment of Hodgkin's disease: current strategies of the German Hodgkin's Lymphoma Study Group. *Ann Oncol* 1999;10(suppl 6):23–29.
29. Eich HT, Staar S, Gossmann A, et al. The HD12 panel of the German Hodgkin Lymphoma Study Group (GHSG): a quality assurance program based on a multidisciplinary panel reviewing all patients' imaging. *Am J Clin Oncol* 2004;27:279–284.
30. Atula TS, Varpula MJ, Kurki TJ, et al. Assessment of cervical lymph node status in head and neck cancer patients: palpation, computed tomography and low field magnetic resonance imaging compared with ultrasound-guided fine-needle aspiration cytology. *Eur J Radiol* 1997;25: 152–161.
31. Hilton S, Herr HW, Teitcher JB, et al. CT detection of retroperitoneal lymph node metastases in patients with clinical stage I testicular nonseminomatous germ cell cancer: assessment of size and distribution criteria. *AJR Am J Roentgenol* 1997;169:521–525.
32. Hogeboom WR, Hoekstra HJ, Mooyaart EL, et al. Magnetic resonance imaging of retroperitoneal lymph node metastases of non-seminomatous germ cell tumours of the testis. *Eur J Surg Oncol* 1993;19:429–437.
33. Weissleder R, Elizondo G, Wittenberg J, et al. Ultrasmall superparamagnetic iron oxide: an intravenous contrast agent for assessing lymph nodes with MR imaging. *Radiology* 1990;175:494–498.
34. Muhler A, Zhang X, Wang H, et al. Investigation of mechanisms influencing the accumulation of ultrasmall superparamagnetic iron oxide particles in lymph nodes. *Invest Radiol* 1995;30:98–103.
35. Vassallo P, Matei C, Heston WD, et al. AMI-227-enhanced MR lymphography: usefulness for differentiating reactive from tumor-bearing lymph nodes. *Radiology* 1994;193:501–506.
36. Chambon C, Clement O, Le Blanche A, et al. Superparamagnetic iron oxides as positive MR contrast agents: in vitro and in vivo evidence. *Magn Reson Imaging* 1993;11:509–519.
37. Harisinghani MG, Dixon WT, Saksena MA, et al. MR lymphangiography: imaging strategies to optimize the imaging of lymph nodes with ferumoxtran-10. *Radiographics* 2004;24:867–878.
38. Harisinghani MG, Saini S, Weissleder R, et al. MR lymphangiography using ultrasmall superparamagnetic iron oxide in patients with primary abdominal and pelvic malignancies: radiographic-pathologic correlation. *AJR Am J Roentgenol* 1999;172:1347–1351.
39. Bellin MF, Lebleu L, Meric JB. Evaluation of retroperitoneal and pelvic lymph node metastases with MRI and MR lymphangiography. *Abdom Imaging* 2003;28:155–163.
40. Mack MG, Balzer JO, Straub R, et al. Superparamagnetic iron oxide-enhanced MR imaging of head and neck lymph nodes. *Radiology* 2002;222:239–244.
41. Harisinghani MG, Barentsz J, Hahn PF, et al. Noninvasive detection of clinically occult lymph-node metastases in prostate cancer. *N Engl J Med* 2003;348:2491–2499.
42. Layer G, Sander W, Traber F, et al. The diagnostic problems in magnetic resonance tomography of the bone marrow in patients with malignomas under G-CSF therapy. *Radiologe* 2000;40:710–715.
43. Daldrup-Link HE, Rummeny EJ, Ihssen B, et al. Iron-oxide-enhanced MR imaging of bone marrow in patients with non-Hodgkin's lymphoma: differentiation between tumor infiltration and hypercellular bone marrow. *Eur Radiol* 2002;12:1557–1566.

CHAPTER 11 ■ FUNCTIONAL IMAGING IN HODGKIN LYMPHOMA

SUKRU MEHMET ERTURK, ANDREA K. NG, AND ANNICK D. VAN DEN ABBEELE

Acknowledgements

The authors gratefully acknowledge the help of Yulia Melenevsky, MD, and Agnieszka Szot-Barnes, MD, in the preparation of the figures.

NUCLEAR MEDICINE IN ONCOLOGY: AN OVERVIEW

Nuclear medicine is an imaging approach that distinguishes itself from those of conventional radiological techniques such as computed tomography (CT) and magnetic resonance imaging (MRI). While conventional imaging focuses on the anatomic structure and is dependent on structural changes in morphology or size, nuclear medicine has the ability to provide unique information on the metabolic function of the investigated organ, tissue, or system, at the molecular level. The nuclear medicine imaging technique involves the injection or ingestion of radiopharmaceuticals designed to track a physiologic or pathophysiologic process. In this context, radiopharmaceuticals are described as radiotracers. The unique potential of nuclear medicine in investigating any particular organ or disease is based on the great diversity and biochemical properties of the available radiotracers. The majority of radiotracers consist of two distinct moieties: a carrier, which is responsible for the biodistribution of the tracer (e.g., fluoro-2-deoxy-D-glucose [FDG], a glucose analog); and a radioactive marker, which enables the external detection of it (e.g., fluorine-18). Some radiotracers do not require a carrier (e.g., gallium-67, an iron analog, or thallium-201, a potassium analog) because of their biochemical properties. Nevertheless, regardless of their structure, the common characteristic of all radiotracers is that they can be metabolized through certain physiologic or pathophysiologic processes that are correlated with physiologic or pathologic conditions of target organs or tissues.[1–3]

In order to comprehensively understand the potential of nuclear medicine in the diagnosis of diseases, one must possess a basic knowledge of the specific methodology that Badawi's review outlines.[4] In short, the simplest nuclear medicine imaging technique is planar imaging, which provides functional images in a two-dimensional format that is similar to that obtained with x-ray imaging in radiology. The planar images are obtained on gamma camera systems that typically contain scintillation detection material, such as sodium iodide crystals. Single photon emission computed tomography (SPECT) is another nuclear medicine imaging technique that has the capability to provide cross-sectional functional images throughout the body. Finally, nuclear medicine imaging may also be performed using positron emission tomography (PET), which allows the use of positron-emitting radionuclides and a range of new radiotracers.

With its unique functional imaging capabilities, nuclear oncology is a rapidly growing field within nuclear medicine and has become an integral part of the multidisciplinary clinical care for patients with cancer. This chapter focuses on nuclear medicine imaging techniques and therapeutic procedures used in the management of patients with Hodgkin lymphoma. The first part of the chapter analyzes the role of FDG-PET in imaging of patients with Hodgkin lymphoma. The second part focuses on gallium-67 citrate imaging. Although this modality has been widely replaced by FDG-PET in this group of patients, gallium-67 citrate still remains a very useful tool in centers where FDG-PET is not available.

FLUORINE-18-FLUORO-2-DEOXY-D-GLUCOSE (FDG) POSITRON EMISSION TOMOGRAPHY

Fluorine-18-fluoro-2-deoxy-D-glucose (FDG) positron emission tomography (FDG-PET) is a rapidly evolving whole-body functional imaging technique. PET with FDG (FDG-PET) takes advantage of the fact that malignant tumors have an increased rate of aerobic glycolysis compared to normal tissues, a phenomenon Warburg first observed in 1931.[5] Most tumors demonstrate an increase in glucose transporters such as GLUT 1 as well as increased hexokinase and decreased glucose-6-phosphatase activity resulting in the retention of the glucose analog FDG.[4,6,7] FDG-PET has proven useful in the characterization of tissues and residual masses, staging and restaging, the evaluation of therapeutic response, and the detection of recurrence in many human cancers.[8,9] The Centers for Medicaid and Medicare Services (CMS) have recognized the utility of FDG-PET in the management of patients with cancer and have approved reimbursement for the diagnosis, staging, and restaging of patients with lymphomas and other malignancies such as non-small cell lung, esophageal, colorectal, breast, head and neck cancers, thyroid cancer, melanoma, and solitary pulmonary nodule characterization.[10] Furthermore, CMS has recently established a National Oncologic PET Registry (NOPR) program to expand coverage for FDG-PET to include cancers and indications not previously eligible for Medicare reimbursement.[11] Cancer imaging with FDG-PET is now one of the most dynamic and rapidly growing areas of contemporary nuclear medicine and clinical imaging.

Physical Properties and Pharmacokinetics

In contrast to single photon emitters used in conventional nuclear medicine imaging, the radionuclides used for radiolabeling in FDG-PET are positron emitters (a type of beta particle, signified by β^+), which will penetrate only a millimeter or so in soft tissues prior to combining with an electron (β^-). The particle pair then undergoes an annihilation reaction in which their masses are entirely converted into the form of two 511-keV annihilation photons, emitted at approximately 180° to each other. Detection of both annihilation photons within a certain time frame (known as a coincidence time window) is termed annihilation coincidence detection; annihilation coincidence represents the basic principle by which FDG-PET scanners operate. The positron emitting radionuclides used for clinical imaging are typically produced by a cyclotron and possess relatively short half-lives. The most widely used tracer in clinical PET applications is a fluorine-18-labeled analog of glucose (FDG). The fluorine-18 has a half-life of 109.8 minutes, allowing acquisition of images over 30 to 120 minutes at reasonable data rates.[12]

FDG is transported into viable cells by facilitative glucose transporter molecules (such as GLUT 1), where it is phosphorylated by hexokinase to FDG-6-phosphate just as glucose is phosphorylated to glucose-6-phosphate.[1] However, unlike glucose-6-phosphate, FDG-6-phosphate does not undergo further metabolism within the cell. Moreover, its dephosphorylation by glucose-6-phosphatase is a relatively slow process compared to that of glucose-6-phosphate. Thus, because FDG-6-phosphate cannot easily cross the cell membrane, it becomes "trapped" within viable cells. The entrapment is very prominent in malignant cells, which typically have higher glucose transport molecules at their surface, higher hexokinase activity, and either low levels of glucose-6-phosphatase or lack it altogether.[5-7]

Physiologic Distribution of FDG

Brain cortex, basal ganglia, and thalami typically show high uptake of FDG. The cortical activity is depressed following the use of sedative or anesthetic drugs, but still remains higher than that seen in other normal tissues.[12]

The uptake of FDG by the normal myocardium is variable, as myocardial metabolism physiologically depends on both glucose and free fatty acids.[13-15] Because intense myocardial FDG uptake may impair the detection of malignant lesions in the mediastinum and lungs during oncologic FDG-PET studies, it is recommended that patients fast for 4 to 6 hours prior to tracer administration. The fast enhances myocardial fatty acid metabolism and reduces myocardial uptake of glucose and FDG. Diabetic patients and insulin-dependent patients need to have their blood glucose level measured prior to the test. Performing the test in a hyperinsulinemic state may result in intense striated muscle uptake and the risk of a false-negative scan.

Accumulation of FDG in skeletal muscle depends predominantly on its metabolic activity; skeletal muscle at rest typically shows low FDG uptake.[14,15] For that reason, patients are asked to refrain from intense exercise 24 hours prior to and on the day of the FDG-PET scan. Simple arrangements aimed at optimizing patient comfort and room temperature may also help to reduce nonspecific brown fat uptake that may impair the interpretation of the study; particularly if it is seen within the neck, pectoral, and axillary regions. Oral sedation with 5 mg of Valium may help reduce muscle uptake if clinically indicated (Fig. 11.1)

Unlike glucose, the kidneys excrete FDG, which means that the renal collecting system, ureters, and urinary bladder visualize on FDG-PET images. In the liver and to a lesser extent in the spleen, a low-grade uptake of FDG is typically

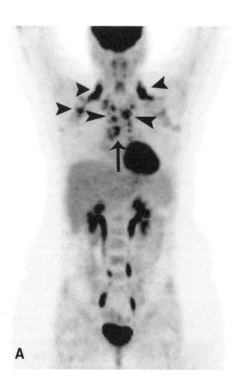
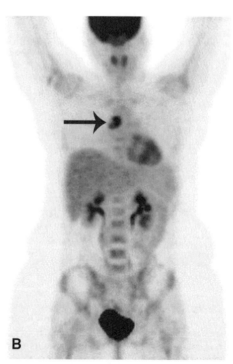

FIGURE 11.1. Patient with Hodgkin lymphoma undergoing FDG-PET for restaging. The initial scan (A) demonstrates intense FDG uptake in regions of brown fat *(arrowheads)* obscuring the uptake in the primary disease site *(arrow)*. Repeat scan (B) after 5 mg Valium p.o. shows resolution of brown fat uptake and clear demonstration of disease site *(arrow)*.

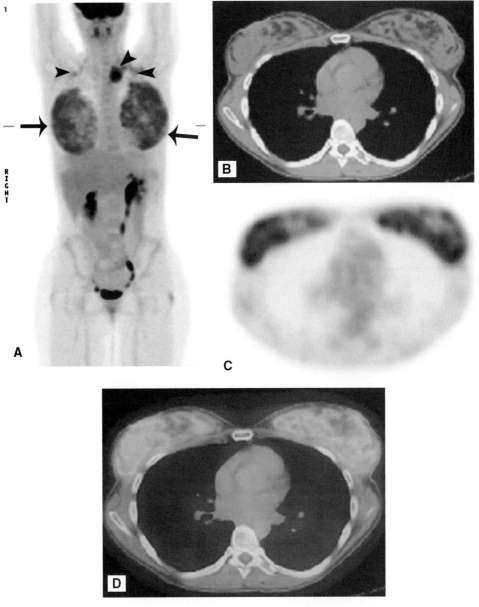

FIGURE 11.2. Patient with Hodgkin lymphoma in recent postpartum status undergoing FDG-PET/CT scan for staging. Coronal PET image (**A**) demonstrates FDG-uptake of lymph nodes in the left paratracheal and supraclavicular *(arrowheads)* regions; in addition, there is bilateral intense FDG-uptake in breast. Axial CT (**B**), PET (**C**), and fused PET/CT (**D**) images clearly demonstrate the FDG-uptake in the breast tissue.

seen in the abdomen. Nevertheless, this uptake is lower than the background uptake seen with gallium-67 scintigraphy and suggests that FDG-PET scanning has a higher sensitivity for detection of disease in these organs than gallium-67 scintigraphy, particularly in the spleen. In the stomach and intestine, normal uptake of FDG is variable. Bowel preparation can be used but requires procedures similar to those used prior to colonoscopy[5,15]and may be too invasive for the oncologic patient population.

Additionally, physiologic FDG uptake can be seen postpartum in the breast tissue, as demonstrated in Figure 11.2. It can be also seen in thymic remnants (thymic rebound), as shown in Figure 11.3.

Benign Pathologic Conditions Accumulating FDG

Various benign diseases and conditions that are usually related to infections or inflammatory changes may show high uptake of FDG and mimic malignancy on PET scans.[15] Granulomatous diseases, including tuberculosis, sarcoidosis, glandular fever, and Epstein-Barr virus infection may cause widespread lymphadenopathy and mimic lymphoma. False-positive FDG uptake may also be seen in histoplasmosis, coccidioidomycosis, pyogenic infections, sites of inflammatory changes post-radiation therapy, and postoperative wound healing.[15]

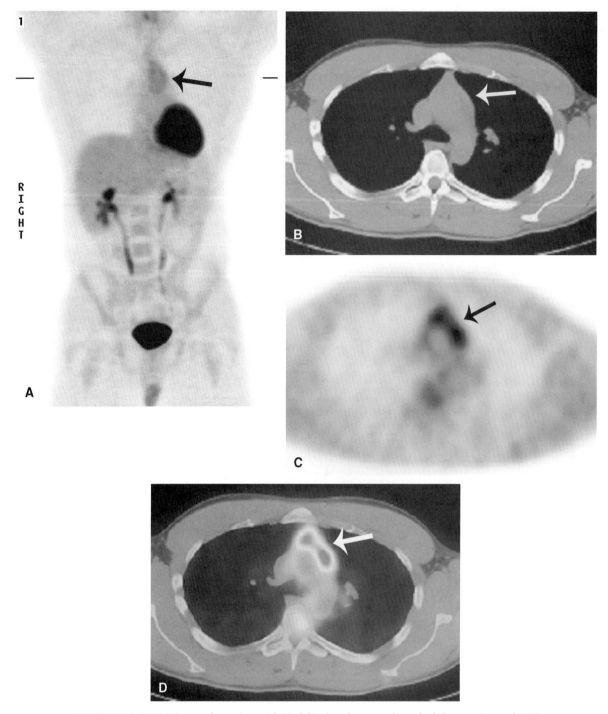

FIGURE 11.3. PET/CT scan of a patient with Hodgkin lymphoma at the end of therapy. Coronal PET image (A) demonstrates mild FDG uptake within the mediastinum. Axial CT (B), PET (C), and fused PET/CT (D) images demonstrate that this uptake is within the thymus gland.

FDG-PET has been reported to correctly detect bone marrow involvement in the majority of lymphoma patients studied before the onset of therapy.[16] Nevertheless, diffuse homogenous bone marrow FDG uptake can also be seen after treatment secondary to physiologic reactive changes and drugs resulting in bone marrow expansion (Fig.11.4).[16] Familiarity with all these benign conditions showing high FDG-uptake is important when interpreting FDG-PET studies.

FDG-PET and Hodgkin Lymphoma

Initial Staging

At one time, a staging laparotomy was the accepted standard of diagnostic procedures in newly diagnosed Hodgkin lymphoma.[17] Later, computed tomography (CT) became the

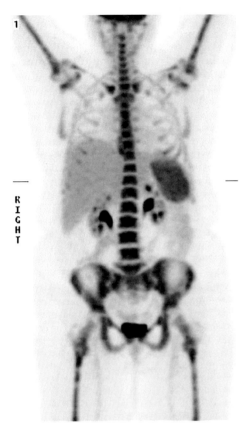

FIGURE 11.4. Patient with Hodgkin lymphoma who was recently treated with a bone marrow expansion drug (Neulasta) showing intense uptake throughout bone marrow and spleen in the context of secondary hematopoiesis.

first-line imaging modality in Hodgkin lymphoma and was essential tool for the Cotswold staging classification process.[18] Occasionally, magnetic resonance imaging (MRI) is used to evaluate suspected extranodal disease or bone marrow involvement.[19] In recent years, FDG-PET has proved to be a very valuable tool in the management of many malignancies, including Hodgkin lymphoma and non-Hodgkin lymphomas. The accuracy of FDG-PET is now considered superior to that of gallium scintigraphy which was introduced in the early 1970s and was incorporated in the management of lymphomas 10 years later due to its relatively high accuracy compared to those of anatomic imaging modalities such as CT or ultrasound.[20]

Currently, cancer hospitals use FDG-PET scanning in lymphomas for staging and restaging, prediction of outcome, evaluation of residual masses seen on CT after treatment, and post-treatment surveillance.

There are many studies reporting high accuracy rates for FDG-PET in initial staging of patients with Hodgkin lymphoma. In their study published in 1998, Bangerter and colleagues[21] discovered that FDG-PET findings led to a change in treatment in 6 of 44 (14%) patients with Hodgkin lymphoma; 5 patients were upstaged and 1 was downstaged. FDG-PET was positive in 38 patients at documented sites, failed to visualize disease in 4 patients, and the FDG-PET results were false-positive in 2 patients. FDG-PET and conventional methods were concordant in 128 (96%) of the 133 diseased lymph node regions. Extranodal lesions were identified in 6 patients. Three patients had involvement of the liver and an additional 3 patients showed involvement of the lung. FDG-PET was able to demonstrate extranodal disease in 4 of these patients, whereas conventional methods found 3 patients with extranodal disease. This study was the first to demonstrate on a reasonably large number of patients that FDG-PET can be used efficiently in the management of patients with Hodgkin lymphoma.[19]

Partridge and associates studied 44 patients with Hodgkin lymphoma and they reported that, because of FDG-PET findings, the disease was upstaged in 41% of patients and downstaged in 7% of patients.[22] Treatment was changed in 25% of patients as the result of metabolic imaging. Of the 18 cases that were upstaged, 6 had occult splenic involvement that was undetected on the CT. In a study by Hueltenschmidt and colleagues, 3 of 25 patients scanned as a part of initial staging were upstaged and 7 patients were downstaged by FDG-PET.[23] In this study, the staging accuracy of FDG-PET was found to be much higher than that of conventional methods (96% versus 56%).

A study by Jerusalem and associates is the first thorough study of region-by-region accuracy in Hodgkin lymphoma.[24] In this study, 33 patients were scanned before initial treatment or before treatment of relapse, and the impact on nodal staging was evaluated. Moreover, this study showed that the sensitivity of FDG-PET for detecting involved lymph node regions was 95% in peripheral regions, 96% in thoracic regions, and 78% in abdominal/pelvic regions. The corresponding sensitivities for conventional methods were 80%, 81%, and 86%. FDG-PET suggested downstaging in 4 patients and upstaging in 3. Using a similar approach, Weihrauch and associates examined 22 patients with Hodgkin lymphoma and found involvement of 72 regions.[25] In 48 lesions in 22 patients, both CT and FDG-PET were positive; 20 lesions in 11 patients were positive on FDG-PET but not detected by CT or other conventional modalities. Six patients had 9 CT-positive, FDG-PET-negative sites. The authors determined a gold standard using all available clinical information at a timepoint at least 6 months after the initial staging procedures. Both FDG-PET and CT have a specificity of 100%; their sensitivities were 88% and 74%, respectively. In a prospective study, Menzel and co-workers discovered a change in staging in 6 of 21 patients with Hodgkin lymphoma (21%).[26] Recently, in a prospective study of 88 patients with Hodgkin lymphoma, Naumann and associates demonstrated a change in staging in 18 patients (20%).[27] The treatment in this study was based on the findings of conventional modalities only. Otherwise, the FDG-PET findings would have led to changes in the management of 16 patients (18%). Munker and associates staged a total of 73 patients with newly diagnosed Hodgkin lymphoma with both conventional methods and whole-body FDG-PET scanning.[17] A total of 21% patients (28.8%) were upstaged by FDG-PET compared with conventional methods. In two cases (2.7%), a lower stage was suggested by FDG-PET scanning.

Finally, Isasi and colleagues conducted a metaanalysis of the published literature to evaluate the diagnostic performance of FDG-PET in the staging and restaging of patients with lymphoma.[28] They reported a median sensitivity and specificity of 93.2% and 87.7% among patients with Hodgkin lymphoma. They concluded that FDG-PET is a very accurate imaging modality for the staging and restaging of patients with lymphoma with a high sensitivity and specificity reported.

To date, FDG-PET is becoming the first instead of the final test performed for staging patients with newly diagnosed Hodgkin lymphoma.[29] The major advantage of FDG-PET over conventional imaging modalities is its ability to detect disease in structures without any morphologic abnormality. In short, the existing evidence shows that in patients with Hodgkin lymphoma, FDG-PET improves the accuracy of initial staging, especially if it results in upstaging.

Early Treatment Response

Today, more aggressive but also more toxic treatments are available for patients with Hodgkin lymphoma. Patients with Hodgkin lymphoma are examined regularly during as well as after the treatment to determine if the desired treatment outcome is being reached.[19,30–32] To date, the response monitoring is mainly based on morphologic criteria and a reduction in tumor size on CT is the most important determinant. Nevertheless, morphologic imaging techniques such as CT are inefficient at differentiating responders from nonresponders in terms of early monitoring. In fact, using CT findings as criteria for early response may label an unacceptable number of patients as nonresponders or poor responders and consequently expose them to more aggressive or experimental therapies. However, these patients could benefit from conventional chemotherapy regimens and achieve durable complete responses.[30] Similarly, when evaluating the initial treatment response, a reduction in tumor size of 50% should not be expected before the fourth cycle of chemotherapy is completed. Indeed, during this time to response, the nonresponders wait a long and costly time before the appropriate changes of treatment are made while they receive a suboptimal therapy.[19]

Promising results with FDG-PET can be obtained when evaluating treatment response.[33] Because glucose provides the primary source of carbons for the de novo synthesis of nucleic acids, lipids, and amino acids, FDG uptake is closely related to the number and proliferation capacity of viable cells.[30] An example of staging of a patient with Hodgkin lymphoma is shown in Figure 11.5, which demonstrates resolution of all FDG-avid sites including the spleen.

Hoekstra and colleagues presented the first report suggesting a role for FDG in the monitoring of lymphoma therapy in 1993.[34] In this study, 26 patients, 13 of them with Hodgkin lymphoma, were examined with FDG-PET before treatment, following two courses of chemotherapy, and after the full treatment. After two courses, FDG uptake had decreased considerably in most of the patients with Hodgkin lymphoma and the decrease exceeded the tumor volume reduction. Negative FDG-PET scans preceded complete remission in 8 of the 13 Hodgkin lymphoma patients. Two patients with abnormal FDG uptake were also clinically suspected of therapeutic inefficacy and shifted to more intensive treatment. This early investigation showed that FDG imaging possesses strong prognostic capabilities.

Kostakoglu and associates[35] performed FDG-PET scans before and after one cycle of chemotherapy in 13 patients with Hodgkin lymphoma. Results after one course were correlated with disease status at completion of treatment. All those patients who had a positive FDG-PET scan after one cycle of chemotherapy had progressive disease except one patient who had thymic rebound, a condition known to cause false-positive

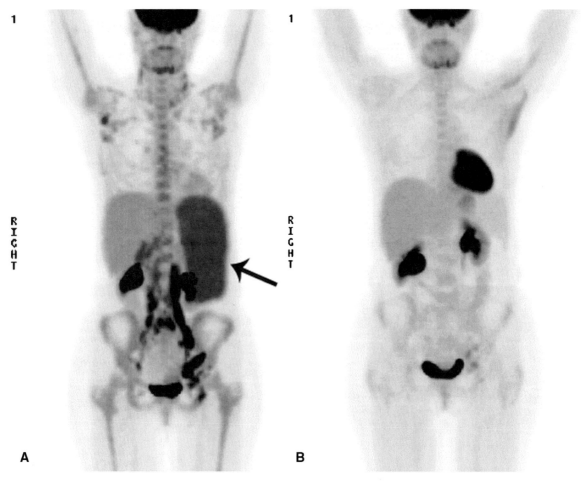

FIGURE 11.5. FDG-PPET scan in a patient with Hodgkin lymphoma: Staging scan (**A**) demonstrates intense FDG-uptake within an enlarged spleen *(arrow)* and FDG-avid lymphadenopathy above and below the diaphragm including bilateral cervical, supraclavicular, axillary, paraaortic, iliac, and inguinal lymph nodes. Midtreatment scan (**B**) shows complete resolution including the splenic involvement.

findings.[36,37] Only one patient with a negative FDG-PET scan had disease progression. In a recent study from our institution, Friedberg and associates reported similar results.[38] In this study, 22 patients with Hodgkin lymphoma underwent FDG-PET scanning after three cycles of chemotherapy. After a median follow-up of 24 months, 4 out of 5 interim FDG-PET–positive patients progressed and 15 out of 17 FDG-PET–negative patients were in continued remission.

More recently, Hutchings and associates investigated[39] a total of 85 patients with Hodgkin lymphoma. After two or three cycles of chemotherapy, 63 patients had negative FDG-PET scans, 9 patients had minimal residual uptake, and 13 patients had positive scans. Three FDG-PET–negative patients and one patient with minimal residual uptake have relapsed. In the FDG-PET–positive group, 9 patients progressed and 2 died. Survival analyses showed highly significant associations between early interim FDG-PET and progression free survival ($p < 0.0001$) and overall survival ($p < 0.03$). In this study, all advanced-stage patients with positive interim FDG-PET scans relapsed within 2 years.

In summary, FDG-PET may probably offer a reliable method for early prediction of long-term remission and progression-free survival in Hodgkin lymphoma. In addition, it may guide further therapy based on early FDG-PET responses. Currently, the EORTC/GELA group is planning to conduct a prospective randomized study in patients with early-stage Hodgkin lymphoma, evaluating whether radiation therapy can be omitted in patients with a negative FDG-PET scan after two cycles of ABVD, with the comparison arm being the standard treatment of combined modality therapy. The results of this trial may help to establish the role of FDG-PET in response-adapted therapy for early-stage Hodgkin lymphoma. The ongoing GHSG HL-15 trial on advanced-stage Hodgkin lymphoma is comparing three variations of the bleomycin, etoposide, doxorubicin, cyclophosphamide, vincristine, procarbazine, and prednisone (BEACOPP) regimen. In this study, involved-field radiation therapy is added only for those with residual disease of 2.5 cm or greater and positive FDG-PET at the end of the chemotherapy. Using these criteria, about 10% of patients are receiving radiation therapy on this trial. Results of this study, when available, will provide information on the usefulness of functional imaging post-chemotherapy in guiding the decision for consolidative radiation therapy.

Assessment of Response after First-Line Treatment—Evaluation of a Residual Mass

According to conventional imaging methods, the tumor mass regresses completely in some patients with Hodgkin lymphoma after first-line therapy and these patients are considered in complete remission.[19] Conventional methods can also clearly identify a few patients as definitely non-responders. Nevertheless, in a larger group of patients, there is uncertainty as to whether a truly complete remission has been achieved. In fact, in some series and trials, they use the designation "uncertain complete response."

After the completion of first-line therapy, it is crucial to distinguish the patients who need additional therapy from those who do not.[19] In patients where the residual tumor is still viable, second-line therapy should be initiated immediately to optimize the outcome. In contrast, second-line therapy should be avoided in patients with a non-viable residual mass, because of the therapy-related toxicity. Unfortunately, in approximately two-thirds of Hodgkin lymphoma patients, a residual lymphoma mass is present on the CT after first-line therapy and only 20% will eventually relapse. It is in this setting of the residual mass that to date FDG-PET has been shown to have the greatest utility in several studies (Fig. 11.6).[33,40]

Hueltenschmidt and associates assessed the clinical value of FDG-PET compared with conventional imaging modalities for treatment monitoring and assessment in 51 patients with Hodgkin lymphoma.[23] They reported an accuracy of 91% for FDG-PET compared with 62% for conventional imaging methods. Weihrauch and associates studied 28 patients with Hodgkin lymphoma with a residual mass of at least 2 cm. within four months of therapy.[41] The one-year, progression-free survival was 95% for the FDG-PET negative group, and 40% for FDG-PET positive group. In a study with a similar prospective approach, De Wit and associates studied 37 patients with Hodgkin lymphoma who had a residual mass both before and after additional radiotherapy.[42] In their study, FDG-PET showed a sensitivity and specificity of 91% and 69%, respectively, for the prediction of disease-free survival. Naumann and associates examined 43 patients with Hodgkin lymphoma and with post-treatment residual masses.[43] Within a mean follow-up period of 35.5 months, all 28 patients with negative FDG-PET scans were in continued complete remission. Four patients had positive scans; however, only one of those relapsed whereas three patients entered and remained in complete remission during the follow-up periods of 21, 34, and 50 months, respectively. This study presented the evidence that a post-treatment FDG-PET has a very high negative predictive value at short term, but that a positive FDG-PET does not in itself predict short-term relapse.

Spaepen and associates evaluated 60 patients with Hodgkin lymphoma with or without residual masses at the end of first-line treatment.[44] Fifty-five of these patients had normal scanning results; only five of them have relapsed with a median follow-up of 32 months. All of five patients with abnormal FDG-PET findings have relapsed during follow-up. Two-year, progression-free survival was 91% for FDG-PET negative patients and 0% for FDG-PET positive patients. In a similar retrospective study of Guay et al., 48 patients with Hodgkin lymphoma underwent FDG-PET after the completion of chemotherapy.[45] In this study, the sensitivity and specificity of FDG-PET to predict relapse were 79% and 97% respectively. Moreover, the diagnostic accuracy (92%) of FDG-PET was significantly higher than the accuracy of CT (56%; $p < 0.0005$).

The data from these and other similar studies suggest that FDG-PET has strong prognostic properties for evaluating patients with Hodgkin lymphoma after first-line therapy. Nevertheless, FDG uptake is unfortunately not specific for tumoral tissue.[31,46] In particular, when abnormal FDG uptake is observed outside the initially involved sites, inflammatory or infectious processes need to be ruled out through correlating FDG-PET findings with clinical data and other imaging modalities before starting salvage therapy.[31,46]

Currently, there is a lack of definitive data on the optimal interval from the end of treatment to the first post-therapy follow-up PET scan. To allow time for response and to avoid false-positive results due to therapy-related inflammatory changes, we recommend scanning at approximately 3 months post-treatment, unless there are suspicious clinical findings that warrant earlier evaluation. This recommendation may change, however, when data addressing this question become available.

Follow-Up and Relapse

After a satisfactory response to first-line therapy and the induction of complete remission, 10% to 30% of patients with Hodgkin lymphoma will still experience a relapse,[19] and early recognition of recurrence is crucial for the outcome.[47] Unfortunately, CT or other morphologic imaging methods are not able to precisely differentiate post-therapeutic changes from recurrent disease.[48] Given the fact that FDG uptake depends on the metabolic state of the lesion in question and considering the promising results of FDG-PET studies for

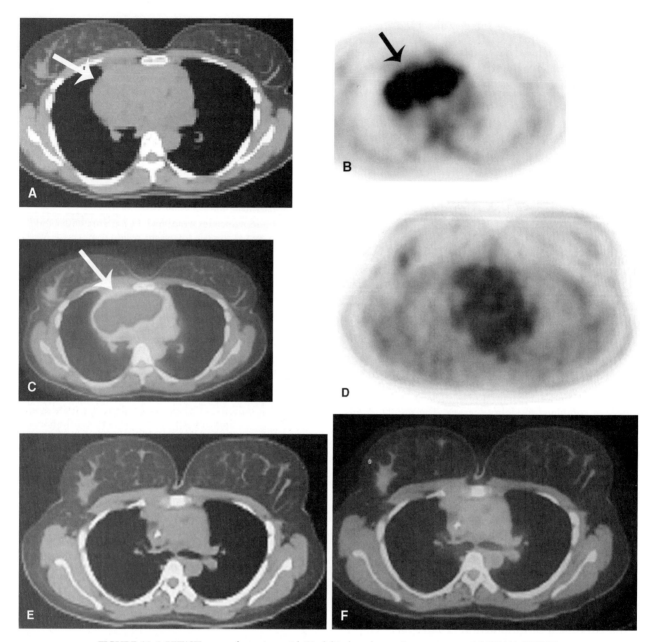

FIGURE 11.6. PET/CT scans of a patient with Hodgkin lymphoma. Pretreatment axial CT (**A**), PET (**B**), and fused PET/CT (**C**) images demonstrate a large FDG-avid anterior mediastinal mass. Follow-up PET scan (**D**) demonstrates complete resolution of the mass despite the presence of a residual mass on CT image (**E**); fused PET/CT image (**F**) confirms the diagnosis of complete resolution.

initial staging as well as treatment monitoring, FDG-PET is considered an important diagnostic tool for follow-up of patients with Hodgkin lymphoma.

Jerusalem and associates examined the value of FDG-PET for detecting preclinical relapse in 36 patients with Hodgkin lymphoma.[49] In this study, the patients were evaluated with FDG-PET just after the procedure and every 4 to 6 months for a 2- to 3-year period after the completion of first-line therapy. Six patients had false-positive initial scans after the end of first-line therapy, but follow-up scans were negative in all of them. Five patients who had residual tumor or relapse had positive FDG-PET findings. One of the most important findings of this study is that only two of the five patients had clinical symptoms at the time of relapse identified with FDG-PET.

The results of the study by Jerusalem and colleagues suggest a role for FDG-PET in detecting relapse in clinically asymptomatic patients or in patients with equivocal conventional radiologic findings. Thus, FDG-PET may enable this group of patients to receive salvage therapy with minimal disease rather than at overt relapse.[50]

Fusion of PET and CT

Fusion of PET image sets that provide functional information with anatomic images sets of CT and MRI systems are of considerable help in numerous clinical circumstances. In the past, visual fusion of the anatomic and functional image sets was typically considered as sufficient. In cases in which a more precise anatomic localization was needed, technologists used software fusion to combine the two sets of images.[51,52] Available data show that fusion of PET and CT images improves the spatial localization of a wide range of foci with increased FDG uptake found within the body.[53–57] Nevertheless, outside of the brain, software fusion is difficult and often unsuccessful as a result of the many factors that occur when using two different modalities to capture the image of the human body on two different occasions.[53] This situation changed dramatically with the introduction of the integrated PET/CT scanners. Today, integrated PET/CT scanners allow technologists to acquire accurately align PET and CT images in a single setting and thus minimize the temporal and spatial differences between the two sets of images. PET/CT image acquisition will be the imaging standard choice in the future; there are continuing efforts to develop combined PET and MRI systems.[51,52]

In fact, PET technology is mostly sold as combined PET/CT scanners and they are now commonplace in most PET centers. The first system of its kind was developed at the University of Pittsburgh (PA); it consisted of a third-generation CT scanner and a rotating partial-ring PET scanner combined in a single gantry.[53,54] Martinelli and associates reviewed the results from over 100 patients studied on this scanner, covering a wide range of malignancies including lung, colorectal, head and neck, and ovarian cancer as well as lymphoma and melanoma.[55] According to this study, the combined PET/CT modality resulted in improved distinction of pathologic from normal physiologic uptake, more accurate localization of functional abnormalities, and enhanced efficacy at monitoring the patient's response to therapy.

GALLIUM-67 CITRATE IMAGING

Gallium-67 citrate was initially developed as a nuclear medicine agent for bone imaging. However, gallium-67 has also proved to accumulate in malignancies other than those originating from bones, including tumors of the lungs, soft tissues, and head and neck. Edward and Hayes reported the role of gallium-67 citrate in lymphoma as early as 1969.[58] During the subsequent years, gallium-67 citrate scanning has been recognized as a valuable and functional tool for the assessment of tumor viability. Consequently, the use of gallium-67 for staging, restaging, and follow-up of patients with lymphomas continued to increase.[1,59,60]

Although, when available, FDG-PET has widely replaced gallium-67 citrate scintigraphy in the staging, restaging, and follow-up of patients with Hodgkin lymphoma, gallium-67 citrate is still considered a very useful tool when FDG-PET or PET/CT technology is not accessible.

Physical Properties and Pharmacokinetics

Gallium-67 is a group IIIA metal with a half-life of 78 hours and behaves as a ferric ion analogue. The bombardment of zinc-68 in a cyclotron produces this metal, and it decays when an electron capture emits a range of gamma rays from 91 to 394 keV. In vivo, because it behaves as a ferric ion analogue, it binds to iron-binding proteins such as transferrin, lactoferrin, haptoglobulin, ferritin, and bacterial siderophores. Although gallium competes with iron for binding to transferrin, it does not form heme because gallium-67 cannot be reduced in vivo from its +3 oxidation state to interact with protoporphyrins.[1,61] Several diverse mechanisms are proposed to explain the penetration of gallium-67 into viable tumor cells, including tumor cell-surface binding via the transferrin receptor CD-71 and active transport into the cytoplasm. After penetrating tumor cells, gallium-67 localizes in lysosomal-like granules. Due to its uptake mechanisms, gallium-67 accumulation can occur in living cells but not in necrotic or scar tissue.

Physiological Distribution of Gallium-67

The normal biodistribution of gallium-67 makes possible the physiologic visualization of the kidneys and urinary bladder between 24 and 48 hours after the injection. During this time period, the kidneys excrete approximately 15% of the gallium-67.[62] The large intestine is a critical organ regarding the radiation-absorbed dose from gallium-67 (0.9 rad/mCi). Furthermore, the presence of activity within the bowel may interfere with the interpretation of gallium scans below the diaphragm on planar images.[63] In fact, when planar imaging is used alone, delayed images up to 14 days after the injection of gallium-67 are required in order to differentiate normal intestinal clearance from pathologic tumor accumulation. The introduction of SPECT has substantially reduced the need for delayed scanning, because the improved anatomic localization that SPECT provides allows differentiating normal physiologic excretion within the bowel from pathologic uptake. The routine use of SPECT for evaluation of the abdomen and pelvis is particularly crucial and increases both the sensitivity and the specificity of the scan, as it does in the chest. Moreover, negative SPECT can rule out disease with a confidence interval of 81% to 96%.[64–67]

Liver, spleen, bone and bone marrow, salivary and lacrimal glands, anterior nasopharynx, thymus and epiphyseal regions in children, soft tissues, external genitalia and female breast (particularly postpartum and during lactation due to gallium-67 binding to lactoferrin) may also show physiologic gallium-67 uptake. On the third day after the injection, splenic uptake is usually mild and less intense compared to that seen in the liver. On days 7 to 14 following the injection, however, the splenic uptake is routinely higher than hepatic uptake. Focal uptake within the spleen at any timepoint should be considered pathologic. Diffuse bone marrow uptake is commonly seen in anemic patients, during chemotherapy, and with bone marrow expansion drugs. Although focal increased bone marrow uptake means worry for pathologic bone marrow involvement, radiotherapy may result in focal decreased bone marrow uptake within the radiation field.

In the postpartum period, gallium-67 scanning is contraindicated in women who wish to breastfeed because gallium-67 is excreted into the milk.

Gallium-67 Scintigraphy and Hodgkin Lymphoma

Gallium-67 uptake indicates the presence of viable lymphoma, and therefore the primary role of gallium-67 scanning is in the follow-up of Hodgkin lymphoma patients for monitoring response to treatment and differentiating between residual viable tumors and residual nontumoral masses after treatment (Fig. 11.7).[68–72]

If gallium-67 scintigraphy is used in the management of a patient with lymphoma, a baseline study prior to therapy is essential in order to demonstrate the initial tumor avidity for gallium and the extent of the disease. Once gallium avidity has been demonstrated at baseline, gallium-67 scintigraphy can be used as a functional imaging tool to determine the viability of that tissue in the course of therapy or in the follow-up. However, a baseline gallium-67 scan may be also of value in the initial staging, detecting up to 10% additional lymphoma sites in normal-size lymph nodes, and also excluding disease in other suspicious lesions.[68,73] Failure to perform baseline gallium-67 scanning prior to initiation of therapy significantly increases the risk of subsequent false-negative scintigraphic findings.[74,75] False-negative gallium-67 scans at baseline may be seen if the patient has received steroid therapy or if therapy

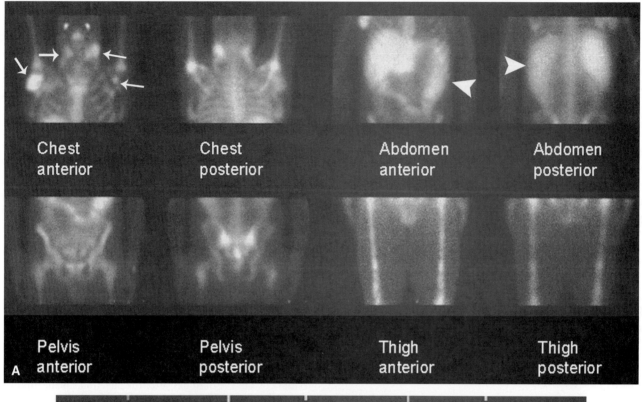

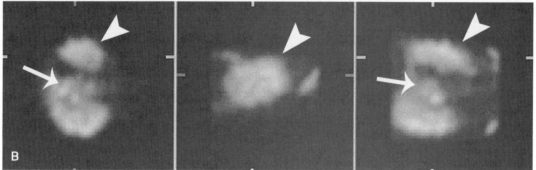

FIGURE 11.7. Staging of a patient with Hodgkin lymphoma. Planar scintigraphy (**A**) of the chest, abdomen, pelvis, and thighs demonstrates abnormal uptake of gallium-67 in the bilateral cervical and axillary lymph nodes *(arrows)* and spleen *(arrowheads)*. (**B**) Axial *(top)*, sagittal *(middle)*, and coronal *(bottom)* SPECT slices through the upper abdomen demonstrate intense uptake within the spleen *(arrowhead)* and within a paraaortic lymph node *(arrow)*.

was initiated prior to the injection of gallium-67 citrate. Therapy may be initiated a few hours, but preferably 24 to 48 hours, following the injection of gallium-67 without resulting in a false-negative scan at the 72-hour timepoint.

Regarding the early assessment of response to therapy in patients with Hodgkin lymphoma, Front and associates evaluated the role of gallium-67 scanning early during treatment in 98 patients with Hodgkin lymphoma.[76] Thirty-one patients underwent gallium-67 scintigraphy after one cycle of chemotherapy and 83 patients after a mean 3.5 cycles (16 patients underwent gallium-67 scintigraphy both after one cycle and at midtreatment). Failure-free survival differed significantly between patients with positive and negative gallium-67 scintigrams after one chemotherapy cycle but, interestingly, not at midtreatment. In this study, 22 of 24 patients (92%) with negative gallium-67 scintigrams after one cycle and 64 of 78 patients (82%) with negative scintigrams at midtreatment remained in complete response. In 4 of 7 patients (57%) with

positive gallium-67 scintigrams after one cycle, treatment failed. The authors concluded that using gallium-67 scintigraphy after one cycle of chemotherapy is a good early predictor of outcome of Hodgkin lymphoma.

Because gallium-67 uptake within a mass reflects uptake within viable cancer cells, gallium-67 scintigraphy has proved to be a suitable indicator of complete response at the end of induction chemotherapy, particularly when a residual mass persists after treatment. Several studies have demonstrated that restaging gallium-67 scans after the therapy could differentiate patients with a high probability of prolonged disease-free survival from patients who fail to respond to initial therapy and who are more likely to have a poor outcome. Persistent positive gallium-67 scans in patients with Hodgkin lymphoma can therefore be used to identify patients who need more aggressive therapy.

In a retrospective study from our institution, Ng and coworkers evaluated 175 patients with Hodgkin lymphoma treated with ABVD chemotherapy with or without radiation therapy. The 5-year overall survival, progression-free survival, and freedom from treatment failure rates among patients with negative mid- and/or immediately post-chemotherapy restaging gallium scans were 97%, 93%, and 95%, respectively. These percentages were significantly superior to the corresponding rates of 53%, 38%, and 45%, respectively, in patients with a positive restaging gallium scan ($p < 0.0001$).[77]

Front and associates compared the predictive value of gallium-67 scintigraphy after treatment with CT in 43 patients with Hodgkin lymphoma.[78] They discovered that there was no difference in the negative predictive value of the two procedures. However, the positive predictive value of gallium-67 scintigraphy was 73% compared to 35% for CT. Moreover, disease-free survival of patients with negative follow-up gallium-67 scintigraphy was significantly better than that of gallium-67–positive patients. In contrast, they did not find much of a difference between patients with positive and negative CT.

Kostakoglu and associates investigated the potential role of gallium-67 SPECT in differentiating active Hodgkin lymphoma from fibrosis in the presence of abnormal mediastinal CT lesions after treatment.[79] Whereas gallium-67 had an accuracy of 93% and correctly identified 96% of biopsy-proven disease sites, CT was not conclusive regarding the presence of active disease in 27% of the patients with positive biopsy results. Moreover, biopsy confirmed the absence of residual disease in all patients with a positive CT and negative gallium-67 scintigraphy. In a study by Brenot-Rossi and colleagues, 61 patients had negative and 13 patients had positive gallium-67 scans after chemotherapy. In the gallium-negative group, 19.7% of the patients relapsed and 91.8% were alive at the end of the follow-up.[80] Relapse occurred in 20% of the patients with residual mass and in 19.6% of the patients without residual mass. In the gallium-positive group, 84.6% of the patients had recurrence disease and 61.5% were alive after intensive chemotherapy. There were statistically significant differences in overall survival and disease-free survival between patients with positive and negative gallium-67 scintigrams. The positive and negative predictive values of gallium-67 scintigraphy for predicting relapse were 85% and 87%, respectively.

Nevertheless, some controversial data have been reported regarding the predictive value of gallium-67 scintigraphy after therapy in patients with Hodgkin lymphoma.[68] Cooper and associates reported recurrence in 12 of 44 patients with mediastinal Hodgkin lymphoma and negative restaging gallium-67 scintigraphy.[81] In addition, Bogart and associates retrospectively studied 60 patients with Hodgkin lymphoma.[82] Based on gallium-67 scintigraphy, 46 patients were in complete remission after initial treatment, 10 were in partial remission, and 4 had persistent or progressive disease. In 34% of patients with complete remission after chemotherapy, relapse occurred subsequently. In a study by Salloum and co-workers, 101 patients with Hodgkin lymphoma underwent gallium-67 scintigraphy after treatment.[83] They reported that 16 out of 97 patients with negative gallium-67 scans relapsed. This group of 16 patients included 5 of 67 (7.5%) with stage I to II disease and 11 of 34 (32.7%) with stage III to IV disease. In this study, recurrence occurred mostly in or adjacent to the original site of diseases, indicating the failure of gallium-67 scintigraphy to detect small-volume residual disease.

It should be noted that the methodology used in gallium-67 scintigraphy has a significant impact on its effectiveness. In the adult population, gallium scans should be performed following the injection of 10 mCi (370 MBq) of gallium-67 citrate. Tomographic techniques (SPECT) of the chest and abdomen/pelvis should be mandatory, as should correlation with anatomic modalities such as CT. SPECT may help to detect disease when planar images appear normal due to superimposition of organs on the 2D images, which results in increased accuracy. SPECT is also particularly valuable in differentiating normal physiologic gallium-67 accumulation within soft tissues, bone, liver, or bowel from pathologic uptake. Combined SPECT/CT gamma cameras are also currently available on the market.

FDG-PET VERSUS GALLIUM-67 SCINTIGRAPHY

FDG-PET can be performed the same day, approximately 45 minutes after the injection of FDG, while there is a delay of 3 days after gallium-67 injection before scanning is performed. FDG has a further advantage over gallium-67 in terms of effective dose. FDG results in an effective patient dose of 27 μSv/MBq, or 5 to 20 mSv, depending on applied adult dose (5–20 mCi; 185–740 MBq). Due to its long half-life, gallium-67 delivers a higher radiation dose of 120 μSv/MBq, or an average adult dose of 44 mSv per standard injection dose (10 mCi; 370 MBq).[84,85] FDG-PET can also be offered as an alternative to gallium-67 scintigraphy to women in the postpartum period who wish to continue breastfeeding. Although FDG is also excreted into breast milk, the shorter half-life of fluorine-18 (109.8 min) allows women to resume breastfeeding within 24 to 48 hours.

The literature is especially sparse regarding studies comparing FDG-PET to gallium-67 scintigraphy in a prospective manner in the same group of patients with Hodgkin lymphoma. In an earlier preliminary study in patients with Hodgkin lymphoma, Wirth and associates suggested improved staging with FDG-PET compared to gallium-67 scintigraphy, although scan interpretation was not performed in an independent, blinded fashion.[86] In a retrospective study of 50 patients with lymphoma (19 with Hodgkin lymphoma) from the same group, FDG-PET identified more disease sites than gallium-67 scintigraphy in 19 patients.[87] Similarly, in a study of 30 patients with lymphoma (14 with Hodgkin lymphoma), FDG-PET upstaged 6 patients in whom gallium-67 scintigraphy partially detected disease sites.[88]

Our group recently conducted a prospective study comparing both modalities in 36 patients with Hodgkin lymphoma at staging, midtherapy, and at the end of treatment. The results show that FDG-PET and gallium scintigraphy findings are largely concordant with the exception of the unique ability of FDG-PET to detect splenic disease, resulting in the upstaging of 3 of 5 patients who demonstrated splenic involvement on FDG-PET alone. Positive FDG-PET findings at midtreatment and at the end of therapy had a higher sensitivity for predicting subsequent relapse than gallium-67 scintigraphy.[38]

In summary, FDG-PET appears superior to gallium-67 scintigraphy in the initial staging and in predicting prognosis during and after chemotherapy. Hence, FDG-PET should be considered the metabolic imaging technique of choice in the management of patients with Hodgkin lymphoma.

References

1. Maisey M. Radionuclide imaging in cancer management. *J R Coll Physicians Lond* 1998;32:525–529.
2. Munley MT, Marks LB, Hardenbergh PH, et al. Functional imaging of normal tissues with nuclear medicine: applications in radiotherapy. *Semin Radiat Oncol* 2001;11:28–36.
3. Valdes Olmos RA, Hoefnagel CA. Nuclear medicine in tailoring treatment in oncology. *Nucl Med Commun* 2001;22:1–4.
4. Badawi RD. Nuclear medicine. *Physics Ed* 2001;36:452–454.
5. Maisey MN, Wahl RL, Barrington SF. *Atlas of clinical positron emission tomography*. London: Arnold; 1999.

6. Brown RS, Wahl RL. Overexpression of Glut-1 glucose transporter in human breast cancer. An immunohistochemical study. *Cancer* 1993;72:2979–2985.
7. Brown RS, Goodman TM, Zasadny KR, et al. Expression of hexokinase II and Glut-1 in untreated human breast cancer. *Nucl Med Biol* 2002;29:443–453.
8. Lacic M, Maisey MN, Kusic Z. Positron emission tomography in oncology: the most sophisticated imaging technology. *Acta Med Croatica* 1997;51:1–9.
9. Lechpammer S, Tetrault RJ, Badawi RD, Van den Abbeele A. PET imaging and treatment evaluation in cancer patients. *Uptake* 2002;8:4–5.
10. Medicare coverage. Available at http://www.cms.hhs.gov. Accessed May 2006.
11. National Oncologic PET Registry. Available at http://www.cancerpetregistry.org. Accessed May 2006.
12. Phelps ME, Mazziotta JC, Schelbert HR. *Positron emission tomography and autoradiography. Principles and applications for the brain and heart.* New York: Raven; 1986.
13. Choi Y, Brunken RC, Hawkins RA, et al. Factors affecting myocardial 2-[F-18]fluoro-2-deoxy-D-glucose uptake in positron emission tomography studies of normal humans. *Eur J Nucl Med* 1993;20:308–318.
14. Cook GJ, Fogelman I, Maisey MN. Normal physiological and benign pathological variants of 18-fluoro-2-deoxyglucose positron-emission tomography scanning: potential for error in interpretation. *Semin Nucl Med* 1996; 26:308–314.
15. Cook GJ, Maisey MN, Fogelman I. Normal variants, artefacts and interpretative pitfalls in PET imaging with 18-fluoro-2-deoxyglucose and carbon-11 methionine. *Eur J Nucl Med* 1999;26:1363–1378.
16. Carr R, Barrington SF, Madan B, et al. Detection of lymphoma in bone marrow by whole-body positron emission tomography. *Blood* 1998;91:3340–3346.
17. Munker R, Glass J, Griffeth LK, et al. Contribution of PET imaging to the initial staging and prognosis of patients with Hodgkin's disease. *Ann Oncol* 2004;15:1699–1704.
18. Schaefer NG, Hany TF, Taverna C, et al. Non-Hodgkin lymphoma and Hodgkin disease: coregistered FDG PET and CT at staging and restaging—do we need contrast-enhanced CT? *Radiology* 2004;232:823–829.
19. Hutchings M, Eigtved AI, Specht L. FDG-PET in the clinical management of Hodgkin lymphoma. *Crit Rev Oncol Hematol* 2004;52:19–32.
20. Schiepers C, Filmont JE, Czernin J. PET for staging of Hodgkin's disease and non-Hodgkin's lymphoma. *Eur J Nucl Med Mol Imaging* 2003;30(suppl 1):S82–S88.
21. Bangerter M, Moog F, Buchmann I, et al. Whole-body 2-[18F]-fluoro-2-deoxy-D-glucose positron emission tomography (FDG-PET) for accurate staging of Hodgkin's disease. *Ann Oncol* 1998;9:1117–1122.
22. Partridge S, Timothy A, O'Doherty MJ, et al. 2-Fluorine-18-fluoro-2-deoxy-D glucose positron emission tomography in the pretreatment staging of Hodgkin's disease: influence on patient management in a single institution. *Ann Oncol* 2000;11:1273–1279.
23. Hueltenschmidt B, Sautter-Bihl ML, Lang O, et al. Whole body positron emission tomography in the treatment of Hodgkin disease. *Cancer* 2001;91:302–310.
24. Jerusalem G, Beguin Y, Fassotte MF, et al. Whole-body positron emission tomography using 18F-fluorodeoxyglucose compared to standard procedures for staging patients with Hodgkin's disease. *Haematologica* 2001;86:266–273.
25. Weihrauch MR, Re D, Bischoff S, et al. Whole-body positron emission tomography using 18F-fluorodeoxyglucose for initial staging of patients with Hodgkin's disease. *Ann Hematol* 2002;81:20–25.
26. Menzel C, Dobert N, Mitrou P, et al. Positron emission tomography for the staging of Hodgkin's lymphoma—increasing the body of evidence in favor of the method. *Acta Oncol* 2002;41:430–436.
27. Naumann R, Beuthien-Baumann B, Reiss A, et al. Substantial impact of FDG PET imaging on the therapy decision in patients with early-stage Hodgkin's lymphoma. *Br J Cancer* 2004;90:620–625.
28. Isasi CR, Lu P, Blaufox MD. A metaanalysis of 18F-2-deoxy-2-fluoro-D-glucose positron emission tomography in the staging and restaging of patients with lymphoma. *Cancer* 2005;104:1066–1074.
29. Hicks RJ, Mac Manus MP, Seymour JF. Initial staging of lymphoma with positron emission tomography and computed tomography. *Semin Nucl Med* 2005;35:165–175.
30. Meyer RM, Ambinder RF, Stroobants S. Hodgkin's lymphoma: evolving concepts with implications for practice. *Hematology* 2004:184—202.
31. Jerusalem G, Hustinx R, Beguin Y, et al. Evaluation of therapy for lymphoma. *Semin Nucl Med* 2005;35:186–196.
32. Front D, Israel O. The role of Ga-67 scintigraphy in evaluating the results of therapy of lymphoma patients. *Semin Nucl Med* 1995;25:60–71.
33. Hoskin PJ. PET in lymphoma: what are the oncologist's needs? *Eur J Nucl Med Mol Imaging* 2003;30(suppl 1):S37–S41.
34. Hoekstra OS, Ossenkoppele GJ, Golding R, et al. Early treatment response in malignant lymphoma, as determined by planar fluorine-18-fluorodeoxyglucose scintigraphy. *J Nucl Med* 1993;34:1706–1710.
35. Kostakoglu L, Coleman M, Leonard JP, et al. PET predicts prognosis after 1 cycle of chemotherapy in aggressive lymphoma and Hodgkin's disease. *J Nucl Med* 2002;43:1018–1027.
36. Bangerter M, Kotzerke J, Griesshammer M, et al. Positron emission tomography with 18-fluorodeoxyglucose in the staging and follow-up of lymphoma in the chest. *Acta Oncol* 1999;38:799–804.
37. Cremerius U, Fabry U, Neuerburg J, et al. Positron emission tomography with 18F-FDG to detect residual disease after therapy for malignant lymphoma. *Nucl Med Commun* 1998;19:1055–1063.
38. Friedberg JW, Fischman A, Neuberg D, et al. FDG-PET is superior to gallium scintigraphy in staging and more sensitive in the follow-up of patients with de novo Hodgkin lymphoma: a blinded comparison. *Leuk Lymphoma* 2004;45:85–92.
39. Hutchings M, Mikhaeel NG, Fields PA, et al. Prognostic value of interim FDG-PET after two or three cycles of chemotherapy in Hodgkin lymphoma. *Ann Oncol* 2005;16:1160–1168.
40. Maisey NR, Hill ME, Webb A, et al. Are 18-fluorodeoxyglucose positron emission tomography and magnetic resonance imaging useful in the prediction of relapse in lymphoma residual masses? *Eur J Cancer* 2000;36:200–206.
41. Weihrauch MR, Re D, Scheidhauer K, et al. Thoracic positron emission tomography using 18F-fluorodeoxyglucose for the evaluation of residual mediastinal Hodgkin disease. *Blood* 2001;98:2930–2934.
42. de Wit M, Bohuslavizki KH, Buchert R, et al. 18FDG-PET following treatment as valid predictor for disease-free survival in Hodgkin's lymphoma. *Ann Oncol* 2001;12:29–37.
43. Naumann R, Vaic A, Beuthien-Baumann B, et al. Prognostic value of positron emission tomography in the evaluation of post-treatment residual mass in patients with Hodgkin's disease and non-Hodgkin's lymphoma. *Br J Haematol* 2001;115:793–800.
44. Spaepen K, Stroobants S, Dupont P, et al. Can positron emission tomography with [(18)F]-fluorodeoxyglucose after first-line treatment distinguish Hodgkin's disease patients who need additional therapy from others in whom additional therapy would mean avoidable toxicity? *Br J Haematol* 2001;115:272–278.
45. Guay C, Lepine M, Verreault J, et al. Prognostic value of PET using 18F-FDG in Hodgkin's disease for posttreatment evaluation. *J Nucl Med* 2003;44:1225–1231.
46. Jerusalem G, Hustinx R, Beguin Y, et al. Positron emission tomography imaging for lymphoma. *Curr Opin Oncol* 2005;17:441–445.
47. Canellos GP, Horwich A. Management of recurrent Hodgkin's disease. In: Mauch P, Armitage JO, Diehl V, et al., eds. *Hodgkin's disease.* Philadelphia: Lippincott Williams & Wilkins; 1999:507–519
48. Kumar R, Maillard I, Schuster SJ, et al. Utility of fluorodeoxyglucose-PET imaging in the management of patients with Hodgkin's and non-Hodgkin's lymphomas. *Radiol Clin North Am* 2004;42:1083–1100.
49. Jerusalem G, Beguin Y, Fassotte MF, et al. Early detection of relapse by whole-body positron emission tomography in the follow-up of patients with Hodgkin's disease. *Ann Oncol* 2003;14:123–130.
50. Burton C, Ell P, Linch D. The role of PET imaging in lymphoma. *Br J Haematol* 2004;126:772–784.
51. Cook GJ, Ott RJ. Dual-modality imaging. *Eur Radiol* 2001;11:1857–1858.
52. Israel O, Keidar Z, Iosilevsky G, et al. The fusion of anatomic and physiologic imaging in the management of patients with cancer. *Semin Nucl Med* 2001;31:191–205.
53. Townsend DW, Carney JP, Yap JT, et al. PET/CT today and tomorrow. *J Nucl Med* 2004;45(suppl 1):4S–14S.
54. Beyer T, Townsend DW, Brun T, et al. A combined PET/CT scanner for clinical oncology. *J Nucl Med* 2000;41:1369–1379.
55. Martinelli M, Townsend D, Meltzer C, et al. Survey of results of whole body imaging using the PET/CT at the University of Pittsburgh Medical Center PET facility. *Clin Positron Imaging* 2000;3:161.
56. D'Amico TA, Wong TZ, Harpole DH, et al. Impact of computed tomography-positron emission tomography fusion in staging patients with thoracic malignancies. *Ann Thorac Surg* 2002;74:160–163; discussion 163.
57. Schaffler GJ, Groell R, Schoellnast H, et al. Digital image fusion of CT and PET data sets–clinical value in abdominal/pelvic malignancies. *J Comput Assist Tomogr* 2000;24:644–647.
58. Edwards CL, Hayes RL. Tumor scanning with 67Ga citrate. *J Nucl Med* 1969;10:103–105.
59. Mansberg R, Wadhwa SS, Mansberg V. Tl-201 and Ga-67 scintigraphy in non-Hodgkin's lymphoma. *Clin Nucl Med* 1999;24:239–242.
60. Waxman AD, Eller D, Ashook G, et al. Comparison of gallium-67-citrate and thallium-201 scintigraphy in peripheral and intrathoracic lymphoma. *J Nucl Med* 1996;37:46–50.
61. Vallabhajosula S, Goldsmith SJ, Lipszyc H, et al. 67Ga-transferrin and 67Ga-lactoferrin binding to tumor cells: specific versus nonspecific glycoprotein-cell interaction. *Eur J Nucl Med* 1983;8:354–357.
62. Tsan MF, Scheffel U. Mechanism of gallium-67 accumulation in tumors. *J Nucl Med* 1988;29:2019–2020.
63. Chen DC, Scheffel U, Camargo EE, et al. The source of gallium-67 in gastrointestinal contents: concise communication. *J Nucl Med* 1980;21:1146–1150.
64. Even-Sapir E, Bar-Shalom R, Israel O, et al. Single-photon emission computed tomography quantitation of gallium citrate uptake for the differentiation of lymphoma from benign hilar uptake. *J Clin Oncol* 1995;13:942–946
65. Holman BL, Tumeh SS. Single-photon emission computed tomography (SPECT). Applications and potential. *JAMA* 1990;263:561–564.

66. Tumeh SS, Rosenthal DS, Kaplan WD, et al. Lymphoma: evaluation with Ga-67 SPECT. *Radiology* 1987;164:111–114.
67. Van den Abbeele AD. Scintigraphy of neoplastic disease. Lymphoma. In: Donohoe KJ, Van den Abbeele AD, eds. *Teaching atlas of nuclear medicine.* New York: Thieme; 2000:199—217.
68. Even-Sapir E, Israel O. Gallium-67 scintigraphy: a cornerstone in functional imaging of lymphoma. *Eur J Nucl Med Mol Imaging* 2003;30(suppl 1): S65–S81.
69. Canellos GP. Residual mass in lymphoma may not be residual disease. *J Clin Oncol* 1988;6:931–933.
70. Front D, Israel O, ben-Haim S. The dilemma of a residual mass in treated lymphoma: the role of gallium-67 scintigraphy. In: Freeman LM, ed. *Nuclear medicine annual, 1991.* New York: Raven; 1991:211—220.
71. McLaughlin AF, Magee MA, Greenough R, et al. Current role of gallium scanning in the management of lymphoma. *Eur J Nucl Med* 1990;16: 755–771.
72. Kaplan WD. Residual mass and negative gallium scintigraphy in treated lymphoma: when is the gallium scan really negative? *J Nucl Med* 1990;31: 369–371.
73. Delcambre C, Reman O, Henry-Amar M, et al. Clinical relevance of gallium-67 scintigraphy in lymphoma before and after therapy. *Eur J Nucl Med* 2000;27:176–184.
74. Israel O, Mor M, Epelbaum R, et al. Clinical pretreatment risk factors and Ga-67 scintigraphy early during treatment for prediction of outcome of patients with aggressive non-Hodgkin lymphoma. *Cancer* 2002;94:873–878.
75. Front D, Bar-Shalom R, Mor M, et al. Aggressive non-Hodgkin lymphoma: early prediction of outcome with 67Ga scintigraphy. *Radiology* 2000; 214:253–257.
76. Front D, Bar-Shalom R, Mor M, et al. Hodgkin disease: prediction of outcome with 67Ga scintigraphy after one cycle of chemotherapy. *Radiology* 1999;210:487–491.
77. Ng AK, Bernardo MV, Silver B, et al. Mid- and post-ABVD gallium scanning predicts for recurrence in early-stage Hodgkin's disease. *Int J Radiat Oncol Biol Phys* 2005;61:175–184.
78. Front D, Ben-Haim S, Israel O, et al. Lymphoma: predictive value of Ga-67 scintigraphy after treatment. *Radiology.* 1992;182:359–363.
79. Kostakoglu L, Yeh SD, Portlock C, et al. Validation of gallium-67-citrate single-photon emission computed tomography in biopsy-confirmed residual Hodgkin's disease in the mediastinum. *J Nucl Med* 1992;33: 345–350.
80. Brenot-Rossi I, Bouabdallah R, Di Stefano D, et al. Hodgkin's disease: prognostic role of gallium scintigraphy after chemotherapy. *Eur J Nucl Med* 2001;28:1482–1488.
81. Cooper DL, Caride VJ, Zloty M, et al. Gallium scans in patients with mediastinal Hodgkin's disease treated with chemotherapy. *J Clin Oncol* 1993; 11:1092–1098.
82. Bogart JA, Chung CT, Mariados NF, et al. The value of gallium imaging after therapy for Hodgkin's disease. *Cancer* 1998;82:754–759.
83. Salloum E, Brandt DS, Caride VJ, et al. Gallium scans in the management of patients with Hodgkin's disease: a study of 101 patients. *J Clin Oncol* 1997;15:518–527.
84. Bartold SP, Donohoe KJ, Fletcher JW, et al. Procedure guideline for gallium scintigraphy in the evaluation of malignant disease. Society of Nuclear Medicine. *J Nucl Med* 1997;38:990–994.
85. Mikhaeel NG, Timothy AR, O'Doherty MJ, et al. 18-FDG-PET as a prognostic indicator in the treatment of aggressive non-Hodgkin's Lymphoma-comparison with CT. *Leuk Lymphoma* 2000;39:543–553.
86. Wirth A, Seymour JF, Ware R, et al. Can F-18 fluorodeoxyglucose positron emission tomography replace gallium-67 scanning for staging of Hodgkin's disease and non-Hodgkin's lymphoma? *Proc Am Soc Clin Oncol* 2000;19:10a.
87. Wirth A, Seymour JF, Hicks RJ, et al. Fluorine-18 fluorodeoxyglucose positron emission tomography, gallium-67 scintigraphy, and conventional staging for Hodgkin's disease and non-Hodgkin's lymphoma. *Am J Med* 2002;112:262–268.
88. Shen YY, Kao A, Yen RF. Comparison of 18F-fluoro-2-deoxyglucose positron emission tomography and gallium-67 citrate scintigraphy for detecting malignant lymphoma. *Oncol Rep* 2002;9:321–325.

CHAPTER 12 ■ PROGNOSTIC FACTORS IN HODGKIN LYMPHOMA

LENA SPECHT AND DIRK HASENCLEVER

HISTORICAL PERSPECTIVE

Early descriptions of the natural history of untreated or palliatively treated patients with Hodgkin's disease showed a highly variable clinical course, although the disease eventually proved fatal in virtually all cases.[1-4] Early on, the concept developed that Hodgkin's disease passes through successive clinical stages with an increasing spread of the disease and progressive worsening of prognosis.[3] Over the years different staging classifications have been proposed based on the anatomic extent of disease.[5-24] A consensus was reached at the Workshop on the Staging of Hodgkin's Disease at Ann Arbor in 1971.[25] The Ann Arbor staging classification has since been universally adopted.[26] Its prognostic significance has been amply demonstrated.[27-40] The Ann Arbor staging classification remains the basis for the evaluation of patients with Hodgkin lymphoma. Survival curves according to Ann Arbor stage for more than 14,000 patients in the International Database on Hodgkin's Disease are shown in Figure 12.1.[33]

Through the years, however, it has become clear that the Ann Arbor staging system cannot be relied upon as the only prognostic tool in Hodgkin lymphoma. New features of prognostic importance have become recognized, many of them related to the extent and volume of disease. The extent of disease may vary considerably in stages other than stage I, and the volume of disease in individual regions is not taken into account at all in the Ann Arbor classification. A modification of the Ann Arbor staging system was devised at the Cotswolds meeting in 1988 to incorporate a designation for number of sites and bulk.[41] However, the recommendations of the Cotswolds meeting have not been universally adopted. A multitude of other prognostic factors for different Ann Arbor stages, presentations, treatments, and outcomes have been examined, and varying combinations of some of these factors are presently being employed by different centers and groups worldwide.

DIFFERENT PROGNOSTIC FACTORS, END-POINTS, AND METHODS OF ANALYSIS

Definition and Use of Prognostic Factors

Prognostic factors are variables measured in individual patients that offer a partial explanation of the heterogeneity observed in the outcome of a given disease.[42] Prognostic factors are important in patient care for selecting management and predicting outcome for individual patients.[43] However, it is important to realize that we cannot predict exactly for individual patients. We can only make statements of probability, and even these will be more accurate for groups of patients than for individuals.[44] Prognostic factors are also important in research for the design and analysis of clinical trials.[42-44] However, prognostic factors are rarely sufficiently explanatory to justify the comparison of treatments by use of nonrandomized data.[45,46]

Types of Prognostic Factors

Prognostic factors can be divided into tumor-related factors, host-related factors, and environment-related factors.[43] Tumor-related factors are directly related to the presence of the tumor or its effect on the host (e.g., tumor pathology, anatomic extent, or tumor biology). Patient- or host-related factors include demographic characteristics (e.g., age and gender), and other factors such as performance status, comorbid conditions, and immune status. Environment-related factors are factors outside of the patient (e.g., socioeconomic and health care status). Although environment-related factors should ideally be easier to modify, usually only tumor-related and host-related factors are analyzed. Both are important, but in many situations it is advisable to keep them separate, especially if they are to form the basis for treatment selection.

For statistical analyses of prognostic factors it is generally assumed that the values of the factors are known at the starting point of the analyses. These factors are called fixed covariates. However, other important prognostic variables are measured later, including time to response, toxicity of treatment, and the value of presumed markers. These are time-dependent covariates, and may help in answering many important biological questions. However, they should never be used for adjustment for treatment comparison, as they may themselves be affected by treatment.[42-44]

Different End-Points

Different outcomes may be of interest in analyses of prognostic factors, including overall survival, disease-specific survival, progression-free survival, event-free survival, and duration of response. For each of these end-points there must be clear specifications of the starting point in time for the analysis and the clinical characteristics of events and censoring. International guidelines have been published,[41,47] and attempts at further international harmonization on this issue are ongoing.[48]

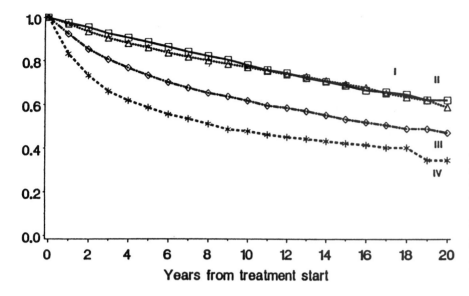

FIGURE 12.1. Overall survival according to clinical Ann Arbor stage for 14,037 patients in the International Database on Hodgkin's Disease treated over the past 25 years. (Reprinted with permission from Henry-Amar M, Aeppli DM, Anderson J, et al. Workshop statistical report. In: Somers R, Henry-Amar M, Meerwaldt JH, et al., eds. *Treatment strategy in Hodgkin's disease.* London: INSERM/John Libbey Eurotext; 1990:169–425.)

Analyzing and Reporting Prognostic Studies

For a patient variable to qualify as a useful prognostic factor, it must be significant, independent, and clinically important.[49] All patient variables are potentially of prognostic significance, and many prove significant in univariate analysis. However, different variables are likely to be interrelated and may thus be partial substitutes for one another. Typically, the relationship between the variables and the clinical end-point is examined by development and testing of a prognostic model.[50,51] Multiple regression analysis is the most common method for examining or adjusting for several prognostic factors in an analysis. The Cox proportional hazards regression model is the preferred method for examining the influence of several prognostic factors when time-to-event outcome is of interest.[52] Other methods such as neural networks and recursive partitioning have also been used, but do not seem to offer better predictions than the Cox regression method.[50,51,53]

Prognostic factor studies may be divided into exploratory and confirmatory studies. Exploratory studies usually have no a priori hypotheses, and generally involve numerous analyses of factors, end-points, and subsets of patients.[54] It is important to realize that one can derive a multiple regression model from any data set, but that its usefulness is determined by how well it works in practice.[50] Different exploratory studies often reveal widely varying results. There are many reasons for these variations; the most common ones are small sample size, adjustment for different variables, different assay techniques, different cut points for variables, inclusion of different subsets of patients, different study end-points, and use of stepwise variable-selection methods.[53,54] The probability that some spurious associations will be found is very high due to multiple testing.[53] Hence, validation of the results of exploratory studies on a different data set is mandatory.[50]

Confirmatory studies, on the other hand, are based on prespecified hypotheses involving one or a few new prognostic factors, and the purpose of the multiple regression analysis is to determine how much the new factor adds to the predictive power of already accepted factors.[53,54] Models are analyzed without and with the new factor to see if it adds prognostic information.

Statistical problems, particularly in exploratory studies, with multiple significance testing leading to spurious conclusions, are becoming even more relevant with the introduction of molecular markers. Powerful technologies to perform high-throughput analysis in genomics and proteomics have led to research in which large quantities of data can be analyzed without a prespecified hypothesis to search for patterns with prognostic significance. When a large number of potential predictors are analyzed on a small number of outcome events, there is a high risk of "over-fitting," leading to promising but nonreproducible results.[55] Selective reporting of positive marker studies may spuriously inflate the importance of postulated prognostic factors, and this has been shown to be a real problem.[56,57] Large studies with adjustment for known prognostic factors and proper validation are needed.[58] To counter some of these problems, guidelines for reporting tumor marker prognostic studies have recently been developed.[59,60]

PROGNOSTIC FACTORS IN EARLY-STAGE HODGKIN LYMPHOMA

Patients with stage I or II disease were previously in many institutions staged further with laparotomy and splenectomy in order to select patients who were suited for radiotherapy alone.[61–68] Today, virtually all patients with early-stage disease are treated with combined chemotherapy and radiotherapy, and laparotomy and splenectomy as part of the staging procedures have been abandoned. However, the information gathered in the past from large series of patients staged with laparotomy and splenectomy has provided us with invaluable data on the intra-abdominal distribution of Hodgkin lymphoma.

The information regarding the extent and anatomic distribution of disease was more accurate in patients staged with laparotomy. Consequently, it would be expected that the prediction of outcome would be relatively precise. From the numerous studies of prognostic factors in early-stage patients who were staged with laparotomy it was clear that the anatomic extent of disease, measured as the number of involved lymph-node regions, was prognostically significant.[69–78] The volume of disease in individual regions was also demonstrated to be prognostically important. This was particularly true for large mediastinal masses, which are common in Hodgkin lymphoma.[73,77,79–91] It is also true for large masses in sites other than the mediastinum, although these are much rarer.[72] An estimate of the total tumor burden, based on a combination of the number of involved regions and the volume of disease in individual regions, was shown to be by far the most important prognostic factor of all.[73,74,92,93] There seems to be no evidence that particular localizations of early-stage disease affect prognosis. Prognosis seems to be determined by the bulk of disease rather than its precise localization.[77,79,82,85,86,89,94–111] Localized extralymphatic lesions, so-called E-lesions, have had a poorer prognosis in some studies[87,91,112] but not in others.[83,86] The prognostic impact of E-lesions is still controversial, which may partly be due to the fact that there is wide disagreement as to what is and what is not an E-lesion.[113,114]

Today, patients are no longer staged with laparotomy. The significant prognostic factors for patients staged without laparotomy are to some extent identical with the ones in patients who were staged with laparotomy. However, our knowledge of the extent and distribution of the disease is less accurate in these patients, and so there is greater variation in outcome. Additional factors, usually providing an indirect or surrogate measure of the total tumor burden and possibly also the growth characteristics of the tumor, are therefore more important in these patients.

Patients Treated with Radiotherapy Alone

Except for patients with lymphocyte-predominant Hodgkin lymphoma, very few patients are treated today with radiotherapy alone. From earlier studies it is clear that both the number of involved regions and the size of a mediastinal mass are independent prognostic factors.[33,40,75,76,115,116] The presence of B-symptoms is correlated with the extent of disease, and B-symptoms are also prognostically significant.[33,40,115,117] Histological subtype is correlated with occult abdominal involvement, which is more common in patients with mixed cellularity, and is therefore prognostically significant.[33,40,115,117–119] Older age is associated with a higher risk for occult abdominal disease. Comorbid conditions that may preclude adequate staging and treatment are also more common in older patients. Hence, older age is a significant prognostic factor.[33,40,116,117,119–121] However, the issue regarding the prognostic importance of age per se is still not settled, and evidence from more recent analyses would seem to indicate that Hodgkin lymphoma in older patients does not have a different natural history from Hodgkin lymphoma in younger patients, but that the reduced tolerance to

staging and treatment may largely explain the differences seen in outcome.[122] Male gender often comes out as an independent adverse prognostic factor, although of minor importance.[33,115,117,118,120] A number of "classical" biologic parameters (hematological, biochemical, immunological) have been shown to be prognostically significant because they provide an indirect indication of disease extent.[123] This is the case for an elevated erythrocyte sedimentation rate (ESR),[33,75,76,115,117,119,124,125] anemia,[23,33,126,127] and a decreased serum albumin.[33,127–129] Many other biologic parameters have been shown to correlate with disease activity, but they have not been shown to possess independent prognostic significance.[130]

Patients Treated with Combined-Modality Therapy

Most patients with early-stage disease are today treated with a combination of chemotherapy and radiotherapy. A meta-analysis of individual patient data showed that combined-modality therapy reduces the risk of relapse compared with radiotherapy alone, but that it does not improve the chance of being cured of Hodgkin lymphoma.[131] However, with very long-term follow–up, survival after combined-modality therapy is superior due to mortality from long-term complications,[132] thus supporting current treatment recommendations. In the meta-analysis the size of the reduction in risk of failure in patients in different stages, with and without B-symptoms, male or female, and of different ages was remarkably similar. Hence, there is no indication that prognostic factors for patients treated with combined-modality therapy are different from the factors for patients treated with radiotherapy alone. As early-stage patients are today treated according to prognostic subgroups, many of the published series are selected, making the detection of prognostic factors difficult. Nevertheless, a number of studies have confirmed the prognostic significance of the same prognostic factors as mentioned above for patients treated with radiotherapy alone.[117,133–138]

As mentioned previously, most of the important prognostic factors are correlated with and provide indirect measures of the patient's total tumor burden.[74,93,130] With modern imaging modalities, in particular CT scans and more recently FDG-PET scans, it is now possible to directly quantitate the individual patient's total tumor volume. Studies employing these

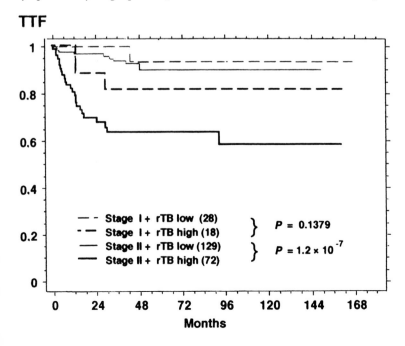

TTF

— - Stage I + rTB low (28)
- - Stage I + rTB high (18)   } *P* = 0.1379
— Stage II + rTB low (129)
— Stage II + rTB high (72)   } *P* = 1.2×10^{-7}

FIGURE 12.2. Time to treatment failure curves for 46 patients with stage I and 201 patients with stage II disease divided according to whether their mean tumor burden normalized to body surface area (rTB) was below or above the mean value for each stage. (Reprinted with permission from Gobbi PG, Broglia C, Di Giulio G, et al. The clinical value of tumor burden at diagnosis in Hodgkin lymphoma. *Cancer* 2004;101:1824–1834.)

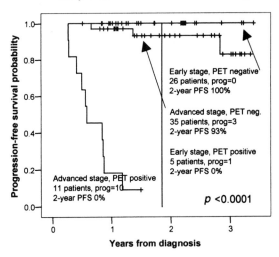

Early interim PET and clinical stage

FIGURE 12.3. Progression-free survival in 31 patients with early-stage and 46 patients with advanced-stage disease divided according to the result of an early interim FDG-PET scan (after two cycles of chemotherapy). (Reprinted with permission from Hutchings M, Loft A, Hansen M, et al. FDG-PET after two cycles of chemotherapy predicts treatment failure and progression-free survival in Hodgkin lymphoma. *Blood* 2006;107:52–59.)

techniques have confirmed the pivotal prognostic role of the total tumor burden.[139–142] Figure 12.2 shows time to treatment failure curves for patient with stage I and II disease according to whether their mean tumor burden normalized to body surface area was below or above the mean value for each stage.[140]

Functional imaging has recently become important in staging and treatment evaluation of lymphomas. Gallium scans during or immediately after treatment have been shown to predict outcome.[143–148] However, FDG-PET is now recognized as being superior to gallium scans in the evaluation of lymphomas, and has largely replaced gallium scans.[149–151] An early interim FDG-PET scan after one or two cycles of chemotherapy has been shown to be highly predictive of outcome,[152–154] and clinical trials are now being initiated testing treatment modification depending on the results of an early interim FDG-PET scan. The result of an early interim FDG-

TABLE 12.1

PROGNOSTIC FACTORS IN EARLY-STAGE HODGKIN LYMPHOMA

Number of involved lymph node regions

Large tumor mass, particularly mediastinal

Tumor burden

B-symptoms

Histologic subtype

Age

Gender

Erythrocyte sedimentation rate (ESR)

Hemoglobin

Serum albumin

Early interim FDG-PET scan (measure of chemosensitivity)

PET scan, although not strictly measured before start of treatment, yields a measure of the chemosensitivity of the disease, a factor of great prognostic value that is likely to become very important for choice of treatment in the future. Figure 12.3 shows progression-free survival curves for early-stage and advanced-stage patients according to the result of an early interim FDG-PET scan (after two cycles of chemotherapy).[153]

Table 12.1 lists the established prognostic factors in early-stage Hodgkin lymphoma. At present, different centers and cooperative groups divide early-stage patients into favorable and unfavorable by varying combinations of these factors (see below).

Rapidly evolving technologies in molecular biology have opened up new possibilities for the discovery of molecular markers that may in the future refine the prognostic evaluation of patients with Hodgkin lymphoma. However, at present none of these markers have gained acceptance in the management of patients.[155–166]

Patients Treated with Chemotherapy Alone

Treatment with chemotherapy as single modality in early-stage Hodgkin lymphoma has been tested in several trials. Relapse-free survival seems inferior compared to combined-modality therapy, but no difference in overall survival has yet been proved.[167–170] However, large cohorts of patients with reasonable follow-up are not yet available.

PROGNOSTIC FACTORS IN ADVANCED HODGKIN LYMPHOMA

The term *advanced disease* is not sharply defined. Pragmatically, advanced-stage patients are those requiring full systemic treatment. Stages IIIB and IV certainly form the core group. Most study groups also generally include stage IIIA and possibly selected patients with stage I or II disease with multiple adverse factors. The role of radiotherapy added to full systemic treatment in advanced stages is limited.[171] Thus, data with these treatment variants may be pooled in prognostic factors analyses.

In the vast literature on prognostic factors in advanced Hodgkin lymphoma, there are two very large data sets that resulted from international cooperation. The International Database on Hodgkin's Disease was set up in 1989, combining individual patient data from 20 study groups in all stages.[33] In addition to early-stage patients it includes data on 5,217 patients in stages CSIII/IV mostly treated with MOPP-type chemotherapy. In 1995 the International Prognostic Factors Project on Advanced Hodgkin's Disease combined data of 5,141 advanced-stage patients mainly treated with a doxorubicin-containing regimen.[172] Large data sets are important to reliably assess the independent contributions of single routinely documented prognostic factors that tend to be small to moderate (5–10% in tumor control).[172]

Patients Treated with Conventional Chemotherapy with or without Additional Radiotherapy

Age is a dominant patient-related prognostic factor for overall survival in advanced Hodgkin lymphoma.[31,173–188] Prevalence of comorbidity increases with age.[189] Therefore about half of the elderly patients (>60 years) are typically excluded from general adult study populations[190] and may require separate studies. Even if included, their risk of treatment-related mortality and toxicity-associated treatment reductions[191] is increased. In patients up to 65 years of age from study populations, age (e.g., >45 years) is an independent prognostic factor for freedom from progression. This may be related to tumor biology, as unfavorable histological subtypes are more frequent in the elderly.[33] The impact of age is much more important on overall survival due to compromised results of salvage treatment in elderly patients who have relapsed: 5-year survival rates after progression/relapse decrease with advancing age from about 40% in patients up to 35 years to less than 5% in patients 55 to 65 years of age at diagnosis.[172]

Gender is correlated with disease stage at presentation, as about two-thirds of patients with advanced stage disease are men.[33,172] Male gender is an independent, although quantitatively moderate, adverse prognostic factor within advanced stages.[31,33,172,179,184,192–195]

Among the tumor-related prognostic factors, the histologic subtype plays a minor role. Some studies report mixed-cellularity or lymphocyte-depletion subtypes as unfavorable prognostic factors,[31,33,179,182,196] but several other studies do not confirm these findings.[172,174,183–185,195,197–200] The prognostic relevance of grading the nodular-sclerosis subtype remains controversial.[201–208] Unfavorable subtypes are correlated with male gender, age, lack of mediastinal involvement, stage, systemic symptoms, and related abnormal blood parameters.[33,127] Given a relatively high reclassification rate under expert pathologic review, histology subtyping does not lend itself to prognostication, at least in multicenter settings.[203]

The principle that a high tumor burden correlates with unfavorable prognosis also holds for advanced disease.[140,184,185] Tumor burden can be quantified directly using CT,[139,209] but this is rarely done routinely. As a surrogate for tumor burden, information on the number of involved areas,[183,185,210] the amount of tumor in the spleen,[211–216] and the subdivision of stage III[212,213,216–222] were established as prognostic in the era of pathologic staging and radiotherapy alone.

Inguinal involvement may be seen as a surrogate marker for maximal nodal spread and was reported as independently prognostic.[186] As described previously, there are various methods of measuring mediastinal bulk.[223] Very large mediastinal bulk (e.g., >0.45 of the thoracic aperture) is relatively rare (<10% of advanced disease[172]), but has been reported as an adverse prognostic factor in some studies[186,224] though not in

others.[225] Large, but not very large (e.g., 0.33 to 0.45 of the thoracic aperture) mediastinal mass is not related to prognosis in advanced Hodgkin lymphoma treated with modern chemotherapy.[172]

Stage IV marks dissemination to extranodal sites and is independently prognostic within advanced disease.[33,172,182] It remains controversial whether a specific organ involvement site carries a particularly bad prognosis within stage IV. Bone marrow involvement was an adverse factor in some studies,[184,186,199,226–230] but not in others.[195,231,232] Pleura, lung, or liver involvement have been reported as prognostically unfavorable,[198,228,231,233] but not in other studies.[184,186,195,199,210,230,234] The number of involved extranodal sites has been reported to be independently prognostic,[175,176,234] but this could not be confirmed in the International Prognostic Factors Project.[172]

Several hematologic and biochemical laboratory parameters carry prognostic information in advanced Hodgkin lymphoma. Decreased serum albumin[172,177,178,235,236] and hemoglobin levels[33,172,175,181,225,237] (or hematocrit[186]) as well as an elevated erythrocyte sedimentation rate[127,238] or alkaline phosphatase[187,238,239] are correlated[33,127,172,237] with one another as well as with the presence of B-symptoms[33,227] and tumor burden.[140] These variables form a cluster of interrelated prognostic indicators that mirror both tumor burden as well as inflammatory processes.[128] They have been variously reported as prognostic, individually or in combination. Serum albumin[172,235] and hemoglobin level[172] show a remarkably monotone relation to prognosis over their full range of variation. Figure 12.4 shows freedom from progression according to serum albumin for 2,239 patients, and Figure 12.5 shows freedom from progression according to hemoglobin for 4,314 patients, in the International Prognostic Factors Project. Moreover, hemoglobin and serum albumin are parameters that change on a scale of weeks and are thus biometrically reliable measurements. This singles them out both as the most informative prognostic factors in advanced Hodgkin lymphoma and as representatives for this prognostic cluster of systemic symptoms. Given hemoglobin and serum albumin, the other members of this cluster, in particular B-symptoms, lose their independent prognostic impact.[172]

Leukocyte and lymphocyte counts form a second cluster of laboratory parameters. These parameters are interrelated, but only weakly correlated to the first cluster mentioned above. Analyzing the joint distribution of leukocyte and lymphocyte counts in advanced Hodgkin lymphoma, there is a simultaneous

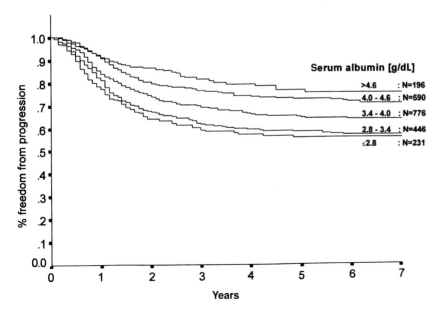

FIGURE 12.4. Freedom from progression according to albumin levels for 2,239 patients with advanced disease in the International Prognostic Factors Project for Advanced Hodgkin's Disease.

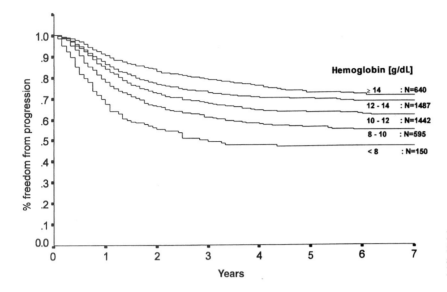

FIGURE 12.5. Freedom from progression according to hemoglobin levels for 4,314 patients with advanced disease in the International Prognostic Factors Project for Advanced Hodgkin's Disease.

shift away from the normal pattern towards both leukocytosis[172] and lymphocytopenia[175,177,178,181,184,187,240] that has an independent prognostic impact.[172] These relatively unspecific measurements may indirectly capture dysregulation of hematopoiesis due to cytokine release by Hodgkin lymphoma cells.

Elevated serum lactic dehydrogenase was found to be independently prognostic by some groups,[175,186] but not in the large data sets of the International Database on Hodgkin Lymphoma and the International Prognostic Factors Project. Serum lactic dehydrogenase probably plays a lesser role in Hodgkin lymphoma than in aggressive non-Hodgkin lymphoma.[241] Elevated β_2-microglobulin is not generally documented, but has been reported as prognostic.[163,242] Table 12.2 summarizes the prognostic factors in advanced disease.

A plethora of biological parameters, including levels of cytokines released by Hodgkin and Reed-Sternberg cells, soluble forms of membrane-derived antigens, and molecular markers, have been investigated for prognostic value.[243] The soluble form of the CD30 molecule is released by Hodgkin and Reed-Sternberg cells, and with sensitive techniques it is detectable in the serum of virtually all untreated patients.[244–247] It maintains independent prognostic significance in multivariate analysis in moderately sized data sets.[246,248,249] Results for further biologic parameters are mostly still immature or controversial.

Prognostic Indices or Scores in Advanced Hodgkin Lymphoma

Prognostic indices or scores for advanced Hodgkin lymphoma may be clinically important, to select patients who may be overtreated and in whom treatment reduction may be considered, or to select patients in whom standard treatment is likely to fail to eliminate the disease and in whom experimental approaches may be indicated.

Several groups developed prognostic indices or scores based on a few hundred cases and defined high-risk groups. Wagstaff and associates[187,195] defined risk groups based on age over 45, male gender, absolute lymphocyte count below $0.75 \times 10^9/L$, and stage IV. Straus and co-workers[186] proposed a five-factor score including age over 45, elevated serum lactic dehydrogenase, low hematocrit, inguinal involvement, and mediastinal mass greater than 0.45 of the thoracic aperture. Proctor and associates[181] developed a numerical index to predict overall survival based on age, stage, hemoglobin level, absolute lymphocyte count, and bulky disease (>10 cm).[181,224] Gobbi and co-workers[31,250] set up a predictive equation based on age, sex, stage, histology, B-symptoms, mediastinal mass, erythrocyte sedimentation rate, hemoglobin, and serum albumin. Low and colleagues[177] defined a score based on age of 45 or above, serum albumin below 35 g/L, and lymphocyte count below 1.5 g/L and validated the score[178] in a large historic BNLI data set. However, none of these indices has received general acceptance.

Gobbi and associates[193] developed a parametrical model to derive numerical estimates of expected survival in all stages. Seven factors were incorporated: stage, age, histology, B-symptoms, serum albumin, sex, and involved area distribution

---

TABLE 12.2

PROGNOSTIC FACTORS IN ADVANCED HODGKIN LYMPHOMA

Age

Gender

Histology

Stage IV disease

Tumor burden

Inguinal involvement

Very large mediastinal mass

B-symptoms

Anemia

Low serum albumin

High erythrocyte sedimentation rate

High serum alkaline phosphatase

Leukocytosis

Lymphocytopenia

High serum lactic dehydrogenase

High serum β_2-microglobulin

TABLE 12.3

ADVERSE PROGNOSTIC FACTORS INCORPORATED IN THE INTERNATIONAL PROGNOSTIC FACTORS PROJECT SCORE FOR FREEDOM FROM PROGRESSION IN ADVANCED HODGKIN LYMPHOMA

Age ≥45 years

Male gender

Stage IV disease

Hemoglobin <10.5 g/dL

Serum albumin <4.0 g/dL

Leukocytosis ≥15 × 10^9/L

Lymphocytopenia <0.6 × 10^9/L or <8% of white blood cell count

(infradiaphragmatic disease or more than three supradiaphragmatic areas). This work was based on 5,023 patients in both early and advanced stages from the International Database on Hodgkin's Disease.[33] They were treated rather heterogeneously with radiotherapy alone or mainly MOPP-type chemotherapy with or without radiotherapy. All of these models used overall survival as main end-point.

The International Prognostic Factors Project on Advanced Hodgkin's Disease[172] focused on the result of first-line treatment. Thus the major end-point was freedom from progression. Individual patient data were collected from 23 centers or study groups on 5,141 patients diagnosed as having advanced-stage Hodgkin lymphoma and treated with (mainly) doxorubicin-containing chemotherapy with and without radiotherapy according to a defined protocol. A prognostic score was developed from this data set in patients up to 65 years of age. The score is the simple count of how many of seven binary adverse prognostic factors (summarized in Table 12.3) of approximately similar prognostic impact are present: age 45 or above, male gender, stage IV, albumin below 4.0 g/dL, hemoglobin below 10.5 g/dL, leukocytosis greater than 15 × 10^9/L, and lymphocytopenia (lymphocyte count <0.6 × 10^9/L, or <8% of leukocytes, or both).

The international prognostic score (IPS) predicts 5-year tumor control rates in the range of 45% to 80%. Each additional factor reduces the prognosis by about 8%. Figure 12.6 shows freedom from progression according to the number of adverse prognostic factors for 1,618 patients in the International Prognostic Factors Project on Advanced Hodgkin's Disease.

Since its publication, the IPS has performed reasonably well in independent data sets,[251–255] in particular to distinguish lower risk (IPS ≤2) and (moderately) higher risk (IPS ≥3) patients. For example, in Italian data (N = 516),[253] about 25% of the patients with an IPS above 2 had a 36% failure rate, whereas patients with an IPS of 2 or less had a failure rate of about 20%. Two trials with significant treatment effects.[251,255] report that prognostic differences were more pronounced with less effective treatments.[172]

Two publications[175,253] compared several prognostic models. None of the models, including the IPS, is able to select either a very low risk group (e.g., <10% failure rate) or a substantial very high risk group (>50%). The prognostic models only discriminate between relatively low risk and relatively high risk patients (e.g., IPS ≤2 versus IPS >2). Because dichotomization always discards information, a small improvement in prognostication[253] may be achieved using a mathematical formula to calculate a prognostic index, but this appears difficult to use in clinical routine. Until new powerful, biologically more specific prognostic markers emerge, the IPS remains the workable method of choice. It is currently used in intergroup trials to select higher-risk advanced-stage patients for treatment intensification.

Several authors tried to extend the IPS beyond advanced stages. The IPS works nicely to predict outcome after autologous hematopoietic stem cell transplantation.[256] It appears to be moderately predictive in early and intermediate stages,[129,257] extending the definition of stage IV to include any extranodal disease.

PROGNOSTIC FACTORS FOR OUTCOME AFTER RELAPSE

Relapses of Hodgkin lymphoma after radiotherapy alone are qualitatively different from relapses after chemotherapy alone or combined-modality therapy. Both freedom from second relapse and overall survival are considerably better for patients relapsing after radiotherapy alone than for the others.[65,131,258] Today, patients are rarely treated with radiotherapy alone except for patients with LP subtype, but patients relapsing after this treatment may still be encountered.

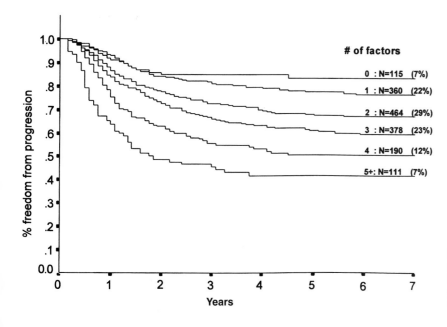

FIGURE 12.6. Freedom from progression according to the number of adverse prognostic factors (see Table 12.3) for 1,618 patients with advanced disease in the International Prognostic Factors Project.

TABLE 12.4

PROGNOSTIC FACTORS FOR OUTCOME AFTER RELAPSE TREATED WITH CONVENTIONAL SALVAGE TREATMENT

Relapse After Radiotherapy Alone

Age

Extent of disease at relapse (relapse stage, extranodal relapse)

Histology

Relapse After Chemotherapy or Combined Modality Therapy

Extent and durability of first remission

Extent of disease at relapse (relapse stage, extranodal relapse, ≥3 sites of relapse)

B-symptoms at relapse

Hemoglobin at relapse

Histology

Age

Performance status

Patients Relapsing after Radiotherapy Alone

From past experience it is known that about 30% of patients with early-stage disease treated with radiotherapy alone relapsed. However, most of these patients could be successfully salvaged with chemotherapy, and durable remissions were achieved in 60% to 80% of cases.[258–270] The extent of disease at relapse has been shown to be important for prognosis.[258,261,264–267,269,271] In early studies, initial stage was important for prognosis, but this correlation was not found in later studies, probably because they included fewer patients with advanced disease at presentation.[262,263,271] Likewise, histologic subtype was significant for prognosis after relapse in earlier but not in later studies.[258,261,263,264,267,269,270] Age has consistently been shown to be independently significant for prognosis after relapse, the efficacy of salvage chemotherapy being much lower in older patients.[117,258–261,263,265,267,270,272] It is possible that a significant part of the impact of age should be ascribed to suboptimal staging and treatment at relapse for some older patients.[272] In contrast to patients relapsing after chemotherapy or combined-modality therapy, the length of the initial disease-free interval has been shown in many studies not to influence prognosis after relapse for patients treated initially with radiotherapy alone.[258,260,261,265–268,271,273] The prognostic factors known to be independently significant for outcome after relapse after primary treatment with radiotherapy alone are summarized in the first part of Table 12.4.

Patients Relapsing after Chemotherapy +/− Radiotherapy

Patients relapsing after initial treatment with chemotherapy or combined-modality therapy, whether for early-stage or advanced disease, have a much poorer prognosis than patients relapsing after radiotherapy alone. With second-line conventional chemotherapy, durable remissions are obtained in only 10% to 30% of cases.[174,258,274–299] The most important prognostic factor for outcome after relapse in these patients has consistently been shown to be the extent and durability of the initial remission, irrespective of the specific initial or second-line treatment employed. Patients who never achieve a complete remission have the poorest prognosis, patients who relapse within 12 months of complete remission have an intermediate prognosis, and patients who relapse more than 12 months after achieving complete remission have the best prognosis.[275–277,279–281,283,285,286,289,295,297–301] However, even for patients relapsing after complete remission lasting more than 12 months, long-term outlook is poor with conventional chemotherapy. Figure 12.7 shows survival curves for patients relapsing after initial chemotherapy divided into these three prognostic groups.[302] Patients relapsing more than once have a dismal prognosis.[282,287,294,295]

The extent of disease at relapse has also been shown to be independently significant for prognosis. Patients with advanced stage at relapse,[276,289,301] with extranodal disease at relapse,[275,282,289,291,292,295,298,299] or with more than three involved sites[298,299] have a significantly poorer prognosis than patients relapsing without these adverse factors. Age,[259] performance status,[280] histology other than nodular sclerosis,[291,298] B-symptoms at relapse,[275,277,283,285,292,298] and a low hemoglobin[299,301] have also been shown to be significant. The prognostic factors known to be independently significant for outcome after relapse after primary treatment with

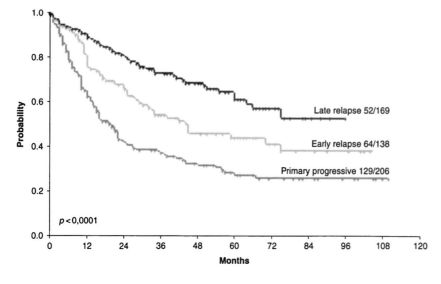

FIGURE 12.7. Overall survival of patients with primary progressive, early relapse, or late relapse of Hodgkin lymphoma, treated in the German Hodgkin Study Group from 1988 to 1999, primarily with conventional salvage. (Reprinted with permission from Josting A, Schmitz N. Insights into 25 years of clinical trials of the GHSG: relapsed and refractory Hodgkin's disease. In: Diehl V, Josting A, eds. *25 years German Hodgkin Study Group*. Munich: Urban & Vogel; 2004:89–99.)

chemotherapy or combined-modality therapy are summarized in the second part of Table 12.4.

A subgroup of patients relapsing after chemotherapy have anatomically limited relapse in nodal sites alone. A number of small series have shown that for selected patients in this subgroup, radiotherapy with or without additional chemotherapy offers some chance of durable disease control.[285,303–314] Prognostic factor analyses in some of the larger series indicate that patients suitable for this kind of relapse treatment are those relapsing exclusively in supradiaphragmatic nodal sites, with no B-symptoms at relapse, with favorable histology (lymphocyte predominance or nodular sclerosis), and after a disease-free interval of 12 months or more.[303,305,310,314] Durable remission with radiotherapy may be obtained in about 50% of cases with these favorable characteristics.

Patients Undergoing High-Dose Chemotherapy and Stem Cell Transplantation for Relapsed or Refractory Disease

High-dose chemotherapy with stem cell transplantation has shown superior outcome in patients relapsing after chemotherapy or combined-modality therapy.[315,316] Several published series have demonstrated a number of independent prognostic factors for outcome of this treatment. The chemosensitivity of the disease is a critical determinant of outcome. Hence, the response to initial or salvage therapy,[317–337] the duration of initial remission,[326,327,330,335,338–340] and the number of prior failed regimens[318,319,323,325,327,332,334,341–345] have been shown to be very important for outcome.

Stage of disease at salvage,[301,319,321,334] bulky disease at salvage,[319,342,345–347] and extranodal relapse,[319,330,331,333,339,344] reflecting the disease burden before transplantation, have been shown to be independently significant. B-symptoms at relapse,[322,330,339,340] a low hemoglobin,[301,326] and an elevated

serum lactic dehydrogenase level at relapse[321,329,348] have also been shown to be significant. As would be expected, a poor performance status is an important adverse prognostic factor.[319,323,339,341,343,348] Most large series have not identified age as a prognostic factor,[341,342,349–351] probably due to the fact that few patients over 45 have been transplanted. Pediatric patients have the same outcome as their adult counterparts.[352]

The seven factors included in IPS for advanced Hodgkin lymphoma were investigated in a cohort of patients treated with high-dose chemotherapy and autologous stem cell transplantation.[256] Only low serum albumin, anemia, age of 45 or older, and lymphocytopenia were independently significant. A simplified prognostic score including these four factors was proposed, but it has not been tested in analyses including chemosensitivity and extent of prior therapy. The prognostic factors known to be independently significant for outcome after high-dose chemotherapy and stem cell transplantation are shown in Table 12.5.

USE OF PROGNOSTIC FACTORS IN CLINICAL TRIALS

Optimizing the treatment strategy for Hodgkin lymphoma is an attempt to make all prognostic factors disappear.[353] Ideally, when the amount and aggressiveness of therapy are adequately tailored to the patient's risk and disease burden, nearly all patients should have the same excellent prognosis. In data from the German Hodgkin Lymphoma Study Group, early, intermediate, and advanced-stage patients have nearly the same failure-free survival rate,[353] with the advanced-stage curve visually in the middle, but many patients are probably overtreated. Thus, with therapeutic progress prognostic factors should be expected to loose their prognostic value and become mere disease burden indicators.

As such, prognostic factors help to stratify the patient population into more homogeneous groups that are then treated with disease burden-adapted treatment options. Together with strategies of response adaptation, this hopefully will lead to increasingly individualized and more adequate treatment.

Prognostic Factor Combinations Currently Used by Major Trial Groups

In clinical trials prognostic factors are primarily used in the definition of the study population (entry and exclusion criteria). Further uses include description of study population and adjustment for prognostic imbalances in the final analysis.

Inclusion criteria that are currently used differ by trial and study group. This is not surprising: prognosis varies on a continuum scale from low-risk minimal disease to high-risk maximally advanced disease. The population of patients with Hodgkin lymphoma does not fall into naturally defined groups that differ in prognosis and clearly require different treatment approaches. The delineation of study populations depends on the prognosis, respective therapeutic challenge, and study history. Any sharp borderline is artificial to a certain degree. Nevertheless, certain clusters of comparable selection criteria have emerged.

The classical Ann Arbor[25] or Cotswold[41] staging systems are based on the anatomic distribution of the disease. Stage correlates reasonably with prognosis, although prognostic factor combinations using additional information show better correlation. The Ann Arbor staging system is well established, universally accepted, and still forms the reference system for most definitions of study entry criteria. However, most study groups currently use hybrid systems to define their study entry

---

TABLE 12.5

PROGNOSTIC FACTORS FOR OUTCOME AFTER HIGH-DOSE CHEMOTHERAPY AND STEM CELL TRANSPLANTATION FOR REFRACTORY OR RECURRENT DISEASE

Chemosensitivity of the disease

    Response to initial or salvage therapy

    Duration of initial remission

    Number of failed prior regimens

Disease burden before salvage

    Stage of disease at salvage

    Bulky disease at salvage

    Extranodal relapse

B-symptoms at relapse

Hemoglobin, serum albumin, and lymphocyte count at relapse

Serum lactic dehydrogenase at relapse

Performance status

(Age ≥45 years)

criteria, basically using stage and in addition presence or absence of unfavorable prognostic factors (also called risk factors in this context). Prognosis of stage groups overlaps considerably; for example, a patient with stage IIB disease with additional risk factors may have a worse prognosis than a patient with limited IIIA disease.

Most study groups partition the population of patients with Hodgkin lymphoma into two (early versus advanced stages) or three (early, intermediate, and advanced stages) separate trial or treatment groups. Attempts to use a fourth "very favorable" early-stage group with minimal treatment have been abandoned by the EORTC.[354] Tables 12.6 and 12.7 describe inclusion criteria currently or recently used by study groups in early-stage and advanced disease, respectively.

Early stages comprise patients from the favorable end of the prognostic distribution in whom full systemic treatment is considered overtreatment. As the prognosis in this group is excellent, study questions focus on how to cure with minimal toxicity or cost. Treatment options comprise radiotherapy alone or increasingly reduced or less toxic chemotherapy with or without minimized involved field radiotherapy. Table 12.6 illustrates that early stages are typically defined as stage I or II without risk factors, with lists of unfavorable prognostic factors that vary by study group and were mainly derived from radiotherapy-alone relapse data.

Studies in advanced stage include patients from the unfavorable end of the prognostic scale in which full systemic treatment is required. Trials either focus on improving results in high-risk advanced stages or minimizing side effects of treatments felt to be satisfactory. Most study groups have stages IIIB/IV as the core group of advanced disease (Table 12.7). Studies differ in whether they include all stage IIIA patients, none, or only selected stage IIIA patients with unfavorable prognostic factors. Some groups also include stages I and II with "systemic" risk factors.

Stages I and II with risk factors and stage IIIA form what may be called intermediate stages. "Intermediate stage" essentially denotes a gray zone between early and advanced disease. Study aims and the treatment modalities therefore overlap. Study groups either have a separate trial for intermediate stages or split this group up including parts of it in early or advanced-stage trials depending on available accrual and the particular question under study.

Two groups (the Scotland and Newcastle Lymphoma Group[244] and Grupo Argentino de Tratamiento de la Leucemia Aguda[355]) have abandoned what was above called

TABLE 12.6

ELIGIBILITY CRITERIA FOR RECENT OR CURRENT STUDIES IN EARLY STAGES[a]

Study group	Early-stage[a] versus intermediate-stage/advanced disease
EORTC (H7 study,[356] H8 study, H9 study)	Age >50 4+ involved nodal sites Erythrocyte sedimentation rate >50 mm/h or B-symptoms and erythrocyte sedimentation rate >30 mm/h Bulky mediastinum (mediastinal thoracic ratio ≥ .35) (Infra-diaphragmatic disease)
Cancer research UK FDG-PET	B-symptoms Infradiaphragmatic disease Large mediastinal mass (>0.33 of the thoracic aperture)
GHSG (HD7 study, HD10 study, HD13 study)	Large mediastinal mass (>0.33 of the thoracic aperture) Massive spleen involvement E-lesions Erythrocyte sedimentation rate >50 mm/h or B-symptoms and erythrocyte sedimentation rate >30 mm/h 3+ involved lymph-node areas
SWOG (9133) CALGB (9391)	B-symptoms Mediastinal mass ≥1/3 maximum thoracic diameter Infra-diaphragmatic presentation
NCI-C[168]	B-symptoms Mixed cellularity or lymphocyte depletion Age >40 years Erythrocyte sedimentation rate >50 mm/h 4+ disease sites
Stanford (G1 study,[357] G5 study)	Constitutional (B) symptoms present at diagnosis Mediastinal mass equal to or greater than one-third the maximum intrathoracic diameter on a standing posteroanterior chest x-ray Any lymph node mass >10 cm in greatest trans-axial diameter Two or more extranodal sites of disease

[a]"Early-stage" disease is typically defined by stage I or II and the absence of certain unfavorable prognostic factors.
EORTC, European Organization for Research and Treatment of Cancer; GHSG, German Hodgkin's Disease Study Group; SWOG, Southwest Oncology Group; CALGB, Cancer and Leukemia Group B; NCI-C, National Cancer Institute of Canada; ECOG, Eastern Cooperative Oncology Group.

TABLE 12.7

ELIGIBILITY CRITERIA FOR RECENT OR CURRENT STUDIES IN ADVANCED DISEASE

Study group	Eligibility criteria for trials in advanced disease
EORTC (H34 study[358])	III/IV
BNLI Stanford V protocol	Stage IB, IIB, IIIA, IIIB, or IV Stage IA or IIA with locally extensive disease (e.g., bulky mediastinal disease greater than 0.33 of the maximum transthoracic diameter on routine chest x-ray or at least 2 extranodal sites of disease) or "other poor risk features"
Manchester Lymphoma Group (VAPEC-B study)[255]	I/II with B-symptoms or bulk, III, IV
GHSG (HD9 study, HD12 study, HD 15 study)	IIB with bulk, massive spleen, or E-lesion PS IIIA S PS IIIA N with bulk, E-lesion, or elevated erythrocyte sedimentation rate CS IIIA bulk, massive spleen, E lesions, elevated erythrocyte sedimentation rate or ≥3 lymph node areas IIIB/IV
Milano (MAMA study[359])	IB, IIA bulk, IIB, III, IV
GELA (H89 study[360])	IIIB, IV
Stanford V study ECOG-2496 NCT00003389, CALGB-59905, CAN-NCIC-HD7, SWOG- E2496 Stanford	Stage I-IIA/B with massive mediastinal adenopathy Stage III or IV
"BEACOPP" intergroup study EORTC-20012 NCT00049595, ALLG-HD04, BNLI-EORTC-20012, CAN-NCIC-EORTC-20012, GELA-EORTC-20012, GELCAB-EORTC-20012, NORDICLG-EORTC-20012	Only higher-risk advanced stages: III, IV with International Prognostic Score >2

EORTC, European Organization for Research and Treatment of Cancer; BNLI, British National Lymphoma Group; GHSG, German Hodgkin Study Group; GELA, Groupe d'Etudes des Lymphomes de l'Adulte; NCI-US, National Cancer Institute of the United States; SWOG, Southwest Oncology Group; CALGB, Cancer and Leukemia Group B; ECOG, Eastern Cooperative Oncology Group; NCI-C, National Cancer Institute of Canada.

the hybrid system and currently use prognostic indices or scores covering the whole range of Hodgkin lymphoma to define trial entry criteria. In these approaches, stage has become one factor among others, and has ceased to form the backbone of the system. Indeed, if predicting outcome is the only task, stage information is not privileged, and the best available predictor, possibly numerical, should be used. On the other hand, entry criteria do not depend on prognosis only. Stage codes the anatomic distribution of the disease and may thus be particularly important to define the applicability of radiotherapy. If group-specific prognostic indices are used, intergroup comparability may be compromised. As stage is well established, at least a population description in terms of stage with and without risk factors should be provided.

CONCLUSION AND FUTURE ASPECTS

As demonstrated in this chapter, a large number of variables have been shown to possess prognostic significance in Hodgkin lymphoma, both at presentation and later in the course of the disease. Today, treatment is often tailored to prognostic factors, decreasing treatment intensity for patients with favorable

prognostic factors to reduce toxicity, and increasing treatment intensity for patients with unfavorable prognostic factors to increase the chance of cure. Unfortunately, different centers and groups worldwide currently use varying combinations of factors when allocating patients to different treatments and clinical trials. This makes comparisons between different patient series difficult. Some form of international harmonization regarding which combinations of prognostic factors should be employed in the future would be highly valuable.

References

1. Craft CB. Results with roentgen ray therapy in Hodgkin's disease. *Bull Staff Meet Univ Minnesota Hosp* 1940;11:391–409.
2. Peters MV. The need for a new clinical classification in Hodgkin's disease: keynote address. *Cancer Res* 1971;31:1713–1722.
3. Reed DM. On the pathological changes in Hodgkin's disease, with especial reference to its relation to tuberculosis. *Johns Hopkins Hosp Rep* 1902;10: 133–196.
4. Sahyoun PF, Eisenberg SJ. Hodgkin's disease. A histopathological and clinical classification with radiotherapeutic response. *Am J Roentgenol* 1949;61:369–379.
5. Banfi A, Bonadonna G, Buraggi G, et al. Proposta di classificazione e terapia della malattia di Hodgkin. *Tumori* 1965;51:97–112.
6. Easson EC, Russell MH. The cure of Hodgkin's disease. *BMJ* 1963;1963:1704–1707.
7. Easson EC. Possibilities for the cure of Hodgkin's disease. *Cancer* 1966;19: 345–350.

8. Hilton G, Sutton PM. Malignant lymphomas: classification, prognosis and treatment. *Lancet* 1962;1:283–287.

9. Hohl K, Sarasin P, Bessler W. Therapie und prognose der lymphogranulomatose Zürcher erfahrungen von 1922-1950. *Oncologia* 1951;4:1–20.

10. Jelliffe AM, Thomson AD. The prognosis in Hodgkin's disease. *Br J Cancer* 1955;9:21–36.

11. Kaplan HS, Bagshaw MA, Rosenberg SA. Présentation du protocole d'essai radiotherapique des lymphomes malins de l'universitéde Stanford. *Nouv Rev Fr Hematol* 1964;4:95–100.

12. Kaplan HS. Long-term results of palliative and radical radiotherapy of Hodgkin's disease. *Cancer Res* 1966;26:1250–1252.

13. Kaplan HS. On the natural history, treatment and prognosis of Hodgkin's disease. In: *Harvey Lectures 1968-1969.* New York: Academic Press; 1970:215–259.

14. Longcope WT, McAlpin KR. Hodgkin's disease. In: *The Oxford Medicine.* New York: Oxford University Press; 1920:1–43.

15. Meighan SS, Ramsay JD. Survival in Hodgkin's disease. *Br J Cancer* 1963;17:24–36.

16. Musshoff K, Stamm H, Lummel G, et al. Zur prognose der lymphogranulomatose. Klinisches bild un strahlentherapie. Freiburger Krankengut 1938–1958. In: Keiderling W, ed. *Beiträge zur inneren medizin.* Stuttgart: FK Schattauer-Verlag; 1964:549–561.

17. Musshoff K, Boutis L. Therapy results in Hodgkin's disease Freiburg i. Br., 1948–1966. *Cancer* 1968;21:1100–1113.

18. Peters MV. A study of survivals in Hodgkin's disease treated radiologically. *Am J Roentgenol* 1950;63:299–311.

19. Peters MV, Middlemiss KCH. A study of Hodgkin's disease treated by irradiation. *Am J Roentgenol* 1958;79:114–121.

20. Peters MV, Hasselback R, Brown TC. The natural history of the lymphomas related to the clinical classification. In: Zarafonetis CJD, ed. *Proceedings of the International Conference on Leukemia-Lymphoma.* Philadelphia: Lea & Febiger; 1968:357–371.

21. Rosenberg SA. Report of the committee on the staging of Hodgkin's disease. *Cancer Res* 1966;26:1310–1310.

22. Rosenberg SA, Kaplan HS. Hodgkin's disease and other malignant lymphomas. *Calif Med* 1970;113:23–38.

23. Westling P. Studies of the prognosis in Hodgkin's disease. *Acta Radiol* 1965;245 (suppl):5–125.

24. Ziegler K. *Die Hodgkinsche krankheit.* Jena: Gustav Fischer Verlag; 1911.

25. Carbone PP, Kaplan HS, Musshoff K, et al. Report of the committee on Hodgkin's disease staging classification. *Cancer Res* 1971;31:1860–1861.

26. Sobin LH, Wittekind C, eds. *TNM classification of malignant tumours.* 1997.

27. Aisenberg AC, Qazi R. Improved survival in hodgkin's disease. *Cancer* 1976;37:2423–2429.

28. Bjorkholm M, Holm G, Mellstedt H, et al. Prognostic factors in Hodgkin's disease. I. Analysis of histopathology, stage distribution and results of therapy. *Scand J Haematol* 1977;19:487–495.

29. Davis S, Dahlberg S, Myers MH, et al. Hodgkin's disease in the United States: a comparison of patient characteristics and survival in the Centralized Cancer Patient Data System and the Surveillance, Epidemiology, and End Results Program. *J Natl Cancer Inst* 1987;78:471–478.

30. Fischer P, Franken T. Ein multivariates prognosemodell für den morbus Hodgkin. *Strahlentherapie* 1984;160:535–542.

31. Gobbi PG, Cavalli C, Federico M, et al. Hodgkin's disease prognosis: a directly predictive equation. *Cancer* 1988;1:675–679.

32. Hancock BW, Aitken M, Martin JF, et al. Hodgkin's disease in Sheffield (1971–76) (with computer analysis of variables). *Clin Oncol* 1979;5:283–297.

33. Henry-Amar M, Aeppli DM, Anderson J, et al. Workshop statistical report. In: Somers R, Henry-Amar M, Meerwaldt JH, Carde P, eds. *Treatment strategy in Hodgkin's disease.* London: INSERM/John Libbey Eurotext; 1990:169–425.

34. Kaplan HS. Survival and relapse rates in Hodgkin's disease: Stanford experience, 1961–71. *Monogr Natl Cancer Inst* 1973;36:487–496.

35. Kaplan HS. *Hodgkin's disease.* Cambridge, MA: Harvard University Press; 1980.

36. Kennedy BJ, Loeb V, Jr., Peterson VM, et al. National survey of patterns of care for Hodgkin's disease. *Cancer* 1985;56:2547–2556.

37. Musshoff K, Hartmann C, Niklaus B, et al. Results of therapy in Hodgkin's disease: Freiburg i. Br. 1964–1971. In: Musshoff K, ed. *Diagnosis and therapy of malignant lymphoma.* Berlin: Springer-Verlag; 1974:206–220.

38. Nordentoft AM, Pedersen-Bjergaard J, Brincker H, et al. Hodgkin's disease in Denmark. A national clinical study by the Danish Hodgkin Study Group, LYGRA. *Scand J Haematol* 1980;24:321–334.

39. Patchefsky AS, Brodovsky H, Southard M, et al. Hodgkin's disease. A clinical and pathologic study of 235 cases. *Cancer* 1973;32:150–161.

40. Sutcliffe SB, Gospodarowicz MK, Bergsagel DE, et al. Prognostic groups for management of localized Hodgkin's disease. *J Clin Oncol* 1985;3:393–401.

41. Lister TA, Crowther D, Sutcliffe SB, et al. Report of a committee convened to discuss the evaluation and staging of patients with Hodgkin's disease: Cotswolds meeting. *J Clin Oncol* 1989;7:1630–1636.

42. George SL. Identification and assessment of prognostic factors. *Semin Oncol* 1988;15:462–471.

43. Gospodarowicz MK, O'Sullivan B. Prognostic factors: principles and application. In: Gospodarowicz MK, Henson DE, Hutter RVP, et al., eds. *Prognostic factors in cancer,* 2nd ed. New York: dWiley-Liss; 2001:17–35.

44. Byar DP. Identification of prognostic factors. In: Buyse ME, Staquet MJ, Sylvester RJ, eds. *Cancer clinical trials. Methods and practice.* Oxford: Oxford University Press; 1988:423–443.

45. Byar DP. Problems with using observational databases to compare treatments. *Stat Med* 1991;10:663–666.

46. Simon R. Importance of prognostic factors in cancer clinical trials. *Cancer Treat Rep* 1984;68:185–192.

47. Cheson BD, Horning SJ, Coiffier B, et al. Report of an international workshop to standardize response criteria for non-Hodgkin's lymphomas. NCI sponsored international working group. *J Clin Oncol* 1999;17:1244–1253.

48. Cheson BD, Pfistner B, Juweid ME, et al. Revised response criteria for malignant lymphomas. *J Clin Oncol* (in press).

49. Burke HB, Henson DE. The American Joint Committee on Cancer. Criteria for prognostic factors and for an enhanced prognostic system. *Cancer* 1993;72:3131–3135.

50. Altman DG, Royston P. What do we mean by validating a prognostic model? *Stat Med* 2000;19:453–473.

51. McShane LM, Simon R. Statistical methods for the analysis of prognostic factor studies. In: Gospodarowicz MK, Henson DE, Hutter RVP, et al., eds. *Prognostic factors in cancer,* 2nd ed. New York: Wiley-Liss; 2001:37–48.

52. Cox DR. Regression models and life-tables. *J R Stat Soc B* 1972;34:187–220.

53. Altman DG, Lyman GH. Methodological challenges in the evaluation of prognostic factors in breast cancer. *Breast Cancer Res Treat* 1998;52:289–303.

54. Simon R. Evaluating prognostic factor studies. In: Gospodarowicz MK, Henson DE, Hutter RVP, et al., eds. *Prognostic factors in cancer,* 2nd ed. New York: Wiley-Liss; 2001:49–56.

55. Ransohoff DF. Rules of evidence for cancer molecular-marker discovery and validation. *Nat Rev Cancer* 2004;4:309–314.

56. Kyzas PA, Loizou KT, Ioannidis JP. Selective reporting biases in cancer prognostic factor studies. *J Natl Cancer Inst* 2005;97:10431055.

57. McShane LM, Altman DG, Sauerbrei W. Identification of clinically useful cancer prognostic factors: what are we missing? *J Natl Cancer Inst* 2005;97:1023–1025.

58. Ntzani EE, Ioannidis JP. Predictive ability of DNA microarrays for cancer outcomes and correlates: an empirical assessment. *Lancet* 2003;362:14391444.

59. McShane LM, Altman DG, Sauerbrei W, et al. REporting recommendations for tumour MARKer prognostic studies (REMARK). *Br J Cancer* 2005;93:387–391.

60. McShane LM, Altman DG, Sauerbrei W, et al. Reporting recommendations for tumor marker prognostic studies (REMARK). *J Natl Cancer Inst* 2005;97:1180–1184.

61. The value of laparotomy and splenectomy in the management of early Hodgkin's disease. A report from the British National Lymphoma Investigation. *Clin Radiol* 1975;26:151–157.

62. Host H, Abrahamsen AF, Jorgensen OG, et al. Laparotomy and splenectomy in the management of Hodgkin's disease. *Scand J Haematol* 1973;10:327–336.

63. Kaplan HS, Dorfman RF, Nelsen TS, et al. Staging laparotomy and splenectomy in Hodgkin's disease: analysis of indications and patterns of involvement in 285 consecutive, unselected patients. *Natl Cancer Inst Monogr* 1973;36:291–301.

64. Kinsella TJ, Glatstein E. Staging laparotomy and splenectomy for Hodgkin's disease: current status. *Cancer Invest* 1983;1:87–91.

65. Mauch PM. Controversies in the management of early stage Hodgkin's disease. *Blood* 1994;83:318–329.

66. Piro AJ, Hellman S, Moloney WC. The influence of laparotomy on management decisions in Hodgkin's disease. *Arch Intern Med* 1972;130:844–848.

67. Rosenberg SA. Exploratory laparotomy and splenectomy for Hodgkin's disease: a commentary. *J Clin Oncol* 1988;6:574–575.

68. Rutherford CJ, Desforges JF, Davies B, et al. The decision to perform staging laparotomy in symptomatic Hodgin's disease. *Br J Haematol* 1980;44:347–358.

69. Barton M, Boyages J, Crennan E, et al. Radiation therapy for early stage Hodgkin's disease: Australasian patterns of care. Australasian Radiation Oncology Lymphoma Group. *Int J Radiat Oncol Biol Phys* 1995;31:227–236.

70. Horwich A, Easton D, Nogueira-Costa R, et al. An analysis of prognostic factors in early stage Hodgkin's disease. *Radiother Oncol* 1986;7:95–106.

71. Lee CK, Aeppli DM, Bloomfield CD, et al. Curative radiotherapy for laparotomy-staged IA, IIA, IIIA Hodgkin's disease: an evaluation of the gains achieved with radical radiotherapy. *Int J Radiat Oncol Biol Phys* 1990;19:547–559.

72. Mendenhall NP, Cantor AB, Barre DM, et al. The role of prognostic factors in treatment selection for early-stage Hodgkin's disease. *Am J Clin Oncol* 1994;17:189–195.

73. Specht L, Nordentoft AM, Cold S, et al. Tumour burden in early stage Hodgkin's disease: the single most important prognostic factor for outcome after radiotherapy. *Br J Cancer* 1987;55:535–539.

74. Specht L, Nordentoft AM, Cold S, et al. Tumor burden as the most important prognostic factor in early stage Hodgkin's disease. Relations to other prognostic factors and implications for choice of treatment. *Cancer* 1988;61:1719–1727.

75. Tubiana M, Henry-Amar M, Hayat M, et al. Prognostic significance of the number of involved areas in the early stages of Hodgkin's disease. *Cancer* 1984;54:885–894.

76. Tubiana M, Henry-Amar M, Hayat M, et al. The EORTC treatment of early stages of Hodgkin's disease: the role of radiotherapy. *Int J Radiat Oncol Biol Phys* 1984;10:197–210.

77. Verger E, Easton D, Brada M, et al. Radiotherapy results in laparotomy-staged Hodgkin's disease. *Clin Radiol* 1988;39:428–431.

78. Willett CG, Linggood RM, Meyer J, et al. Results of treatment of stage IA and IIA Hodgkin's disease. *Cancer* 1987;59:1107–1111.

79. Anderson H, Crowther D, Deakin DP, et al. A randomised study of adjuvant MVPP chemotherapy after mantle radiotherapy in pathologically staged IA-IIB Hodgkin's disease:10-year follow-up. *Ann Oncol* 1991; 2(suppl 2):49–54.

80. Crnkovich MJ, Leopold K, Hoppe RT, et al. Stage I to IIB Hodgkin's disease: the combined experience at Stanford University and the Joint Center for Radiation Therapy. *J Clin Oncol* 1987;5:1041–1049.

81. Fuller LM, Madoc-Jones H, Hagemeister FB Jr., et al. Further follow-up of results of treatment in 90 laparotomy-negative stage I and II Hodgkin's disease patients: significance of mediastinal and non-mediastinal presentations. *Int J Radiat Oncol Biol Phys* 1980;6:799–808.

82. Hagemeister FB, Fuller LM, Velasquez WS, et al. Stage I and II Hodgkin's disease: involved-field radiotherapy versus extended-field radiotherapy versus involved-field radiotherapy followed by six cycles of MOPP. *Cancer Treat Rep* 1982;66:789–798.

83. Hoppe RT, Coleman CN, Cox RS, et al. The management of stage I–II Hodgkin's disease with irradiation alone or combined modality therapy: the Stanford experience. *Blood* 1982;59:455–465.

84. Hughes-Davies L, Tarbell NJ, Coleman CN, et al. Stage IA-IIB Hodgkin's disease: management and outcome of extensive thoracic involvement. *Int J Radiat Oncol Biol Phys* 1997;39:361–369.

85. Lee CK, Bloomfield CD, Goldman AI, et al. Prognostic significance of mediastinal involvement in Hodgkin's disease treated with curative radiotherapy. *Cancer* 1980;46:2403–2409.

86. Leslie NT, Mauch PM, Hellman S. Stage IA to IIB supradiaphragmatic Hodgkin's disease. Long-term survival and relapse frequency. *Cancer* 1985;55:2072–2078.

87. Liew KH, Easton D, Horwich A, et al. Bulky mediastinal Hodgkin's disease management and prognosis. *Hematol Oncol* 1984;2:45–59.

88. Mauch P, Tarbell N, Weinstein H, et al. Stage IA and IIA supradiaphragmatic Hodgkin's disease: prognostic factors in surgically staged patients treated with mantle and paraaortic irradiation. *J Clin Oncol* 1988;6:1576–1583.

89. Mazza P, Lauria F, Sciascia R, et al. Prognostic significance of large mediastinal involvement in Hodgkin's disease. *Scand J Haematol* 1983;31: 315–321.

90. Willett CG, Linggood RM, Leong JC, et al. Stage IA to IIB mediastinal Hodgkin's disease: three-dimensional volumetric assessment of response to treatment. *J Clin Oncol* 1988;6:819–824.

91. Zagars G, Rubin P. Laparotomy-staged IA versus IIA Hodgkin's disease. A comparative study with evaluation of prognostic factors for stage IIA disease. *Cancer* 1985;56:864–873.

92. Enblad G. Hodgkin's disease in young and elderly patients. Clinical and pathological studies. Minireview based on a doctoral thesis. *Ups J Med Sci* 1994;99:1–38.

93. Specht L. Tumour burden as the main indicator of prognosis in Hodgkin's disease. *Eur J Cancer* 1992;28A:1982–1985.

94. Barrett A, Gregor A, McElwain TJ, et al. Infradiaphragmatic presentation of Hodgkin's disease. *Clin Radiol* 1981;32:221–224.

95. Cionini L, Magrini S, Mungai V, et al. Stage I and II Hodgkin's disease presenting in infradiaphragmatic nodes. *Tumori* 1982;68:519–525.

96. Dorreen MS, Wrigley PF, Jones AE, et al. The management of localized, infradiaphragmatic Hodgkin's disease: experience of a rare clinical presentation at St Bartholomew's Hospital. *Hematol Oncol* 1984;2:349–357.

97. Enrici RM, Osti MF, Anselmo AP, et al. Hodgkin's disease stage I and II with exclusive subdiaphragmatic presentation. The experience of the Departments of Radiation Oncology and Hematology, University "La Sapienza" of Rome. *Tumori* 1996;82:48–52.

98. Frassica DA, Schomberg PJ, Banks PM, et al. Management of subdiaphragmatic early-stage Hodgkin's disease. *Int J Radiat Oncol Biol Phys* 1989;16: 1459–1463.

99. Givens SS, Fuller LM, Hagemeister FB, et al. Treatment of lower torso stages I and II Hodgkin's disease with radiation with or without adjuvant mechlorethamine, vincristine, procarbazine, and prednisone. *Cancer* 1990;66:69–74.

100. Hoppe RT, Horning SJ, Rosenberg SA. The concept, evolution and preliminary results of the current Stanford clinical trials for Hodgkin's disease. *Cancer Surv* 1985;4:459–475.

101. Krikorian JG, Portlock CS, Mauch PM. Hodgkin's disease presenting below the diaphragm: a review. *J Clin Oncol* 1986;4:1551–1562.

102. Leibenhaut MH, Hoppe RT, Varghese A, et al. Subdiaphragmatic Hodgkin's disease: laparotomy and treatment results in 49 patients. *J Clin Oncol* 1987;5:1050–1055.

103. Mai DH, Peschel RE, Portlock C, et al. Stage I and II subdiaphragmatic Hodgkin's disease. *Cancer* 1991;68:1476–1481.

104. Mauch P, Gorshein D, Cunningham J, et al. Influence of mediastinal adenopathy on site and frequency of relapse in patients with Hodgkin's disease. *Cancer Treat Rep* 1982;66:809–817.

105. Mauch P, Greenberg H, Lewin A, et al. Prognostic factors in patients with subdiaphragmatic Hodgkin's disease. *Hematol Oncol* 1983;1:205–214.

106. Prosnitz LR, Curtis AM, Knowlton AH, et al. Supradiaphragmatic Hodgkin's disease: significance of large mediastinal masses. *Int J Radiat Oncol Biol Phys* 1980;6:809–813.

107. Roos DE, O'Brien PC, Wright J, et al. Treatment of subdiaphragmatic Hodgkin's disease: is radiotherapy alone appropriate only for inguino-femoral presentations? *Int J Radiat Oncol Biol Phys* 1994;28:683–691.

108. Schomberg PJ, Evans RG, O'Connell MJ, et al. Prognostic significance of mediastinal mass in adult Hodgkin's disease. *Cancer* 1984;53:324–328.

109. Specht L, Nissen NI. Hodgkin's disease stages I and II with infradiaphragmatic presentation: a rare and prognostically unfavourable combination. *Eur J Haematol* 1988;40:396–402.

110. Tarbell NJ, Thompson L, Mauch P. Thoracic irradiation in Hodgkin's disease: disease control and long-term complications. *Int J Radiat Oncol Biol Phys* 1990;18:275–281.

111. Vlachaki MT, Hagemeister FB, Fuller LM, et al. Long-term outcome of treatment for Ann Arbor Stage I Hodgkin's disease: prognostic factors for survival and freedom from progression. *Int J Radiat Oncol Biol Phys* 1997;38:593–599.

112. Levi JA, Wiernik PH. Limited extranodal Hodgkin's disease. Unfavorable prognosis and therapeutic implications. *Am J Med* 1977;63:365–372.

113. Connors JM, Klimo P. Is it an E lesion or stage IV? An unsettled issue in Hodgkin's disease staging. *J Clin Oncol* 1984;2:1421–1423.

114. Prosnitz LR. The Ann Arbor staging system for Hodgkin's disease: does E stand for error? *Int J Radiat Oncol Biol Phys* 1977;2:1923–1924.

115. Tubiana M, Henry-Amar M, Werf-Messing B, et al. A multivariate analysis of prognostic factors in early stage Hodgkin's disease. *Int J Radiat Oncol Biol Phys* 1985;11:23–30.

116. Vaughan HB, MacLennan KA, Easterling MJ, et al. The prognostic significance of age in Hodgkin's disease: examination of 1500 patients (BNLI report no. 23). *Clin Radiol* 1983;34:503–506.

117. Tubiana M, Henry-Amar M, Carde P, et al. Toward comprehensive management tailored to prognostic factors of patients with clinical stages I and II in Hodgkin's disease. The EORTC Lymphoma Group controlled clinical trials: 1964–1987. *Blood* 1989;73:47–56.

118. Radiotherapy of stage I and II Hodgkin's disease. A collaborative study. *Cancer* 1984;54:1928–1942.

119. Gospodarowicz MK, Sutcliffe SB, Clark RM, et al. Analysis of supradiaphragmatic clinical stage I and II Hodgkin's disease treated with radiation alone. *Int J Radiat Oncol Biol Phys* 1992;22:859–865.

120. Meerwaldt JH, van Glabbeke M, Vaughan Hudson B. Prognostic factors for stage I and II Hodgkin's disease. In: Somers R, Henry-Amar M, Meerwaldt JH, Carde P, eds. *Treatment strategy in Hodgkin's disease. Proceedings of the Paris International Workshop and Symposium held on June 28-30, 1989.* London: INSERM/John Libbey Eurotext; 1989: 37–50.

121. Kim HK, Silver B, Li S, et al. Hodgkin's disease in elderly patients (>or = 60): clinical outcome and treatment strategies. *Int J Radiat Oncol Biol Phys* 2003;56:556–560.

122. Guinee VF, Giacco GG, Durand M, et al. The prognosis of Hodgkin's disease in older adults. *J Clin Oncol* 1991;9:947–953.

123. Tubiana M. Hodgkin's disease: historical perspective and clinical presentation. *Baillieres Clin Haematol* 1996;9:503–530.

124. Haybittle JL, Hayhoe FG, Easterling MJ, et al. Review of British National Lymphoma Investigation studies of Hodgkin's disease and development of prognostic index. *Lancet* 1985;1:967–972.

125. Tubiana M, Henry-Amar M, Burgers MV, et al. Prognostic significance of erythrocyte sedimentation rate in clinical stages I–II of Hodgkin's disease. *J Clin Oncol* 1984;2:194–200.

126. Tubiana M, Attie E, Flamant R, et al. Prognostic factors in 454 cases of Hodgkin's disease. *Cancer Res* 1971;31:1801–1810.

127. Vaughan HB, MacLennan KA, Bennett MH, et al. Systemic disturbance in Hodgkin's disease and its relation to histopathology and prognosis (BNLI report no. 30). *Clin Radiol* 1987;38:257–261.

128. Gobbi PG, Gendarini A, Crema A, et al. Serum albumin in Hodgkin's disease. *Cancer* 1985;55:389–393.

129. Franklin J, Paulus U, Lieberz D, et al. Is the international prognostic score for advanced stage Hodgkin's disease applicable to early stage patients? German Hodgkin Lymphoma Study Group. *Ann Oncol* 2000;11: 617–623.

130. Specht L. Prognostic factors in Hodgkin's disease. *Cancer Treat Rev* 1991; 18:21–53.

131. Specht L, Gray RG, Clarke MJ, et al. Influence of more extensive radiotherapy and adjuvant chemotherapy on long-term outcome of early-stage Hodgkin's disease: a meta-analysis of 23 randomized trials involving 3,888 patients. International Hodgkin's Disease Collaborative Group. *J Clin Oncol* 1998;16:830–843.

132. Specht L. Very long-term follow-up of the Danish National Hodgkin Study Group's randomized trial of radiotherapy (RT) alone vs. combined modality treatment (CMT) for early stage Hodgkin lymphoma, with special reference to second tumours and overall survival. *Blood* 2003;102: 637A.

133. Bonfante V, Santoro A, Viviani S, et al. Early stage Hodgkin's disease: ten-year results of a non-randomised study with radiotherapy alone or combined with MOPP. *Eur J Cancer* 1993;29A:24–29.

134. Colonna P, Jais JP, Desablens B, et al. Mediastinal tumor size and response to chemotherapy are the only prognostic factors in supradiaphragmatic Hodgkin's disease treated by ABVD plus radiotherapy: ten-year results of the Paris-Ouest-France 81/12 trial, including 262 patients. *J Clin Oncol* 1996;14:1928–1935.

135. Lagarde P, Eghbali H, Bonichon F, et al. Brief chemotherapy associated with extended field radiotherapy in Hodgkin's disease. Long-term results in a series of 102 patients with clinical stages I-IIIA. *Eur J Cancer Clin Oncol* 1988;24:1191–1198.

136. Longo DL, Glatstein E, Duffey PL, et al. Alternating MOPP and ABVD chemotherapy plus mantle-field radiation therapy in patients with massive mediastinal Hodgkin's disease. *J Clin Oncol* 1997;15:3338–3346.

137. Pavlovsky S, Maschio M, Santarelli MT, et al. Randomized trial of chemotherapy versus chemotherapy plus radiotherapy for stage I-II Hodgkin's disease. *J Natl Cancer Inst* 1988;80:1466–1473.

138. Glimelius I, Molin D, Amini RM, et al. Bulky disease is the most important prognostic factor in Hodgkin lymphoma stage IIB. *Eur J Haematol* 2003;71:327–333.

139. Gobbi PG, Ghirardelli ML, Solcia M, et al. Image-aided estimate of tumor burden in Hodgkin's disease: evidence of its primary prognostic importance. *J Clin Oncol* 2001;19:1388–1394.

140. Gobbi PG, Broglia C, Di Giulio G, et al. The clinical value of tumor burden at diagnosis in Hodgkin lymphoma. *Cancer* 2004;101:1824–1834.

141. Grow A, Quon A, Graves EE, et al. Metabolic tumor volume as an independent prognostic factor in lymphoma. *J Clin Oncol* 2005;23(suppl.):583S.

142. Hutchings M, Berthelsen AK, Jakobsen AL, et al. Volume of abnormal tumour tissue on FDG-PET—a predictor of progression-free survival in Hodgkin lymphoma? *Int J Radiat Oncol Biol Phys* 2005;63:S45.

143. Delcambre C, Reman O, Henry-Amar M, et al. Clinical relevance of gallium-67 scintigraphy in lymphoma before and after therapy. *Eur J Nucl Med* 2000;27:176–184.

144. Hagemeister FB, Purugganan R, Podoloff DA, et al. The gallium scan predicts relapse in patients with Hodgkin's disease treated with combined modality therapy. *Ann Oncol* 1994;5(suppl 2):59–63.

145. Ionescu I, Brice P, Simon D, et al. Restaging with gallium scan identifies chemosensitive patients and predicts survival of poor-prognosis mediastinal Hodgkin's disease patients. *Med Oncol* 2000;17:127–134.

146. Ng AK, Bernardo MV, Silver B, et al. Mid- and post-ABVD gallium scanning predicts for recurrence in early-stage Hodgkin's disease. *Int J Radiat Oncol Biol Phys* 2005;61:175–184.

147. Front D, Bar-Shalom R, Mor M, et al. Hodgkin disease: prediction of outcome with 67Ga scintigraphy after one cycle of chemotherapy. *Radiology* 1999;210:487–491.

148. Salloum E, Brandt DS, Caride VJ, et al. Gallium scans in the management of patients with Hodgkin's disease: a study of 101 patients. *J Clin Oncol* 1997;15:518–527.

149. Hutchings M, Eigtved AI, Specht L. FDG-PET in the clinical management of Hodgkin lymphoma. *Crit Rev Oncol Hematol* 2004;52:19–32.

150. Specht L. Staging systems and staging investigations at presentation. In: Magrat I, ed. *The lymphoid neoplasms*, 3rd ed. London: Hodder Arnold; 2006 (in press).

151. Friedberg JW, Fischman A, Neuberg D, et al. FDG-PET is superior to gallium scintigraphy in staging and more sensitive in the follow-up of patients with de novo hodgkin lymphoma: A blinded comparison. *Leuk Lymphoma* 2004;45:85–92.

152. Hutchings M, Mikhaeel NG, Fields PA, et al. Prognostic value of interim FDG-PET after two or three cycles of chemotherapy in Hodgkin lymphoma. *Ann Oncol* 2005;16:1160–1168.

153. Hutchings M, Loft A, Hansen M, et al. FDG-PET after two cycles of chemotherapy predicts treatment failure and progression-free survival in Hodgkin lymphoma. *Blood* 2006;107:52–59.

154. Kostakoglu L, Coleman M, Leonard JP, et al. PET predicts prognosis after 1 cycle of chemotherapy in aggressive lymphoma and Hodgkin's disease. *J Nucl Med* 2002;43:1018–1027.

155. Bohlen H, Kessler M, Sextro M, et al. Poor clinical outcome of patients with Hodgkin's disease and elevated interleukin-10 serum levels. Clinical significance of interleukin-10 serum levels for Hodgkin's disease. *Ann Hematol* 2000;79:110–113.

156. Chronowski GM, Wilder RB, Tucker SL, et al. An elevated serum beta-2-microglobulin level is an adverse prognostic factor for overall survival in patients with early-stage Hodgkin disease. *Cancer* 2002;95:2534–2538.

157. Hohaus S, Di Ruscio A, Di Febo A, et al. Glutathione S-transferase P1 genotype and prognosis in Hodgkin's lymphoma. *Clin Cancer Res* 2005;11:2175–2179.

158. Portlock CS, Donnelly GB, Qin J, et al. Adverse prognostic significance of CD20 positive Reed-Sternberg cells in classical Hodgkin's disease. *Br J Haematol* 2004;125:701–708.

159. Smolewski P, Robak T, Krykowski E, et al. Prognostic factors in Hodgkin's disease: multivariate analysis of 327 patients from a single institution. *Clin Cancer Res* 2000;6:1150–1160.

160. ten Berge RL, Oudejans JJ, Dukers DF, et al. Percentage of activated cytotoxic T-lymphocytes in anaplastic large cell lymphoma and Hodgkin's disease: an independent biological prognostic marker. *Leukemia* 2001;15:458–464.

161. Tzankov A, Krugmann J, Fend F, et al. Prognostic significance of CD20 expression in classical Hodgkin lymphoma: a clinicopathological study of 119 cases. *Clin Cancer Res* 2003;9:1381–1386.

162. Vassilakopoulos TP, Nadali G, Angelopoulou MK, et al. Serum interleukin-10 levels are an independent prognostic factor for patients with Hodgkin's lymphoma. *Haematologica* 2001;86:274–281.

163. Vassilakopoulos TP, Nadali G, Angelopoulou MK, et al. The prognostic significance of beta(2)-microglobulin in patients with Hodgkin's lymphoma. *Haematologica* 2002;87:701–708.

164. von Wasielewski R, Seth S, Franklin J, et al. Tissue eosinophilia correlates strongly with poor prognosis in nodular sclerosing Hodgkin's disease, allowing for known prognostic factors. *Blood* 2000;95:1207–1213.

165. Benharroch D, Levy A, Prinsloo I, et al. Apoptotic index as a prognostic factor in Hodgkin's disease. *Leuk Lymphoma* 1999;33:351–359.

166. Smolewski P, Niewiadomska H, Los E, et al. Spontaneous apoptosis of Reed-Sternberg and Hodgkin cells; clinical and pathological implications in patients with Hodgkin's disease. *Int J Oncol* 2000;17:603–609.

167. Laskar S, Gupta T, Vimal S, et al. Consolidation radiation after complete remission in Hodgkin's disease following six cycles of doxorubicin, bleomycin, vinblastine, and dacarbazine chemotherapy: is there a need? *J Clin Oncol* 2004;22:62–68.

168. Meyer RM, Gospodarowicz MK, Connors JM, et al. Randomized comparison of ABVD chemotherapy with a strategy that includes radiation therapy in patients with limited-stage Hodgkin's lymphoma: National Cancer Institute of Canada Clinical Trials Group and the Eastern Cooperative Oncology Group. *J Clin Oncol* 2005;23:4634–4642.

169. Nachman JB, Sposto R, Herzog P, et al. Randomized comparison of low-dose involved-field radiotherapy and no radiotherapy for children with Hodgkin's disease who achieve a complete response to chemotherapy. *J Clin Oncol* 2002;20:3765–3771.

170. Shahidi M, Kamangari N, Ashley S, et al. Site of relapse after chemotherapy alone for stage I and II Hodgkin's disease. *Radiother Oncol* 2006;78:1–5.

171. Loeffler M, Brosteanu O, Hasenclever D, et al. Meta-analysis of chemotherapy versus combined modality treatment trials in Hodgkin's disease. International Database on Hodgkin's Disease Overview Study Group. *J Clin Oncol* 1998;16:818–829.

172. Hasenclever D, Diehl V. A prognostic score for advanced Hodgkin's disease. International Prognostic Factors Project on Advanced Hodgkin's Disease. *N Engl J Med* 1998;339:1506–1514.

173. Austin-Seymour MM, Hoppe RT, Cox RS, et al. Hodgkin's disease in patients over sixty years old. *Ann Intern Med* 1984;100:13–18.

174. Canellos GP, Anderson JR, Propert KJ, et al. Chemotherapy of advanced Hodgkin's disease with MOPP, ABVD, or MOPP alternating with ABVD. *N Engl J Med* 1992;327:1478–1484.

175. Ferme C, Bastion Y, Brice P, et al. Prognosis of patients with advanced Hodgkin's disease: evaluation of four prognostic models using 344 patients included in the Group d'Etudes des Lymphomes de l'Adulte Study. *Cancer* 1997;80:1124–1133.

176. Jaffe HS, Cadman EC, Farber LR, et al. Pretreatment hematocrit as an independent prognostic variable in Hodgkin's disease. *Blood* 1986;68:562–564.

177. Low SE, Horsman JM, Hancock H, et al. Prognostic markers in malignant lymphoma: an analysis of 1,198 patients treated at a single centre. *Int J Oncol* 2001;19:1203–1209.

178. Low SE, Horsman JM, Walters SJ, et al. Risk-adjusted prognostic models for Hodgkin's disease (HD) and grade II non-Hodgkin's lymphoma (NHL II): validation on 6728 British National Lymphoma Investigation patients. *Br J Haematol* 2003;120:277–280.

179. Löffler M, Dixon DO, Swindell R. Prognostic factors of stage III and IV Hodgkin's disease. In: Somers R, Henry-Amar M, Meerwaldt JH, Carde P, eds. *Treatment strategy in Hodgkin's disease. Proceedings of the Paris International Workshop and Symposium held on June 28–30, 1989.* London: INSERM/John Libbey Eurotext; 1990:89–103.

180. Peterson BA, Pajak TF, Cooper MR, et al. Effect of age on therapeutic response and survival in advanced Hodgkin's disease. *Cancer Treat Rep* 1982;66:889–898.

181. Proctor SJ, Taylor P, Donnan P, et al. A numerical prognostic index for clinical use in identification of poor-risk patients with Hodgkin's disease at diagnosis. Scotland and Newcastle Lymphoma Group (SNLG) therapy working party. *Eur J Cancer* 1991;27:624–629.

182. Ranson MR, Radford JA, Swindell R, et al. An analysis of prognostic factors in stage III and IV Hodgkin's disease treated at a single centre with MVPP. *Ann Oncol* 1991;2:423–429.

183. Somers R, Carde P, Henry-Amar M, et al. A randomized study in stage IIIB and IV Hodgkin's disease comparing eight courses of MOPP versus an alteration of MOPP with ABVD: a European Organization for Research and Treatment of Cancer Lymphoma Cooperative Group and Groupe Pierre-et-Marie-Curie controlled clinical trial. *J Clin Oncol* 1994;12:279–287.

184. Specht L, Nissen NI. Prognostic factors in Hodgkin's disease stage IV. *Eur J Haematol* 1988;41:359–367.

185. Specht L, Nissen NI. Prognostic factors in Hodgkin's disease stage III with special reference to tumour burden. *Eur J Haematol* 1988;41:80–87.

186. Straus DJ, Gaynor JJ, Myers J, et al. Prognostic factors among 185 adults with newly diagnosed advanced Hodgkin's disease treated with alternating potentially noncross- resistant chemotherapy and intermediate-dose radiation therapy. *J Clin Oncol* 1990;8:1173–1186.

187. Wagstaff J, Gregory WM, Swindell R, et al. Prognostic factors for survival in stage IIIB and IV Hodgkin's disease: a multivariate analysis comparing two specialist treatment centres. *Br J Cancer* 1988;58:487–492.

188. Yelle L, Bergsagel D, Basco V, et al. Combined modality therapy of Hodgkin's disease:10-year results of National Cancer Institute of Canada Clinical Trials Group multicenter clinical trial. *J Clin Oncol* 1991;9: 1983–1993.

189. van Spronsen DJ, Janssen-Heijnen ML, Lemmens VE, et al. Independent prognostic effect of co-morbidity in lymphoma patients: results of the population-based Eindhoven Cancer Registry. *Eur J Cancer* 2005;41: 1051–1057.

190. Proctor SJ, Rueffer JU, Angus B, et al. Hodgkin's disease in the elderly: current status and future directions. *Ann Oncol* 2002;13(suppl 1):133–137.

191. Engert A, Ballova V, Haverkamp H, et al. Hodgkin's lymphoma in elderly patients: a comprehensive retrospective analysis from the German Hodgkin's Study Group. *J Clin Oncol* 2005;23:5052–5060.

192. Dienstbier Z, Chytry P, Hermanska Z, et al. A multivariate analysis of prognostic factors in adult Hodgkin's disease. *Neoplasma* 1989;36:447–456.

193. Gobbi PG, Comelli M, Grignani GE, et al. Estimate of expected survival at diagnosis in Hodgkin's disease: a means of weighting prognostic factors and a tool for treatment choice and clinical research. A report from the International Database on Hodgkin's Disease (IDHD). *Haematologica* 1994;79:241–255.

194. Klimm B, Reineke T, Haverkamp H, et al. Role of hematotoxicity and sex in patients with Hodgkin's lymphoma: an analysis from the German Hodgkin Study Group. *J Clin Oncol* 2005;23:8003–8011.

195. Wagstaff J, Steward W, Jones M, et al. Factors affecting remission and survival in patients with advanced Hodgkin's disease treated with MVPP. *Hematol Oncol* 1986;4:135–147.

196. Rodgers RW, Fuller LM, Hagemeister FB, et al. Reassessment of prognostic factors in stage IIIA and IIIB Hodgkin's disease treated with MOPP and radiotherapy. *Cancer* 1981;47:2196–2203.

197. Hancock BW, Vaughan HG, Vaughan HB, et al. LOPP alternating with EVAP is superior to LOPP alone in the initial treatment of advanced Hodgkin's disease: results of a British National Lymphoma Investigation trial. *J Clin Oncol* 1992;10:1252–1258.

198. Longo DL, Young RC, Wesley M, et al. Twenty years of MOPP therapy for Hodgkin's disease. *J Clin Oncol* 1986;4:1295–1306.

199. Moore MR, Jones SE, Bull JM, et al. MOPP chemotherapy for advanced Hodgkin's disease. Prognostic factors in 81 patients. *Cancer* 1973;32:52–60.

200. Sutcliffe SB, Wrigley PF, Peto J, et al. MVPP chemotherapy regimen for advanced Hodgkin's disease. *Br Med J* 1978;1:679–683.

201. d'Amore ES, Lee CK, Aeppli DM, et al. Lack of prognostic value of histopathologic parameters in Hodgkin's disease, nodular sclerosis type. A study of 123 patients with limited stage disease who had undergone laparotomy and were treated with radiation therapy. *Arch Pathol Lab Med* 1992;116:856–861.

202. Ferry JA, Linggood RM, Convery KM, et al. Hodgkin disease, nodular sclerosis type. Implications of histologic subclassification. *Cancer* 1993;71: 457–463.

203. Georgii A, Fischer R, Hubner K, et al. Classification of Hodgkin's disease biopsies by a panel of four histopathologists. Report of 1,140 patients from the German National Trial. *Leuk Lymphoma* 1993;9:365–370.

204. Hess JL, Bodis S, Pinkus G, et al. Histopathologic grading of nodular sclerosis Hodgkin's disease. Lack of prognostic significance in 254 surgically staged patients. *Cancer* 1994;74:708–714.

205. MacLennan KA, Bennett MH, Tu A, et al. Relationship of histopathologic features to survival and relapse in nodular sclerosing Hodgkin's disease. A study of 1659 patients. *Cancer* 1989;64:1686–1693.

206. Masih AS, Weisenburger DD, Vose JM, et al. Histologic grade does not predict prognosis in optimally treated, advanced-stage nodular sclerosing Hodgkin's disease. *Cancer* 1992;69:228–232.

207. Norum J, Wist E, Nordoy T, et al. Subclassification of Hodgkin's disease, nodular sclerosis type. Prognostic value? *Anticancer Res* 1995;15: 1569–1572.

208. van Spronsen DJ, Vrints LW, Hofstra G, et al. Disappearance of prognostic significance of histopathological grading of nodular sclerosing Hodgkin's disease for unselected patients, 1972–92. *Br J Haematol* 1997;96:322–327.

209. Torricelli P, Grimaldi PL, Fiocchi F, et al. Hodgkin's disease: a quantitative evaluation by computed tomography of tumor burden. *Clin Imaging* 2004;28:239–244.

210. Selby P, Patel P, Milan S, et al. ChlVPP combination chemotherapy for Hodgkin's disease: long-term results. *Br J Cancer* 1990;62:279–285.

211. Hoppe RT, Rosenberg SA, Kaplan HS, et al. Prognostic factors in pathological stage IIIA Hodgkin's disease. *Cancer* 1980;46:1240–1246.

212. Hoppe RT, Cox RS, Rosenberg SA, et al. Prognostic factors in pathologic stage III Hodgkin's disease. *Cancer Treat Rep* 1982;66:743–749.

213. Mauch P, Goffman T, Rosenthal DS, et al. Stage III Hodgkin's disease: improved survival with combined modality therapy as compared with radiation therapy alone. *J Clin Oncol* 1985;3:1166–1173.

214. Mazza P, Miniaci G, Lauria F, et al. Prognostic significance of lymphography in stage IIIs Hodgkin's disease (HD). *Eur J Cancer Clin Oncol* 1984;20: 1393–1399.

215. Powlis WD, Mauch P, Goffman T, et al. Treatment of patients with "minimal" stage IIIA Hodgkin's disease. *Int J Radiat Oncol Biol Phys* 1987;13: 1437–1442.

216. Stein RS, Golomb HM, Wiernik PH, et al. Anatomic substages of stage IIIA Hodgkin's disease: followup of a collaborative study. *Cancer Treat Rep* 1982;66:733–741.

217. Brada M, Ashley S, Nicholls J, et al. Stage III Hodgkin's disease—long-term results following chemotherapy, radiotherapy and combined modality therapy. *Radiother Oncol* 1989;14:185–198.

218. Desser RK, Golomb HM, Ultmann JE, et al. Prognostic classification of Hodgkin disease in pathologic stage III, based on anatomic considerations. *Blood* 1977;49:883–893.

219. Farah R, Golomb HM, Hallahan DE, et al. Radiation therapy for pathologic stage III Hodgkin's disease with and without chemotherapy. *Int J Radiat Oncol Biol Phys* 1989;17:761–766.

220. Golomb HM, Sweet DL, Ultmann JE, et al. Importance of substaging of stage III Hodgkin's disease. *Semin Oncol* 1980;7:136–143.

221. Levi JA, Wiernik PH. The therapeutic implications of splenic involvement in stage IIIA Hodgkin's disease. *Cancer* 1977;39:2158–2165.

222. Levi JA, Wiernik PH, O'Connel MJ. Patterns of relapse in stages I, II and IIIA Hodgkin's disease: influence of initial therapy and implications for the future. *Int J Radiat Oncol Biol Phys* 1977;2:853–862.

223. Hopper KD, Diehl LF, Lynch JC, et al. Mediastinal bulk in Hodgkin disease. Method of measurement versus prognosis. *Invest Radiol* 1991;26: 1101–1110.

224. Proctor SJ, Taylor P, Mackie MJ, et al. A numerical prognostic index for clinical use in identification of poor-risk patients with Hodgkin's disease at diagnosis. The Scotland and Newcastle Lymphoma Group (SNLG) therapy working party. *Leuk Lymphoma* 1992;7(suppl):17–20.

225. Hasenclever D, Schmitz N, Diehl V. Is there a rationale for high-dose chemotherapy as first line treatment of advanced Hodgkin's disease? German Hodgkin's Lymphoma Study Group (GHSG). *Leuk Lymphoma* 1995;15(suppl 1):47–49.

226. Bartl R, Frisch B, Burkhardt R, et al. Assessment of bone marrow histology in Hodgkin's disease: correlation with clinical factors. *Br J Haematol* 1982;51:345–360.

227. Brusamolino E, Orlandi E, Morra E, et al. Analysis of long-term results and prognostic factors among 138 patients with advanced Hodgkin's disease treated with the alternating MOPP/ABVD chemotherapy. *Ann Oncol* 1994;5(suppl 2):53–57.

228. Carde P, MacKintosh FR, Rosenberg SA. A dose and time response analysis of the treatment of Hodgkin's disease with MOPP chemotherapy. *J Clin Oncol* 1983;1:146–153.

229. Gibbs GE, Peterson BA, Kennedy BJ, et al. Long-term survival of patients with Hodgkin's disease. Treatment with cyclophosphamide, vinblastine, procarbazine, and prednisone. *Arch Intern Med* 1981;141:897–900.

230. Hoffken K, Ippisch A, Pfeiffer R, et al. Chemotherapie der fortgeschrittenen lymphogranulomatose. *Dtsch Med Wochenschr* 1985;110:618–623.

231. DeVita VT, Jr., Simon RM, Hubbard SM, et al. Curability of advanced Hodgkin's disease with chemotherapy. Long-term follow-up of MOPP-treated patients at the National Cancer Institute. *Ann Intern Med* 1980;92: 587–595.

232. Munker R, Hasenclever D, Brosteanu O, et al. Bone marrow involvement in Hodgkin's disease: an analysis of 135 consecutive cases. German Hodgkin's Lymphoma Study Group. *J Clin Oncol* 1995;13:403–409.

233. Bonadonna G, Valagussa P, Santoro A. Alternating non-cross-resistant combination chemotherapy or MOPP in stage IV Hodgkin's disease. A report of 8-year results. *Ann Intern Med* 1986;104:739–746.

234. Pillai GN, Hagemeister FB, Velasquez WS, et al. Prognostic factors for stage IV Hodgkin's disease treated with MOPP, with or without bleomycin. *Cancer* 1985;55:691–697.

235. Gobbi PG, Cavalli C, Gendarini A, et al. Prognostic significance of serum albumin in Hodgkin's disease. *Haematologica* 1986;71:95–102.

236. Straus DJ. High-risk Hodgkin's disease prognostic factors. *Leuk Lymphoma* 1995;15(suppl 1):41–42.

237. MacLennan KA, Vaughan HB, Easterling MJ, et al. The presentation haemoglobin level in 1103 patients with Hodgkin's disease (BNLI report no. 21). *Clin Radiol* 1983;34:491–495.

238. Loeffler M, Pfreundschuh M, Hasenclever D, et al. Prognostic risk factors in advanced Hodgkin's lymphoma. Report of the German Hodgkin Study Group. *Blut* 1988;56:273–281.

239. Aviles A, Talavera A, Garcia EL, et al. La fosfatasa alcalina como factor pronóstico en enfermedad de Hodgkin (Alkaline phosphatase as a prognostic factor in Hodgkin's disease). *Rev Gastroenterol Mex* 1990;55: 211–214.

240. MacLennan KA, Hudson BV, Jelliffe AM, et al. The pretreatment peripheral blood lymphocyte count in 1100 patients with Hodgkin's disease: the prognostic significance and the relationship to the presence of systemic symptoms. *Clin Oncol* 1981;7:333–339.

241. A predictive model for aggressive non-Hodgkin's lymphoma. The International Non-Hodgkin's Lymphoma Prognostic Factors Project. *N Engl J Med* 1993;329:987–994.

242. Dimopoulos MA, Cabanillas F, Lee JJ, et al. Prognostic role of serum beta 2-microglobulin in Hodgkin's disease. *J Clin Oncol* 1993; 11:1108–1111.

243. Zander T, Wiedenmann S, Wolf J. Prognostic factors in Hodgkin's lymphoma. *Ann Oncol* 2002;13(suppl 1):67–74.

244. Gause A, Jung W, Keymis S, et al. The clinical significance of cytokines and soluble forms of membrane-derived activation antigens in the serum of patients with Hodgkin's disease. *Leuk Lymphoma* 1992;7:439–447.

245. Gause A, Jung W, Schmits R, et al. Soluble CD8, CD25 and CD30 antigens as prognostic markers in patients with untreated Hodgkin's lymphoma. *Ann Oncol* 1992;3(suppl 4):49–52.

246. Nadali G, Vinante F, Ambrosetti A, et al. Serum levels of soluble CD30 are elevated in the majority of untreated patients with Hodgkin's disease and correlate with clinical features and prognosis. *J Clin Oncol* 1994;12: 793–797.

247. Pizzolo G, Vinante F, Chilosi M, et al. Serum levels of soluble CD30 molecule (Ki-1 antigen) in Hodgkin's disease: relationship with disease activity and clinical stage. *Br J Haematol* 1990;75:282–284.

248. Axdorph U, Sjoberg J, Grimfors G, et al. Biological markers may add to prediction of outcome achieved by the International Prognostic Score in Hodgkin's disease. *Ann Oncol* 2000;11:1405–1411.

249. Zanotti R, Trolese A, Ambrosetti A, et al. Serum levels of soluble CD30 improve International Prognostic Score in predicting the outcome of advanced Hodgkin's lymphoma. *Ann Oncol* 2002;13:1908–1914.

250. Gobbi PG, Gobbi PG, Mazza P, et al. Multivariate analysis of Hodgkin's disease prognosis. Fitness and use of a directly predictive equation. *Haematologica* 1989;74:29–8.

251. Diehl V, Franklin J, Pfreundschuh M, et al. Standard and increased-dose BEACOPP chemotherapy compared with COPP-ABVD for advanced Hodgkin's disease. *N Engl J Med* 2003;348:2386–2395.

252. Duggan DB, Petroni GR, Johnson JL, et al. Randomized comparison of ABVD and MOPP/ABV hybrid for the treatment of advanced Hodgkin's disease: report of an intergroup trial. *J Clin Oncol* 2003;21:607–614.

253. Gobbi PG, Zinzani PL, Broglia C, et al. Comparison of prognostic models in patients with advanced Hodgkin disease. Promising results from integration of the best three systems. *Cancer* 2001;91:1467–1478.

254. Johnson PW, Radford JA, Cullen MH, et al. Comparison of ABVD and alternating or hybrid multidrug regimens for the treatment of advanced Hodgkin's lymphoma: results of the United Kingdom Lymphoma Group LY09 trial (ISRCTN97144519). *J Clin Oncol* 2005;23:9208–9218.

255. Radford JA, Rohatiner AZ, Ryder WD, et al. ChlVPP/EVA hybrid versus the weekly VAPEC-B regimen for previously untreated Hodgkin's disease. *J Clin Oncol* 2002;20:2988–2994.

256. Bierman PJ, Lynch JC, Bociek RG, et al. The International Prognostic Factors Project score for advanced Hodgkin's disease is useful for predicting outcome of autologous hematopoietic stem cell transplantation. *Ann Oncol* 2002;13:1370–1377.

257. Gisselbrecht C, Mounier N, Andre M, et al. How to define intermediate stage in Hodgkin's lymphoma? *Eur J Haematol Suppl* 2005;111–114.

258. Healey EA, Tarbell NJ, Kalish LA, et al. Prognostic factors for patients with Hodgkin disease in first relapse. *Cancer* 1993;71:2613–2620.

259. Amini RM, Glimelius B, Gustavsson A, et al. A population-based study of the outcome for patients with first relapse of Hodgkin's lymphoma. *Eur J Haematol* 2002;68:225–232.

260. Cooper MR, Pajak TF, Gottlieb AJ, et al. The effects of prior radiation therapy and age on the frequency and duration of complete remission among various four-drug treatments for advanced Hodgkin's disease. *J Clin Oncol* 1984;2:748–755.

261. Horwich A, Specht L, Ashley S. Survival analysis of patients with clinical stages I or II Hodgkin's disease who have relapsed after initial treatment with radiotherapy alone. *Eur J Cancer* 1997;33:848–853.

262. Mauch P, Ryback M, Rosenthal D, et al. The influence of initial pathologic stage on the survival of patients who relapse from Hodgkin's disease. *Blood* 1980;56:892–897.

263. Ng AK, Li S, Neuberg D, et al. Comparison of MOPP versus ABVD as salvage therapy in patients who relapse after radiation therapy alone for Hodgkin's disease. *Ann Oncol* 2004;15:270–275.

264. Olver IN, Wolf MM, Cruickshank D, et al. Nitrogen mustard, vincristine, procarbazine, and prednisolone for relapse after radiation in Hodgkin's disease. An analysis of long-term follow-up. *Cancer* 1988;62:233–239.

265. Roach M, III, Brophy N, Cox R, et al. Prognostic factors for patients relapsing after radiotherapy for early- stage Hodgkin's disease. *J Clin Oncol* 1990;8:623–629.

266. Santoro A, Viviani S, Villarreal CJ, et al. Salvage chemotherapy in Hodgkin's disease irradiation failures: superiority of doxorubicin-containing regimens over MOPP. *Cancer Treat Rep* 1986;70:343–348.

267. Specht L, Horwich A, Ashley S. Salvage of relapse of patients with Hodgkin's disease in clinical stages I or II who were staged with laparotomy and initially treated with radiotherapy alone. A report from the international database on Hodgkin's disease. *Int J Radiat Oncol Biol Phys* 1994;30:805–811.

268. Timothy AR, Sutcliffe SB, Wrigley PF, et al. Hodgkin's disease: combination chemotherapy for relapse following radical radiotherapy. *Int J Radiat Oncol Biol Phys* 1979;5:165–169.

269. Tubiana M, Werf-Messing B, Laugier A, et al. Survival after recurrence: prognostic factors and spread patterns in clinical stages I and II of Hodgkin's disease. *Natl Cancer Inst Monogr* 1973;36:513–530.

270. Vinciguerra V, Propert KJ, Coleman M, et al. Alternating cycles of combination chemotherapy for patients with recurrent Hodgkin's disease following radiotherapy. A prospectively randomized study by the Cancer and Leukemia Group B. *J Clin Oncol* 1986;4:838–846.

271. Portlock CS, Rosenberg SA, Glatstein E, et al. Impact of salvage treatment on initial relapses in patients with Hodgkin disease, stages I-III. *Blood* 1978;51:825–833.

272. Specht L, Nissen NI. Hodgkin's disease and age. *Eur J Haematol* 1989;43: 127–135.

273. Herman TS, Hoppe RT, Donaldson SS, et al. Late relapse among patients treated for Hodgkin's disease. *Ann Intern Med* 1985;102:292–297.

274. Biti GP, Cimino G, Cartoni C, et al. Extended-field radiotherapy is superior to MOPP chemotherapy for the treatment of pathologic stage I-IIA Hodgkin's disease: eight-year update of an Italian prospective randomized study. *J Clin Oncol* 1992;10:378–382.

275. Bonfante V, Santoro A, Viviani S, et al. Outcome of patients with Hodgkin's disease failing after primary MOPP-ABVD. *J Clin Oncol* 1997;15: 528–534.

276. Brice P, Bastion Y, Divine M, et al. Analysis of prognostic factors after the first relapse of Hodgkin's disease in 187 patients. *Cancer* 1996;78:1293–1299.

277. Canellos GP, Petroni GR, Barcos M, et al. Etoposide, vinblastine, and doxorubicin: an active regimen for the treatment of Hodgkin's disease in relapse following MOPP. Cancer and Leukemia Group B. *J Clin Oncol* 1995;13: 2005–2011.

278. Enblad G, Glimelius B, Hagberg H, et al. Methyl-GAG, ifosfamide, methotrexate and etoposide (MIME) as salvage therapy for Hodgkin's disease and non-Hodgkin's lymphoma. The Swedish Lymphoma Study Group. *Acta Oncol* 1990;29:297–301.

279. Fairey AF, Mead GM, Jones HW, et al. CAPE/PALE salvage chemotherapy for Hodgkin's disease patients relapsing within 1 year of ChlVPP chemotherapy. *Ann Oncol* 1993;4:857–860.

280. Ferme C, Bastion Y, Lepage E, et al. The MINE regimen as intensive salvage chemotherapy for relapsed and refractory Hodgkin's disease. *Ann Oncol* 1995;6:543–549.

281. Fisher RI, DeVita VT, Hubbard SP, et al. Prolonged disease-free survival in Hodgkin's disease with MOPP reinduction after first relapse. *Ann Intern Med* 1979;90:761–763.

282. Hagemeister FB, Tannir N, McLaughlin P, et al. MIME chemotherapy (methyl-GAG, ifosfamide, methotrexate, etoposide) as treatment for recurrent Hodgkin's disease. *J Clin Oncol* 1987;5:556–561.

283. Harker WG, Kushlan P, Rosenberg SA. Combination chemotherapy for advanced Hodgkin's disease after failure of MOPP: ABVD and B-CAVe. *Ann Intern Med* 1984;101:440–446.

284. Krikorian JG, Portlock CS, Rosenberg SA. Treatment of advanced Hodgkin's disease with adriamycin, bleomycin, vinblastine, and imidazole carboxamide (ABVD) after failure of MOPP therapy. *Cancer* 1978;41: 2107–2111.

285. Lohri A, Barnett M, Fairey RN, et al. Outcome of treatment of first relapse of Hodgkin's disease after primary chemotherapy: identification of risk factors from the British Columbia experience 1970 to 1988. *Blood* 1991;77: 2292–2298.

286. Longo DL, Duffey PL, Young RC, et al. Conventional-dose salvage combination chemotherapy in patients relapsing with Hodgkin's disease after combination chemotherapy: the low probability for cure. *J Clin Oncol* 1992;10:210–218.

287. Perren TJ, Selby PJ, Milan S, et al. Etoposide and adriamycin containing combination chemotherapy (HOPE-Bleo) for relapsed Hodgkin's disease. *Br J Cancer* 1990;61:919–923.

288. Pfreundschuh MG, Schoppe WD, Fuchs R, et al. Lomustine, etoposide, vindesine, and dexamethasone (CEVD) in Hodgkin's lymphoma refractory to cyclophosphamide, vincristine, procarbazine, and prednisone (COPP) and doxorubicin, bleomycin, vinblastine, and dacarbazine (ABVD): a multicenter trial of the German Hodgkin Study Group. *Cancer Treat Rep* 1987;71: 1203–1207.

289. Radman I, Basic N, Labar B, et al. Long-term results of conventional-dose salvage chemotherapy in patients with refractory and relapsed Hodgkin's disease (Croatian experience). *Ann Oncol* 2002;13:1650–1655.

290. Richards MA, Waxman JH, Man T, et al. EVA treatment for recurrent or unresponsive Hodgkin's disease. *Cancer Chemother Pharmacol* 1986;18: 51–53.

291. Salvagno L, Soraru M, Aversa SM, et al. Late relapses in Hodgkin's disease: outcome of patients relapsing more than twelve months after primary chemotherapy. *Ann Oncol* 1993;4:657–662.

292. Santoro A, Bonfante V, Bonadonna G. Salvage chemotherapy with ABVD in MOPP-resistant Hodgkin's disease. *Ann Intern Med* 1982;96: 139–143.

293. Schulman P, McCarroll K, Cooper MR, et al. Phase II study of MOPLACE chemotherapy for patients with previously treated Hodgkin's disease: a CALGB study. *Med Pediatr Oncol* 1990;18:482–486.

294. Straus DJ, Passe S, Koziner B, et al. Combination chemotherapy salvage of heavily pretreated patients with Hodgkin's disease: an analysis of prognostic factors in two chemotherapy trials and the literature. *Cancer Treat Rep* 1981;65:207–211.

295. Straus DJ, Myers J, Koziner B, et al. Combination chemotherapy for the treatment of Hodgkin's disease in relapse. Results with lomustine (CCNU), melphalan (Alkeran), and vindesine (DVA) alone (CAD) and in alternation with MOPP and doxorubicin (Adriamycin), bleomycin, and vinblastine (ABV). *Cancer Chemother Pharmacol* 1983;11:80–85.

296. Sutcliffe SB, Wrigley PF, Stansfeld AG, et al. Adriamycin, bleomycin, vinblastine and imidazole carboxamide (ABVD) therapy for advanced Hodgkin's disease resistant to mustine, vinblastine, procarbazine and prednisolone (MVPP). *Cancer Chemother Pharmacol* 1979;2:209–213.

297. Tannir N, Hagemeister F, Velasquez W, et al. Long-term follow-up with ABDIC salvage chemotherapy of MOPP-resistant Hodgkin's disease. *J Clin Oncol* 1983;1:432–439.

298. Viviani S, Santoro A, Negretti E, et al. Salvage chemotherapy in Hodgkin's disease. Results in patients relapsing more than twelve months after first complete remission. *Ann Oncol* 1990;1:123–127.

299. Vassilakopoulos TP, Angelopoulou MK, Siakantaris MP, et al. Hodgkin's lymphoma in first relapse following chemotherapy or combined modality therapy: analysis of outcome and prognostic factors after conventional salvage therapy. *Eur J Haematol* 2002;68:289–298.

300. Josting A, Rueffer U, Franklin J, et al. Prognostic factors and treatment outcome in primary progressive Hodgkin lymphoma: a report from the German Hodgkin Lymphoma Study Group. *Blood* 2000;96:1280–1286.

301. Josting A, Franklin J, May M, et al. New prognostic score based on treatment outcome of patients with relapsed Hodgkin's lymphoma registered in the database of the German Hodgkin's Lymphoma Study Group. *J Clin Oncol* 2001;20:221–230.

302. Josting A, Schmitz N. Insights into 25 years of clinical trials of the GHSG: Relapsed and refractory Hodgkin's disease. In: Diehl V, Josting A, eds. *25 years German Hodgkin Study Group.* Munich: Urban & Vogel; 2004: 89–99.

303. Brada M, Eeles R, Ashley S, et al. Salvage radiotherapy in recurrent Hodgkin's disease. *Ann Oncol* 1992;3:131–135.

304. Fox KA, Lippman SM, Cassady JR, et al. Radiation therapy salvage of Hodgkin's disease following chemotherapy failure. *J Clin Oncol* 1987;5:38–45.

305. Josting A, Nogova L, Franklin J, et al. Salvage radiotherapy in patients with relapsed and refractory Hodgkin's lymphoma: a retrospective analysis from the German Hodgkin Lymphoma Study Group. *J Clin Oncol* 2005;23:1522–1529.

306. Kirkove C, Timothy AR. Radiotherapy as salvage treatment in patients with Hodgkin's disease or non-Hodgkin's lymphoma relapsing after initial chemotherapy. *Hematol Oncol* 1991;9:163–167.

307. Leigh BR, Fox KA, Mack CF, et al. Radiation therapy salvage of Hodgkin's disease following chemotherapy failure. *Int J Radiat Oncol Biol Phys* 1993;27:855–862.

308. MacMillan CH, Bessell EM. The effectiveness of radiotherapy for localized relapse in patients with Hodgkin's disease (IIB-IVB) who obtained a complete response with chemotherapy alone as initial treatment. *Clin Oncol (R Coll Radiol)* 1994;6:147–150.

309. Mauch P, Tarbell N, Skarin A, et al. Wide-field radiation therapy alone or with chemotherapy for Hodgkin's disease in relapse from combination chemotherapy. *J Clin Oncol* 1987;5:544–549.

310. O'Brien PC, Parnis FX. Salvage radiotherapy following chemotherapy failure in Hodgkin's disease—what is its role? *Acta Oncol* 1995;34:99–104.

311. Pezner RD, Lipsett JA, Vora N, et al. Radical radiotherapy as salvage treatment for relapse of Hodgkin's disease initially treated by chemotherapy alone: prognostic significance of the disease-free interval. *Int J Radiat Oncol Biol Phys* 1994;30:965–970.

312. Roach M III, Kapp DS, Rosenberg SA, et al. Radiotherapy with curative intent: an option in selected patients relapsing after chemotherapy for advanced Hodgkin's disease. *J Clin Oncol* 1987;5:550–555.

313. Uematsu M, Tarbell NJ, Silver B, et al. Wide-field radiation therapy with or without chemotherapy for patients with Hodgkin disease in relapse after initial combination chemotherapy. *Cancer* 1993;72:207–212.

314. Wirth A, Corry J, Laidlaw C, et al. Salvage radiotherapy for Hodgkin's disease following chemotherapy failure. *Int J Radiat Oncol Biol Phys* 1997;39:599–607.

315. Linch DC, Winfield D, Goldstone AH, et al. Dose intensification with autologous bone-marrow transplantation in relapsed and resistant Hodgkin's disease: results of a BNLI randomised trial. *Lancet* 1993;341:1051–1054.

316. Schmitz N, Pfistner B, Sextro M, et al. Aggressive conventional chemotherapy compared with high-dose chemotherapy with autologous haemopoietic stem-cell transplantation for relapsed chemosensitive Hodgkin's disease: a randomised trial. *Lancet* 2002;359:2065–2071.

317. Ager S, Wimperis JZ, Tolliday B, et al. Autologous bone marrow transplantation for Hodgkin's disease—a five-year single centre experience. *Leuk Lymphoma* 1994;13:263–272.

318. Akpek G, Ambinder RF, Piantadosi S, et al. Long-term results of blood and marrow transplantation for Hodgkin's lymphoma. *J Clin Oncol* 2001;19:4314–4321.

319. Anderson JE, Litzow MR, Appelbaum FR, et al. Allogeneic, syngeneic, and autologous marrow transplantation for Hodgkin's disease: the 21-year Seattle experience. *J Clin Oncol* 1993;11:2342–2350.

320. Anselmo AP, Cavalieri E, Meloni G, et al. Dose intensification with autologous stem cell transplantation in relapsed and resistant Hodgkin's disease. *Haematologica* 2002;87:507–511.

321. Argiris A, Seropian S, Cooper DL. High-dose BEAM chemotherapy with autologous peripheral blood progenitor-cell transplantation for unselected patients with primary refractory or relapsed Hodgkin's disease. *Ann Oncol* 2000;11:665–672.

322. Ferme C, Mounier N, Divine M, et al. Intensive salvage therapy with high-dose chemotherapy for patients with advanced Hodgkin's disease in relapse or failure after initial chemotherapy: results of the Groupe d'Etudes des Lymphomes de l'Adulte H89 Trial. *J Clin Oncol* 2002;20:467–475.

323. Hahn T, Benekli M, Wong C, et al. A prognostic model for prolonged event-free survival after autologous or allogeneic blood or marrow transplantation for relapsed and refractory Hodgkin's disease. *Bone Marrow Transplant* 2005;35:557–566.

324. Harding M, Selby P, Gore M, et al. High-dose chemotherapy and autologous bone marrow transplantation for relapsed and refractory Hodgkin's disease. *Eur J Cancer* 1992;28A:1396–1400.

325. Jones RJ, Piantadosi S, Mann RB, et al. High-dose cytotoxic therapy and bone marrow transplantation for relapsed Hodgkin's disease. *J Clin Oncol* 1990;8:527–537.

326. Josting A, Rudolph C, Mapara M, et al. Cologne high-dose sequential chemotherapy in relapsed and refractory Hodgkin lymphoma: results of a large multicenter study of the German Hodgkin Lymphoma Study Group (GHSG). *Ann Oncol* 2005;16:116–123.

327. Josting A. Autologous transplantation in relapsed and refractory Hodgkin's disease. *Eur J Haematol Suppl* 2005;141–145.

328. Lavoie JC, Connors JM, Phillips GL, et al. High-dose chemotherapy and autologous stem cell transplantation for primary refractory or relapsed Hodgkin lymphoma: long-term outcome in the first 100 patients treated in Vancouver. *Blood* 2005;106:1473–1478.

329. Lazarus HM, Loberiza FR Jr., Zhang MJ, et al. Autotransplants for Hodgkin's disease in first relapse or second remission: a report from the autologous blood and marrow transplant registry (ABMTR). *Bone Marrow Transplant* 2001;27:387–396.

330. Moskowitz CH, Nimer SD, Zelenetz AD, et al. A 2-step comprehensive high-dose chemoradiotherapy second-line program for relapsed and refractory Hodgkin disease: analysis by intent to treat and development of a prognostic model. *Blood* 2001;97:616–623.

331. Neben K, Hohaus S, Goldschmidt H, et al. High-dose therapy with peripheral blood stem cell transplantation for patients with relapsed or refractory Hodgkin's disease: long-term outcome and prognostic factors. *Ann Hematol* 2000;79:547–555.

332. O'Brien ME, Milan S, Cunningham D, et al. High-dose chemotherapy and autologous bone marrow transplant in relapsed Hodgkin's disease—a pragmatic prognostic index. *Br J Cancer* 1996;73:1272–1277.

333. Poen JC, Hoppe RT, Horning SJ. High-dose therapy and autologous bone marrow transplantation for relapsed/refractory Hodgkin's disease: the impact of involved field radiotherapy on patterns of failure and survival. *Int J Radiat Oncol Biol Phys* 1996;36:3–12.

334. Popat U, Hosing C, Saliba RM, et al. Prognostic factors for disease progression after high-dose chemotherapy and autologous hematopoietic stem cell transplantation for recurrent or refractory Hodgkin's lymphoma. *Bone Marrow Transplant* 2004;33:1015–1023.

335. Sureda A, Constans M, Iriondo A, et al. Prognostic factors affecting long-term outcome after stem cell transplantation in Hodgkin's lymphoma autografted after a first relapse. *Ann Oncol* 2005;16:625–633.

336. Yahalom J, Gulati SC, Toia M, et al. Accelerated hyperfractionated total-lymphoid irradiation, high-dose chemotherapy, and autologous bone marrow transplantation for refractory and relapsing patients with Hodgkin's disease. *J Clin Oncol* 1993;11:1062–1070.

337. Zinzani PL, Tani M, Gabriele A, et al. High-dose therapy with autologous transplantation for Hodgkin's disease: the Bologna experience. *Haematologica* 2003;88:522–528.

338. Bierman PJ, Anderson JR, Freeman MB, et al. High-dose chemotherapy followed by autologous hematopoietic rescue for Hodgkin's disease patients following first relapse after chemotherapy. *Ann Oncol* 1996;7:151–156.

339. Reece DE, Phillips GL. Intensive therapy and autologous stem cell transplantation for Hodgkin's disease in first relapse after combination chemotherapy. *Leuk Lymphoma* 1996;21:245–253.

340. Rodriguez J, Rodriguez MA, Fayad L, et al. ASHAP: a regimen for cytoreduction of refractory or recurrent Hodgkin's disease. *Blood* 1999;93:3632–3636.

341. Bierman PJ, Bagin RG, Jagannath S, et al. High dose chemotherapy followed by autologous hematopoietic rescue in Hodgkin's disease: long-term follow-up in 128 patients. *Ann Oncol* 1993;4:767–773.

342. Chopra R, McMillan AK, Linch DC, et al. The place of high-dose BEAM therapy and autologous bone marrow transplantation in poor-risk Hodgkin's disease. A single-center eight-year study of 155 patients. *Blood* 1993;81:1137–1145.

343. Jagannath S, Armitage JO, Dicke KA, et al. Prognostic factors for response and survival after high-dose cyclophosphamide, carmustine, and etoposide with autologous bone marrow transplantation for relapsed Hodgkin's disease. *J Clin Oncol* 1989;7:179–185.

344. Nademanee A, O'Donnell MR, Snyder DS, et al. High-dose chemotherapy with or without total body irradiation followed by autologous bone marrow and/or peripheral blood stem cell transplantation for patients with relapsed and refractory Hodgkin's disease: results in 85 patients with analysis of prognostic factors. *Blood* 1995;85:1381–1390.

345. Stewart DA, Guo D, Gluck S, et al. Double high-dose therapy for Hodgkin's disease with dose-intensive cyclophosphamide, etoposide, and cisplatin (DICEP) prior to high-dose melphalan and autologous stem cell transplantation. *Bone Marrow Transplant* 2000;26:383–388.

346. Crump M, Smith AM, Brandwein J, et al. High-dose etoposide and melphalan, and autologous bone marrow transplantation for patients with advanced Hodgkin's disease: importance of disease status at transplant. *J Clin Oncol* 1993;11:704–711.

347. Rapoport AP, Rowe JM, Kouides PA, et al. One hundred autotransplants for relapsed or refractory Hodgkin's disease and lymphoma: value of pretransplant disease status for predicting outcome. *J Clin Oncol* 1993;11:2351–2361.

348. Lumley MA, Milligan DW, Knechtli CJ, et al. High lactate dehydrogenase level is associated with an adverse outlook in autografting for Hodgkin's disease. *Bone Marrow Transplant* 1996;17:383–388.

349. Brice P, Bouabdallah R, Moreau P, et al. Prognostic factors for survival after high-dose therapy and autologous stem cell transplantation for patients with relapsing Hodgkin's disease: analysis of 280 patients from the French registry. Societe Francaise de Greffe de Moelle. *Bone Marrow Transplant* 1997;20:21–26.

350. Horning SJ, Chao NJ, Negrin RS, et al. High-dose therapy and autologous hematopoietic progenitor cell transplantation for recurrent or refractory Hodgkin's disease: analysis of the Stanford University results and prognostic indices. *Blood* 1997;89:801–813.

351. Wheeler C, Eickhoff C, Elias A, et al. High-dose cyclophosphamide, carmustine, and etoposide with autologous transplantation in Hodgkin's disease: a prognostic model for treatment outcomes. *Biol Blood Marrow Transplant* 1997;3:98–106.

352. Williams CD, Goldstone AH, Pearce R, et al. Autologous bone marrow transplantation for pediatric Hodgkin's disease: a case-matched comparison with adult patients by the European Bone Marrow Transplant Group Lymphoma Registry. *J Clin Oncol* 1993;11:2243–2249.

353. Hasenclever D. The disappearance of prognostic factors in Hodgkin's disease. *Ann Oncol* 2002;13(suppl 1):75–78.

354. Cosset JM, Mauch PM. The role of radiotherapy for early stage Hodgkin's disease: limitations and perspectives. *Ann Oncol* 1998;9(suppl 5):S57–S62.

355. Pavlovsky S, Schvartzman E, Lastiri F, et al. Randomized trial of CVPP for three versus six cycles in favorable- prognosis and CVPP versus AOPE plus radiotherapy in intermediate- prognosis untreated Hodgkin's disease. *J Clin Oncol* 1997;15:2652–2658.

356. Noordijk EM, Carde P, Mandard AM, et al. Preliminary results of the EORTC-GPMC controlled clinical trial H7 in early-stage Hodgkin's disease. EORTC Lymphoma Cooperative Group. Groupe Pierre-et-Marie-Curie. *Ann Oncol* 1994;5(suppl 2):107–112.

357. Horning SJ, Hoppe RT, Mason J, et al. Stanford-Kaiser Permanente G1 study for clinical stage I to IIA Hodgkin's disease: subtotal lymphoid irradiation versus vinblastine, methotrexate, and bleomycin chemotherapy and regional irradiation. *J Clin Oncol* 1997;15:1736–1744.

358. Raemaekers J, Burgers M, Henry-Amar M, et al. Patients with stage III/IV Hodgkin's disease in partial remission after MOPP/ABV chemotherapy have excellent prognosis after additional involved-field radiotherapy: interim results from the ongoing EORTC-LCG and GPMC phase III trial. The EORTC Lymphoma Cooperative Group and Groupe Pierre-et-Marie-Curie. *Ann Oncol* 1997;8(suppl 1):111–114.

359. Viviani S, Bonadonna G, Santoro A, et al. Alternating versus hybrid MOPP and ABVD combinations in advanced Hodgkin's disease: ten-year results. *J Clin Oncol* 1996;14:1421–1430.

360. Ferme C, Sebban C, Hennequin C, et al. Comparison of chemotherapy to radiotherapy as consolidation of complete or good partial response after six cycles of chemotherapy for patients with advanced Hodgkin's disease: results of the groupe d'etudes des lymphomes de l'Adulte H89 trial. *Blood* 2000;95:2246–2252.

TREATMENT PRINCIPLES AND TECHNIQUES

CHAPTER 13 ■ PRINCIPLES AND TECHNIQUES OF RADIATION THERAPY FOR HODGKIN LYMPHOMA

JOACHIM YAHALOM, RICHARD T. HOPPE, AND PETER M. MAUCH

Radiation therapy (RT) is a major component of the current successful treatment of Hodgkin lymphoma. For decades, radiation was used alone to cure the majority of patients with Hodgkin lymphoma; radiation therapy is still the most effective single agent in the the the oncologic armamentarium for this disease. Currently, in most patients with Hodgkin lymphoma, radiation therapy is used as consolidative therapy after chemotherapy, For some patients, such as those with early-stage lymphocyte-predominant Hodgkin lymphoma (LPHL), and for selected patients with classical Hodgkin lymphoma with contraindications to chemotherapy, radiation alone is still the primary curative modality of choice.[1] There are only a few situations in Hodgkin lymphoma where radiation therapy is not employed as part of the treatment program.[2] As the role of radiation therapy has transformed over the years from a single modality into a component of combined-modality therapy, the classic principles of radiation therapy fields, dose, and technique have fundamentally changed.

The following principles guide the current strategy for the use of radiation therapy in Hodgkin lymphoma:

1. Radiation therapy as a part of a combined-modality program is radically different from the extended-field radiation therapy that was used in the past as a single modality. The volume that requires radiation therapy after chemotherapy is significantly smaller and the dose is markedly reduced. Furthermore, the planning and delivery of radiation therapy has considerably improved over the last two decades.
2. Adding radiation therapy to chemotherapy not only improves disease control, but also allows the administration of shorter and less toxic chemotherapy for all stages of Hodgkin lymphoma, including programs of salvage therapy.
3. The new "mini-radiotherapy" for Hodgkin lymphoma is well-tolerated and is unlikely to result in the same extent of long-term morbidities that were associated with wide-field radiation therapy, often used as a single therapy for Hodgkin lymphoma in the 1960s through the 1980s.

This chapter will review the evolution of radiotherapy for Hodgkin lymphoma, principles of the new role of radiation therapy in Hodgkin lymphoma, current concepts of field and dose, radiation fields commonly used, technical aspects of planning and delivering radiation therapy for Hodgkin lymphoma, care and side effects during treatments, and implementation of new technology. The long-term complications of treatment for Hodgkin lymphoma, including those attributable to radiation therapy, are reviewed in Chapters 23 to 27.

EVOLUTION OF RADIOTHERAPY FOR HODGKIN LYMPHOMA

The discovery of x-rays by Roentgen, radioactivity by Becquerel, and radium by the Curies in the late 19th century led to the early treatment of Hodgkin lymphoma with crude x-rays in 1901. Within one to two years there were reports of dramatic shrinkage of enlarged lymph nodes with x-ray treatments in patients with Hodgkin's disease and other lymphomas.[3,4]

During the first two decades of the 20th century, crude x-ray equipment was used to treat patients with lymphoma. Although there was initial shrinkage of nodes, the superficial characteristics of the radiation therapy deposited high doses in the skin and subcutaneous tissues, causing skin burns and ulceration; and under-dosed deep nodes, resulting in less than optimal control.

Two technical advances in the 1920s, an improved cathode tube and deep therapy transformers capable of delivering higher voltage x-rays, produced more deeply penetrating x-ray beams. However, even with the more powerful x-rays, adequate treatment of tumors deep in the abdomen or chest frequently was associated with complications to the skin, muscles, heart, or bowel. Machines powerful enough to treat deep tumors without delivering excessive dose to more superficial normal tissues would not be available until the late 1950s, when high-activity cobalt sources were first produced.

The development of modern radiation therapy techniques for the treatment of Hodgkin lymphoma began with the work of Gilbert, a Swiss radiotherapist in 1925.[5] Gilbert was one of the first physicians to point out predictable clinical patterns in the spread of Hodgkin's disease. Initial treatment was concentrated on the regions involved by Hodgkin's disease, after which additional fields were used to encompass apparently healthy regions until low blood counts precluded further radiation. Gilbert and Babaiantz, in 1931, reported on 15 patients treated with involved and adjacent site fractionated irradiation. Seven of the 15 were still alive with an average survival time of 4.3 years for all patients,[6] a survival rate that was unprecedented at that time.

Vera Peters, in 1950, was the first physician to present definitive evidence that radiation therapy was a curative modality for early-stage Hodgkin's disease.[7,8] She did this by identifying patients with limited-stage disease who were cured with high-dose, fractionated radiation therapy. Patients received 1800 to 5000 R to areas of involvement, with the highest dose given to patients with early-stage disease. She reported 5-year and 10-year survival rates of 88% and 79%, respectively, for patients with stage I Hodgkin's disease, rates that were notably high for a disease in which virtually no one survived 10 years.

At Stanford, Henry S. Kaplan, building on the work of Rene Gilbert and Vera Peters, helped pioneer a new technology for cancer treatment—the linear accelerator. Kaplan became aware of the work in linear accelerator technology being conducted at the Stanford Microwave Laboratory by Edward Ginzton, William Hansen, and others. Kaplan and Ginzton both realized that the features of the linear accelerator made it ideally suitable for cancer therapy.[9] They secured funding from the United States Public Health Service, the Office of Naval Research, and the American Cancer Society to develop a linear accelerator suitable for clinical radiation therapy.[10] The unit was completed and installed in 1956.

The development of the linear accelerator facilitated the evolution of high-dose, extended-field irradiation concepts in the management of Hodgkin's disease. Immediately after the Stanford linear accelerator was commissioned, Kaplan began to treat patients with Hodgkin's disease utilizing these concepts of high-dose extended-field treatment and, in 1962, published his first observations on the radical radiotherapy of regionally localized Hodgkin's disease.[10,11] In this paper, he compared his results (using 30 to 40 Gy, to extended fields) with the results of patients who were being treated palliatively (4 to 12 Gy, involved field) by other physicians at Stanford during the same period of time. He demonstrated dramatic improvement with the more aggressive approach. At 2 years, the freedom from recurrence or extension was 85% in the radically treated group but only 20% in the palliatively treated group ($p <0.01$). Thirteen of the 16 patients treated radically were alive at the time of analysis, compared to only one of nine patients treated palliatively.

In 1962, Henry Kaplan and Saul Rosenberg initiated one of the first prospective randomized clinical trials for Hodgkin's disease. At first, patients with both Hodgkin's disease and non-Hodgkin lymphoma were treated on the same protocols. The L1 study, for patients with stage I to II disease, randomized treatment between involved-field (40 Gy) (the standard treatment arm) and extended-field (40 Gy) (the experimental arm) irradiation. The L2 study, for patients with stage III disease, randomized between involved-field (15 Gy) (the standard palliative treatment at that time) and total lymphoid (40 Gy) irradiation. This was the first successful experimental treatment for patients with stage III Hodgkin's disease. Some of those patients remain alive today.

As outlined above, the development of the linear accelerator, which allowed higher doses and larger radiation fields to be used, the initiation of randomized clinical trials, the proposal of new classification systems for histologic subtyping[12] and staging,[13] the pioneering of methods for more precise radiographic and surgical staging (bipedal lymphangiography and staging laparotomy),[14] and the development of an effective multiagent chemotherapy regimen,[15] all contributed to the development of curative treatment for early-stage Hodgkin lymphoma. Because of these advances and the advent of effective and less toxic chemotherapy combinations (like ABVD), the philosophy and practice for managing Hodgkin lymphoma changed dramatically from no treatment in the early 1960s; to extensive staging, and wide-field, high-dose radiation therapy by the late 1960s; to the current use of combined-modality therapy.[2]

INDICATIONS FOR RADIATION THERAPY IN HODGKIN LYMPHOMA

It is important to distinguish between the two well-defined entities of Hodgkin lymphoma: classical Hodgkin lymphoma and the less common nodular lymphocyte-predominant Hodgkin lymphoma (LPHL). The radiation approach to each entity is different. Most patients with LPHL are potentially curable with radiation alone, whereas combined-modality therapy is the standard approach for the majority of patients with classical Hodgkin lymphoma.

Lymphocyte-Predominant Hodgkin Lymphoma (LPHL)

Most (>75%) patients with LPHL present at an early stage; the disease is commonly limited to one peripheral site (neck, axilla, or groin); and involvement of the mediastinum is extremely rare. The treatment recommendations for LPHL differ markedly from those for classical Hodgkin lymphoma. The American National Comprehensive Cancer Network (NCCN) guidelines,[1] the German Hodgkin Lymphoma Study Group (GHSG),[16] and the European Organization for Research and Treatment of Cancer (EORTC) currently recommend *involved-field radiation alone* as the treatment of choice for early-stage LPHL. It should be emphasized that even if regional radiation fields are selected, the uninvolved mediastinum should not be irradiated, thus avoiding the site most prone for radiation-related short- and long-term morbidity. In a recent retrospective study of 131 patients with stage IA LPHL, 98% of patients achieved a complete response; 98% after extended-field RT alone, 100% after involved-field RT alone, and 95% after combined-modality therapy.[17] With a median follow-up of 43 months there were 5% relapses and only 3 patients died. Toxicity of treatment was generally mild, with most events observed if combined-modality treatment was used.

Although there has not been a study that prospectively compared extended-field with involved-field radiation therapy, retrospective data suggest that involved-field therapy is sufficient.[17,18] The radiation dose recommended is 30 to 36 Gy, with an optional additional boost of 4 Gy to a (rare) bulky site.

CLASSICAL HODGKIN LYMPHOMA

Early-Stage (Favorable and Unfavorable)

Over the last two decades, the treatment of favorable and unfavorable (for definition, see Chapters 16 and 17) early-stage classical Hodgkin lymphoma has changed markedly. Combined-modality therapy consisting of short-course chemotherapy (most often ABVD), followed by reduced-dose radiation carefully directed only to the involved lymph node site(s), has replaced radiation alone as the treatment of choice. Combined modality is the standard treatment for favorable and unfavorable early-stage Hodgkin lymphoma in Europe, including the EORTC/GELA and GHSG. In the United States, chemotherapy followed by involved-field radiation therapy (IFRT) is the preferred treatment recommended by the NCCN guidelines.[1,16] Subtotal lymphoid irradiation (STLI) alone remains an effective choice for favorable early-stage Hodgkin lymphoma, but is recommended by NCCN only to highly selected patients who cannot tolerate chemotherapy.[1] Although radiotherapy alone is no longer the primary treatment for classical Hodgkin lymphoma due to its potential long-term risks, consolidation IFRT of smaller volumes, at a reduced dose and by better techniques of planning and delivery, remains an important component of an effective treatment program following chemotherapy.

EVOLUTION OF CURRENT PRINCIPLES OF TREATMENT FOR EARLY-STAGE HODGKIN LYMPHOMA

Because in earlier years (1950s to 1980s) radiation therapy was considered the only curative modality for early-stage Hodgkin lymphoma, treatment was designed to maximize both the field size and dose and was termed "radical radiotherapy." Even in later years, radiotherapy remained extensive in order to minimize the necessity to use relatively toxic chemotherapy, such as MOPP.

Radical radiotherapy alone cured most patients with early-stage disease. As an example, long-term follow-up of 392 pathologically staged patients without large mediastinal adenopathy treated by the Harvard group demonstrated 10- and 20-year freedom-from treatment failure rates of 84% and 82%, respectively. The 10- and 20-year overall survival rates were 92% and 82%, respectively. The Harvard group, like many others, found the late increase in the incidence of second solid tumors as the main cause for decrease in survival rate after 10 years.[19,20] Although recognition of late morbidity and mortality secondary to treatments such as radical radiotherapy or MOPP chemotherapy is important, it must be remembered that radiotherapy alone as a "single agent" remains a highly effective modality for curing Hodgkin lymphoma. In combination with chemotherapy, its use can be modified to maximize cure while avoiding toxicity.

Table 13.1 summarizes studies that compare radiation therapy alone to combined-modality therapy for patients with favorable presentations of Hodgkin lymphoma. The improved efficacy of combining doxorubicin-based chemotherapy with traditional large-field or involved-field radiotherapy is demonstrated in most studies.

The studies summarized in Table 13.2 show that when combined with chemotherapy, involved-field irradiation is as effective as a combination of the same chemotherapy followed by extended-field irradiation.

Chemotherapy Alone for Favorable Early-Stage Hodgkin Lymphoma

The idea of eliminating radiotherapy from the treatment program in all stages of Hodgkin lymphoma has been advocated by some.[21,22] Several groups tested the hypothesis that anthracycline-based chemotherapy alone could provide equivalent disease control to that achieved with combined-modality therapy. The studies from Europe,[23] Asia,[24] and North America[25–27] targeted mostly early-stage favorable and unfavorable patients and were conducted in adults, children, and adolescents. In some, the randomization was up front[25,26]; in others, it was limited to patients who achieved a clear CR with chemotherapy.[24,27,28] The detailed results are discussed in Chapters 16 and 17.

All studies (with the exception of an underpowered small study from the Memorial Sloan-Kettering Cancer Center) showed a significantly superior EFS or freedom-from-progression for combined-modality therapy compared to chemotherapy alone. Only in the study with the longest follow-up (8 years), has superior initial disease control translated into a significantly better overall survival.[24] This is despite the fact that, in Hodgkin lymphoma, most randomized studies have not been able to document a significant survival advantage for the treatment arm that achieves superior disease control, even when one arm was clearly more effective. There are several reasons for this phenomenon: good salvage for patients who relapse, long survival with disease, and possibly more toxic events in the more effective arm. Most studies have not reported the very long-term survival of patients treated for Hodgkin lymphoma, and thus the treatment providing the best freedom from treatment failure without excessive morbidity was accepted as the standard. Indeed, salvage with high-dose therapy is often effective, but it is associated with a very high risk of acute and late toxicity and is physically and psychologically difficult for the patient. Chemotherapy alone for early favorable or unfavorable Hodgkin lymphoma should thus be considered investigational and employed only in carefully conducted IRB-approved trials or in situations where there is a clear contraindication to the use of radiation therapy.[2]

TABLE 13.1

STUDIES COMPARING RADIATION THERAPY ALONE TO COMBINED-MODALITY THERAPY IN PATIENTS WITH FAVORABLE PRESENTATIONS OF STAGE I–II HODGKIN LYMPHOMA

Study	Treatment regimens	FFTF/RFS	OS (years)
GHSG HD7[75]	EF	75%	94% (5)
(617 pts)	ABVD (2) + EF	91%	94%
		p <0.001	NS
SWOG 9133[76]	STLI	81%	96% (3)
(326 pts)	AV (3) + STLI	94%	98%
		p <0.001	NS
EORTC/GELA H7F[77]	STLI	81%	95% (5)
(333 pts)	EBVP (6) + IFRT	90%	98%
		p = 0.0001	NS
EORTC/GELA H8F[78]	STLI	80%	95%(4)
(543 pts)	MOPP/ABV (3) + IFRT	99%	99%
		p <0.0001	p <0.02

FFTF, freedom from treatment failure; RFS, relapse-free survival; OS, overall survival; EFRT, extended-field radiotherapy; IFRT, involved-field radiotherapy; STLI, subtotal lymphoid irradiation.

TABLE 13.2

STUDIES COMPARING INVOLVED-FIELD IRRADIATION WITH EXTENDED-FIELD IRRADIATION IN COMBINED-MODALITY PROGRAMS FOR STAGE I–II HODGKIN LYMPHOMA

Study	Treatment regimens	FFTF/RFS	OS (years)
Milan[79]	ABVD (4) + STLI	97%	93% (5)
(133 pts)	ABVD (4) + IFRT	94%	94%
		NS	NS
GHSG HD8[80]	COPP/ABVD (4) + EFRT	86%	91% (5)
(1,064 pts)	COPP/ABVD (4) + IFRT	84%	92%
		NS	NS
EORTC/GELA H8U[81]	MOPP/ABV (6) + IFRT	94%	90% (4)
(995 pts)	MOPP/ABV (4) + IFRT	95%	95%
	MOPP/ABV (4) + STLI	96%	93%
		NS	NS

FFTF, freedom from treatment failure; RFS, relapse-free survival; OS, overall survival; EFRT, extended-field radiotherapy; IFRT, involved-field radiotherapy; STLI, subtotal lymphoid irradiation.

Advanced-Stage Hodgkin Lymphoma

Although the role of consolidation radiotherapy after induction chemotherapy remains controversial,[29] irradiation is often added in patients with advanced-stage Hodgkin lymphoma who present with bulky disease or remain in uncertain complete remission after chemotherapy. When advanced-stage Hodgkin lymphoma is treated with the highly effective and less toxic Stanford V program, it is imperative to follow the brief chemotherapy program with involved-field radiotherapy to sites originally larger than 5 cm or to a clinically involved spleen.[30] When radiotherapy is used in advanced-stage disease, it should be limited to the involved site (IFRT).

Salvage Programs for Refractory and Relapsed Hodgkin Lymphoma

High-dose therapy supported by autologous stem-cell transplantation (ASCT) has become a standard salvage treatment for patients who relapse or remain refractory to chemotherapy or to combined-modality therapy. Many of the patients who enter these programs have not received prior radiotherapy or have relapsed in sites outside the original radiation field. These patients could benefit from integrating radiotherapy into the salvage regimen, as demonstrated by several retrospective studies.[31] See also Chapters 19 and 20.

Radiation Fields: Principles and Design

In the past, radiation-field design attempted to include multiple involved and uninvolved lymph node sites. The large fields known as "mantle," "inverted Y," and "total lymphoid irradiation (TLI)" were synonymous with the radiation treatment of Hodgkin's disease. These fields should rarely be used nowadays. The involved field, or its slightly larger version, the regional field, encompasses a significantly smaller, but adequate volume when radiotherapy is used as consolidation after chemotherapy in Hodgkin lymphoma (Figs. 13.1 to 13.4). Even when radiation is used as the only treatment in lymphocyte-predominant Hodgkin lymphoma, the field should be limited to the involved site or to the involved sites and immediately adjacent lymph node groups. Even more limited radiation fields, restricted to the originally involved

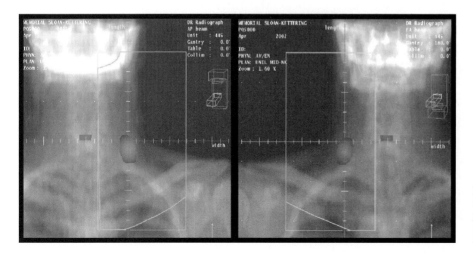

FIGURE 13.1. Involved-field irradiation for a patient with stage I Hodgkin lymphoma involving the left neck. The GTV (PET+ node) is displayed in red. See color insert.

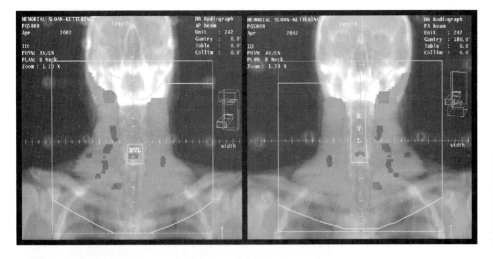

FIGURE 13.2. Involved-field irradiation for a patient with stage II Hodgkin lymphoma extensively involving the right neck and with a solitary node in the left neck. The GTV (PET+ disease) is displayed in red; the CTV (involved lymph node regions) is displayed in green. See color insert.

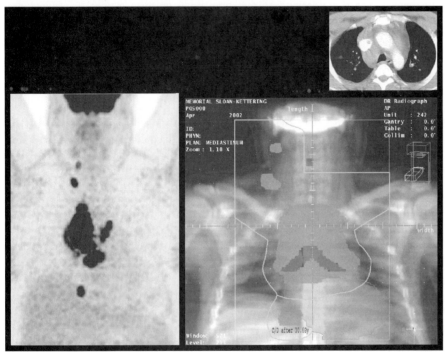

FIGURE 13.3. Involved-field irradiation for a patient with stage II Hodgkin lymphoma who has a large mediastinal mass and involvement of the right neck, right hilum, and right cardiophrenic region. The image at the left shows the FDG-PET localization of disease. The image at the top is an axial CT slice through the mediastinum. The GTV (PET+ disease) is displayed in green. See color insert.

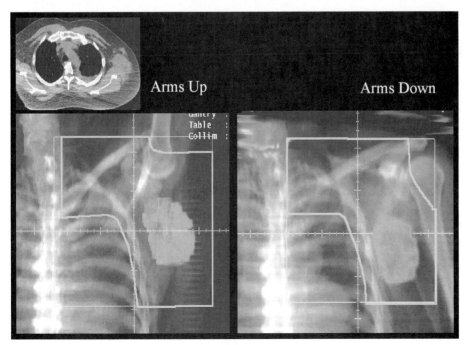

FIGURE 13.4. Involved-field irradiation for a patient with stage I Hodgkin lymphoma involving the left axilla. The image at the top shows an axial CT cut with the involved node outlined. The image on the left shows the field configuration with patient in an "arms-up" position. The image on the right shows the field configuration with the patient in an "arms-akimbo" position. The GTV (PET+ node) is displayed in green. See color insert.

181

lymph node(s) only, are currently under study by several European groups.

The many terminologies given to radiation field variations in Hodgkin lymphoma caused significant confusion and difficulties in comparing treatment programs. Although the final determination of the field may vary from patient to patient and depends on many clinical, anatomic, and normal tissue-tolerance considerations, general definitions and guidelines are available and should be followed.

The following are definitions of types of radiation fields used in Hodgkin lymphoma:

Involved Field

An involved field is limited to the site of the clinically involved lymph node group. For extranodal sites, the field includes the affected area of the involved organ alone (if there is no evidence for lymph node involvement). The "grouping" of lymph nodes is not clearly defined, and involved-field borders for common presentation of Hodgkin lymphoma will be discussed later (Figs. 13.1 to 13.4).

Regional Field

A regional field includes the involved lymph node region *plus* at least one adjacent clinically uninvolved region. For extranodal disease, it includes the involved organ plus the clinically uninvolved lymph nodes region.

Extended Field

An extended field includes *multiple* involved and uninvolved lymph node groups. If the multiple sites are limited to one side of the diaphragm, the upper field is called the *mantle* field. The extended field that includes all lymph nodes sites below the diaphragm (with or without the spleen) is named after its shape: *inverted Y*.

When radiation treatment includes all lymph nodes on both sides of the diaphragm, these large fields are combined, and the resulting field is called *total lymphoid irradiation (TLI)* or *total nodal irradiation (TNI)*; if the pelvic lymph nodes are excluded, the field is called *subtotal lymphoid irradiation (STLI)*.

Involved Lymph Node(s) Field

The involved lymph node field is the most limited radiation field that has just recently been introduced.[32] The clinical treated volume (CTV) includes only the originally involved lymph node(s) volume (pre-chemotherapy) with the addition of 1 cm margin to create planning treatment volume (PTV). Several groups have begun to evaluate the potential advantages and risks of this minimal RT volume approach, but only short outcome data are available and treatment techniques and guidelines are still evolving. At present, IFRT, as described in more detail later, remains the standard treatment field in combined chemo-radiotherapy programs.

Considerations in Designing Involved-Field Radiotherapy

Although it is understood that the involved field should address an area smaller than the classical extended fields of mantle or inverted Y, it is not entirely clear how small the field should remain. Should only the area of the enlarged lymph node (with margins) be irradiated? Should a region of lymph nodes be addressed? And if yes, what are the borders of this region? Many use the lymph node region diagram that was adopted for staging purposes at the Rye symposium (1966) to define a region of lymph nodes.[33] (See Chapter 9, Figure 9.1) However, this diagram was not developed for individual radiation field design, separates the mediastinal and hilar regions, has a separate infraclavicular region, and does not provide borders of the individual sites. Another question relates to the impact on field design related to change in size (or complete resolution) of lymph node enlargement after chemotherapy, especially in the mediastinum. Should the pre-chemotherapy volume be irradiated? Or should we spare the tissues (such as lung) that are no longer involved by the disease, and irradiate the post-chemotherapy residual abnormality alone?

There are no definitive answers to these questions, and it is often the individual clinical situation that affects the field design. At the same time, uniform general guidelines are important for assuring a high standard of treatment and are essential for collaborative group studies.

Guidelines for Delineating the Involved Field for Nodal Sites[34]

1. IFRT is treatment of a region, not of an individual lymph node.
2. The main involved-field nodal regions are the neck (unilateral), mediastinum (including the hilar regions bilaterally), axilla (including the supraclavicular and infraclavicular lymph nodes), spleen, para-aortic lymph nodes, and inguinal lymph nodes (including the femoral and iliac nodes).
3. In general, the fields include the involved pre-chemotherapy sites and volume, with an important exception that involves the transverse diameter of the mediastinal and para-aortic lymph nodes. For the field width of these sites, it is recommended to use the reduced post-chemotherapy diameter. In these areas the regression of the lymph nodes is easily confirmed by CT imaging, and critical normal tissue may be spared by reducing the irradiated volume.
4. The supraclavicular lymph nodes are considered part of the cervical region. If involved alone (based on CT and PET imaging, when appropriate), only the low neck need be treated (to the top of the larynx). This is to avoid irradiating the salivary glands when the risk for the area is low. If other cervical nodes are involved, the whole neck is treated unilaterally.
5. All borders should be easy to outline (most are bony landmarks) and plan with a conventional 2D simulation unit. CT data are required for outlining the mediastinal and para-aortic region, and will also help in designing the axillary field.
6. Pre-chemotherapy and post-chemotherapy information (both CT and PET) regarding lymph node localization and size is critical and should be available at the time of treatment planning.

Involved-Field Guidelines for Common Nodal Sites

Unilateral Cervical/Supraclavicular Region (Fig. 13.1). Involvement at any cervical level with or without involvement of the supraclavicular (SCL) nodes.

Arm Position: Akimbo or at sides. *Upper Border:* 1 to 2 cm above the lower tip of the mastoid process and midpoint through the chin. If only the supraclavicular nodes are involved, the upper border of the field may be placed at the top of the larynx. *Lower Border:* 1 to 2 cm below the bottom of the clavicle. *Lateral Border:* To include the medial two-thirds of the clavicle. *Medial Border:* (a) If the supraclavicular nodes are not involved, the border is placed at the ipsilateral transverse processes, except when medial nodes close to the vertebral bodies are seen on the initial staging neck CT scan. For medial nodes, the entire vertebral body is included. (b) When the supraclavicular nodes are involved, the border should be placed at the contralateral traverse processes. For patients with stage I disease, the larynx and vertebral bodies above the larynx can be blocked (assuming no medial cervical nodes). *Blocks:* A posterior cervical cord block is required only if the cord dose exceeds 40 Gy. Mid-neck calculations should be performed to determine the maximum cord dose, especially when the central axis is in the mediastinum. A laryngeal block should be used unless lymph nodes were present in that location. In that case, the block should be added at 20 Gy.

Bilateral Cervical/Supraclavicular Region (Fig. 13.2). Both cervical and supraclavicular regions should be treated as described above regardless of the extent of disease on each side. Posterior cervical cord and larynx blocks should be used as described above. Use a posterior mouth block if treating the patient supine (preferably with an extended travel couch at greater than 100 cm FSD) to block the upper field divergence through the mouth.

Mediastinum. Involvement of the mediastinum and/or the hilar nodes. In Hodgkin lymphoma, this field includes also the medial SCL nodes even if not clinically involved.

Arm Position: Akimbo or at sides. The arms-up position is optional if the axillary nodes are involved. *Upper Border:* C5–C6 interspace. If supraclavicular nodes were also involved, the upper border should be placed at the top of the larynx and the lateral border should be adjusted as described in the section on treating neck nodes. *Lower Border:* The lower of (a) 5 cm below the carina or (b) 2 cm below the *pre-chemotherapy* inferior border. *Lateral Border:* The *post-chemotherapy* volume with a 1- to 1.5-cm margin. *Hilar Area:* To be included with 1-cm margin unless initially involved, in which case the margin should be 1.5 cm.

If paracardiac lymph nodes are involved, they should be treated either as an extension of the mediastinal field, or if significantly lower than the mediastinal field, as a separate targeted involved lymph node area. Irradiation of the whole heart (for even a lower dose) is not recommended in most cases (Fig. 13.3).

Mediastinum with Involvement of the Cervical Nodes (Fig. 13.3). When both cervical regions are involved, the field is a mantle without the axilla, using the guidelines described above. If only one cervical chain is involved, the vertebral bodies, contralateral upper neck and larynx can be blocked as previously described. Because the isocenter is in the upper mediastinum, this field will usually require the use of wedges, compensators, or selective field blocking to adjust for the differential dose to the neck and mediastinum.

Axillary Region (Fig. 13.4). The ipsilateral axillary, infra-clavicular, and supraclavicular areas are treated when the axilla is involved. Whenever possible, use CT-based planning for this region.

Arm Position: Arms akimbo or arms up. *Upper Border:* C5–C6 interspace or bottom of the larynx. *Lower Border:* The lower of (a) the tip of the scapula or (b) 2 cm below the lowest axillary node. *Medial Border:* Ipsilateral cervical transverse process. Include the vertebral bodies only if the SCL are involved. *Lateral Border:* Flash axilla.

Spleen. The spleen is treated only if abnormal imaging was suggestive of involvement. The post-chemotherapy volume is treated with 1.5-cm margins. Treatment with respiratory gating may facilitate reduction in the lung and kidney doses.

Abdomen (Paraaortic Nodes). Upper Border: Top of T11 and at least 2 cm above pre-chemotherapy volume. Lower Border: Bottom of L4 and at least 2 cm below pre-chemotherapy volume. Lateral Borders: The edge of the transverse processes and at least 2 cm from the post-chemotherapy volume.

Inguinal/Femoral/External Iliac Region. These ipsilateral lymph node groups are treated together if any of the nodes are involved. Upper Border: Middle of the sacroiliac joint Lower Border: 5 cm below the lesser trochanter. Lateral Border: The greater trochanter and 2 cm lateral to initially involved nodes. Medial Border: Medial border of the obturator foramen with at least 2 cm medial to involved nodes. If common iliac nodes are involved, the field should extend to the L4–L5 interspace and at least 2 cm above the initially involved nodal border.

Involved-Field Radiotherapy of Extranodal Sites

Either the whole involved organ or the affected portion is the target, and draining lymph nodes are not included unless involved. The optimal plan is 3D-conformal and CT-simulation based. The margins for the planned treatment volume depend on quality of imaging and reliability of immobilization, and most importantly, should account for organ motion during respiration. Typically, organs in the head and neck require margins of 1 cm and organs in the mediastinum, abdomen, and pelvis require margins of 2 cm.

TECHNICAL ASPECTS OF RADIOTHERAPY FOR HODGKIN LYMPHOMA

Choice of Equipment

The linear accelerator is the machine of choice for radiotherapy of Hodgkin lymphoma. The desired energy is 6 mV for treatment of peripheral nodal sites; but higher energies, such as 10 or 15 mV, may be used for abdominal and thoracic tumors, depending on anatomy and choice of treatment plan. A 6-mV beam is sufficiently penetrating to produce good dose homogeneity throughout most treatment fields. The maximum dose point of 6 mV is close enough to the skin surface to avoid under-dosing superficially located lymph nodes, such as the cervical or inguinal nodes. The dose inhomogeneity measured in fields treated with a 6-mV beam may be as high as 10%, due primarily to differences in patient separation within the field and to large separations in big patients. For patients with large nodes near the skin surface, tissue equivalent bolus may be needed to increase the subcutaneous dose.

Linear accelerators at 4 mV and cobalt-60 are less desirable than higher-energy equipment. Greater dose inhomogeneity within the field is seen with 4-mV beams. Cobalt-60 units, while seldom used in North America today, are still common in other areas of the world. With cobalt-60, the dose falls off toward the edge of the field, so that there is a risk of under-dosing the tumor.[35] To compensate, a larger field size may be needed. With both 4 MV and cobalt-60, skin reactions will be greater than with 6-mV. Also, field sizes and ability to treat at extended source to skin distance are restricted with cobalt-60.

Positioning, Immobilization, and Simulation

For most anatomic sites selected for IFRT as primary or complementary treatment of Hodgkin lymphoma, CT simulation will provide essential information for determining treatment volume and optimal plan. This is particularly important as the recommended radiotherapy fields have become smaller. In current practice, most radiation oncologists will incorporate indirectly acquired or direct CT-simulation information into the treatment planning process. In selective cases, FDG- PET imaging and/or MRI performed in the same treatment position with fiduciary markers is also incorporated into the simulation and treatment planning process.

One of the important lessons learned from three-dimensional treatment planning is that radiotherapy accuracy during a course of fractionated radiation is only as good as the immobilization of the patient. With Cerrobend blocks attached to a standard machine block-holding tray or automated multi-leaf collimator blocks, very small changes in patient position may result in considerable field variations. Accurate positioning requires reproducible neck and arm positioning, and reproducible alignment and rotation of the torso and pelvis. Reproducible knee and foot positioning may also be required under certain circumstances.

The following techniques can be used for immobilization of the head position. Most patients will be treated in the supine position. Although resting the head on a soft sponge (or alternatively in a head rest or cup) with tape used to fix the chin position allows good visualization of the light field and subtle adjustment of the head position, we are increasingly recommending the use of an Aquaplast mask, especially when the cervical nodes are to be treated. This mask can be molded to the shape of the head and chin at treatment planning, and is fixed to the table at simulation and treatment, allowing patient comfort but very little movement. Furthermore, if the fields are limited to the head and neck region, marks can be placed on the mask, eliminating the need to permanently mark the patient. On occasion, with very large tumors, the patient may need to undergo a new simulation and mask midtreatment to adjust for tumor shrinkage. One tremendous advantage of the mask is the immobilization achieved that is needed for the use of conformal fields or intensity-modulated radiation therapy designed to avoid irradiation of the salivary glands and other crucial structures.

An alternative method of immobilization is a customized upper-body Styrofoam mold or an alpha cradle in conjunction with a chin band. The patient is simulated and treated in the cradle. A disadvantage of this system is that some bolus effect of the back results when the posterior field is treated through the cradle, resulting in an increase in the skin reaction posteriorly.[36] Arm position varies according to the age of the patient and institutional preference. The akimbo arm position can be reproduced by simply having the patient place his or her thumbs in the waistband or belt or on the table at that level. The arms-up position can be secured with an alpha cradle or customized upper body mold with hand grips for reproducible position,[37] although in a cooperative patient the arm position may be secured with a less rigorous setup. The arms-up position may especially be used when treating the axilla, or when oblique or lateral thoracic field approaches are planned. An upper body mold is useful for the treatment of lower neck and thoracic fields.

Wall-mounted lasers in the simulation and treatment rooms can aid in reproducing torso and pelvic alignment and rotation. Leveling tattoos, one pair of lateral tattoos on each side of the central axis, will aid in lining up with the side lasers.

Techniques to assure reproducibility of the knee and foot position are especially important for patients treated to fields below the diaphragm. One technique is to place a standard wedge under the knees that can be used each day. The ankles can be immobilized with tape or a bandage with a reproducible ankle separator that maintains ankle separation and thereby precludes knee or hip rotation. Many patients prefer a small amount of knee flexion for comfort.

If the patient is to be treated with sequential radiation fields, positioning for the two fields must be as consistent as possible to avoid inadvertent overlap with the previously treated field, created by shifts in patient position. The previous field position must be clearly documented. Inconspicuous tattoos placed at the field borders, use of the same patient position, radiographic documentation, and knowledge of previous field size and source-to-skin distance will allow calculation of an appropriate skin gap, so that sequential fields may be treated safely. Although it is now unusual to use matching fields in the initial treatment of patients with Hodgkin lymphoma, it is not uncommon when managing relapse that fields are used that overlap a previously treated area. In this case, the prior details of treatment and simulation films must be obtained so that doses to crucial organs such as the spinal cord can be limited.

Custom shielding blocks are essential to the delivery of high-quality radiation therapy. Divergent blocks are generally cast from an alloy with a low melting point such as Cerrobend and mounted on the collimator of the linear accelerator. Most modern linear accelerators, as an alternative, have multi-leaf collimators that allow blocking within the head of the machine itself. In either case, the blocks are of a thickness calculated to reduce the transmitted beam by 5 half-values, that is, to approximately 3% of the prescribed dose.

In addition to the 3% transmitted from the primary beam directly through the block, there is some dose delivered to the shielded areas from radiation scattered internally from other tissues within the direct path of the radiation beam. The amount of scatter depends on the amount of surrounding tissue within the primary beam (width of the area contributing scatter), width of the block, radiation energy (less scatter with higher energy beams), and distance from the edge of the protective block. Of the normal tissues, the testes are the most sensitive to low-dose fractionated radiation. A total dose of 3 to 3.5 Gy may result in sterility in over 50% of patients. Thus, the 3% received from the primary beam through the block may significantly add to the scattered dose and bring the total dose into this range. This is of importance in patients receiving external iliac, inguinal, and femoral irradiation where the testes are within the radiation field borders but under the block. One way to reduce the primary beam dose to the testes is to utilize both the templated blocks and the multi-leaf collimators. This should provide 10 half layers of protection and reduce the primary dose component to 0.01% of the total dose.

Further, the testicles must be shielded from as much internally scattered radiation as possible by using a special clamshell-like testicular shield.[38–40] It is important that the testicles are positioned behind the front wall of the shield. These shields will provide a 3- to 10-fold reduction in scatter dose to the testes.[39] Loss of fertility is also significantly reduced by limiting the radiation field to one side of the pelvis. With bilateral pelvic nodal irradiation, the internal scatter component increases greatly.

Normally, the ovaries lie just medial to the external iliac nodes and within a standard pelvic radiation field. The tolerance of the ovaries to radiation is well below the doses employed for lymphoma. If preservation of ovarian function, including fertility, is desired, the ovaries must be transposed to a location outside the primary radiation beam, or to a location over which sufficient secondary shielding can be provided to prevent ovarian ablation. Surgical transposition or oophoropexy may be accomplished through a laparoscopic procedure. Careful coordination between surgeon and radiation oncologist is required so that the surgeon understands exactly where the ovaries must be placed, marks them with radio-opaque clips, and takes radiographs at the time of surgery on the operating room table to ensure that the placement is correct. With unilateral pelvic irradiation, one ovary should remain outside of the field and should have normal function. In some patients with lymphoma, the age at onset is beyond childbearing age. In the young patient receiving whole pelvic irradiation, transposition of the ovaries is the only way to preserve hormonal function and fertility.

Treatment Verification and Documentation

A number of studies have documented difficulty with accurate daily delivery of treatment.[41–46] With the frequent use of imaging films, which document the volume of tissue actually exposed to radiation during a treatment, it is clear that both systematic errors and random errors may occur. Systematic errors result from a flawed simulation, perhaps because the patient was tense and later relaxed on the actual treatment table, or because the initial simulation position was uncomfortable and not sustainable.[41,43,45] Typically, systematic errors can be identified with an imaging film on the first day of treatment. Random errors are related to malposition of the patient or shielding blocks in daily treatment setups. The use of better positioning tools such as immobilization devices and lasers have aided in securing more accurate setups, and the use of frequent imaging films has focused attention on accuracy and identified systematic problems.[41,43,44]

There is limited information specific to patients with lymphoma on the accuracy of radiation treatment planning. In a study from the Netherlands, the accuracy of patient positioning was prospectively evaluated in 13 patients receiving mantle radiation therapy.[47] Patients were treated in the supine position for the anterior field and prone position for the posterior field. Larger discrepancies between simulation films and portal films were found in the posterior fields than for the anterior fields. The authors concluded that attention should be directed to increasing the stability of patients in the prone position in order to minimize systemic and random error rates. Naida and associates from the University of Michigan evaluated the localization error rate of four experienced radiation oncologists on their lung blocks for mantle-field irradiation, with or without consideration of the diagnostic CT scans.[48] A three-dimensional treatment planning system displaying tumor volumes was used as reference. Localization errors were defined as touching or overlap of the shielding blocks onto enlarged nodes. The overall error rates in the absence and presence of the diagnostic computed tomography were 18% and 13%, respectively ($p = 0.038$). The axillary region was found to be associated with the highest error rate while the superior mediastinum had the lowest error rate. Localization errors were also more likely with increasing tumor volume. These results showed that even with the benefit of diagnostic CT, the error rate can still be considerable, and that the use of three-dimensional planning in mantle-field definition may reduce the incidence of geographic misses.

Quality Control

Quality control and assurance are critical to the interpretation of clinical trial results and ensuring uniformly optimal patient care. The quality of radiation treatment depends on the successful completion of each of the following steps.

1. Identification of sites of involvement and sites at significant risk for microscopic disease. This requires an ability to perform an accurate and complete physical examination, to interpret the diagnostic images used in staging, and to understand the regions at risk and patterns of spread of lymphoma.
2. Selection and design of treatment fields that will adequately cover all areas requiring treatment and adequately spare normal tissues.
3. Prescription of the optimal dose for disease control and normal tissue preservation.
4. Meticulous delivery of the treatment plan.

Proper execution of each of these steps is important in ensuring the quality and success of overall treatment. Quality control

programs for radiation treatment have been established by European cooperative groups for Hodgkin lymphoma. In the EORTC H8 protocol,[49] a quality control program for verification of radiation technical files was implemented. Among 161 files reviewed, major deviations in radiation volumes and dose were observed in 13.6% and 39.7% of the cases, respectively. The number of major deviations was felt to justify such a radiation quality control program. In the German Hodgkin Lymphoma Study Group HD4 trial,[50] all planning and verification films as well as dose charts were prospectively reviewed. Cases with protocol violations were found to have a significantly lower 5-year freedom from treatment failure (70% versus 82%, $p <0.04$), illustrating the importance of quality assurance. Ongoing cooperative trials on non-Hodgkin lymphoma treatment may provide an opportunity to collect similar data. The GHSG has established a special central pretreatment review mechanism to ensure adequate field selection to improve the quality of radiation therapy in the large number of centers participating in the group studies.[51,52]

The Patterns of Care studies in the United States have reported extensively on Hodgkin lymphoma. The results demonstrated that patients with adequate portal margins had significantly fewer in-field or marginal recurrences, or relapses of any type.[53] Furthermore, the experience of the radiation oncologist; use of a dedicated simulator; performance of routine port films to ensure set-up accuracies; and use of individually shaped blocks, linear accelerators, and extended-field treatments were all associated with an improved treatment outcome.[53,54] In the Patterns of Care study published in 1995, discrepancies between the consensus guidelines developed in 1993 and the surveyed United States practice were noted in a number of areas.[55] The authors suggested that specific changes in treatment techniques, and utilization of appropriate equipment and services, may improve the quality of treatment planning and delivery.

The National Comprehensive Cancer Network (NCCN) Outcomes Database measures the adherence of clinicians to NCCN guidelines, and provides clinical and other outcomes data to evaluate the quality of cancer care.[56] The first disease site studied was breast cancer, although the final results have not yet been published. Non-Hodgkin lymphoma is the next disease site to be measured by the NCCN Outcomes Database. The results, when available, will hopefully provide information on patterns of care, and allow integration of quality control into improved care in patients with lymphoma.

DOSE CONSIDERATIONS AND RECOMMENDATIONS

The relationship between radiation dose and probability of tumor control has been the subject of an interesting and lengthy debate in the past. The recommended tumoricidal dose for Hodgkin lymphoma of 40 Gy is based on a classic paper by Kaplan[57] and the excellent results reported in the 1960s and 1970s from Stanford University. These results were obtained with a dose of 44 Gy. Other studies questioned the need for this relatively high dose and showed that the dose–response curve for Hodgkin lymphoma is sigmoid in nature and relatively flat with doses exceeding 30 Gy.[58–62]

Modern dose data support the efficacy of using lower doses for uninvolved regions than originally recommended by the Stanford group. The German Hodgkin's Study Group (GHSG) conducted a prospectively randomized dose evaluation study in 376 pathologically staged patients with stage I or II disease who were without risk factors (large mediastinal mass, extranodal lesions, massive splenic disease, elevated erythrocyte sedimentation rate, or three or more involved areas).[50] These patients were treated with a radiation-alone program. All patients received 40 Gy total fractionated dose to the involved field areas but were randomly assigned to receive either 40 Gy (arm A) or 30 Gy (arm B) total fractionated dose for the *clinically uninvolved* extended field. No chemotherapy was given Complete remission was attained in 98% of patients in each arm. With a median follow-up of 86 months, 7-year relapse-free survival (RFS) rates were 78% (arm A) and 83% (arm B) (*p* = 0.093). Corresponding overall survival rates were 91% (arm A) and 96% (arm B) (*p* = 0.16): Extended-field RT alone achieves good survival rates in favorable early-stage HD and 30 Gy is an adequate dose for *clinically uninvolved* areas. Based on this study, the recommended radiation dose for patients treated with extended-field radiation alone is 40 Gy to involved sites and 30 Gy to uninvolved sites.

More relevant to current practice is the determination of the adequate radiation dose after treatment with chemotherapy. Although in many studies, radiation doses were kept at the 40-Gy level following a complete response to chemotherapy, others reduced the dose in the combined-modality setting to 20 to 24 Gy with excellent overall results.[63] Studies of combined modality in advanced-stage disease also used reduced doses of radiation for patients achieving a complete response to chemotherapy and increased the dose to 30 Gy for patients who achieved only a partial response.[64] The pediatric groups addressing the concern of radiation effects on skeletal and muscular development also effectively reduced the dose of radiation after combination chemotherapy to 21 to 24 Gy.[65]

The GHSG randomized patients with intermediate-stage (unfavorable early-stage) disease who responded to chemotherapy and were to receive extended-field irradiation to either a full dose of 40 Gy or to a dose of only 20 Gy with an additional 20-Gy boost to the bulky site (HD 1 trial). No differences in freedom from treatment frailure or in overall survival were found. The outcome was similar in a group of patients treated to 30 Gy in nonbulky and 40 Gy in bulky sites in a later program (HD 5).[66] A more recent GHSG randomized study (HD 10) addressed the radiation dose question after short-course chemotherapy. Patients with favorable stage I to II were randomized to receive either 4 or only 2 cycles of ABVD followed by involved-field irradiation of either 30 or 20 Gy. At a median follow-up of 4 years, the overall results are excellent (FFTF of 94%, OS of 97%), with no difference between the four arms.[67] Reducing chemotherapy appeared safe, and at this point there was no difference between the different RT doses. In a companion study, HD11 targeted patients with unfavorable early-stage disease and randomized them to either ABVD × 4 or BEACOPP × 4; either program was followed by either 20 Gy or 30 Gy to the involved field. The interim analysis at 3 years has shown no difference between the arms, with a FFTF of 87% and OS of 96%.

Significance of Reducing the Radiation Dose

Recent studies clearly indicate that the risk of secondary solid tumor induction is radiation dose-related. This was carefully analyzed for secondary breast and lung cancers as well as for other tumors.[68–71] Although it will take more years of careful follow-up of patients in randomized studies to display the full magnitude of risk reduction by the decrease in radiation field size and dose, recent data suggest that this is likely to be the case. In a recent Duke University study, two groups of patients with early-stage Hodgkin lymphoma were treated with different radiation approaches over the same period. One group received radiotherapy alone, given to extended fields with a median dose of 38 Gy; the second group received chemotherapy followed by involved-field low-dose (median of 25 Gy) radiotherapy. Although 12 patients developed second tumors in the first group and 8 of them died, no second tumors were detected in the second group. The median follow-up was 11.7 and 8.1 years, respectively.[72] Similar observations with an even longer follow-up were made by the Yale group.[73]

Dose Recommendations

Radiation Alone (As Primary Treatment)

Clinically involved sites: 36 to 40 Gy.
  Clinically uninvolved sites (when regional or extended fields are used): 30 Gy.

Radiation Following Chemotherapy in a Combined-Modality Program

Patients in CR or CRu after chemotherapy: 20 to 30 Gy. Most guidelines recommend 30 Gy for adults, until lower-dose (20-Gy) data mature.
  For pediatric or adolescent patients: 21 to 24 Gy.
  In some programs of short chemotherapy for bulky or advanced-stage disease (e.g., Stanford V), the recommended RT dose is 36 Gy.
  Patients in PR after chemotherapy: 30 to 40 Gy.

NEW ASPECTS OF RADIATION FIELD DESIGN AND DELIVERY

As the notion of treating large areas of involved and uninvolved areas has changed in favor of treating only the involved lymph node group or extranodal organ, new options of more conformal radiotherapy have opened up. The old extensive radiation fields like mantle or inverted Y included multiple sites at various depths (from the body surface) and each site had different limitations of access and tolerance of normal tissue. The only way to include these sites in one radiation field (and thus avoid overlaps and gaps when radiation fields were matched) was to treat the whole field from only two opposed directions, anterior and posterior. This technique assured the inclusion of most lymph nodes in one field, yet it also resulted in exposure of large volumes of normal organs (e.g., heart, lungs, breasts, and spinal cord) to the full prescribed radiation dose.

The radiotherapy of the involved-field alone as is practiced today avoids this shortcoming in most cases by allowing the use three-dimensional conformal radiotherapy (3-D CRT). For example, 3-D CRT of an anterior mediastinal mass could potentially avoid irradiation of the spine and much of the heart and lung tissue located behind the mass.

The change in the lymphoma radiotherapy paradigm coincided with substantial improvement in imaging and treatment planning technology, which has revolutionized the field of radiotherapy over the last 15 years. The integration of fast high-resolution CT into the simulation and planning systems of radiation oncology has changed the way treatment volumes and relationship to normal critical structures are defined and planned. In the recent past, tumor volume determinations were made with conventional simulators that required the inclusion of wide "safety margins" that detracted from accuracy and sparing of critical organs. Most modern simulators are actually high-resolution CT scanners with capabilities and software that allow accurate conformal treatment planning with detailed information on the dose and volume delivered to normal structures and the homogeneity of dose delivered to the target. More recently, these simulators have also been integrated with a PET scanner that provides additional tumor volume information for consideration during radiation planning.

Intensity-modulated radiotherapy (IMRT) is the most advanced planning and radiation delivery mode and is used primarily for small-volume cancers that require high radiation doses (e.g., prostate and head neck cancers) or are adjacent to critical organs. With IMRT, the volume of interest can be accurately encompassed in all dimensions, permitting higher doses to the tumor volume or greater sparing of normal tissues. In the radiotherapy of lymphoma, there are several clinical situations where IMRT may provide a benefit, including the treatment of complicated tumor volumes in the mediastinum and abdomen, and lymphomas of the head and neck. IMRT also allows re-irradiation of sites prior to high-dose salvage programs that otherwise will be prohibited by normal tissue tolerance, particularly of the spinal cord.[74]

COMMON SIDE EFFECTS AND SUPPORTIVE CARE DURING RADIOTHERAPY

Side effects of radiotherapy depend on the irradiated volume, dose administered, and technique employed. They are also influenced by the extent and type of prior chemotherapy, if any, and by the patient's age. Most of the information that we use today to estimate risk of radiotherapy is derived from strategies that used radiation alone. The field size and configuration, doses, and technology have all drastically changed over the last decade. It is probably misleading to judge the risks associated with current radiotherapy programs for Hodgkin lymphoma and inform patients solely based on the risks of past practice of radiotherapy alone in treating Hodgkin lymphoma.

It is of interest that most of the data on long-term complications associated with radiotherapy and particularly second solid tumors and coronary heart disease were reported from databases of Hodgkin lymphoma patients treated more than 25 years ago. It is also important to note that we have very limited long-term follow-up data on patients with Hodgkin lymphoma who were treated with chemotherapy alone.

Acute Effects

Radiation, in general, may cause fatigue, and areas of the irradiated skin may develop mild sun-exposure-like dermatitis. The acute side effects of irradiating the full neck include mouth dryness, change in taste, and pharyngitis. These side effects are usually mild and transient. If treatment involves the upper neck and/or lower mandible and mouth, attention to dental care is advised. If dryness is a concern, it is advised to arrange for an expert dental appointment for overall dental evaluation prior to treatment and supplemental fluoride treatment during and after radiotherapy.

Soreness of the throat and mild to moderate difficulty swallowing solid and dry food may also occur during neck irradiation at doses exceeding 20 Gy. These side effects are almost always mild, self-limited, and subside shortly after completion of radiotherapy. Skin care using moisturizers and sunscreen is advised for all patients undergoing radiotherapy. Temporary hair loss is expected in irradiated areas, and recovery is observed after several months. The main potential side effects of subdiaphragmatic irradiation are loss of appetite, nausea, and increased bowel movements. These reactions are usually mild and can be minimized with standard antiemetic medications.

Irradiation of more than one field, particularly after chemotherapy, can cause myelosuppression, which may necessitate short treatment interruption and, very rarely, administration of G-CSF, erythropoietin-type drugs, or platelet transfusion.

Early Side Effects

Fewer than 5% of patients may note an electric shock sensation radiating down the backs of both legs when the head is flexed (*Lhermitte sign*) 6 weeks to 3 months after mantle-field irradiation. Possibly secondary to transient demyelinization of the spinal cord, Lhermitte sign resolves spontaneously after a few months and is not associated with late or permanent spinal cord damage.

During the same period, radiation *pneumonitis* and/or acute *pericarditis* may occur in fewer than 5% of patients; these side effects occur more often in those who have extensive mediastinal disease. Both inflammatory processes have become rare with modern irradiation techniques.

The consideration and discussion of potential complications and late effects following radiotherapy and chemotherapy is of prime importance and is detailed in Chapters 23 to 27.

It is important to prepare the patient for the potential side effects of treatment. Many organizations and cancer centers provide written patient information regarding radiotherapy of lymphomas.

We normally recommend a first post-RT follow-up visit 6 weeks after the end of treatment, and obtain post-RT baseline blood count, standard biochemistry tests, TSH levels, and a lipid profile (if applicable) at that visit. Follow-up imaging studies normally commence 3 months after completion of treatment. Other follow-up studies are included in the NCCN guidelines for Hodgkin lymphoma[1] and in Chapter 9.

References

1. Hoppe RT, Advani RH, Bierman PJ, et al. NCCN physician guidelines: Hodgkin disease 2006 v.1. www.nccn.org; 2006.
2. Hoppe RT, Advani RH, Bierman PJ, et al. Hodgkin disease/lymphoma. Clinical practice guidelines in oncology. *J Natl Compr Cancer Netw* 2006;4:210–230.
3. Pusey WE. Cases of Sarcoma and of Hodgkin's Disease Treated by Exposures to x-rays—a Preliminary Report. *JAMA* 1902;38:166–169.
4. Senn N. Therapeutical value of Roentgen ray in treatment of pseudoleukemia. *New York Medical Journal* 1903;77:665–668.
5. Gilbert R. La roentgentherapie de la granulomatose maligne. *J Radiol Electrol* 1925;9:509–514.
6. Gilbert R, Babaiantz L. Notre methode de roentgentherapie de la lymphogranulomatose (Hodgkin): resultats eloignes. *Acta Radiol* 1931; 12: 523–529.
7. Peters M. A study of survivals in Hodgkin's disease treated radiologically. *Am J Roentgenol* 1950;63:299–311.
8. Peters M, Middlemiss K. A study of Hodgkin's disease treated by irradiation. *Am J Roentgenol* 1958;79:114–121.
9. Fuks Z, Feldman M. Henry S. Kaplan 1918–1984: A physician, a scientist, a friend. *Cancer Surv* 1985;4:295–311.
10. Ginzton E, Mallory K, Kaplan H. The Stanford medical linear accelerator I: design and development. *Stanford Med Bull* 1957;15:123–140.
11. Kaplan HS. The radical radiotherapy of regionally localized Hodgkin's disease. *Radiology* 1962;78:553.
12. Lukes R, Butler J, Hicks E. Natural history of Hodgkin's disease as related to pathological picture. *Cancer* 1966;19:317–344.
13. Carbone PP, Kaplan HS, Musshoff K, et al. Report of the Committee on Hodgkin's Disease Staging Classification. *Cancer Res* 1971;31:1860–1861.
14. Glatstein E, Guernsey JM, Rosenberg SA, et al. The value of laparotomy and splenectomy in the staging of Hodgkin's disease. *Cancer* 1969; 24:709–718.
15. Devita VT Jr., Serpick AA, Carbone PP. Combination chemotherapy in the treatment of advanced Hodgkin's disease. *Ann Intern Med* 1970;73: 881–895.
16. Diehl V, Thomas RK, Re D. Part II: Hodgkin's lymphoma—diagnosis and treatment. *Lancet Oncol* 2004;5:19–26.
17. Nogova L, Reineke T, Eich HT, et al. Extended field radiotherapy, combined modality treatment or involved field radiotherapy for patients with stage IA lymphocyte-predominant Hodgkin's lymphoma: a retrospective analysis from the German Hodgkin Study Group (GHSG). *Ann Oncol* 2005;16:1683–1687.
18. Schlembach PJ, Wilder RB, Jones D, et al. Radiotherapy alone for lymphocyte-predominant Hodgkin's disease. *Cancer J* 2002;8:377–383.
19. Ng AK, Bernardo MP, Weller E, et al. Long-term survival and competing causes of death in patients with early-stage Hodgkin's disease treated at age 50 or younger. *J Clin Oncol* 2002;20:2101–2108.
20. Ng AK, Bernardo MV, Weller E, et al. Second malignancy after Hodgkin disease treated with radiation therapy with or without chemotherapy: long-term risks and risk factors. *Blood* 2002;100:1989–1996.
21. DeVita VT Jr. Hodgkin's disease—clinical trials and travails. *N Engl J Med* 2003;348:2375–2376.
22. Longo DL. Radiation therapy in the treatment of Hodgkin's disease—do you see what I see? *J Natl Cancer Inst* 2003;95:928–929.
23. Eghbali H, Raemaekers J, Carde P. The EORTC strategy in the treatment of Hodgkin's lymphoma. *Eur J Haematol Suppl* 2005;135–140.
24. Laskar S, Gupta T, Vimal S, et al. Consolidation radiation after complete remission in Hodgkin's disease following six cycles of doxorubicin, bleomycin, vinblastine, and dacarbazine chemotherapy: is there a need? *J Clin Oncol* 2004;22:62–68.

25. Meyer RM, Gospodarowicz M, Connors JM, et al. Randomized comparison of ABVD chemotherapy with a strategy that includes radiation therapy in patients with limited-stage Hodgkin's lymphoma: National Cancer Institute of Canada Trials Group and the Eastern Cooperative Oncology Group. *J Clin Oncol* 2005;23:4634–4642.

26. Straus DJ, Portlock CS, Qin J, et al. Results of a prospective randomized clinical trial of doxorubicin, bleomycin, vinblastine, and dacarbazine (ABVD) followed by radiation therapy (RT) versus ABVD alone for stages I, II, and IIIA nonbulky Hodgkin disease. *Blood* 2004;104:3483–3489.

27. Nachman JB, Sposto R, Herzog P, et al. Randomized comparison of low-dose involved-field radiotherapy and no radiotherapy for children with Hodgkin's disease who achieve a complete response to chemotherapy. *J Clin Oncol* 2002;20:3765–3771.

28. Noordijk EM, Thomas J, Ferme C, et al. First results of the EORTC-GELA H9 randomized trials: the H9-F trial (comparing 3 radiation dose levels) and H9-U trial (comparing 3 chemotherapy schemes) in patients with favorable or unfavorable early stage Hodgkin's lymphoma. *Proc Am Soc Clin Oncol* 2005;23:561s.

29. Prosnitz LR, Wu JJ, Yahalom J. The case for adjuvant radiation therapy in advanced Hodgkin's disease. *Cancer Invest* 1996;14:361–370.

30. Horning SJ, Hoppe RT, Breslin S, et al. Stanford V and radiotherapy for locally extensive and advanced Hodgkin's disease: mature results of a prospective clinical trial. *J Clin Oncol* 2002;20:630–637.

31. Poen JC, Hoppe RT, Horning SJ. High-dose therapy and autologous bone marrow transplantation for relapsed/refractory Hodgkin's disease: the impact of involved field radiotherapy on patterns of failure and survival [see comments]. *Int J Radiat Oncol Biol Phys* 1996;36:3–12.

32. Girinsky T, van der Maazen R, Specht L, et al. Involved-node radiotherapy (INRT) in patients with early Hodgkin lymphoma: concepts and guidelines. *Radiother Oncol* 2006;79:270–277.

33. Kaplan HS, Rosenberg SA. The treatment of Hodgkin's disease. *Med Clin North Am* 1966;50:1591–1610.

34. Yahalom J, Mauch P. The involved field is back: issues in delineating the radiation field in Hodgkin's disease. *Ann Oncol* 2002;13(suppl 1):79–83.

35. Gray L, Prosnitz L. Dosimetry of Hodgkin's disease therapy using a 4 MV linear accelerator. *Radiology* 1975;116:423–428.

36. Bentel GC, Marks LB, Krishnamurthy R, et al. Comparison of two repositioning devices used during radiation therapy for Hodgkin's disease. *Int J Radiat Oncol Biol Phys* 1997;38:791–795.

37. Bentel G. Positioning and immobilization of patients undergoing radiation therapy for Hodgkin's disease. *Med Dosim* 1991;16:111–117.

38. Fraass BA, van de Geijn J. Peripheral dose from megavolt beams. *Med Phys* 1983;10:809–818.

39. Fraass B, Kinsella T, Harrington F, et al. Peripheral dose to the testes: the design and clinical use of practical and effective gonadal shield. *Int J Radiat Biol Phys* 1985;11:609.

40. Kubo H, Shipley WU. Reduction of the scatter dose to the testicle outside the radiation treatment fields. *Int J Radiat Oncol Biol Phys* 1982; 8:1741–1745.

41. McCord DL, Million RR, Northrop MF, et al. Daily reproducibility of lung blocks in the mantle technique. *Radiology* 1973;109:735–736.

42. Marks J, Haus A, Sutton H, et al. Localization error in the radiotherapy of Hodgkin's disease and malignant lymhoma with extended mantle fields. *Cancer* 1974;34:83–90.

43. Griffiths S, Pearcey R. The daily reproducibility of large complex-shaped radiotherapy fields to the thorax and neck. *Clin Radiol* 1986;37:39.

44. Taylor BW, Jr., Mendenhall NP, Million RR. Reproducibility of mantle irradiation with daily imaging films. *Int J Radiat Oncol Biol Phys* 1990;19:149–151.

45. Hulshof M, Vanuytsel L, Van Den Bogaert W, et al. Localization errors in mantle-field irradiation for Hodgkin's disease. *Int J Radiat Oncol Biol Phys* 1989;17:679–683.

46. Rabinowitz I, Broomberg J, Goitein M, et al. Accuracy of radiation field alignment in clinical practice. *Int J Radiat Oncol Biol Phys* 1985;11:1857–1867.

47. Creutzberg C, Visser A, De Porre P, et al. Accuracy of patient positioning in mantle field irradiation. *Radiother Oncol* 1992;23:257–264.

48. Naida J, Eisbruch A, Schoeppel S, et al. Analysis of localization errors in the definition of the mantle field using a beam's eye view treatment-planning system. *Int J Radiat Oncol Biol Phys* 1996;35:377–382.

49. Hennequin C, Carrie C, Hofstetter S, et al. A quality control program for radiotherapy in Hodgkin's disease. *Cancer Radiother* 1999;3:187–190.

50. Duhmke E, Diehl V, Loeffler M, et al. Randomized trial with early-stage Hodgkin's disease testing 30 Gy vs. 40 Gy extended field radiotherapy along. *Int J Radiat Oncol Biol Phys* 1996;36:305–310.

51. Muller RP, Eich HT. The development of quality assurance programs for radiotherapy within the German Hodgkin Study Group (GHSG). Introduction, continuing work, and results of the radiotherapy reference panel. *Strahlenther Onkol* 2005;181:557–566.

52. Eich HT, Muller RP. The radiotherapy reference panel—experiences and results of the German Hodgkin Study Group (GHSG). *Eur J Haematol Suppl* 2005:98–105.

53. Kinzie JJ, Hanks GE, MacLean CJ, et al. Patterns of care study: Hodgkin's disease relapse rates and adequacy of portals. *Cancer* 1983;52: 2223–2226.

54. Hoppe R, Hanlon A, Hanks G, et al. Progress in the treatment of Hodgkin's disease in the United States, 1973 versus 1983: the Patterns of Care Study. *Cancer* 1994;74:3198–3203.

55. Hughes DB, Smith AR, Hoppe R, et al. Treatment planning for Hodgkin's disease: a Pattern of Care Study. *Intl J Radiat Oncol Biol Phys* 1995; 33:519–524.

56. Weeks J. Outcomes assessment in the NCCN. *Oncology (Huntingt)* 1997; 11:137–140.

57. Kaplan HS. Evidence for a tumoricidal dose level in the radiotherapy of Hodgkin's disease. *Cancer Res* 1966;26:1221–1224.

58. Hanks GE, Kinzie JJ, White RL, et al. Patterns of care outcome studies. Results of the national practice in Hodgkin's disease. *Cancer* 1983; 51:569–573.

59. Thar TL, Million RR, Hausner RJ, et al. Hodgkin's disease, stages I and II: relationship of recurrence to size of disease, radiation dose, and number of sites involved. *Cancer* 1979;43:1101–1105.

60. Mendenhall NP, Rodrigue LL, Moore-Higgs GJ, et al. The optimal dose of radiation in Hodgkin's disease: an analysis of clinical and treatment factors affecting in-field disease control. *Int J Radiat Oncol Biol Phys* 1999;44:551–561.

61. Schewe KL, Reavis J, Kun LE, et al. Total dose, fraction size, and tumor volume in the local control of Hodgkin's disease. *Int J Radiat Oncol Biol Phys* 1988;15:25–28.

62. Vijayakumar S, Myrianthopoulos LC. An updated dose–response analysis in Hodgkin's disease. *Radiother Oncol* 1992;24:1–13.

63. Prosnitz LR, Farber LR, Fischer JJ, et al. Long term remissions with combined modality therapy for advanced Hodgkin's disease. *Cancer* 1976; 37:2826–2833.

64. Aleman BM, Raemaekers JM, Tirelli U, et al. Involved-field radiotherapy for advanced Hodgkin's lymphoma. *N Engl J Med* 2003;348: 2396–2406.

65. Donaldson SS, Link MP. Combined modality treatment with low-dose radiation and MOPP chemotherapy for children with Hodgkin's disease. *J Clin Oncol* 1987;5:742–749.

66. Loeffler M, Diehl V, Pfreundschuh M, et al. Dose-response relationship of complementary radiotherapy following four cycles of combination chemotherapy in intermediate-stage Hodgkin's disease. *J Clin Oncol* 1997;15:2275–2287.

67. Diehl V, Brillant C, Engert A, et al. HD10: investigating reduction of combined modality treatment intensity in early stage Hodgkin's disease. Interim analysis of a randomized trial of the German Hodgkin Study Group (GHSG). *J Clin Oncol* 2005;21(suppl 1):abstract 6506.

68. Dores GM, Metayer C, Curtis RE, et al. Second malignant neoplasms among long-term survivors of Hodgkin's disease: a population-based evaluation over 25 years. *J Clin Oncol* 2002;20:3484–3494.

69. van Leeuwen FE, Klokman WJ, Stovall M, et al. Roles of radiation dose, chemotherapy, and hormonal factors in breast cancer following Hodgkin's disease. *J Natl Cancer Inst* 2003;95:971–980.

70. Travis LB, Hill DA, Dores GM, et al. Breast cancer following radiotherapy and chemotherapy among young women with Hodgkin disease. *JAMA* 2003;290:465–475.

71. Kuttesch JF, Jr., Wexler LH, Marcus RB, et al. Second malignancies after Ewing's sarcoma: radiation dose-dependency of secondary sarcomas. *J Clin Oncol* 1996;14:2818–2825.

72. Koontz B, Kirkpatrick J, Clough R, et al. Combined modality therapy versus radiotherapy alone for treatment of early stage Hodgkin disease: cure versus complications. *J Clin Oncol* 2006;24:605–611.

73. Salloum E, Doria R, Schubert W, et al. Second solid tumors in patients with Hodgkin's disease cured after radiation or chemotherapy plus adjuvant low-dose radiation. *J Clin Oncol* 1996;14:2435–2443.

74. Goodman KA, Toner S, Hunt M, et al. Intensity-modulated radiotherapy for lymphoma involving the mediastinum. *Int J Radiat Oncol Biol Phys* 2005;62:198–206.

75. Sieber M, Franklin J, Tesch H, et al. Two cycles ABVD plus extended field radiotherapy is superior to radiothearpy alone in early stage Hodgkin's disease: results of the German Hodgkin's Lymphoma Study Group (GHSG) trial HD7. *Blood* 2002;100:A341.

76. Press OW, LeBlanc M, Lichter AS, et al. Phase III randomized intergroup trial of subtotal lymphoid irradiation versus doxorubicin, vinblastine, and subtotal lymphoid irradiation for stage IA to IIA Hodgkin's disease. *J Clin Oncol* 2001;19:4238–4244.

77. Carde P, Noordijk E, Hagenbeek A. Superiority of EBVP chemotherapy in combination with involved field irradiation over subtotal nodal irradiation in favorable clinical stage I-II Hodgkin's disease: The EORTC-GPMC H7F randomized trial. *Proc ASCO* 1997;16:13.

78. Hagenbeek A, Eghbali H, Ferme C, et al. Three cycles of MOPP/ABV hybrid and involved-field irradiation is more effective than subtotal nodal irradiation in favorable supradiaphragmatic clinical stages I-II Hodgkin's disease: prelinary results of the EORTC-GELA H9-F randomized trial in 543 patients. *Blood* 2000;96:A575.

79. Bonadonna G, Bonfante V, Viviani S, et al. ABVD plus subtotal nodal versus involved-field radiotherapy in early-stage Hodgkin's disease: long-term results. *J Clin Oncol* 2004;22:2835–2841.

80. Engert A, Schiller P, Josting A, et al. Involved-field radiotherapy is equally effective and less toxic compared with extended-field radiotherapy after four cycles of chemotherapy in patients with early-stage unfavorable Hodgkin's lymphoma: results of the HD8 trial of the German Hodgkin's Lymphoma Study Group. *J Clin Oncol* 2003;21:3601–3608.

81. Ferme C, Eghbali H, Hagenbeek A, et al. MOPP/ABV hybrid and irradiation in unfavorable supradiaphragmatic clinical stages I-II Hodgkin's disease: comparison of three treatment modalities. Preliminary results of the EORTC-GELA H8-U randomized trial in 995 patients. *Blood* 2000;96:A576.

CHAPTER 14 ■ PRINCIPLES OF CHEMOTHERAPY IN HODGKIN LYMPHOMA

RACHEL E. HOUGH AND BARRY W. HANCOCK

HISTORY OF CHEMOTHERAPY IN HODGKIN LYMPHOMA

The advances made in the use of chemotherapy in Hodgkin lymphoma over the past half-century have been considerable, providing both the potential for cure in patients with advanced Hodgkin lymphoma and also a springboard for the development of modern chemotherapy in other malignancies.

By the early 1900s, it was recognized that arsenicals had some activity against Hodgkin's disease. However, the first real breakthrough came by way of an accident in World War II. Seamen exposed to mustard gas following the explosion of a military ship were found to have marrow and lymphoid hypoplasia. In the latter years of the war, nitrogen mustard was given to patients with Hodgkin's disease, and it resulted in a dramatic, albeit short-lived, clinical regression of disease.[1] Development of mustard derivatives and other agents, including antifolate antimetabolites, corticosteroids, vinca alkaloids, nitrosoureas, and procarbazine, followed quickly. In 1964, the outlook for patients with Hodgkin's disease was dramatically improved with the development of the MOPP regimen (mechlorethamine, oncovin, procarbazine, and prednisone),[2] which achieved a complete remission in 84% of patients. Furthermore, unlike any treatment before it, these remissions were durable, with a 66% relapse-free survival at 20 years.[3] From a historial perspective it is interesting to note that the original combination used at the NCI (dubbed "combination 1") was actually MOMP (methotrexate instead of procarbazine), and 14 patients were treated on this regimen prior to the introduction of MOPP ("combination 2").

Since then, researchers have looked for ways of improving survival while minimizing both the short- and long-term side effects of treatment. Various MOPP-like and other combination regimens have been developed and given alone or as alternating or hybrid regimens. With the clear efficacy of radiotherapy in localized disease, a combined-modality approach has also been investigated in advanced Hodgkin lymphoma, using combination chemotherapy with radiotherapy to sites of bulky disease or slowly responding lymph nodes.

Today, the great success of these early researchers means that around 70% of patients with Hodgkin lymphoma will be cured. Regimens designed in the light of MOPP have provided some reduction in side effects but no significant gain in overall survival. Improving outcome and minimizing toxicity remain the challenges of today.

BASIC PRINCIPLES OF CHEMOTHERAPY AS APPLIED TO HODGKIN LYMPHOMA

The ultimate aim of a cytotoxic drug is tumor cell death. This is achieved by a variety of mechanisms, which include causing structural change in the DNA, interference with enzymes central to DNA synthesis, and damage to the mitotic spindle.

The DNA structure can be altered by alkylation or intercalation of base pairs or by strand breakage. Nitrogen mustard and other alkylating agents form covalent bonds between the alkyl groups of the drug and the base pairs of the two DNA strands resulting in interstrand cross-links.[4] These prevent the normal separation of DNA during mitosis. Intercalating agents such as the anthracyclines cause distortion of the DNA molecule by intercalation between adjacent nucleotide base pairs and prevent the action of DNA and RNA polymerases. Anthracyclines also cause double DNA strand breakage via inhibition of topoisomerase II.[5,6]

Antimetabolite drugs inhibit DNA synthesis by binding to key enzymes in the purine or pyrimidine synthetic pathways. A number of enzymes may be targeted, including thymidylate synthetase (fluorouracil), DNA polymerase (cytosine arabinoside), and dihydrofolate reductase (methotrexate).[7]

The vinca alkaloids[8] and taxanes[9] cause disruption of the mitotic spindle. The spindle is vital in the sorting and movement of chromosomes during mitosis, and these drugs result in metaphase arrest of dividing tumor cells.

Cytotoxic drugs are rarely, if ever, entirely selective for tumor cells, and will inevitably affect normal cells passing through their cycle, particularly those in the bone marrow and gastrointestinal tract. Although normal cells are effective in repairing drug-induced DNA damage, they never develop drug resistance,[10] and the maximum dose of any agent will be limited by its toxicity to normal tissues.

As our understanding of the biology of Hodgkin lymphoma increases, new drugs and strategies are developed. Initial efficacy is assessed using human tumor cell lines, and pharmacokinetic and toxicology data are obtained from animal studies. If a drug appears promising on the basis of these tests, it must be thoroughly investigated in at least three phases of human clinical trials before it can become widely available. In Hodgkin lymphoma, as with other cancers, phase I and II studies are performed in patients with refractory, advanced disease for whom there is no effective alternative therapy.

TABLE 14.1

EFFICACY AND TOXICITY OF SINGLE AGENTS IN HODGKIN LYMPHOMA

Drug	Any response (%)	Complete remission (%)	Toxicity
Chlorambucil	60	16	Myelosuppression, teratogenesis
Cyclophosphamide	54	12	Myelosuppression, hemorrhagic cystitis, nausea, sterility, pulmonary fibrosis, alopecia
Nitrogen mustard	63	13	Nausea, vomiting, myelosuppression, thrombophlebitis, alopecia
Prednisolone	61	10	Cushing syndrome, peptic ulceration, psychiatric disturbance, diabetes
Procarbazine	69	38	Nausea, myelotoxicity, neuropsychiatric disturbance, teratogenesis
Vinblastine	68	30	Myelotoxicity, neurotoxicity (infrequent)
Vincristine	64	36	Neurotoxicity

Phase I trials are primarily concerned with drug safety. Initially a low dose of drug (as predicted from animal data) is used, and the dose is then escalated. Pharmacokinetic, pharmacodynamic, and toxicity data are analyzed to determine the optimum dose for further evaluation. A phase II trial is employed to determine whether the drug is effective against a particular malignancy. The optimum dose (determined in a phase I trial) is given to at least 14 patients with measurable disease. The principal end-point is tumor shrinkage.

Any drug that has been shown to be both safe and effective must finally be compared to the standard treatment for that disease in a large number of patients by means of a prospective, randomized, controlled trial (phase III). This chapter focuses on data accrued from such studies. The incorporation of a new drug or drug regimen into standard practice must be based on data from all available clinical trials. This can be a difficult process, as trials often differ in patient selection, indices of response and survival, drug delivery, and lengths of follow-up; thus, only broad comparisons can be made. Patients should be carefully staged before and after treatment, and response recorded in accordance with standard criteria, as follows:

- A *complete response* is achieved when there is disappearance of all known disease on two identical evaluations not less than 4 weeks apart. A *partial response* is defined as a 50% or greater decrease in the sum of products of the largest perpendicular diameters of measurable lesions.
- *Stable disease* describes less than a 50% decrease or 25% increase in measurable disease.
- *Progressive disease* is defined as a 25% or greater increase in one or more of the measurable lesions or the appearance of a new lesion.

No cure can be achieved without the patient having first achieved a complete response, and this is an important goal for all cytotoxic drugs. However, the durability of this remission is central to long-term outcome, and progression-free survival following completion of chemotherapy is now considered to be an important measure of the quality of a response. In Hodgkin lymphoma, the cause-specific survival plateaus at between 5 and 10 years; such patients can be considered "cured." However, overall survival is, of course, influenced by other factors (second malignancy, increased heart and lung disease), and survival curves still show a downward trend even 20 to 25 years after treatment.

SINGLE AGENTS

Using the murine leukemia L1210, Skipper and colleagues provided a kinetic model for tumor growth and response to treatment.[11,12] All the cells in this tumor were proliferating, and tumor growth was found to be logarithmic with a constant doubling time. It was seen that cell kill by drug administration was also logarithmic, following first-order kinetics; the proportion of tumor cells killed by a given dose of drug was constant irrespective of the number of tumor cells present initially. All tumor cells needed to be killed before cure could be achieved, as any remaining cells would inevitably proliferate. From these experiments, it was predicted that tumor eradication would be dependent on initial tumor burden, drug dose, and doubling time of residual tumor cells.

Following the discovery of the effects of nitrogen mustard in 1946,[1] a number of different drugs were developed and shown to be effective in Hodgkin lymphoma. Table 14.1 summarizes the response rates and toxicities associated with these agents when given to previously untreated patients.[13,14] The majority of patients had regression of disease, with some achieving a complete remission. However, relapse was inevitable,[14] and there have been no reports of cure of advanced Hodgkin lymphoma following administration of a single agent alone.

At least 10^9 to 10^{12} tumor cells must be present before disease becomes clinically detectable. It was clear that the drugs available by the early 1960s could reduce the tumor burden below this threshold. However, if they were used within the confines of acceptable toxicity, the tumor was not totally eradicated and quickly relapsed. To date, with the exceptions of choriocarcinoma[15] and Burkitt lymphoma, human malignancies have proved to be incurable by single-agent chemotherapy.[16]

COMBINATION CHEMOTHERAPY

Based on Skipper's model, it was postulated that the simultaneous use of more than one drug with different biological actions might have an additive killing effect. The combination of drugs could be tolerated if drugs with different toxicity profiles were used. DeVita has subsequently outlined principles that facilitate the selection of new effective combination regimens (Table 14.2).[16,17]

TABLE 14.2

IMPORTANT PRINCIPLES IN THE SELECTION OF COMBINATION CHEMOTHERAPY REGIMENS

- Only drugs known to cause tumor regression (partial or complete) when used alone should be included.
- When several equally effective drugs of the same class are available, the drug selection should be based on minimizing overlapping toxicities with the other elements of the regimen.
- Drugs should be used in their optimal doses and schedules.
- Drug combinations should be given at consistent intervals; these intervals should be as short as possible for renewal of normal tissue, usually the bone marrow.

The first indication that such an approach was superior came in 1965. Lacher and Durant treated 16 patients with advanced Hodgkin lymphoma with a combination of chlorambucil and vinblastine.[18] Thirteen had remissions (81%), which were complete in 10 (63%). Median relapse-free survival was 7.5 months, a modest improvement from those previously treated with single agents, although the trial included no formal control group.

However, the true potential of combination chemotherapy in advanced Hodgkin's disease was first realized in 1967, when the effects of the quadruple regimen MOPP were first reported by DeVita and co-workers at the National Cancer Institute (NCI).[19] Of the 188 patients with histologically proven Hodgkin's disease receiving treatment, 157 (84%) achieved a complete remission. Subsequent follow-up has shown that this regimen gives a relapse-free survival of 66% and overall survival of 48% after more than 20 years.[2,3] Patients received at least 6 cycles of MOPP or treatment to complete response followed by a further 2 cycles. Higher complete remission rates and longer survival were associated with the absence of B-symptoms and with a higher dose of vincristine. Disease relapse tended to occur within 4 years of achieving a complete response and was uncommon after this time. Associated side effects were significant. Nausea, vomiting, phlebitis, myelosuppression, and reversible vincristine-related neuropathies were common acute toxicities. Long-term side effects included infertility and secondary malignancy. All men became azoospermic, and 41% of women over the age of 26 years became amenorrheic.[3] Acute leukemia developed in 13 patients from the NCI series, but in all but one patient, radiotherapy had also been given. The efficacy of MOPP has been confirmed in a number of other studies,[20–22] and this regimen quickly became the "gold standard" treatment in advanced Hodgkin's disease.

Since the development of the MOPP regimen, clinical research has striven to improve outcome while minimizing short- and long-term toxicity. A number of researchers attempted to improve MOPP by adding, removing, or substituting elements of the regimen (Table 14.3).[23] Mechlorethamine (nitrogen mustard) was replaced by less toxic agents including chlorambucil,[24–26] cyclophosphamide,[27] lomustine,[28] and carmustine.[29–32] Reduction in neurotoxicity was achieved by the substitution of vinblastine for vincristine, although none of the neurologic complications seen in the patients given MOPP caused permanent disability.[3] Substitution of vinblastine for vincristine in the MVPP regimen reduced neurotoxicity at the expense of myelotoxicity.[33] Efficacy was comparable to that with MOPP. McElwain and colleagues found that substituting chlorambucil for nitrogen mustard in the MVPP regimen (ChlVPP) provided a better-tolerated, equally efficacious combination.[24] Substitution of chlorambucil (Leukeran) for nitrogen mustard in the MOPP regimen in a randomized British National Lymphoma Investigation (BNLI) study confirmed that

toxicity could be reduced without compromising efficacy.[34–36] The Eastern Cooperative Oncology Group (ECOG) reported the only prospective randomized study in which there was any improved therapeutic benefit when compared to MOPP.[20,37] They demonstrated an increase in disease-free survival following complete response with BCVPP (BCNU, cyclophosphamide, vinblastine, procarbazine, prednisone), although overall survival was no better. However, BCVPP was associated with a higher incidence of secondary acute leukemia. In a Southwest Oncology Group (SWOG) study, addition of bleomycin to MOPP was associated with no additional benefit.[38,39] Although the role of prednisone had been debated, the prospective BNLI trial in which prednisolone was omitted from the MOPP regimen demonstrated significant reduction in the attainment of complete response and overall survival.[40–42]

MOPP-like combination regimens significantly reduced some of the acute toxicities associated with MOPP but have failed to improve overall or disease-free survival.

A different approach was taken by Bonadonna and the Milan Cancer Institute Group. The ABVD regimen was developed as a non–cross-resistant alternative, initially for MOPP failures.[43] It comprised Adriamycin, bleomycin, vinblastine, and dacarbazine, agents that had all been shown to have single-agent activity in Hodgkin lymphoma relapsing after MOPP. The regimen was shown to have good activity in patients with MOPP-resistant disease, causing less myelotoxicity, sterility, or acute leukemia. Side effects associated with ABVD included acute severe nausea and vomiting and long-term cardiac and pulmonary damage.[44,45] The Cancer and Leukemia Group B (CALGB) investigated the efficacy of this regimen in previously untreated patients with advanced Hodgkin lymphoma in a prospective randomized clinical trial.[46,47] Complete remission rates were 82% in the ABVD arm compared with 66% for MOPP. Failure-free survival was also superior for ABVD (61% for ABVD and 50% for MOPP). However, no improvement in overall survival has been demonstrated. The lower response rate to MOPP probably resulted from drug delivery at a lower dose intensity than that originally described by the NCI, and this has led to some criticism of the trial.[48]

Other alternative combination regimens have been shown to have activity as salvage regimens in relapsed or refractory Hodgkin lymphoma following MOPP and are summarized in Table 14.4. These include ABDIC (Adriamycin, bleomycin, DTIC, prednisolone, CCNU),[49] CABS (CCNU, Adriamycin, bleomycin, streptozocin),[53] CEP (CCNU, etoposide, prednimustine),[55] and MIME (methyl-GAG, ifosfamide, methotrexate, etoposide).[58] Their role in previously untreated patients has not yet been established in prospective randomized studies.

The use of maintenance chemotherapy to prevent regrowth of any residual tumor cells after complete remission has been achieved has not been shown to be beneficial in Hodgkin lymphoma. A number of studies have consistently failed to

TABLE 14.3

EFFICACY AND TOXICITY OF MOPP VARIANTS IN ADVANCED HODGKIN LYMPHOMA

	Modification	Regimens compared	Complete remission	Freedom from relapse	Overall survival	Efficacy compared to MOPP	Toxicity compared to MOPP	Center regimen (reference)
MVPP	Substitution of vinblastine for vincristine		76%		65% (5 yr)	Equivalent	Less neurotoxicity	St Bartholomew's, London[33]
ChlVPP	Substitution of chlorambucil for nitrogen mustard and vinblastine for vincristine		85%	71% (10 yr)	65% (10 yr)	Equivalent	Less nausea, vomiting, alopecia, and neurotoxicity	Royal Marsden, London[24-26]
LOPP	Substitution of chlorambucil for nitrogen mustard	LOPP MOPP	57% 63%	55% (10 yr) 60%	54% 52%	Equivalent	Less nausea, vomiting, and myelosuppression	BNLI[34-36]
BOPP	Substitution of BCNU for nitrogen mustard	BOPP MOPP	67% 63%	Approx 55% (5 yr) Approx 55%	Approx 50% Approx 50%	Equivalent	Equivalent	CALBG[29]
MOP	Deletion of prednisolone	MOP MOPP	36% 69%		30% (5 yr)[a] 60%	Reduced complete response rate and overall survival	Equivalent	BNLI[42]
BCVPP	Substitution of vinblastine for vincristine and BCNU and cyclophosphamide for nitrogen mustard	BCVPP MOPP	77% 73%	65% (5 yr)[a] 50%	65% 61%	Increased relapse-free survival Overall survival unchanged	Less nausea, vomiting, and neurotoxicity More myelotoxicity and leukemia	ECOG[20,37]
Bleo-MOPP	Addition of bleomycin	Bleo-MOPP MOPP	84% 70%	64% (3 yr) 53%	78% 58%	Equivalent		SWOG[38,39]

[a]Statistically significant.

TABLE 14.4

EFFICACY AND TOXICITY OF OTHER COMBINATION CHEMOTHERAPY REGIMENS USED IN ADVANCED HODGKIN LYMPHOMA

Regimen	Trial design and patients included	Complete remission	Freedom from relapse	Overall survival	Toxicity	Center (reference)
ABDIC	Phase II. Patients refractory to MOPP	35%	47 months in complete responders (median)	24 months (median)	Myelosuppression, vomiting, alopecia	MD Anderson[49]
B-CAVe	Phase II. Patients refractory to MOPP	44%	24 months (median)	—	Thrombocytopenia	Stanford[50]
BCNU-VPP	Randomized trial comparing BCNU-VPP to BCNU alone as primary chemotherapy	83%	67% at 51+ months	92% at 51+ months	Myelosuppression, vomiting, peripheral neuropathy, encephalopathy	Northwest Oncology Group[51]
CABS	Phase II. Previously untreated patients	80%	8.6 years in complete responders (median)	—	—	Albert Einstein Center[52]
CCNU-VP	Randomized controlled trial comparing CCNU-VP to MOPP	72%	—	60% at 89+ months	Less nausea and emesis compared to MOPP	Western Cancer Study Group[53]
CEP	Phase II. Patients refractory to MOPP and ABVD	40%	15 months (median)	17 months (median)	Nausea, alopecia, myelosuppression	NCI[54]
CVPP	Randomized controlled trial comparing CVPP to MOPP, MVPP, or COPP	69%	71% of complete responders at 56 months	36% at 60 months	Myelosuppression; less gastrointestinal and neurotoxicity compared to MOPP	CALBG[55]
CVPP	Phase II. Previously untreated patients	74%	27 months (median)	—	Nausea, alopecia, myelosuppression	Minnesota[56]
EVA	Phase II. Previously untreated patients	54%	44% at 2 years	86% at 2 years leukemogenic	Myelosuppression,	Duke[57]
MIME	Phase II. Patients refractory to MOPP and ABVD	23%	25 months (median)	50 weeks (median)	Infections, hemorrhagic cystitis, neutropenia	MD Anderson[58]
MOP-BAP	Randomized controlled trial comparing MOP-BAP to MOPP-Bleomycin	77%	—	Superior to MOPP-Bleo in low risk patients	—	SWOG[39]
NOVP	Phase II. Early-stage disease with poor prognostic factors. Given with RT	40% / 44% (CRu)	93% at 1 year	100% at 1 year	Nausea, alopecia, myelosuppression, myalgia	MD Anderson[59]
PACEBOM	Phase II. Previously untreated patients	40% / 16% (CRu)	64% at 3 years	92% at 3 years	Myelosuppression, skin reactions, mucositis, alopecia	CRC[60]
PAVe	Randomized controlled trial comparing PAVe+RT to MOPP+RT or ABVD+RT	93%	78% at 15 years	75% at 15 years	Myelosuppression, secondary malignancies	Stanford[61]
VAPEC B	Phase II. Patients refractory to Adriamycin-containing regimens, principally MVPP	30%	—	—	Myelosuppression	Christie[62]

RT, radiotherapy.

demonstrate any improvement in either disease-free or overall survival,[37,63–65] and so maintenance chemotherapy is not routinely given in Hodgkin lymphoma.

ALTERNATING CHEMOTHERAPY

None of the combination regimens developed for the treatment of advanced Hodgkin lymphoma has shown clear superiority in efficacy when delivered close to the original intended dose and schedule. Goldie and Coldman hypothesized that this observation was a consequence of the development of chemotherapy resistance.[66] They proposed that spontaneous mutations arise in tumor cells at a specific mutation rate related to the inherent genetic instability of a particular malignancy. The number of resistant cells in any tumor is therefore related to the total number of mitotic divisions that have occurred. Because at least 10^9 cells must be present before a tumor is clinically detectable, it is likely that cells resistant to at least one agent are present at the time of diagnosis. Further spontaneous mutations arising during treatment may result in additional resistance to other drugs. Goldie and Coldman predicted that the early introduction of as many effective agents as possible, before resistant clones emerged, would be more likely to eradicate the tumor.[67] Taking into account acceptable toxicity, they advocated the use of alternating non–cross-resistant chemotherapy regimens.

The efficacy of ABVD in disease relapsing after treatment with MOPP is suggestive of non–cross-resistance between the two regimens. Bonadonna and colleagues in Milan randomized 88 patients with previously untreated stage IV Hodgkin lymphoma to monthly cycles of MOPP or MOPP alternating with ABVD.[45,68–70] Relapse-free survival was better for the alternating regimen (Table 14.5), but the complete response rate was not significantly improved, and long-term follow-up has shown no overall survival advantage. A number of criticisms have been made of this study.[48,71] MOPP was not administered in the standard manner described by the NCI group. A total of 12 cycles were given, rather than 6, and the dose intensity was significantly reduced in more than half the patients. The outcome of patients on MOPP alone was worse than that described by other studies. In addition, half of the MOPP patients ultimately received ABVD.

The CALBG randomized a further 361 patients with stage III and IV Hodgkin lymphoma to 6 to 8 cycles of MOPP or ABVD alone or 12 cycles of MOPP alternating with ABVD.[46,47] Complete response rates and freedom from progression were equivalent for ABVD alone and the alternating regimen, both of which were superior to MOPP. No difference in overall survival was observed. Again, the dose intensity of MOPP was compromised.

A number of other studies, using a variety of alternating regimens, have failed to demonstrate a dramatic improvement in outcome when compared with properly administered four-drug combinations (Table 14.3). In fact, only the BNLI LOPP/EVAP versus LOPP study has shown a persisting advantage in overall survival for the alternating regimen.[36]

However, these studies do not necessarily refute the Goldie–Coldman hypothesis, as the regimens used have not all been shown to be truly non–cross-resistant and have not always been administered at their optimal dose intensities.

HYBRID CHEMOTHERAPY

A further application of the Goldie-Coldman hypothesis was the development of hybrid chemotherapy, in which seven or eight drugs from effective non–cross-resistant regimens were consolidated into monthly cycles.

In 1982, the Milan group developed the MA/MA regimen, which consisted of half-cycles of MOPP on day 1 and half-cycles of ABVD on day 15 of a 28-day cycle. Four hundred and fifteen patients were randomized to receive either 6 cycles of MA/MA or 6 cycles of MOPP alternating with ABVD.[68] After 9 years of follow-up, no significant difference between the two regimens could be demonstrated (Table 14.5).[83,84]

The MOPP/ABV regimen of Connors and Klimo comprised MOPP on day 1 and ABV on day 8 of a 28-day cycle. Dacarbazine was omitted, and the dose of doxorubicin was increased from 25 to 35 mg/m². Three hundred and one patients were randomized to receive 8 cycles of MOPP/ABV or 8 cycles of MOPP alternating with ABVD. Although the hybrid regimen initially appeared superior,[85] long-term follow-up has shown that both regimens are equally effective (Table 14.5).[86]

Table 14.6 summarizes the efficacy and toxicity associated with other hybrid regimens that have been investigated. In general, these regimens appear to have equivalent efficacy to four-drug or alternating therapies but may be associated with increased toxicity. It has recently been confirmed that using conventional multidrug regimens (whether by hybrid or alternation) does not improve efficacy over ABVD, and their toxicity is greater.[87]

DOSE INTENSITY

Skipper's laws were based on the L13210 mouse leukemia, in which 100% of the tumor cells were actively dividing and in cell cycle.[11,12] In most human tumors there is a nonproliferating cell population as well as the proliferating population.[95] As a result, most tumors follow a sigmoid-shaped Gompertzian growth curve rather than the logarithmic growth seen by Skipper.[10] In this model, tumor growth is initially slow as the total number of cells is small. Growth rate reaches a maximum during the middle part of the curve and then slows to a plateau as the tumor reaches its maximum size. The concept of kinetic resistance in tumor response to chemotherapy was developed by Norton and Simon.[96] They proposed that tumor cell kill also follows Gompertzian regression and is related to the dose of drug administered and the tumor growth rate at the start of treatment. Failure of a chemotherapy regimen to cure could reflect inadequate drug delivery, insufficient duration of treatment, or rapid doubling time of remaining tumor cells.

The dose intensity of a treatment was defined by Hryniuk and colleagues as the amount of drug delivered per unit of time, in milligrams per square meter per week.[97] Dose intensity is therefore dependent on the dose of drug and the interval between successive cycles of treatment. The importance of dose intensity in determining outcome has been demonstrated in both animal studies and prospective clinical trials.

Based on data from experiments performed by Skipper and colleagues with the Ridgeway osteogenic sarcoma in mice,[98] DeVita has emphasized that a reduction in dose intensity of the two-drug regimen cyclophosphamide and L-PAM by 27% reduces the cure rate by 80%, although the complete remission rate is unaffected.[99] The results of these murine experiments become available in 90 days. The effects of delivering suboptimal therapy to humans in clinical trials may take up to 10 years to be realized.

The effects of altered dose intensity on outcome in the Skipper model are indeed paralleled in prospective clinical trials. DeVita and co-workers have calculated the actual dose intensities of MOPP delivered in published prospective clinical trials.[99] In keeping with the animal data, reduction in dose intensity had no consistent effect on complete response rate but significantly reduced ongoing disease-free survival. In the

TABLE 14.5

EFFICACY AND TOXICITY OF ALTERNATING CHEMOTHERAPY IN ADVANCED HODGKIN LYMPHOMA

Regimen (no. cycles)	Complete remission	Freedom from relapse	Overall survival	Efficacy	Toxicity	Center (reference)
MOPP (12)	74%	46% (10 yr)[a]	58%	No overall survival advantage MOPP given at reduced dose intensity	Greater alopecia and gastrointestinal disturbance with MOPP/ABVD; greater myelotoxicity with MOPP alone	Milan[45,68,69,70]
MOPP (6)/ABVD (6)	89%	68%	69%			
MOPP (6)	67%[a]	50% (5 yr)[a]	66%	MOPP had inferior CR and FFR to ABVD alone and alternating regimen; MOPP given at reduced dose intensity	Increased myelotoxicity in MOPP-containing regimens; pulmonary and cardiac toxicity with ABVD; increased gastrointestinal toxicity with MOPP/ABVD	CALBG[46,47]
ABVD (6)	82%	61%	73%			
MOPP (6)/ABVD (6)	83%	65%	75%			
MOPP (6)	91%	65% (12 yr)	68%	Equivalent	Greater gastrointestinal toxicity; increased risk of secondary leukemia	NCI[72]
MOPP (3)/CABS (3)	92%	72%	54%			
MOPP (8)	57%	61% (6 yr)	57%	Alternating therapy had improved progression-free survival	Less secondary malignancy with MOPP/ABVD	EORTC[73]
MOPP (2)/ABVD (2)	59%	69%	65%			
MOPP (3)/ABV (3)/ CAD (3) + RT	76%	Approx 90% (3 yr)	80%	Equivalent	Increased myelosuppression but less nausea and vomiting in MOPP/ABV/CAD+RT arm	MSKCC[74]
MOPP (5)/ABVD (4) + RT	83%	Approx 90%	90%			
BVCPP-Bleo (6)	Approx 73%	68% (5 yr)	62%	Equivalent Not truly cross-resistant regimens	Equivalent	SECSG[75,76]
BVCPP-Bleo (3)/ABVD (3)	Approx 73%	77%	64%			
CVPP (12)	72%	50% (5 yr)	55%	Equivalent	Increased myelosuppression with CVPP	CALBG[77,78]
BAVS (12)	70%	59%	61%			
CVPP (6)/BAVS (6)	82%	57%	68%			
LOPP (8)	57%	52% (5 yr)[a]	66%[a]	Alternating regimen superior	Increased alopecia and myelosuppression with	BNLI[36,79]
LOPP (4)/EVAP (4) LOPP/EVAP	64%	66%	75%			
ChlVPP (6)	80%	68% (5 yr)	81%	Equivalent	Increased life-threatening myelosuppression in elderly with ChlVPP	Norwegian Lymphoma Group[80]
ChlVPP (3)/ABOD (3)	80%	69%	80%			
PABLOE (6)	64%	58% (3yr)[a]	85%	PABLOE inferior	Increased treatment mortality with PABLOE	BNLI/CLG[81,82]
ChlVPP (3)/PABIOE (3)	78%	77%	91%			

[a]Statistically significant.
CR, complete response; FFR, freedom from relapse; FFP, freedom from progression.

195

TABLE 14.6

EFFICACY AND TOXICITY OF HYBRID CHEMOTHERAPY REGIMENS IN ADVANCED HODGKIN LYMPHOMA

Regimen (no. Cycles)	Complete remission	Freedom from relapse	Overall survival	Efficacy	Toxicity	Center (reference)
MOPP (3)/ABVD (3) MA MA (6)	91% 89%	76% (10 yr) 78%	74% 75%	Equivalent	Equivalent	Milan[68,83,84]
MOPP (4)/ABVD (4) MOPP ABV (8)	83% 81%	67% (5 yr) 71%	83% 81%	Equivalent	Increased myelotoxicity with the hybrid	NCI, Canada [85,86]
MVPP (6) ChlVPP EVA (6)	55% 68%		71% (5 yr) 80%	Freedom from progression significantly better with hybrid	Equivalent	Christie/Barts[88]
MOPP (6)/ABVD (3)[a] MOPP ABV	73%[b] 82%	65% (8 yr)[b] 77%	82%[b] (3 yr) 89%	Hybrid superior	Increased risk of pulmonary toxicity and severe myelotoxicity but reduced incidence of secondary leukemia or myelodysplasia with hybrid	Intergroup, USA[89]
LOPP (3)/EVAP (3) LOPP EVA (6)	65%[b] 40%	85% (2 yr) 79%	88% 78%	Trial terminated early because of significantly inferior complete response for hybrid	Increased myelotoxicity with alternating regimen	BNLI[36,90]
ABVD (8) MOPP ABV (8)	76% 80%	63% (5 yr) 66%	82% (5 yr) 81%	Equivalent	Trial stopped early in view of excess deaths because of sepsis, pulmonary toxicity, and secondary malignancies in hybrid arm	Intergroup USA[91,92]
COPP/ABVD COPP/ABV/IMEP	78% 77%	56% (7 yr) 54%	73% (7 yr) 73%	Equivalent	Acute toxicity worse with hybrid regimen	GHDSG[93]
ABVD Multidrug	68% 67%	75%[c] (3 yr) 75%	90% (3yr) 88%	Equivalent	Increased infection, mucositis and neuropathy with multidrug regimen	UK Lymphoma Group[87]
ChlVPP/EVA VAPEC-B	62% 47%	82% (5 yr) 62%	89% (5 yr) 79%	Hybrid superior	Equivalent	Christie/Barts[94]

[a]Sequential therapy.
[b]Statistically significant.
[c]Event-free survival.

NCI study, the rate of delivery of vincristine was found to be the most important variable in predicting outcome.[3] The Stanford group found that the dose and dose rate of nitrogen mustard, vincristine, and procarbazine were important in the attainment of a complete remission, and reduction in the dose of nitrogen mustard was associated with a significantly poorer outcome[100] DeVita and associates point out that the loss of life to disease resulting from suboptimal therapy could far exceed the morbidity and mortality associated with a properly administered regimen.[99]

Dose intensity of chemotherapy regimens can be increased by shortening the interval between cycles and escalating the dose of individual agents. Intensified (escalated) chemotherapy regimens and high-dose chemotherapy supported by hematopoietic stem-cell transplants are practical applications of this theory and are currently under evaluation. Also chemotherapy-treated patients with advanced Hodgkin lymphoma differ considerably in acute hematotoxicity, which probably reflects pharmacologic and metabolic heterogeneity. Patients with low hematologic toxicity during chemotherapy seem to have significantly higher failure rates despite higher doses and dose intensity. It has been suggested that this should lead to a strategy of indivudualized dosing adopted to hematotoxicity.[101]

INTENSIFIED (ESCALATED) CHEMOTHERAPY

One of the major dose-limiting toxicities of chemotherapy is myelosuppression. The recent advent of hematologic growth factors[102] to support treatment may allow regimens with higher dose intensity to be tolerated. According to the models of kinetic and genetic resistance previously discussed, this approach should, theoretically, increase the likelihood of total tumor eradication or cure. Indeed, Goldie and Coldman hypothesized that the most effective treatment strategies would be those that allowed the minimum amount of regrowth of residual cells between cycles of treatment.[67]

Intensified regimens may have the additional advantage of reduced long-term morbidity. Most late side effects of chemotherapy agents are a function of the total dose delivered.[103–105] Increasing the dose intensity of specific drugs can reduce the overall cumulative dose. Starting in May 1989, the Stanford group treated 65 previously untreated patients with an intensified approach.[106] The Stanford V regimen included weekly chemotherapy for 12 weeks, alternating myelosuppressive and nonmyelosuppressive drugs (Table 14.7). All patients received prophylactic, daily oral trimethoprim and, from May 1991, all patients with significant hematologic toxicity received granulocyte colony-stimulating factor (G-CSF). In the first 25 patients, consolidative radiotherapy was given to sites of initial bulky disease or persistent radiologic abnormalities following chemotherapy. Subsequently, radiotherapy was limited to sites of bulky disease alone. Radiotherapy was given at an attenuated dose to prevent unacceptable toxicity. Bartlett and colleagues[106] reported preliminary results in 1995 after a median of 2 years follow-up. The 3-year failure-free survival was 100% for stage II patients with bulky mediastinal disease and 82% with stage III and IV disease. Overall survival was 96%, and failure-free survival was 87% at 3 years. Fertility appeared to be preserved, and no symptomatic pulmonary or cardiac toxicities were observed. More mature results confirmed Stanford V to be highly effective[107]; freedom from progression and overall survival at 5 years were 89% and 96% respectively. Definitive radomized trials comparing this with ABVD are ongoing in the United States and the United Kingdom.

TABLE 14.7

THE STANFORD V CHEMOTHERAPY REGIMEN[a]

Doxorubicin 25 mg/m^2 day 1 + 15

Vinblastine 6 mg/m^2 day 1 + 15

Mechlorethamine 6 mg/m^2 day 1

Vincristine 1.4 mg/m^2 (max. dose 2 mg) day 8 + 22

Bleomycin 5 U/m^2 day 8 + 22

Etoposide 60 mg/m^2 day 15 + 16

Prednisolone 40 mg/m^2 (reducing from week 10) alternate days

[a]Vinblastine dose decreased to 4 mg/m^2 and vincristine dose to 1 mg/m^2 during cycle 3 in those 50 years or older. Treatment repeated every 28 days for a total of 3 cycles.

Seventy-three patients with stage IIB to IV Hodgkin lymphoma were treated with the Milan group's VEBEP regimen (Table 14.8).[108] Eight cycles were given every 21 days, followed by involved-field radiotherapy. All patients received prophylactic antibacterial and antifungal therapy. Complete response was achieved in 94%. After 6 years of follow-up, freedom from progression was 78%, with an overall survival of 82%.

The German Hodgkin Lymphoma Study Group developed an alternative intensified regimen.[109] Thirty untreated patients with stage IIB to IV Hodgkin lymphoma were treated with 8 cycles of a seven-drug BEACOPP regimen every 21 days (Table 14.9). Consolidative radiotherapy was restricted to sites of bulky disease pretreatment and residual tumor following chemotherapy. Complete response was achieved in 93%, and freedom from treatment failure was 89% at a median follow-up of 40 months. Moderate toxicity was observed, particularly hematologic, but there were no treatment-related deaths.

BEACOPP was shown to be more effective than COPP/ABVD in a multicenter randomized trial.[110] Patients were randomized to receive 4 double cycles of COPP/ABVD or BEACOPP at standard dose or escalated dose. An interim analysis of the first 321 patients showed a nonsignificantly poorer complete response rate in the alternating arm compared with the BEACOPP arm (76% versus 89%). Progression rates and overall survival were significantly worse in the alternating arm, which was closed early.[110] The most recent analysis, with a median follow-up of 6.9 years, included 1,195 patients and demonstrated impressive and superior freedom from treatment failure and overall survival at 5 years (87% and 91%, respectively) for those treated with escalated BEACOPP ± radiotherapy.[111]

The risk of long-term complications in dose-intense regimens remains uncertain. An interim analysis of the BEACOPP regimens at 7 years from the start of trials gave an incidence of 0.7%

TABLE 14.8

THE VEBEP REGIMEN

VP16 120 mg/m^2 days 1 + 2

Epidoxorubicin 40 mg/m^2 days 1 + 2

Bleomycin 10 mg/m^2 day 1

Cyclophosphamide 500 mg/m^2 days 1 + 2

Prednisolone 50 mg days 1–7

TABLE 14.9

THE BEACOPP REGIMENS

BEACOPP 1 from August 1991 to May 1992
Cyclophosphamide 650 mg/m^2 day 1
Doxorubicin 40 mg/m^2 day 1
Etoposide 50 mg/m^2 days 3–12
Procarbazine 100 mg/m^2 days 1–7
Prednisolone 40 mg/m^2 days 1–14
Vincristine 1.4 mg/m^2 (max. dose 2 mg) day 8
Bleomycin 10 mg/m^2 day 8

BEACOPP 2 from May 1992 to January 1993 as growth factor support became available
Cyclophosphamide 650 mg/m^2 day 1
Doxorubicin 25 mg/m^2 day 1
Etoposide 100 mg/m^2 days 1–3
Procarbazine 100 mg/m^2 days 1–7
Prednisolone 40 mg/m^2 days 1–14
Vincristine 1.4 mg/m^2 (max. dose 2 mg) day 8
Bleomycin 10 mg/m^2 day 8

for secondary neoplasia. Nine cases of acute leukaemia were seen after escalated BEACOPP. Escalated BEACOPP is undoubtedly more toxic, and whether this can be justified for all patients with advanced Hodgkin lymphoma is uncertain.[112] There is an ongoing EORTC study comparing this regimen with ABVD, particularly in poor risk patients.

HIGH-DOSE CHEMOTHERAPY

Throughout the development of chemotherapy strategies in advanced Hodgkin lymphoma, bone marrow suppression has been the major dose-limiting toxicity. However, dose intensity can be maximized by administering myeloblative doses of effective agents, if rescued by the infusion of hematopoietic stem cells (see Chapter 20).

COMBINED-MODALITY THERAPY

Approximately one-third of patients achieving a complete response with conventional combination chemotherapy will subsequently relapse, most often at sites of previous bulk disease.[113] Radiotherapy is curative in early-stage Hodgkin lymphoma and appears to be non–cross-resistant with the chemotherapy regimens currently used in widespread disease. It would be reasonable to anticipate that combining chemotherapy with radiotherapy to involved nodes would improve the potential for cure in advanced Hodgkin lymphoma.

A number of retrospective studies support this hypothesis, demonstrating improved disease-free and overall survival with this approach. However, the majority of prospective studies have been unable to substantiate these observations (Table 14.10). Current philosophies still range from the routine administration of radiotherapy to all initially involved sites once chemotherapy is complete to the restriction of radiotherapy to bulky mediastinal involvement or poorly responding nodes.

Loeffler and associates have reported a meta-analysis on the outcome of 1,740 patients treated in 14 randomized trials comparing chemotherapy with combined-modality treatment.[125] Additional radiotherapy showed a significant improvement in tumor control rate but no difference in overall survival. In contrast, when compared with extended chemotherapy, combined-modality treatment had a significantly inferior long-term survival; there were significantly more deaths unrelated to Hodgkin lymphoma in this group.

The combined use of radiotherapy and chemotherapy is also associated with an increased risk of both short- and long-term side effects including mucositis, neuropathies, secondary leukemia, other cancers,[126] and cardiac and pulmonary toxicity. Attempts to minimize toxicity by reducing the dose of radiation delivered have been ineffective.[48] The role of the combined-modality approach in the treatment of advanced Hodgkin lymphoma therefore remains a controversial issue. Current advice is to avoid radiotherapy in those patients who attain complete remission with chemotherapy.[112,127]

The use of neoadjuvant chemotherapy before radiotherapy in localized disease, in an attempt to reduce the toxicity of combined modality programs and eliminate any need for staging by laparotomy, is also subject to debate[128] and ongoing investigation. This "minimal invasive treatment" philosophy will be difficult to validate given the long-term favorable natural history in this group of patients.

Bonadonna and associates considered that brief ABVD followed by involved-field radiotherapy was an effective and safe in early Hodgkin lymphoma.[129] Other studies have confirmed this.[128] Reducing the radiation field and giving lower doses is another option, but most recently good evidence has emerged that chemotherapy alone with ABVD can be an option in the treament of localized nonbulky disease.[130] In an NCIC/ECOG study no difference in overall survival was seen between patients randomized to treatment including radiotherapy or ABVD alone.[131] Freedom from disease progression was better for those receiving radiotherapy, but the advantage may be offset by deaths from treatment-related toxicity. It is possible that with more accurate functional imaging (such as PET scanning) it may be possible to identify early complete responders to chemotherapy, thus sparing these patients more prolonged treament.

See Table 14.11 for a listing of chemotherapy agent synonyms.

PATIENT SELECTION

Several groups have attempted to identify prognostic groupings for advanced Hodgkin lymphoma, with limited success. Such studies have not yet managed to define a wide separation of risk categories using conventional prognostic indices. Even with the International Prognostic Score,[132] only a relatively small number of patients can be identified as having a very poor prognosis (fewer than 10% of patients were expected to have a progression-free survival of less than 5 years). If it were possible to identify patient groups with significant difference in survival, it would be feasible to devise different strategies for initial treatments. For example, in those with a favorable prognosis, therapy could be kept to a minimum with the least possible number of courses of relatively nontoxic chemotherapy or short-course chemotherapy (with or without minimum-field radiotherapy) as an extension of the principles already being applied to localized Hodgkin lymphoma. For those with poor prognosis, very intensive chemotherapy regimens such as escalated BEACOPP might be employed up front. As we have seen, however, as yet the

TABLE 14.10

EFFICACY AND TOXICITY OF COMBINED–MODALITY THERAPY IN ADVANCED HODGKIN LYMPHOMA

Regimens (no. cycles)	Complete response	Freedom from relapse	Overall survival	Efficacy	Toxicity	Center (reference)
TNI TNI + BOPP (6) BOPP(6) + TNI BOPP (6)	60–96% 79–84% 88–94% 74–77%	60% (3 yr)[a] 80% 55%		FFR superior for TNI + BOPP; no significant differences in overall survival		CALGB[77]
TNI TNI + LOPP	86% 86%	55% (15 yr)[a] 75%	60% 60%	FFR superior for TNI + LOPP		BNLI[114,114]
MOPP-Bleo (10) MOPP-Bleo (3) + TNI	89% 96%	84% (5 yr) 70%	87% 89%	Equivalent	Increased risk of infection, pulmonary toxicity and possibly secondary leukemia with combined modality; increased neurotoxicity with MOPP alone	SWOG[116]
CVPP (6 or 12) CVPP (6) + low dose RT CVPP (3)/RT/CVPP (3)	68% or 59% 57% 65%	60% or 55% (3 yr) 55% 65%		Possible survival advantage to sandwich therapy arm		CALGB[77]
MVPP (6) MVPP (6) + RT	88% 100%	80% (5 yr) 80%	85% 85%	Equivalent	Equivalent	Christie[117]
MOPP-Bleo (6) + ABVD (3) MOPP-Bleo (6) + RT	74% 74%	68% (5 yr) 66%	92%[a] 83%	Survival advantage to chemotherapy alone	Increased hematological toxicity with combined modality; increased emesis with ABVD	ECOG[37,118]
CVPP (6) CVPP (6) + RT	73% 86%	23% (7 yr)[a] 51%	58% 71%	FFR superior for CVPP + RT	Equivalent	GATLA[119]
MOP-BAP (6) MOP-BAP (6) + RT	CR with MOPP-BAP prerequisite for entry	66% (5 yr) 74%	79% 86%	Equivalent	Increased risk of secondary malignancy with combined modality approach	SWOG[120]
COPP/ABVD (6) + COPP/ABVD (2) COPP/ABVD (6) + RT	CR with COPP/ABVD (6) prerequisite for entry	81% (21 mo) 87%	87% (5 yr) 95%	Equivalent	Equivalent	GHSG[121]
MOPP-ABV or ABVPP (6) +2 Ditto + RT	CR with chemotherapy prerequisite for entry	68–80% (5yr) 75–82%	85–94% 78–88%	Equivalent	Equivalent	GELA[122]
MOPP-ABV (6–8) MOPP/ABV (6–8) + RT	CR with MOPP/ABV prerequisite for entry	84% (5 yr) 74%	91% (5 yr) 85%	Equivalent	More second cancers after added radiotherapy	EORTC[123]
ABVD (6) ABVD + RT	CR with ABVD prerequisite for entry	76% (8 yr)[a] 88%	89% (8 yr)[a] 100%	Advantage to RT	Equivalent	Mumbai, India[124]

[a]Statistically significant.
TNI, total nodal irradiation; RT, radiotherapy; CR, complete response; FFR, freedom from relapse.

TABLE 14.11

CHEMOTHERAPY AGENT SYNONYMS

Bleomycin, blenoxane

Carmustine, BCNU

Cyclophosphamide, cytoxan

Cytarabine, cytosine arabinoside, ara-C

Dacarbazine, DTIC

Doxorubicin, adriamycin

Etoposide, VP16

Lomustine, CCNU

Mechlorethamine, nitrogen mustard, mustine

Methotrexate, mexate

Procarbazine, matulane, natulan

Streptozocin, zanosar

Vinblastine, velban, velbe

Vincristine, oncovin

numbers of patients that can be identified in these very good and very poor prognostic groups are relatively small, and therapies can only be validated by international collaboration in clinical trials.

SPECIAL SITUATIONS

Elderly Patients

Although it is no longer appropriate to withhold or limit treatments for the elderly with Hodgkin lymphoma because they can achieve responses comparable to those in younger patients, credance must be taken of chronological age and associated comorbidity factors that may lead to reduced tolerance of conventional therapy and more serious toxicity- and treatment-related deaths. This, together with biological differences in the nature of the disease, means that elderly patients have a significantly poorer survival They have a higher mortality during treatment as well as lower dose intensity,[133] and more aggressive chemotherapy therefore may not be appropriate.[134] In an effort to improve results by minimizing toxicities, specific regimens for the elderly have been introduced. For example, VEPEMB (piloted by the Italian Group)[135] gave similar results to ABVD when compared to historical cases, but was better tolerated.

Pregnancy

Hodgkin lymphoma mandating chemotherapy during pregnancy can pose a real dilemma. Usually it is possible to deal effectively with the disease and allow the pregnancy to go to full or near term.[112] If symptomatic or threatening disease develops, single-agent chemotherapy with vinblastine (which is not associated with major teratogenicity or carcinogenicity) at infrequent controlling doses can be given, and the regimen can then be changed to multiagent therapy after delivery.

Rarely, aggressive disease mandates full-dose combination chemotherapy. ABVD given after the first trimester of pregnancy is appropriate and effective; any danger to the fetus is largely related to neutropenic maternal sepsis, although there may be growth retardation. The role of restricted-field radiotherapy (with very little risk to the fetus) should be kept in mind.[136]

CHEMOTHERAPY ADMINISTRATION

Patients with Hodgkin lymphoma should be treated by multidisciplinary teams. Certain skills and resources are mandatory to their optimal care. The senior clinicians directing care should have a clear understanding of treatment protocols, the importance of maintaining dose intensity, the acute and chronic side effects of treatment, and what action should be taken if the disease does not respond or complications of therapy arise. Expert nursing support is essential, as patients with Hodgkin lymphoma are often sick and have very specific needs. Specialist knowledge and experience of intravenous drug administration (including indwelling catheters), complications of chemotherapy, and the associated emotional difficulties are central to good patient care.

Dedicated pharmacy facilities are also important for the preparation and checking of drug doses and schedules. Radiotherapy presence is important from the start, and other oncologists should be aware of the crucial importance of radiotherapy as part of the planned management of patients.

MANAGEMENT OF PATIENTS RECEIVING CHEMOTHERAPY FOR HODGKIN LYMPHOMA

The dose intensity of chemotherapy in Hodgkin lymphoma has clearly been shown to influence outcome. Inappropriate dose reductions or delays potentially reduce disease-free and overall survival. Deviations from drug protocols are usually in response to side effects but may occasionally anticipate expected side effects. In a less well-supported and experienced setting, the risk of delivering a suboptimal regimen may be greater.

Therefore, every effort should be made to deliver chemotherapy regimens at the intended dose and schedule. A thorough clinical assessment should be performed before any treatment. Simple noninvasive tests should be used to monitor for toxicity; for example, full blood count for marrow suppression, pulmonary function tests in regimens incorporating bleomycin and those receiving mantle radiotherapy, and echocardiography for those receiving anthracyclines (particularly if there is a history of cardiac disease). A male patient to be treated with an alkylating agent should be offered sperm storage, and in female patients the possibility of cryopreservation of ovarian tissue or embryo should be discussed.

When toxicity occurs, the following should be considered:

- Hematopoietic growth factors to prevent neutropenia.
- Prophylactic antibiotics during periods of neutropenia, particularly following a previous episode of neutropenic sepsis, or in those at high risk of infection (those who are elderly and/or have poor performance status).
- Substitution of vinblastine for vincristine in neuropathy.
- Dose reduction or delay in therapy may be inevitable but should be as minimal as possible; it may be necessary to consider adopting an alternative regimen that does not include the likely offending drug.

CLINICAL SETTING

There is no cause for complacency in the management of Hodgkin lymphoma; over one-fourth of patients still die of their disease. Where possible, patients should be offered treatment in the context of a well-designed clinical trial.[137] Even where this is not feasible, they should be managed by a skilled multidisciplinary team; optimal resources include facilities for high-dose chemotherapy, state-of-the-art radiotherapy, specialized nursing, and other supporting resources. Such criteria are more likely to be met in comprehensive cancer treatment centers, and these centers are more likely to offer their patients involvement in clinical trials. It does seem (though it is still much debated) that patients treated at such centers are likely to have a better outcome than those treated elsewhere.[138] For example, Davis and associates found that survival in 3,607 patients entered into the Surveillance, Epidemiology and End Results program of the National Cancer Institute was about 1.5 times better than in the 2,278 patients treated in community general hospitals.[139]

FOLLOW-UP

We are now starting to learn more about the long-term toxicity of treatment. With chemotheapy this is mainly sterility, cardiopulmonary damage, and second malignancy. Although routine, infrequent long-term follow-up will not usually pick up relapse (far more likely the patient will self-report relevant symptoms or signs),[140] a planned approach to certain late effects might be feasible. For example, the role for cardiac and pulmonary monitoring needs to be assessed prospectively, because there is no sense in pursuing earlier diagnosis if the clinical management is no different from that of later diagnosis.

FUTURE PROSPECTS FOR CHEMOTHERAPY IN HODGKIN LYMPHOMA

It is nearly 40 years since cyclic combination chemotherapy (MOPP or MVPP) was established as effective treatment for Hodgkin lymphoma. Long-term survival was observed in approximately one-half of patients treated with these regimens. The substitution of chlorambucil for mustine gave each equally favorable results with less toxicity. However, such regimens and others containing alkylating agents (such as the nitrosoureas) have given concern regarding long-term toxicities. ABVD appeared at least as efficacious with less gonadal toxicity and second cancers. Alternating or hybrid regimens appeared to give promising results in terms of overall survival, but they have proved no better than ABVD, which remains the gold stadard against which new regimens have to be tested. The role of combined-modality therapy is now less controversial; radiotherapy is almost cettainly unnecessary if there is complete remission after full-course chemotherapy.

In general, the regimens that have been most widely adopted are those shown in prospective, randomized clinical trials to be equally efficacious or better than MOPP, with less short- and long-term toxicity and that can be successfully administered in a number of centers (not only at heavily resourced academic units); the most popular is ABVD.

It is unlikely that the introduction of new chemotherapeutic agents will dramatically improve the outlook in Hodgkin lymphoma, although new salvage regimens have been devised using combinations containing drugs such as gemcitabine. More likely, raising the doses or intensifying the schedules of established agents will lead to further modest improvement in

overall survival. Hence, escalated, intensified regimens such as Stanford V and BEACOPP (often growth factor supported) are being evaluated in randomized studies.

High-dose chemotherapy with stem-cell rescue is finding its niche, particularly for relapsed or chemoresistant patients; however, the role for high-dose chemotherapy up front or in first remission remains to be established. It would be nice to be able to identify and select patients for different approaches on the basis of prognostic factors; unfortunately, this is still not possible except for a small proportion of very-high-risk patients.

For localized Hodgkin lymphoma, radiotherapy can be curative. The use of minimally invasive approaches, usually in the form of a short course of relatively nontoxic chemotherapy before involved-field radiotherapy, is likely to reduce relapse and long-term toxicity but unlikely to have a major effect on survival (given the already recognized excellent prognosis in this group). Chemotherapy alone can also now be considered an option in localized nonbulky disease.

The majority of patients with Hodgkin lymphoma can now be cured; however, a significant percentage still die. For this reason, patients should be given the opportunity to be involved in clinical trials whenever possible. They should be treated by multidisciplinary teams working in well-resourced centers.

References

1. Goodman LS, Wintrobe MM, Dameshek W, et al. Nitrogen mustard therapy. *JAMA* 1946;132:126–132.
2. De Vita VT, Serpick AA, Carbone PP. Combination chemotherapy in the treatment of advanced Hodgkin's disease. *Ann Intern Med* 1970;73:881–895.
3. Longo DL, Young RC, Wesley M, et al. 20 years of MOPP therapy for Hodgkin's disease. *J Clin Oncol* 1986;4:1295–1306.
4. Bubley GJ, Ogata GK, Dupuis NP, et al. Detection of sequence specific antitumor alkylating agent DNA damage from cells treated in culture and from a patient. *Cancer Res* 1994;54:6325–6329.
5. D'Incalci M. DNA topoisomerase inhibitors. *Curr Opin Oncol* 1993;5:1023–1028.
6. Smith PJ, Soues S. Multilevel therapeutic targeting by topoisomerase inhibitors. *Br J Cancer* 1994;23(suppl):47–51.
7. Bleyer WA. The clinical pharmacology of methotrexate: new applications of an old drug. *Cancer* 1978;41:36–51.
8. Jordan MA, Thrower D, Wilson L. Mechanisms of inhibition of cell proliferation by vinca alkaloids. *Cancer Res* 1991;51:2212–2222.
9. Schiff PB, Fant J, Horwitz SB. Promotion of microtubule assembly in vitro by taxol. *Nature* 1979;277:665–667.
10. Yarbro JW. The scientific basis of cancer chemotherapy. In: Perry MC, ed. *The chemotherapy source book.* Baltimore: Williams & Wilkins, 1992:2–15.
11. Skipper HE, Schabel FM, Wilcox WS. Experimental evaluation of potential anti-cancer agents. XII. On the criteria and kinetics associated with "curability" of experimental leukemia. *Cancer Chemother Rep* 1964;35:1–111.
12. Skipper HE. Historic milestones in cancer biology: a few that are important to cancer treatment (revisited). *Semin Oncol* 1979;6:506–514.
13. Carter SK, Livingstone RB. Single-agent therapy for Hodgkin's disease. *Arch Intern Med* 1973;131:377–387.
14. Coltman CA. Chemotherapy of advanced Hodgkin's disease. *Semin Oncol* 1980;7:155–173.
15. Sheridan E, Hancock BW, Smith SC. Gestational trophoblastic disease: Experience of the Sheffield (United Kingdom) supraregional screening and treatment service (review). *Int J Oncol* 1993;3:149–155.
16. DeVita VT Jr, DeVita VT. Principles of cancer management: chemotherapy. In: DeVita VT, Hellman S, Rosenberg SA, eds. *Cancer, principles and practice of oncology,* 5th ed. Philadelphia: Lippincott-Raven, 1997:333–348.
17. De Vita VT, Schein PS. The use of drugs in combination for the treatment of patients with cancer: rationale and results. *N Engl J Med* 1973;288:998–1006.
18. Lacher MU, Durant JR. Combined vinblastine and chlorambucil therapy of Hodgkin's disease. *Ann Intern Med* 1965;62:468–476.
19. DeVita VT, Serpick A. Combination chemotherapy in the treatment of advanced Hodgkin's disease. *Proc Am Assoc Cancer Res* 1967;8:13. Abstract.
20. Bakemeier RF, Anderson JR, Costello W, et al. BCVPP chemotherapy for advanced Hodgkin's disease: evidence for greater duration of complete remission, greater survival, and less toxicity than with a MOPP regimen. *Ann Intern Med* 1984;101:447–456.

21. Bonadonna G, Valagussa P, Santoro A. Alternating non-cross-resistant combination chemotherapy or MOPP in stage IV Hodgkin's disease. A report of 8 year results. *Ann Intern Med* 1986;104:739–746.

22. Rosenberg SA, Kaplan HS, Hoppe RT, et al. The Stanford randomized trials of the treatment of Hodgkin's disease 1967–1980. In: Rosenberg SA, Kaplan HS, eds. *Malignant lymphomas*. New York: Academic Press, 1982:513–522.

23. Longo DL, Young RC, DeVita VT Jr. Chemotherapy for Hodgkin's disease: the remaining challenges. *Cancer Treat Rep* 1982;66:925–936.

24. McElwain TJ, Toy J, Peckham MJ, et al. A combination of chlorambucil, vinblastine, procarbazine and prednisolone for treatment of Hodgkin's disease. *Br J Cancer* 1977;36:276–280.

25. Selby P, Patel P, Milan S, et al. ChlVPP combination chemotherapy for Hodgkin's disease; long-term results. *Br J Cancer* 1990;62:279–285.

26. The International ChlVPP Treatment Group. ChlVPP therapy for Hodgkin's disease: Experience of 960 patients. *Ann Oncol* 1995;6:167–172.

27. Bloomfield CS, Weiss RB, Fortuny I, et al. Combined chemotherapy with cyclophosphamide, vinblastine, procarbazine and prednisone (CVPP) for patients with advanced Hodgkin's disease: An alternative program to MOPP. *Cancer* 1976;38:42–48.

28. Cooper MR, Pajak TF, Nissen NI, et al. A new effective four-drug combination of CCNU (1-[2-chloroethyl]-3-cyclohexyl-1-nitrosourea) (NSC-79038), vinblastine, prednisone and procarbazine for the treatment of advanced Hodgkin's disease. *Cancer* 1980;46:654–662.

29. Nissen NI, Pajak TF, Glidewell O, et al. A comparative study of a BCNU containing 4-drug programme versus 3-drug combinations in advanced Hodgkin's disease. A comparative study by the Cancer and Leukaemia Group B. *Cancer* 1979;43:31–40.

30. Bennett JM, Bakemeier RF, Carbone PP, et al. Clinical trials with BCNU (NSC-409962) in malignant lymphomas by the Eastern Cooperative Oncology Group. *Cancer Treat Rep* 1976;60:739–745.

31. Durant JR, Gams RA, Velez-Garcia E, et al. BCNU, velban, cyclophosphamide, procarbazine and prednisone (BVCPP) in advanced Hodgkin's disease. *Cancer* 1978;42:2101–2110.

32. Harrison DT, Neiman PE. Primary treatment of disseminated Hodgkin's disease with BCNU alone and in combination with vincristine, procarbazine and prednisone. *Cancer Treat Rep* 1977;61:789–795.

33. Sutcliffe SB, Wrigley RF, Peto J, et al. MVPP chemotherapy regimen for advanced Hodgkin's disease. *Br Med J* 1978;1:679–683.

34. Hancock BW. Randomised study of MOPP (mustine, oncovin, procarbazine, prednisone) against LOPP (leukeran substituted for mustine) in advanced Hodgkin's disease. British National Lymphoma Investigation. *Radiother Oncol* 1986;7:215–221.

35. Hancock BW, Vaughan Hudson G, Vaughan Hudson B, et al. British National Lymphoma Investigation randomised study of MOPP (mustine, oncovin, procarbazine, predisolone) against LOPP (leukeran substituted for mustine) in advanced Hodgkin's disease—long term results. *Br J Cancer* 1991;63:579–582.

36. Hancock BW, Vaughan Hudson G, Vaughan Hudson B, et al. British National Lymphoma Investigation (BNLI) randomised trial in advanced Hodgkin's disease: update of the MOPP v LOPP (1979–1983), LOPP v LOPP/EVAP (1983–1989), and LOPP/EVAP v LOPP/EVA (1990–1991) studies. *Proc XVI Int Cancer Cong New Dehli* 1994;2611–2615.

37. Glick JH, Barnes JM, Bakemeier RF, et al. Treatment of advanced Hodgkin's disease:10 years experience in the Eastern Cooperative Oncology Group. *Cancer Treat Rep* 1982;66:855–870.

38. Coltman CA, Jones SE, Grozea P, et al. Bleomycin in combination with MOPP for the management of Hodgkin's disease: Southwest Oncology Group experience. In: Carter SK, Crooke ST, Umezawa H, eds. *Bleomycin: Current status and new developments*. New York: Academic Press, 1978:227–242.

39. Jones SE, Coltman CA, Grozea PN, et al. Conclusions from clinical trials of the Southwest Oncology Group. *Cancer Treat Rep* 1982;66:847–853.

40. Goldman JM. Combination chemotherapy for stage IV Hodgkin's disease. *Clin Radiol* 1981;32:531–536.

41. Hancock BW. Advanced Hodgkin's disease—British National Lymphoma Investigation results. Oncology section of Royal Society of Medicine. British Institute of Radiology and Royal College of Radiologists. *J R Soc Med* 1986;80:122–123.

42. British National Lymphoma Investigation. Value of prednisolone in combination chemotherapy of stage IV Hodgkin's disease. *Br Med J* 1975;3:413–414.

43. Santoro A, Bonfante V, Bonadonna G. Salvage chemotherapy with ABVD in MOPP-resistant Hodgkin's disease. *Ann Intern Med* 1982;96:139–143.

44. Bonnadonna G, Zucali R, Monfardini S, et al. Combination chemotherapy of Hodgkin's disease with adriamycin, bleomycin, vinblastine, and imidazole carboxamide versus MOPP. *Cancer* 1975;36:252–259.

45. Bonadonna G. Modern treatment of malignant lymphomas: a multidisciplinary approach? *Ann Oncol* 1994;5(suppl 2):S5–S16.

46. Canellos GP, Propert K, Cooper R, et al. Cancer and leukemia group B. MOPP vs ABVD vs MOPP alternating with ABVD in advanced Hodgkin's disease: a prospective randomized CALGB trial (abstract 888). *Proc Am Soc Clin Oncol* 1988;7:230.

47. Canellos GP, Anderson JR, Propert KJ, et al. Chemotherapy of advanced Hodgkin's disease with MOPP, ABVD, or MOPP alternating with ABVD. *N Engl J Med* 1992;327:1478–1484.

48. Urba WJ, Longo DL. Hodgkin's disease in adults: part I. *Invest Radiol* 1993;28:737–752.

49. Tannir N, Hagemeister F, et al. Long-term follow-up with ABDIC salvage chemotherapy of MOPP-resistant Hodgkin's disease. *J Clin Oncol* 1983;1:432–438.

50. Harker GW, Kushlan P, Rosenberg SA. Combination chemotherapy for advanced Hodgkin's disease after failure of MOPP: ABVD and B-CAVe. *Ann Intern Med* 1984;101:440–446.

51. Harrison DT, Neiman PE. Primary treatment of disseminated Hodgkin's disease with BCNU alone and in combination with vincristine, procarbazine and prednisone. *Cancer Treat Rep* 1977;61:789–795.

52. Wiernik PH, Schiffer CA. Long-term follow-up of advanced Hodgkin's disease patients treated with a combination of streptozotocin, lomustine (CCNU) and bleomycin (SCAB). *J Cancer Res Clin Oncol* 1988;114:105–107.

53. Liebman HA, Hum GJ, Sheehan WW, et al. Randomized study for the treatment of adult advanced Hodgkin's disease: mechlorethamine, vincristine, procarbazine and prednisolone (MOPP) versus lomustine, vinblastine and prednisolone. *Cancer Treat Rep* 1983;67:413–419.

54. Santoro A, Viviani S, Valagussa P, et al. CCNU, etoposide and prednimustine (CEP) in refractory Hodgkin's disease. *Semin Oncol* 1986;13:23–26.

55. Cooper MR, Pajak TF, Nissen NI, et al. A new effective four-drug combination of CCNU, vinblastine, prednisolone and procarbazine for the treatment of advanced Hodgkin's disease. *Cancer* 1980;46:654–662.

56. Bloomfield CD, Weiss RB, Fortuny I, et al. Combined chemotherapy with cyclophosphamide, vinblastine, procarbazine and prednisolone (CVPP) for patients with advanced Hodgkin's disease. *Cancer* 1976;38:42–48.

57. Brizel DM, Gockerman JP, Crawford J, et al. A pilot study of etoposide, vinblastine, and doxorubicin plus involved field irradiation in advanced, previously untreated Hodgkin's disease. *Cancer* 1994;74:159–163.

58. Hagemeister FB, Tannir N, McLaughlin P, et al. MIME chemotherapy (methyl-GAG, ifosfamide, methotrexate, etoposide) as treatment for recurrent Hodgkin's disease. *J Clin Oncol* 1987;5:556–561.

59. Hagemeister FB, Cabanillas F, Velasquez WS, et al. NOVP: a novel chemotherapeutic regimen with minimal toxicity for treatment of Hodgkin's disease. *Semin Oncol* 1990;17:34–40.

60. Simmonds PD, Mead GM, Sweetenham JW, et al. PACEBOM chemotherapy: a twelve week alternating regimen for advanced Hodgkin's disease. *Ann Oncol* 1997;8:259–266.

61. Horning SJ, Ang PT, Hoppe RT, et al. The Stanford experience with combined procarbazine, alkeran and vinblastine (PAVe) and radiotherapy for locally extensive and advanced stage Hodgkin's disease. *Ann Oncol* 1992;3:747–754.

62. Radford JA, Crowther D. Treatment of relapsed Hodgkin's disease using a weekly chemotherapy of short duration: results of a pilot study in 20 patients. *Ann Oncol* 1991;2:505–509.

63. Coltman CA, Frei E III, Delaney FC. Effectiveness of actinomycin (A), methotrexate (MTX) and vinblastine (V) in prolonging the duration of combination chemotherapy (MOPP) induced remission in advanced Hodgkin's disease (HD). *Proc Am Soc Clin Oncol* 1973;9:78.

64. Medical Research Council's Working Party on Lymphomas. Randomised trial of two-drug and four-drug maintenance chemotherapy in advanced or recurrent Hodgkin's disease. *Br Med J* 1979;1:1105–1108.

65. Young RC, Canellos GP, Chabner BA, et al. Maintenance chemotherapy for advanced Hodgkin's disease in remission. *Lancet* 1973;1:1339–1343.

66. Goldie JH, Coldman AJ. A mathematical model for relating the drug sensitivity of tumors to their spontaneous mutation rate. *Cancer Treat Rep* 1979;63:1727–1733.

67. Goldie JH, Coldman AJ, Gudauskas GA. Rationale for the use of alternating non-cross-resistant chemotherapy. *Cancer Treat Rep* 1982;66:439–449.

68. Bonadonna G, Santoro A, Valagussa P, et al. Current status of the Milan trials for Hodgkin's disease in adults. In: Cavalli F, Bonadonna G, Rozencweig M, eds. *Malignant lymphomas and Hodgkin's disease: experimental and therapeutic advances. Proceedings of the Second International Conference on Malignant Lymphomas, Lugano, Switzerland, June 13–16, 1984.* Boston: Martinus Nijhoff, 1985:299–307.

69. Santoro A, Bonadonna G, Bonfante V, et al. Alternating drug combinations in the treatment of advanced Hodgkin's disease. *N Engl J Med* 1982;306:770–775.

70. Bonadonna G, Valagussa P, Santoro A. Alternating non-crossresistant combination chemotherapy or MOPP in stage IV Hodgkin's disease: a report of 8-year results. *Ann Intern Med* 1986;104:739–746.

71. Longo DL. The use of chemotherapy in the treatment of Hodgkin's disease. *Semin Oncol* 1990;6:716–735.

72. Longo DL, Duffey PL, DeVita VT, et al. Treatment of advanced-stage Hodgkin's disease: alternating non-cross-resistant MOPP/CABS is not superior to MOPP. *J Clin Oncol* 1991;9:1409–1420.

73. Somers R, Carde P, Henry-Amar M, et al. A randomised study in stage IIIB and IV Hodgkin's disease comparing eight courses of MOPP versus an alternation of MOPP with ABVD: a European Organisation for Research and Treatment of Cancer Lymphoma Co-operative Group and Groupe Pierre et Marie Curie controlled clinical crial. *J Clin Oncol* 1994;12:279–287.

74. Straus DJ, Myers J, Lee BJ, et al. Treatment of advanced Hodgkin's disease with chemotherapy and irradiation. Controlled trial of two versus three alternating, potentially non-cross-resistant drug combinations. *Am J Med* 1984;76:270–278.

75. Gams RA, Omura GA, Velez-Garcia E, et al. Alternating sequential combination chemotherapy in the management of advanced Hodgkin's disease. A Southeastern Cancer Study Group trial. *Cancer* 1986;58:1963–1986.

76. Gams RA, Durant JR, Bartolucci AA. Chemotherapy for advanced Hodgkin's disease: conclusions from the Southeastern Cancer Study Group. *Cancer Treat Rep* 1982;66:899–905.

77. Bloomfield CD, Pajak TF, Glicksman AS, et al. Chemotherapy and combined modality therapy for Hodgkin's disease: a progress report on Cancer And Leukaemia Group B studies. *Cancer Treat Rep* 1982;66:835–846.

78. Vinciguerra V, Propert KJ, Coleman M, et al. Alternating cycles of combination chemotherapy for patients with recurrent Hodgkin's disease following radiotherapy. A prospectively randomized study by the Cancer and Leukaemia Group B. *J Clin Oncol* 1986;4:838–846.

79. Hancock BW, Vaughan Hudson G, Vaughan Hudson B, et al. LOPP alternating with EVAP is superior to LOPP alone in the initial treatment of advanced Hodgkin's disease: results of a British National Lymphoma Investigation Trial. *J Clin Oncol* 1992;10:1252–1258.

80. Holte H, Mella O, Telhaug R, et al. Randomised study in stage III—IV Hodgkin's disease: ChlVPP is as effective as alternating ChlVPP/ABOD chemotherapy. In *3rd International Symposium on Hodgkin's Lymphoma, September 18–23, Köln, Germany.* 1995:113.

81. Cullen BW, Stuart NSA, Woodroffe C, et al. ChlVPP/PABlOE and radiotherapy in advanced Hodgkin's disease. *J Clin Oncol* 1994;12:779–787.

82. Hancock BW, Gregory WM, Cullen MH, et al. ChlVPP alternating with PABIOE alone in the initial treatment of advanced Hodgkin's disease: results of a British National Lymphoma Investigation/Central Lymphoma Group randomized controlled trial. *Br J Cancer* 2001;84:1293–1300.

83. Viviani S, Bonadonna G, Devizzi L, et al. Ten year results of alternating vs hybrid administration of MOPP—ABVD in Hodgkin's disease (HD). In *3rd International Symposium on Hodgkin's Lymphoma. September 18–23, Köln, Germany.* 1995:74.

84. Viviani S, Bonadonna G, Santoro A, et al. Alternating versus hybrid MOPP and ABVD combinations in advanced Hodgkin's disease: ten-year results. *J Clin Oncol* 1996;14:1421–1430.

85. Klimo P, Connors JM. MOPP/ABV hybrid program: combination chemotherapy based on early introduction of seven effective drugs for advanced Hodgkin's disease. *J Clin Oncol* 1985;3:1174–1182.

86. Connors JM, Klimo P, Adams G, et al. Treatment of advanced Hodgkin's disease with chemotherapy—comparison of MOPP/ABV hybrid regimen with alternating courses of MOPP and ABVD: a report from the National Cancer Institute of Canada Clinical Trials Group. *J Clin Oncol* 1997; 15:1638–1645.

87. Johnson PWM, Radford JA, Cullen MH, et al. Comparison of ABVD and alternating or hybrid multiddrug regimens for the treatment of advanced Hodgkin's Lymphoma: results of the United Kingdom Lymphoma Group LY09 trial (ISRCTN97144519). *J Clin Oncol* 2005;36:1–13.

88. Radford JA, Crowther D, Rohatiner AZS, et al. Results of a randomised trial comparing MVPP chemotherapy with a hybrid regimen, ChlVPP/EVA, in the initial treatment of Hodgkin's disease. *J Clin Oncol* 1995;13: 2379–2385.

89. Glick J, Tsiatis R, Schilsky T, et al. A randomised phase III trial of MOPP/ABV hybrid vs sequential MOPP/ABVD in advanced Hodgkin's disease: results of the intergroup trial (abstract 59). In *Fifth International Conference on Malignant Lymphoma, Lugano, 1993.*

90. Hancock BW, Vaughan Hudson G, Vaughan Hudson B, et al. Hybrid LOPP/EVA is not better than LOPP alternating with EVAP: a prematurely terminated British National Lymphoma Investigation randomized trial. *Ann Oncol* 1994;5(suppl 2):S117–S120.

91. Duggan D, Petroni G, Johnson J, et al. MOPP/ABV versus ABVD for advanced Hodgkin's disease—a preliminary report of CALGB 8952 (with SWOG, ECOG, NCIC) (abstract 43). *Proc Am Soc Clin Oncol* 1997;16:12a.

92. Duggan D, Petroni GR, Johnson JL, et al. The treatment of advanced Hodgkin's disease: report of an intergroup trial. *J Clin Oncol* 2003;4:607–614.

93. Sieber M, Tesch H, Pfistner B, et al. Treatment of advanced Hodgkin's disease with COPP/ABV/IMEP versus COPP/ABVD and consolidating radiotherapy: final results of the German Hodgkin's Lymphoma Study Group HD6 trial. *Ann Oncol* 2004;15:276–282.

94. Radford JA, Rohatiner AZS, Ryder WDJ, et al. ChlVPP/EVA hybrid versus the weekly VAPEC-B regimen for previously untreated Hodgkin's disease. *J Clin Oncol* 2002;20:2988–2994.

95. Tannock IF. The relationship between proliferation and the vascular system in a transplanted mouse mammary tumor. *Br J Cancer* 1968;22:258–273.

96. Norton L, Simon R. The Norton–Simon hypothesis revisited. *Cancer Treat Rep* 1986;70:163–169.

97. Hryniuk W, Bush H. The importance of dose intensity in chemotherapy of metastatic breast cancer. *J Clin Oncol* 1984;2:1281–1288.

98. Skipper HS. *Analyses of 42 arms of 4 multiarmed trials in which animals bearing 2–3g ROS tumors were treated with simultaneous cyclophosphamide and L-PAM with systemic variations of the relative dose intensity of each drug and the average relative dose intensity.* Booklet 5, AL. Southern Research Institute, 1986.

99. DeVita VT, Hubbard SM, Longo DL. The chemotherapy of lymphomas: looking back, moving forward—-the Richard and Hinda Rosenthal Foundation award lecture. *Cancer Res* 1987;47:5810–5824.

100. Carde P, MacKintosh R, Rosenberg SA. A dose and time response analysis of the treatment of Hodgkin's disease with MOPP therapy. *J Clin Oncol* 1983;1:146–153.

101. Brosteanu O, Hansenclever D, Loeffler M, et al. Low acute haematological toxicity during chemotherapy predicts reduced disease control in advanced Hodgkin's disease. *Ann Hematol* 2004;83:176–182.

102. Clark SC, Kamen R. The human hematopoietic colony-stimulating factors. *Science* 1987;236:1229–1237.

103. Bristow MR, Billingham ME, Mason JW, et al. Clinical spectrum of anthracycline cardiotoxicity. *Cancer Treat Rep* 1978;62:873–879.

104. Schaeppi U, Phelan R, Stadnicki SW, et al. Pulmonary fibrosis following multiple treatment with bleomycin (NSC-125066) in dogs. *Cancer Chemother Rep* 1974;58:301–310.

105. Pedersen-Bjergaard J, Larsen SO, Struck J, et al. Risk of therapy-related leukaemia and pre-leukaemia after Hodgkin's disease: relation to age, cumulative dose of alkylating agents, and time for chemotherapy. *Lancet* 1987;2:83–88.

106. Bartlett NL, Rosenberg SA, Hoppe RT, et al. Brief chemotherapy, Stanford V, and adjuvant radiotherapy for bulky or advanced-stage Hodgkin's disease: a preliminary report. *J Clin Oncol* 1995;13:1080–1088.

107. Horning AJ, Hoppe RT, Breslin S, et al. Stanford V and radiotherapy for locally extensive and advanced Hodgkin's disease: mature results of a prospective clinical trial. *J Clin Oncol* 2002;3:630–637.

108. Viviani S, Bonfante V, Santoro A, et al. Long-term results of an intensive regimen: VEBEP plus involved-field radiotherapy in advanced Hodgkin's disease: *Cancer J Sci Am* 1999;5:275–282.

109. Diehl V, Sieber M, Rüffler U, et al. BEACOPP: An intensified chemotherapy regimen in advanced Hodgkin's disease. *Ann Oncol* 1997;8:143–148.

110. Diehl V, Tesch H, Lathan B, et al. BEACOPP, a new intensified hybrid regimen, is at least equally effective compared with COPP/ABVD in patients with advanced stage Hodgkin's lymphoma (abstract 5). *Proc Am Soc Clin Oncol* 1997;16:2a.

111. Diehl V, Franklin J, Pfreundschuh M, et al. Standard and increased-dose BEACOPP chemotherapy compared with COPP-ABVD for advanced Hodgkin's disease. *N Eng J Med* 2003;348:2386–2395.

112. Connors JM. State-of-the-art therapeutics: Hodgkin's lymphoma. *J Clin Oncol* 2005;23:6400–6408.

113. Young RC, Canellos GP, Bruce A, et al. Patterns of relapse in advanced Hodgkin's disease treated with combination chemotherapy. *Cancer* 1978; 42:1001–1007.

114. Strickland P. Radiotherapy or chemotherapy as the initial treatment for stage IIIA Hodgkin's disease. *Clin Radiol* 1981;32:527–530.

115. Hancock BW, Vaughan Hudson G, Vaughan Hudson B, et al. British National Lymphoma Investigation studies of pathological stage IIIA Hodgkin's disease: long term follow up. No role for total nodal irradiation? *Br J Cancer* 1990;62(suppl 11):9. Abstract.

116. Grozea PN, Depersio EJ, Coltman CA Jr, et al. Chemotherapy alone versus combined modality therapy for stage III Hodgkin's disease: a five-year follow-up of a Southwest Oncology Group study (SWOG-7518). In *Proceedings of the Second International Conference on Malignant Lymphomas, Lugano, Switzerland, June 13–16.* 1984:345–351.

117. Crowther D, Wagstaff J, Deakin D, et al. A randomized study comparing chemotherapy alone with chemotherapy followed by radiotherapy in patients with pathologically stage IIIA Hodgkin's disease. *J Clin Oncol* 1984;2:892–897.

118. Glick J, Tsiatis A, Prosnitz L, et al. Improved survival with sequential Bleo-MOPP followed by ABVD for advanced Hodgkin's disease (abstract 926). *Proc Am Soc Clin Oncol* 1984;3:237.

119. Pavlovsky S, Santarelli MT, Sackmann MF, et al. Randomized trial of chemotherapy versus chemotherapy plus radiotherapy for stage III–IV A & B Hodgkin's disease. *Ann Oncol* 1992;3:533–537.

120. Fabian CJ, Mansfield CM, Dahlberg S, et al. Low dose involved field radiation after chemotherapy in advanced Hodgkin's disease. A Southwest Oncology Group randomised study. *Ann Intern Med* 1994; 120: 903–912.

121. Diehl V, Pfreundschuh M, Löffler M, et al. Further chemotherapy versus low-dose involved-field radiotherapy as consolidtion of complete remission after six cycles of alternating chemotherapy in patients with advanced Hodgkin's disease. *Ann Oncol* 1995;6:901–910.

122. Fermé C, Sebban C, Hennequin C, et al. Comparison of chemotherapy to radiotherapy as consolidation of complete or good partial response after six cycles of chemotherapy for patients with advanced Hodgkin's disease: results of the Groupe d'études des Lymphomes de l'Adulte H89 trial. *Blood* 2000;95:2246–2252.

123. Aleman B, Raemaekers J, Tierlli U, et al. Involved-field radiotherapy for advanced Hodgkin's lymphoma. *N Eng J Med* 2003;348:2396–2406.

124. Laskar S, Gupta S, Vimal MA, et al. Consolidation radiation after complete remission in Hodgkin's disease following six cycles of Doxorubicin, Bleomycin, Vinblastine and Dacarbazine chemotherapy: is there a need? *J Clin Oncol* 2004;22:62–68.

125. Loeffler M, Brosteanu O, Hasenclever D, et al. Meta-analysis of chemotherapy versus combined modality treatment trials in Hodgkin's disease. *J Clin Oncol* 1998;6:818–829.

126. Tucker M, Coleman CN, Cox RS, et al. Risk of second cancers after treatment for Hodgkin's disease. *N Engl J Med* 1988;318:76–81.

127. Diehl V. Chemotherapy of combined modality treatment: the optimal treatment for Hodgkin's disease. *J Clin Oncol* 2004;22:15–18.

128. Connors JM. Evolving approaches to primary treatment of Hodgkin lymphoma. *Hematol (Am Soc Hematol Educ Program)* 2005;239–244.

129. Bonadonna G, Bonfante V, Viviani S, et al. ABVD plus subtotal nodal versus involved-field radiotherapy in early-stage Hodgkin's disease: long term results. *J Clin Oncol* 2004;22:2835–2841.
130. Canellos GP. Chemotherapy alone for early Hodgkin's lymphoma: an emerging option. *J Clin Oncol* 2005;23:4574–4576.
131. Meyer RM, Gospadarowicz MK, Connors JM, et al. Randomised comparison of ABVD chemotherapy with a strategy that includes radiation therapy in patients with limited-stage Hodgkin's lymphoma: National Cancer Institute of Canada Clinical Trials Group and the Eastern Co-operative Oncology Group. *J Clin Oncol* 2005;23:4634–4642.
132. Hasenclever D, Diehl V. A propgnostic score for advanced Hodgkin's disease. International Prognostic Factors Project on advanced Hodgkin's disease. *N Engl J Med* 1998;19:1506–1514.
133. Engert A, Vallova V, Haverkamp H, et al. Hodgkin's lymphoma in elderly patients: A comprehensive retrospective analysis from the German Hodgkin's Study Group. *J Clin Oncol* 2005;22:5052–5060.
134. Ballova V, Rüffer JU, Haverkamp H, et al. A prospectively randomised trial carried out by the German Hodgkin Study Group (GHSG) for elderly patients with advanced Hodgkin's disease comparing BEACOPP baseline and COPP-ABVD (study HD9 elderly). *Ann Oncol* 2005;16:124–131.
135. Levis A, Anselmo AP, Ambrosetti A, et al. VEPEMB in elderly Hodgkin's lymphoma patients. Results from an Intergruppo Italiano Linfomi (IIL) study. *Ann Oncol* 2004;15:123–128.
136. Kal HB, Struikmans H. Radiotherapy during pregnancy: fact and fiction. *Lancet Oncol* 2005;6:328–333.
137. Hancock BW, Aitken M, Radstone C, et al. Why don't cancer patients get entered into clinical trials? Experience of the Sheffield Lymphoma Group's collaboration in British National Lymphoma Investigation studies. *Br Med J* 1997;314:36–37.
138. Selby P, Gillis C, Haward R. Benefits of specialised cancer care. *Lancet* 1996;348:313–318.
139. Davis S, Dahlberg S, Myers M, et al. Hodgkin's disease in the United States: comparison of patient characteristics and survival in the centralized cancer patient data system and the Surveillance, Epidemiology and End Results program. *J Natl Cancer Inst* 1987;78:471–478.
140. Radford JA, Eardley A, Woodman C, et al. Follow up policy after treatment for Hodgkin's disease: too many clinic visits and routine tests? A review of hospital records. *BMJ* 1997;314:343–346.

CHAPTER 15 ■ NOVEL TREATMENT TECHNIQUES FOR HODGKIN LYMPHOMA

JAN OLIVER STAAK, ROLAND SCHNELL, PETER BORCHMANN, AND ANDREAS ENGERT

Polychemotherapy and extended-field radiotherapy in the early stages of Hodgkin lymphoma have improved the long-term remission rates from less than 5% in 1963 to about 80% at the present time.[1] Nevertheless, 30% to 50% of patients with advanced-stage Hodgkin lymphoma will relapse and finally die from their disease.[2] A new era of intensified chemotherapy regimens beginning in the 1990s has significantly improved clinical outcome for patients with advanced disease.[3,4] Currently, the majority of patients with relapsed Hodgkin lymphoma are treated with high-dose chemotherapy and autologous bone marrow or hematopoietic cell transplantation, and recent data from the German Hodgkin Study Group (GHSG) confirm that some of these patients with chemosensitive disease can be successfully salvaged,[5,6] but outcome for patients with primary refractory disease remains poor. Patients who are cured face the risk of developing late toxicities such as cardiovascular disease and secondary malignancies including acute myeloid leukemia, myelodysplastic syndrome, and solid tumors, in up to 11% within 15 years after treatment.[7-9] However, only patients younger than 60 years without major organ dysfunction are eligible for high-dose therapy. Patients relapsing after second-line treatment rarely achieve long-term remission. The development of cell clones escaping conventional therapy is considered the major cause of relapse. These cells might be eradicated using targeting approaches with high specificity, such as monoclonal antibodies (MAbs), or cytokines to modulate host response, or cell-based immunotherapy. In addition, targeted drugs, including molecules that interfere with critical intracellular functions, could substantially contribute to decreasing acute toxicities, in particular late toxicities, which currently jeopardize the initial success of cytoreductive combined-modality treatment.

HODGKIN AND REED-STERNBERG CELLS AS TARGETS FOR SELECTIVE IMMUNOTHERAPY

Systemic chemotherapy kills rapidly dividing cells, whereas the concept of immunotherapy comprises the application of anticancer agents such as monoclonal antibodies and other biological compounds that are designed to selectively target tumor cells. Normal cells lacking the specific tumor antigen or target are spared.

Hodgkin lymphoma seems to be an ideal candidate for treatment approaches involving MAbs for the following reasons:

- Hodgkin/Reed-Sternberg cells express a variety of specific surface antigens such as CD15, CD25, CD30, CD40, and CD80 (B7-1), which are present only on a minority of normal cells. Due to low cross-reactivity with healthy human tissue, side effects are expected to be minimal.
- The number of malignant cells is relatively small (<1%) with the majority of cells found in involved lymph nodes surrounded by lymphoid (so-called bystander) cells.
- Hodgkin lymphoma tumors are well vascularized with high accessibility of intravenously administered MAbs/conjugates to target antigens due to favorable vascularity.
- Hodgkin lymphoma is known to respond very well to conventional therapeutic regimens; bulky disease can be eliminated by chemotherapy and/or radiotherapy, with the options of targeting the remaining cells with immunotherapeutics.

Other promising treatment strategies derive from the presence of Epstein-Barr virus (EBV) in approximately 50% of patients with Hodgkin lymphoma. The expression of EBV nuclear antigens or latent membrane proteins (e.g., LMP1, 2) on Hodgkin/Reed-Sternberg cells provides attractive targets for adoptive cellular immunotherapy using viral antigen-specific cytotoxic T-cells. Despite the lack of definitive evidence for the extracellular accessibility of LMP1 and LMP2A, antibody-based targeting of LMP1 and LMP2 extracellular domains on EBV-positive Hodgkin/Reed-Sternberg cells may also have therapeutic (and diagnostic) potential. Advances in molecular biology techniques over the past two decades have resulted in a better understanding of malignant transformation, a more distinct classification of subtypes on the basis of molecular markers, and a better characterization of eligible molecular targets. This knowledge has allowed for rapid progress in rational drug design of targeted therapies. Many immunotherapeutic concepts, especially MAb-based constructs, have been or are currently being tested in clinical phase I/II trials for toxicity and efficacy in patients with Hodgkin lymphoma. Strategies using new targets that exploit critical functions or genetic abnormalities in tumor cells continue to emerge for a variety of hematologic malignancies and other diseases. Next-generation novel chemical or biological compounds directed against key proteins or genes responsible for various aspects of cell proliferation, differentiation, and function, as well as angiogenesis and invasion, should be on the verge of entering clinical evaluation in the near future.

INTERLEUKIN-2 (IL-2)

IL-2 was one of the first immunotherapeutic agents used for anticancer therapy, since it augments the cytotoxicity of natural killer (NK) cells, induces lymphokine-activated killer (LAK) cells, and activates T- and B-lymphocytes as well as monocytes. Antitumor effects have been demonstrated in vitro and in various animal models. Several clinical trials have studied the efficacy of IL-2 alone or in combination with autologous LAK cells (adoptive immunotherapy) or other cytokines in patients with Hodgkin lymphoma.[10–15] Various cytokine-dosing regimens and cell-infusion schedules failed to produce convincing treatment results, with most patients progressing in the face of immune activation following IL-2 administration. Side effects were moderate and transient and included renal and hepatic dysfunction, dyspnea, fatigue, fever, hypotension, edema, mucositis, anemia, and thrombocytopenia.

With the intention of reducing relapse rates following autologous transplant, 24 Hodgkin lymphoma patients with minimal residual disease (MRD) after high-dose chemotherapy and autologous hematopoietic cell transplantation (AHCT) were treated in a phase II clinical trial with a combination of IL-2 and interferon-alpha (IFN-α).[16] IL-2 and IFN-α were administered in two cycles beginning 2.5 to 10 months post-transplant. Each cycle consisted of 3×10^6 U/d of IFN-α combined with 3 to 6 IU/m² of IL-2 given 5 days per week for 4 consecutive weeks. The overall survival at 48 months for patients receiving the cytokine-mediated immunotherapy was higher (100%) compared to a historical control group (57%). Less encouraging results were obtained from a study conducted in 11 patients with Hodgkin lymphoma when IL-2 administration (160×10^6 IU/m²) was started 6 to 8 weeks post-transplantation consisting of 1 cycle of 5 days followed by 4 cycles of 2 days every other week.[17] None of the patients responded to the treatment. Considering the fact that IL-2 was mainly administered to heavily pretreated patients, some reports may be promising, but somewhat inconsistent outcomes were noted in these phase I/II trials with low patient numbers. The results may sufficiently justify prospectively randomized phase III trials to determine the true impact of IL-2 on survival after transplant.

INTERFERON-α

The mechanism of action of IFN-α is multifaceted and includes immunoregulatory activity as well as antiproliferative effects that may be due to modulation of certain oncogenes.[18,19] Single-agent IFN-α has been reported to induce remissions in patients with low-grade lymphoma.[20] A recent meta-analysis evaluated the role of IFN-α2 in combination with chemotherapy for follicular lymphoma.[21] Despite considerable heterogeneity between studies, IFN-α2 was found to not significantly improve response rates. Analyses for survival and remission duration favored IFN-α2 treatment when it was given in conjunction with intensive initial chemotherapy, at a single dose of at least 5 million units (and at a cumulative dose of 36 million units per month), and in combination with chemotherapy rather than maintenance therapy. However, experience with IFN in patients with Hodgkin lymphoma is limited. Case reports of a few patients who received IFN for treatment of viral infections observed minor responses of Hodgkin lymphoma, and some pilot studies investigated the efficacy of IFN in the salvage therapy of Hodgkin lymphoma.[22–28] Overall, results were disappointing and further clinical trials of single-agent IFN-α in patients with advanced Hodgkin lymphoma appear not to be indicated. Treatment approaches in conjunction with other biologically active agents were more promising, as demonstrated in a phase II trial in 24 patients with Hodgkin lymphoma treated with repeated doses of IFN-α in combination with IL-2 following AHCT.[16] The median time from transplantation until the onset of immunotherapy was 4 months. Overall and disease-free survivals were significantly higher in the group treated with combined cytokine maintenance therapy compared with historical controls (see also the IL-2 section earlier in the chapter). Three out of 24 patients in the treatment group relapsed after transplant and immunotherapy, as opposed to 8 out of 25

control patients. Side effects were as expected from IFN-α and IL-2 when given as single agents. An interesting report on a pilot study was published by Streetly and associates to evaluate the feasibility of sequential cyclosporine A (CsA) and IFN-α treatment to induce autologous graft versus host-disease (GvHD) following a second autologous transplant.[29] This GvHD reaction is less severe than that seen after allogeneic transplant and usually self-limited. Two of three patients with Hodgkin lymphoma achieved a complete remission. Median overall survival for all patients (including 7 patients with non-Hodgkin lymphoma) was 13.5 months, and median relapse-free survival had not been reached at 42 months. This approach with low toxicity and promising data appears to be encouraging and warrants further evaluation.

MONOCLONAL ANTIBODIES (MABS)

The concept of targeted antibody therapy to attack cancer cells emerged at the beginning of the last century. A few years after the discovery of antiserum against diphtheria by Behring, Hericourt and Richet reported in 1895 on their efforts to treat cancer patients with antiserum produced in dogs or donkeys.[30] In 1906, Paul Ehrlich introduced the term "magic bullet" for compounds, such as antibodies, with selective toxicity. In 1953, Pressman and Korngold showed that antibodies could specifically target tumor cells.[31] Attempts to use these concepts clinically were hindered by the lack of monospecificity. It was not until 1975, when Köhler and Milstein described their Nobel Prize-winning work in hybridoma technology, that a continuous supply of specifically targeting MAbs became available.[32] By 1979, Nadler and colleagues treated the first patient with a MAb directed against a lymphoma-associated antigen.[33] The antibody, which had shown to lyse the patient's tumor cells in vitro, turned out to be clinically ineffective due to large amounts of circulating target antigen, but the therapy was safe and well-tolerated. However, it still took almost another 20 years until the first MAb was approved by the FDA for the treatment of cancer (anti-CD20 MAb; rituximab).

Ideally, the MAb targets an antigen that is only present on the tumor cell with high specificity and without cross-reactivity with normal human tissues. The mechanisms of action of native MAbs include complement activation, antibody-dependent cellular cytotoxicity (ADCC), phagocytosis of antibody-coated target cells, inhibition of cell-cycle sequences, and induction of apoptosis. MAbs can kill tumor cells by blocking essential structures that play key roles in signal transduction or cell proliferation, such as growth factor receptors. The activity of an individual MAb depends on various different aspects such as specificity and affinity of the MAb, density of the antigen on the cell membrane, magnitude of antigen shedding (cleavage from the cell membrane) into the bloodstream, antigen modulation and internalization after antibody binding including metabolism, homogeneity of antigen expression on tumor cells versus normal tissues, average number of antigen copies per cell, and tumor size.

Native MAbs

In contrast to non-Hodgkin lymphoma and chronic lymphocytic leukemia (CLL), which are sensitive to the humanized anti-CD52 MAb alemtuzumab[34] and the chimeric anti-CD20 MAb rituximab,[35] showing remission rates of approximately 50% in clinical trials, the evaluation of MAbs in Hodgkin lymphoma was less promising. Preclinical studies with two murine anti-CD30 antibodies (HeFi-1, M44) had distinct suppressive effects on cells derived from anaplastic large-cell lymphoma (ALCL), whereas there was no cytotoxicity observed toward Hodgkin lymphoma cells.[36,37] Engert and associates analyzed the potential use of 40 new MAbs directed against CD25, CD30, and IRac against Hodgkin/Reed-Sternberg cells in vitro without evidence of significant cytotoxic activity.[38] Through advances in MAb technology, remarkable progress has been made with improved affinities and enhanced effector functions.

CD30

Among the different available and investigated target antigens, CD30 seems to be most promising, because it is specifically up-regulated on Hodgkin/Reed-Sternberg cells as well as on ALCL and adult T-cell leukemia.[39] CD30 is a member of the tumor necrosis factor receptor (TNF) superfamily and physiologically involved in the negative selection process of autoreactive lymphocytes. Similar to other members of the TNF family, CD30 seems to play a role in cell-cycle regulation.[40] The targeting of this receptor with humanized/human anti-CD30 MAbs might recruit effector mechanisms including CDC and ADCC. Currently, there are two anti-CD30 MAbs being investigated in clinical trials. SGN-30, a chimeric anti-CD30 MAb, showed minimal toxicity and antitumor activity was seen in 2 of 13 patients[41] (see Table 15.1). In a phase I/II dose-escalation study of 6 weekly infusions of SGN-30 at doses of up to 12 mg/kg, 24 heavily pretreated patients were enrolled (21 Hodgkin lymphoma, 2 ALCL, 1 diffuse large B-cell lymphoma).[42,43] The MAb was very well tolerated, with fatigue being the major drug-related adverse event. Preliminary response data (up to the 8 mg/kg cohort) include one complete remission in a patient with ALCL and 5 patients with Hodgkin lymphoma who had disease stabilization. 5F11 (MDX-060) is a fully human MAb that recognizes CD30 with nanomolar affinity.[44] It induces Fc-receptor–mediated killing of Hodgkin lymphoma and ALCL cell lines in vitro including ADCC and in xenograft tumor models. In a phase I/II dose-escalation study of MDX-060 in patients with relapsed or refractory Hodgkin lymphoma, ALCL, or other CD30-expressing lymphomas, MDX-060 was administered intravenously at dose levels of up to 10 mg/kg weekly for 4 weeks.[45] Forty-eight patients (40 Hodgkin lymphoma, 6 ALCL, 2 other) have been treated without significant infusion-related reactions. Objective responses have been reported in 5 patients. Two patients had a complete remission, including one with Hodgkin lymphoma with 4 months duration. Interestingly, the retreatment of the ALCL patients resulted in a second complete remission. Another 3 patients (2 Hodgkin lymphoma, 1 ALCL) achieved partial responses; 17 patients had stable disease.

CD20

Lymphocyte-predominant Hodgkin lymphoma (LPHL) accounts for 3% to 8% of all cases of Hodgkin lymphoma and has the most favorable prognosis among all Hodgkin lymphoma subtypes.[46] Whereas only a small minority of classical Hodgkin lymphoma is CD20 positive, all patients with LPHL express this B-cell marker in high density on their malignant cell population. Information on feasibility and activity of the anti-CD20 chimeric MAb rituximab in this subpopulation is limited to reports of single cases or small patient groups, due to the infrequency of patients with CD20+ Hodgkin lymphoma.[47,48] The first prospective clinical trial investigating rituximab in patients with LPHL was conducted by the German Hodgkin Study Group (GHSG). Patients with refractory Hodgkin lymphoma and CD20-positive histology were treated at the standard dose of 375 mg/m² weekly for 4 consecutive weeks.[49] Of 14 included patients, 8 achieved a complete remission and 4 patients had a partial remission; 2 patients showed progressive disease. The median time of response duration was 14 months, with 10 patients remaining in remission at the time of analysis. Similar results were seen in another trial involving 22 patients with recurrent LPHL, with an overall response rate of 100% including 10 complete remissions and a second remission in one patient after tumor progression.[50] Toxicity was limited to mild infusion-related reactions. Responses were in general short-lived, with 9 patients relapsing after a median of 9 months. Eight patients relapsed exclusively at sites previously involved with LPHL. It was noted that the quality of response to rituximab correlated with relapse. Two patients with recurrent disease following rituximab treatment were found to have transformed to a large-cell lymphoma on re-biopsy, raising the concern that rituximab might facilitate transformation. However, LPHL represents a rare histologic subtype, restricting the use of rituximab to a small group of patients with Hodgkin lymphoma. Further trials could focus on its application in first-line therapy and possible combination with established regimens.

IMMUNOTOXINS

Immunotoxins (ITs) generally consist of cell-selective ligands covalently linked to peptide toxins of bacterial or plant origin (Fig. 15.1). The ligand delivers the molecule to specific cell-surface receptors on malignant cells. The toxin triggers cell death either by reaching the cytosol and catalytically inactivating vital cell processes or by modifying the tumor cell-surface membrane. The ligand is usually a MAb, a MAb fragment (Fab-fragment or single-chain variable fragment), or a cytokine. The covalent connection of toxin and ligand for clinical applicability requires high stability of the construct in the bloodstream and interstitial fluids. It should also not interfere with ligand affinity to its receptor, toxin translocation, or enzymatic activity. Conjugation of ligand and toxin has been achieved using chemical linkers and, more recently, genetic fusion technology.

All toxins used for the treatment of hematologic tumors have been cytotoxins, which can directly induce cell death upon internalization of the construct. In theory, one toxin molecule is sufficient to kill a given single cell.[51] Almost all ITs used for hematologic malignancies have been made with intracellular enzymes, because these conjugates damage cells only upon ligand-receptor internalization, which provides an additional safety precaution. The majority of ITs inactivate cytosolic protein synthesis either by altering elongation factor 2 (e.g., diphtheria toxin, or *Pseudomonas* exotoxin), or by degrading ribosomal RNA (e.g., ricin, abrin, viscumin, saporin) or total RNA (ribonuclease, angiogenin) (Fig. 15.2). Among the several hundred ITs developed and engineered for the treatment of hematologic malignancies, more than 20 have been tested in phase I to III clinical trials. A number of these compounds have shown significant activity in patients with leukemia and lymphoma. ITs with the highest response rates in clinical studies have been active in tissue culture in the picomolar range and have been fully recombinant molecules, with one ($DAB_{389}IL2$, Ontak) being approved by the FDA in 1999 for the therapy of cutaneous T-cell lymphoma.

Ricin A-Chain ITs Against CD25

The low-affinity IL-2 receptor (IL-2Rα, CD25, Tac) is another attractive target on Hodgkin/Reed-Sternberg cells,[52] and has been explored for its suitability using anti-CD25 conjugated ITs.

TABLE 15.1

CLINICAL TRIALS WITH VARIOUS IMMUNOCONJUGATES IN HODGKIN LYMPHOMA

Group	Antigen	Construct	Application (dose, MTD)	Toxicity	Immune response	Response	Reference
MAb	CD20	Rituximab	4 × 1 bolus infusion/w (given dose: 375 mg/m²)	Rhinitis, fever, chills, nausea	None	8/14 CR 4/14 PR	49
MAb	CD20	Rituximab	4 × 1 bolus infusion/w (given dose: 375 mg/m²)	No grade 3 or 4 toxicities	ND	10/22 CR 12/22 PR	50
MAb	CD20	Rituximab	6 × 1 bolus infusion/w (given dose: 375 mg/m²)	ND	ND	1/22 CR 4/22 PR	129
MAb	CD30	SGN-30	6 × 1 bolus infusion/w (given dose: 2–12 mg/kg)	Fatigue	ND	None of 21	42, 43
MAb	CD30		6 × 1 bolus infusion/w (given dose: 6 mg/kg)			1/9 PR	41
MAb	CD30	MDX060	4 × 1 bolus infusion/w (given dose: 0.1–15 mg/kg)	2 grade 3 toxicities (elevated transaminases, pneumonia)	ND	1/40 CR 2/40 PR	45
IT	CD30	Ki-4.dgA	4-h infusion, days 1-3-5-7 (5 mg/m²)	VLS, myalgia, nausea, fatigue	1/17 HAMA 7/17 HARA	1/17 PR, 1/17 MR	54
IT	CD30	BerH2-Sap6	1 bolus infusion (0.8 mg/kg)	Elevated transaminases, VLS, myalgia, fever, fatigue	12/12 HAMA	4/12 PR 3/12 MR	55
IT	CD25	RFT5.dgA	4-h infusion, days 1-3-5-7 (15 mg/m²)	VLS, myalgia, nausea, fatigue	6/15 HAMA 7/15 HARA	2/15 PR, 1/15 MR	53
rIT	CD25	DAB₃₈₉IL-2	Bolus infusion days 1–5 (27 μg/kg/d)	Elevated transaminases, chills, fever, fatigue	50% anti-DT-A pre-therapy, 89% anti-DT-A post-therapy	No response 17 patients	57
rIT	CD25	DAB₄₈₆IL-2	Bolus infusions days 1–5 (up to 0.3 mg/kg/d)	Elevated transaminases, chills, fever, fatigue	50% anti-DT-A	1/7 CR	56
rIT	CD25	DAB₄₈₆IL-2	10 bolus infusions (0.1 mg/kg/d)	Elevated transaminases, elevated creatinine, nausea, rash, fever, fatigue	2/2 anti-DT-A 1/2 anti-IL-2-A 1/2 anti-DAB-A	No response 3 patients	130

(*continued*)

Type	Target	Agent	Dosing	Toxicity	HAMA	Response	Ref
rIT	CD25	DAB$_{486}$IL-2	Bolus infusion, days 1–5 (0.2 mg/kg/d)	Elevated transaminases, elevated creatinine, rash, proteinuria, hypoalbuminemia	2/4 anti-DT-A, 2/4 anti-DAB-A	1/4 CR	131
rIT	CD25	anti-Tac(Fv)-PE38	Bolus infusion QOD × 3 (40 µg/kg)	Elevated transaminases, fever	5/11 HAMA, 7/11 anti-PE38	1/11 PR, 3/11 MR	58
Bi-MAb	CD30XCD16	HRS-3/A9	4 bolus infusions, every 3 or 4 days (not reached, max given dose 64 mg/m^2)	Fever, rash, pain (in lymph nodes)	60% HAMA	1/15 CR, 1/15 PR, 3/15 MR	72
Bi-MAb	CD30XCD16	HRS-3/A9	4 bolus infusions every other day or continuous infusion (2.5mg/m^2) ± IL-2	Fever	38% HAMA	1/16 CR, 3/16 PR	73
Bi-Fab	CD30XCD64	Ki-4XH22	4-h infusion, days 1-3-5-7 (not reached, max given dose 20 mg/m^2)	Hypotension, tachycardia, chills, fever, fatigue	n.e.	1/10 CR, 3/10 PR	74
RAb	anti-ferritin	^{131}I-antiferritin	Bolus IV 30 mCi day 1, Bolus IV 20 mCi day 5	Myelosuppression	ND	1/37 CR, 14/37 PR	64
RAb	anti-ferritin	^{90}Y-antiferritin	Bolus IV 20–50 mCi day 1 ± ABMT	Myelosuppression	None	9/29 CR, 9/29 PR	132
RAb	anti-ferritin	^{90}Y-antiferritin	Bolus IV 20–50 mCi day 1 CX + ABMT	Myelosuppression	ND	1/12 CR, 3/12 PR	68
RAb	anti-ferritin	^{90}Y-antiferritin	Bolus IV 20–50 mCi day 1	Myelosuppression, mild fever and fatigue	None	10/39 CR, 10/39 PR	67
RAb	anti-ferritin	^{90}Y-antiferritin	Bolus IV 0.3–0.5 mCi/kg day 1 or 2 × 0.25 mCi/kg day 1 + 8	Myelosuppression, mild fever and fatigue	ND	15/90 CR, 29/90 PR	65
RAb	CD30	^{131}I-Ki-4	Bolus IV 20–100 mCi day 1	Myelosuppression, fever, fatigue	18% HAMA	1/22 CR, 5/22 PR	66

ABMT, autologous bone marrow transplantation; MAb, monoclonal antibody; IT, immunotoxin; rIT, recombinant immunotoxin; Bi-MAb, bispecific antibody; RAb, radiolabeled antibody; CR, complete remission; PR, partial remission; MR, minor response; VLS, vascular leak syndrome; HAMA, human anti-mouse antibodies; HARA, human anti-ricin antibodies; anti-DT-A, anti-diphtheria toxin antibodies; anti-DAB-A, anti-DAB antibodies; anti-IL-2-A, anti-IL-2 antibodies; ND, not done.

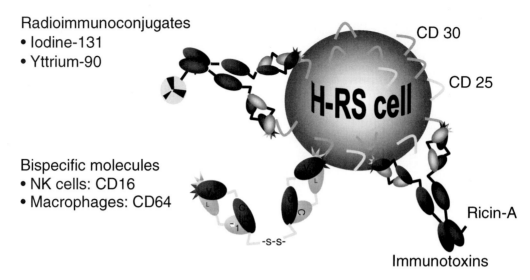

Radioimmunoconjugates
- Iodine-131
- Yttrium-90

Bispecific molecules
- NK cells: CD16
- Macrophages: CD64

CD 30

CD 25

H-RS cell

Ricin-A

Immunotoxins

FIGURE 15.1. Examples of Mab-based constructs for immunotherapy of Hodgkin lymphoma. See color insert.

The anti-CD25 IT RFT5.dgA, with potent preclinical antitumor activity, is derived from the deglycosylated ricin A-chain (dgA), a ribosome-inactivating protein extracted from the seeds of *Ricinus communis* (castor bean), and was tested in a phase I/II clinical trial in heavily pretreated patients with refractory Hodgkin lymphoma.[53] The MTD (maximum tolerated dose) was 15 mg/m^2, and the response of 15 evaluable patients treated at the MTD included 2 partial remissions, 1 minor response, and 5 patients had stable disease. Seven of 15 patients produced human anti-ricin antibodies (HARA). Side effects were related to transient vascular leak syndrome, a typical phenomenon observed with most ITs.

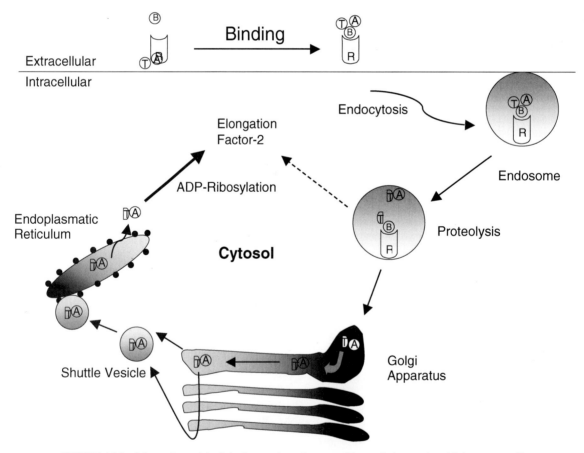

FIGURE 15.2. Schematic model of the interaction of a recombinant fusion toxin with its target cell. After binding of the immunotoxin (IT) to a specific cell-surface receptor, the toxin–receptor complex is internalized into an endosome. Low pH induces unfolding of the IT followed by specific proteolytic cleavage. The released-37kD carboxy-terminal fragment finally reaches the cytosol and inhibits protein synthesis by adenosine diphosphate (ADP)-ribosylation of elongation factor 2. (R, specific receptor on target cell surface; B, binding moiety (cytokine, MAb); T, translocation domain of *Pseudomonas* exotoxin A; A, catalytically active component of the exotoxin.)

Ricin A-Chain ITs Against CD30

Ki-4.dgA, consisting of the murine anti-CD30 MAb Ki-4 and dgA, demonstrated superior preclinical potency compared to previously tested anti-CD30 dgA-ITs, and was selected for a clinical phase-I trial in 17 patients with refractory CD30-positive Hodgkin lymphoma and non-Hodgkin lymphoma.[54] The IT was given as a 30-minute infusion every other day in escalating doses for a total of 4 doses per cycle. Administration of multiple cycles was possible, unless patients experienced toxicity or developed antibodies against the construct. Side effects were related to VLS, which occurred in almost all patients at early dose levels; thus MTD was already reached at 5 mg/m^2. Four patients responded to IT treatment (one partial remission), and 2 patients had stable disease. Immune responses to the construct were observed in 7 patients, 6 against the ricin (HARA) and 1 against the murine MAb (HAMA, or human anti-mouse antibodies).

ITs Containing Saporin

Saporin-S6 (Sap6), extracted from the seeds of *Saponaria officinalis* (soapworth), is another plant-derived ribosome-inactivating single-chain toxin used for IT construction. Saporin-S6 ITs were constructed by linkage with the anti-CD30 MAb Ber-H2 for a phase I/II trial. 12 patients with advanced refractory disease were treated with 1 or 2 infusions of 0.8mg/kg Ber-H2-Sap6 over 4 hours. Four patients achieved a partial remission with substantial decrease of tumor mass, although short-lived, and 3 patients had a minor response with a median duration of 2 months.[55] Common adverse events included fever, malaise, anorexia, fatigue, mild myalgias, weight gain, and a reversible 4- to 5-fold increase in liver enzymes. The MTD of 0.8 mg/kg was established by grade 3 VLS and liver toxicity.

ITs Containing Diphtheria Toxin (DT)

DAB$_{486}$IL-2 is a fusion protein composed of a truncated deletion mutant of DT in which the native receptor-binding domain of DT has been replaced with human IL-2 as the binding moiety. In a phase I/II study for CD25 expressing hematologic malignancies including CLL, T-cell lymphoma, and Hodgkin lymphoma, one patient with Hodgkin lymphoma achieved a complete remission after the IT had been administered as a 90-minute IV infusion at daily doses of 0.2 mg/kg for 5 consecutive days.[56] However, 6 other patients with Hodgkin lymphoma did not respond. Side effects were hypersensitivity-like symptoms, reversible elevated liver function tests, and fatigue as the major toxicity. A refined version termed DAB$_{389}$IL-2 (now known as Ontak) bound 5-fold more avidly to the high-affinity IL-2 receptor and showed 10-fold improved cytotoxicity compared to DAB$_{486}$IL-2. Of 73 patients suffering from various refractory lymphomas including 21 patients with Hodgkin lymphoma treated on a phase II trial with DAB$_{389}$-IL-2 at a similar schedule, none responded to IT administration.[57] It was recognized that the formation of anti-IT antibodies by the patient's functioning immune system also poses a problem when recombinant fusion proteins are used, because previous studies demonstrated a correlation of anti-IT antibody titers and the incidence of side effects. Immunogenicity may also impede efficacy, because patients with anti-toxin antibodies clear ITs more rapidly from the bloodstream. Also, with most people being immunized with DT in early childhood, there is a significant titer present in the blood of many patients prior to treatment and an amnestic response occurs in additional patients treated with DT conjugates.

ITs Containing Pseudomonas Exotoxin A

In a clinical phase I trial, the recombinant anti-CD25 IT anti-Tac (Fv)-PE38 (LMB-2), containing a single-chain Fv fragment of the anti-Tac MAb to the IL-2 receptor alpha subunit (CD25) fused to a truncated form of the bacterial toxin *Pseudomonas* exotoxin, was administered to 35 patients with chemotherapy-refractory hematologic malignancies.[58] In the phase II trial, 11 patients with Hodgkin lymphoma were treated with 30-minute infusions at doses of 2 to 63 µg/kg IV on alternating days for a total of 3 doses. The MTD was 40 µg/kg, with transient elevation of transaminases and fever being the most common side effects. Vascular leak syndrome was not observed. Interestingly, most of the patients did not produce neutralizing antibodies, which allowed for repeated cycles of LMB-2. Responses included 1 partial remission, 3 minor responses, and 6 patients experienced disease stabilization.

Overall, clinical outcome with regard to toxicity and response is not markedly auspicious when compared with promising experimental data obtained for many engineered ITs and calls for examination of the underlying matters in greater detail to explain these discrepancies. Notably, factors influencing immune response cascades in humans, which are difficult to simulate in animal models, may significantly limit IT efficacy and therefore compromise clinical application. In addition, toxin-related side effects may derive from unspecific binding of ITs to organs such as liver or endothelium and aggravate the toxicity profile. Much effort will be necessary to overcome these obstacles.

RADIOIMMUNOCONJUGATES

Radioimmunoconjugates consist of an MAb linked to a radioactive isotope with the MAb targeting radiation to tumor cells. Radiolabeled MAbs (RAbs) are a particularly promising approach for targeted therapy as they induce reliable and specific killing of tumor cells. Antitumor activity of radioimmunotherapy (RIT) primarily derives from the radioactivity of the nuclide attached to the antibody, which emits continuous, exponentially decreasing radiation with heterogeneous dose deposition (Fig. 15.1). In some cases, as is evidenced in lymphoma, the antibody itself may contribute to tumor destruction.[59] Several limitations of native MAbs may be potentially overcome with RIT. To induce cell death, the isotope is not required to internalize or to dissociate from the MAb, unlike toxin-conjugates or chemotherapeutic agents. In addition, RAbs can also destroy bystander cells (cells contiguous to an RAb-bound cell) due to the cytotoxicity of β-particles (1–5 mm) emitted by commonly used radioisotopes such as 131-iodine (^{131}I), 90-yttrium (^{90}Y), 212-bismuth (^{212}Bi), or 67-copper (^{67}Cu) over many cell diameters. One β-particle from ^{90}Y, for instance, can reach more than 200 cells. The so-called crossfire-effect does not require binding of the RAb to each individual tumor cell and helps to overcome low or heterogeneous antigen expression on target cells as well as the limited accretion of antibody in poorly vascularized or bulky tumors. Crucial factors for RIT efficacy include the nature of the antibody (specificity, affinity, avidity, dose, immunoreactivity, mechanism of action), the nuclide (emission properties, half-life, stability), the antigen (distribution, modulation), and the nature of the targeted tumor (radiosensitivity, location, size, vascularization, proliferation rate). Various radionuclides have been investigated clinically, but only few appear to meet the requirements for clinical practice and commercial development, such as ^{131}I and ^{90}Y, the two most widely used.

Clinical investigations of RIT in cancer patients started in the 1950s when radioiodine-labeled quinoline derivatives were administered to 14 patients with metastatic melanoma and achieved a pathologically documented complete remission in one patient.[60] After efforts during more than four decades to implement the use of radiolabeled antibodies for cancer therapy, two RAbs targeting the CD20 antigen were approved by the FDA for the treatment of chemotherapy and rituximab-refractory low-grade non-Hodgkin lymphome: ibritumomab (tiuxetan, Zevalin) murine yttrium-90-anti-CD20 in 2002; and iodine-131-tositumomab (Bexxar) murine iodine-131-anti-CD20 in 2003). Randomized studies evaluating these agents at non-myeloablative doses have demonstrated superior response rates compared to unlabeled MAbs.[61] Alternative approaches explored the use of RAbs in conjunction with AHCT to augment radiation doses delivered to the tumor sites.[62,63] High-dose RIT was well tolerated with only low non-hematologic toxicity and yielded improved survival. However, most patients eventually developed recurrent lymphoma. Both non-myeloablative (low-dose) as well as myeloablative (high-dose) therapeutic strategies with RAbs have also been investigated in Hodgkin lymphoma patients.

LOW-DOSE RADIOIMMUNOTHERAPY

In the mid-1980s, Lenhard and colleagues treated 38 patients with advanced Hodgkin lymphoma in a phase I trial using ^{131}I-labeled polyclonal antibodies directed against ferritin, a tumor-associated protein.[64] The drug was administered IV at an initial dose of 30 mCi followed by an additional 20 mCi 5 days later. Forty percent of patients experienced objective tumor regression. Side effects were mostly related to myelosuppression. Another trial evaluated the use of single-dose (0.3–0.5 mCi/kg)

versus fractionated (2 × 0.25 mCi/kg) ^{90}Y-labeled anti-ferritin antibodies.[65] Eleven patients received 0.3 mCi/kg, 39 patients 0.4 mCi/kg, 7 patients 0.5 mCi/kg, and 33 patients the fractionated regimen. The most significant toxicity was thrombocytopenia. Tumor response was dose related, with a response rate of 86% in the 0.5-mCi/kg group. Response in patients undergoing the fractionated schedule was only 45%, in contrast to what was expected from the experience with external-beam irradiation. In summary, 15 of 90 patients had a complete remission and 29 had a PR with a median duration of 6 months. Recently, the use of the first specific RAb for RIT in 22 patients with advanced relapsed Hodgkin lymphoma was reported from a phase I trial utilizing the anti-CD30 MAb Ki-4 labeled with [131]I.[66] A dose of 250 to 300 MBq ^{131}I-Ki-4 was administered at escalating individual total body doses of up to 0.35 Gy. Acute toxicity was mild, but 8 patients experienced grade 4 hematotoxicity 3 to 5 weeks after treatment, particularly thrombocytopenia, which was prolonged and lasted for a median of 8 weeks. The number of previous therapies and a platelet count below 150,000/μL before RIT were identified as the main risk factors. Overall response was 27% including 1 complete remission and 5 partial remissions. Positive tumor imaging was not predictive of good response in this trial, and only one patient with a positive scintigraphy responded to treatment (Fig. 15.3). The study suggested that targeting the CD30 antigen with ^{131}I-Ki-4 in multiply relapsed patients can be effective but is associated with unpredictable myelosuppression. This might be due the fact that CD30, unlike CD20, is internalized upon binding of the iodinated construct with subsequent release of radioiodine catabolites causing undesired side effects. Residualizing radiolabels (e.g., ^{90}Y) may help reduce toxicity.

MYELOABLATIVE RADIOIMMUNOTHERAPY

The approach with high-dose RIT involves Rabs as part of the conditioning regimen and stem cell support for hematopoietic recovery. Herpst and associates infused 39 patients, who had previously failed multiple chemotherapy regimens, with anti-

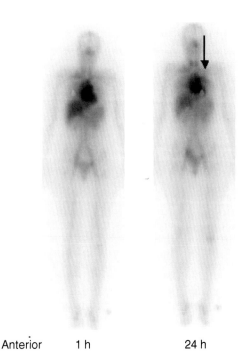

Anterior   1 h   24 h

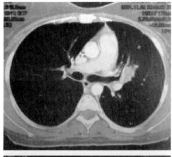

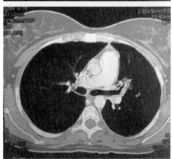

FIGURE 15.3. Scintigraphic and CT scans from patients treated with the anti-CD30 radioimmunoconjugate ^{131}I-Ki-4. Twenty-one-year-old female patient with pulmonary Hodgkin lymphoma (2.5 cm in diameter on CT scan) demonstrating specific tumor uptake of ^{131}I-Ki-4. Treatment resulted in a partial remission with major improvement of clinical symptoms. The duration of response was 5 months.

ferritin polyclonal antibodies radiolabeled with ^{90}Y in multiple doses at 10 to 50 mCi.[67] Overall response rate was 20 of 39 patients (51%), including 10 patients with a complete remission. Two patients had stable disease. The small amount of labeled protein (2–5 mg) suggested that responses were radiation induced rather than MAb induced. Fifty percent of patients survived for at least 6 months. Patients received autologous bone marrow cells (5×10^7 cells/kg) due to severe myelosuppression. Another group examined the feasibility of combining RIT with high-dose chemotherapy followed by autologous marrow transplantation.[68] Twelve patients received ^{90}Y-labeled anti-ferritin infusions on 3 consecutive days, followed by high-dose chemotherapy 5 days later, and then bone marrow infusion. Four patients died early of transplant-related causes, another 4 were alive more than 2 years following transplantation, and 3 were free from disease progression at >24, >25, and >28 months. The progression-free survival rate at 1 year was estimated to be 21%. Considering the poor prognostic characteristics of these patients, toxicity on this protocol was not greater than that observed with high-dose chemotherapy alone.

Reviewing the studies with anti-ferritin it was noted that results obtained with ^{90}Y-labeled anti-ferritin were significantly better than with ^{131}I-labeled antiferritin.[69] Responses were more common in patients with longer disease histories (>3 years), smaller tumor volumes (<30 cm^3), and in patients receiving at least 0.4 mCi ^{90}Y-labeled anti-ferritin/kg body weight. Complete responders survived significantly longer than partial responders. Despite results suggesting that a transplant approach using ^{90}Y-anti-ferritin alone provides objective responses in approximately half of patients with chemotherapy-refractory disease, the majority of survivors had developed recurrent disease. Relapse following RIT mainly occurred in previously uninvolved areas. It may be speculated that improved outcomes would be seen in a similar population of patients treated earlier in the course of their disease.

So far, the few available studies have gathered some evidence of activity of RIT in relapsed Hodgkin lymphoma, but were associated with severe toxicities in the majority of trials. The role of RIT in Hodgkin lymphoma remains to be defined. Having the achievements of RIT for non-Hodgkin lymphoma in mind, efforts to improve outcome for Hodgkin lymphoma patients are currently underway and focus on the choice of alternative radionuclides, new targets and carriers, and the definition of markers that allow a better identification of Hodgkin lymphoma patients who may benefit from RIT.

BI-SPECIFIC MONOCLONAL ANTIBODIES (BI-MABS)

Bi-MAbs contain two distinct recognition sites. One binds to tumor-associated antigens on tumor cells, and the other to a trigger antigen on immune effector cells such as macrophages, T-cells, or natural killer (NK) cells, therefore combining the advantages of MAb specificity with cytotoxic capabilities of immunocompetent cells (Fig. 15.1). The most extensively used trigger molecules are CD3 on T-cells, FcγRI (CD64) on granulocytes and monocytes, FcγRIII (CD16) on NK-cells, and FcαRI (CD89) on macrophages. Bi-MAbs can be obtained by chemically cross-linking two MAbs or Fab fragments with different specificity, by somatic fusion of two hybridoma cell lines (hybrid-hybridoma, tetradoma), or by using recombinant technology. Unfortunately, problems of large-scale manufacturing in the past have significantly hampered research and development as well as limited clinical application of Bi-MAbs.

The fact that patients with Hodgkin lymphoma both at diagnosis and after therapy generally have underlying immunodeficiency, especially of cellular immunity, can make approaches that require full T-cell recognition and effector function difficult. In contrast, NK-cell function in patients with Hodgkin lymphoma is usually intact and competent. Many Bi-MAbs involve the T-cell receptor (TCR)/CD3 complex, thus activating and recruiting cytotoxic T-cells at the tumor site. Full T-cell activation and proliferation requires the presence of antigen-presenting cells and co-stimulatory signals. Absence of these factors may cause unresponsiveness and clonal anergy or deletion. Co-stimulation can be provided by a variety of cytokines or membrane-bound molecules, such as members of the B7 family, which represent natural ligands for the CD28 and CTLA-4 counterreceptors on T-cells. Therefore, preactivation via cytokines or antigen-presenting cells is necessary before T-cells, attracted and stimulated by Bi-MAbs, can fully exert their cytotoxic activity in vivo.

NK-cells represent another frequently used cell type in studies involving Bi-MAbs. Unlike T-cells, NK-cells do not require specific activation as they constitutively exert cytolytic functions against a number of NK-susceptible tumor target cells, although some activation is needed for effective tumor lysis. CD16 is a surface marker for NK-cells and serves as Fc part receptor for IgG (FcγRIII). Engagement of CD16 with anti-CD16 MAbs leads to NK-cell–mediated cytotoxicity, which is not major histocompatibility complex (MHC) gene product restricted.[70] There is evidence that additional administration of cytokines such as IL-2 and IL-12 to pre-stimulate NK-cells may help reduce relapse rates and the amount of MAb needed to induce augmented tumor cell lysis.[71]

Bi-MAbs Activating Natural Killer Cells

The first clinical trial using Bi-MAbs for the treatment of Hodgkin lymphoma was initiated in 1995. In a phase-I/II study 15 patients with refractory Hodgkin lymphoma received 4 infusions of the CD30/CD16 Bi-MAb (HRS-3/A9) every 3 to 4 days.[72] Escalating doses were administered up to 64 mg/m^2 without reaching the MTD because of limited drug supply. This was also the reason why only 15 patients could be treated and illustrates the drawbacks of Bi-MAb production when large amounts of antibody are needed for clinical trials. Responses included a complete and a partial remission lasting for 6 and 3 months, respectively. There was no clear correlation of administered dose and observed antitumor effects or toxicities, nor was an immunologic parameter identified that was predictive for treatment outcome in that study. Side effects occurred in 6 patients and were mild to moderate. The majority of patients developed HAMA, and retreatment with the Bi-MAb was prevented by allergic reactions in all 5 attempted cases. In a subsequent trial, a modified Bi-MAb application schedule with prolonged infusion time was used to potentially provide higher antitumor efficacy and better tolerance of retreatment attempts.[73] Patients with objective response after the first course were eligible to receive another Bi-MAb cycle with concomitant IL-2 and GM-CSF application to stimulate NK-cells, which was crucial for this immunotherapeutic strategy. The first treatment cycle yielded 2 partial remissions and 6 patients with stable disease. Responders received further treatment with HRS-3/A9 without additional cytokines, whereas patients with stable disease received the second Bi-MAb course after pretreatment with IL-2 followed by GM-CSF at the end of the cycle. Two of the five patients with stable disease converted to remission (one complete, one partial), accompanied by an increase of peripheral blood NK-cells, raising the cumulative response rate to HRS-3/A9 treatment to 25%. The complete remission lasted for 6 months and the 3 partial remissions for 3 to 9 months. NK-cell counts prior to treatment start appeared to be higher in the blood of the 4 responders as compared with patients who experienced stable or progressive disease. In all 5 patients with cytokine co-stimulation, at least doubling of circulating NK-cells was observed. Overall, despite some immunologic evidence of benefit from cytokine pretreatment, clinical outcome was not significantly different compared to previously treated patients. In contrast to the initial study, a weak HAMA response was seen in 6 patients, three of whom were retreated without adverse reactions.

Bi-MAbs Activating Monocytes

The Bi-MAb H22×Ki-4 consists of the Fab' fragment derived from the humanized anti-CD64 MAb H22, which was chemically linked to the Fab' fragment of the murine anti-CD30 Ki-4. CD64 serves as a trigger molecule for cytotoxic effector cells expressing FcγRI. Binding of IgG-antigen complexes to FcγRI results in increased cytotoxic activity, including cytolysis, respiratory burst, and production of oxidative enzymes.[70] The BiMAb binds to H-RS cells and CD64-positive immune effector cells such as monocytes and macrophages mediating ADCC. Ten patients with refractory Hodgkin lymphoma received escalating doses (1–20 mg/m²) of H22×Ki-4 on alternating days for a total of 4 doses per cycle.[74] Treatment was well tolerated with only mild and transient side effects. There were no dose-limiting toxicities, and the MTD of this construct was not reached with one patient receiving a total dose of 740mg. Response to H22×Ki-4 in this population of heavily pretreated patients was seen over a broad range of doses without clear dose–response correlation and included a complete remission, 3 partial remissions, and 4 patients with stable disease. The observed duration of responses was only 1 to 5 months.

Although generally well tolerated, the use of Bi-MAbs in clinical trials with patients suffering from multiply relapsed or refractory disease showed augmented biological and immunologic antitumor activity, but objective responses occurred only in few patients. However, production of Bi-MAbs is cumbersome and expensive, and marked improvement of clinical outcome may be required to justify the further development of this approach.

VASCULAR TARGETING

Malignant cells are highly dependent on a sufficient blood supply, and local interruption of the tumor vasculature would result in tumor cell death due to the inability to obtain oxygen and nutrients. The main advantages of targeting tumor vessels versus targeting tumor cells directly are (a) the immediate accessibility of tumor endothelial cells to intravenously administered therapeutic drugs, permitting rapid localization of a high percentage of the injected dose; (b) occlusion of larger vessels results in an amplifying effect; (c) the lower likelihood of developing treatment-induced resistance due to higher genetic stability in contrast to tumor cells; and (d) tumor vessels share common morphologic and biochemical properties, suggesting that this strategy should be applicable to different tumor types. Targeting the vasculature is of particular interest in the treatment of solid tumors, but also in patients with bulky lymphoma. In general, there are two conceptually distinct groups of "anti-vasculature" reagents, vascular targeting agents (VTAs) and angiogenesis inhibitors. Although VTAs appear to be more effective in large tumors, angiogenesis inhibitors exhibit higher efficacy in smaller lesions.

Vascular Targeting Agents (VTAs)

VTAs are designed to selectively bind to components of tumor vasculature and deliver an effector molecule that causes occlusion of the tumor vessels. VTAs can be divided into two types, small-molecule VTAs and ligand-directed VTAs. Small-molecule VTAs do not localize selectively to tumor vessels but exploit pathophysiologic differences between tumor and normal tissue endothelium. Ligand-based VTAs use a targeting ligand to achieve selective binding to tumor vasculature, and to cause vascular collapse with subsequent massive central necrosis. A ligand could act by directly thrombosing tumor blood vessels, by inducing vascular injury that leads to coagulation, or by causing shape changes in the tumor endothelium that physically block the vessels. MAbs directed against a specific marker of tumor endothelium are usually used as targeting moieties. Alternatively, ligands that bind to high-affinity receptors that are over-expressed on tumor vessels can be used. Effector moieties include coagulant proteins, liposomally encapsulated drugs, toxins, or cytokines that induce thrombosis on the injured vasculature. The main challenge is to identify a surface marker that is specifically and homogeneously expressed on the majority of tumor vessels. Most tumor endothelial markers are expressed at low levels in some normal tissues or are heterogeneously distributed within the tumor. Up-regulated markers on tumor vessels include molecules involved in angiogenesis and vascular remodeling (e.g., VEGF, PSMA, endoglin, $\alpha_v\beta_3$ integrin); cell adhesion molecules (e.g., VCAM-1), which are released by tumor cells and tumor-infiltrating normal cells; and molecules associated with prothrombotic changes that occur on tumor vascular endothelium (e.g., phosphatidylserine, tissue factor). Most potential target molecules were studied in solid tumors. However, Hodgkin lymphoma has well-vascularized tumors and feature a variety of vascular surface markers such as vascular cell adhesion molecule-1(VCAM-1), endoglin (CD105), or phosphatidylserine. VTAs directed against these surface molecules have shown some evidence of activity in preclinical Hodgkin lymphoma mouse models.[75–77] Evidence that VTAs may have enhanced therapeutic benefit in combination with chemotherapy, radiation, or other biological agents would warrant additional efforts to define the most appropriate therapeutic setting in human cancer and to potentially translate promising preclinical data into clinical applications.

ANGIOGENESIS INHIBITORS

Inhibitors of angiogenesis prevent vascular endothelial cell division and inhibit tumor growth in areas of neovascularization but do not prevent tumor proliferation along existing, nonproliferating vessels. Angiogenesis inhibitors are probably most effective against tumors and metastases at their early stage when angiogenesis is occurring vigorously. Recent clinical trials have shown that treatment of patients with advanced and bulky tumors with anti-angiogenic drugs results in stabilization but usually not in shrinkage of the tumor.

THALIDOMIDE

The re-emergence of thalidomide as a therapeutic drug derives from its wide range of anti-inflammatory, immunomodulatory, and antiangiogenic properties and coincided with the emerging importance of angiogenesis in tumor growth and progression. Its mechanism of action is complex and probably comprises different molecular targets including the interruption of processes mediated by basic fibroblast growth factor (bFGF) or vascular endothelial growth factor

(VEGF) and inhibition of TNF-α synthesis.[78,79] Human studies suggest that thalidomide undergoes activation to metabolites with antiangiogenic activity. Thalidomide has been investigated in a variety of solid and hematologic cancers. Despite evidence of antitumor activity, a clear clinical benefit has only been demonstrated so far in patients with recurrent and refractory multiple myeloma with an overall response rate of 30%.[80]

To evaluate the single-agent activity of thalidomide in lymphoma, 19 heavily pretreated patients with recurrent or multiply relapsed lymphoma were treated with escalating doses (200–800 mg/day, orally).[81] Treatment was tolerated, with the most common side effects being peripheral neuropathy in 76%, fatigue in 52%, edema in 52%, and constipation in 41% of patients. Overall, 1 complete remission was observed (19+ months) and 3 patients achieved stable disease The 2 patients with Hodgkin lymphoma in this trial did not respond. Although this report is not clearly supportive of antitumor activity in lymphoma, the combination with chemotherapy or biological compounds may help improve outcome. It was reported that thalidomide might sensitize lymphoma cells to other agents by modulating intracellular resistance pathways such as NFκB. When rituximab was given to patients with mantle-cell lymphoma following thalidomide treatment, 10 responses out of 11 patients were obtained.[82] Current research focuses on the development of new analogues and derivatives of thalidomide with improved efficacy and reduced toxicity, with some of these drugs showing 1,000-fold higher potency than thalidomide.

MOLECULAR TARGETING USING SMALL MOLECULES

In the past few years, extensive research has allowed for a better understanding of the complex biology of Hodgkin lymphoma. The application of genomic technology might even more facilitate the endeavor to clarify molecular changes that underlie malignant transformation and cellular proliferation of this malignancy. These findings could form the basis for a more fundamental approach in the generation of novel strategies for molecular treatment of Hodgkin lymphoma. Although the pathogenesis of Hodgkin lymphoma is still not entirely resolved, it is now recognized that constitutively aberrant activation of signaling pathways, such as the NFκB pathway, is essential for Hodgkin/Reed-Sternberg cell survival.[83] The implementation of knowledge derived from recently discovered biological characteristics and pathways in Hodgkin cells led to the design of novel agents to specifically target molecular pathways that are critical for cell growth and survival in Hodgkin lymphoma.

Bortezomib (PS-341, Velcade)

Nuclear factor κB (NFκB) plays an essential role in regulating the expression of various genes involved in cell survival and apoptosis, making it an attractive therapeutic target. In resting cells, NFκB is present in the cytoplasm in an inactive form, bound to inhibitors of NFκB (IκBα, IαBβ, and IκBε). IκB is rapidly phosphorylated upon activation, undergoes ubiquination, and is subsequently degraded by the proteasome pathway.[84] As a transcription factor, NFκB increases the production of growth factors, cell-adhesion molecules, and anti-apoptotic factors, all of which contribute to tumor cell growth and protection from apoptosis.

Bortezomib is a novel dipeptide boronic acid and a specific, selective inhibitor of the ubiquitin-proteasome pathway, which plays a crucial role in the degradation of most intracellular proteins, including those that regulate cell cycle, cell survival, and apoptosis. By inhibiting the degradation of IκBα, bortezomib suppresses NFκB activation and antagonizes anti-apoptotic cascades. Bortezomib has also been reported to modify levels of other regulator proteins such as Bcl-2, Bax, XIAP, and p53, leading to cell-cycle arrest and apoptosis in several tumor types. It was the first proteasome inhibitor to enter clinical trials, where it showed evidence of antitumor activity in patients with hematologic cancers; it was approved by the FDA in 2003 for patients with relapsed multiple myeloma.[85] However, information on the activity of bortezomib in Hodgkin lymphoma is scarce. Preclinical data suggested strong anti-proliferative activity in four different Hodgkin-lymphoma–derived cell lines that occurred independently of the IκBα gene mutation status.[86] Another set of experiments investigated the potential of bortezomib in conjunction with an anti-CD30 MAb (5F11).[87] CD30 signaling is pleiotropic, and MAbs that bind CD30 can induce cell death in ALCL cells and stimulate proliferation of some, but not all, CD30-positive Hodgkin lymphoma cell lines.[88] The resistance in Hodgkin lymphoma has been attributed, at least in part, to NFκB activation upon CD30 triggering.[89] It was found that the anti-CD30 MAb stimulated NFκB activation in vitro, which could subsequently be down-regulated by bortezomib administration. When Hodgkin lymphoma tumor-bearing mice were coinjected with 5F11 and bortezomib, tumor growth inhibition was significantly more pronounced and sustained compared to either reagent alone.

Clinical data on the efficacy of bortezomib as a single agent in Hodgkin lymphoma come from two recent reports. Eleven patients with recurrent Hodgkin lymphoma were treated with 3 cycles of bortezomib, each consisting of 4 infusions (1.3 mg/m^2) of bortezomib every 3 days.[90] Treatment was generally well tolerated, with cumulative thrombocytopenia being the major hematologic toxicity. Of 8 patients who completed 3 cycles, 1 achieved a partial remission and another a minor response. In the second report, bortezomib was administered to 32 lymphoma patients including 3 with Hodgkin lymphoma using the same treatment schedule.[91] Most common grade 3 and 4 toxicities included thrombocytopenia, fatigue, anemia, and peripheral neuropathy. Although 4 of 11 patients with mantle-cell lymphoma responded (including 1 complete and 3 partial remissions) to bortezomib treatment, no other lymphoma entity including Hodgkin lymphoma showed a clinical response. These early data may indicate some clinical activity of bortezomib in Hodgkin lymphoma patients as a single agent, but warrant the investigation of bortezomib in less pretreated patients or in combination with chemotherapy or biological compounds.

In summary, bortezomib represents an excellent example of how the translation of biological progress impacts clinical advances toward a new era of rational therapeutics. Its mechanism of action and nonoverlapping toxicity profile with other therapeutics make it a very attractive compound for combined therapeutic approaches and holds promise for future integrated strategies.

CELLULAR IMMUNOTHERAPY

Patients with chemotherapy-refractory or radiation-refractory disease, especially after AHCT, have few options for a long-term remission. Cell-based strategies have been developed to augment immune responses against tumor cells through in vivo vaccination or ex vivo expansion of antigen-specific effector cells followed by adoptive transfer. Both modalities share many features, and antigen-presenting cells to induce effector responses in vivo and in vitro represent a crucial element for shaping the specificity and phenotype of the intended immune response. The cytokines necessary for augmentation and maintenance of the immune effector function and survival, the required co-stimulatory factors, and regulatory as well as inhibitory mechanisms that must be overcome to achieve tumor eradication, must be taken into consideration, whether vaccine strategies or adoptive T-cell therapy is used. However, the behavior and fate of effector cells generated in vivo can be substantially different from those generated in vitro.

Unfortunately, it is impossible to completely simulate in vivo conditions by in vitro manipulation, and there may be effector cells of a desired phenotype and function that can only or more easily be generated in vivo. On the other hand, effector cells can be generated in vitro with higher specificity and magnitude, as well as with better-defined functional phenotype. Adoptive immunotherapy may have the advantage of anticipating underlying mechanisms responsible for successful or ineffective results of a given strategy with higher precision.

Adoptive Immunotherapy

Adoptive T-cell therapy provides highly selected T-cells of a defined phenotype, specificity, and function that may influence their biological behavior in vivo. Depending on the method of ex vivo selection, stimulation, and expansion, varying degrees of uniformity with respect to antigen specificity and phenotype may be obtained, ranging from a diverse polyclonal population to highly selected T-cell clones of defined phenotype, specificity, and tumor avidity.

Epidemiologic evidence supports an Epstein-Barr virus (EBV)-related etiology in approximately 50% of patients with Hodgkin lymphoma. Immunohistochemical and molecular examination of Hodgkin/Reed-Sternberg cells revealed EBV detection in approximately 80% of patients with mixed-cellularity and 20% with nodular-sclerosing Hodgkin lymphoma, but rarely in lymphocyte-predominant Hodgkin lymphoma.[92] Adoptive immunotherapy with EBV cytotoxic T-lymphocytes (CTL) has therapeutic value, due to the association of Hodgkin lymphoma with immune deficiency including impairment of NK-cell function and cytokine production as well as in delayed type hypersensitivity and diminished responses to T-cell mitogens.[93] The transforming potential of EBV induces expression of different sets of viral genes in EBV-positive tumors such as EBV nuclear antigen 1 (EBNA1) and latent membrane proteins 1 and 2 (LMP1, LMP2), indicating a type II latency gene

expression pattern (Fig. 15.4).[94] Successful T-cell–based immunotherapy for EBV-positive Hodgkin lymphoma requires the host immune system to recognize infected cells. It has been shown that the essential components for CTL recognition are present, and viral antigens expressed in Hodgkin lymphoma are recognized by CD8 T-cells.[95]

Adoptive transfer of polyclonal EBV-specific autologous CTL into patients with advanced Hodgkin lymphoma was reported by Roskrow and associates.[96] Nine patients with relapsed Hodgkin lymphoma and 4 in complete remission after first or subsequent therapy were treated. All patients had measurable biologic responses, including 100-fold reduction of EBV-DNA, and resolution of B-symptoms with transient stabilization of disease. One limitation of this approach was the expansion of CTLs by stimulating peripheral blood lymphocytes with autologous LCL (patient-derived B-lymphoblastoid cell lines), which are known to preferentially stimulate EBNA-specific T-cells (especially EBNA3) rather than cells specific for LMP1 and LMP2. In spite of these limitations, short-term therapeutic effects appear encouraging, and further improvement of the CTL-activation strategy may allow for selective expansion of T-cells that are specific for a limited range of viral antigens expressed in Hodgkin lymphoma.

Selective expansion of LMP1-specific CTLs by stimulation of T-cells with autologous dendritic cells (DCs) as antigen-presenting cells (APCs), which were transduced with an LMP1-encoding adenoviral vector, has been successfully demonstrated.[97] However, the clinical use of LMP1 may be confined on the basis of its oncogenic and immunosuppressive potential, as well as its heterogeneity between virus strains, so that LMP1 tumor variants may not be recognized by specifically raised CTLs. Recent approaches have focused on LMP2A, which is consistently expressed on Hodgkin/Reed-Sternberg cells, and its epitopes are stably conserved between viral strains and Hodgkin lymphoma biopsy specimens. Bollard and co-workers generated high levels of LMP2A-specific CTLs by stimulation through LMP2-transduced DCs followed by LCLs overexpressing LMP2 from the same vector.[98] This approach allowed the activation of both CD8+ T-cells specific for multiple LMP2 epitopes as well as CD4+ T-cells, which favor long-term persistence in the host, which was demonstrated recently in a pilot study of 14 patients with Hodgkin lymphoma.[99] Nine patients received 4×10^7 cells/m^2, and 5 patients received 1.2×10^8 cells/m^2. Infused cells persisted for up to 12 months and homed to tumor sites. Five patients achieved a remission lasting up to 40 months, 1 had a partial

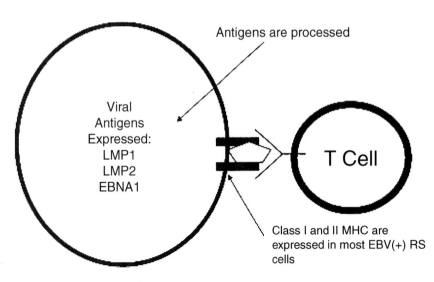

FIGURE 15.4. Epstein-Barr virus–positive Hodgkin lymphoma as immunotherapeutic target.

remission, and another 5 had stable disease. Nonresponders included 3 patients with bulky disease. CTLs were well tolerated, controlled B-symptoms, and decreased virus load.

Although adoptive transfer of autologous LMP-specific CTLs appears promising, this technique of cell-based immunotherapy is technically demanding, with extensive preclinical testing of autologous cells for each individual patient. It will also be difficult to produce sufficient amounts of cells for large patient numbers. An alternative way for the future might be to use human leukocyte antigen (HLA)-partially matched allogeneic EBV-specific CTL, the rationale being that patients with Hodgkin lymphoma have defects in cellular immunity, thus limiting tumor control. In addition, CTLs from healthy donors can be cultured in less time. On the other hand, problems with allogeneic CTLs include the risk of cell rejection and the lack of establishment of donor lymphoid chimerism, which in turn may impair efficacy. Other potential problems include graft-versus-host disease and the need to find a matched donor, because EBV antigens are recognized in the context of shared HLA molecules.

Based on studies demonstrating the clinical efficacy of allogeneic CTLs in organ transplantation, a phase I pilot study was conducted to examine the effects of allogeneic, partially matched EBV CTLs in patients with recurrent/refractory, EBV-positive Hodgkin lymphoma.[100] A group of 3 patients received 3 separate infusions of CTL (5.0×10^6 CTL/kg per dose), a second group received fludarabine (30 mg/m^2/day) for 3 days followed by a single CTL infusion (1.5×10^7 EBV CTL/kg). All 3 patients who received CTLs showed disease regression, with 1 patient remaining disease free for 22 months after infusion. Of the 3 fludarabine recipients, 2 had tumor regression, even though it was not determined whether those decreases were related to fludarabine or to CTLs, and 1 patient had stable disease for 7 months. The study demonstrates the safety and antitumor activity of allogeneic CTLs, although most patients eventually experienced disease progression. It was noted that fludarabine recipients did not have increases in antidonor CTL responses, indicating the absence of detectable donor hematopoietic chimerism, which may be required to improve clinical outcomes.

Vaccination

Tumor vaccination can be defined as an active immunotherapy, where the host is induced to generate an immune response against autologous tumor cells. The types of vaccines are variable and include those directed towards known tumor specific antigens, such as idiotype vaccines, and those that attempt to induce an immune response against presumed tumor-specific antigens by increasing tumor-specific immunogenicity. The latter include transducing genes encoding for GM-CSF into tumor cells or genes encoding for molecules such as CD40 ligand (CD40L) that enhance or induce tumor self-antigen presentation. As adoptive transfer of ex vivo generated LMP-specific CTLs has produced only transient responses in EBV+ Hodgkin lymphoma patients, multiple infusions may be required to provide long-term protection against progressive disease. Vaccination strategies to activate LMP-specific CTLs in vivo have been developed to enhance regression of LMP-expressing tumors. Evidence of clinical activity for this approach derives from an initial study that was conducted in patients with nasopharyngeal carcinoma (NPC), which represents another classic example of virus-infected malignancy characterized by expression of EBNA1, LMP1, and LMP2. Two of 16 patients immunized with autologous dendritic cells (DCs), that were pulsed with HLA A1101, A2402, or B40011-restricted peptides from LMP 2A and injected into the inguinal lymph node weekly for a month, achieved partial tumor reduction, indicating that a CD8+ driven immune response may have been induced.[101] Alternatively, a recombinant polyepitope vaccine encoding 6 adjacent LMP1 HLA A2-restricted epitopes was constructed for the treatment of EBV+ Hodgkin lymphoma and NPC.[102] The LMP polyepitope vaccine induced LMP1 epitope-specific CTLs of multiple specificities in EL4-A2/Kb tumor (express LMP1 as transgene) bearing HLA-A2/Kb transgenic mice, which were used as a quasi-Hodgkin lymphoma/NPC tumor model. The epitopes were recognized by CTL lines from HLA A2-positive healthy donors. These findings indicate efficient epitope processing by antigen-presenting cells. Immunization of HLA A2/Kb mice with the polyepitope vaccine resulted in a high degree of protection from tumor outgrowth. Ex vivo CTL analysis indicated that this protection was coincident with the generation of strong LMP1 epitope-specific responses. More importantly, the LMP1 polyepitope vaccine was not only efficient as a prophylactic therapy but also successfully reversed the outgrowth of pre-existing tumors. Besides the promising activity seen in this study, the use of a recombinant polyepitope vaccine may also overcome two major limitations of using the intact LMP1 protein as a vaccine to induce antigen-specific T-cells: (a) the risk of LMP1-induced normal cell transformation and (b) the restricted accessibility of LMP1 to cytosolic degradation pathways and therefore limited presentation through the classic MHC class I pathway. Clinical trials will be required to further validate the therapeutic value of polyepitope vaccination. Considering the immunosuppressive nature of the malignant cells in Hodgkin lymphoma, LMP1, and LMP2, CTL induction may be facilitated by co-administration of cytokines or prime boost strategies involving the consecutive use of DNA vaccines and attenuated poxvirus vectors encoding similar heterologous antigens.

PERSPECTIVES

The past few decades have seen enormous advances in the treatment of Hodgkin lymphoma. And yet therapeutic challenges still remain, particularly with respect to minimizing long-term side effects. Designing an effective salvage strategy for relapsed and refractory disease and the need to identify better prognostic markers to enable patients with poor-risk disease to be stratified towards novel therapies will be major tasks for the future. That MAb treatment can be highly efficient in Hodgkin lymphoma has been demonstrated, for example, by the use of the anti-CD20 MAb rituximab for the treatment of LPHL and rare forms of CD-20–positive classical Hodgkin lymphoma for first- and second-line treatment.[49,50] Although in these two studies high response rates have been observed, freedom from treatment failure rates might be improved by incorporating rituximab or another anti-CD20 MAb such as radiolabeled ibritumomab tiuxetan (Zevalin) or tositumomab (Bexxar) in future combined-modality treatment regimens.

Extensive research led to a better understanding of the complex biology of Hodgkin lymphoma, and the knowledge gained has already begun to form the basis for a more fundamental approach in the generation of novel strategies for molecular treatment on both the extracellular and intracellular level. The targeting of cell surface markers such as CD20 or CD30 using MAbs could be extended in the near future by several other novel compounds, which were developed for the treatment of various benign and malignant diseases. They target specific molecular pathways in order to interfere with signaling cascades critical for cell growth and survival. Because some of these pathways as well as pathophysiologic and biological features are apparently also present in Hodgkin lymphoma, interesting novel reagents, which may be of potential use for the treatment of Hodgkin lymphoma, are briefly described.

The malignant Hodgkin/Reed-Sternberg cells of Hodgkin lymphoma express several tumor necrosis factor (TNF) family receptors, including CD30, CD40, tumor necrosis factor-related apoptosis-inducing ligand receptor 1 (TRAIL-1), and receptor activator of nuclear factor κB (RANK) (Fig. 15.5).[103] Many of these survival and apoptotic pathways are currently under investigation for targeted therapy of cancer. CD40 is a member of the tumor necrosis factor (TNF) family and represents another potential target for Hodgkin lymphoma. It is expressed by malignant cells that originate from normal CD40-expressing cells, including B- and T-cell lymphoma and Reed-Sternberg cells of Hodgkin lymphoma. Besides enhancing antigen presentation and regulating cytokine and chemokine production, the activation of CD40 through its natural ligand CD40L on B-cells stimulates proliferation and Ig class switching in conjunction with other cytokines such as IL-13.[104] Several reports indicate a promotional role for resistance of B-cell lymphoma to chemotherapy. CD40 and CD40L can be co-expressed on the cell surface, and an autocrine/paracrine CD40/CD40L survival loop has been proposed to be involved in the pathogenesis and survival of B-cell derived neoplasms.[105] A fully human antagonistic anti-CD40 MAb (CHIR-12.12) has been shown to mediate potent antitumor activity by blocking CD40L binding and CD40 signaling as well as by ADCC.[106] The MAb induced stronger cytotoxic effects on CD40-expressing malignancies compared to rituximab in preclinical models of lymphoma.[107–109] In addition, these studies demonstrate the MAb's ability to work synergistically with rituximab and to ablate rituximab-resistant tumors.[110] The results from preclinical toxicology testing so far have been encouraging.

Tumor necrosis factor-related apoptosis-inducing ligand receptor 1 (TRAIL-R1) is a death receptor and another member of the TNF receptor family expressed in Hodgkin/Reed-Sternberg cells. Activation through its natural ligand TRAIL induces apoptosis, resulting in antitumor activity against many cancer cell lines including lymphoma.[111] It also acts synergistically with chemotherapeutic agents. Normal tissues usually do not express TRAIL-R1, which protects them from TRAIL-induced apoptosis and makes TRAIL-R1 an attractive therapeutic target. TRM-1 (HGS-ETR1) is an agonistic human MAb that specifically binds to the TRAIL-R1 protein, inducing apoptosis in a broad range of TRAIL-R1–expressing primary and cultured human tumor cells including cells of hematologic origin, both as a single agent and in combination with chemotherapy.[112] Early stage clinical trials are currently ongoing in patients with multiple myeloma, NHL, and solid tumors, to provide information on this novel MAb's safety and efficacy in humans.

Another target for MAb-based treatment is the receptor activator of NFκB (RANK) signaling pathway that regulates activation, differentiation, proliferation, and apoptosis of RANK-expressing cells including dendritic cells, CD4+ and CD8+ T-cells, as well as various cancer cells including Hodgkin lymphoma.[113] Signaling through the ligand (RANKL) in bone diseases has been associated with increased bone resorption, such as osteoporosis, multiple myeloma, and bone metastasis derived from various cancers. A human MAb (AMG162) that binds and neutralizes RANKL induced marked and sustained suppression of RANKL-driven osteoclast activity.[114] The MAb is currently under clinical evaluation for the treatment of postmenopausal osteoporosis, treatment-related osteoporosis in prostate cancer, and bone metastases. Engagement of RANK with RANKL has been shown to be involved in NFκB-dependent proliferation and survival of Hodgkin lymphoma cells,[115] and may therefore represent another valuable target to be investigated for the treatment of Hodgkin lymphoma.

Studies of IL-13 expression on Hodgkin lymphoma cells have suggested a key function of IL-13 as an important autocrine growth factor inducing the antiapoptotic phenotype.[116] Both IL-13 and its receptor are expressed in the majority of Hodgkin lymphoma cases almost exclusively, which is consistent with a role as autocrine growth stimulator. In fact, antibody-mediated neutralization of IL-13 in two IL-13–positive cell lines induced dose-dependent growth inhibition and apoptosis.[116,117] Currently, a human anti-IL-13 MAb (CAT-354) is being investigated in early clinical trials in patients with severe asthma, but it may also be of potential interest for the treatment of Hodgkin lymphoma.

Intracellular approaches include the application of small molecules that modulate protein function of targets or prevent expression of a respective protein using antisense technology or RNA interference (RNAi). Novel compounds have been designed to aim at intracellular pathways or cascades such as the IKK-IκBα-NFκB cascade, particularly IKK inhibitors, proteasome inhibitors, and direct NFκB inhibitors. The earlier discussed proteasome inhibitor bortezomib (PS-341) may be the most prominent reagent in this new class, holding promise for future implementation into clinical treatment concepts. Another proteasome inhibitor currently under preclinical investigation for Hodgkin lymphoma is MG-182, which was

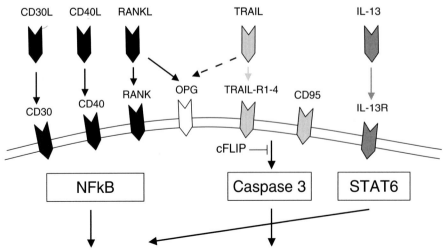

FIGURE 15.5. Members of the tumor necrosis factor (TNF) receptor family (CD30, CD40, RANK, TRAIL) and other cel-surface receptors with their respective ligands and intracellular mediators as potential molecular targets for therapy of Hodgkin lymphoma.

effective in Hodgkin/Reed-Sternberg cell lines by inhibiting critical steps of the Jak/STAT pathway.[118]

Most selective IKK inhibitors target IKKβ and are active in preclinical testing series in the nanomolar range. Well-studied molecules include the reversible ATP-competitive inhibitor SPC-839, which is a quinazoline analog, and the imidazo-quinoxaline BMS-345541, which acts as an ATP-noncompetitive inhibitor.[119,120] Effective inhibition via these compounds relies on the presence of functional IκBα molecules and might be compromised by mutational events in about one-third of cases, rendering IκBα nonfunctional. Further studies will help to identify feasible and promising strategies.

NFκB is a heterodimer composed of p50 and RelA subunits. Expression of NFκB target genes is under the influence of co-activators (e.g., p300/CBP) and co-repressors (e.g., histone deacetylases, or HDACs) that post-translationally acetylate or deacetylate the RelA molecule regulating different functions of NFκB, including transcriptional activation, DNA-binding affinity, IκBα assembly, and subcellular localization. Reversible acetylation of RelA apparently serves as an important intranuclear regulatory mechanism that further provides dynamic control of NFκB action. Direct inhibition of NFκB activity can be achieved by aiming at intranuclear events regulating the duration and level of NF B binding to respective DNA elements. Novel compounds such as MS-275, depsipeptide (FR901228), or suberoylanilide hydroxamic acid (SAHA) inhibit HDAC enzymes, interfere with NFκB-transactivating potential, and mediate apoptosis induction via p21 up-regulation, inhibition of cFLIP, or the generation of reactive oxygen species.[121–123] These compounds also favor the assembly of NFκB with its repressor IκBβ and the shift of NFκB from the nucleus towards the cytoplasm, which finally leads to down-regulation of NFκB activity. Recent data suggest that the combination of SAHA with bortezomib might act synergistically.[124] Depsipeptide and SAHA are currently under investigation in clinical trials in patients with lymphoma including Hodgkin lymphoma, and early clinical data indicate promising antitumor activity.[125]

Signal transducer and activator of transcription 3 (STAT-3) is constitutively activated in many human cancers including Hodgkin lymphoma, functions as a critical mediator of oncogenic signaling, and apparently plays an important role in cell development and death. Gene targeting represents a novel approach to inhibit expression of critical molecules involved in intracellular signaling. Ablation of STAT-3 expression was achieved with an antisense oligonucleotide (ISIS 345794), which impaired and delayed the growth of human and mouse lymphoma tumors in vivo.[126] This second-generation antisense drug has been selected for clinical trials in patients with advanced malignancies and may also serve as a valuable and promising therapeutic target for patients with Hodgkin lymphoma.

As the anti-apoptotic phenotype is one of the major characteristics of Hodgkin/Reed-Sternberg cells, implementing anti–anti-apoptotic compounds into preclinical and early clinical studies appears to be promising and a challenging task for the future. Besides acting as a caspase inhibitor, the X-linked inhibitor of apoptosis (XIAP) seems to be another attractive target for Hodgkin lymphoma, as it influences cell-cycle progression and enhances NFκB activity. Its overexpression results in a blockade of cell death arising from a number of different triggers including cytotoxic drugs, ionizing radiation, and growth factor deprivation, and antagonizes both the mito-chondria-regulated (intrinsic) and death-receptor–mediated (extrinsic) apoptotic pathway.[127] In clinical investigations, the protein has been shown to be overexpressed in a number of different tumors relative to normal tissues, and high expression was often associated with poor patient outcome and resistance to chemotherapy. A second-generation 19-mer antisense chimeric oligonucleotide targeting XIAP, constructed as a mixed backbone of chemically modified DNA/RNA nucleotides

(AEG35156), has recently entered phase I clinical evaluation in patients with malignant diseases.[128]

It seems to be clear that aberrant activation of several signaling pathways is of key importance for cell survival, and this knowledge has led to novel biologically based reagents with anticipated clinical activity in Hodgkin lymphoma. Although the pathogenesis of Hodgkin lymphoma is still largely unresolved, much has been learned in biology on transcriptional programs governing the anti-apoptotic and proproliferative phenotype of Hodgkin/Reed-Sternberg cells as well as genetic characteristics and cellular networks. The above-mentioned examples of new and fascinating strategies in the constantly evolving fields of immunotherapy and molecular biology will soon have to prove their clinical applicability in patients. Not only do these strategies represent innovative technologies and promising tools in cancer therapy, but they also serve basic science in augmenting the understanding of pathophysiologic pathways and critical regulation mechanisms of tumor cell proliferation and survival. In other malignancies, such as chronic myelogenous leukemia, small molecules such as the tyrosine kinase inhibitor STI571 (Gleevec), as the first approved drug to directly turn off the signal of a protein known to induce malignant transformation, exemplify both success and limitations of targeted therapies.

The further development of effective agents such as specific enzyme inhibitors for a variety of hematologic and solid cancers has already resulted in preclinical and some clinical investigations. Efforts to determine the appropriate sequencing and combination of these agents for the optimal treatment setting will be a crucial task. During the next several years, the exciting field of oncology drug development will thrive hand in hand with new biological findings, and will see numerous reagents emerge and pass through the different stages of the approval process. Biologically based concepts will give rise to new treatment options and will hopefully translate into improved and intertwined clinical concepts and strategies for Hodgkin lymphoma in the near future. The implementation of drugs with well-defined molecular targets may be of particular importance for patients who may be cured at high rates by standard chemotherapeutic regimens, but continue to suffer from treatment-related late toxicities.

References

1. Diehl V. Hodgkin lymphoma: a curable disease: what comes next? *Eur J Haematol* 2005: (suppl 66):6–13.
2. Canellos GP, Anderson JR, Propert KJ, et al. Chemotherapy of advanced Hodgkin's disease with MOPP, ABVD, or MOPP alternating with ABVD. *N Engl J Med* 1992;327:1478–1484.
3. Diehl V, Franklin J, Pfreundschuh M, et al. Standard and increased-dose BEACOPP chemotherapy compared with COPP-ABVD for advanced Hodgkin's disease. *N Engl J Med* 2003;348(24):2386–2395.
4. Horning SJ, Hoppe RT, Breslin S, et al. Stanford V and radiotherapy for locally extensive and advanced Hodgkin's disease: mature results of a prospective clinical trial. *J Clin Oncol* 2002;20(3):630–637.
5. Josting A, Rudolph C, Reiser M, et al. Time-intensified dexamethasone/cisplatin/cytarabine: an effective salvage therapy with low toxicity in patients with relapsed and refractory Hodgkin's disease. *Ann Oncol* 2002;13(10):1628–1635.
6. Schmitz N, Pfistner B, Sextro M, et al. Aggressive conventional chemotherapy compared with high-dose chemotherapy with autologous haemopoietic stem-cell transplantation for relapsed chemosensitive Hodgkin's disease: a randomised trial. *Lancet* 2002;359(9323):2065–2071.
7. Josting A, Wiedenmann S, Franklin J, et al. Secondary myeloid leukemia and myelodysplastic syndromes in patients treated for Hodgkin's disease: a report from the German Hodgkin's Lymphoma Study Group. *J Clin Oncol* 2003;21(18):3440–3446.
8. Behringer K, Josting A, Schiller P, et al. Solid tumors in patients treated for Hodgkin's disease: a report from the German Hodgkin Lymphoma Study Group. *Ann Oncol* 2004;15(7):1079–1085.
9. Bhatia S, Yasui Y, Robison LL, et al. High risk of subsequent neoplasms continues with extended follow-up of childhood Hodgkin's disease: report from the Late Effects Study Group. *J Clin Oncol* 2003;21(23):4386–4394.

10. Paciucci PA, Holland JF, Glidewell O, et al. Recombinant interleukin-2 by continuous infusion and adoptive transfer of recombinant interleukin-2-activated cells in patients with advanced cancer. *J Clin Oncol* 1989;7(7): 869–878.

11. Margolin KA, Aronson FR, Sznol M, et al. Phase II trial of high-dose interleukin-2 and lymphokine-activated killer cells in Hodgkin's disease and non-Hodgkin's lymphoma. *J Immunother* 1991;10(3):214–220.

12. Bernstein ZP, Vaickus L, Friedman N, et al. Interleukin-2 lymphokine-activated killer cell therapy of non-Hodgkin's lymphoma and Hodgkin's disease. *J Immunother* 1991;10(2):141–146

13. Tourani JM, Levy V, Briere J, et al. Interleukin-2 therapy for refractory and relapsing lymphomas. *Eur J Cancer* 1991;27(12):1676–1680.

14. Lim SH, Worman CP, Callaghan T, et al. Continuous intravenous infusion of high dose recombinant interleukin 2 for advanced lymphomas—a phase II study. *Leuk Res* 1991;15(6):435–440.

15. Gisselbrecht C, Maraninchi D, Pico JL, et al. Interleukin-2 treatment in lymphoma: a phase II multicenter study. *Blood* 1994;83(8):2081–2085.

16. Nagler A, Ackerstein A, Or R, et al. Immunotherapy with recombinant human interleukin-2 and recombinant interferon-a in lymphoma patients postautologous marrow or stem cell transplantation. *Blood* 1997;89(11):3951–3959.

17. Vey N, Blaise D, Tiberghien P, et al. A pilot study of autologous bone marrow transplantation followed by recombinant interleukin-2 in malignant lymphomas. *Leuk Lymphoma* 1996;21(1–2):107–114.

18. Baron S, Tyring SK, Fleischmann WR Jr., et al. The interferons. Mechanisms of action and clinical applications. *JAMA* 1991;266(10):1375–1383.

19. Einat M, Resnitzky D, Kimchi A. Close link between reduction of c-myc expression by interferon and, G0/G1 arrest. *Nature* 1985;313(6003):597–600.

20. McLaughlin P. The role of interferon in the therapy of malignant lymphoma. *Biomed Pharmacother* 1996;50(3–4):140–148.

21. Rohatiner AZ, Gregory WM, Peterson B, et al. Meta-analysis to evaluate the role of interferon in follicular lymphoma. *J Clin Oncol* 2005;23(10): 2215–2223.

22. Janssen JT, Ludwig H, Scheithauer W, et al. Phase I study of recombinant human interferon alpha-2C in patients with chemotherapy-refractory malignancies. *Oncology* 1985;42(suppl 1):3–6.

23. Koziner B. Alpha interferon in patients with progressive and/or recurrent Hodgkin's disease. *Eur J Cancer* 1991;27(suppl 4):S79–S80.

24. Leavitt RD, Ratanatharathorn V, Ozer H, et al. Alfa-2b interferon in the treatment of Hodgkin's disease and non-Hodgkin's lymphoma. *Semin Oncol* 1987;14(2 suppl 2):18–23.

25. Horning SJ, Merigan TC, Krown SE, et al. Human interferon alpha in malignant lymphoma and Hodgkin's disease. Results of the American Cancer Society trial. *Cancer* 1985;56(6):1305–1310.

26. Clark RH, Dimitrov NV, Axelson JA, et al. Leukocyte interferon as a possible biological response modifier in lymphoproliferative disorders resistant to standard therapy. *J Biol Response Mod* 1984;3(6):613–619.

27. Rybak ME, McCarroll K, Bernard S, et al. Interferon therapy of relapsed and refractory Hodgkin's disease: Cancer and Leukemia Group B Study 8652. *J Biol Response Mod* 1990;9(1):1–4.

28. Redman J, Hagemeister F, McLaughlin P, et al. Alpha-interferon treatment of Hodgkin's disease. *Proc Am Soc Clin Oncol* 1990;256.

29. Streetly M, Kazmi M, Radia D, et al. Second autologous transplant with cyclosporin/interferon alpha-induced graft versus host disease for patients who have failed first-line consolidation. *Bone Marrow Transplant* 2004; 33(11):1131–1135.

30. Hericourt J, Richet C. "Physologie pathologique"—de la serotherapie dans la traitement du cancer. *C R Hebd Seanc Acad Sci* 1895;121:567–569.

31. Pressman D, Korngold L. The in vivo localization of anti-Wagner-osteogenic-sarcoma antibodies. *Cancer* 1953;6(3):619–623.

32. Kohler G, Milstein C. Continuous cultures of fused cells secreting antibody of predefined specificity. *Nature* 1975;256(5517):495–497.

33. Nadler LM, Stashenko P, Hardy R, et al. Serotherapy of a patient with a monoclonal antibody directed against a human lymphoma-associated antigen. *Cancer Res* 1980;40(9):3147–3154.

34. Osterborg A, Fassas AS, Anagnostopoulos A, et al. Humanized CD52 monoclonal antibody Campath-1H as first-line treatment in chronic lymphocytic leukaemia. *Br J Haematol* 1996;93(1):151–153.

35. Maloney DG, Grillo-Lopez AJ, White CA, et al. IDEC-C2B8 (Rituximab) Anti-CD20 monoclonal antibody therapy in patients with relapsed low-grade non-Hodgkin's lymphoma. *Blood* 1997;90(6):2188–2195.

36. Hsu SM, Ho YS, Hsu PL. Effect of monoclonal antibodies anti-2H9, anti-IRac, and anti-HeFi-1 on the surface antigens of Reed-Sternberg cells. *J Natl Cancer Inst* 1987;79(5):1091–1099.

37. Pfeifer W, Levi E, Petrogiannis-Haliotis T, et al. A murine xenograft model for human CD30+ anaplastic large cell lymphoma. Successful growth inhibition with an anti-CD30 antibody (HeFi-1). *Am J Pathol* 1999;155(4):1353–1359.

38. Engert A, Burrows F, Jung W, et al. Evaluation of ricin A chain-containing immunotoxins directed against the CD30 antigen as potential reagents for the treatment of Hodgkin's disease. *Cancer Res* 1990;50(1): 84–88.

39. Stein H, Mason DY, Gerdes J, et al. The expression of the Hodgkin's disease associated antigen Ki-1 in reactive and neoplastic lymphoid tissue: evidence that Reed-Sternberg cells and histiocytic malignancies are derived from activated lymphoid cells. *Blood* 1985;66(4):848–858.

40. Horie R, Watanabe T. CD30: Expression and function in health and disease. *Semin Immunol* 1998;10(6):457–470.

41. Bartlett NL, Younes A, Carabasi MA, et al. Phase I study of SGN-30, a chimeric monoclonal antibody (MAb) in patients with refractory or recurrent CD30(+) hematologic malignancies. *Blood* 2002;100(suppl):362a–363a. Abstract 1403.

42. Leonard JP, Rosenblatt JD, Bartlett NL, et al. Phase II study of SGN-30 (anti-CD30 monoclonal antibody) in patients with refractory or recurrent Hodgkin's disease. *Blood* 2004;104(11):2635.

43. Bartlett NL, Bernstein SH, Leonard JP, et al. Safety, antitumor activity and pharmacokinetics of six weekly doses of SGN-30 (anti-CD30 monoclonal antibody) in patients with refractory or recurrent CD30+ hematologic malignancies. *Blood* 2003;102(11):2390.

44. Borchmann P, Treml JF, Hansen H, et al. The human anti-CD30 antibody 5F11 shows in vitro and in vivo activity against malignant lymphoma. *Blood* 2003;102(10):3737–3742.

45. Ansell SM, Byrd JC, Horwitz SM, et al. Phase I/II study of a fully human anti-CD30 monoclonal antibody, (MDX-060) in Hodgkin's disease and anaplastic large cell lymphoma. *Blood* 2004;104(11):632.

46. Diehl V, Sextro M, Franklin J, et al. Clinical presentation, course, and prognostic factors in lymphocyte-predominant Hodgkin's disease and lymphocyte-rich classical Hodgkin's disease: report from the European Task Force on Lymphoma Project on Lymphocyte-Predominant Hodgkin's Disease. *J Clin Oncol* 1999;17(3):776–783.

47. Boulanger E, Meignin V, Leverger G, et al. Rituximab monotherapy in nodular lymphocyte-predominant Hodgkin's disease. *Ann Oncol* 2003; 14(1):171.

48. Keilholz U, Szelenyi H, Siehl J, et al. Rapid regression of chemotherapy refractory lymphocyte predominant Hodgkin's disease after administration of rituximab (anti-CD 20 monoclonal antibody) and interleukin-2. *Leuk Lymphoma* 1999;35(5–6):641–642. Letter.

49. Rehwald U, Schulz H, Reiser M, et al. Treatment of relapsed CD20+ Hodgkin lymphoma with the monoclonal antibody rituximab is effective and well tolerated: results of a phase 2 trial of the German Hodgkin Lymphoma Study Group. *Blood* 2003;101(2):420–424.

50. Ekstrand BC, Lucas JB, Horwitz SM, et al. Rituximab in lymphocyte-predominant Hodgkin disease: results of a phase 2 trial. *Blood* 2003; 101:4285–4289.

51. Eiklid K, Olsnes S, Pihl A. Entry of lethal doses of abrin, ricin and modeccin into the cytosol of HeLa cells. *Exp Cell Res* 1980;126(2):321–326.

52. Strauchen JA, Breakstone BA. IL-2 receptor expression in human lymphoid lesions. Immunohistochemical study of 166 cases. *Am J Pathol* 1987; 126(3):506–512.

53. Engert A, Diehl V, Schnell R, et al. A phase-I study of an anti-CD25 ricin A-chain immunotoxin (RFT5-SMPT-dgA) in patients with wefractory Hodgkin's lymphoma. *Blood* 1997;89(2):403–410.

54. Schnell R, Staak O, Borchmann P, et al. A phase I study with an anti-CD30 ricin A-chain immunotoxin (Ki-4.dgA) in patients with refractory CD30(+) Hodgkin's and non-Hodgkin's lymphoma. *Clin Cancer Res* 2002;8(6): 1779–1786.

55. Falini B, Bolognesi A, Flenghi L, et al. Response of refractory Hodgkin's disease to monoclonal anti-CD30 immunotoxin. *Lancet* 1992;339(8803): 1195–1196.

56. LeMaistre CF, Craig FE, Meneghetti C, et al. Phase I trial of a 90-minute infusion of the fusion toxin DAB₄₈₆IL-2 in hematological cancers. *Cancer Res* 1993;53(17):3930–3934.

57. Foss F, Nichols J, Parker K, et al. Phase I/II trial of DAB₃₈₉IL-2 in patients with NHL, HD and CTCL. In: Abstracts of the Fourth International Symposium on Immunotoxins, Myrtle Beach, South Carolina, June 8–14, 1991, 159.

58. Kreitman RJ, Wilson WH, White JD, et al. Phase I trial of recombinant immunotoxin anti-Tac(Fv)-PE38 (LMB-2) in patients with hematologic malignancies. *J Clin Oncol* 2000;18(8):1622–1636.

59. Du Y, Honeychurch J, Cragg MS, et al. Antibody-induced intracellular signaling works in combination with radiation to eradicate lymphoma in radioimmunotherapy. *Blood* 2004;103(4):1485–1494.

60. Beierwaltes WH. Radioiodine-labelled compounds previously or currently used for tumour localization. In: Beierwaltes WH, ed. Tumor localization with radioactive agents Vienna, Austria: International Atomic Agency; 1974:47.

61. Witzig TE, Gordon LI, Cabanillas F, Energy et al. Randomized controlled trial of yttrium-90-labeled ibritumomab tiuxetan radioimmunotherapy versus rituximab immunotherapy for patients with relapsed or refractory low-grade, follicular, or transformed B-cell non-Hodgkin's lymphoma. *J Clin Oncol* 2002;20(10):2453–2463.

62. Gopal AK, Gooley TA, Maloney DG, et al. High-dose radioimmunotherapy versus conventional high-dose therapy and autologous hematopoietic stem cell transplantation for relapsed follicular non-Hodgkin's lymphoma: a multivariable cohort analysis. *Blood* 2003;102(7):2351–2357.

63. Press OW, Eary JF, Appelbaum FR, et al. Myeloablative radiolabeled antibody therapy with autologous bone marrow transplantation for relapsed B cell lymphomas. *Cancer Treat Res* 1995;76:281–297.

64. Lenhard REJ, Order SE, Spunberg JJ, et al. Isotopic immunoglobulin: a new systemic therapy for advanced Hodgkin's disease. *J Clin Oncol* 1985; 3(10):1296–1300.

65. Vriesendorp HM, Quadri SM, Wyllie CT, et al. Fractionated radiolabeled antiferritin therapy for patients with recurrent Hodgkin's disease. *Clin Cancer Res* 1999;5(10 suppl):3324s–3329s.

66. Schnell R, Dietlein M, Staak JO, et al. Treatment of refractory Hodgkin's lymphoma patients with an iodine-131-labeled murine anti-CD30 monoclonal antibody. *J Clin Oncol* 2005;23(21):4669–4678.

67. Herpst JM, Klein JL, Leichner PK, et al. Survival of patients with resistant Hodgkin's disease after polyclonal yttrium 90-labeled antiferritin treatment. *J Clin Oncol* 1995;13(9):2394–2400.
68. Bierman PJ, Vose JM, Leichner PK, et al. Yttrium 90-labeled antiferritin followed by high-dose chemotherapy and autologous bone marrow transplantation for poor-prognosis Hodgkin's disease. *J Clin Oncol* 1993;11(4):698–703.
69. Vriesendorp HM, Morton JD, Quadri SM. Review of five consecutive studies of radiolabeled immunoglobulin therapy in Hodgkin's disease. *Cancer Res* 1995;55(23 suppl):5888s–5892s.
70. Fanger MW, Shen L, Graziano RF, et al. Cytotoxicity mediated by human Fc receptors for IgG. *Immunol Today* 1989;10(3):92–99.
71. Sahin U, Kraft-Bauer S, Ohnesorge S, et al. Interleukin-12 increases bispecific-antibody-mediated natural killer cell cytotoxicity against human tumors. *Cancer Immunol Immunother* 1996;42(1):9–14.
72. Hartmann F, Renner C, Jung W, et al. Treatment of refractory Hodgkin's disease with an anti-CD16/CD30 bispecific antibody. *Blood* 1997;89(6):2042–2047.
73. Hartmann F, Renner C, Jung W, et al. Anti-CD16/CD30 bispecific antibody treatment for Hodgkin's disease: role of infusion schedule and costimulation with cytokines. *Clin Cancer Res* 2001;7(7):1873–1881.
74. Borchmann P, Schnell R, Fuss I, et al. Phase I trial of the novel bispecific molecule H22×Ki-4 in patients with refractory Hodgkin lymphoma. *Blood* 2002;100(9):3101–3107.
75. Ran S, Gao B, Duffy S, et al. Infarction of solid Hodgkin's tumors in mice by antibody-directed targeting of tissue factor to tumor vasculature. *Cancer Res* 1998;58(20):4646–4653.
76. Schiefer D, Huang X, Trieu V, et al. Enhanced expression of endoglin on blood vessels of human Hodgkin's lymphoma xenografted in SCID mice. *Ann Hematol* 1995;73(suppl).
77. Ran S, He J, Huang X, et al. Antitumor effects of a monoclonal antibody that binds anionic phospholipids on the surface of tumor blood vessels in mice. *Clin Cancer Res* 2005;11(4):1551–1562.
78. D'Amato RJ, Loughnan MS, Flynn E, et al. Thalidomide is an inhibitor of angiogenesis. *Proc Natl Acad Sci USA* 1994;91(9):4082–4085.
79. Keifer JA, Guttridge DC, Ashburner BP, et al. Inhibition of NF-kappa B activity by thalidomide through suppression of IkappaB kinase activity. *J Biol Chem* 2001;276(25):22382–22387.
80. Singhal S, Mehta J, Desikan R, et al. Antitumor activity of thalidomide in refractory multiple myeloma. *N Engl J Med* 1999;341(21):1565–1571.
81. Pro B, Younes A, Albitar M, et al. Thalidomide for patients with recurrent lymphoma. *Cancer* 2004;100(6):1186–1189.
82. Drach J, Kaufmann H, Puespoek A, et al. Marked antitumor activity of rituximab plus thalidomide in patients with relapsed/resistant mantle cell lymphoma. *Blood* 2002;100(11).
83. Kuppers R, Hansmann ML. The Hodgkin and Reed/Sternberg cell. *Int J Biochem Cell Biol* 2005;37(3):511–517.
84. Karin M, Lin A. NF-kappaB at the crossroads of life and death. *Nat Immunol* 2002;3(3):221–227.
85. Richardson PG, Barlogie B, Berenson J, et al. A phase 2 study of bortezomib in relapsed, refractory myeloma. *N Engl J Med* 2003;348(26):2609–2617.
86. Zheng B, Georgakis GV, Li Y, et al. Induction of cell cycle arrest and apoptosis by the proteasome inhibitor PS-341 in Hodgkin disease cell lines is independent of inhibitor of nuclear factor-kappaB mutations or activation of the CD30, CD40, and RANK receptors. *Clin Cancer Res* 2004;10(9):3207–3215.
87. Boll B, Hansen H, Heuck F, et al. The fully human anti-CD30 antibody 5F11 activates NF-kB and sensitizes lymphoma cells to bortezomib-induced apoptosis. *Blood* 2005;106(5):1839–1842.
88. Mir SS, Richter BW, Duckett CS. Differential effects of CD30 activation in anaplastic large cell lymphoma and Hodgkin disease cells. *Blood* 2000;96(13):4307–4312.
89. Horie R, Higashihara M, Watanabe T. Hodgkin's lymphoma and CD30 signal transduction. *Int J Hematol* 2003;77(1):37–47.
90. Younes A, Pro B, Romaguera J, et al. Safety and efficacy of bortezomib (Velcade) for the treatment of relapsed classical Hodgkin's disease. *Blood* 2004;104(11):2638.
91. Strauss SJ, Maharaj L, Stec J, et al. Phase II clinical study of bortezomib (VELCADE) in patients with relapsed /refractory non-Hodgkin's lymphoma (NHL) and Hodgkin's disease (HD). *Blood* 2004;104(11):1386.
92. Thomas RK, Re D, Wolf J, et al. Part I: Hodgkin's lymphoma—molecular biology of Hodgkin and Reed-Sternberg cells. *Lancet Oncol* 2004;5(1):11–18.
93. Levy R, Kaplan HS. Impaired lymphocyte function in untreated Hodgkin's disease. *N Engl J Med* 1974;290(4):181–186.
94. Murray RJ, Kurilla MG, Brooks JM, et al. Identification of target antigens for the human cytotoxic T cell response to Epstein-Barr virus (EBV): implications for the immune control of EBV-positive malignancies. *J Exp Med* 1992;176(1):157–168.
95. Yang J, Lemas VM, Flinn IW, et al. Application of the ELISPOT assay to the characterization of CD8(+) responses to Epstein-Barr virus antigens. *Blood* 2000;95(1):241–248.
96. Roskrow MA, Suzuki N, Gan Y, et al. Epstein-Barr virus (EBV)-specific cytotoxic T lymphocytes for the treatment of patients with EBV-positive relapsed Hodgkin's disease. *Blood* 1998;91(8):2925–2934.
97. Gottschalk S, Edwards OL, Sili U, et al. Generating CTLs against the subdominant Epstein-Barr virus LMP1 antigen for the adoptive immunotherapy of EBV-associated malignancies. *Blood* 2003;101(5):1905–1912.
98. Bollard CM, Straathof KC, Huls MH, et al. The generation and characterization of LMP2-specific CTLs for use as adoptive transfer from patients with relapsed EBV-positive Hodgkin disease. *J Immunother* 2004;27(4):317–327.
99. Bollard CM, Aguilar L, Straathof KC, et al. Cytotoxic T lymphocyte therapy for Epstein-Barr virus + Hodgkin's disease. *J Exp Med* 2004;200(12):1623–1633.
100. Lucas KG, Salzman D, Garcia A, et al. Adoptive immunotherapy with allogeneic Epstein-Barr virus (EBV)-specific cytotoxic T-lymphocytes for recurrent, EBV-positive Hodgkin disease. *Cancer* 2004;100(9):1892–1901.
101. Lin CL, Lo WF, Lee TH, et al. Immunization with Epstein-Barr virus (EBV) peptide-pulsed dendritic cells induces functional CD8+ T-cell immunity and may lead to tumor regression in patients with EBV-positive nasopharyngeal carcinoma. *Cancer Res* 2002;62(23):6952–6958.
102. Duraiswamy J, Sherritt M, Thomson S, et al. Therapeutic LMP1 polyepitope vaccine for EBV-associated Hodgkin disease and nasopharyngeal carcinoma. *Blood* 2003;101(8):3150–3156.
103. Clodi K, Younes A. Reed-Sternberg cells and the TNF family of receptors/ligands. *Leuk Lymphoma* 1997;27(3–4):195–205.
104. Banchereau J, Bazan F, Blanchard D, et al. The CD40 antigen and its ligand. *Annu Rev Immunol* 1994;12:881–922.
105. Younes A, Carbone A. CD30/CD30 Ligand and CD40/CD40 ligand in malignant lymphoid disorders. *Int J Biol Markers* 1999;14(3):135–143.
106. Long L, Tong X, Patawaran M, et al. Antagonist anti-CD40 antibody CHIR-12.12 causes tumor regression and prolongs survival in multiple myeloma xenograft models. *Blood* 2004;104(11):4888.
107. Tong X, Georgakis GV, Long L, et al. In vitro activity of a novel fully human anti-CD40 antibody CHIR-12.12 in chronic lymphocytic leukemia: blockade of CD40 activation and induction of ADCC. *Blood* 2004;104(11):2504.
108. Weng WK, Tong X, Luqman M, et al. A fully human anti-CD40 antagonistic antibody, CHIR-12.12, inhibits the proliferation of human B-cell non-Hodgkin's lymphoma. *Blood* 2004;104(11):3279.
109. Tai YT, Li XF, Tong X, et al. A fully human antagonist anti-CD40 antibody triggers significant antitumor activity against human multiple myeloma. *Blood* 2004;104(11):2414.
110. Long L, Tong X, Patawaran M, et al. Antagonist anti-CD40 monoclonal antibody, CHIR-12.12, inhibits growth of a rituximab-resistant NHL xenograft model and achieves synergistic activity when combined with ineffective rituximab. *Blood* 2004;104:3281.
111. Younes A, Kadin ME. Emerging applications of the tumor necrosis factor family of ligands and receptors in cancer therapy. *J Clin Oncol* 2003;21(18):3526–3534.
112. Georgakis GV, Li Y, Humphreys R, et al. Activity of selective agonistic monoclonal antibodies to TRAIL death receptors R1 and R2 in primary and cultured tumor cells of hematological origin. *Blood* 2003;102(11):799.
113. Fiumara P, Snell V, Li Y, et al. Functional expression of receptor activator of nuclear factor kappaB in Hodgkin disease cell lines. *Blood* 2001;98(9):2784–2790.
114. Bekker PJ, Holloway DL, Rasmussen AS, et al. A single-dose placebo-controlled study of AMG 162, a fully human monoclonal antibody to RANKL, in postmenopausal women. *J Bone Miner Res* 2004;19(7):1059–1066.
115. Zheng B, Fiumara P, Li YV, et al. MEK/ERK pathway is constitutively active in Hodgkin disease: a shared signaling pathway among CD30, CD40, and RANK that regulates cell proliferation and survival. *Blood* 2003;102(3):1019–1027.
116. Kapp U, Yeh WC, Patterson B, et al. Interleukin 13 is secreted by and stimulates the growth of Hodgkin and Reed-Sternberg cells. *J Exp Med* 1999;189(12):1939–1946.
117. Skinnider BF, Mak TW. The role of cytokines in classical Hodgkin lymphoma. *Blood* 2002;99(12):4283–4297.
118. Izban KF, Ergin M, Huang Q, et al. Characterization of NF-kappaB expression in Hodgkin's disease: inhibition of constitutively expressed NF-kappaB results in spontaneous caspase-independent apoptosis in Hodgkin and Reed-Sternberg cells. *Mod Pathol* 2001;14(4):297–310.
119. Re D, Thomas RK, Behringer K, et al. From Hodgkin disease to Hodgkin lymphoma: biologic insights and therapeutic potential. *Blood* 2005;105(12):4553–4560.
120. Karin M, Yamamoto Y, Wang QM. The IKK NF-kappa B system: a treasure trove for drug development. *Nat Rev Drug Discov* 2004;3(1):17–26.
121. Rosato RR, Almenara JA, Grant S. The histone deacetylase inhibitor MS-275 promotes differentiation or apoptosis in human leukemia cells through a process regulated by generation of reactive oxygen species and induction of p21CIP1/WAF1 1. *Cancer Res* 2003;63(13):3637–3645.
122. Aron JL, Parthun MR, Marcucci G, et al. Depsipeptide (FR901228) induces histone acetylation and inhibition of histone deacetylase in chronic lymphocytic leukemia cells concurrent with activation of caspase 8-mediated apoptosis and down-regulation of c-FLIP protein. *Blood* 2003;102(2):652–658.
123. Ruefli AA, Ausserlechner MJ, Bernhard D, et al. The histone deacetylase inhibitor and chemotherapeutic agent suberoylanilide hydroxamic acid (SAHA) induces a cell-death pathway characterized by cleavage of Bid and production of reactive oxygen species. *Proc Natl Acad Sci USA* 2001;98(19):10833–10838.
124. Yu C, Rahmani M, Conrad D, et al. The proteasome inhibitor bortezomib interacts synergistically with histone deacetylase inhibitors to induce

apoptosis in Bcr/Abl+ cells sensitive and resistant to STI571. *Blood* 2003;102(10):3765–3774.

125. Kelly WK, Richon VM, O'Connor O, et al. Phase I clinical trial of histone deacetylase inhibitor: suberoylanilide hydroxamic acid administered intravenously. *Clin Cancer Res* 2003;9(10 pt 1):3578–3588.

126. Chiarle R, Simmons WJ, Cai H, et al. Stat3 is required for ALK-mediated lymphomagenesis and provides a possible therapeutic target. *Nat Med* 2005;11(6):623–629.

127. Holcik M, Korneluk RG. XIAP, the guardian angel. *Nat Rev Mol Cell Biol* 2001;2(7):550–556.

128. Cummings J, Ward TH, LaCasse E, et al. Validation of pharmacodynamic assays to evaluate the clinical efficacy of an antisense compound (AEG 35156) targeted to the X-linked inhibitor of apoptosis protein XIAP. *Br J Cancer* 2005;92(3):532–538.

129. Younes A, Romaguera J, Hagemeister F, et al. A pilot study of rituximab in patients with recurrent, classic Hodgkin disease. *Cancer* 2003;98(2):310–314.

130. LeMaistre CF, Meneghetti C, Rosenblum M, et al. Phase I trial of an interleukin-2 (IL-2) fusion toxin (DAB_{486}IL-2) in hematologic malignancies expressing the IL-2 receptor. *Blood* 1992;79(10):2547–2554.

131. Tepler I, Schwartz G, Parker K, et al. Phase I trial of an interleukin-2 fusion toxin (DAB_{486}IL-2) in hematologic malignancies: complete response in a patient with Hodgkin's disease refractory to chemotherapy. *Cancer* 1994;73(4):1276–1285.

132. Vriesendorp HM, Herpst JM, Germack MA, et al. Phase I-II studies of yttrium-labeled antiferritin treatment for end-stage Hodgkin's disease, including radiation therapy oncology group 87-01. *J Clin Oncol* 1991;9(6):918–928.

SELECTION
OF
TREATMENT

CHAPTER 16 ■ TREATMENT OF FAVORABLE-PROGNOSIS, STAGE I–II HODGKIN LYMPHOMA

PETER M. MAUCH, THEODORE GIRINSKY, KAROLIN BEHRINGER, JOSEPH M. CONNORS, AND SANTIAGO PAVLOVSKY

The development of modern radiation therapy techniques for the treatment of Hodgkin lymphoma is due to the contributions of many individuals in the 20th century; only a few of these key contributors are listed below. Modern radiation therapy techniques began in the 1920s with the work of Gilbert, a Swiss radiotherapist. One of the first physicians to point out certain clinical patterns in the behavior of Hodgkin's disease, Gilbert attempted to adopt his radiation therapy techniques to these patterns. He began to advocate not only treatment of the evident sites of lymph node involvement but also of the apparently uninvolved adjacent lymph node chains that might contain suspected microscopic disease, and demonstrated that patients survived longer when using these techniques.[1]

Vera Peters, in 1950,[2] was the first physician to publish definitive data supporting the curability of early-stage Hodgkin's disease. Prior to that time Hodgkin's disease invariably had been considered a fatal illness. Treatment was mainly palliative—given to patients with advanced disease to shrink large nodes that were painful or that interfered with movement, eating, or breathing. Limited disease was not treated at all, or only with small doses of radiation. Peters reviewed the records of 113 patients treated at the Ontario Institute of Radiotherapy from 1924 to 1942 and reported 5-year and 10-year survival rates of 88% and 79%, respectively, for patients with stage I Hodgkin's disease. The similar 5- and 10-year survival rates demonstrated that patients with limited disease could be cured with a treatment approach using high doses of fractionated radiation therapy. In Peters' report, patients likely to be cured with radiation therapy had disease limited to a single lymph node region of involvement.

Dr. Henry Kaplan at Stanford University Medical Center pioneered work on the development of the linear accelerator, defined radiation field sizes and doses for a curative approach for early Hodgkin's disease, refined and improved diagnostic staging techniques, and promoted early randomized clinical trials in the United States.[3,4] His contributions lead to the standardization of modern curative approaches for Hodgkin's disease.

The development of new classification systems for histologic subtyping[5] and staging,[6] the pioneering of methods for more precise radiographic and surgical staging (bipedal lymphangiography and staging laparotomy), and the development of effective multiagent chemotherapy[7] all contributed to the curative treatment of early-stage Hodgkin's disease. From these advances, the philosophy and practice of managing early-stage Hodgkin's disease changed dramatically by the late 1960s. Early-stage patients who 10 years earlier would not have been treated now received extensive staging and radiation therapy with wide fields and high doses, resulting in the cure of a high proportion of patients.

This chapter discusses current approaches to the staging and treatment of favorable-prognosis stage I–II Hodgkin lymphoma (defined further in this chapter). Although clinical practice has based the amount of treatment on stage and extent of disease since the late 1960s, the concept of identifying prognostic factors, often independent of stage, to determine or modify treatment is a relatively new concept that has been employed since the 1980s. Chapter 17 discusses current approaches to the staging and treatment of unfavorable prognosis stage I–II disease. Both chapters examine the role of radiation field size and dose, the use of chemotherapy alone, and approaches with combined chemotherapy and radiation therapy. Prognostic factors and their influence on treatment and outcome, factors for development of late complications, and details of ongoing clinical trials are also evaluated.

RANDOMIZED CLINICAL TRIALS: META-ANALYSES OF TRIALS FROM THE 1970'S

Significant advances in the treatment of early-stage Hodgkin lymphoma have been derived from information obtained from clinical trials. These trials were first organized in the 1960s. Stanford University School of Medicine and the European Organization for the Research and Treatment of Cancer (EORTC) pioneered some of the first approaches in treating early-stage Hodgkin lymphoma, and many other groups made significant contributions. Specht and colleagues[8] reported on the influence of radiation field size and separately on the impact of adjuvant chemotherapy on long-term outcome in early stage disease in a meta-analysis of 23 randomized trials involving 3,888 patients treated in the1970s and 1980s. Some of these data had been analyzed in a previous meta-analysis by Shore and colleagues.[9] Early-stage Hodgkin lymphoma in these trials was defined as patients with clinically or laparotomy staged I–II disease, although in some cases patients with stage III disease were included. The randomized trials were divided into two groups: 8 trials compared more extensive radiation therapy to less extensive radiation therapy, and 13 trials compared multiagent chemotherapy and radiotherapy to radiotherapy alone (see meta-analysis[8] for specific referenced trials). Individual patient data including age, stage, date of entry, treatment allocation, date of recurrence, and date and cause of death or date last seen were collected for each patient randomized.

Meta-Analysis of Studies of More-Extensive Versus Less-Extensive Radiation Therapy

Eight trials evaluated treatment with larger versus smaller radiation field sizes.[8] Larger fields included subtotal nodal (mantle and upper abdomen) or total nodal irradiation; smaller fields included involved fields or in some cases a mantle field. Although approximately half the trials showed a significant advantage in disease-free survival favoring larger-field over smaller-field irradiation, survival differences were not seen in any of the studies. Figure 16.1 shows the combined risk of failure and survival by treatment in the eight trials of more extensive versus less extensive radiation therapy. At 10 years, the risk of recurrence was 43.4% for patients treated with less-extensive radiation therapy compared to 31.3% for those treated with more-extensive radiation therapy ($p < 0.00001$). Similar results were seen in subgroup analyses by stage, by use of staging laparotomy, by age at diagnosis, and by gender.

Ten-year actuarial survival rates were 77% for both groups ($p = NS$). The lack of a survival difference suggests that salvage chemotherapy for relapse after initial radiation therapy is effective enough to minimize the impact of any increase in relapse on survival. In addition, increased mortality from recurrent Hodgkin lymphoma in patients receiving smaller-field irradiation appeared to be balanced by increased mortality from treatment-related causes in patients receiving more extensive radiation therapy. Data from the metaanalysis supported this

premise; the annual death rate for patients who died of causes other than Hodgkin lymphoma was 1.18% in the more-extensive radiation group compared to 0.89% in the less-extensive radiation group.

Meta-Analysis of Studies of Multiagent Chemotherapy and Radiotherapy Versus Radiotherapy Alone

Thirteen trials compared treatment with multiagent chemotherapy and radiotherapy to radiotherapy alone for early-stage Hodgkin lymphoma.[8] Approximately half the individual trials showed a significant advantage in disease-free survival with combined chemotherapy and radiation therapy compared to radiation therapy alone; survival differences were not seen in any of the individual 13 studies. Figure 16.2 shows the combined risk of failure and survival by treatment for the 13 trials for multiagent chemotherapy and radiotherapy versus radiotherapy alone. At 10 years, the risk of recurrence was 32.7% for patients treated with radiation therapy alone and 15.8% for those treated with chemotherapy and radiation therapy ($p < 0.00001$). Similar results were seen by subgroup analysis. The 10-year actuarial survival rates were 76.5% for patients treated with radiation therapy alone and 79.4% for those treated with chemotherapy and radiation therapy ($p > 0.1$). As in the trials of radiation field size, salvage chemotherapy for relapse after initial radiation therapy appeared to minimize the impact of any increase in relapse on survival. In addition, increased mortality from recurrent Hodgkin lymphoma in patients receiving radiation therapy alone was offset by

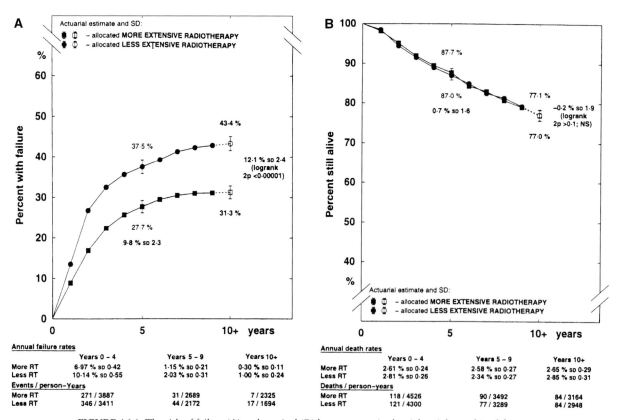

FIGURE 16.1. The risk of failure (**A**) and survival (**B**) by treatment in the eight trials combined for more extensive versus less extensive radiation therapy. (Reprinted with permission from Specht L, Gray R, Clarke M, et al. The influence of more extensive radiotherapy and adjuvant chemotherapy on long-term outcome of early stage Hodgkin's disease: a meta-analysis of 23 randomized trials involving 3888 patients. *J Clin Oncol* 1998;16:830–843.)

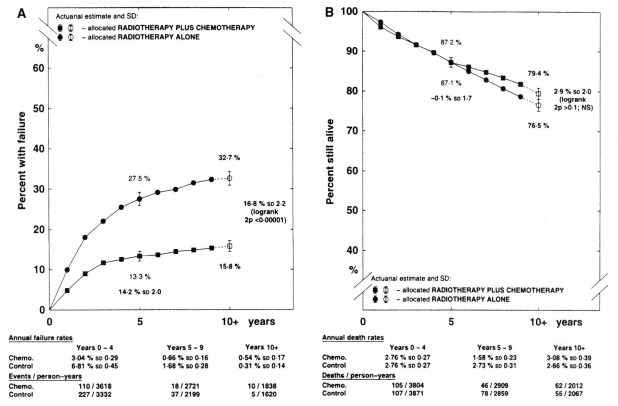

FIGURE 16.2. The risk of failure (**A**) and survival (**B**) by treatment for the 13 trials combined for multi-agent chemotherapy and radiotherapy versus radiotherapy alone. (Reprinted with permission from Specht L, Gray R, Clarke M, et al. The influence of more extensive radiotherapy and adjuvant chemotherapy on long-term outcome of early stage Hodgkin's disease: a meta-analysis of 23 randomized trials involving 3888 patients. *J Clin Oncol* 1998;16:830–843.

increased mortality from treatment-related causes in patients receiving initial radiation therapy and chemotherapy.

Most patients received alkylating agent chemotherapy (usually MOPP—mechlorethamine, Oncovin [vincristine], procarbazine, prednisone—or an equivalent) in the trials analyzed in this meta-analysis. Thus, these results are not directly reflective of current practice in which MOPP has been replaced by more effective and safer treatment regimens such as ABVD (Adriamycin [doxorubicin], bleomycin, vinblastine, dacarbazine) and by improved radiation techniques that include the use of smaller fields and lower doses.

There are also a number of potential problems with the meta-analysis format. The quality of the data, including the details of cause of death and the length of follow-up, varies from center to center. In addition, definitions were not always consistent between studies. For example, in the more-extensive versus less-extensive radiation therapy studies, the size of the radiation therapy field varied greatly in both groups. In addition, the extent of staging differed (i.e., laparotomy versus no laparotomy), patients with more advanced stage (IIB–III) were included in some studies but not in others, and there was no randomization for bulk disease. Therefore, the influence of prognostic factors (i.e., dose, age, stage, bulk of disease, number of sites of disease) on outcome cannot be addressed by the metaanalysis. However, the analysis is a powerful and important tool in addressing the general question of how the extent of treatment affects the disease-free and overall survival of patients. In all these trials, there is one consistent observation: more extensive treatment results in fewer recurrences, but does not affect long-term survival in stage I–II Hodgkin lymphoma. This observation continues to be seen in the more modern trials.

LONG-TERM OUTCOME OF TREATMENT FOR EARLY-STAGE HODGKIN LYMPHOMA USING WIDE-FIELD IRRADIATION AFTER A NEGATIVE LAPAROTOMY

Many of the long-term follow-up data for early-stage Hodgkin lymphoma are derived from laparotomy staged patients treated with radiation therapy alone in the 1970s and 1980s. Large, single institutional studies demonstrated approximately an 80% actuarial 10- to 20-year freedom from relapse and less than a 10% mortality rate from Hodgkin lymphoma following mantle and para-aortic irradiation for laparotomy staged (PS) IA-IIA patients who did not have the adverse feature of large mediastinal adenopathy.[10] Radiation therapy alone was used in many centers because MOPP chemotherapy was associated with significant toxicity (sterility, immune suppression, marrow toxicity, development of leukemia), and felt by many physicians to be too toxic to be used routinely in patients with early-stage disease. In order to identify patients suitable for radiation alone, staging with laparotomy and splenectomy was frequently performed to rule out abdominal involvement. The risk of abdominal involvement not detected by radiographic imaging was known to be 20% to 35% in patients with clinical stage (CS) I–II Hodgkin lymphoma.[11,12] Thus, staging laparotomy allowed selection of patients for radiation alone if the laparotomy was negative, and for MOPP chemotherapy and radiation if it was positive, and resulted in the cure of the majority of patients treated with these approaches.

With longer follow-up after Hodgkin lymphoma, reports began to emerge in the 1980s on the increased risk of leukemia and lung cancer from the MOPP regimen and the increase in solid tumors from the large radiation fields. During this same time, the ABVD regimen, first described in the 1970s by Bonadonna and colleagues,[13] began to be used in clinical trials and found to be both more effective and less toxic than the MOPP regimen, allowing it to be used routinely in early-stage patients.

The routine use of combined ABVD chemotherapy and radiation therapy in patients with early-stage disease also allowed radiologic staging to replace staging laparotomy. In addition, the randomized EORTC H6 trial, which evaluated the role of staging laparotomy and subsequent treatment modification in early-stage Hodgkin lymphoma, demonstrated no significant advantage in disease-free or overall survival for patients who were laparotomy staged.[14] Long-term follow-up data now demonstrate that the treatment of early-stage Hodgkin lymphoma in these studies was so successful that at 15 to 20 years post-treatment, the overall mortality rate from causes other than Hodgkin lymphoma exceeds that seen from Hodgkin lymphoma.[15–17] Thus, it is in the second and third decades after Hodgkin lymphoma that improved survival of patients with early-stage disease might be seen with modern-era reduced-treatment regimens.

There are a number of published reports that detail causes of mortality after Hodgkin lymphoma[15,17–19] (see also Chapter 23). Deaths from Hodgkin lymphoma occur most frequently in the first 5 to 10 years; causes of death other than Hodgkin lymphoma are most common after 5 to 10 years (Fig. 16.3). In one recent study, the absolute excess risk of mortality by 5-year interval ranged from 87 to 158 per 10,000 person-years.[15] Thus, on average, these patients had approximately a 1% excess risk of mortality per year over the first 25 to 30 years after Hodgkin lymphoma (Table 16.1).[15] Most of these results are from laparotomy-staged patients treated with wide-field radiation therapy with or without MOPP or MOPP-like regimens. There are some data to suggest that reduction of field size and dose of radiation and the use of modified chemotherapy regimens often without containing alkylating agents will result in a reduction of this late mortality incidence.

The three most common causes of death after treatment for Hodgkin lymphoma (Hodgkin lymphoma, secondary malignancy, cardiac disease) are discussed briefly below. These causes of death are also presented in more detail in Chapters 24 and 25. Patients who develop recurrent Hodgkin lymphoma after radiation therapy alone are as likely to be cured with combination

TABLE 16.1

EXCESS MORTALITY AFTER HODGKIN LYMPHOMA

Time after Hodgkin lymphoma (yr)	Absolute excess risk per 10,000 person–years
0–5	117
5–10	89
10–15	87
15–20	100
≥20	158

Adapted with permission from Ng A, Bernardo M, Weller E, et al. Long-term survival and competing causes of death in patients with early stage Hodgkin's disease treated at age 50 or younger. *J Clin Oncol* 2002;20:2101–2108.

chemotherapy as if the chemotherapy were used as part of initial treatment. The 10-year actuarial survival rate of patients initially treated with radiation therapy alone after relapse and treatment with multiagent chemotherapy ranges from 57% to 89%.[20,21] Survival rates appear significantly worse for patients who relapse after chemotherapy alone or combined radiation therapy and chemotherapy. Treatment with similar or alternative chemotherapy regimens after relapse from chemotherapy alone for more advanced-stage disease yields 5- to 10-year survival rates of only 20% to 32%,[22,23] suggesting cross-resistance among different chemotherapy regimens. Most of these data are from patients who initially had advanced Hodgkin lymphoma. Although few data are available, perhaps the results may be better in patients with more favorable initial stages. However, a recent study of outcomes of patients relapsing after two cycles of ABVD and radiation therapy in the early-stage German Hodgkin Study Group HD7 and HD10 trials suggests that the response to subsequent chemotherapy is inferior when compared to that seen in patients relapsing after radiation therapy alone.[24]

Because of the poor overall prognosis of patients who relapse after standard chemotherapy, many centers recommend high-dose chemotherapy (HDCT) and autologous stem cell rescue at first relapse for patients initially treated with chemotherapy or combined chemotherapy and radiation therapy. Although the

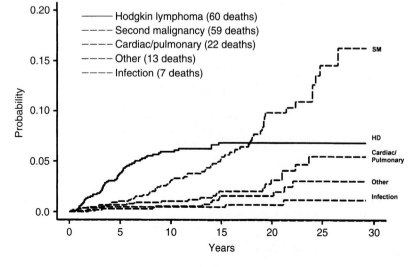

FIGURE 16.3. Competing causes of death over time in 1,080 patients with early-stage Hodgkin lymphoma treated at age 50 or younger (Reprinted with permission from Ng A, Bernardo M, Weller E, et al. Long-term survival and competing causes of death in patients with early stage Hodgkin's disease treated at age 50 or younger. *J Clin Oncol* 2002;20:2101–2108.

results of high-dose therapy are promising, some patients with recurrent disease are not eligible for this approach because of poor tumor response, co-morbid disease, or advanced age. Patients who undergo HDCT and who are subsequently cured of Hodgkin lymphoma face significant long-term treatment-related morbidity and mortality risks. Until more data are available, current information suggests that when chemotherapy is used as definitive treatment for early-stage Hodgkin lymphoma, treatment should be designed to minimize relapse. This is probably best achieved with the combined use of both chemotherapy and radiation therapy or perhaps with chemotherapy alone in selected circumstances (currently being defined in trials).

Years after chemotherapy and/or radiation therapy, patients with Hodgkin lymphoma have an increased risk of developing acute non-lymphoblastic leukemia, non-Hodgkin lymphoma, and secondary solid tumors.[25–28] This increased risk may be multifactorial, resulting both from the immune dysregulation associated with Hodgkin lymphoma and/or its treatment and the carcinogenic effects of radiation therapy and chemotherapy. Certain cytotoxic agents, especially those contained in the MOPP and ChlVPP (chlorambucil, vinblastine, procarbazine, and prednisone) regimens, are associated with a marked increase in acute non-lymphoblastic leukemia after Hodgkin lymphoma.[29,30] The total incidence of acute leukemia after these regimens, usually occurring within 10 years of treatment, ranges from 2% to 6%.[30,31] The routine use of ABVD has dramatically reduced the risk of leukemogenesis, but there remains concern for secondary leukemia with alternating or hybrid regimens. Regimens that contain significant amounts of alkylating agents known to cause leukemia should not be used in treating favorable-prognosis CS I–II patients.

Nearly all cases of non-Hodgkin lymphoma occurring after Hodgkin lymphoma are of intermediate or high-grade histology. The histologies represented are similar to lymphomas seen in patients with immunodeficiency diseases or under chronic immunosuppression for organ transplantation or autoimmune disorders. These lymphomas have a cumulative risk of 1.2% to 2.1% at 15 years.[31,32] The risk does not appear to be treatment related.

The absolute excess risk of developing a solid tumor is greater than that of developing leukemia or non-Hodgkin lymphoma after Hodgkin lymphoma. Solid tumors constitute 55% to 75% of the second malignancies in long-term studies.[25,27,30–32] The relative risk of solid tumors continues to be elevated more than 20 years after Hodgkin lymphoma.[25] Risk factors for developing a solid tumor after treatment for Hodgkin lymphoma include initial treatment with radiation therapy (solid tumors), treatment with chemotherapy (lung cancer), age at treatment (female patients younger than 35 years of age at treatment and increased breast cancer risk), and environmental factors (i.e., smoking and lung cancer).[33] Volume and dose of radiation therapy and type of chemotherapy appear to be independent risk factors for the development of second tumors. Additional data are needed to determine the extent to which current treatment reduction strategies will result in a lower second tumor mortality. However, reduction in the radiation field size will almost certainly result in a lower second tumor risk, as many of the treatment-induced tumors occur within or on the edge of the radiation field. Reduction of radiation field size is being studied in stage I–II trials that use combined radiation therapy and chemotherapy. In addition, prevention and surveillance strategies are becoming increasingly important in the routine follow-up of long-term survivors of Hodgkin lymphoma, and a number of efforts are ongoing to help define these strategies.[34]

Long-term cardiac complications have been carefully documented after radiation therapy to the mediastinum. In many of the earlier studies, these complications were related to treatment techniques that resulted in a high radiation dose to the anterior mediastinum and heart (lower-energy machines, anterior weighted fields, doses per fraction of greater than 2 Gy, treatment with one field per day). Current practice using involved-field radiation restricts the dose and volume of radiation to the heart, and has resulted in less long-term cardiac morbidity and mortality. However, even with these advances in treatment, patients will continue to be at some increased risk for cardiac disease years after Hodgkin lymphoma. Three recent studies detail cardiac risks in long-term survivors of Hodgkin lymphoma and provide recommendations for surveillance.[35–37] Although many of the patients in these studies were treated with higher doses and larger fields of radiation therapy than current practice, the data do provide guidelines for late follow-up care. Data are now emerging that indicate that patients who received mediastinal irradiation and have other classic cardiac risk factors are at significantly increased risk for cardiac disease compared to patients without risk factors.[38] This may allow development of prevention strategies to reduce the development of long-term cardiac disease.

PROGNOSTIC FACTORS

With the increasing use of combination chemotherapy in patients with early-stage disease and reliance on clinical and radiographic staging in place of staging laparotomy, it has become important to use prognostic factors to determine eligibility for clinical trials. Clinical trials in patients with stage I–II disease have increasingly evaluated treatment reduction as a strategy to reduce late morbidity and mortality for patients likely to be cured of Hodgkin lymphoma. These trials have, over the last 2 decades, defined and refined prognostic factors for favorable- and unfavorable-prognosis stage I–II Hodgkin lymphoma. Trials initially adopted prognostic factors from studies that correlated extent of initial disease with clinical outcome (see Chapter 12 for a more comprehensive review). Although many of the adverse prognostic factors have lost significance as more intensive combined radiation therapy and chemotherapy regimens have been used, these factors continue to be very important in the design of clinical trials that evaluate reduction of treatment.

Prognostic factors have been identified for stage I–II Hodgkin lymphoma that predict for a higher risk of relapse or a lower rate of survival. Many factors predict for recurrence after treatment with radiation therapy alone; fewer predict for relapse after chemotherapy and radiation therapy. Only older age at diagnosis has been consistently reported as a significant adverse factor for survival, both after radiation therapy alone and after combined radiation therapy and chemotherapy.

A number of studies have identified prognostic factors for patients with stage I–II disease, presenting an analysis of significance adjusted for other factors.[39–41] All studies report large mediastinal adenopathy or large tumor burden as a major factor predicting an increased risk of relapse; in one study a lower survival rate was seen as well.[39]

Most reports have identified B-symptoms as an important factor for recurrence and survival. A large retrospective study combining data from laparotomy staged (PS) IB–IIB patients treated at Stanford University School of Medicine and Harvard Medical School suggested that patients with night sweats without other B–symptoms treated with radiation therapy alone had a prognosis similar to that of patients with PS IA–IIA disease. However, the presence of fevers, weight loss, large mediastinal adenopathy, and age 40 years or older all independently predicted for an increased risk of relapse, and survival was impaired in patients who had both fevers and weight loss.[42] Other studies evaluating clinically staged patients have also identified B-symptoms as a risk factor for relapse.

Two other factors, large number of regions involved and elevated erythrocyte sedimentation rate (ESR), have been identified

TABLE 16.2

FAVORABLE PROGNOSIS STAGE I–II HODGKIN LYMPHOMA

EORTC	GHSG
No large mediastinal adenopathy	No large mediastinal adenopathy
ESR <50 without B-symptoms	ESR <50 without B-symptoms
ESR <30 with B-symptoms	ESR <30 with B-symptoms
Age ≤50	No E-disease
1–3 lymph node sites involved	1–2 lymph node sites involved

EORTC, European Organization for the Research and Treatment of Cancer; GHSG, German Hodgkin's Study Group.

as adverse factors for freedom from treatment failure in clinically staged patients.[40,41] Many factors, including B-symptoms (similar to ESR), male sex, number of sites of involvement, and, to a lesser extent, age, also predict for an increased risk of occult abdominal involvement in clinical stage (CS) I–II patients. This may in part explain why some of these factors are identified for clinically staged, but not for laparotomy-staged, patients. In current clinical trials, B-symptoms are often combined with an elevated ESR in defining an unfavorable prognosis.

Older patients appear to have a lower survival rate, but if treated as younger patients, do not have a higher recurrence rate. Older patients appear to be less successfully treated at relapse,[20,43] and they have a greater absolute excess risk of mortality from causes other than Hodgkin lymphoma, such as second tumors and cardiac disease. Thus, their reduced survival is both disease and treatment related. Age older than 50 years is used as the criteria for unfavorable prognosis in some current stage I–II trials.

Prognostic factors for the current European Organization for the Research and Treatment of Cancer (EORTC) and the German Hodgkin Study Group (GHSG) are listed in Table 16.2 for favorable prognostic factors and in Table 16.3 for

TABLE 16.3

UNFAVORABLE-PROGNOSIS STAGE I–II HODGKIN LYMPHOMA

EORTC	GHSG
Large mediastinal adenopathy	Large mediastinal adenopathy
ESR ≥50 without B-symptoms	ESR ≥50 without B-symptoms
ESR ≥30 with B-symptoms	ESR ≥30 with B-symptoms
Age >50	E-disease
≥4 lymph node sites involved	≥3 lymph node sites involved

EORTC, European Organization for the Research and Treatment of Cancer; GHSG, German Hodgkin's Study Group.

unfavorable prognostic factors. For the EORTC and GHSG, favorable prognosis means the absence of each of the factors listed in Table 16.2. Approximately 55% of patients with CS I–II Hodgkin lymphoma will fall into the favorable-prognosis group. For the EORTC and GHSG, unfavorable prognosis means the presence of any of the factors listed in Table 16.2. Approximately 35% of patients with CS I–II Hodgkin lymphoma will have either B-symptoms or large mediastinal adenopathy, and approximately 10% will have 4 or more sites involved without B-symptoms or large mediastinal disease. The EORTC and GHSG prognostic factor guidelines are the most commonly used factors for early-stage disease. The International Prognostic Factor Project analyzed additional prognostic factors in patients with advanced-stage Hodgkin lymphoma to determine poor prognostic groups of patients who might need more aggressive initial treatment.[44] The prognostic index is especially valuable in determining treatment for patients with advanced Hodgkin lymphoma.

Many of the ongoing and recently completed studies in stage I–II Hodgkin lymphoma were developed in an attempt to reduce the long-term complications of treatment without increasing mortality from Hodgkin lymphoma. These include studies that (a) evaluate combined radiation therapy and chemotherapy and attempt to identify the optimal chemotherapy regimen, identify the optimum number of cycles of chemotherapy, or determine the optimal radiation volume and dose when combined with chemotherapy; (b) evaluate combination chemotherapy alone; (c) and define circumstances for radiation therapy alone and define radiation dose and field size in this setting. Most of the studies discussed in the following sections have relatively short follow-up or are ongoing and would not be expected to demonstrate survival differences. High relapse rates and significant acute toxicity are the main criteria for adverse outcome.

Patients with stage I–II Hodgkin lymphoma with favorable prognostic factors are candidates for modified chemotherapy and involved-field irradiation, or in some cases for chemotherapy alone or radiation therapy alone. Patients with unfavorable prognostic factors should almost always receive chemotherapy and radiation therapy as initial treatment.

COMBINATION RADIATION THERAPY AND CHEMOTHERAPY

Randomized Clinical Trials Using Modified Chemotherapy and Radiation Therapy in Favorable-Prognosis Stage I–II Hodgkin Lymphoma

Randomized trials of combined-modality therapy are based on the premise that this approach results in a very high freedom from recurrence in early stage Hodgkin lymphoma, and that the efficacy of combined chemotherapy and radiation can be maintained even when using modified and less toxic regimens. Listed in Table 16.4 are selected trials using modified chemotherapy regimens and radiation therapy.

The first set of trials used limited chemotherapy (1–3 months) and radiation therapy. In the Southwest Oncology Cancer Group 9133 (SWOG)/Cancer and Leukemia Group B 9391 (CALGB) trial and the German Hodgkin Study Group (GHSG) HD7 trial, subtotal nodal and splenic irradiation was used in the combined chemotherapy and radiation therapy arm in part because STLI was the standard treatment at the time the trial was developed.

TABLE 16.4

CLINICAL TRIALS IN FAVORABLE-PROGNOSIS STAGE I–II HODGKIN LYMPHOMA USING MODIFIED CHEMOTHERAPY AND RADIATION THERAPY

Trial	Eligibility	Treatment regimens	No. patients	Outcome
SWOG 9133/ CALGB 9391[45]	CS IA–IIA *without:* age <16, or large mediastinal disease	A. doxorubicin and vinblastine for 3 cycles and STLI (S) (36–40 Gy) B. STLI (S) (36–40 Gy)	348	Failure-free survival (3-year) A = 94%; B = 81%, $p <0.001$ Overall survival (3-year) No difference
GHSG HD7[46]	CS IA-IIB *without:* large mediastinal mass, massive splenic disease, localized extranodal disease, ESR ≥50 mm in A, ≥30 mm in B, ≥3 involved areas	A. RT alone (STLI-spleen (30 GY) + IFRT (40 Gy) B. ABVD × 2 + RT (RT regimen as in A)	617	FFTF (2-year) A = 75%; B = 91%; $p <0.0001$ Survival (2-year) A = 98%; B = 98%; $p = NS$
Stanford V[48] for favorable prognosis CS IA-IIA HD	CS I-II *without:* B symptoms, large mediastinal disease, ≥2 extranodal sites. age >16 and ≤60	Stanford V for 8 weeks and modified FRT	87 (open)	Event-free survival (8-year) 96% (5.7 yr med fu) Overall Survival (8-year) 98%
EORTC H7-F (1988–1993)[49,50]	CS IA-IIB *without:* age >50, ESR ≥50 mm in A; ≥30 mm in B, 4 or more sites of disease, large mediastinal disease (≥0.35 M/T ratio), CS IA, NS/LP, < 40, ESR <50	A. EBVP X 6 + IFRT (36 Gy) B. STLI (S)	168 165	Relapse-free survival (6 yr): A = 92%; B = 81%; $p = 0.004$ Survival (6 year): A = 98%; B = 96%; $p = 0.156$
EORTC/ GELA H8-F	CS IA-IIB *without:* age ≥50, ESR ≥50 mm in A, ≥30 mm in B, 4 or more sites of disease, large mediastinal disease	A. MOPP/ABV × 3 + IFRT (36 Gy) B. STLI (S)	543	FFS (4-year) A = 99%; B = 80%; $p =0.001$ (52) Survival (4-year) A = 99%; B = 96%; $p = NS$
GHSG HD10[53]	CS IA-IIB *without:* large mediastinal mass, massive splenic disease, localized extranodal disease, ESR ≥ 50 mm in A, ≥30 mm in B, ≥3 involved areas	A. ABVD × 2 + IFRT (30 Gy) B. ABVD × 2 + IFRT (20 Gy) C. ABVD × 4 + IFRT (30 Gy) D. ABVD × 4 + IFRT (20 Gy)	1131	FFTF (28 mo) 96.6% (all arms) OS (28 mo) 98.5% (no indiv arm data)
GHSG HD 13	Favorable-prognosis patients	A. ABVD × 2 + 30 Gy IFRT B. AVD × 2 + 30 Gy IFRT C. ABV × 2 + 30 Gy IFRT D. AV × 2 + 30 Gy IFRT		Ongoing

RT, radiation therapy; STLI/TLI (S), subtotal nodal/total nodal irradiation (splenic irradiation); CS, clinical stage; EORTC, European Organization for the Research and Treatment of Cancer; EBVP, epirubicin, bleomycin, vinblastine, and prednisone; IF, involved field; NS, nodular sclerosis histology; LP, lymphocyte predominant histology; BNLI, British National Lymphoma Investigation; Stanford V regimen, mechlorethamine, doxorubicin, vinblastine, prednisone, vincristine, bleomycin, VP-16; GHSG, German Hodgkin's Study Group; FFTF, freedom from treatment failure; FU, follow-up; IF, involved field; MOPP, mechlorethamine, vincristine, procarbazine, prednisone; ABVD, doxorubicin, vinblastine, bleomycin, dacarbazine; GELA, French Adult Lymphoma Group; FFS, failure-free survival; NS, no significant difference.

SWOG/CALGB Study of Three Cycles of Adjuvant Doxorubicin and Vinblastine Plus Subtotal Nodal and Splenic Irradiation Versus Subtotal Nodal and Splenic Irradiation Alone in CS IA–IIA Hodgkin Lymphoma Patients

This trial met stopping rules at the second interim analysis after 348 of the initially planned 420 patients had been enrolled, with the radiation alone group having significantly more recurrences than the combined chemotherapy and radiation group (3-year failure-free survival [FFS] 81% versus 94%, p <0.001, Table 16.4). No overall survival differences were seen. There was significantly higher grade 3–4 hematologic toxicity in the patients receiving both radiation therapy and chemotherapy.[45]

The German Hodgkin Study Group HD7 Trial (1994–1998)

The GHSG HD7 study randomized patients to subtotal nodal and splenic irradiation alone or to two courses of ABVD and the same radiation therapy regimen. Among the 617 patients available for analysis, there was a significantly improved 5-year freedom from treatment failure in the radiation therapy and chemotherapy arm (91%) versus radiation therapy alone (75%, p <0.0001). No survival difference was seen.[46]

Two recent trials and two more mature trials have restricted the radiation fields to the involved regions when combined with chemotherapy. The newer short-course British LY05 trial randomized 4 weeks of VAPEC-B (vincristine, doxorubicin [Adriamycin], prednisolone, etoposide [VP-16], cyclophosphamide, and bleomycin) plus involved-field irradiation versus mantle irradiation alone and reported a 5-year FFTF of 87% (median follow-up 51 months) for the combined-modality arm.[47] The modified 8-week Stanford V (mechlorethamine, doxorubicin, vinblastine, prednisone, vincristine, bleomycin, and etoposide [VP-16]) and involved-field irradiation[48] has resulted in a freedom-from-progression (FFP) of 96% and overall survival (OS) of 98% (median follow-up 5.7 years).

European Organization for the Research and Treatment of Cancer (EORTC) H7-F Trial (1988–1993)

The EORTC H7-F trial compared EBVP (epirubicin, bleomycin, vinblastine, and prednisone) plus involved field irradiation (n = 168) to mantle and paraaortic–splenic irradiation (n = 165) for favorable-prognosis CS IA–IIA patients. Subtotal lymphoid irradiation was the standard treatment of the time and served as the control both in this trial and in the H8-F trial. The EORTC EBVP (epirubicin, bleomycin, vinblastine, prednisone) regimen (one dose per cycle or half the equivalent ABVD dose) was proposed as a potentially less toxic but similar regimen in design to ABVD. At 6 years, the relapse-free survival rate was significantly higher for patients on the combined chemotherapy and radiation therapy arm than for those on the radiation therapy alone arm (92% versus 81%, respectively, p = 0.004). The 6-year survival rate was excellent in both treatment arms (98% vs. 96%, respectively, p = 0.156).[49,50] In contrast, in the H7-U trial for patients with unfavorable disease, EBVP plus involved-field radiation therapy was inferior to MOPP/ABV (Adriamycin [doxorubicin], bleomycin, and vinblastine) plus involved-field radiation therapy, suggesting that defining prognostic factors is crucial in selecting patients for modified chemotherapy and radiation therapy regimens.[51]

EORTC/Groupe d'Etude des Lymphomes de l'Adulte (GELA) H8-F Trial (1993–1998)

This trial compared three cycles of MOPP/ABV hybrid and involved-field irradiation to mantle and para-aortic–splenic irradiation for favorable-prognosis CS IA–IIA patients. Completed in 1998, this trial shows a significant advantage in failure-free survival with three cycles of MOPP/ABV and involved-field radiation (99% at 4 years) as compared to subtotal nodal and splenic irradiation alone (80%, p = 0.001). No survival differences were seen.[52] Although very effective, the trial used a hybrid regimen, which conferred some risk of sterility and leukemogenesis in the favorable-prognosis Hodgkin lymphoma patients. In part, because of this concern, most current trials use ABVD or ABVD-like regimens.

The German Hodgkin Study Group HD10 Trial (1998–2003)

This study randomized 1,370 patients to four treatment arms: two cycles of ABVD followed by 30 Gy involved-field radiation therapy; two cycles of ABVD followed by 20 Gy involved-field radiation therapy; four cycles of ABVD followed by 30 Gy involved-field radiation therapy; and four cycles of ABVD followed by 20 Gy involved-field radiation therapy. The questions being asked in this trial are how many cycles of ABVD are needed to control occult Hodgkin lymphoma outside of known sites of disease, and what dose of radiation is needed to control Hodgkin lymphoma when combined with limited chemotherapy? This trial should give physicians further guidelines for reduction of treatment in early-stage favorable-prognosis Hodgkin lymphoma. At a median follow-up of 28 months, the 2-year freedom from treatment failure was 96.6% and the 2-year overall survival was 98.5%, with no significant differences between the number of cycles of chemotherapy or in the involved-field radiation dose (median follow-up 28 months).[53] However, in a third interim analysis with 41-month median follow-up, although there were no differences in the FFTF curves at 4 years, there appears to be a near significant increase in the recurrence rates in the 20 Gy arms (versus the 30-Gy arms) with separation of the curves after 4 years (p = 0.076) (data presented in the plenary session of the American Society of Therapeutic Radiation Oncology meeting held in Denver, Colorado, October 2005). Comparison data between the four individual arms are not available.

The GHSG 13 trial is a newly opened four-arm study comparing two cycles of ABVD, AVD, ABV and AV, all followed by 30 Gy of involved-field irradiation in CS I–II patients without risk factors. This trial is designed to determine the most important drugs in the ABVD regimen, focusing especially on the dacarbazine and the bleomycin.

Randomized Clinical Trials Identifying the Appropriate Radiation Volume and Dose When Combined with Chemotherapy

There are four trials comparing involved-field versus extended-field irradiation when combined with chemotherapy in stage I–II Hodgkin lymphoma. All the trials are in unfavorable-prognosis stage I–II patients with no differences in recurrence rates or survival seen by radiation field size.[54-57]

Two trials in favorable-prognosis early-stage Hodgkin lymphoma evaluate radiation dose to involved-field sites after chemotherapy. The GHSG HD10 trial (Table 16.4) evaluated the number of cycles of chemotherapy and radiation dose. Patients in complete remission after two or four cycles of ABVD were randomized to either 20 Gy or 30 Gy involved-field radiation (see discussion of preliminary results). The EORTC H9F trial is evaluating 36 Gy, 20 Gy, or no radiation to involved sites in patients who have achieved a complete remission after six cycles of EBVP. At July 2005, the 4-year event-free survival was 88%, 85% and 69% for the 36 Gy and 20 Gy involved-field irradiation and no-radiotherapy groups, respectively (p <0.001).

No difference was observed in overall survival at 4 years (98% vs. 100%).[58] The no-radiation arm has been closed as a high recurrence rate met stopping rules in the interim analysis and suggested that EBVP is not a sufficiently intense chemotherapy regimen to be used in favorable-prognosis stage I–II disease without the addition of involved-field irradiation. The median follow-up time (33 months) in the EORTC trial is shorter than in the GHSG trial (41 months) and is probably too short to assess potential differences between the two radiation doses.

Involved-Field Versus Involved-Node Radiation Therapy

Several groups are beginning to evaluate the use of involved-nodal versus the standard involved-field irradiation in combination with chemotherapy in order to further reduce the long-term risks from the radiation therapy component of treatment. Only very short outcome data are available and the treatment techniques are still being defined. The techniques to deliver involved nodal irradiation will likely need more technical expertise due to the need to deliver radiation therapy to a much smaller treatment volume. At present, involved field-radiation therapy remains the standard treatment technique in combined chemoradiotherapy programs (see Chapter 13 for definitions of involved-field irradiation).

Summary of Combined Chemotherapy and Radiation Therapy Alone Trials

Combined radiation therapy and chemotherapy trials have focused on maintaining a low risk of relapse while minimizing late complications of treatment through systematic reduction of both modalities in clinical trials. The success of these trials depends in part on the careful selection of patients with favorable prognostic features. Quality control in the details of delivery of radiation therapy will be increasingly important with the reduction in the amount of chemotherapy and both the EORTC and the GHSG have built quality controls into their early-stage trials. There is a tendency to publish interim analyses of ongoing trials. One must be careful not to rely too heavily on these data as the follow-up times are short and with reduction in treatment, the time to recurrence may be delayed beyond that seen with more aggressive treatment. Early results from the GHSG HD10 trial suggest that this may be the case with increased recurrences seen after 4 years in the arms that use the lower 20 Gy radiation doses.

CHEMOTHERAPY ALONE

Randomized Clinical Trials of Chemotherapy Alone Versus Radiation Therapy Alone

Two randomized trials in patients with PS I-II disease have been published evaluating MOPP chemotherapy alone versus subtotal lymph node irradiation alone. The National Cancer Institute (NCI) study was initially designed to include patients with both favorable- and unfavorable-prognosis early-stage Hodgkin lymphoma. However, the most favorable patients with PS IA Hodgkin lymphoma in peripheral sites were not included in the trial and were treated with radiation therapy alone, and patients with an unfavorable prognosis (B-symptoms, large mediastinal adenopathy, and limited-stage III disease) were included in the trial so that many of the patients did not have favorable-prognosis early-stage disease.[59] Patients were randomized to 6 months of MOPP chemotherapy alone or subtotal nodal irradiation alone. After researchers recognized that patients with massive mediastinal involvement and PS IIIA disease were not optimal candidates for the radiation therapy alone arm, the eligibility criteria were changed while the study was ongoing. Table 16.5

TABLE 16.5

RANDOMIZED CLINICAL TRIALS IN FAVORABLE-PROGNOSIS STAGE I–II HODGKIN LYMPHOMA: TRIALS OF CHEMOTHERAPY ALONE VERSUS RADIATION THERAPY ALONE

Trial	Eligibility	Treatment regimens	No. patients	Outcome
Italian prospective randomized trial[60]	PS IA–IIA	A. STLI	45	FFP (8 year): A = 76%; B = 64%; $p > 0.05$
		B. MOPP × 6	44	Survival (8 year): A = 93%; B = 56%; $p < 0.001$
NCI242[59]	PS IA-IIB *without* large mediastinal disease			
	PS IA peripheral nodes	STLI	30	30/30 FFFR; 28/30 alive
	PS IA (central), IB, IIA, IIB	A. STLI	41	FFP (10 year) A = 67%; B = 82%; $p = 0.27$
		B. MOPP × 6	41	Survival (10 year) A = 85%; B = 90%; $p = 0.68$
NCIC CTG HD6[61]	CS IA-IIA *without* MC or LD histology, age ≥40, ESR ≥50, ≥4 sites of involvement	A. STLI (S) or inverted-Y RT B. ABVD × 4–6		Interim analysis not analyzed by prognostic group. Progression-free survival was 87% with CT; 93% with RT or CMT ($p = 0.006$)

RT, radiation therapy; STLI (S), subtotal nodal irradiation + (splenic irradiation); CS, clinical stage; PS, laparotomy staged; FFFR, freedom from first relapse; MC, mixed-cellularity histology; LD, lymphocyte-depletion histology; MOPP, mechlorethamine, vincristine, procarbazine, prednisone; ABVD, doxorubicin, vinblastine, bleomycin, dacarbazine; NCI, National Cancer Institute; NCIC, National Cancer Institute of Canada; CT, chemotherapy; RT, radiation therapy; CMT, combined chemotherapy and radiation therapy.

TABLE 16.6

SELECTED RANDOMIZED CLINICAL TRIALS IN FAVORABLE-PROGNOSIS STAGE I–II HODGKIN LYMPHOMA: TRIALS OF CHEMOTHERAPY ALONE VERSUS COMBINED MODALITY THERAPY

Trial	Eligibility	Treatment regimens	No. patients	Outcome
EORTC H9-F[58]	CS IA-IIB *without* age ≥50, ESR ≥50 mm in A, ≥30 mm in B, 4 or more sites of disease, large mediastinal disease (≥0.35 m/t ratio)	A. EBVP × 6 + IFRT (36 Gy) B. EBVP × 6 + IFRT (20 Gy) C. EBVP × 6 alone (closed due to stopping rules)	229 209 130	88% 85% 69% (p <0.001)
	Trial ongoing for arms A and B; Interim 4-yr EFS data presented			
CCG 5942[62]	All stages	Patients stratified by stage into one of 3 treatment regimens. Patients in CR randomized to A. IFRT or B. no radiation	501	EFS: A = 93%; B = 85%, p = 0.0024
MSKCC[63]	CS/PS IA-IIB, IIIA *without* large mediastinal disease, peripheral or retroperitoneal nodes >10 cm	A. ABVD × 6 B. ABVD × 6 + Mantle or Inverted-Y (36 Gy); STLI/TLI for stage IIIA		FFP: A 81%; B 86% OS: A 90%; B 97% p = NS
	Trial closed early due to poor accrual			

RT, radiation therapy; STLI/TLI (S), subtotal nodal/total nodal irradiation; CS, clinical stage; PS, laparotomy staged; CVPP, cyclophosphamide, vincristine, procarbazine, prednisone; ABVD, doxorubicin, vinblastine, bleomycin, dacarbazine; EBVP, epirubicin, bleomycin, vinblastine, prednisone; MSKCC, Memorial Sloan-Kettering Cancer Center.

shows the data for the IA (central sites), IB, IIA, and IIB patients without large mediastinal adenopathy. No difference in disease-free or overall survival was seen at 10 years.

The Italian prospective trial randomized patients with PS IA–IIA Hodgkin lymphoma to receive either 6 months of MOPP alone or subtotal nodal irradiation alone.[60] There were no differences in freedom from progression (see Table 16.6). However, the survival rate was significantly higher in patients treated with radiation therapy alone (93%) than in those treated with chemotherapy alone (56%). The difference in survival was attributed to the inability to salvage patients relapsing after MOPP chemotherapy. These results are similar to the poor results of salvage ABVD in patients who relapsed after MOPP for advanced Hodgkin lymphoma (see earlier discussion in this chapter).

Both the NCI and the Italian studies demonstrated greater acute toxicities in patients who received MOPP chemotherapy. In the NCI study, more than 50% of patients treated with MOPP had at least one hospital admission for fever and neutropenia. Both trials demonstrate freedom from treatment failure rates of only 64% to 82% with MOPP alone. More modern trials are being conducted in clinically staged patients using ABVD or similar regimens without alkylating agent chemotherapy. These are discussed in the following paragraphs.

The National Cancer Institute of Canada (NCIC) and Eastern Cooperative Oncology Group CTG HD6 study is a modification of the NCI and Italian studies with the randomization of clinically staged patients and the use of ABVD as the chemotherapy regimen. Patients with nonbulky CS I–II disease were stratified into low-risk (LP/NS, age <40, ESR <50, and <3 sites of disease) and high-risk groups.[61] Low-risk patients were randomized to extended-field irradiation versus four to six cycles of ABVD, and high-risk patients were randomized to two cycles of ABVD followed by radiation therapy versus four to six cycles of ABVD. At a median follow-up of 4.2 years,

patients treated with chemotherapy alone had a significantly inferior 5-year progression-free survival of 87% versus 93% in patients treated with either extended-field irradiation or combined-modality therapy (p = 0.006). There were no significant differences in event-free or overall survival. The trial has not reported separately the results among favorable-prognosis versus unfavorable-prognosis patients. A criticism of this trial is the long time to completion of the patient accrual, so that the "standard arm," defined as extended-field irradiation, is currently no longer viewed as standard treatment. An important observation, but needing further follow-up, is that in the group of patients treated with ABVD alone who reached a complete remission after two cycles of chemotherapy, the progression-free survival rate was greater than 95%.

Randomized Clinical Trials of Chemotherapy Alone Versus Combined Modality Therapy

The *EORTC three-armed trial (H9-F)* for favorable-prognosis CS I–II patients compares six cycles of the EBVP regimen alone to the same regimen with different doses of involved-field irradiation. Patients who achieve a complete remission or complete remission undetermined after the chemotherapy are randomized to 36 Gy involved-field irradiation versus 20 Gy involved-field irradiation versus no radiation therapy (Table 16.6). This trial is designed to evaluate the role of involved-field irradiation in favorable-prognosis early-stage Hodgkin lymphoma and to evaluate potential differences in the dose of radiation delivered. At the time of the most recent interim analysis, the chemotherapy-alone arm was closed due to a higher than expected number of relapses that met stopping rules.[58] A potential criticism of this study is that inadequate chemotherapy was employed because EBVP has been shown to be inferior to ABVD when used for more advanced disease. However, this study was restricted to selected patients with favorable features, and the EBVP regimen was chosen because its efficacy in combination with involved-field radiation therapy had been proven in the earlier EORTC H7-F trial.

The Children's Cancer Group (CCG) randomized 501 patients who received a complete response to chemotherapy to involved-field radiation or no further treatment. All stages were included. The chemotherapy-alone arm in this trial has been stopped. The interim analysis showed increased recurrences in the no-radiation arm that met the stopping rules.[62] At 3 years, based on treatment received, the event-free survival was 93% with involved-field radiation and 85% without radiation ($p = 0.024$).

The Memorial Sloan-Kettering Cancer Center trial randomized CS I–IIIA patients who achieved a complete remission after six cycles of ABVD to either mantle irradiation (36 Gy) or no further treatment. Patients with large mediastinal adenopathy and nodes greater than 10 cm were not eligible; however, CS IIB and CS IIA patients were included, and so this trial was not restricted to early-stage favorable-prognosis Hodgkin lymphoma. After 152 patients were accrued at 10 years, the trial was closed due to slow accrual. No significant differences for the combined-modality versus chemotherapy-alone arm were seen in freedom from progression (86% versus 81%, respectively) or overall survival (97% versus 90%, respectively) at a median follow-up of 60 months. The trial, however, was underpowered to determine if the two treatment approaches are truly equivalent, but preliminary analysis predicts no greater than an 18% difference in recurrence-free survival favoring the radiation arm.[63]

Pavlovsky and colleagues from the *Grupo Argentino de Tratamiento de la Leucemia Aguda (GATLA)* randomized 277 patients with CS I–II Hodgkin lymphoma to receive six monthly cycles of cyclophosphamide, vinblastine, procarbazine, and prednisone (CVPP) followed by involved-field radiation therapy to 30 Gy, versus six cycles of modified CVPP alone (omission of cyclophosphamide on day 8).[64] At 84 months, the disease-free survival (DFS) of the combined-modality therapy arm was significantly higher than that of the chemotherapy-alone arm (71% versus 62%, $p = 0.01$). On subgroup analysis, the difference between the two arms was highly significant among patients with unfavorable features (age >45, >2 sites or bulky disease), with DFS of 75% in the combined-modality therapy arm versus 34% in the chemotherapy-alone arm ($p = 0.001$). Among favorable patients, the difference in DFS was not significant (77% versus 70%).

Laskar and colleagues reported results of a randomized trial from *Tata Memorial Hospital* with 6 cycles of ABVD. Complete responders were randomized to involved-field radiation therapy or no further treatment (65). Patients of all stages were included; 55% had CS I–II disease. Significant differences in 6-year event-free survival (88% versus 76%, $p = 0.01$) and overall survival (100% versus 89%, $p = 0.002$) were observed, favoring the combined-modality therapy arm. The trial contained a high proportion of pediatric patients. Seventy-one percent of cases were of mixed-cellularity histology, reflecting the high proportion of Epstein Barr Virus-related cases in developing countries.

Summary of chemotherapy-alone trials: Nearly all of the chemotherapy-alone trials are in favorable-prognosis patients. These trials have had a number of problems in design, in patient accrual, and in variations in the type of chemotherapy and field size of radiation therapy utilized. Nevertheless, most of the trials have demonstrated significantly higher recurrence rates in the chemotherapy-alone arms versus the chemotherapy and radiation therapy arms. One recent retrospective study demonstrates that the majority of recurrences after chemotherapy alone are in initial sites of involvement and that planned involved-field irradiation would have treated the site of recurrence in nearly half of the recurrences.[66] Another recent publication argues that low-dose involved-field radiation therapy is considerably safer than the higher-dose larger-field treatments used in the past, and that on balance the use of the use of adjuvant radiation may reduce toxicity by limiting the risk of relapse and allowing a shorter course of chemotherapy.[67] Given the relatively short follow-up, and the relatively small numbers of patients entered in many of the trials, significant survival differences have not been seen in most of the trials. More data are needed to understand the long-term impact of the approximately 10% to 15% increased recurrence risks with the use of chemotherapy alone in these trials.

One area of future investigation will be trials evaluating the use of response-adapted treatment in stage I–II patients.[68] Such trials would use FDG-PET to assess the response to chemotherapy and to determine whether patients should go onto radiation therapy. This approach is being used in pediatric Hodgkin lymphoma[69] and will be studied in the EORTC H10 trial.

RADIATION THERAPY ALONE TRIALS

Combination chemotherapy and limited-field irradiation or in some cases chemotherapy alone have largely replaced radiation therapy for early-stage Hodgkin lymphoma. This has occurred due to the availability of safer chemotherapy (such as ABVD), and because of the concerns for the increased risk of late second malignancies and cardiac disease after high-dose wide-field irradiation. The routine use of chemotherapy has allowed a reduction of both the dose and field size of radiation therapy. The additional benefits of the approach have been the replacement of surgical staging with radiographic staging, and the improved freedom from treatment failure with the use of both chemotherapy and radiation therapy. Included below is a discussion of the use of radiation therapy alone in the modern era, especially as it pertains to very-early-stage disease and to nodular lymphocyte-predominant Hodgkin lymphoma.

Historically, the results of STLI and splenic irradiation in favorable-prognosis early-stage patients results in a low risk of recurrence, and thus this provided the background for the clinical use of this approach as the control arm in many of the early-stage studies in the 1980s and early 1990s. Princess Margaret Hospital reported results of treating CS I–II Hodgkin lymphoma with radiation therapy alone. In a report of 250 patients, the 8-year actuarial freedom from relapse rate was 71.6%, with a median follow-up time of 6.3 years.[70] Patients with CS I–II Hodgkin lymphoma with favorable prognostic features (age <50 years, ESR <40 mm/h, and lymphocyte- predominant/nodular-sclerosis histology) treated with mantle and para-aortic–splenic irradiation had only a 12.7% actuarial risk of relapse at 8 years.

Dose–Response Data

Only one prospective randomized study has been completed.[71] The multicenter trial by the GHSG evaluated the tumoricidal doses for subclinical involvement in favorable-prognosis early-stage Hodgkin lymphoma. Patients were randomized to receive either 40 Gy extended-field radiation therapy or 30 Gy extended-field radiation therapy followed by an additional 10 Gy to involved lymph node regions. The 5-year freedom from treatment failure results favored the 30 Gy extended field plus 10 Gy arm over the 40 Gy extended field arm (81% vs. 70%, respectively, $p = 0.026$). The 5-year survival results also favored the 30 Gy extended-field arm (98% vs. 93%, respectively, $p = 0.067$). Several other retrospective and modeling studies have also suggested that 30 Gy may be sufficient for patients treated with radiation therapy alone without bulky disease.[72,73]

Field Size: Mantle Irradiation Alone in PS IA–IIA Patients

To determine the role of prophylactic subdiaphragmatic irradiation in early-stage Hodgkin lymphoma, the EORTC H-5 trial (1977–1982) compared the use of mantle and para-aortic–splenic pedicle irradiation to mantle irradiation alone in laparotomy-negative patients with favorable early-stage Hodgkin lymphoma.[74,75] This study included only patients with nodular-sclerosis or lymphocyte-predominant histology, age 40 years or younger, PS I or PS II with mediastinal adenopathy, and an ESR less than 70 mm/h. With 15-year follow-up, no differences were seen between the two treatment arms, either for cumulative treatment failure probability or overall survival. These excellent results with mantle irradiation alone in laparotomy-staged patients have been corroborated in another retrospective study.[76] In the single-arm Harvard University Medical School trial for patients with laparotomy-staged IA–IIA Hodgkin lymphoma the freedom from treatment failure at 5 years was 89% for stage IA and 80% for stage IIA disease (Fig. 16.4).[77] The 10-year survival rate was 98%.

Mantle Irradiation Alone in CS IA–IIA Patients

Results from prospective and retrospective studies of mantle irradiation alone for unselected CS I–II patients have been disappointing. The EORTC H-1 trial, one of the first studies to evaluate the role of chemotherapy in early-stage Hodgkin lymphoma, randomized clinically staged I–II patients to receive mantle irradiation alone or followed by vinblastine chemotherapy. All CS I–II patients were enrolled. Fewer recurrences were seen in patients who received both mantle irradiation and vinblastine chemotherapy. However, relapse rates were high in both groups (freedom from recurrence was only 38% in the mantle irradiation alone group, and the 15-year survival rate was only 58%), suggesting that mantle irradiation alone was not adequate treatment for unselected patients with CS I–II Hodgkin lymphoma.[70] Similarly, the Toronto series reported a 10-year rate of freedom from recurrence of only 54%.[78] These high recurrence rates in unselected patients are not surprising, as more than 20% of CS I–II patients have occult abdominal involvement, and absence of treatment (with radiation therapy or chemotherapy) to cover potential abdominal disease therefore results in higher recurrence rates than achieved with more extensive treatment. When mantle irradiation was restricted to clinically staged, asymptomatic patients with a single lymph node region involved (CS IA), better results have been seen, with 10- to 15-year freedom-from-recurrence rates of 58 to 81%.[76,78,79]

Mantle Irradiation Alone in Patients with a Low Risk of Abdominal Involvement

The EORTC defined a subgroup of CS I–II patients (women younger than 40 years of age with CS IA nodular-sclerosis Hodgkin lymphoma or nodular lymphocyte-predominant Hodgkin lymphoma and an ESR <50 mm/h) that were treated with mantle irradiation alone without staging laparotomy in the EORTC H7-VF (VF, very favorable) and H8-VF trials. This was a group of patients that would have been expected to have a low risk of abdominal involvement by prognostic factors.[11,12] In the H7VF trial, 40 patients were treated according to this concept and complete remission was reached in 95%. However, 23% of patients relapsed, yielding a 6-year event-free survival rate of 66%, a relapse-free survival rate of 73%, and overall and cause-specific survival rates of 96%.[80] The relapse rates were thought to be unacceptably high in this selected subgroup of stage IA patients. Most patients relapsed primarily in the abdomen.

In summary, in most trials the freedom from treatment failure with mantle irradiation alone in clinically staged patients is inferior to results with more extensive radiation therapy or combined radiation therapy and chemotherapy. In contrast, following a negative laparotomy, patients with early-stage disease have a very good outcome after mantle irradiation alone. In an era when staging laparotomy is rarely performed, most patients should be treated with combined radiation therapy and chemotherapy.

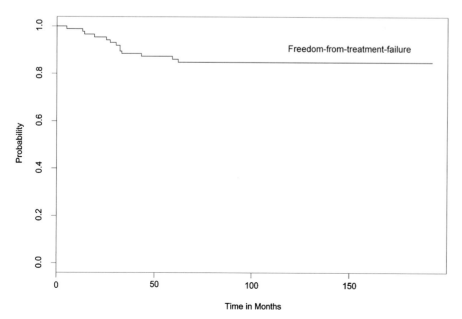

FIGURE 16.4. Freedom from first recurrence and survival of patients enrolled in the Harvard Joint Center for Radiation Therapy prospective trial for mantle irradiation alone in selected patients with PS IA–IIA Hodgkin lymphoma (unpublished data).

Regional Irradiation Alone for Nodular Lymphocyte-Predominant Hodgkin Lymphoma (NLPHL)

The preferred treatment for NLPHL is regional radiation alone (see Chapter 22). This subtype of Hodgkin lymphoma has the lowest disease-related mortality[81,82] of all the subtypes, and studies suggest that ABVD may not be as effective for NLPHL as in classic Hodgkin lymphoma.[82] In an attempt to reduce the risk of treatment-related second cancers, we and others have suggested treatment with radiation therapy alone with limited fields, usually defined as the involved nodal and adjacent prophylactic nodal regions.[82] For patients with disease above the diaphragm, it may be feasible to avoid treating the mediastinal nodes as the mediastinum is rarely involved.

INFRADIAPHRAGMATIC HODGKIN LYMPHOMA

The incidence of infradiaphragmatic Hodgkin lymphoma is very low and accounts for only 4% to 13% of cases of stage I–II disease.[83–85] Patients with Hodgkin lymphoma presenting below the diaphragm appear to have a similar prognosis to patients with supradiaphragmatic Hodgkin lymphoma when the results are adjusted for risk factors. In a study conducted by Iannitto and colleagues,[84] poorer overall survival was documented in patients with Hodgkin lymphoma below the diaphragm, but when the outcome data were adjusted for age, overall survival and RFS rates were the same for supra- and infradiaphragmatic presentations. Similar observations have just been published by Darabi and colleagues.[86] In their study, a group of 1,013 patients with supradiaphragmatic stage I–II Hodgkin lymphoma was compared to a group of 101 patients with infradiaphragmatic Hodgkin lymphoma. The group with infradiaphragmatic disease was older, predominantly male, had more frequent involvement of ≥3 lymph node areas, and mixed-cellularity or lymphocyte-depletion histology. Overall there was a higher recurrence rate in the group of patients presenting with infradiaphragmatic disease, but the adjusted hazard ratio correcting for risk factors determined that infradiaphragmatic disease presentation was not an independent adverse prognostic factor for survival or treatment failure.[86]

We recommend treating infradiaphragmatic stage I–II Hodgkin lymphoma is a manner similar to supradiaphragmatic Hodgkin lymphoma, mainly with combination chemotherapy and involved-field irradiation. In young patients, with inguinal/femoral/pelvic presentations, special blocking techniques may be needed to minimize loss of fertility.

HODGKIN LYMPHOMA IN THE ELDERLY

Elderly patients (>60 years old) have a poorer prognosis than younger patients. Although age by itself is an important prognostic factor, frailty in the aged (which can be assessed by the Comprehensive Geriatric Assessment[87]) and age-associated co-morbidities are important prognostic factors. Patients over 60 years of age presenting with Hodgkin lymphoma are more likely to have advanced disease and mixed-cellularity or lymphocyte-depletion histology. In addition, elderly patients are less able to tolerate aggressive treatment, and at recurrence have a lower freedom from second relapse and survival than younger patients. In advanced-stage Hodgkin lymphoma the expected 5-year survival rate is only about 30% to 35%. This discussion will focus on early-stage Hodgkin lymphoma in the elderly. Advanced-stage disease in the elderly will be covered in Chapter 18.

Only an international multicenter study might be able to determine the best treatment for patients in different prognostic groups and avoid either excessive toxicity or a lower dose intensity. Such a study is unlikely, as only 8% to 15% of patients with Hodgkin lymphoma are over 60 at presentation, making it unlikely such a study would be adequately powered.

Certain recommendations can be provided based on a careful analysis of available retrospective data. First, the use of combined-modality treatment is worth considering in the elderly patient because excessive toxicity, which can occur with a single modality, can be avoided. Most studies using either radiotherapy or chemotherapy alone demonstrate poor clinical outcomes. Proctor and co-workers[88] demonstrated a 40% 5-year overall survival rate in 361 patients with early-stage disease mostly treated with radiotherapy or chemotherapy (86% of patients). In that study, 40% of deaths were due to Hodgkin lymphoma. Kim and associates[89] reported a 46% and a 33% relapse rate respectively in 52 patients, also with early-stage disease and mostly treated with radiotherapy or chemotherapy (88% of the patients). In contrast, only a 20% relapse rate was observed with combined-modality therapy (used in just 5 patients). Encouraging 5-year disease-specific survival rates (73% and 97%) were also reported by Engert and associatges[90] and Levis and co-workers[91] using combined-modality therapy.

There are some data to suggest that the use of doxorubicin in the treatment regimen may benefit the prognosis of elderly patients. Weekes and colleagues,[92] in a small group of patients (15) most of whom had a good performance status, showed that adding doxorubicin to their chemotherapy regimen (ChlVPP; chlorambucil, vinblastine, procarbazine, prednisone) yielded a two-fold increase in overall and event-free survival. Engert and associates[90] showed that two cycles of ABVD or COPP (cyclophosphamide, vincristine, procarbazine, prednisone)/ABVD and involved-field radiotherapy (IF-RT) led to a disease-specific survival rate of 73%. In 59 patients, Levis and co-workers[91] used an alternative option, the VEPEMB (vinblastine, cyclophosphamide, procarbazine, prednisone, etoposide, mitoxantrone, bleomycin) regimen up front before involved-field radiotherapy (IF); 5-year overall survival and disease-specific survival rates of 95% were obtained. Engert and associates[90] showed that the percentage of patients receiving full treatment decreased drastically as the number of cycles increased (95%, 78%, and 67% for 2, 4, and 8 cycles respectively). Although compliance with treatment is not always reported, two studies[90,91] seem to suggest that two to three cycles of chemo-radiotherapy may sufficient in early-stage disease.

RECOMMENDATIONS AND FUTURE DIRECTIONS

Standard care currently provides a number of treatment options for patients with early-stage favorable-prognosis Hodgkin lymphoma (see the NCCN guidelines on Hodgkin lymphoma). These options include combination chemotherapy and radiation therapy, often with a modified number of cycles of chemotherapy and some modification of radiation field sizes and doses (preferred option); the use of mantle irradiation alone or mantle–para-aortic and splenic irradiation without laparotomy in selected patients; and chemotherapy alone. With modified combined-modality therapy, reasonable modification of chemotherapy off-study includes giving ABVD for three or four cycles. Reasonable modifications of radiation therapy off-study include involved fields to 30 Gy after a complete remission or an uncertain complete remission. Although clinical trials have demonstrated an increased risk of recurrence in early-stage

Hodgkin lymphoma after chemotherapy alone compared to combined chemotherapy and radiation therapy, trials using risk-adapted therapy with FDG-PET to select patients in early complete remission for treatment with chemotherapy alone may provide a way to reduce the recurrence risk in this subgroup of early-stage patients. Mature trial data are needed before this approach can be recommended as standard practice.

Current clinical trials are evaluating the use of alternative chemotherapy combinations, shortened courses of chemotherapy, chemotherapy with smaller radiation fields or lower radiation doses, and chemotherapy without radiation therapy. Fortunately, death from Hodgkin lymphoma in favorable-prognosis early-stage patients is unusual and mortality from causes other than Hodgkin lymphoma occurs many years later; however, this means that survival is not a useful parameter to evaluate short- to intermediate-term results in early-stage Hodgkin lymphoma. Current trials must be judged by rates of freedom from first recurrence, acute morbidity, quality of life, and cost-effectiveness while awaiting the long-term overall survival results. Trial objectives to obtain the highest freedom from first recurrence may not provide the optimum treatment once long-term (10- to 20-year) data are available; thus every effort must be taken to reanalyze trials as data become more mature. New methods in decision analysis should also help in the design of trials and in the analysis of retrospective data.

Despite the increasing availability of guidelines for the treatment of Hodgkin lymphoma, there must remain room for individualization of treatment. With different treatment options, some of which may result in a higher recurrence risk at the gain of less toxic initial treatment (without any difference in long-term survival), patient preferences must be assessed. In addition, treatment should be individualized when a particular treatment approach might result in a higher risk of serious late complications, even when these complications may not influence overall survival (e.g., treatment of young female patients with large radiation fields and the risk of late breast cancer; heavy smoking history, and risk of lung cancer).

References

1. Gilbert R. Radiotherapy in Hodgkin's disease (malignant granulomatosis): anatomic and clinical foundations; governing principles: results. *Am J Roentgenol Radium Ther Nucl Med* 1939;41:198–241.
2. Peters M. A study in survivals in Hodgkin's disease treated radiologically. *Am J Roentgenol* 1950;63:299–311.
3. Kaplan H. The radical radiotherapy of regionally localized Hodgkin's disease. *Radiology* 1962;78:553–561.
4. Kaplan HS. Role of intensive radiotherapy in the management of Hodgkin's disease. *Cancer* 1966;19:356.
5. Lukes R, Butler J, Hicks E. Natural history of Hodgkin's disease as related to pathological picture. *Cancer* 1966;19:317–344.
6. Carbone P, Kaplan H, Musshoff K, et al. Report of the committee on Hodgkin's Disease staging classification. *Cancer Res* 1971;31:1860–1861.
7. DeVita V, Serpick A, Carbone P. Combination chemotherapy in the treatment of advanced Hodgkin's disease. *Ann Intern Med* 1970;73:881–895.
8. Specht L, Gray R, Clarke M, et al. The influence of more extensive radiotherapy and adjuvant chemotherapy on long-term outcome of early-stage Hodgkin's disease: a meta-analysis of 23 randomized trials involving 3888 patients. *J Clin Oncol* 1998;16:830–843.
9. Shore T, Nelson N, Weinerman B. A meta-analysis of stages I and II Hodgkin's disease. *Cancer* 1990;65:1155–1160.
10. Mauch P: Controversies in the management of early stage Hodgkin's disease. *Blood* 1994; 83:318–329.
11. Leibenhaut M, Hoppe R, Efron B, et al. Prognostic indicators of laparotomy findings in clinical stage I–II supradiaphragmatic Hodgkin's disease. *J Clin Oncol* 1989;7:81–91.
12. Mauch P, Larson D, Osteen R, et al. Prognostic factors for positive surgical staging in patients with Hodgkin's disease. *J Clin Oncol* 1990; 8:257–265.
13. Bonadonna G, Zucali R, Monfardini S, et al. Combination chemotherapy of Hodgkin's disease with adriamycin, bleomycin, vinblastine, and imidazole carboxamide versus MOPP. *Cancer* 1975;36:252–259.
14. Carde P, Hagenbeek A, Hayat M, et al. Clinical staging versus laparotomy and combined modality with MOPP versus ABVD in early-stage Hodgkin's disease: the H6 twin randomized trials from the European Organization for Research and Treatment of Cancer Lymphoma Cooperative Group. *J Clin Oncol* 1993;11:2258.
15. Ng A, Bernardo M, Weller E, et al. Long-term survival and competing causes of death in patients with early stage Hodgkin's disease treated at age 50 or younger. *J Clin Oncol* 2002;20:2101–2108.
16. Cosset J, Henry-Amar M, Meerwaldt J. Long-term toxicity of early stages of Hodgkin's disease therapy: the EORTC experience. *Ann Oncol* 1991;2:77–82.
17. Hancock S, Hoppe R, Horning S, et al. Intercurrent death after Hodgkin's disease therapy in radiotherapy and adjuvant MOPP trials. *Ann Intern Med* 1988;109:183–189.
18. Ng AK, Hoppe RT, Mauch PM. Life expectancy of patients with Hodgkin's disease. In: Mauch PM, Armitage JO, Diehl V, et al., eds. *Hodgkin's disease.* Philadelphia: Lippincott Williams & Wilkins; 1999:585–605.
19. Hoppe RT. Hodgkin's disease: complications of therapy and excess mortality. *Ann Oncol* 1997;8:S115–S118.
20. Roach M III, Brophy N, Cox R, et al. Prognostic factors for patients relapsing after radiotherapy for early stage Hodgkin's disease. *J Clin Oncol* 1990;8:623–629.
21. Ng AK, Li S, Neuberg D, et al. Comparison of MOPP versus ABVD as salvage therapy in patients who relapse after radiation therapy alone for Hodgkin's disease. *Ann Oncol* 2004; 15:270–275.
22. Santoro A, Bonfante V, Bonadonna G. Salvage chemotherapy with ABVD in MOPP-resistant Hodgkin's disease. *Ann Intern Med* 1982;96:139–143.
23. Longo D, Duffey P, Young R, et al. Conventional-dose salvage combination chemotherapy in patients relapsing with Hodgkin's disease after combination chemotherapy: the low probability for cure. *J Clin Oncol* 1992;10:210–218.
24. Josting A, Franklin J, Sieniawski M, et al. Outcome of patients progressing or relapsing after primary treatment with two cycles of chemotherapy and radiotherapy for early stage favorable Hodgkin's disease. *Blood* 2005;106:241a
25. Ng A, Bernardo M, Weller E, et al. Second malignancy after Hodgkin's disease treated with radiation therapy with or without chemotherapy: long-term risks and risk factors. *Blood* 2002;100:1989.
26. Swerdlow A, Barber J, Hudson F, et al. Risk of second malignancy after Hodgkin's disease in collaborative British cohort: the relation to age at treatment. *J Clin Oncol* 2000;18:498–509.
27. van Leeuwen F, Klokman W, Veer M, et al. Long-term risk of second malignancy in survivors of Hodgkin's disease treated during adolescence or young adulthood. *J Clin Oncol* 2000;18:487–497.
28. Cutuli B, Borel C, Dhermain F, et al. Breast cancer occurred after treatment for Hodgkin's disease: analysis of 133 cases. *Radiother Oncol* 2001;59:547–555.
29. van Leeuwen F, Chorus A, van den Belt-Dusebout A, et al. Leukemia risk following Hodgkin's disease: relation to cumulative dose of alkylating agents, treatment with teniposide combinations, number and episodes of chemotherapy, and bone marrow damage. *J Clin Oncol* 1994;12:1063–1073.
30. van Leeuwen FE, Swerdlow AJ, Valagussa P, et al. Hodgkin's disease. In: Mauch PM, Armitage JO, Diehl V, et al., eds. *Hodgkin's disease.* Philadelphia: Lippincott Williams & Wilkins; 1999:607–632.
31. Tucker M, Coleman C, Cox R, et al. Risk of second cancers after treatment for Hodgkin's disease. *N Engl J Med* 1988;318:76–81.
32. Swerdlow A, Douglas A, Hudson G, et al. Risk of second primary cancers after Hodgkin's disease by type of treatment: analysis of 2846 patients in the British National Lymphoma Investigation. *Br Med J* 1992;304:1137–1148.
33. Swerdlow A, Schoemaker M, Allerton R, et al. Lung cancer after Hodgkin's disease: a nested case-control study of the relation to treatment. *J Clin Oncol* 2001;19:1610–618.
34. Mauch P. Late effects after Hodgkin's disease: recommendations from the Rockefeller Foundation sponsored workshop on reducing mortality and improving quality of life in long-term survivors of Hodgkin's disease (held in Bellagio, Italy, July 9 through July 16th, 2003). *Eur J Haematol* 2004; 73(suppl 65):23–24.
35. Adams MJ, Lipsitz SR, Colan SD, et al. Cardiovascular status in long-term survivors of Hodgkin's disease treated with chest radiotherapy. *J Clin Oncol* 2004; 22:3139–3148.
36. Heidenreich PA, Hancock SL, Lee BK, et al: Asymptomatic cardiac disease following mediastinal irradiation. *J Am Coll Cardiol* 2003;42:743–749.
37. Hull, M.C., et al., Valvular dysfunction and carotid, subclavian, and coronary artery disease in survivors of Hodgkin lymphoma treated with radiation therapy. *JAMA* 2003; 290:2831–2837.
38. Strasser JF, Li S, Neuberg D, et al. Late cardiac toxicity after mediastinal radiation therapy for Hodgkin's disease. *Int J Radiat Oncol Biol Phys* 2004;60(suppl 1):S216–S217.
39. Specht L, Nordentoft A, Cold S, et al. Tumor burden as the most important prognostic factor in early stage Hodgkin's disease. Relations to other prognostic factors and implications for choice of treatment. *Cancer* 1988;61:1719–1727.
40. Tubiana M, Henry-Amar M, Carde P, et al. Toward comprehensive management tailored to prognostic factors of patients with clinical stages I and II in Hodgkin's disease. The EORTC Lymphoma Group controlled clinical trials:1964–1987. *Blood* 1989;73:47–56.
41. Gospodarowicz M, Sutcliffe S, Clark R, et al. Analysis of supradiaphragmatic clinical stage I and II Hodgkin's disease treated with radiation alone. *Int J Radiat Oncol Biol Phys* 1992;22:859–865.
42. Crnkovich M, Leopold K, Hoppe R, et al. Stage I to IIB Hodgkin's disease: the combined experience at Stanford University and the Joint Center for Radiation Therapy. *J Clin Oncol* 1987;5:1041–1049.

43. Healey E, Tarbell N, Kalish L, et al. Prognostic factors for patients with Hodgkin's disease in first relapse. *Cancer* 1993;71:2613–2620.
44. Hasenclever D, Diehl V. A prognostic score for advanced Hodgkin's disease. International Prognostic Factors Project on Advanced Hodgkin's Disease. *N Engl J Med* 1998;339:1506–1514.
45. Press O, LeBlanc M, Lichter A, et al. Phase III randomized intergroup trial of subtotal lymphoid irradiation versus doxorubicin, vinblastine, and subtotal lymphoid irradiation for stage IA to IIA Hodgkin's disease. *J Clin Oncol* 2001;19:4238–4244.
46. Sieber M, Franklin J, Tesch H, et al. Two cycles ABVD plus extended field radiotherapy is superior to radiotherapy alone in early stage Hodgkin's disease: results of the German Hodgkin's Lymphoma Study Group (GHSG) trial HD7. *Blood* 2002;100:A341.
47. Radford JA, Williams MV, Hancock BW, et al. Minimal initial chemotherapy plus involved field radiotherapy (RT) vs mantle field RT for clinical stage IA/IIA supradiaphragmatic Hodgkin's disease (HD). Results of the UK Lymphoma Group LY07 trial. *Eur J Haematol* 2004;73:E08a.
48. Horning SJ, Hoppe RT, Advani R, et al. Efficacy and late effects of Stanford V chemotherapy and radiotherapy in untreated Hodgkin's disease: mature data in early and advanced stage patients. *Blood* 2004;104:308.
49. Noordijk E, Carde P, Hagenbeek A, et al. Combination of radiotherapy and chemotherapy is advisable in all patients with clinical stage I-II Hodgkin's disease. Six-year results of the EORTC-GPMC controlled clinical trials "H7-VF," "H7-F," and "H7-U." *Int J Radiat Oncol Biol Phys* 1997;39:173. Abstract.
50. Carde P, Noordijk E, Hagenbeek A, et al. Superiority of EBVP chemotherapy in combination with involved field irradiation over subtotal nodal irradiation in favor-able clinical stage I-II Hodgkin's disease: The EORTCGPMC H7F randomized trial. *Proc Am Soc Clin Oncol* 1997;16:13.
51. Carde P, Noordijk N, Hagenbeek A, et al. Superiority of MOPP/ABV over EBVP in combination with involved field irradiation in unfavorable clinical stage I-II Hodgkin's disease: the EORTC H7U randomized trial. *Proc Am Soc Clin Oncol* 1993;12:362.
52. Hagenbeek A, Eghbali H, Ferme C, et al. Three cycles of MOPP/ABV (M/A) hybrid and involved-field irradiation is more effective than subtotal nodal irradiation (STNI) in favorable supradiaphragmatic clinical stages (CS) I-I Hodgkin's disease (HD): preliminary results of the EORTC-GELA H8-F randomized trial in 543 patients. *Blood* 2000;96:575a.
53. Diehl V, Brilliant C, Engert A, et al: Reduction of combined modality treatment intensity in early stage Hodgkin's lymphoma, interim analysis of HD10 trial of GHSG. *Eur J Haematol* 2004;73:E03a.
54. Ferme C, Eghabali H, Hagenbeek A, et al. MOPP/ABV (M/A) hybrid and irradiation in unfavorable supradiaphragmatic clinical stages (CS) I-II Hodgkin's disease (HD): comparison of three treatment modalities. Preliminary results of the EORTC-GELA H8-U randomized trial in 995 patients. *Blood* 2000;96:576a.
55. Zittoun R, Audebert A, Hoerni B, et al. Extended versus involved field irradiation combined with MOPP chemotherapy in early clinical stages of Hodgkin's disease. *J Clin Oncol* 1985;3:207–214.
56. Bonadonna G, Bonfante V, Viviane S, et al. ABVD plus subtotal nodal versus involved field radiotherapy in early stage Hodgkin's disease: long term results. *J Clin Oncol* 2004; 22:2835–2841.
57. Engert A, Schiller P, Josting A, et al. Involved field radiotherapy is equally effective and less toxic compared with extended field radiotherapy after four cycles of chemotherapy in patients with early stage unfavorable Hodgkin's lymphoma. Results of the trial of the German Hodgkin's Lymphoma Study Group. *J Clin Oncol* 2003; 21:3601–3608.
58. Thomas J, Ferme C, Noordijk E, et al: Six cycles of EBVP followed by 36Gy involved-field irradiation vs. no irradiation in favourable supradiaphragmatic clinical stage I-II Hodgkin's lymphoma: the EORTC-GELA strategy in 771 patients. *Eur J Haematol* 2004;73:40.
59. Longo D, Glatstein E, Duffey P, et al. Radiation therapy versus combination chemotherapy in the treatment of early stage Hodgkin's disease: seven-year results of a prospective randomized trial. *J Clin Oncol* 1991;9: 906–917.
60. Biti G, Cimino G, Cartoni C, et al. Extended-field radio-therapy is superior to MOPP chemotherapy for the treatment of pathologic stage I-IIA Hodgkin's disease: eight-year update of an Italian prospective randomized study. *J Clin Oncol* 1992;10:378–382.
61. Meyer R, Gospodarowicz M, Connors J, et al. A randomized phase III comparison of single-modality ABVD with a strategy that includes radiation therapy in patients with early-stage Hodgkins disease: the HD-6 trial of the National Cancer Institute of Canada Clinical Trials Group (Eastern Cooperative Oncology Group trial JHD06). *Blood* 2004;102:A81.
62. Nachman J, Sposto R, Herzog P, et al. Randomized comparison of low-dose involved-field radiotherapy and no radiotherapy for children with Hodgkin's disease who achieve a complete response to chemotherapy. *J Clin Oncol* 2002;20:3755–3767.
63. Straus DJ, Portlock CS, Qin J, et al. Results of a prospective randomized clinical trial of doxorubicin, bleomycin, vinblastine and dacarbazine (ABVD) followed by radiation therapy (RT) vs. ABVD alone for stages I, II and IIIA non bulky Hodgkin's disease. *Blood* 2004;104:3483–3489.
64. Pavlovsky S, Maschio M, Santarelli MT, et al. Randomized trial of chemotherapy versus chemotherapy plus radiotherapy for stage I-II Hodgkin's disease. *J Natl Cancer Inst* 1988;80:1466–1473.
65. Laskar S, Gupta T, Vimal S, et al. Consolidation radiation after complete remission in Hodgkin's disease following six cycles of doxorubicin, bleomycin, vinblastine, and dacarbazine chemotherapy: is there a need? *J Clin Oncol* 2004; 22:62–68.
66. Shahidi M, Kamangari N, Ashley S, et al. Site of relapse after chemotherapy alone for stage I and II Hodgkin's disease. *Radiother Oncol* 2006;78: 1–5.
67. Yahalom J. Don't throw out the baby with the bathwater: on optimizing cure and reducing toxicity in Hodgkin's lymphoma. *J Clin Oncol* 2006;24: 544–548.
68. Hutchings M, Loft A, Hansen, et al. FDG-PET after 2 cycles of chemotherapy predicts treatment failure and progression free survival in Hodgkin lymphoma. *Blood* 2006;107:52–62.
69. Mauz-Koerholz CG, Kluge R, Sorge R, et al. Response adapted therapy: using FDG-PET after chemotherapy in order to restrict indication for radiotherapy in children and adolescents with early stages of Hodgkin's lymphoma. *Blood* 2005;106:750a.
70. Gospodarowicz MK, Sutcliffe SB, Bergsagel DE, et al. Radiation therapy in clinical stage I and II Hodgkin's disease. The Princess Margaret Hospital Lymphoma Group. *Eur J Cancer* 1992;28A:1841–1846.
71. Duhmke E, Diehl V, Loeffler M, et al. Randomized trial with early-stage Hodgkin's disease testing 30 Gy vs. 40 Gy extended field radiotherapy alone. *Int J Radiat Oncol Biol Phys* 1996;36:305–310.
72. Schewe K, Reavis J, Kun L, et al. Total dose, fraction size, and tumor volume in the local control of Hodgkin's disease. *Int J Radiat Oncol Biol Phys* 1988;15:25–28.
73. Vijayakumar S, Myrianthopoulos L. An updated dose-response analysis in Hodgkin's disease. *Radiother Oncol* 1992;24:1–13.
74. Tubiana M, Henri-Amar M, Hayat M, et al. The EORTC treatment of early stages of Hodgkin's disease: the role of radiotherapy. *Int J Radiat Oncol Biol Phys* 1984;10:197–210.
75. Carde P, Burgers J, Henry-Amar M, et al. Clinical stages I and II Hodgkin's disease: a specifically tailored therapy according to prognostic factors. *J Clin Oncol* 1988;6:239–252.
76. Ganesan T, Wrigley P, Murray P, et al. Radiotherapy for stage I Hodgkin's disease:20 years of experience at St Bartholomew's Hospital. *Br J Cancer* 1990;62:314–318.
77. Ng A, Li S, Neuberg D, et al. Long-term results of a prospective trial of mantle irradiation alone for early stage Hodgkin's disease. *Int J Radiat Oncol Biol Phys* 2005;63:S45–S46.
78. Sutcliffe SB, Gospodarowicz MK, Bush RS, et al. Role of radiation therapy in localized non-Hodgkin's lymphoma. *Radiother Oncol* 1985;4:211–223.
79. Wirth A, Byram D, Chao M, et al. Long-term results of mantle irradiation alone in 261 patients with clinical stage I-II supradiaphragmatic Hodgkin's disease. *Int J Radiat Oncol Biol Phys* 1997;39:174.
80. Noordijk E, Carde P, Hagenbeek A, et al. Combination of radiotherapy and chemotherapy is advisable in all patients with clinical stage I-II Hodgkin's disease. Six-year results of the EORTC-GPMC controlled clinical trials "H7-VF," "H7-F." and "H7-U." *Int J Radiat Oncol Biol Phys* 1997;39:173.
81. Diehl V, Franklin J, Sextro M, et al. Clinical presentation and treatment of lymphocyte predominance Hodgkin's disease. In: Mauch PM, Armitage JO, Diehl V, et al., eds. *Hodgkin's disease*. Philadelphia: Lippincott Williams & Wilkins; 1999:563–582.
82. Bodis S, Kraus M, Pinkus G, et al. Low mortality from lymphocyte predominant Hodgkin's disease with long-term follow-up. *J Clin Oncol* 1997;15:3060–3066.
83. Ifrah N, Hunault M, Jais JP, et al. Infradiaphragmatic Hodgkin's disease: long term results of combined modality therapy. *Leuk Lymphoma* 1996;21:79–84.
84. Iannitto E, Accurso V, Federico M, et al. Hodgkin's disease presenting below the diaphragm. The experience of the Gruppo Italiano Studio Linfomi (GISL). *Haematologica* 1997;82:676–682.
85. Mauch P, Greenberg H, Lewin A, et al. Prognostic factors in patients with subdiaphragmatic Hodgkin's disease. *Hematol Oncol* 1983;1: 205–214.
86. Darabi K, Sieber M, Chaitowitz, et al. Infradiaphragmatic versus supradiaphragmatic Hodgkin lymphoma: a retrospective review of 1114 patients. *Leuk Lymphoma* 2005;46:1715–1720.
87. Monfardini S, Ferruci L, Fratino, L et al. Validation of a multidimensional evaluation scale for use in elderly patients. *Cancer* 1995;77: 395–401.
88. Proctor SJ, White J, Jones GL. An international approach to the treatment of Hodgkin's disease in the ederly: launch of the SHIELD programme. *Eur J Haematol* 2005;75:63–67.
89. Kim HK, Silver B, Li S, et al. Hodgkin's disease in elderly patients (>60): clinical outcome and treatment strategies. *Int J Radiat Oncol Biol Phys* 2003;56:556–560.
90. Engert A, Ballova V, Haverkamp H, et al. Hodgkin's lymphoma in elderly patients: a comprehensive retrospective analysis from the German Hodgkin's Study Group. *J Clin Oncol* 2005;23:5052–5060.
91. Levis A, Anselmo AP, Ambrosetti A, et al. VEPEMB in elderly Hodgkin's lymphoma patients. Results from an Intergruppo Italiano Linfomi (IIL) study. *Ann Oncol* 2004;15:123–128.
92. Weekes CD, Vose JM, Lynch JC, et al. Hodgkin's disease in the elderly: improved treatment outcome with a doxorubicin-containing regimen. *J Clin Oncol* 2002;20:1087–1093.

CHAPTER 17 ■ TREATMENT OF UNFAVORABLE-PROGNOSIS, STAGE I–II HODGKIN LYMPHOMA

RICHARD T. HOPPE, ANDREAS ENGERT, AND EVERT M. NOORDIJK

The Ann Arbor staging system for Hodgkin's disease defines important prognostic subgroups of patients based on the anatomic distribution of disease (stage I to IV) and the presence or absence of systemic (B) symptoms. In the years immediately following the introduction of this staging system, its stage groupings provided a reasonable means for categorizing patients in clinical trials. At that time, important advances in radiation therapy techniques, including the use of high-dose extended-field irradiation, had resulted in dramatic increases in the proportion of patients with early-stage Hodgkin's disease who were being cured. The era of combination chemotherapy was still in its infancy. Although the initial clinical trials of the European Organization for the Research and Treatment of Cancer (EORTC) had used single-agent chemotherapy in combination with radiation therapy for early-stage disease,[1,2] there was little experience using combination chemotherapy in patients with stage I–II disease. It was not until the late 1960s and early 1970s, after initial favorable experience with MOPP (mechlorethamine, vincristine, procarbazine, prednisone) in advanced-stage disease had been reported,[3] that trials including combination chemotherapy were introduced for patients with stage I–II disease as well. Poised with two very effective treatments for Hodgkin's disease, investigators began to combine extended-field irradiation and combination chemotherapy for patients with relatively limited disease. In stage I–II Hodgkin's disease, the early results of these trials, often reporting only freedom from relapse as an end-point, demonstrated an improved outcome after combined-modality therapy.[4–6] Long-term outcome of these same studies, however, failed to demonstrate any differences in survival. A large metaanalysis of 23 randomized trials (3,888 patients) conducted by Specht and associates[7] confirmed this observation.

A reason for the lack of survival differences in these trials is that patients with stage I–II disease who relapsed after treatment with radiation therapy alone were quite often salvaged successfully with combination chemotherapy (with or without additional radiation) (see Chapter 19). In addition, patients who were treated initially with combined-modality therapy had a greater likelihood of mortality from treatment-related causes compared to patients treated initially with radiation therapy alone (see Chapter 23). Nevertheless, as single institutions and clinical trial groups began to evaluate the outcome of these studies in more detail, it became apparent that there were certain subsets of patients who benefited from more aggressive treatment, whereas others could be treated effectively with conventional radiation therapy alone. During the 1970s and 1980s, this led to numerous analyses of clinical prognostic factors for patients with stage I–II Hodgkin's disease.[8] The details of these studies, including the impact of treatment type and measured end-points, are discussed in great detail in Chapter 12. Based on these prognostic factors, clinical investigators have defined favorable and unfavorable (and occasionally very favorable) prognostic groups of patients with stage I–II disease in an effort to be more refined in the design of clinical trials and to tailor treatment in accordance with these prognostic factors. The challenge is to define for each prognostic group the precise amount of therapy that will achieve cure reliably, but with the least risk for long-term toxicity—that is, to optimize the therapeutic ratio. Patients with unfavorable-prognosis stage I–II disease have a somewhat worse underlying prognosis than patients with favorable-prognosis stage I–II disease and in general require more aggressive treatment. However, the likelihood of cure of patients with unfavorable stage I–II disease is still quite high, and therefore consideration of long-term toxicity remains an important issue for these patients.

As noted in the analyses in Chapter 12, individual studies of prognostic factors vary in their conclusions. These differences may be explained by patient selection, subtle variations in staging and treatment policies, and even statistical quirks. Factors that have been cited as important in multiple studies and have been used to identify prognostic groups for clinical trials include the number of involved sites,[9–12] the presence of bulky disease (especially in the mediastinum)[4,13–19] the presence of B-symptoms,[4,13,20,21] patient age,[22–24] gender,[22,23] and erythrocyte sedimentation rate (ESR).[25,26]

BULKY DISEASE

One factor of overriding importance in stage I–II disease is the presence of bulky disease, especially in the mediastinum.[4,13–19,27] Bulky disease has been identified as important in nearly all studies that have examined it as a potential prognostic factor in stage I–II disease, especially when freedom from relapse or event-free survival is the endpoint.[4,14,15,18,19,27] The presence of mediastinal bulk is incorporated as a prognostic factor for differentiating favorable- from unfavorable-prognosis stage I–II Hodgkin lymphoma in nearly all contemporary clinical trials. Unfortunately, when the original analyses were performed evaluating the extent of mediastinal disease, multiple definitions of bulk were used, including absolute measurements in centimeters, surface area, volumetric calculations, and ratios of the mass size to thoracic measurements.[19,28,29] As a result, the definition of mediastinal bulk in current clinical trials varies. The two most common definitions are (a) the maximum width of the mediastinal mass divided by the maximum intrathoracic diameter [mediastinal mass ratio (MMR)], with a ratio greater than 0.33 being bulky[30]; and (b) the maximum width of the mediastinal mass divided by the intrathoracic diameter at the T5-6 interspace [mediastinal tumor ratio (MTR)], with a ratio greater than 0.35 being bulky (Fig. 17.1).[18] This difference in definition may result in a marked difference in distribution of patients in favorable versus unfavorable subgroups. For this reason, it is often difficult to compare the results of different clinical trials for patients with large mediastinal adenopathy, as the inclusion criteria may vary widely. In fact, neither of these definitions is exactly consistent with the definition of mediastinal bulk according to the Cotswolds modification of the Ann Arbor staging system, in which a large mediastinal mass is defined as a ratio exceeding *one-third* of the intrathoracic measurement at the T5-6 interspace.[31]

The initial report that defined the prognostic impact of large mediastinal adenopathy among patients treated with radiation therapy alone was that of Mauch and co-workers.[13] In this report, patients who had mediastinal disease less than or equal to one-third of the maximum intrathoracic diameter (MMR ≤0.33) had a relapse risk of 2% within the mediastinum, whereas patients who had mediastinal disease that exceeded one-third of the maximum intrathoracic diameter (MMR >0.33) had a relapse risk of 40% in the mediastinum. Using the same definition of mediastinal bulk, Hoppe and associates,[14] reporting the Stanford data, showed that patients with large mediastinal masses had a 10-year freedom from

relapse of only 45% compared to 83% for patients with smaller mediastinal disease. However, the long-term survival for these two cohorts was equivalent (83% at 10 years). In the Stanford series, the freedom from relapse for patients with large mediastinal adenopathy was improved by the addition of adjuvant chemotherapy (usually MOPP). The 10-year freedom from relapse was 45% after treatment with radiation therapy alone versus 81% after combined-modality treatment. These general results were confirmed at a number of other centers, although varying definitions of bulky mediastinal involvement sometimes led to different interpretations of the data.[4,15–19,27,32]

The data with respect to the impact on outcome of bulk disease outside the mediastinum are limited. In one study of patients treated with radiation therapy alone from the University of Florida, Mendenhall and associates[11] were able to demonstrate a higher relapse rate when peripheral nodes exceeded 6 cm in diameter. However, Bonadonna and co-workers[33] failed to identify an impact of peripheral bulk when disease exceeded 7 cm, despite the fact that large mediastinal adenopathy was associated with a worse outcome in the same series of patients. In that report, all patients were treated with chemotherapy with or without irradiation. Currently, measurement of peripheral bulk is only occasionally included as a prognostic factor to define patients as unfavorable for the purpose of clinical trials.

CONSTITUTIONAL SYMPTOMS

Constitutional symptoms (unexplained fever >38°C, drenching night sweats, and weight loss >10% in the preceding 6 months) are often coincident with other prognostic factors, such as number of sites of disease, Ann Arbor stage, total tumor burden, and ESR. B-symptoms are usually easy to define clinically and have been associated with a worse prognosis for patients with stage I–II disease in most analyses.[21,34–40] However, each B-symptom does not have an equivalent impact. In a pooled analysis from the Joint Center for Radiation Therapy (JCRT) and Stanford University of 180 patients with pathologic stage (PS) I–IIB Hodgkin lymphoma,[41] all of whom had undergone staging laparotomy, the presence of night sweats alone was inconsequential, because the freedom from relapse in that group of stage I–IIB patients was identical to that in asymptomatic stage I–IIA patients. The presence of unexplained fevers or significant weight loss each had an equivalent impact, and those patients who had both unexplained fevers and significant weight loss had an even worse prognosis, with only 48% of patients free of disease 7 years after treatment with radiation therapy alone or radiation therapy followed by adjuvant chemotherapy. In a multivariate analysis of patients with single B-symptoms, the relative relapse risk was 4.3 for fevers, 2.4 for weight loss, and 0.8 for night sweats.

Acknowledging the adverse impact of B-symptoms reported in many studies, clinical trial groups include consideration of B-symptoms, either alone or in combination with ESR, in defining favorable versus unfavorable cohorts of patients with stage I–II disease.

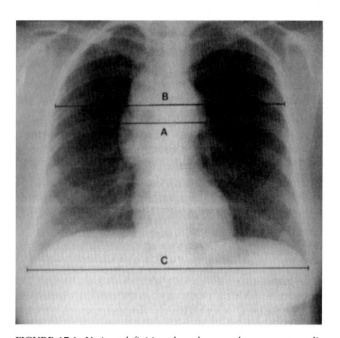

FIGURE 17.1. Various definitions have been used to measure mediastinal bulk. The MTR is the ratio of the maximum mediastinal mass width (**A**) divided by the intrathoracic diameter at the T5-6 interspace (**B**), with an MTR ≥0.35 generally considered bulky. In this example, the ratio is 9.0 cm/23.7 cm, or 0.38, so the mass is bulky. For the MMR, the maximum mediastinal mass measurement (**A**) is divided by the maximum intrathoracic diameter (**C**). In this example, the ratio is 9.0 cm/29 cm, or 0.31, so the mass is nonbulky. (Reprinted with permission from Hoppe RT. The management of bulky mediastinal Hodgkin's disease. *Hematol Oncol Clin North Am* 1989;3:265–276.)

OTHER UNFAVORABLE FACTORS IN STAGE I–II DISEASE

Among other prognostic factors that have been included in defining patient subgroups for clinical trials are patient age, histology, erythrocyte sedimentation rate, number of sites of disease, and presence of E-lesions. Table 17.1 summarizes the

TABLE 17.1

DEFINITION OF "UNFAVORABLE" STAGE I–II HODGKIN LYMPHOMA IN RECENT CLINICAL TRIALS

Factors[a]	EORTC	GHSG	NCIC	Stanford
Age (years)	≥50	—	≥40	—
Histology	—	—	MC/LD	—
ESR/B-symptoms	≥30 mm with any B ≥50 mm without B	≥30 mm with any B ≥50 mm without B	≥50 mm *or* any B	any B
Mediastinal mass	MTR ≥0.35	MMR >0.33	10 cm *or* MMR >0.33	MMR >0.33
No. nodal sites	≥4	≥3	≥4	—
E-lesion	—	Present	—	—

[a]Patients with one or more of these factors were considered unfavorable.
EORTC, European Organization for Research and Treatment of Cancer; GHSG, German Hodgkin Study Group; NCIC, National Cancer Institute, Canada; MC, mixed cellularity; LD, lymphocyte depleted; ESR, erythrocyte sedimentation rate; MTR, maximum mediastinal width/chest width at T5-T6 on chest x-ray; MMR, maximum mediastinal width/maximum chest width on chest x-ray; E, extralymphatic.

current criteria for defining favorable and unfavorable presentations of stage I–II disease used by the European Organization for the Research and Treatment of Cancer (EORTC) and German Hodgkin Study Group (GHSG the National Cancer Institute, Canada (NCIC) and Stanford).

In addition, there are well-established prognostic factors for stage III-IV Hodgkin lymphoma, as detailed in Chapter 12. The International Prognostic Score (IPS) for advanced Hodgkin lymphoma[42] may be applied to patients with stage I–II disease with just slight modification. For example, Gisselbrecht and associates[43] applied the prognostic factors of the IPS, as well as the additional factors used by the EORTC and GHSG, to patients with stage I–II disease enrolled on the EORTC-GELA H9 trial and confirmed independent prognostic significance for age over 45 years, male gender, hemoglobin below 10.5 g/dL, absolute lymphocyte count below 600/mm^3, B-symptoms with ESR above 50, and presence of extranodal disease. Overall survival was estimated to be 99%, 98%, 92%, 82%, and 73% for patients with an increasing number of adverse factors (p <0.0001). The greatest impact on outcome appeared among patients who had three or more adverse factors; however, this accounted for fewer than 10% of the patients in the H9 trial.

EORTC TRIALS FOR UNFAVORABLE-PROGNOSIS STAGE I–II DISEASE (TABLE 17.2)

The EORTC has made elegant use of prognostic factors in defining patient subgroups for clinical trials. However, in the very first trials (H1 and H2), conducted between 1964 and 1976, all patients with clinical stage (CS) I–II Hodgkin's disease were treated without distinction as to favorable or unfavorable characteristics. The long-term outcome of patients in these trials was evaluated and this led to the development of prognostic models.[8] Therefore, in the H5 trial, initiated in 1977, patients were stratified for the first time into favorable and unfavorable groups based on initial disease characteristics.[44] Patients were defined as unfavorable if they had any of the following characteristics: age 40 years or over; ESR 70 mm (at 1 hour) or greater; mixed-cellularity or lymphocyte-depletion histology; or clinical stage II without mediastinal involvement. Patients with these unfavorable characteristics were assigned to the H5-U (unfavorable) trial and were randomized to treatment with total nodal radiation alone (excluding the pelvis in

women younger than 40 years) or combined-modality therapy. The combined-modality therapy consisted of split-course MOPP and mantle irradiation, with three cycles of MOPP followed by mantle irradiation, and then another three cycles of MOPP; 296 patients were randomized. At 15 years the overall survival was 69% in both arms of the trial (p = 0.36), but the rate of treatment failure was 35% versus 16% (p <0.001), favoring treatment with combined-modality therapy.[44] In subsequent trials (H6–H9), the criteria for favorable and unfavorable groups were refined further.

In these trials, patients were considered unfavorable and entered into the H6-U, H7-U, and H8-U studies if they had any of the following characteristics: an ESR of 50 mm or above; an ESR of 30 mm or above in the presence of B-symptoms; a mediastinal mass of 0.35 or more of the intrathoracic diameter at T5-6 (MTR ≥0.35); or three or more sites of disease (four or more in the H7, H8, and H9). In all of these trials, patients in the unfavorable groups were treated with programs of combined modality therapy (Table 17.2). In the H6-U study (no. 20822, 1982–1988), all patients received split-course chemotherapy and mantle irradiation. Treatment consisted of three cycles of chemotherapy, followed by mantle irradiation (35 Gy with an optional 5- to 10-Gy boost), and then three more cycles of chemotherapy. The chemotherapy was randomized between MOPP and ABVD.[45] The trial included 316 patients, and at 10 years the survival in both arms was 87% (p = 0.5); however, the risk of treatment failure was 24% for MOPP versus only 12% for ABVD (p <0.01).[6] With respect to complications, there was less hematologic and late gonadal toxicity with ABVD than MOPP. However, an early decrement in pulmonary vital capacity was more common after ABVD than MOPP (12% versus 2%, p = 0.08), and there were two respiratory deaths in the combined-modality ABVD arm.[45] There were no significant differences in changes in left ventricular ejection fractions following treatment in the two different arms of the trial. In general, given the lower hematologic and gonadal toxicity, ABVD would appear to be the preferred of these two combinations in these young patients. However, careful attention must be paid to the pulmonary status of patients who receive ABVD, especially when mantle irradiation is contemplated (see Chapters 25 and 26).

In the H7-U trial (no. 20881), conducted from 1988 to 1992, combined-modality therapy using two different non-MOPP combinations was compared. Treatment was with either EBVP chemotherapy followed by involved-field irradiation (36–40 Gy) or six cycles of MOPP/ABV chemotherapy[46]

TABLE 17.2

EUROPEAN ORGANIZATION FOR RESEARCH AND TREATMENT OF CANCER (EORTC) RANDOMIZED TRIALS FOR UNFAVORABLE-PROGNOSIS STAGE I–II HODGKIN LYMPHOMA

Study	Dates	Eligibility	Treatment arms
H5-U	1977–1982	CS II with negative mediastinum *or* MC/LD histology *or* age ≥40 *or* ESR ≥70	A. Total nodal irradiation (40–45 Gy) B. 3 MOPP + mantle (35 Gy) + 3 MOPP
H6-U	1982–1988	≥3 regions *or* A and ESR ≥50 *or* B and ESR ≥30 *or* bulky mediastinum	A. 3 MOPP + mantle (35 Gy) + 3 MOPP B. 3 ABVD + mantle (35 Gy) + 3 ABVD
H7-U	1988–1993	Age ≥50 *or* A and ESR ≥50 *or* B and ESR ≥30 *or* ≥4 sites *or* bulky mediastinum	A. 6 EBVP + involved field (36–40 Gy) B. 6 MOPP/ABV + involved field (36–40 Gy)
H8-U	1993–1998	Age ≥50 *or* A and ESR ≥50 *or* B and ESR ≥30 *or* ≥3 sites *or* bulky mediastinum	A. 6 MOPP/ABV + involved field (36 Gy) B. 4 MOPP/ABV + involved field (36 Gy) C. 4 MOPP/ABV + subtotal nodal irradiation (36 Gy)
H9-U	1998–2004	Same as H8-U	A. 6 ABVD + involved field (30 Gy) B. 4 ABVD + involved field (30 Gy) C. 4 BEACOPP + involved field (30 Gy)
H10-U	2006–	Same as H8U	A. 4 ABVD + "involved node" (30 Gy) B. 2 ABVD, PET a. PET negative – 4 ABVD b. PET positive – 2 BEACOPP esc + "involved node" (30 Gy)

H5U study also included patients from H5F trial who were identified as stage IIIA after laparotomy. Bulky mediastinum defined as MTR ≥0.35 at T5-6. H8U and H9U trials were in collaboration with GELA.

CS, clinical stage; LD, lymphocyte depletion; MC, mixed cellularity; ESR, erythrocyte sedimentation rate; MOPP, mechlorethamine, vincristine, procarbazine, prednisone; ABVD, Adriamycin bleomycin, vinblastine, docarbazine; BEACOPP, bleomycin, etoposide, Adriamycin, cyclophosphamide, vincristine, procarbazine, prednisone.

followed by involved-field irradiation. The EBVP combination was a less intense (and presumably safer) drug combination for early-stage Hodgkin lymphoma developed by Hoerni and associates.[47] However, significant differences in 10-year event-free survival (88% vs. 68%, *p* <0.001) and overall survival (87% versus 79%) have been reported, favoring the MOPP/ABV combination.[48] This is one of only very few recent clinical trials in Hodgkin lymphoma that shows a survival difference among the treatment arms. These unexpectedly poor results for EBVP in combined-modality programs for early-stage disease led to its abandonment in the next generation of clinical trials, except for patients with favorable presentations.

The H8-U trial (no. 20931), a collaborative study between the EORTC and the French Adult Lymphoma Group (GELA), was a three-arm trial conducted from 1993 to 1998. Based on the H7-U results, MOPP/ABV was selected as the standard chemotherapy. A three-arm trial was designed to evaluate both the number of cycles of chemotherapy required and the extent of the radiation fields. The treatment options were MOPP/ABV × 6 plus involved-field irradiation (36 Gy), MOPP/ABV × 4 plus involved-field irradiation, and MOPP/ABV × 4 plus subtotal nodal irradiation. 995 patients were accrued, and thus far no differences in relapse-free, event-free, or overall survival have been detected.[49]

The H9-U trial was also a three-arm study, two arms of which were common with the German Hodgkin Study Group (GHSG) HD11 trial (discussed later). In this trial, ABVD replaced MOPP/ABV chemotherapy based on the comparison of those two regimens in advanced disease, where MOPP/ABV was associated with a greater incidence of acute toxicity (pulmonary and hematologic), myelodysplastic syndrome, and acute leukemia.[50] One treatment arm tested the BEACOPP (bleomycin, etoposide, Adriamycin, cyclophosphamide, Oncovin [vincristine], procarbazine, and prednisone) regimen of the GHSG.[51] The treatments in this trial included ABVD × 6 plus

involved-field irradiation (now reduced to 30 Gy), ABVD × 4 plus involved field (30 Gy), and BEACOPP × 4 plus involved field (30 Gy). In the first results reported from this trial, there are no differences in complete response rate, event-free survival, or overall survival among the three treatment arms.[52] The chemotherapy-related toxicity (need for antibiotic coverage, transfusions, and hospitalizations) was greater with BEACOPP than with ABVD.

The proposal for the new H10 trial is to randomize patients to four cycles of ABVD plus 30-Gy involved-node irradiation versus two cycles of ABVD followed by PET. If the PET is negative, four more cycles of ABVD alone would be administered. If the PET is positive, patients would receive two cycles of BEACOPP escalated plus 30-Gy involved-node irradiation.

Table 17.2 summarizes the results of the EORTC trials of combined-modality therapy for patients with unfavorable presentations of stage I–II Hodgkin lymphoma.

GERMAN HODGKIN STUDY GROUP TRIALS FOR UNFAVORABLE-PROGNOSIS STAGE I–II DISEASE (TABLE 17.3)

The GHSG initiated prospective randomized clinical trials in 1983, and from the outset considered prognostic subgroupings in its assignment of patients to clinical protocols. The HD1 trial was open from 1983 to 1988 and accrued 180 patients (148 of whom were randomized). Laparotomy staging was performed routinely. Patients were eligible for this trial if they had stage I–IIA/B or IIIA disease with bulky mediastinal disease (MMR ≥0.33), extranodal involvement, or massive splenic disease (diffuse involvement or more than five

TABLE 17.3

GERMAN HODGKIN STUDY GROUP (GHSG) RANDOMIZED TRIALS FOR UNFAVORABLE-PROGNOSIS STAGE I–II HODGKIN LYMPHOMA

Study	Dates	Eligibility	Treatment arms
HD1	1983–1988	PS I–II with bulky mediastinal mass *or* E involvement *or* massive splenic disease	A. 2 (COPP/ABVD) + extended field (40 Gy) B. 2 (COPP/ABVD) + extended field (20 Gy) plus 20-Gy boost to initially bulky (>5 cm) sites
HD5	1988–1993	CS I–II with bulky mediastinal mass *or* A and ESR ≥50 *or* B and ESR ≥30 *or* ≥3 sites *or* E involvement *or* massive splenic disease	A. 2 (COPP/ABVD) + extended field (30 Gy) plus 10-Gy boost to initially bulky (>5 cm) sites B. 2 (COPP/ABV/IMEP) + extended field (30 Gy) plus 10-Gy boost to initially bulky (>5 cm) sites
HD8	1993–1998	CS IA–IB *or* CS IIA with bulky mediastinal mass *or* E involvement *or* ESR ≥50 *or* >2 sites; CS IIB with ESR ≥30 *or* >2 sites; CS IIIA without any risk factors; massive splenic disease	A. 2 (COPP/ABVD) + extended field (30 Gy) plus 10-Gy boost to initially bulky sites B. 2 (COPP/ABVD) + involved field (30 Gy) plus 10-Gy boost to initially bulky sites
HD11	1998–2002	CS IA–IB *or* CS IIA with bulky mediastinal mass *or* E involvement *or* ESR ≥50 *or* ≥2 sites; CS IIB with ESR ≥30 *or* >2 sites; Same as HD8, except massive splenic disease no longer included; excludes stage IIIA	A. 4 ABVD + involved field (30 Gy) B. 4 ABVD + involved field (20 Gy) C. 4 BEACOPP + involved field (30 Gy) D. 4 BEACOPP + involved field (20 Gy)
HD14	2002	Same as HD11	A. 4 ABVD + involved field (30 Gy) B. 2 BEACOPP escalated + 2 ABVD + involved field (30 Gy)

Bulky mediastinal mass defined as MMR ≥0.33 at maximum transthoracic diameter. Massive splenic disease defined as diffuse involvement or >5 nodules. Patients on the HD1 and HD5 trials underwent staging laparotomy and splenectomy. HD5 trial also included patients who were eligible for the HD4 (favorable) trial, but were found to have PS IIIA disease at the time of laparotomy.

COPP, cyclophosphamide, vincristine, procarbazine, prednisone; IMEP, ifosfamide, methotrexate, etoposide, prednisone; MMR, ratio of mediastinal mass width to maximum intrathoracic measurement; PS, pathologic stage.

nodules).[53] This was a combined-modality therapy trial in which the question related to radiation therapy dose. All patients were treated with two cycles of COPP (cyclophosphamide, Oncovin, procarbazine, prednisone)/ABVD (4 months) followed by irradiation to extended fields. The dose was 20 Gy on one arm and 40 Gy on the other arm of the trial; however, sites of bulky disease (≥5 cm) were always treated to 40 Gy.

A separate analysis of the HD1 study has not been reported, but results have been published together with one of the arms of the HD5 trial.[53] The HD5 trial, open from 1988 to 1993, included patients who had a MMR of 0.33 or above; an ESR of 50 mm or above; B-symptoms in combination with an ESR of 30 mm or above; more than two sites of disease; extranodal involvement; or massive splenic disease. In addition, patients who had stage IIIA in the absence of risk factors were included. The treatment randomization was between combined modality with COPP/ABVD (two double cycles) or COPP/ABV/IMEP (two triple cycles) plus extended-field irradiation (40 Gy to bulky sites, 30 Gy to nonbulky or uninvolved sites).[54] The COPP/ABVD arm included 111 patients who had eligibility criteria identical to patients in the HD1 trial, and the results for these patients were compared to the two arms of the HD1 trial. In effect, this became a comparison of combined-modality therapy (2 COPP/ABVD) in which extended fields were irradiated to three different doses: 20, 30, and 40 Gy. Bulky sites (≥5 cm in any axis) were always irradiated to 40 Gy. The 4-year survival rates were 93%, 94%, and 88% for 20, 30, and 40 Gy, respectively ($p = 0.8$). The corresponding freedom from treatment failure rates were 86%, 80%, and 90% ($p = 0.5$). This suggests that in a combined-modality program that includes the equivalent of at least 4 months of COPP/ABVD chemotherapy, as little as 20 Gy irradiation in extended-field technique to nonbulky sites and 40 Gy to bulky sites (>5 cm) is adequate.[53]

The HD8 trial, conducted between 1993 and 1998, enrolled 1,204 patients with CS IA–B or CS IIA with any of the following risk factors: MMR above 0.33, massive splenic disease, extranodal disease, ESR of 50 or more, or three or more sites of disease. It also included patients with CS IIB disease who had an ESR of 30 or more or three or more sites of disease and patients with CS IIIA without any risk factors. Staging laparotomy was not performed. Patients with stage IIB who had an MMR of 0.33 or above, extranodal involvement, or massive splenic disease were treated on the HD9 study. The HD8 trial used the same chemotherapy as the HD1 and HD5 trials (2 COPP/ABVD) and a radiation field size question was posed. Patients were randomly assigned to involved-field (30 Gy, 40 Gy to bulky sites) or extended-field (30 Gy, 40 Gy to bulky sites) irradiation following the completion of chemotherapy. With a median follow-up of 54 months and 1,064 evaluable patients, there were no significant differences for involved-field (IF) versus extended-field (EF) radiation therapy (overall survival 92% versus 91%, freedom from treatment failure 84% versus 86% for IF versus EF, respectively).[55] There was significantly greater acute toxicity, including leukopenia, thrombocytopenia, nausea, and gastrointestinal toxicity in the extended-field treatment group. However, thus far there is no difference in the risk for secondary neoplasia (4.5% for EF, 2.8% for IF).

The HD9 trial, intended primarily for patients with advanced disease, also included patients with stage IIB or IIIA disease who had an MMR of 0.33 or above, extranodal involvement, or massive splenic disease (with diffuse infiltration or more than five focal lesions, as determined by CT and sonography). A subset analysis of patients who were stage II and had both B-symptoms and large mediastinal adenopathy or extranodal extension has not been reported. The overall results of the HD9 trial are reviewed in Chapter 18.

The HD11 study (1998–2002) succeeded the HD8 study. This was a four-arm trial of combined-modality therapy, testing chemotherapy type and radiation dose. The four arms were four cycles of ABVD plus involved field (30 Gy), four cycles of ABVD plus involved field (20 Gy), four cycles of BEACOPP plus involved field (30 Gy), and four cycles of BEACOPP plus involved field (20 Gy).[56] The first and third arms of this trial were identical to the EORTC H_9U trial discussed earlier in the chapter. A total of 1,363 patients were enrolled in this trial. With a median follow-up of 2 years, the overall survival of all patients was 97.4% and the freedom from treatment failure was 89.9%, with no significant differences between arms of the study. Leukopenia and infection were reported more frequently among the patients treated with BEACOPP.[56]

The current trial of the GHSG for unfavorable-prognosis stage I–II patients, opened in 2003, is the HD 14. In this trial, four cycles of ABVD plus 30 Gy IF is compared to four cycles of BEACOPP escalated followed by two cycles of ABVD plus 30 Gy involved-field irradiation (Table 17.3).

THE STANFORD CLINICAL TRIALS FOR UNFAVORABLE-PROGNOSIS STAGE I–II DISEASE (TABLE 17.4)

The initial Stanford clinical trial for stage I–II lymphoma, the L1 study, initiated in 1962, did not distinguish between favorable and unfavorable presentations, and all patients were randomized to treatment with involved-field or extended-field irradiation. Based on the early results of this trial, patients with B-symptoms were identified as having a poorer prognosis and subsequently included in separate clinical trials. Somewhat later, other factors, including multiple sites of extranodal involvement (stage IV according to the criteria of many other investigators), and a large mediastinal mass, that is, MMR greater than 0.33, were identified as unfavorable prognostic signs. From 1968 to 1980, the Stanford trials primarily addressed the question of radiation therapy alone versus combined-modality therapy. The results, as noted earlier, showed differences in freedom from relapse but equivalent overall survival.

In 1980, specific trials were initiated for patients who had stage I–II A/B disease with a large mediastinal mass (MMR >0.33) or multiple extranodal sites of disease that focused on efforts to refine the combined-modality approach. Between 1980 and 1990, patients were randomized to combined-modality therapy with either PAVe,[57] a MOPP-like combination that included procarbazine, l-phenylalanine mustard, and vinblastine; or ABVD. The treatment was administered in a split-course fashion: three cycles (months) of chemotherapy, followed by mantle irradiation (44 Gy), followed by three more cycles of chemotherapy. At 15 years, both the survival (73% versus 100%, $p = 0.06$) and freedom from relapse (56% versus 83%, $p = 0.1$) were superior in the ABVD arm.

In 1990, a nonrandomized pilot study was initiated for patients with large mediastinal masses (MMR >0.33) using the Stanford V management approach of brief intensive chemotherapy followed by irradiation (at first 44 Gy, later 36 Gy) to initially bulky sites (greater than 5 cm) (see Chapter 18).[58,59] The most recent report included 87 patients, with a median follow-up of nearly 6 years.[60] The 8-year overall survival was 95% and freedom from progression was 96%. Based on these data, a phase III intergroup trial was initiated in the Eastern Cooperative Oncology Group (ECOG) (E2496), randomizing patients between ABVD and Stanford V chemotherapy followed in either case by 36 Gy to initially bulky sites of disease (Stanford V) or large mediastinal masses only (ABVD). This trial has recently reached accrual goals and has closed.

TABLE 17.4

STANFORD CLINICAL TRIALS FOR UNFAVORABLE-PROGNOSIS STAGE I–II HODGKIN LYMPHOMA

Study	Dates	Eligibility	Treatment arms
H2	1968–1980	PS I–IIB (B-symptoms)	A. Total lymphoid irradiation (44 Gy/35 Gy) B. Total lymphoid irradiation + 6 MOP(P)
K1, H4	1968–1974	PS IIEA/B, E-lesion	A. Total lymphoid irradiation (44 Gy/35 Gy) B. Total lymphoid irradiation + 6 MOP(P)
S2, S3	1974–1980	PS IIEA/B, E-lesion	A. Total lymphoid irradiation (44 Gy) + 6 MOP(P) B. Total lymphoid irradiation (44 Gy) + 6 PAVe
C4, C5	1980–1990	CS I–IIA/B, bulky mediastinum *or* multiple E-lesions	A. 3 PAVe + mantle (44 Gy) + 3 PAVe B. 3 ABVD + mantle (44 Gy) + 3 ABVD
G2	1990	CS I–IIA/B, bulky mediastinum	12-week Stanford V chemotherapy plus 36 Gy to initially bulky (>5 cm) sites

Radiation dose (involved/uninvolved) portions of field. Prednisone was deleted from the MOP(P) combination whenever there was prior mediastinal irradiation. Patients on the H, K, and S trials underwent staging laparotomy and splenectomy. Pelvic irradiation was not used on the K1 or S2 (PS IIEA) trials. Bulky mediastinum defined as MMR more than one-third of *maximum* intrathoracic diameter. The G2 study was nonrandomized, but the ECOG E2496 randomizes these patients between ABVD and Stanford V (Table 5).
PAVe, procarbazine, l-phenylalanine mustard, vinblastine.

REFINEMENTS OF COMBINED-MODALITY THERAPY FOR UNFAVORABLE-PROGNOSIS STAGE I– II DISEASE

Trials to Identify the Best Chemotherapy Combination (Table 17.5)

The evolution of studies to identify the best chemotherapy combination for unfavorable early-stage Hodgkin lymphoma have paralleled trials to identify the best chemotherapy in advanced Hodgkin lymphoma (see Chapters 14 and 18). Early trials evaluated MOPP versus MOPP-like combinations; later trials compared MOPP or MOPP-like combinations with ABVD, alternating, or hybrid regimens. In virtually every situation, ABVD-containing treatment programs proved somewhat better than MOPP or MOPP-like treatment programs, although the differences were often not statistically significant.

The concept of rapid alternation of non-cross-resistant drug combinations was tested in the GHSG HD5 trial. Patients with stage I–II and risk factors were randomized to the conventional COPP/ABVD (4 months) versus COPP/ABV/IMEP, a 10-drug regimen administered in a rapid alternating fashion over a 35-day period and repeated after 6 weeks, for a total duration also of 4 months. This was followed in each arm by extended-field irradiation (30 Gy) plus a 10-Gy boost to initial sites that were greater than 5 cm.[54] The complete response rates were similar for the two different management approaches (93% and 94%) and at a median observation period of 7 years, there were no differences in freedom from treatment failure (80% and 79%) or overall survival (88% for both regimens).

The failure of the ABVD-containing regimens to show more convincing advantage over the MOPP or MOPP-like combinations was in contrast to the results observed in trials of chemotherapy alone for patients with advanced Hodgkin lymphoma.[61] This may be due to the fact that the studies for patients with unfavorable presentations of stage I–II always included irradiation, and the use of combined-modality therapy may obscure the differences that are observed after treatment with chemotherapy alone. However, an important factor that led to the adoption of ABVD was that the secondary leukemia risk and frequency of sterility were much lower after ABVD than after MOPP.

In patients with unfavorable prognosis who receive combined-modality therapy, especially those patients with large mediastinal masses, it is important to consider the potential risk due to the overlapping pulmonary toxicities of bleomycin and irradiation and the potential overlapping cardiac toxicities of doxorubicin and irradiation. Careful delineation of the radiation fields is required (discussed later in the chapter). Recognition of these risks has led to attempts to develop less toxic drug combinations for these patients.

At Stanford, the concept for alternative chemotherapy was to reduce total drug dosage, especially of Adriamycin and bleomycin, by reducing the duration and increasing the intensity of treatment. The Stanford V regimen (nitrogen mustard, doxorubicin, vincristine, vinblastine, etoposide, bleomycin, and prednisone) is administered for 12 weeks. This program includes only 50% of the Adriamycin dosage and 25% of the bleomycin dosage that would be included in six cycles of ABVD. The chemotherapy is followed by mediastinal/supraclavicular irradiation to 36 Gy. The most recent results show a 4-year survival of 95% and freedom from relapse of 96%.[60] In the ECOG 2496 study of combined modality therapy, six cycles of ABVD are being compared to 3 months of Stanford V, in each case followed by irradiation of bulky mediastinal disease. This trial has reached its accrual goals and was closed in June 2006.

Significant reductions in chemotherapy intensity for patients with unfavorable presentations of stage I–II disease have not met with success. The Grupo Argentino de Tratamiento de la

TABLE 17.5

RECENT RANDOMIZED CLINICAL TRIALS IN UNFAVORABLE-PROGNOSIS STAGE I–II HODGKIN LYMPHOMA: IDENTIFICATION OF THE OPTIMAL CHEMOTHERAPY COMBINATION

Trial	Treatment regimens	No. patients	Outcome	
EORTC H7-U[48]	A. 6 EBVP + IF (36 Gy) B. 6 MOPP/ABV + IF (36 Gy)	183 182	10-year:	EFS: A = 68%, B = 88%, p <0.001 OS: A = 79%, B = 87%, p = 0.0175
EORTC/GELA H9-U[52]	A. 6 ABVD + IF (30 Gy) B. 4 ABVD + IF (30 Gy) C. 4 BEACOPP + IF (30 Gy)	277 276 255	4-year:	RFS: A = 86%, B = 88%, C = 84% EFS: A = 89%, B = 94%, C = 91% OS: A = 95%, B = 96%, C = 93%
ECOG 2496	A. 6 ABVD + RT (36 Gy) to large mediastinal mass B. 12 week Stanford V + RT (36 Gy)	Closed 6/06		
GHSG HD 5[54]	A. 2 (COPP/ABVD) + extended field (30 Gy) + 10-Gy boost to initially bulky sites B. 2 (COPP/ABV/IMEP) + extended field (30 Gy) + 10-Gy boost to initially bulky sites	487 486	7-year:	CR: A = 93%, B = 94% FFTF: A = 80%, B = 79% OS: A = 88%, B = 88%
GHSG HD11[56]	A. 4 ABVD + IF (30 Gy) B. 4 ABVD + IF (20 Gy) C. 4 BEACOPP + IF (30 Gy) D. 4 BEACOPP + IF (20 Gy)	264 257 262 268	2-year:	FFTF: 90% (all arms combined, p = ns) OS: 97% (all arms combined, p = ns)
GHSG HD14	A. 4 ABVD + IF (30 Gy) B. 2 BEACOPP esc + 2 ABVD + IF (30 Gy)	Open		

Leucemia Aguda (GATLA) identified an unfavorable impact on event-free survival (85% versus 66%; $p = 0.009$) when they substituted AOPE (Adriamycin [doxorubicin], Oncovin [vincristine], prednisone, and etoposide) for CVPP (cyclophosphamide, vincristine, procarbazine, and prednisone)[62] in patients with an intermediate prognosis.

The EORTC attempted to reduce drug intensity in the H7-U trial, randomizing patients between six cycles of EBVP (plus involved-field irradiation) and six cycles of MOPP/ABV (plus involved-field irradiation). The 10-year survival (79% versus 87%; $p = 0.0175$), event-free survival (68% versus 88%; $p < 0.001$), and risk of treatment failure (31% versus 12%; $p < 0.001$) were all worse in the EBVP arm.[48]

Finally, the SWOG 9051 study tested three cycles of EVA (etoposide, vinblastine, and doxorubicin) followed by subtotal lymphoid irradiation in patients with CS I–III disease. A large mediastinal mass (>9 cm) was present in 55%. The 3-year failure-free survival was only 67%, with most patients failing in sites of initial bulk.[63] Therefore, in contrast to studies for patients with favorable-prognosis stage I–II Hodgkin lymphoma (see Chapter 16), where less toxic and less intense chemotherapy regimens have been effective in combined-modality therapy programs, significant reduction of chemotherapy intensity has led to an increased risk for relapse among patients with unfavorable disease presentations.

Largely based on trials in advanced Hodgkin lymphoma,[61] ABVD became the standard regimen employed in this group of patients with large mediastinal adenopathy. Therefore, in 1998 trials were designed to compare combined-modality therapy using ABVD with more intense, newer regimens. Both the EORTC H9-U and GHSG HD11 studies of combined-modality therapy compared four cycles of ABVD with four cycles of BEACOPP baseline, followed by irradiation. As noted previously, current results from these trials fail to indicate any differences in outcome, but somewhat greater toxicity among patients treated with BEACOPP compared to ABVD.[52,56] The successor HD 14 of the GHSG compares four cycles of ABVD plus radiation to two cycles of BEACOPP escalated plus two cycles of ABVD plus radiation.

Trials to Identify the Optimal Number of Cycles of Chemotherapy (Table 17.6)

There are no conclusive trials regarding the optimal number of cycles of contemporary chemotherapy for patients with intermediate-prognosis Hodgkin lymphoma. The EORTC H8-U study randomized patients to combined-modality therapy with four or six cycles of MOPP/ABV, and the failure to observe any differences in outcome suggests that four cycles of MOPP/ABV may be sufficient when followed by irradiation;[49] however, this drug combination has now been abandoned in clinical trials. The EORTC H9-U trial randomized patients to four or six cycles of ABVD plus irradiation. The absence of any differences in outcome thus far suggests that four cycles of ABVD may be sufficient when combined with irradiation.[52]

Nonrandomized Trials of Brief-Duration (Less than 6 Months) Chemotherapy

A number of trials incorporating brief-duration chemotherapy have been reported in which the duration of chemotherapy was not the question being studied.

Brusamolino and colleagues,[64] from Pavia, Italy, treated patients with bulky mediastinal disease (not otherwise defined) with combined-modality therapy, including three cycles of ABVD. The 10-year survival rate was 70% and freedom from relapse 74%, somewhat less than would be expected.

The Hôpital St.-Louis trial H85, conducted between 1985 and 1994, treated patients who had a variety of unfavorable prognostic factors with three cycles of ABVD (vindesine substituted for vinblastine) followed by subtotal nodal irradiation.[65] Patients with large mediastinal masses (MTR >0.33) had a 5-year survival rate of 82%.

Finally, the Milan study of four cycles of ABVD plus irradiation (involved-field versus extended-field) included 32% of patients with unfavorable risk factors (large mediastinal mass, E-lesion, hilar disease, or B-symptoms), most commonly bulky disease (Table 17.7). The 12-year freedom-from-progression rate was 88% among these patients.[66]

Based on these retrospective data, it appears that patients with unfavorable disease by virtue of age, histology, number of sites of disease, or B-symptoms may be treated adequately in combined-modality programs with as little as 3 months of conventional chemotherapy. For patients with large mediastinal masses, the data are less clear, and may depend somewhat on the definition of large mediastinal adenopathy; however, it appears that at least 4 months of chemotherapy is required in this group. If one looks simply at duration of chemotherapy (ignoring intensity), the Stanford V program is attractive, because the 87 patients with an MMR above 0.33 who were treated with just 3 months of chemotherapy had a 4-year survival of 95% and freedom from relapse of 96%.[60]

TABLE 17.6

RECENT RANDOMIZED CLINICAL TRIALS IN UNFAVORABLE-PROGNOSIS STAGE I–II HODGKIN LYMPHOMA: TRIALS TO IDENTIFY THE OPTIMAL NUMBER OF CYCLES OF CHEMOTHERAPY

Trial	Treatment regimens	No. patients	Outcome	
EORTC/GELA H8-U[49]	A. 6 MOPP/ABV + IF (36 Gy)	995 total	4-year:	RFS: A = 94%; B = 95%; C = 96%
	B. 4 MOPP/ABV + IF (36 Gy)			EFS: A = 80%; B = 80%; C = 80%
	C. 4 MOPP/ABV + STLI			OS: A = 85%; B = 85%; C = 85%
EORTC/GELA H9-U[52]	A. 6 ABVD + IF (30 Gy)	277	4-year:	RFS: A = 86%, B = 88%, C = 84%
	B. 4 ABVD + IF (30 Gy)	276		EFS: A = 89%, B = 94%, C = 91%
	C. 4 BEACOPP + IF	255		OS: A = 95%, B = 96%, C = 93%

TABLE 17.7

RANDOMIZED CLINICAL TRIALS IN UNFAVORABLE-PROGNOSIS STAGE I–II HODGKIN LYMPHOMA: TRIALS TO IDENTIFY THE APPROPRIATE RADIATION VOLUME

Trial	Eligibility	Treatment regimens	No. patients	Outcome	
French Cooperative 1976–1981[67]	Age ≥40 *or* MC/LD *or* CS II without mediastinum involved *or* E-involvement *or* B-symptoms	A. 3 MOPP + IF (40 Gy) + 3 MOPP B. 3 MOPP + EF (40 Gy) + 3 MOPP	109 109	6-year results:	DFS: A = 87%, B = 93%, $p = 0.15$
INT, Milan[66] 1990–	All CS I–II includes age >40, bulky disease, E-involvement, >3 sites, bulky disease	A. 4 ABVD + STNI (36/30 Gy) B. 4 ABVD + IF (36 Gy)	65 68	12-years results:	FFP: A = 93%, B = 94%, p = ns EFS: A = 85%; B = 91%, p = ns OS: A = 100%, B = 96%, p = ns
EORTC/GELA H8-U[49]	See Table 17.2	(A. 6 MOPP/ABV + IF [36 Gy]) B. 4 MOPP/ABV + IF C. 4 MOPP/ABV + STLI	995 Total	4-year results:	RFS: A = 94%; B = 95%; C = 96% EFS: A = 80%; B = 80%; C = 80% OS: A = 85%; B = 85%; C = 85%
GHSG HD8[55]	See Table 17.3	A. 2 (COPP/ABVD) + EF (30 Gy, 40 Gy to bulk) B. 2 (COPP/ ABVD) + IF	532 evaluable 532 evaluable	54-mo results:	FFTF: A = 86%; B = 84% OS: A = 91%; B = 92%

DFS, disease free survival; FFP, freedom from progression; RDF, relapse free survival; OS, overall survival.

Trials to Identify the Appropriate Radiation Therapy Volume

Several randomized trials have addressed the question of radiation therapy volumes in combined-modality programs for intermediate-prognosis patients. Without exception these have demonstrated that involved-field irradiation is sufficient when administered in the combined-modality setting. The first was a French trial reported by Zittoun and associates[67] that included 209 patients with stage I–II and a variety of unfavorable factors who were treated with six cycles of MOPP sandwiched around involved-field (40 Gy) or extended-field (40 Gy) irradiation. The 6-year disease-free survival rates were 87% and 93%, respectively ($p = 0.15$).

The Milan study incorporated 4 months of ABVD, followed by involved-field (36 Gy) or subtotal nodal irradiation (30–36 Gy); 136 patients were treated, 20% of whom had bulky disease. The 12-year freedom-from-progression rates were 93% and 94%.

In the EORTC/GELA study, open from 1993 to 1998, two of the three arms were 4 × MOPP/ABV plus involved-field (36 Gy) and 4 × MOPP/ABV plus subtotal nodal irradiation. The most recent report of outcome (4-year data) showed no difference for IF versus STNI.[49]

The GHSG HD8 trial, also conducted between 1993 and 1998, used two cycles (4 months) of COPP/ABVD followed by either involved-field or extended-field irradiation (30 Gy to involved or uninvolved sites, 40 Gy to initially bulky sites). Again, there was no difference in outcome. With a median follow-up of 54 months, the 5-year survival rate for all patients was 91% and freedom-from treatment failure was 83%.[55]

The evidence from these randomized trials, as well as from numerous nonrandomized studies, indicates that radiation fields may be safely limited to involved regions (variably defined) in most combined-modality programs. A question remains whether the fields can be reduced any further, such as restricting irradiation to bulky sites as in the Stanford V program.

Trials to Identify the Appropriate Radiation Therapy Dose

Initial studies of combined-modality therapy for Hodgkin lymphoma generally used doses that were similar to doses used for radiation treatment alone (36–44 Gy). The GHSG HD1 tested 40 Gy versus 20 Gy extended-field irradiation (bulky sites >5 cm were always treated to 40 Gy) following two cycles (4 months) of COPP/ABVD. Because the HD5 trial used the same chemotherapy plus 30-Gy extended field (40 Gy to bulky sites), the data could be pooled for analysis, providing a comparison of 20, 30, and 40 Gy for the nonbulky and uninvolved portions of the field. Loeffler and associates[53] reported no significant differences for the three different radiation doses when employed in the treatment of nonbulky sites after 4 months of conventional chemotherapy. However, this did not provide an answer to dose for bulky sites of disease.

The GHSG HD11 trial compared involved-field doses of 30 Gy versus 20 Gy following either 4 × ABVD or 4 × BEACOPP-baseline. Unlike the HD1 and HD5 trials, bulky sites will no longer be boosted to 40 Gy. Thus far, no differences are reported (median 2-year follow-up).[56]

Trials of Chemotherapy Alone

Combined-modality therapy has become the mainstay of treatment for patients with intermediate-prognosis Hodgkin lymphoma, and chemotherapy alone has not generally been included as a treatment option in clinical trials. An exception is the planned EORTC H10-U trial. This is a trial of response-adapted therapy. In the conventional arm, patients are treated with four cycles of ABVD plus 30 Gy involved-node irradiation. Involved-node irradiation is a more strictly defined volume, based on the initial CT abnormalities, rather than on the more generous conventional anatomic lymph node regions. The alternative arm of this trial is two cycles of ABVD followed by PET imaging. If the PET scan is negative, those patients will receive four cycles of ABVD (total six cycles of ABVD), with no radiation. If the PET scan is positive, treatment will be completed with two cycles of BEACOPP escalated plus 30 Gy involved-node irradiation.

SPECIAL ISSUES IN THE MANAGEMENT OF PATIENTS WITH LARGE MEDIASTINAL MASSES

Radiation Therapy Treatment Planning

Historically, special radiation therapy techniques evolved to optimize treatment outcomes for patients with large mediastinal adenopathy and enable them to be treated with irradiation alone. These included the "shrinking field" technique, partial transmission lung blocks, treatment in the sitting position, and decreased fraction size.[68] However, contemporary management mandates the use of combined-modality therapy in virtually every situation.

After completion of a course of chemotherapy, the volume remaining to be irradiated is almost always substantially smaller than it would have been at the time of diagnosis. It is important to take advantage of this tumor regression and design fields that conform to the residual disease, as this will reduce the risk of pulmonary complications related to the radiation. Treatment of the original tumor volume will lead to additional risk. For example, at the National Cancer Institute, patients underwent radiation therapy simulation and treatment planning prior to being treated with 6 months of MOPP/ABVD. Following the completion of chemotherapy they were irradiated to the initial tumor volume to a dose of 10 to 15 Gy, followed by treatment to the residual volume of disease to an additional 25 to 35 Gy[69]; 16% of patients developed symptomatic or radiographic changes of radiation pneumonitis and 6 required management with systemic glucocorticoids. This complication was fatal in one instance.

Ideally, radiation volumes can be reduced as a correlate to chemotherapy response. These more restricted fields will result in smaller radiation volumes and reduced risk of complications. In the Stanford V program, for example, only initially bulky sites (>5 cm) are irradiated. Commonly, this will include only the mediastinum. Even if the supraclavicular areas are treated concurrently, the volume proportional to an entire mantle is much less. This may be especially beneficial, for example, in a young woman who has minimal axillary adenopathy, for whom the elimination of axillary irradiation may markedly reduce the risk for developing subsequent breast cancer.

Residual Mediastinal Abnormalities

It is common for patients who present with large mediastinal adenopathy to have residual mediastinal abnormalities on chest x-rays or CT scans after the completion of therapy. Historically, these patients were considered to be in an "unconfirmed complete response" (CRu) according to the Cotswald criteria[31] and were followed with serial radiographic studies. For the patient, there followed a period of uncertainty until there was evidence of disease progression in the mediastinum or elsewhere, and relapse could be documented, or else after a period of stable or slowly regressing abnormality they were declared free of disease.

Functional imaging with 67-Ga SPECT scanning and more recently with 18-FDG PET scanning has demonstrated significant untility in the management of patients with Hodgkin lymphoma (see Chapter 11). Interim PET scanning after two to three cycles of chemotherapy has been shown to correlate with both progression-free survival and overall survival.[70,71] Several investigators have looked specifically at the value of FDG-PET in assesment of residual mediastinal abnormalities.[72,73] The relapse risk for patients with negative PET scans was only 15% to 20%, while those with positive scans had a relapse risk of 60% to 75%. Biopsy documentation of relapse is important, however, because salvage therapy such as high-dose chemotherapy and hematopoietic cell rescue may be associated with significant morbidity. False-positive PET scans in this setting have been reported to be associated with thymic hyperplasia, infection, granulomatous lymphadenitis, and massive histiocytic reactions.[72,73]

UNFAVORABLE PRESENTATIONS OF INFRADIAPHRAGMATIC STAGE I–II HODGKIN LYMPHOMA

Approximately 10% of patients with stage I–II Hodgkin lymphoma present with disease limited to infradiaphragmatic sites. In general, these patients have a higher frequency of adverse prognostic factors, including older age, male predominance, more lymph node regions involved, mixed cellularity histology, B-symptoms, and higher international prognostic score.[74,75] Although these patients have a higher treatment failure rate, when subjected to multivariate analysis the infradiaphragmatic location is not an independent factor predictive of outcome. The poorer outcome is attributable to the other recognized adverse factors.[74,75] The same general treatment principles as applied for patients with supradiapragmatic disease are appropriate for patients with infradiaphragmatic involvement.

UNFAVORABLE PRESENTATIONS OF STAGE I–II HODGKIN LYMPHOMA IN THE ELDERLY

There are no substantial data related to the management of unfavorable presentations of stage I–II Hodgkin lymphoma restricted to the elderly. The same general principles apply as for patients with favorable presentations of stage I–II (see Chapter 16) and stage III–IV (see Chapter 18).

RECOMMENDATIONS AND FUTURE DIRECTIONS

The outcome of treatment for patients with unfavorable-prognosis stage I–II Hodgkin lymphoma has improved dramatically in the past three decades. This is due primarily to the more common use of combined-modality therapy. The introduction of combined-modality therapy permits a reduction of radiation field size, radiation dose, and chemotherapy duration.

The combined-modality approach enhances the likelihood of local tumor control and addresses the problem of occult extranodal or distant disease. With the effective reduction in the use of radiation and duration of chemotherapy, an ideal safe combination of chemotherapy and irradiation that leads to a high likelihood of cure with minimal long-term toxicity is likely to be identified.

Our ability to monitor response to treatment has been enhanced with FDG-PET and PET/CT scanning. New protocols will be devised that adapt treatment to response measured by FDG-PET, and this is likely to improve outcomes even further. The improved prognosis and long-term survival of these patients will increase the importance of monitoring for late effects.

References

1. Tubiana M, Henry-Amar M, Hayat M, et al. Long-term results of the E.O.R.T.C. randomized study of irradiation and vinblastine in clinical stages I and II of Hodgkin's disease. *Eur J Cancer* 1979;15:645–657.
2. Tubiana M, Henry-Amar M, Carde P, et al. Toward comprehensive management tailored to prognostic factors of patients with clinical stages I and II in Hodgkin's disease. The EORTC Lymphoma Group controlled clinical trials: 1964–1987. *Blood* 1989;73:47–56.
3. Frei EIII, DeVita VT, Moxley JHIII, et al. Approaches to improving the chemotherapy of Hodgkin's disease. *Cancer Res* 1966;26:1284–1289.
4. Anderson H, Crowther D, Deakin DP, et al. A randomised study of adjuvant MVPP chemotherapy after mantle radiotherapy in pathologically staged IA-IIB Hodgkin's disease:10-year follow-up. *Ann Oncol* 1991;2(suppl 2):49–54.
5. Nordentoft AM. Radiotherapy in 50 cases of Hodgkin's disease in stages I and II. Report from the Lymphogranulomatosis Committee (LYGRA). *Ugeskr Laeger* 1972;134:2382–2385.
6. Cosset JM, Henry-Amar M, Noordijk P, et al. The EORTC trials for adult patients with early stage Hodgkin's disease. A 1997 update, 39th Annual Scientific Meeting of ASTRO, Orlando, FL. 1997.
7. Specht L, Gray RG, Clarke MJ, et al. Influence of more extensive radiotherapy and adjuvant chemotherapy on long-term outcome of early-stage Hodgkin's disease: a meta-analysis of 23 randomized trials involving 3,888 patients. International Hodgkin's Disease Collaborative Group. *J Clin Oncol* 1998;16:830–843.
8. Tubiana M, Henry-Amar M, van der Werf-Messing B, et al. A multivariate analysis of prognostic factors in early stage Hodgkin's disease. *Int J Radiat Oncol Biol Phys* 1985;11:23–30.
9. Tubiana M, Henry-Amar M, Hayat M, et al. Prognostic significance of the number of involved areas in the early stages of Hodgkin's disease. *Cancer* 1984;54:885–894.
10. Lee CK, Aeppli DM, Bloomfield CD, et al. Hodgkin's disease: a reassessment of prognostic factors following modification of radiotherapy. *Int J Radiat Oncol Biol Phys* 1987;13:983–991.
11. Mendenhall NP, Cantor AB, Barre DM, et al. The role of prognostic factors in treatment selection for early-stage Hodgkin's disease. *Am J Clin Oncol* 1994;17:189–195.
12. Barton M, Boyages J, Crennan E, et al. Radiation therapy for early stage Hodgkin's disease: Australasian patterns of care. Australasian Radiation Oncology Lymphoma Group. *Int J Radiat Oncol Biol Phys* 1995;31:227–236.
13. Mauch P, Goodman R, Hellman S. The significance of mediastinal involvement in early stage Hodgkin's disease. *Cancer* 1978;42:1039–1045.
14. Hoppe RT, Coleman CN, Cox RS, et al. The management of stage I–II Hodgkin's disease with irradiation alone or combined modality therapy: the Stanford experience. *Blood* 1982;59:455–465.
15. Prosnitz LR, Curtis AM, Knowlton AH, et al. Supradiaphragmatic Hodgkin's disease: significance of large mediastinal masses. *Int J Radiat Oncol Biol Phys* 1980;6:809–813.
16. Fuller LM, Madoc-Jones H, Hagemeister FB Jr., et al. Further follow-up of results of treatment in 90 laparotomy-negative stage I and II Hodgkin's disease patients: significance of mediastinal and non-mediastinal presentations. *Int J Radiat Oncol Biol Phys* 1980;6:799–808.
17. Liew KH, Easton D, Horwich A, et al. Bulky mediastinal Hodgkin's disease management and prognosis. *Hematol Oncol* 1984;2:45–59.
18. Lee CK, Bloomfield CD, Goldman AI, et al. Prognostic significance of mediastinal involvement in Hodgkin's disease treated with curative radiotherapy. *Cancer* 1980;46:2403–2409.
19. Willett CG, Linggood RM, Leong JC, et al. Stage IA to IIB mediastinal Hodgkin's disease: three-dimensional volumetric assessment of response to treatment. *J Clin Oncol* 1988;6:819–824.
20. Lagarde P, Eghbali H, Bonichon F, et al. Brief chemotherapy associated with extended field radiotherapy in Hodgkin's disease. Long-term results in a series of 102 patients with clinical stages I-IIIA. *Eur J Cancer Clin Oncol* 1988;24:1191–1198.
21. Hagemeister FB, Fuller LM, Velasquez WS, et al. Stage I and II Hodgkin's disease: involved-field radiotherapy versus extended-field radiotherapy versus involved-field radiotherapy followed by six cycles of MOPP. *Cancer Treatment Rep* 1982;66:789–798.
22. Jelliffe AM, Thomson AD. The prognosis in Hodgkin's disease. *Br J Cancer* 1955;9:21–36.
23. Peters V. A study of Hodgkin's disease treated radiologically. *Am J Roentgenol* 1950;63:299–311.
24. Bjorkholm M, Holm G, Mellstedt H. Immunologic profile of patients with cured Hodgkin's disease. *Scand J Haematol* 1977;18:361–368.
25. Henry-Amar M, Friedman S, Hayat M, et al. Erythrocyte sedimentation rate predicts early relapse and survival in early-stage Hodgkin disease. The EORTC Lymphoma Cooperative Group. *Ann Intern Med* 1991;114:361–365.
26. Vaughan Hudson B, Maclennan KA, Bennett MH, et al. Systemic disturbance in Hodgkin's disease and its relation to histopathology and prognosis (BNLI report No. 30). *Clin Radiol* 1987;38:257–261.
27. Schomberg PJ, Evans RG, O'Connell MJ, et al. Prognostic significance of mediastinal mass in adult Hodgkin's disease. *Cancer* 1984;53:324–328.
28. Hoppe RT. The management of bulky mediastinal Hodgkin's disease. *Hematol Oncol Clin North Am* 1989;3:265–276.
29. Hopper KD, Diehl LF, Lynch JC, et al. Mediastinal bulk in Hodgkin disease. Method of measurement versus prognosis. *Invest Radiol* 1991;26:1101–1110.
30. Piro AJ, Weiss DR, Hellman S. Mediastinal Hodgkin's disease: a possible danger for intubation anesthesia. Intubation danger in Hodgkin's disease. *Int J Radiat Oncol Biol Phys* 1976;1:415–419.
31. Lister TA, Crowther D, Sutcliffe SB, et al. Report of a committee convened to discuss the evaluation and staging of patients with Hodgkin's disease: Cotswolds meeting. *J Clin Oncol* 1989;7:1630–1636.
32. Cosset JM, Henry-Amar M, Carde P, et al. The prognostic significance of large mediastinal masses in the treatment of Hodgkin's disease. The experience of the Institut Gustave-Roussy. *Hematol Oncol* 1984;2:33–43.
33. Bonadonna G, Valagussa P, Santoro A. Prognosis of bulky Hodgkin's disease treated with chemotherapy alone or combined with radiotherapy. *Cancer Surv* 1985;4:439–458.
34. Anderson H, Deakin DP, Wagstaff J, et al. A randomised study of adjuvant chemotherapy after mantle radiotherapy in supradiaphragmatic Hodgkin's disease PS IA-IIB: a report from the Manchester lymphoma group. *Br J Cancer* 1984;49:695–702.
35. Tubiana M, Henry-Amar M, Hayat M, et al. The EORTC treatment of early stages of Hodgkin's disease: the role of radiotherapy. *Int J Radiat Oncol Biol Phys* 1984;10:197–210.
36. Timothy AR, Sutcliffe SB, Stansfeld AG, et al. Radiotherapy in the treatment of Hodgkin's disease. *Br Med J* 1978;1:1246–1249.
37. Mintz U, Miller JB, Golomb HM, et al. Pathologic stage I and II Hodgkin's disease, 1968–1975: relapse and results of retreatment. *Cancer* 1979;44: 72–79.
38. Coltman CA, Fuller LA, Fisher R, et al. Extended field radiotherapy versus involved field radiotherapy plus MOPP in stage I and II Hodgkin's disease. In: Jones S, Salmon S, eds. *Adjuvant therapy of cancer.* Vol II. New York: Grune and Stratton; 1979:129–136.
39. Stoffel TJ, Cox JD. Hodgkin's disease stage I and II. A comparison between two different treatment policies. *Cancer* 1977;40:90–97.
40. Aisenberg AC, Linggood RM, Lew RA. The changing face of Hodgkin's disease. *Am J Med* 1979;67:921–928.
41. Crnkovich MJ, Leopold K, Hoppe RT, et al. Stage I to IIB Hodgkin's disease: the combined experience at Stanford University and the Joint Center for Radiation Therapy. *J Clin Oncol* 1987;5:1041–1049.
42. Hasenclever D, Diehl V. A prognostic score for advanced Hodgkin's disease. International Prognostic Factors Project on Advanced Hodgkin's Disease. *N Engl J Med* 1998;339:1506–1514.
43. Gisselbrecht C, Mounier N, Andre M, et al. How to define intermediate stage in Hodgkin's lymphoma? *Eur J Haematol Suppl* 2005:111–114.
44. Carde P, Burgers JM, Henry-Amar M, et al. Clinical stages I and II Hodgkin's disease: a specifically tailored therapy according to prognostic factors. *J Clin Oncol* 1988;6:239–252.
45. Carde P, Hagenbeek A, Hayat M, et al. Clinical staging versus laparotomy and combined modality with MOPP versus ABVD in early-stage Hodgkin's disease: the H6 twin randomized trials from the European Organization for Research and Treatment of Cancer Lymphoma Cooperative Group. *J Clin Oncol* 1993;11:2258–2272.
46. Klimo P, Connors JM. MOPP/ABV hybrid program: combination chemotherapy based on early introduction of seven effective drugs for advanced Hodgkin's disease. *J Clin Oncol* 1985;3:1174–1182.
47. Hoerni B, Orgerie MB, Eghbali H, et al. New combination of epirubicine, bleomycin, vinblastine and prednisone (EBVP II) before radiotherapy in localized stages of Hodgkin's disease. Phase II trial in 50 patients. *Bull Cancer* 1988;75:789–794.
48. Noordijk EM, Carde P, Dupouy N, et al. Combined-modality therapy for clinical stage I or II Hodgkin's lymphoma: long-term results of the European Organisation for Research and Treatment of Cancer H7 randomized controlled trials. *J Clin Oncol* 2007:32–41.
49. Eghbali H, Raemaekers J, Carde P. The EORTC strategy in the treatment of Hodgkin's lymphoma. *Eur J Haematol Suppl* 2005;75:135–140.
50. Duggan DB, Petroni GR, Johnson JL, et al. Randomized comparison of ABVD and MOPP/ABV hybrid for the treatment of advanced Hodgkin's disease: report of an intergroup trial. *J Clin Oncol* 2003;21:607–614.
51. Tesch H, Diehl V, Latham B, et al. Interim analysis of the HD9 study of the German Hodgkin Study Group (GHSG)—BEACOPP is more effective than COPP-ABVD in advanced stage Hodgkin's disease. *Leuk Lymphoma* 1998;29:2.

52. Noordijk EM, Thomas J, Ferme C, et al. First results of the EORTC-GELA H9 randomized trials: the H9-F trial (comparing 3 radiation dose levels) and H9-U trial (comparing 3 chemotherapy schemes) in patients with favorable or unfavorable early stage Hodgkin's lymphoma. *Proc Am Soc Clin Oncol* 2005;23:561s. Abstract 6505.

53. Loeffler M, Diehl V, Pfreundschuh M, et al. Dose-response relationship of complementary radiotherapy following four cycles of combination chemotherapy in intermediate-stage Hodgkin's disease. *J Clin Oncol* 1997;15:2275–2287.

54. Sieber M, Tesch H, Pfistner B, et al. Rapidly alternating COPP/ABV/IMEP is not superior to conventional alternating COPP/ABVD in combination with extended-field radiotherapy in intermediate-stage Hodgkin's lymphoma: final results of the German Hodgkin's Lymphoma Study Group Trial HD5. *J Clin Oncol* 2002;20:476–484.

55. Engert A, Schiller P, Josting A, et al. Involved-field radiotherapy is equally effective and less toxic compared with extended-field radiotherapy after four cycles of chemotherapy in patients with early-stage unfavorable Hodgkin's lymphoma: results of the HD8 trial of the German Hodgkin's Lymphoma Study Group. *J Clin Oncol* 2003;21:3601–3608.

56. Klimm BD, Engert A, Brillant C, et al. Comparison of BEACOPP and ABVD chemotherapy in intermediate stage Hodgkin's lymphoma: Results of the fourth interim analysis of the HD 11 trial of GHSG. *Proc Am Soc Clin Oncol* 2005;23:6507. Abstract 6507.

57. Hoppe RT, Portlock CS, Glatstein E, et al. Alternating chemotherapy and irradiation in the treatment of advanced Hodgkin's disease. *Cancer* 1979;43:472–481.

58. Bartlett NL, Rosenberg SA, Hoppe RT, et al. Brief chemotherapy, Stanford V, and adjuvant radiotherapy for bulky or advanced-stage Hodgkin's disease: a preliminary report. *J Clin Oncol* 1995;13:1080–1088.

59. Horning SJ, Rosenberg SA, Hoppe RT. Brief chemotherapy (Stanford V) and adjuvant radiotherapy for bulky or advanced Hodgkin's disease: an update. *Ann Oncol* 1996;7(suppl 4):105–108.

60. Horning SJ, Hoppe RT, Advani R, et al. Efficacy and late effects of Stanford V chemotherapy and radiotherapy in untreated Hodgkin's disease: mature data in early and advanced stage patients. *Blood* 2004;104:92a. Abstract 308.

61. Canellos GP, Anderson JR, Propert KJ, et al. Chemotherapy of advanced Hodgkin's disease with MOPP, ABVD, or MOPP alternating with ABVD. *N Engl J Med* 1992;327:1478–1484.

62. Pavlovsky S, Schvartzman E, Lastiri F, et al. Randomized trial of CVPP for three versus six cycles in favorable-prognosis and CVPP versus AOPE plus radiotherapy in intermediate-prognosis untreated Hodgkin's disease. *J Clin Oncol* 1997;15:2652–2658.

63. Wasserman T, Petroni GR, Millard F, et al. Etoposide, vinblastine, and doxorubicin (EVA) chemotherapy plus subtotal nodal irradiation for early stage, high risk Hodgkin's disease. In: Program/Proceeding of the American Society of Clinical Oncology. ASCO annual meeting. 1996;15.

64. Brusamolino E, Lazzarino M, Orlandi E, et al. Early-stage Hodgkin's disease: long-term results with radiotherapy alone or combined radiotherapy and chemotherapy. *Ann Oncol* 1994;5(suppl 2):101–106.

65. Andre M, Brice P, Cazals D, et al. Results of three courses of adriamycin, bleomycin, vindesine, and dacarbazine with subtotal nodal irradiation in 189 patients with nodal Hodgkin's disease (stage I, II and IIIA). *Hematol Cell Ther* 1997;39:59–65.

66. Bonadonna G, Bonfante V, Viviani S, et al. ABVD plus subtotal nodal versus involved-field radiotherapy in early-stage Hodgkin's disease: long-term results. *J Clin Oncol* 2004;22:2835–2841.

67. Zittoun R, Audebert A, Hoerni B, et al. Extended versus involved fields irradiation combined with MOPP chemotherapy in early clinical stages of Hodgkin's disease. *J Clin Oncol* 1985;3:207–214.

68. Hoppe RT, Cosset JM, Santoro A, et al. Treatment of unfavorable prognosis stage I-II Hodgkin's disease. In: Mauch P, Armitage JO, Diehl V, et al., eds. *Hodgkin's disease.* Philadelphia: Lippincott Williams & Wilkins; 1999:459–482.

69. Longo DL, Glatstein E, Duffey PL, et al. Alternating MOPP and ABVD chemotherapy plus mantle-field radiation therapy in patients with massive mediastinal Hodgkin's disease. *J Clin Oncol* 1997;15:3338–3346.

70. Hutchings M, Mikhaeel NG, Fields PA, et al. Prognostic value of interim FDG-PET after two or three cycles of chemotherapy in Hodgkin lymphoma. *Ann Oncol* 2005;16:1160–1168.

71. Hutchings M, Loft A, Hansen M, et al. FDG-PET after two cycles of chemotherapy predicts treatment failure and progression-free survival in Hodgkin lymphoma. *Blood* 2006;107:52–59.

72. Weihrauch MR, Re D, Scheidhauer K, et al. Thoracic positron emission tomography using 18F-fluorodeoxyglucose for the evaluation of residual mediastinal Hodgkin disease. *Blood* 2001;98:2930–2934.

73. Panizo C, Perez-Salazar M, Bendandi M, et al. Positron emission tomography using 18F-fluorodeoxyglucose for the evaluation of residual Hodgkin's disease mediastinal masses. *Leuk Lymphoma* 2004;45:1829–1833.

74. Darabi K, Sieber M, Chaitowitz M, et al. Infradiaphragmatic versus supradiaphragmatic Hodgkin lymphoma: a retrospective review of 1,114 patients. *Leuk Lymphoma* 2005;46:1715–1720.

75. Vassilakopoulos TP, Angelopoulou MK, Siakantaris MP, et al. Pure infradiaphragmatic Hodgkin's lymphoma. Clinical features, prognostic factor and comparison with supradiaphragmatic disease. *Haematologica* 2006;91:32–39.

CHAPTER 18 ■ TREATMENT OF STAGE III–IV HODGKIN LYMPHOMA

VOLKER DIEHL, KAROLIN BEHRINGER, JOHN RAEMAEKERS, RANJANA ADVANI, AND SANDRA J. HORNING

With current management programs, the majority of patients with Hodgkin lymphoma can be cured, even those with advanced-stage disease. New dose- and time-intensified or time-dense regimens, aided by hematopoietic growth factors, facilitate the delivery of higher and more prolonged concentrations of cytotoxic drugs, ensuring more effective tumor control. Longer-term follow-up data support that these strategies also offer an improved long-term survival. A final judgment, however, regarding their overall benefit, considering treatment-related complications, awaits longer-term follow-up from recent and current clinical trials.

The improvements in the systemic management of Hodgkin lymphoma have been remarkable. Prior to the mid-1960s, patients with stage III–IV Hodgkin's disease were treated with single-agent chemotherapy, resulting in a median survival of approximately 1 year and a 5-year overall survival less than 5%.[1] In 1964, investigators at the National Cancer Institute (NCI) developed a four-drug combination chemotherapy program, MOPP (nitrogen mustard, Oncovin [vincristine], procarbazine, and prednisone) (Table 18.1). This landmark study established the curability of about 50% of patients with stage III and IV disease.[2] Furthermore, the seminal observations regarding prognostic features, patterns of relapse, and toxicities have greatly influenced clinical practice and investigation to the present time.

However, the failure of approximately 20% of patients to enter complete remission, and the relapse of about one-third of patients following complete remission with MOPP chemotherapy, encouraged the development of strategies to decrease treatment failures through the investigation of alternate primary therapies. Patterns of failure with MOPP demonstrated the inverse relationship between tumor burden and rate of cure, and indicated that over 90% of patients failed in sites of initial disease, especially previously involved lymph nodes.[3] Failure in bulky disease sites, especially the mediastinum, was often observed. These observations provided the rationale for the integration of radiation therapy in advanced-stage disease.

As new effective agents in the treatment of Hodgkin lymphoma were identified, the MOPP regimen and its derivatives were abandoned and nearly completely replaced by ABVD, which today is considered the gold standard to which all new therapies for the treatment of stage III–IV Hodgkin lymphoma must be compared.

In the 40 years since MOPP was introduced, histopathologic, immunopathologic, and radiographic techniques have become increasingly sophisticated, and there have been significant advances in supportive care. There has been a virtual disappearance of the lymphocyte-depletion histology from clinical series. Staging laparotomy as a routine staging technique has become obsolete. We now rely upon more sensitive anatomic and functional imaging studies to enumerate the sites of disease and assign an overall Ann Arbor stage. With more sensitive radiographic examinations and the advent of functional imaging with FDG-positron emission tomography (PET) to assess treatment response, it is likely that "complete remission" will be defined more precisely and allow for the use of more adapted treatments that vary with individual response.

The availability of potent anti-emetics and the more routine use of venous access devices have changed the perception of acute chemotherapy toxicity. With the use of granulocytic growth factors to support dose intensity, deviations from optimal drug doses and schedules can be minimized. In addition, there has been a move toward the use of absolute neutrophil count rather than total white blood cell count in dose adjustment and greater tolerance of grade III–IV neutropenia. These subtleties in diagnosis, staging, and clinical practice must be considered in the interpretation of the studies discussed in this chapter, which were conducted over a period of more than four decades.

The definition of advanced Hodgkin lymphoma warrants comment. In contrast to the original NCI study, recent investigations have included patients with bulky stage I and II or IIB disease under the rubric of "advanced" Hodgkin lymphoma. Clinical studies also vary with respect to the inclusion of patients who have progressed after primary radiation therapy. Reported end-points also vary. The NCI investigators have traditionally expressed their results as "relapse-free survival," which excluded the subset of patients who did not achieve a complete remission, whereas more recent trials have included all patients in their end-points of "freedom from recurrence," "freedom from treatment failure," or "freedom from progression." Likewise, the NCI data were expressed as "tumor-specific mortality," which excluded patients who were thought to have died from causes other than Hodgkin lymphoma. Currently, many clinical investigators specify "event-free survival" or "failure-free survival," which score both relapse and death as adverse events. Comparisons across studies must consider and attempt to translate these terms. The recent International Harmonization Project attempts to standardize response assessment and outcome measurements and will facilitate comparison of results in clinical trials.[4]

COMBINATION CHEMOTHERAPY

MOPP

In 1964, NCI investigators developed the four-drug MOPP program, in which each drug was given at full dose over 2 weeks, followed by a 2-week recovery period. Patients were treated for two additional monthly cycles after a complete

TABLE 18.1

MOPP AND MOPP DERIVATIVE COMBINATION CHEMOTHERAPY

Drug combination	Dose (mg/m^2)	Route	Schedule (days)	Cycle length (days)
MOPP				21
Mechlorethamine	6	IV	1, 8	
Oncovin(vincristine)	1.4	IV	1, 8	
Procarbazine	100	PO	1–14	
Prednisone	40	PO	1–14	
BCVPP				28
Carmustine	100	IV	1	
Cyclophosphamide	600	IV	1	
Vinblastine	5	IV	1	
Procarbazine	50	PO	1	
	100	PO	2–10	
Prednisone	60	PO	1–10	
ChlVPP				28
Chlorambucil	6	PO	1–14	
Vinblastine	6	IV	1, 8	
Procarbazine	100	PO	1–14	
Prednisone	40 total	PO	1–14	
COPP				28
Cyclophosphamide	650	IV	1, 8	
Oncovin (vincristine)	1.4	IV	1, 8	
Procarbazine	100	PO	1–14	
Prednisone	40	PO	1–14	
MVPP				42
Nitrogen mustard	6	IV	1, 8	
Vinblastine	6	IV	1, 8	
Procarbazine	100	PO	1–14	
Prednisone	40 total	PO	1–14	
LOPP				28
Chlorambucil	10 total	PO	1–10	
Oncovin (vincristine)	1.4	IV	1, 8	
Procarbazine	100	PO	1–10	
Prednisone	25	PO	1–14	
CVPP				28
Lomustine	75	PO	1	
Vinblastine	4	IV	1, 8	
Procarbazine	100	PO	1–14	
Prednisone	40	PO	1–14	

Some studies capped vincristine at 2 mg. Prednisone was given in cycles 1 and 4 only by some groups. Chlorambucil and vinblastine were capped at 10 mg and procarbazine was capped at 200 mg in some studies.
IV, intravenous; PO, oral.

remission was achieved, but all received a minimum of six monthly cycles unless there was disease progression. Dose reductions were prospectively defined based on objective criteria, and the doses of vincristine were not capped at 2 mg. The results of the complete NCI studies were published by DeVita and associates[2] in 1980 and have been updated subsequently[5] with a median follow-up of 14 years. The complete remission rate was 81% and 36% of the complete responders relapsed, yielding a 52% freedom-from-progression rate at 10 years. The overall survival was estimated to be 50% at 10 years. The ability of MOPP to cure advanced-stage Hodgkin lymphoma was subsequently confirmed by multiple investigators in both single-institution and cooperative group trials, often as the standard arm of a randomized clinical trial. The major toxicities were generally reversible bone marrow suppression, neuropathy, and sterility.

NCI investigators also made important observations regarding the ability to treat patients who relapsed after initial treatment with MOPP.[6] The success of retreatment with MOPP correlated with the duration of initial remission, an observation that has been confirmed with a variety of second-line treatments.[7,8] The low probability of an effective outcome with a second course of MOPP chemotherapy was largely related to relapse, but toxicity was a significant cause of failure as well, particularly second malignancy related to the total doses of alkylating agents.[9,10]

MOPP Derivatives

Despite the excellent results achieved with MOPP, investigation of alternative regimens was motivated by the desire to obtain equivalent or improved results with less toxicity, particularly gastrointestinal and neurologic toxicity. Early studies conducted by CALGB demonstrated that omission of mechlorethamine or procarbazine from the MOPP regimen resulted in inferior complete remission rates and overall survival.[11] Based on these data, chemotherapy regimens for advanced Hodgkin lymphoma generally have adhered to the four-drug principle established by the initial MOPP studies.

Table 18.1 details the composition of MOPP and established MOPP-like regimens. In several regimens, vinblastine, a vinca alkaloid with more myelosuppressive but fewer neuropathic effects, was substituted for vincristine. Alternate alkylating agents such as cyclophosphamide or chlorambucil and the nitrosourea agents lomustine and carmustine were incorporated into four or five drug regimens.[12–18] In some cases, however, these derivative regimens also altered the doses and duration of procarbazine and prednisone.

In brief, multiple MOPP-like alternatives proved to have efficacy equivalent to MOPP with less gastrointestinal and neurologic toxicity. Lower cure rates were achieved with MOPP delivered outside of the NCI, and this spurred lively debates for a number of years. Indeed, it was difficult to interpret the significance of patient selection variables (previous treatment with chemotherapy or radiotherapy, referral versus population-based practice); planned treatment variables (mandated dose reduction, vincristine capping, shortened schedules of procarbazine, maintenance therapies); and individual practice variables (dose adjustments and treatment delays based on subjective and objective toxicities). However, this phase of the quest for more optimal treatment of advanced Hodgkin lymphoma was ended due to two constant features: the failure of treatment in about half of patients with advanced-stage disease, and the routine association of alkylating agent-based chemotherapy regimens with an increased risk of sterility and acute leukemia.

ABVD

In 1973 Bonadonna and colleagues introduced the novel ABVD (Adriamycin [doxorubicin], bleomycin, vinblastine, and dacarbazine) regimen for patients who had failed MOPP chemotherapy (Table 18.2).[19] ABVD was specifically developed for MOPP resistance, incorporating four different, individually effective compounds. Vinblastine was one of the most active single agents in advanced Hodgkin lymphoma and lacked cross-resistance with vincristine in human tumors.[20] Doxorubicin and bleomycin were also very active drugs, producing objective responses through a wide variety of treatment schedules in about 40% to 60% of patients.[21–23] The single-agent activity of dacarbazine reported by Frei and associates[22] was confirmed in Milan and, in experimental systems, dacarbazine showed synergy with doxorubicin without additional toxicity.[19]

TABLE 18.2

ABVD AND ABV(D)-CONTAINING COMBINATION CHEMOTHERAPY

Drug combination	Dose (mg/m²)	Route	Schedule (days)	Cycle length (days)
ABVD				28
Adriamycin (doxorubicin)	25	IV	1, 15	
Bleomycin	10	IV	1, 15	
Vinblastine	6	IV	1, 15	
Dacarbazine	375	IV	1, 15	
MOPP/ABVD alternating (Milan)				28
Alternate cycles of MOPP with ABVD				
COPP/ABVD alternating (GHSG)				28
Alternate cycles of COPP with ABVD				
MOPP→ABVD sequential (ECOG)				28
MOPP × 6–8 followed by ABVD × 3				
MOPP-ABVD hybrid (Milan)				28
Mechlorethamine	6	IV	1	
Oncovin (vincristine)	1.4[a]	IV	1	
Procarbazine	100	PO	1–7	
Prednisone	40	PO	1–7	
Adriamycin (doxorubicin)	25	IV	15	
Bleomycin	10	IV	15	
Vinblastine	6	IV	15	
Dacarbazine	375	IV	15	
MOPP-ABV hybrid (Vancouver)				28
Mechlorethamine	6	IV	1	
Oncovin (vincristine)	1.4[a]	IV	1	
Procarbazine	100	PO	1–7	
Prednisone	40	PO	1–14	
Adriamycin (doxorubicin)	35	IV	8	
Bleomycin	10	IV	8	
Vinblastine	6	IV	8	

[a]Vincristine dose capped at 2 mg.
GHSG, German Hodgkin Study Group; ECOG, Eastern Cooperative Oncology Group; IV, intravenous; PO, oral.

The efficacy of ABVD was initially compared with MOPP in a prospective randomized trial in previously untreated patients with stage IIB, III, and IV Hodgkin lymphoma or in those in first relapse after radiotherapy.[19] The study design included irradiation for responding patients and a crossover design for patients failing to achieve complete remission or relapsing within 12 months. The complete remission rate favored ABVD over MOPP, 80% versus 71%. A trend at 4 years toward superior freedom from progression (53% MOPP versus 65% ABVD) and overall survival (88% MOPP versus 90% ABVD) was noted for ABVD. Because of the small number of patients in this study and the confounding treatment variables, the authors were only able to conclude that ABVD was at least as effective as MOPP in the remission induction of advanced Hodgkin lymphoma, alone or with irradiation. Table 18.3 shows the 10-year results of this study, which, in retrospect, predicted the outcome of larger cooperative group studies initiated a decade or more later.[19]

The Milan group followed their initial study with a larger trial involving 232 patients with pathologic stage IIB, IIIA, and IIIB Hodgkin lymphoma (Table 18.3).[24] Patients were randomized to three cycles of MOPP or ABVD followed by subtotal or total lymphoid irradiation and concluding with three additional cycles of the same chemotherapy. Outcomes in this study at 7 years were statistically significant in favor of ABVD, with freedom from progression (63% MOPP versus 81% ABVD, $p < 0.02$) and overall survival (68% MOPP versus 77% ABVD, $p < 0.03$) as end-points.[25] This study demonstrated the difficulty in delivery of planned doses of MOPP following irradiation, a factor that led to criticism of the conclusions. Of major significance, ABVD was associated with a reduction in serious late effects[24,26]

The acute toxicities of ABVD included a higher incidence of alopecia and vomiting compared with MOPP. Prior to the current era of potent anti-emetics, anticipatory nausea and vomiting complicated the delivery of ABVD. Relative to MOPP, the neurotoxicity of ABVD was mild but the administration of dacarbazine often required prolonged infusion in small peripheral vessels. Severe myelosuppression was rare when ABVD was administered alone and, therefore, ABVD could be delivered in more optimal doses in a combined-modality setting.[24]

In contrast to MOPP, ABVD was not associated with a high incidence of permanent azoospermia or amenorrhea.[26] Azoospermia and oligospermia were recorded with an incidence of 36% and 20% with recovery to normal values in all patients in the Milan trial.[24] However, a significant proportion of patients in this combined modality trial did not receive six cycles of treatment and/or had dose modifications subsequent to irradiation. In a smaller study of ABVD alone, the incidence of azoospermia was 33%.[27] Of major importance, secondary leukemia and myelodysplasia were not observed after ABVD.[28] The rate of secondary leukemia within 10 years of MOPP plus irradiation was 6.5% compared to 0 among patients treated with ABVD plus irradiation.[24]

There is, however, mounting evidence that ABVD may cause late cardiopulmonary toxicity, with or without mediastinal irradiation. In the Milan trial, the only adverse factor noted among ABVD recipients was an increase in pulmonary fibrosis on chest radiograph.[24] However, in prospective studies conducted at Stanford and the European Organization for the Research and Treatment of Cancer (EORTC), ABVD in combination with irradiation resulted in definable abnormalities on formal pulmonary function testing.[29,30] Although many of these laboratory abnormalities were not clinically significant, fatal pulmonary complications related to bleomycin have occurred after ABVD alone.[30,31] Children appear to be more susceptible to both the cardiotoxicity of doxorubicin and the pulmonary toxicity of bleomycin.[32,33] For a full discussion of this topic, see Chapters 21, 25, and 26.

The superior outcomes with ABVD compared to MOPP in the Milan trials set the stage for the definitive large randomized trials of chemotherapy alone in advanced Hodgkin lymphoma that would follow. The CALGB led a trial in advanced Hodgkin lymphoma comparing ABVD with MOPP and MOPP alternating with ABVD (see below).[31] The results from this study suggested that ABVD was superior to MOPP and

TABLE 18.3

RANDOMIZED TRIALS WITH ABVD CHEMOTHERAPY

Group and treatment	No. cycles	RT	No. patients	Stage	% FFP (p)	% FFS (p)	% OS (p)	Time analyzed (years)
Milan[19]	6	IF	76	IIB, III, IV				10
ABVD	6				63		54	
MOPP	6				50		39	
					(NS)		(NS)	
Milan[24]		STLI	232	IIB, III				7
ABVD	6				81		77	
MOPP	6				63		68	
					(<0.002)		(<0.03)	
CALGB[31]	—		361	III, IV prior RT				5
ABVD	6–8					61	73	
MOPP	6–8					50	66	
MOPP/ABVD	12					65	75	
						(0.03)	(NS)	
CALGB[130]	—		856	III, IV prior RT				3
ABVD	8–10					65	87	
MOPP-ABV	8–10					67	85	
						(NS)	(NS)	

RT, radiotherapy; FFP, freedom from progression; FFS, failure-free survival; OS, overall survival; IF, involved field; STLI, subtotal lymphoid irradiation; NS, not significant; CALGB, Cancer and Leukemia Group B.

could be substituted for MOPP/ABVD combination therapy in advanced Hodgkin lymphoma , eliminating a source of serious late morbidity. The efficacy of ABVD and its favorable toxicity profile, relative to that of the MOPP-ABV hybrid combination, was confirmed in a subsequent trial, also led by the CALGB, as detailed below.[34] These studies established the ABVD regimen as the standard treatment for advanced Hodgkin lymphoma.

Alternating Therapy

In 1974 the Milan group initiated a treatment strategy to alternate cycles of MOPP and ABVD in patients with stage IV disease, based on the therapeutic limitations of MOPP and the efficacy of ABVD in patients refractory to MOPP (Table 18.2).[35] Patients with stage IV disease were randomized to MOPP or MOPP/ABVD, which in the absence of disease progression was given for 12 cycles. In this small study of 88 patients, 25 had received previous irradiation. Despite the small numbers, the results in favor of the alternating program were striking and statistically significant for freedom from progression at 8 years (36% MOPP versus 65% MOPP/ABVD, $p <0.005$). The overall survival was likewise superior for MOPP/ABVD (64% MOPP versus 84% MOPP/ABVD), but this difference did not achieve statistical significance. An important aspect of this trial was the superiority of MOPP/ABVD in subsets considered to be prognostically unfavorable with MOPP: age over 40 years, systemic symptoms, nodular sclerosis histology, and bulky disease.

Three large cooperative group trials have confirmed the Milan results and established the superiority of combination treatment with MOPP and ABVD over treatment with MOPP or a MOPP derivative alone in advanced Hodgkin lymphoma. Based on their previous clinical trial and the emerging data regarding the efficacy of ABVD, ECOG randomized patients to BCVPP, BCVPP plus low-dose irradiation, or MOPP followed by ABVD.[36] The complete remission rate was significantly higher with the sequential delivery of MOPP and ABVD, and overall survival favored the sequential regimen as well.

The Milan trial suggested the superiority of MOPP/ABVD over MOPP in patients with stage IV disease, whereas the trials from this group testing MOPP or ABVD in combined-modality programs demonstrated an advantage for ABVD in other stages. Therefore, the CALGB designed a three-arm comparative trial to test the relative efficacy and toxicity of six to eight cycles of MOPP, six to eight cycles of ABVD, and 12 cycles of MOPP alternating with ABVD in advanced Hodgkin lymphoma (Table 18.3).[31] Patients failing prior irradiation were eligible for this study also. A total of 361 eligible patients were randomized to MOPP ($n = 123$), ABVD ($n = 115$), or alternating ($n = 123$) therapy. Figure 18.1 demonstrates that at 10 years, the failure-free survival rates were 38% for MOPP, 55% for ABVD, and 50% for MOPP/ABVD, $p = 0.02$. There was a trend for superior overall survival with ABVD (68%) or MOPP/ABVD (65%) compared with MOPP alone (58%, $p = 0.15$) (Table 18.3).

The power of numbers in cooperative clinical trials was demonstrated in this trial. The differences in outcome mirror the Bonadonna trial of MOPP versus ABVD initiated in 1974, but the statistical significance in the CALGB trial was appropriately termed a definitive advance in the treatment of Hodgkin lymphoma.[31]

The EORTC and the Groupe Pierre-et-Marie-Curie initiated a study in 1981 in which MOPP chemotherapy was compared with two courses of MOPP alternating with two courses of ABVD to a total of eight courses.[37] Radiotherapy was given to initial nodal sites of 5 cm or more in diameter or residual masses after four courses of chemotherapy. Freedom from progression data for this trial were not provided. Failure-free survival at 6 years significantly differed between the treatment arms (43% MOPP, 60% MOPP/ABVD, $p = 0.01$). There were more deaths in the MOPP arm ($n = 40$) compared to MOPP/ABVD ($n = 29$) and more patients in the MOPP arm died from Hodgkin lymphoma ($n = 29$) than in the MOPP/ABVD arm ($n = 20$).

Five years following the initiation of the MOPP versus MOPP/ABVD trial in Milan, Goldie and Coldman[38] proposed a mathematical model relating the drug sensitivity of tumors to their spontaneous mutation rate. The model predicted that alternation of treatments with quantitative antitumor equivalence and absence of cross-resistance would yield superior results. This hypothesis was frequently cited to support studies

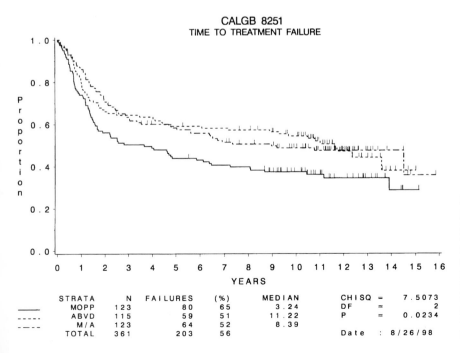

CALGB 8251
TIME TO TREATMENT FAILURE

STRATA	N	FAILURES	(%)	MEDIAN		
MOPP	123	80	65	3.24	CHISQ =	7.5073
ABVD	115	59	51	11.22	DF =	2
M/A	123	64	52	8.39	P =	0.0234
TOTAL	361	203	56		Date :	8/26/98

FIGURE 18.1. Failure-free survival in 131 patients with stage III–IV Hodgkin lymphoma randomized in Cancer and Leukemia Group B (CALGB) study 8251 to six to eight cycles of MOPP (mechlorethamine, Oncovin [vincristine], procarbazine, and prednisone) (*solid line, n = 123*), six to eight cycles of ABVD (Adriamycin [doxorubicin], bleomycin, vinblastine, and dacarbazine) (broken line, *n = 115*), or 12 cycles of MOPP alternating with ABVD (*dotted line, n = 123*). (Data updated by George Canellos, MD.)

in advanced Hodgkin lymphoma, although the basic tenets of the model were rarely satisfied by the clinical designs.[39–41]

Hybrid Regimens

The theoretic basis for multidrug regimens is the predicted advantage of the earliest possible introduction of all active agents to address heterogeneous tumor cell populations. The SWOG conducted one of the first clinical trials incorporating elements of MOPP with doxorubicin in a hybrid regimen.[42] Working independently, the groups in Vancouver and Milan created the first true hybrids of MOPP and ABVD designed to prospectively test the Goldie-Coldman[38] hypothesis (Table 18.2). In 1985, Klimo and Connors[43] reported the preliminary results of a MOPP-ABV

hybrid in which MOPP was given on days 1 to 7 and ABV was given on day 8.

Dacarbazine was omitted and doxorubicin was increased from 25 to 35 mg/m^2. Prednisone was given for a full 14 days. Selected partial responders also received involved-field irradiation. A complete remission rate of 88% and an overall survival rate of 90% were reported at 4 years in previously untreated patients with stage IIEA, III, and IV disease.

Based on these encouraging data, the National Cancer Institute of Canada embarked on a trial comparing MOPP-ABV hybrid with alternating MOPP/ABVD in patients with IIIB or IV Hodgkin lymphoma or those who had previously received wide-field irradiation (Table 18.4).[44] Responding patients received a minimum of eight cycles of chemotherapy, and those with residual disease in a localized region received irradiation

TABLE 18.4

EFFICACY AND TOXICITY OF MOPP AND ABV(D) COMBINATION CHEMOTHERAPY

Group and treatment	No. cycles	No. patients	Stage	% FFS (p)	% OS (p)	Time analyzed (years)	Toxicity
NCI-Canada[44]		301	III, IV prior RT				
Alternating MOPP/ABVD ± RT[a]	8–12			67	83	5	More febrile neutropenia and mucositis with MOPP/ABV
Hybrid MOPP-ABV ± RT[a]	8–12			71 (NS)	81 (NS)		No difference in toxic deaths or second malignancy
Milan[45]		427	I–IIB[b], III, IV prior RT				
Alternating MOPP/ABVD ± RT[c]	6–8			67[d]	74	10	6% incidence of second malignancy in all treated patients
Hybrid MOPP-ABVD ± RT[c]	6–8			65 (NS)	72 (NS)		
ECOG[46]		737	III, IV prior RT				
Hybrid MOPP-ABV	8–12			64	79	8	More neutropenia and pulmonary toxicity with hybrid; more leukemia/MDS with sequential
Sequential MOPP→ABVD	9–11			54 (0.01)	71 (0.02)		
CALGB[130]		856	III, IV prior RT				
Hybrid MOPP-ABV	8–10			67	85	3	More neutropenia and pulmonary toxicity with hybrid; more leukemia/MDS with sequential
ABVD	8–10			65 (NS)	87 (NS)		

[a]RT given for residual disease.
[b]IIA bulky also included.
[c]RT given for bulky disease.
[d]Freedom from progression.
RT, radiation therapy; FFS, failure-free survival; OS, overall survival, NS, not significant; ECOG, Eastern Cooperative Oncology Group; MDS, myelodysplastic syndrome; CALGB, Cancer and Leukemia Group B.

between the sixth and seventh cycle. The overall survival rates at 5 years in the 301 randomized patients were similar (81% MOPP-ABV hybrid, 83% alternating MOPP/ABVD; $p = 0.74$). Failure-free survivals were also similar (71% MOPP-ABV hybrid, 67% alternating MOPP/ABVD; $p = 0.87$). The hybrid regimen proved to be more toxic with a higher incidence of febrile neutropenia and stomatitis. Of note, in planned subset analyses, the alternating regimen yielded superior 5-year failure-free survival in patients with prior irradiation (73% MOPP-ABV hybrid, 94% alternating MOPP/ABVD; $p = 0.01$).

The hybrid regimen developed by the Milan group was initially tested in a randomized trial comparing MOPP-ABVD given in a day 1 and 15 hybrid fashion with the conventional alternating schedule (Table 18.2). Patients were treated for two consolidation cycles to a maximum of eight cycles. The mature data from this study were published in 1996 (Table 18.4).[45] A total of 427 patients with stages IB, IIA bulky, IIB, III, and IV Hodgkin lymphoma were enrolled. Patients relapsing after subtotal or total nodal irradiation were also eligible. Radiotherapy was planned for nodal sites of initial bulky lymphoma. At 10 years the freedom-from-progression rate showed no difference between the hybrid (69%) and alternating (67%) treatment arms. Similarly, the overall survival at 10 years in the two regimens was nearly identical: 72% for hybrid and 74% for alternating MOPP/ABVD. A total of 17 patients died of second malignancies, including 10 with secondary leukemia. However, 9 of these 10 patients had received salvage chemotherapy in addition to MOPP/ABVD.

ECOG led an intergroup trial of 737 patients with advanced Hodgkin lymphoma or in relapse after radiotherapy.[46] Patients were randomized to best response to MOPP (six to eight cycles) followed by three cycles of ABVD or MOPP-ABV hybrid as described by the Vancouver group (Table 18.2). At 8 years, failure-free survival significantly favored MOPP-ABV hybrid (64%) over MOPP followed by ABVD (54%), $p = 0.01$ (Table 18.4). Overall survival was statistically ($p = 0.02$) prolonged after MOPP-ABV. More life-threatening or fatal neutropenia and pulmonary toxicity were seen with MOPP-ABV, whereas the sequential treatment had more significant thrombocytopenia. Of note, in this study, which used higher cumulative doses of MOPP and no radiotherapy, the incidence of acute leukemia and myelodysplasia was greater on the sequential arm (Table 18.4).

The superior outcome for MOPP-ABV hybrid in the ECOG trial, together with the efficacy of ABVD in the CALGB trial, formed the basis of an intergroup comparison of ABVD with MOPP/ABV hybrid led by CALGB. A total of 856 patients with stage III or IV Hodgkin lymphoma or recurrent disease following irradiation were randomized to a minimum of eight cycles of chemotherapy (Table 18.4).[34] At 5 years, there was no difference in failure-free survival for ABVD (63%) or MOPP-ABV (66%), $p = 0.42$. However, this study was prematurely stopped by the Data and Safety Monitoring Board due to excess treatment-related deaths and second malignancies with the hybrid regimen (Table 18.4). Although no difference in overall survival was seen, 82% for ABVD and 81% for MOPP-ABV ($p = 0.82$), hematologic and pulmonary toxicities were significantly greater with hybrid treatment ($p = 0.06$ and 0.001). Overall, there were 24 treatment-related deaths. There were 9 second malignancies with ABVD (including myelodysplasia/leukemia in 2 patients who received MOPP-like salvage regimens) compared with 28 second cancers with MOPP-ABV (including 11 cases of myelodysplasia/leukemia; $p = 0.011$). Based on this analysis, the study was closed and the authors concluded that ABVD was equivalent in efficacy and less toxic than hybrid treatment.

Another test of the hybrid concept was in the design of the GHSG HD6 trial. The efficacy of the hybrid regimen COPP/ABV/IMEP was compared with the standard COPP/ABVD in 584 patients with advanced disease. There was no significant difference between the two arms with respect to 7-year survival (73% in both arms) or freedom from treatment failure (54% versus 56%). Grade 3 to 4 thrombocytopenia was more common in the COPP/ABV/IMEP arm.[47] Taken together, these studies of alternating and hybrid therapy, as well as the groundbreaking work of Bonadonna and colleagues, established ABV(D)-containing chemotherapy as the treatment of choice for advanced Hodgkin lymphoma to which new treatments would need to be compared.

Duration of Therapy

As noted previously, patients in the original studies of MOPP chemotherapy conducted by the NCI were treated for two additional monthly cycles after a complete remission was achieved.[2] All received a minimum of six monthly cycles unless they progressed before that time such that the vast majority of patients received six to eight cycles of MOPP. Bonadonna and associates lengthened the treatment to 12 cycles of MOPP such that equal time periods of chemotherapy would be compared in alternating MOPP (six cycles) and ABVD (six cycles).[35] However, the subsequent trial from the Milan group shortened the alternating program to eight cycles without apparent reduction in efficacy.[45] Subsequently, the CALGB trial demonstrated that the efficacy of eight cycles of ABVD was comparable to 12 cycles of alternating MOPP/ABVD.[31] A total of 8 to 12 cycles of chemotherapy was delivered in the more recent randomized phase III trials described in Table 18.4. It should be noted, however, that both the more recent Milan trial and the Canadian study also incorporated selective, consolidative radiotherapy.

The EORTC Lymphoma Group has adopted a treatment strategy that restricts the number of cycles to six when an early complete remission—e.g, after four cycles—is reached, whereas those who achieve a complete remission only after six cycles receive a total of eight cycles.[37] Recently, there has been interest in using even fewer cycles of chemotherapy in combination with radiation therapy in early-stage Hodgkin lymphoma.[48] Extrapolation of this approach to advanced disease is not recommended. Mathematical modeling suggests that cumulative dose as well as dose intensity may be important to the successful treatment of advanced disease.[49]

The NCI recommendation of treating patients with two cycles beyond best response is still applicable in many situations. However, the definition of complete response, and the interpretation of residual radiographic abnormalities and their impact on the length of therapy, frequently challenge physicians. If stable radiographic abnormalities remain, it may be extremely difficult to determine whether they represent residual disease or fibrosis. As discussed below, even though randomized trials have not been conducted, consolidation of chemotherapy-induced remissions with radiation therapy is generally accepted for patients with massive mediastinal Hodgkin lymphoma, regardless of stage.[50,51] Functional imaging with FDG-PET scanning may improve the ability to define a true complete remission (see Chapter 11). A positive PET scan after the completion of therapy is highly predictive of residual disease, although false-positive studies have been reported. Conversely, the negative predictive value of PET is estimated to be only 92%.[52] At the completion of all therapy, if there is suspicion of residual disease and the site is accessible, biopsy is recommended. Patients for whom a major surgical exploration would be required to confirm residual disease should be closely monitored, undergoing pathologic confirmation at the first sign of disease progression.

There is no role for maintenance therapy in advanced Hodgkin lymphoma. None of the older randomized trials that studied chemotherapy maintenance identified a therapeutic benefit.[53,54] Based on the available data, it is recommended that patients with stage III and IV disease be monitored for response during treatment and receive two courses of chemotherapy beyond best response, with six cycles considered to be a minimum duration.

PROGNOSTIC FACTORS IN ADVANCED DISEASE

It is imperative to identify patients who may profit most from dose intensification. An international effort involving more than 5,000 patients, led by Hasenclever and Diehl[55] identified prognostic factors in advanced Hodgkin lymphoma. Seven factors were recognized—stage IV, male sex, age, hemoglobin, white blood count, lymphocyte count, and albumin—each of which contributed about a 7% reduction in freedom from progression at 5 years (Table 18.5). When five to seven adverse factors were present, one of which included age over 45 years, freedom from progression at 5 years fell to 45%.[55] However, this subgroup constituted only 7% of the total patient population, indicating that randomized trials would require international collaboration to evaluate new therapies in this group.

In clinical practice, the benefits of dose intensification, often theoretical, must be balanced against the established risks of cumulative drug doses with serious adverse effects such as second malignancies, sterility, neuropathy, and cardiopulmonary toxicity. Newer treatments for advanced Hodgkin lymphoma, discussed below, have generally focused on these issues, with the objective of increasing efficacy through dose intensification and/or the introduction of new drugs or the reduction of toxicity by lowering cumulative drug and radiation exposure, drug addition, and drug substitution.

BEACOPP

Drug delivery may be intensified by increasing individual drug dose, shortening the interval between treatments, or both. The German Hodgkin Study Group (GHSG) has completed a series of studies that address these issues of dose intensity. A mathematical model of tumor growth and chemotherapy effects fitted to the data from 705 patients treated by the GHSG served as the basis for these studies.[49] This model predicted that moderate dose escalation would improve failure-free survival by 10% to 15% at 5 years. The BEACOPP (bleomycin, etoposide, Adriamycin [doxorubicin], cyclophosphamide, Oncovin [vincristine], procarbazine, and prednisone) regimen (see Table 18.6) was devised to serve as a standard combination for dose escalation.[56] After establishing excellent tolerance as well as efficacy, a second study of escalated BEACOPP was performed in which doxorubicin was increased to a fixed level (140%) and doses of cyclophosphamide and etoposide were increased in a stepwise fashion with growth factor support.[57] Maximum doses, with hematologic toxicity as an end-point, were found to be 190% of cyclophosphamide and 200% of etoposide.

With the design of standard and escalated BEACOPP in place, the GHSG embarked upon a three-arm trial (HD-9) in which these combinations were prospectively tested together with COPP/ABVD in advanced Hodgkin lymphoma.[57] All three arms of this randomized trial included 30 Gy consolidative radiotherapy for initially bulky (>5 cm) or residual disease, which was administered to 61% to 70% of patients. The pooled BEACOPP arms were superior to COPP/ABVD with regard to progression rate and freedom from treatment failure in the interim analyses, and the COPP/ABVD arm was closed early to further accrual. In the most recent report, which included 1,186 evaluable patients with a median follow-up of 7 years, the freedom-from-treatment failure rate was 67% in the COPP/ABVD group, 75% in the BEACOPP group, and 85% in the increased-dose BEACOPP group.[57]

The induction-failure rates were 25%, 12%, and 4%. Overall survival rates were 79%, 84%, and 90% for COPP/ABVD, BEACOPP, and the increased-dose BEACOPP, respectively, with the difference between COPP/ABVD and increased-dose BEACOPP being significant ($p < 0.002$). Although the two BEACOPP regimens were superior to COPP/ABVD in all prognostic groups, the most pronounced differences were in the poor-risk group of patients with four to seven adverse factors according to the International Prognostic Score (Table 18.7). As expected, the escalated BEACOPP was associated with greater hematologic toxicity, including red blood cell and platelet transfusions, neutropenia, and time in hospital, although patients were generally treated in the outpatient setting. The high cumulative doses of alkylating agents and etoposide predicted that both sterility and an increased risk of leukemia/myelodysplasia would complicate the use of BEACOPP. Indeed, there were 4 cases of acute leukemia/MDS after standard BEACOPP, 9 after increased-dose BEACOPP, and 1 after COPP/ABVD. Nevertheless, these results from a large, cooperative group are outstanding.

The next trial of the GHSG, HD-12, assigned patients to treatment with eight cycles of escalated BEACOPP or four cycles of escalated BEACOPP plus four cycles of baseline BEACOPP. Following chemotherapy, patients were randomized to receive 30 Gy irradiation to initial bulky or residual disease, versus no further therapy. After a median follow-up of 2 years with 908 evaluable patients, FFTF and OS for the whole cohort were 88% and 94%, respectively. For the group getting four cycles of escalated BEACOPP plus four cycles of baseline BEACOPP, FFTF was 88% and OS 94%, respectively; for the patient cohort getting eight cycles of escalated BEACOPP, FFTF was 90% and OS 96%. There was no statistical difference between the two different treatment arms for either outcome measure and the toxicity profile was similar to that seen in the HD9 trial.[57]

Experience with the toxicity of the escalated BEACOPP regimen, especially the risk for AML/MDS, next led the GHSG to develop a BEACOPP variant in which the drug dosage and timing of administration was calculated to achieve the same efficacy with reduced toxicity, according to the dose model of Hasenclever and colleagues.[49] The result was a time-intensified BEACOPP-baseline regimen given in 14-day intervals, and facilitated by the use of granulocyte colony stimulating factor (G-CSF), BEACOPP-14 (Table 18.6).

TABLE 18.5

INTERNATIONAL PROGNOSTIC FACTORS FOR HODGKIN LYMPHOMA[55]

No. factors[a]	Population (%)	Estimated freedom from disease progression at 5 years (%)
0	7	84
1	22	77
2	29	67
3	23	60
4	12	51
5+	7	42

[a]Factors: stage IV; male sex; age >45 years; hemoglobin <10.5 g/dL; WBC ≥15,000/μL; lymphocytes <8% or <600/μL; albumin <4 g/dL.

TABLE 18.6

ETOPOSIDE-CONTAINING COMBINATION CHEMOTHERAPY FOR ADVANCED HODGKIN LYMPHOMA

Drug combination	Dose (mg/m^2)	Route	Schedule (days)	RT	cycle/length (days)
Alkylating agent-containing					
BEACOPP (Escalated BEACOPP)				Bulky, residual	21
Bleomycin	10	IV	8		
Etoposide	100 (200)	IV	1–3		
Adriamycin (doxorubicin)	25 (35)	IV	1		
Cyclophosphamide	650 (1250)	IV	1		
Oncovin (vincristine)	1.4[a]	IV	8		
Procarbazine	100	PO	1–7		
Prednisone	40	PO	1–14		
G-CSF		SQ	8+		
BEACOPP-14				Bulky, residual	14
Cyclophosphamide	650	IV	1		
Adriamycin	25	IV	1		
Etoposide	100	IV	1–3		
Procarbazine	100	PO	1–7		
Prednisone	80	PO	1–7		
Vincristine	1.4 (max. 2)	IV	8		
Bleomycin	10	IV	8		
G-CSF		SC	from day 8		
Stanford V				Bulky	12 weeks
Mechlorethamine	6	IV	Wk 1, 5, 9		
Adriamycin (doxorubicin)	25	IV	Wk 1, 3, 5, 7, 9, 11		
Vinblastine	6	IV	Wk 1, 3, 5, 7, 9, 11		
Vincristine	1.4[a]	IV	Wk 2, 4, 6, 8, 10, 12		
Bleomycin	5	IV	Wk 2, 4, 6, 8, 10, 12		
Etoposide	60 × 2	IV	Wk 3, 7, 11		
Prednisone	40	PO	Wk 1–10 qod		
G-CSF			Dose reduction or delay		
OEPA/COPP[b]				IF	28
Oncovin (vincristine)	1.5[a]	IV	1, 8, 15		
Etoposide	125	IV	3–6		
Prednisone	60	PO	1–15		
Adriamycin (doxorubicin)	40	IV	1, 15		
ChlVPP/EVA				—	28
Chlorambucil	10 total	PO	1–7		
Vinblastine	10 total	IV	1		
Procarbazine	150 total	PO	1–7		
Prednisolone	50 total	PO	1–7		
Etoposide	200	IV	8		
Vincristine	2 total	IV	8		
Adriamycin (doxorubicin)	50	IV	8		
ChlVPP/PABLOE				Bulky	50
Chlorambucil	6	PO	1–14		
Vinblastine	6	IV	1, 8		
Procarbazine	100	PO	1–14, 29–43		
Prednisolone	30	PO	1–14		
Adriamycin (doxorubicin)	40	IV	29		
Bleomycin	10	IV	29, 36		
Vincristine	1.4[a]	IV	29, 36		
Etoposide	200	PO	30–32		
VAPEC-B				Bulky, residual	11 weeks
Vincristine	1.4[a]	IV	Wk 2, 4, 6, 8, 10		
Adriamycin (doxorubicin)	35	IV	Wk 1, 3, 5, 7, 9, 11		
Prednisolone	50	PO	Wk 1–6		
Etoposide	75–100 × 5	PO	Wk 3, 7, 11		
Cyclophosphamide	350	IV	Wk 1, 5, 9		
Bleomycin	10	IV	Wk 2, 4, 6, 8, 10		

(continued)

TABLE 18.6

CONTINUED

Drug combination	Dose (mg/m²)	Route	Schedule (days)	RT	Cycle/length (days)
Non–alkylating agent-containing					
EVA				Bulky, residual	28
Etoposide	100	IV	1–3		
Vinblastine	6	IV	1		
Adriamycin (doxorubicin)	50	IV	1		
VEPA				IF	28
Vinblastine	6	IV	1, 15		
Etoposide	200	IV	1, 15		
Prednisone	40	PO	1–14		
Adriamycin (doxorobucin)	25	IV	1,15		

[a]Vincristine dose capped at 2 mg.
[b]Two cycles of OEPA followed by two to four cycles of COPP.
RT, radiation therapy; G-CSF, granulocyte colony-stimulating factor; IV, intravenous; PO, oral; SQ, subcutaneous; IF, involved field.

In a multicenter pilot study, the GHSG tested the feasibility, toxicity, and efficacy of BEACOPP-14 in 99 patients with advanced disease.[58] All eight cycles were completed by 91% of the patients; 77% of courses were completed within 16 days and 94% of courses within 22 days. Consolidative irradiation was administered to 70% of patients. A complete response was achieved by 94% of patients, and only 4 patients had progressive disease. The overall survival and FFTF at 5 years were 95% and 90%, respectively. The acute hematologic toxicity was moderate, intermediate between that of the escalated and the baseline BEACOPP-21 regimens, with 80% of patients experiencing WHO grade 3 or 4 leukopenia, 27% thrombocytopenia, and 70 % anemia. There were 13% of patients with documented WHO grade III infection.

Based on the results of this pilot study, BEACOPP-14 was introduced in the HD15 trial. In this three-arm trial, patients are treated with eight cycles of escalated BEACOPP, six cycles of escalated BEACOPP, or eight cycles of BEACOPP-14. Patients who achieve only a partial response receive radiotherapy to PET-positive residual disease.

Other cooperative clinical trials groups have also tested BEACOPP for advanced-stage Hodgkin lymphoma. The EORTC/GELA joined with the Nordic group, NCI Canada, British BNLI, the Australian Lymphoma Group, and two Spanish groups to initiate the 20012 trial. This trial compares eight cycles of ABVD to four cycles of escalated BEACOPP followed by four cycles of standard BEACOPP. An ongoing Italian trial compares the same two chemotherapy programs with MEC, an Italian 10-drug regimen.

THE STANFORD V PROGRAM

The Stanford group took another approach to the concern for late toxicity in the management of Hodgkin lymphoma.[59–61] They devised Stanford V, a 7-drug regimen (doxorubicin, vinblastine, mustard, bleomycin, vincristine, etoposide, prednisone) that includes weekly treatment given over 12 weeks for patients with locally extensive or advanced Hodgkin lymphoma (Table 18.6). Compared with ABVD or hybrid regimens, Stanford V maintains or increases the dose intensity of individual drugs but reduces the cumulative doses of doxorubicin, mechlorethamine, and bleomycin compared to the doses in MOPP/ABV(D) or ABVD alone, and omits procarbazine. An important feature of Stanford V is the use of consolidative radiotherapy (36 Gy) to sites of disease 5 cm or larger at diagnosis and macroscopic splenic involvement. Radiotherapy is initiated 1 to 3 weeks after completion of chemotherapy. It was postulated that pulmonary and cardiac dysfunction, sterility, and the incidence of secondary leukemia might be reduced or avoided with this regimen. With the intent of reducing the risks of breast cancer and long-term cardiac or vascular toxicity, radiotherapy fields were also reduced, omitting the axillae and high neck from treatment unless they were sites of bulky disease. Chemotherapy intensity was supported by growth factor use after the first dose reduction or treatment delay. Mature results from a phase II study of 162 patients at Stanford report a FFP of 89% and OS 96%, with a median follow-up of 5.4 years. The 71% of patients with 0 to 2 risk factors according to the IPS had a FFP of 94%, compared to 75% for patients with 3 or more risk factors.[61]

TABLE 18.7

SEVEN-YEAR RESULTS OF GHSG HD9 TRIAL ACCORDING TO INTERNATIONAL PROGNOSTIC SCORE[131]

	IPS = 0–1; N = 306		IPS = 2–3; N = 465		IPS ≥4; N = 169	
	FFTF	OS	FFTF	OS	FFTF	OS
COPP/ABVD	78%	89%	64%	78%	59%	66%
BEACOPP	83%	91%	73%	84%	74%	79%
BEACOPP-escalated	91%	93%	83%	90%	81%	83%
P	0.023	0.53	0.0017	0.042	0.23	0.6

GHSG, German Hodgkin Study Group; IPS, International Prognostic Score; FFTF, freedom from treatment failure; OS, overall survival.

The OS for this high-risk group was still greater than 90%, due to effective salvage therapy. The main toxicities were neutropenia and constipation. No cases of bleomycin toxicity or radiation pneumonitis were observed. In addition, no cases of secondary MDS/leukemia or lymphoma have been reported to date.[62] Unlike alkylator-intense regimens, Stanford V also preserves fertility. In a recent update, 72 post-treatment conceptions were reported (excluding pre-treatment semen or embryo cryopreservation) with 65 live births.[63]

Similar outcomes with Stanford V have been reported in a phase II study from Memorial Sloan-Kettering Cancer Center (MSKCC),[64] a pilot study by the Eastern Cooperative Oncology Group (ECOG),[60] a pilot study from the UK,[65] and a multicenter study from Italy.[66]

In both the Stanford and MSKCC series, approximately 50% to 60% of patients who failed Stanford V were salvaged successfully with secondary treatment. Two recent randomized trials compare Stanford V to ABVD in patients with advanced disease. The ECOG 2496 intergroup trial (recently closed, accrual goals met) compared the Stanford V program (chemotherapy plus radiation as defined above) with ABVD plus radiation for bulky mediastinal disease. An ongoing UK study compares Stanford V plus radiation with ABVD plus radiation (a follow-up to the pilot study noted above). Mature results from both these trials are awaited to evaluate the long-term effects both for cure and for complications.

Recently, another group from Italy (Intergruppo Italiano Linfomi) compared ABVD to a "modified Stanford V" program and a multiagent chemotherapy regimen consisting of mechlorethamine, vincristine, procarbazine, prednisone, epidoxirubicin, bleomycin, vinblastine, lomustine, doxorubicin, and vindesine (MOPPEBVCAD).[67] In this study, the 5-year FFS and PFS rates for the modified Stanford V arm were inferior to the other two regimens, with no differences in overall survival. The interpretation of these results is confounded for several reasons. First, the response evaluation, which determined whether patients continued on the study arm, was completed at different times: after 8 weeks of Stanford V chemotherapy, 16 weeks for ABVD, and 24 weeks for MOPPEBVCAD. Second, the modifications to radiotherapy were substantial, including a limit on the number of treated sites, a different definition of bulk, and a delay in initiating radiotherapy to a median of 6 weeks. The proportion of patients who received consolidative irradiation was substantially less than in the series reported from Stanford and ECOG (66% versus 90%). It is difficult to compare the outcomes of these different studies because patient selection and prognostic variables varied. However, one possible explanation for the different outcomes in the abbreviated chemotherapy programs is the variable use of radiotherapy as a consolidative therapy.

OTHER CHEMOTHERAPY REGIMENS

The success of ABVD indicated that alkylating agents were not an essential component of curative treatment for advanced Hodgkin lymphoma. However, the pulmonary toxicity of bleomycin, which was more pronounced in children and in combination with mediastinal irradiation, remained a concern with ABVD.[29,30,68] Meanwhile, a 20% to 60% response rate in refractory Hodgkin lymphoma was reported with single-agent etoposide.[69] These factors led to the development of a number of new etoposide-containing drug regimens (Table 18.6).

Groups in Boston and the United Kingdom initially tested the EVA (etoposide, vinblastine, Adriamycin [doxorubicin]) regimen in disease recurrent after MOPP or MVPP.[70] The Yale group conducted a study in 26 previously untreated patients with locally extensive, symptomatic, or advanced Hodgkin lymphoma in which six cycles of EVA were followed by low-dose involved-field radiotherapy in responding patients.[71] The estimated 2-year failure-free survival in these patients was just 44%. Results with EVA plus radiotherapy were also reported by the Boston group in bulky stage II ($n = 20$) and advanced ($n = 20$) disease.[72] With a median follow-up of 111 months, the failure-free survival was 57%. A group of 66 pediatric patients with unfavorable or advanced Hodgkin lymphoma was enrolled in a collaborative study of VEPA (vinblastine, etoposide, prednisone, Adriamycin [doxorubicin]) and low-dose consolidative radiotherapy conducted at Stanford University, Dana-Farber Cancer Institute, and St. Jude Children's Research Hospital.[73] This study was stopped when, with 15 months of follow-up, a projected failure-free survival of 66% was observed, a result inferior to historical controls.

These data suggest that etoposide-based regimens that do not include alkylating agents may be inferior treatments for advanced Hodgkin lymphoma. The fact that all three components in the EVA-type regimens are natural products that share the multidrug resistance phenotype may provide an explanation for these poor results.[74] In contrast, chemotherapy combinations that incorporate both etoposide and alkylating agents (BEACOPP, OEPA [Oncovin, etoposide, prednisone, Adriamycin]-COPP, ChlVPP/EVA, and Stanford V), as noted previously, have been associated with excellent results.

The Manchester group developed an abbreviated, 11-week chemotherapy program, VAPEC-B (vincristine, doxorubicin, prednisone, etoposide, cyclophosphamide, bleomycin).[75] In a four-center trial VAPEC-B and ChlVPP/EVA (chlorambucil, etoposide, vincristine, procarbazine, prednisone, vinblastine, doxorubicin) were compared. ChlVPP/EVA, a hybrid regimen, was found to be well tolerated and superior to MVPP in a previous study in patients with locally extensive or symptomatic or advanced disease.[76,77] Radiotherapy was given to sites of previous bulk disease or significant residual radiographic disease. This study was stopped after 26 months due to a threefold increase in the rate of disease progression after VAPEC-B. After a median follow-up time of 4.9 years, FFP, EFS, and OS were significantly better with ChlVPP/EVA than with VAPEC-B (82% versus 62%; 78% versus 58%; and 89% versus 79%).

Another abbreviated, weekly chemotherapy program was developed in the United Kingdom by the Southampton group, PACE-BOM (prednisone, doxorubicin, cyclophosphamide, etoposide, bleomycin, vincristine, methotrexate) and studied in 83 patients with stage II–IV disease.[78] Radiotherapy was applied if residual disease was demonstrable by chest x-ray. At 5 years, a 64% failure-free survival was reported.

In boys, two cycles of the OEPA combination followed by two to four cycles of COPP and low-dose radiotherapy have been a highly successful treatment for patients with stage IIB–IV Hodgkin lymphoma.[79] The Central Lymphoma Group used the same drugs, with the addition of bleomycin, in a combination termed PABIOE (prednisone, Adriamycin [doxorubicin], bleomycin, Oncovin [vincristine], etoposide), which was studied in an alternating fashion with ChlVPP.[80] Based on promising failure-free survival and overall survival data at 5 years, the Central Lymphoma Group and the BNLI collaborated in a randomized trial of ChlVPP/PABIOE versus PABIOE.[81] Radiotherapy was not used in this trial. A marked advantage in complete remission rate was noted with the alternating regimen (78% ChlVPP/PABIOE versus 64% PABIOE, $p < 0.0001$). A statistically significant benefit in progression-free survival and overall survival was also seen for the alternating regimen. This study again found that an etoposide-containing combination without alkylating agents yielded disappointing results. Table 18.6 illustrates that there are potentially important differences with regard to drug dosing and scheduling, particularly the vinca alkaloids and etoposide, in addition to alkylating agents, that may have relevance to these findings.

In the LY09 trial, the United Kingdom Lymphoma Group LY09 compared ABVD with two multidrug regimens: (a) the alternating regimen, ChlVPP/PABIOE; and (b) the hybrid regimen, ChlVPP/EVA. A total of 807 patients were evaluable. After a median observation time of 3 years, EFS was 75% for patients receiving ABVD and 75% for patients receiving one of the multidrug regimens. The 3-year OS for the ABVD regimen and for the multidrug regimens were 90% and 88%, respectively. Patients receiving the multidrug regimens experienced more severe infections, mucositis, and neuropathy. These results fail to support a multidrug approach in preference to ABVD, and the alternating regimens have been abandoned by the UKLG.[82]

The potential importance of dose intensity and scheduling was exemplified in a recent BNLI study in which a significant difference in outcomes was found between two regimens (LOPP/EVA hybrid and LOPP alternating with EVA that contained identical total doses).[83] The complete remission rate was significantly less in the hybrid arm, and the trial was prematurely terminated. This outcome emphasizes the potential impact of individual drug doses and scheduling.

It is hazardous to compare outcomes between studies, because patient selection variables (prognostic factors) have often proved to be of greater significance than design and drug usage. Randomized trials continue to be the only reliable method of determining the relative contributions of individual drugs, doses, and scheduling. As noted above, application of the international prognostic factors may serve to identify those patients who benefit most from a dose-intense approach as well as indicating those patients who may be successfully treated with less morbidity.[55]

HEMATOPOIETIC GROWTH FACTORS

Interest in the use of hematopoietic growth factors to support optimal drug delivery or to facilitate dose escalation was stimulated by the dose-limiting neutropenia associated with most combination chemotherapy regimens for advanced Hodgkin lymphoma. The Stanford V regimen used granulocyte colony-stimulating factor (G-CSF) at the first occurrence of neutropenia requiring a dose reduction or delay.[59,60] The escalated BEACOPP regimens were among the first conventional combinations in which the design was dependent on the use of growth factors. Growth factors are also routinely employed in the BEACOPP-14 regimen. Apart from these treatment programs, adherence to the guidelines of the American Society of Clinical Oncology for the use of growth factors is advised in practice.[84]

HIGH-DOSE THERAPY WITH HEMATOPOIETIC CELL SUPPORT

Numerous phase II studies in Hodgkin lymphoma recurrent after primary chemotherapy have shown benefit for high-dose chemotherapy or chemoradiotherapy supported by autologous hematopoietic stem cell transplantation.[85–87] (See Chapter 20.) Based in part upon these results, two groups have extended the concept of high-dose chemotherapy and transplantation to previously untreated patients with poor risk features. Carella and associates[88] conducted a phase II trial of myeloablative therapy and autografting among patients with poor risk features as defined by Straus and coworkers.[89] Based on encouraging results in the pilot study, the European Bone Marrow Transplant Registry conducted a prospective study in poor-risk patients who were randomized to receive high-dose chemotherapy and autografting or an additional four cycles of conventional chemotherapy after achieving complete remission or partial remission with four initial cycles of an ABVD-containing chemotherapy. After a median follow-up of 48 months, the 5-year failure-free survival rate was 75% in the high-dose arm and 82% in the conventional arm, and the 5-year overall survival rate was 88% in both arms. In conclusion, no benefit from an early intensification for these poor-risk patients was demonstrated.[90]

At this time, considering the outcome of the trials noted above, the use of myeloablative therapy and transplantation should be considered investigational for patients with advanced Hodgkin lymphoma, regardless of prognostic features.

COMBINED-MODALITY THERAPY

The appropriate role of radiation therapy in advanced Hodgkin lymphoma has sparked lively debate and remains controversial.[91–94] Confidence in the contribution of radiotherapy is evidenced by its inclusion in most of the large phase III trials discussed above. The potential contribution of radiation therapy is dependent on multiple factors, including patient characteristics, the chemotherapy program, duration of chemotherapy, and response to drug therapy. Field size and dose influence both efficacy and toxicity. Radiation therapy in advanced Hodgkin lymphoma may be considered in three clinical settings. First, it may be used as an adjuvant after complete remission with standard chemotherapy. Second, it may be an integrated component of a combined-modality program, possibly with reduced or brief chemotherapy. Finally, it can serve as a non–cross-resistant treatment for patients with partial or uncertain response after chemotherapy.

The rationale for combined-modality therapy in advanced Hodgkin lymphoma is based on the data discussed above, which indicated that a subset of patients treated with chemotherapy alone failed to respond completely or progressed, primarily in previously involved nodal sites. In 42 patients who relapsed after MOPP/ABVD or MOPP/ABV alternating with CAD (lomustine, melphalan, and vindesine), reported from Memorial Sloan-Kettering Cancer Center (MSKCC), 26 (62%) did so exclusively in unirradiated sites.[95] Similarly, 80% of relapses after MOP-BAP chemotherapy in the SWOG study were restricted to initially involved sites.[96] Although high-dose therapy and transplantation (see Chapter 20) have improved prospects for second-line cure, the success of this treatment is limited to a subset of patients and is associated with substantial cost and morbidity. Thus, there is continued interest in the selective application of radiotherapy in advanced Hodgkin lymphoma.

The ability of radiation therapy to provide local control in Hodgkin lymphoma is well established.[97] Further, radiotherapy is non–cross-resistant with standard combination chemotherapy. A number of authors have reported that approximately 30% of selected patients who relapsed after chemotherapy achieved durable remissions after irradiation.[98,99] However, the benefits of consolidative radiotherapy must be balanced against the potential for serious late effects, particularly second malignancy.

Single-institution studies provided a rationale for testing the concept of combined-modality therapy in advanced disease.[95,100,101] Table 18.8 details the randomized trials designed to test the role of radiotherapy in a more rigorous fashion. In the SWOG 7808 Trial, 322 of 530 patients (61%) who achieved complete remission with MOP-BAP chemotherapy, were randomized to low-dose (20 Gy) involved-field radiotherapy or to no further treatment.[96] No significant differences in remission duration or overall survival were seen in the

TABLE 18.8

MAJOR RANDOMIZED TRIALS IN ADULT STAGE III–IV HODGKIN LYMPHOMA TESTING THE VALUE
OF COMBINED-MODALITY THERAPY VERSUS CHEMOTHERAPY ALONE

	Dates	No. patients	Chemotherapy	Radiotherapy
SWOG 7808	1978–1988	590	MOP-BAP × 6	IF 20 Gy nodal 10–15 other
GHSG HD3	1984–1988	288	COPP/ABVD × 6	IF 20 Gy nodal
GELA H89	1989–1996	559	MOPP/ABVD × 6 ABVPP × 6	STNI/TNI 30 Gy nodal 5–10 Gy boosts
EORTC 20884	1989–2000	739	MOPP-ABV × 6-8	IF 24 Gy nodal 16–24 other

SWOG, Southwest Oncology Group; GHSG, German Hodgkin Study Group; GELA, Group d'Etude des Lymphome d'Adulte; EORTC, European Organization for the Research and Treatment of Cancer; MOP-BAP, nitrogen mustard, vincristine, procarbazine, bleomycin, doxorubicin, and prednisone; COPP, cyclophosphamide, vincristine, procarbazine, and prednisone; ABVD, doxorubicin, bleomycin, vinblastine, and dacarbazine; ABVPP, doxorubicin, bleomycin, vinblastine, procarbazine, and prednisone; ABV, doxorubicin, bleomycin, vinblastine; IF, involved-field irradiation; STNI/TNI, subtotal/total nodal irradiation.

intent-to-treat analysis (Table 18.9). Subset analyses restricted to the patients who actually received irradiation (104 of 135) showed that remission duration was significantly prolonged with combined-modality treatment (85% versus 67% disease-free survival at 5 years, $p = 0.002$). The rate of relapse was also linked to the quality of the irradiation received. Of the 86 patients irradiated without a major protocol violation, only 7 relapses were recorded. When the analysis was confined to nodular-sclerosis histology, significant differences were seen in favor of the combined-modality group (82% versus 60% disease-free survival at 5 years, $p = 0.002$). There were no survival differences in this study.

The GHSG conducted a randomized multicenter study designed to evaluate the role of low-dose (20 Gy) involved-field radiotherapy versus chemotherapy consolidation of complete remission in 288 patients with advanced Hodgkin lymphoma (Table 18.8).[102] After six cycles of COPP/ABVD, 59% of patients achieved a complete response and 58% of these (34% of the total accrued to study) were randomized to 20 Gy involved-field radiotherapy or two additional cycles of chemotherapy. No significant differences were noted in the

study arms either for freedom from progression or overall survival (Table 18.9). The study had sufficient power to detect a 20% difference after 7 years. The majority of relapses in both arms of this study were confined to nodal sites of disease. Of interest, the relapse rate was greatest among patients who refused further treatment on either arm of the study.

Another study that compared consolidation after complete remission with chemotherapy versus radiation therapy was the GELA H89 trial. Patients with stage IIIB–IV were randomized to MOPP/ABV × 6 or ABVPP (doxorubicin, bleomycin, vinblastine, procarbazine, and prednisone) × 6 (Table 18.8). Those who achieved a complete remission were randomized to two additional cycles of the same chemotherapy or to 30 Gy subtotal lymphoid irradiation. The 5-year disease-free and overall survival estimates did not differ between the chemotherapy and radiation therapy consolidation arms (Table 18.9).[103]

The ECOG conducted a study in which patients received six cycles of MOPP plus bleomycin followed by a randomization to 15 to 20 Gy involved-field radiotherapy or three cycles of ABVD.[36] Both freedom from progression and overall

TABLE 18.9

MAJOR RANDOMIZED TRIALS IN ADULT STAGE III–IV HODGKIN LYMPHOMA TESTING THE VALUE
OF COMBINED-MODALITY THERAPY VERSUS CHEMOTHERAPY ALONE

	CR	5-year EFS[a]	5-year survival
SWOG 7808	61%	40% CT[b] / 45% CMT[b]	79% / 86%
GHSG HD3	59%	61% CT / 61% CMT	95% / 88%
GELA H89	50%	61% CT[b] / 62% CMT[b]	90% / 83%
EORTC 20884	57%	48% CT / 48% CMT	91% / 85%

[a]EFS for all patients accrued to trial.
[b]Estimated based upon published complete response rates.
SWOG, Southwest Oncology Group; GHSG, German Hodgkin Study Group; GELA, Group d'Etude des Lymphome d'Adulte; EORTC, European Organization for the Research and Treatment of Cancer; CT, chemotherapy alone; CMT, combined chemotherapy and irradiation.

survival favored the sequential chemotherapy arm. As described above, a second ECOG study evaluated the curative potential of BCVPP, BCVPP plus low-dose radiotherapy, and sequential MOPP/ABVD.[36] Outcomes in the BCVPP arms were not different and, when the data were pooled, outcome was statistically inferior to MOPP/ABVD. These studies demonstrated the superior contribution of ABVD relative to low-dose radiotherapy after MOPP-like therapy, but do not address the additional benefit of irradiation to a more effective induction regimen.

This question was addressed in a recent Pediatric Oncology Group study in which children received eight cycles of MOPP alternating with ABVD followed by no further treatment or low-dose total nodal irradiation.[104] It is important to note that patients were randomized at study entry. Of 186 patients accrued to the study, 161 were randomized. At 5 years, estimates for failure-free survival were no different for patients treated with radiotherapy (80%) or observation (79%). In like manner, there were no survival differences. However, in a study from India reported by Laskar and colleagues, 179 patients with all stages of Hodgkin lymphoma who achieved a CR to ABVD were randomized to no further treatment or to 30-Gy involved field irradiation.[105] The 8-year event-free survivals (76% versus 88%, $p = 0.01$) and overall survivals (89% versus 100%, $p = 0.002$) both favored radiation consolidation. Unfortunately, these randomized trials generally fell short of the 180+ patients needed for the detection of an estimated 15% survival benefit from irradiation.[91] Thus, as a group, they suffer from possible false-negative outcome (type 2 error) resulting from insufficient power. This predicament is magnified by the attrition of patients failing to achieve complete remission or refusing randomization after chemotherapy or the assigned treatment, as well as by technical errors in the prescribed irradiation.

In the EORTC/GELA 20884 trial, patients with stage III–IV HD were treated with six to eight cycles of MOPP/ABV.[106] Those who achieved a complete remission were randomly assigned to receive either involved-field radiotherapy (24 Gy to all initially involved nodal areas, 16 to 24 Gy to all initially involved extranodal sites) or no further treatment (Table 18.8). Among the patients who achieved a complete remission, 172 received involved-field radiotherapy and 161 received no further treatment. The 250 patients with partial remission were all treated with radiotherapy, 30 Gy to partial remission nodal sites, 24 Gy to complete remission nodal sites, and 18 to 24 Gy to extranodal sites. The 5-year event-free survival and 5-year overall survival rates were 84% and 91% for patients with no further treatment and 79% and 85% in the group with complete remission assigned to involved-field irradiation ($p = 0.35$ for event-free and $p = 0.07$ for overall survival) (Table 18.9). The difference in survival was largely attributed to an increase in secondary leukemia/MDS in the combined-modality group (8 cases among 172 patients with consolidative irradiation, 1 case among 161 patients after chemotherapy alone).

Among the patients with PR after chemotherapy, the 5-year event free survival rate was 97% and the 5-year overall survival was 87%, very similar to the group of patients who achieved an initial complete response. Interestingly, in this group of 250 patients, there were only 2 instances of secondary leukemia/MDS.[106]

These results fail to support the routine use of consolidative irradiation in patients with stage III–IV who achieve a complete response to a full course of conventional irradiation, but suggest a beneficial role for those who achieve only a partial remission.[107]

Another large trial that addressed the specific question of the role of radiation therapy for patients with initially bulky (>5 cm) or residual disease after chemotherapy was the GHSG HD12 study. In this trial, patients were randomized to eight cycles of intensified BEACOPP or four cycles of intensified BEACOPP plus four cycles of standard BEACOPP followed by either radiotherapy to initial bulky and residual disease or no further treatment. The third interim analysis with 908 patients and a median observation time of more than 24 months showed an FFTF of 90% and an OS of 94%, with no significant differences between the treatment arms. In this study, less than 35% of the total cohort of patients received consolidative involved-field radiation.[108] However, analysis of the comparison between the radiotherapy arms and the no-radiotherapy arms was compromised, because 13% of patients in the "no-radiotherapy" arms of the trial were assigned by a review panel to receive 30 Gy involved-field radiotherapy due to either minor response or residual disease greater than 2.5 cm.

The new HD15 trial of the GHSG compares eight cycles of BEACOPP escalated to six cycles of BEACOPP escalated and eight cycles of BEACOPP-14. In this trial, local radiation therapy is given only to PET-positive residual disease.[109]

DOSE AND VOLUME

Only a few studies have addressed the important issues of radiation dose and volume in combination with chemotherapy for Hodgkin lymphoma. As a single modality, a radiation dose of 35 Gy provides local control in 95% of cases, while lower doses of 20 to 25 Gy result in local control of 50% to 60% of involved sites.[110,111] Low-dose irradiation (15–30 Gy) has been employed in many combined-modality studies in adults and children, based on the hypothesis that a lower dose would suffice in the adjuvant setting.[96,112] In fact, the in-field relapse rate has generally been below 10% in these studies.

Two studies have addressed the issue of dose of irradiation in consolidation after chemotherapy. At the University of Pennsylvania, a retrospective analysis was performed among 121 children who received low-dose (17.5–22.5 Gy) or high-dose (>32 Gy) irradiation following chemotherapy.[113] The failure-free and overall survival rates at 10 years were not significantly different. Further, the in-field failure rates in the two groups (2% high dose, 7% low dose) were similar. The GHSG evaluated the effect of 20 Gy versus 40 Gy irradiation to non-bulky disease sites following four cycles of COPP-ABVD chemotherapy in patients with stage I–III disease.[114] All patients received 40 Gy to bulky disease sites in this study. No difference in freedom from progression was seen between the two randomized groups, and most relapses occurred in sites receiving full-dose irradiation.

Many studies have defined radiation fields as involved fields, although in most patients with advanced-stage Hodgkin lymphoma such a definition would require large volumes. This is an important point, because a large international collaborative effort to define prognostic factors in advanced disease confirmed that stage IV is a significant adverse factor.[55] As noted above, authors of the MSKCC study concluded that it was necessary to treat all involved disease sites. In contrast, studies from the GHSG (HD9 and HD12) and Stanford University report excellent outcomes with new chemotherapy combinations (Table 18.6) in combination with radiotherapy restricted to disease sites of 5 cm or more.[57,61]

TOXICITY

A major concern in combined-modality therapy is the potential increase in risk of serious side effects, particularly second malignancy. Difficulties in quantifying the magnitude of risk include the long latency for solid tumors, the important contribution of drug combinations and cumulative doses, and the radiation variables of field size and dose.

Although the risk of secondary leukemia in advanced Hodgkin lymphoma is primarily dependent on the cumulative dose of alkylating agents, some groups have found an added risk when MOPP-like chemotherapy was combined with radiotherapy.[28,115] In contrast, a large-scale epidemiologic study found no significantly increased risk with the addition of radiation.[10] Some data indicate that the risk of leukemia may be larger when chemotherapy is given as salvage therapy after radiation failure or when wide-field radiotherapy is used.[28,116]

The main concern regarding the additional risk of radiotherapy is the potential for induction of solid tumors. Treatment of early-stage disease with radiotherapy alone has been associated with a significant and continuing risk of secondary solid tumors, particularly those involving lung, breast, gastrointestinal tract, and skin (see Chapter 24). Van Leeuwen and colleagues report a 25-year cumulative risk of solid tumors of 23.3%.[117] Data focusing on secondary breast cancer in women receiving chest irradiation to a dose of 40 Gy or more at age 25 years demonstrate estimated cumulative absolute risks of breast cancer by age 35, 45, and 55 years of 1.4%, 11.1%, and 29.0%, respectively.[118]

The additional impact of radiotherapy, given after induction chemotherapy, on the risk of second malignancy in advanced patients is less obvious. This is because published series have lacked a sufficient number of patients or adequate follow-up to accurately determine the risk associated with chemotherapy, usually alkylating-agent based, alone. Indeed, series that include a large number of patients treated with chemotherapy alone suggest that the risk of secondary solid tumors may be as high as the risk with combined-modality treatment or radiotherapy alone.[119]

The BNLI study of 2,864 patients, of whom 1,002 were treated with chemotherapy alone, showed that the relative risk for lung cancer after chemotherapy alone was 4.2 compared with 4.0 after combined-modality therapy and 3.3 after radiotherapy alone.[119] A case-control study conducted by the international Hodgkin lymphoma registries confirmed this observation.[120] In an analysis of 25,000 treated patients, the risk of lung cancer after chemotherapy alone was twice that of the risk after radiotherapy alone. In two other studies in which the relative risk of second cancers in adults and children was evaluated, no increase in relative risk for combined-modality therapy was found.[121,122] Again, it should be remembered that these data are primarily based on MOPP or MOPP-like chemotherapy regimens and their relevance to ABVD or new combinations is speculative. Further, there are particular clinical circumstances, such as increased risk of breast cancer in girls and women under the age of 30 treated with mantle radiotherapy, that require careful consideration in the risks and benefits of combined-modality treatment.[123,124]

The use of lower doses of radiotherapy, as well as the obvious impact of limited fields, may reduce the risk of second cancers. This notion is supported by the retrospective analyses of second cancer risk in the Yale series and the Late Effects Study Group.[125,126] In addition, dose may be critical in cardiac morbidity related to thoracic radiotherapy. An increased risk of cardiac-related mortality, particularly related to coronary artery disease, was documented at Stanford University in both adults and children.[127] However, this risk was confined to patients receiving 42 Gy or more. Similarly, the excess risks of other causes of cardiac death, including pericarditis, valvular heart disease, and congestive heart failure, were not observed in patients receiving less than 30 Gy.

Pulmonary complications of combined-modality therapy are likewise related to volume and dose. Radiotherapy delivered in reduced dose and delivered to smaller mediastinal volumes as a consolidation to cytoreduction with chemotherapy showed no increased pulmonary complications compared to chemotherapy alone in the Duke series.[101] Hirsch and associates[128] reported no significant clinical sequelae for a cohort of patients treated at MSKCC with ABVD alone or ABVD followed by mediastinal irradiation.

SELECTED CLINICAL SETTINGS

Combined-modality treatment is currently favored for patients with massive mediastinal disease, regardless of stage, based on improved disease-free survival compared with radiotherapy or chemotherapy alone (see Chapter 17). A small retrospective study from the NCI evaluated the role of irradiation in advanced-stage Hodgkin lymphoma with massive mediastinal involvement.[51] Thirteen of 26 patients achieving complete remission relapsed after MOPP alone compared with 1 of 9 who received consolidative irradiation ($p = 0.055$). Although the study was small, it provided support for combined-modality treatment.

Many patients, particularly those with massive mediastinal disease, have residual abnormalities on CT scanning after chemotherapy. The Canadian study of alternating versus hybrid chemotherapy discussed above included radiotherapy for such patients.[44] In this study, there was no difference in outcome for patients with a very good partial response compared to those achieving complete remission. In the EORTC study of MOPP-ABV ± radiotherapy for advanced Hodgkin lymphoma, a significant proportion of patients were not randomized, but rather received irradiation based on failure to achieve a complete response.[129] Outcomes for these partial-remission patients were indistinguishable from those of complete-remission patients, indicating that residual radiographic abnormalities either did not represent active disease or that radiation therapy was truly effective in this setting. The role of radiotherapy as a consolidation for patients with positive FDG-PET scans after chemotherapy also remains a question and is being addressed in the GHSG HD15 trial, noted previously. These issues, together with those discussed above, indicate that the role of adjuvant radiation therapy in selected situations in advanced-stage Hodgkin lymphoma requires clarification in ongoing studies.

SUMMARY AND CONCLUSIONS

In 2006, patients with Hodgkin lymphoma, even in advanced stages, have a better than 80% chance of being cured of their disease if appropriate and adequate therapy is given at the outset. Adequate therapy today should consider two major principles: risk adaptation and response adaptation.

1. Risk Adaptation

Risk adaptation means treating the patient according to his or her individual risk of failing to achieve a complete response or relapsing after having obtained a complete remission. The globally used measurement of risk assessment is the IPS.[55]

2. Response Adaptation

Response-adapted therapy implies modulating the intensity of treatment according to the treatment response, measured by morphologic and/or functional criteria such as FDG-PET or CT/PET after just a partial course of chemotherapy. This enables the oncologist to ameliorate or intensify the treatment according to the outcome of those studies.

Most ongoing or planned international studies use these two principles to tailor therapy according to the needs of the individual patient, also accounting for anatomic stage, tumor burden, age, gender, and biologic host factors that affect prognosis. With this approach it might be possible to use less aggressive treatment regimens such as for the lower-risk groups and limit the use of the more aggressive dose- and time-intensified/dense regimen like BEACOPP-escalated for the higher IPS risk groups. With this individualized approach, it might be possible to yield higher cure rates and simultaneously reduce the risk of late complications and mortality. The remaining question of whether consolidative irradiation should be given may be answered by ongoing studies using FDG-PET as a predictor of a true complete response after chemotherapy. A positive PET scan in this setting demands further therapy, either irradiation or possibly high-dose chemotherapy, followed by stem-cell transplantation.

These issues will only be resolved through well-planned and well-controlled prospective, collaborative clinical trials. This compels all oncologists to offer to all patients with Hodgkin lymphoma, regardless of clinical stage, the opportunity to participate in clinical trials, in order to improve the outcome for the generations of patients to come.

References

1. DeVita VT Jr., Hubbard SM. Hodgkin's disease. N Engl J Med 1993;328:560–565.
2. DeVita VT Jr., Simon RM, Hubbard SM, et al. Curability of advanced Hodgkin's disease with chemotherapy. Long-term follow-up of MOPP-treated patients at the National Cancer Institute. Ann Intern Med 1980;92:587–595.
3. Young RC, Canellos GP, Chabner BA, et al. Patterns of relapse in advanced Hodgkin's disease treated with combination chemotherapy. Cancer 1978;42:1001–1007.
4. Cheson BD. CLL response criteria. Clin Adv Hematol Oncol 2006;4(suppl 12):4–5; discussion 10.
5. Longo DL, Young RC, Wesley M, et al. Twenty years of MOPP therapy for Hodgkin's disease. J Clin Oncol 1986;4:1295–1306.
6. Fisher RI, DeVita VT, Hubbard SP, et al. Prolonged disease-free survival in Hodgkin's disease with MOPP reinduction after first relapse. Ann Intern Med 1979;90:761–763.
7. Viviani S, Santoro A, Negretti E, et al. Salvage chemotherapy in Hodgkin's disease. Results in patients relapsing more than twelve months after first complete remission. Ann Oncol 1990;1:123–127.
8. Bonadonna G, Santoro A, Gianni AM, et al. Primary and salvage chemotherapy in advanced Hodgkin's disease: the Milan Cancer Institute experience. Ann Oncol 1991;2(uppl 1):9–16.
9. Longo DL, Duffey PL, Young RC, et al. Conventional-dose salvage combination chemotherapy in patients relapsing with Hodgkin's disease after combination chemotherapy: the low probability for cure. J Clin Oncol 1992;10:210–218.
10. Kaldor JM, Day NE, Clarke EA, et al. Leukemia following Hodgkin's disease. N Engl J Med 1990;322:7–13.
11. Nissen NI, Pajak TF, Glidewell O, et al. A comparative study of a BCNU containing 4-drug program versus MOPP versus 3-drug combinations in advanced Hodgkin's disease: a cooperative study by the Cancer and Leukemia Group B. Cancer 1979;43:31–40.
12. Bakemeier RF, Anderson JR, Costello W, et al. BCVPP chemotherapy for advanced Hodgkin's disease: evidence for greater duration of complete remission, greater survival, and less toxicity than with a MOPP regimen. Results of the Eastern Cooperative Oncology Group study. Ann Intern Med 1984;101:447–456.
13. McElwain TJ, Toy J, Smith E, et al. A combination of chlorambucil, vinblastine, procarbazine and prednisolone for treatment of Hodgkin's disease. Br J Cancer 1977;36:276–280.
14. Nicholson WM, Beard ME, Crowther D, et al. Combination chemotherapy in generalized Hodgkin's disease. Br Med J 1970;3:7–10.
15. Sutcliffe SB, Wrigley PF, Peto J, et al. MVPP chemotherapy regimen for advanced Hodgkin's disease. Br Med J 1978;1:679–683.
16. Hancock BW. Randomised study of MOPP (mustine, Oncovin, procarbazine, prednisone) against LOPP (Leukeran substituted for mustine) in advanced Hodgkin's disease. British National Lymphoma Investigation. Radiother Oncol 1986;7:215–221.
17. Bloomfield CD, Weiss RB, Fortuny I, et al. Combinaed chemotherapy with cyclophosphamide, vinblastine, procarbazine, and prednisone (CVPP) for patients with advanced Hodgkin's disease. An alternative program to MOPP. Cancer 1976;38:42–48.
18. Cooper MR, Pajak TF, Nissen NI, et al. A new effective four-drug combination of CCNU (1-[2-chloroethyl]-3-cyclohexyl-1-nitrosourea) (NSC-79038), vinblastine, prednisone, and procarbazine for the treatment of advanced Hodgkin's disease. Cancer 1980;46:654–662.
19. Bonadonna G, Zucali R, Monfardini S, et al. Combination chemotherapy of Hodgkin's disease with adriamycin, bleomycin, vinblastine, and imidazole carboxamide versus MOPP. Cancer 1975;36:252–259.
20. Carbone PP, Bono V, Frei E III, et al. Clinical studies with vincristine. Blood 1963;21:640–647.
21. Carter SK, Livingston RB. Single-agent therapy for Hodgkin's disease. Arch Intern Med 1973;131:377–387.
22. Frei E III, Luce JK, Talley RW, et al. 5-(3,3-dimethyl-1-triazeno)imidazole-4-carboxamide (NSC-45388) in the treatment of lymphoma. Cancer Chemother Rep 1972;56:667–670.
23. Skibba JL, Beal DD, Ramirez G, et al. N-demethylation of the antineoplastic agent 4(5)-(3,3-dimethyl-1-triazeno)imidazole-5(4)-carboxamide by rats and man. Cancer Res 1970;30:147–150.
24. Santoro A, Bonadonna G, Valagussa P, et al. Long-term results of combined chemotherapy-radiotherapy approach in Hodgkin's disease: superiority of ABVD plus radiotherapy versus MOPP plus radiotherapy. J Clin Oncol 1987;5:27–37.
25. Bonfante V, Santoro A, Viviani S, et al. ABVD in the treatment of Hodgkin's disease. Semin Oncol 1992;19:38–44, discussion 44–35.
26. Viviani S, Santoro A, Ragni G, et al. Gonadal toxicity after combination chemotherapy for Hodgkin's disease. Comparative results of MOPP vs ABVD. Eur J Cancer Clin Oncol 1985;21:601–605.
27. Anselmo AP, Cartoni C, Bellantuono P, et al. Risk of infertility in patients with Hodgkin's disease treated with ABVD vs MOPP vs ABVD/MOPP. Haematologica 1990;75:155–158.
28. Valagussa P, Santoro A, Fossati-Bellani F, et al. Second acute leukemia and other malignancies following treatment for Hodgkin's disease. J Clin Oncol 1986;4:830–837.
29. Horning SJ, Adhikari A, Rizk N, et al. Effect of treatment for Hodgkin's disease on pulmonary function: results of a prospective study. J Clin Oncol 1994;12:297–305.
30. Carde P, Hagenbeek A, Hayat M, et al. Clinical staging versus laparotomy and combined modality with MOPP versus ABVD in early-stage Hodgkin's disease: the H6 twin randomized trials from the European Organization for Research and Treatment of Cancer Lymphoma Cooperative Group. J Clin Oncol 1993;11:2258–2272.
31. Canellos GP, Anderson JR, Propert KJ, et al. Chemotherapy of advanced Hodgkin's disease with MOPP, ABVD, or MOPP alternating with ABVD. N Engl J Med 1992;327:1478–1484.
32. Mefferd JM, Donaldson SS, Link MP. Pediatric Hodgkin's disease: pulmonary, cardiac, and thyroid function following combined modality therapy. Int J Radiat Oncol Biol Phys 1989;16:679–685.
33. Lipshultz SE, Colan SD, Gelber RD, et al. Late cardiac effects of doxorubicin therapy for acute lymphoblastic leukemia in childhood. N Engl J Med 1991;324:808–815.
34. Duggan DB, Petroni GR, Johnson JL, et al. Randomized comparison of ABVD and MOPP/ABV hybrid for the treatment of advanced Hodgkin's disease: report of an intergroup trial. J Clin Oncol 2003;21:607–614.
35. Bonadonna G, Valagussa P, Santoro A. Alternating non-cross-resistant combination chemotherapy or MOPP in stage IV Hodgkin's disease. A report of 8-year results. Ann Intern Med 1986;104:739–746.
36. Glick J, Tsiatis A, Chen M, et al. Radiotherapy (RT) for advanced Hodgkin's disease (HD). Proc Am Soc Clin Oncol 1988;7:A863. Abstract.
37. Somers R, Carde P, Henry-Amar M, et al. A randomized study in stage IIIB and IV Hodgkin's disease comparing eight courses of MOPP versus an alteration of MOPP with ABVD: a European Organization for Research and Treatment of Cancer Lymphoma Cooperative Group and Groupe Pierre-et-Marie-Curie controlled clinical trial. J Clin Oncol 1994;12:279–287.
38. Goldie JH, Coldman AJ. A mathematic model for relating the drug sensitivity of tumors to their spontaneous mutation rate. Cancer Treat Rep 1979;63:1727–1733.
39. Longo DL, Duffey PL, DeVita VT, Jr., et al. Treatment of advanced-stage Hodgkin's disease: alternating noncrossresistant MOPP/CABS is not superior to MOPP. J Clin Oncol 1991;9:1409–1420.
40. Gams RA, Omura GA, Velez-Garcia E, et al. Alternating sequential combination chemotherapy in the management of advanced Hodgkin's disease. A Southeastern Cancer Study Group trial. Cancer 1986;58:1963–1968.
41. Vinciguerra V, Propert KJ, Coleman M, et al. Alternating cycles of combination chemotherapy for patients with recurrent Hodgkin's disease following radiotherapy. A prospectively randomized study by the Cancer and Leukemia Group B. J Clin Oncol 1986;4:838–846.
42. Jones SE, Haut A, Weick JK, et al. Comparison of adriamycin-containing chemotherapy (MOP-BAP) with MOPP-Bleomycin in the management of advanced Hodgkin's disease. A Southwest Oncology Group Study. Cancer 1983;51:1339–1347.
43. Klimo P, Connors JM. MOPP/ABV hybrid program: combination chemotherapy based on early introduction of seven effective drugs for advanced Hodgkin's disease. J Clin Oncol 1985;3:1174–1182.
44. Connors JM, Klimo P, Adams G, et al. Treatment of advanced Hodgkin's disease with chemotherapy—comparison of MOPP/ABV hybrid regimen with alternating courses of MOPP and ABVD: a report from the National Cancer Institute of Canada clinical trials group. J Clin Oncol 1997;15:1638–1645.

45. Viviani S, Bonadonna G, Santoro A, et al. Alternating versus hybrid MOPP and ABVD combinations in advanced Hodgkin's disease: ten-year results. *J Clin Oncol* 1996;14:1421–1430.
46. Glick JH, Young ML, Harrington D, et al. MOPP/ABV hybrid chemotherapy for advanced Hodgkin's disease significantly improves failure-free and overall survival: the 8-year results of the intergroup trial. *J Clin Oncol* 1998;16:19–26.
47. Engert A, Schiller P, Josting A, et al. Involved-field radiotherapy is equally effective and less toxic compared with extended-field radiotherapy after four cycles of chemotherapy in patients with early-stage unfavorable Hodgkin's lymphoma: results of the HD8 trial of the German Hodgkin's Lymphoma Study Group. *J Clin Oncol* 2003;21:3601–3608.
48. Bonadonna G, Bonfante V, Viviani S, et al. ABVD plus subtotal nodal versus involved-field radiotherapy in early-stage Hodgkin's disease: long-term results. *J Clin Oncol* 2004;22:2835–2841.
49. Hasenclever D, Loeffler M, Diehl V. Rationale for dose escalation of first line conventional chemotherapy in advanced Hodgkin's disease. German Hodgkin's Lymphoma Study Group. *Ann Oncol* 1996;7(suppl 4):95–98.
50. Behar RA, Horning SJ, Hoppe RT. Hodgkin's disease with bulky mediastinal involvement: effective management with combined modality therapy. *Int J Radiat Oncol Biol Phys* 1993;25:771–776.
51. Longo DL, Russo A, Duffey PL, et al. Treatment of advanced-stage massive mediastinal Hodgkin's disease: the case for combined modality treatment. *J Clin Oncol* 1991;9:227–235.
52. Hutchings M, Mikhaeel NG, Fields PA, et al. Prognostic value of interim FDG-PET after two or three cycles of chemotherapy in Hodgkin lymphoma. *Ann Oncol* 2005;16:1160–1168.
53. Frei E, 3rd, Luce JK, Gamble JF, et al. Combination chemotherapy in advanced Hodgkin's disease. Induction and maintenance of remission. *Ann Intern Med* 1973;79:376–382.
54. Young RC, Canellos GP, Chabner BA, et al. Maintenance chemotherapy for advanced Hodgkin's disease in remission. *Lancet* 1973;1:1339–1343.
55. Hasenclever D, Diehl V. A prognostic score for advanced Hodgkin's disease. International Prognostic Factors Project on Advanced Hodgkin's Disease. *N Engl J Med* 1998;339:1506–1514.
56. Diehl V. Dose-escalation study for the treatment of Hodgkin's disease. The German Hodgkin Study Group (GHSG). *Ann Hematol* 1993;66:139–140.
57. Diehl V, Franklin J, Pfreundschuh M, et al. Standard and increased-dose BEACOPP chemotherapy compared with COPP-ABVD for advanced Hodgkin's disease. *N Engl J Med* 2003;348:2386–2395.
58. Sieber M, Bredenfeld H, Josting A, et al. 14-day variant of the bleomycin, etoposide, doxorubicin, cyclophosphamide, vincristine, procarbazine, and prednisone regimen in advanced-stage Hodgkin's lymphoma: results of a pilot study of the German Hodgkin's Lymphoma Study Group. *J Clin Oncol* 2003;21:1734–1739.
59. Bartlett NL, Rosenberg SA, Hoppe RT, et al. Brief chemotherapy, Stanford V, and adjuvant radiotherapy for bulky or advanced-stage Hodgkin's disease: a preliminary report. *J Clin Oncol* 1995;13:1080–1088.
60. Horning SJ, Williams J, Bartlett NL, et al. Assessment of the Stanford V regimen and consolidative radiotherapy for bulky and advanced Hodgkin's disease: Eastern Cooperative Oncology Group pilot study E1492. *J Clin Oncol* 2000;18:972–980.
61. Horning SJ, Hoppe RT, Breslin S, et al. Stanford V and radiotherapy for locally extensive and advanced Hodgkin's disease: mature results of a prospective clinical trial. *J Clin Oncol* 2002;20:630–637.
62. Advani R. Incidence of secondary leukemia/myelodysplasia (AML/MDS) in Hodgkin's disease (HD) with three generations of therapy at Stanford University. *J Clin Oncol, Annual Meeting Proceedings Part I* 2006; 24(18S):7516.
63. Horning SJ, Hoppe RT, Advani R, et al. Efficacy and late effects of Stanford V chemotherapy and radiotherapy in untreated Hodgkin's disease: mature data in early and advanced stage patients. *Blood* 2004;104:92a. Abstract 308.
64. Yahalom J, Edwards-Bennet S, Jacobs J, et al. Stanford V and radiotherapy for advanced and locally extensive Hodgkin's disease (HD): the Memorial Sloan-Kettering Cancer Center (MSKCC) experience. *Blood* 2004;104:3483–3489.
65. Johnson P, Hoskin P, Horwich A, et al. Stanford V (SV) regimen versus ABVD for the treatment of advanced Hodgkin lymphoma (HL): results of a UK NCRI/LTO randomised phase II trial. *Blood* 2004;104:311.
66. Aversa SM, Salvagno L, Soraru M, et al. Stanford V regimen plus consolidative radiotherapy is an effective therapeutic program for bulky or advanced-stage Hodgkin's disease. *Acta Haematol* 2004;112:141–147.
67. Gobbi PG, Levis A, Chisesi T, et al. ABVD versus modified stanford V versus MOPPEBVCAD with optional and limited radiotherapy in intermediate- and advanced-stage Hodgkin's lymphoma: final results of a multicenter randomized trial by the Intergruppo Italiano Linfomi. *J Clin Oncol* 2005;23:9198–9207.
68. Brice P, Tredaniel J, Monsuez J, et al. Cardiopulmonary toxicity after three courses of ABVD and mediastinal irradiation in favorable Hodgkin's disease. *Ann Oncol* 1991;2(suppl 2):73–76.
69. Schmoll H. Review of etoposide single-agent activity. *Cancer Treat Rev* 1982;9(suppl):21–30.
70. Richards MA, Waxman JH, Man T, et al. EVA treatment for recurrent or unresponsive Hodgkin's disease. *Cancer Chemother Pharmacol* 1986;18:51–53.
71. Brizel DM, Gockerman JP, Crawford J, et al. A pilot study of etoposide, vinblastine, and doxorubicin plus involved field irradiation in advanced, previously untreated Hodgkin's disease. *Cancer* 1994;74:159–163.
72. Canellos GP, Gollub J, Neuberg D, et al. Primary systemic treatment of advanced Hodgkin's disease with EVA (etoposide, vinblastine, doxorubicin):10-year follow-up. *Ann Oncol* 2003;14:268–272.
73. Friedmann AM, Hudson MM, Weinstein HJ, et al. Treatment of unfavorable childhood Hodgkin's disease with VEPA and low-dose, involved-field radiation. *J Clin Oncol* 2002;20:3088–3094.
74. Yuen AR, Sikic BI. Multidrug resistance in lymphomas. *J Clin Oncol* 1994;12:2453–2459.
75. Radford JA, Whelan JS, Rohatiner AZ, et al. Weekly VAPEC-B chemotherapy for high grade non-Hodgkin's lymphoma: results of treatment in 184 patients. *Ann Oncol* 1994;5:147–151.
76. Radford JA, Crowther D, Rohatiner AZ, et al. Results of a randomized trial comparing MVPP chemotherapy with a hybrid regimen, ChlVPP/EVA, in the initial treatment of Hodgkin's disease. *J Clin Oncol* 1995;13: 2379–2385.
77. Radford JA, Rohatiner AZ, Ryder WD, et al. ChlVPP/EVA hybrid versus the weekly VAPEC-B regimen for previously untreated Hodgkin's disease. *J Clin Oncol* 2002;20:2988–2994.
78. Simmonds PD, Mead GM, Sweetenham JW, et al. PACE BOM chemotherapy: a 12-week regimen for advanced Hodgkin's disease. *Ann Oncol* 1997;8:259–266.
79. Schellong G, Bramswig JH, Hornig-Franz I, et al. Hodgkin's disease in children: combined modality treatment for stages IA, IB, and IIA. Results in 356 patients of the German/Austrian Pediatric Study Group. *Ann Oncol* 1994;5(suppl 2):113–115.
80. Cullen MH, Stuart NS, Woodroffe C, et al. ChlVPP/PABlOE and radiotherapy in advanced Hodgkin's disease. The Central Lymphoma Group. *J Clin Oncol* 1994;12:779–787.
81. Hancock BW, Gregory WM, Cullen MH, et al. ChlVPP alternating with PABlOE is superior to PABlOE alone in the initial treatment of advanced Hodgkin's disease: results of a British National Lymphoma Investigation/Central Lymphoma Group randomized controlled trial. *Br J Cancer* 2001;84:1293–1300.
82. Johnson PW, Radford JA, Cullen MH, et al. Comparison of ABVD and alternating or hybrid multidrug regimens for the treatment of advanced Hodgkin's lymphoma: results of the United Kingdom Lymphoma Group LY09 trial (ISRCTN97144519). *J Clin Oncol* 2005;23:9208–9218.
83. Hancock BW, Vaughan Hudson G, Vaughan Hudson B, et al. Hybrid LOPP/EVA is not better than LOPP alternating with EVAP: a prematurely terminated British National Lymphoma Investigation randomized trial. *Ann Oncol* 1994;5(suppl 2):117–120.
84. Smith TJ, Khatcheressian J, Lyman GH, et al. 2006 update of recommendations for the use of white blood cell growth factors: an evidence-based clinical practice guideline. *J Clin Oncol* 2006;24:3187–3205.
85. Chopra R, McMillan AK, Linch DC, et al. The place of high-dose BEAM therapy and autologous bone marrow transplantation in poor-risk Hodgkin's disease. A single-center eight-year study of 155 patients. *Blood* 1993;81:1137–1145.
86. Horning SJ, Chao NJ, Negrin RS, et al. High-dose therapy and autologous hematopoietic progenitor cell transplantation for recurrent or refractory Hodgkin's disease: analysis of the Stanford University results and prognostic indices. *Blood* 1997;89:801–813.
87. Reece DE, Barnett MJ, Connors JM, et al. Intensive chemotherapy with cyclophosphamide, carmustine, and etoposide followed by autologous bone marrow transplantation for relapsed Hodgkin's disease. *J Clin Oncol* 1991;9:1871–1879.
88. Carella AM, Carlier P, Congiu A, et al. Autologous bone marrow transplantation as adjuvant treatment for high-risk Hodgkin's disease in first complete remission after MOPP/ABVD protocol. *Bone Marrow Transplant* 1991;8:99–103.
89. Straus DJ, Gaynor JJ, Myers J, et al. Prognostic factors among 185 adults with newly diagnosed advanced Hodgkin's disease treated with alternating potentially noncross-resistant chemotherapy and intermediate-dose radiation therapy. *J Clin Oncol* 1990;8:1173–1186.
90. Federico M, Bellei M, Brice P, et al. High-dose therapy and autologous stem-cell transplantation versus conventional therapy for patients with advanced Hodgkin's lymphoma responding to front-line therapy. *J Clin Oncol* 2003;21:2320–2325.
91. Hoppe RT. Hodgkin's disease—the role of radiation therapy in advanced disease. *Ann Oncol* 1996;7(suppl 4):99–103.
92. Prosnitz LR, Wu JJ, Yahalom J. The case for adjuvant radiation therapy in advanced Hodgkin's disease. *Cancer Invest* 1996;14:361–370.
93. Loeffler M, Brosteanu O, Hasenclever D, et al. Meta-analysis of chemotherapy versus combined modality treatment trials in Hodgkin's disease. International Database on Hodgkin's Disease Overview Study Group. *J Clin Oncol* 1998;16:818–829.
94. Mauch P. What is the role for adjuvant radiation therapy in advanced Hodgkin's disease? *J Clin Oncol* 1998;16:815–817.
95. Yahalom J, Ryu J, Straus DJ, et al. Impact of adjuvant radiation on the patterns and rate of relapse in advanced-stage Hodgkin's disease treated with alternating chemotherapy combinations. *J Clin Oncol* 1991;9:2193–2201.
96. Fabian CJ, Mansfield CM, Dahlberg S, et al. Low-dose involved field radiation after chemotherapy in advanced Hodgkin disease. A Southwest Oncology Group randomized study. *Ann Intern Med* 1994;120:903–912.
97. Kaplan HS. Evidence for a tumoricidal dose level in the radiotherapy of Hodgkin's disease. *Cancer Res* 1966;26:1221–1224.

98. Wirth A, Corry J, Laidlaw C, et al. Salvage radiotherapy for Hodgkin's disease following chemotherapy failure. *Int J Radiat Oncol Biol Phys* 1997;39:599–607.

99. Pezner RD, Lipsett JA, Vora N, et al. Radical radiotherapy as salvage treatment for relapse of Hodgkin's disease initially treated by chemotherapy alone: prognostic significance of the disease-free interval. *Int J Radiat Oncol Biol Phys* 1994;30:965–970.

100. Prosnitz LR, Farber LR, Kapp DS, et al. Combined modality therapy for advanced Hodgkin's disease:15-year follow-up data. *J Clin Oncol* 1988;6:603–612.

101. Brizel DM, Winer EP, Prosnitz LR, et al. Improved survival in advanced Hodgkin's disease with the use of combined modality therapy. *Int J Radiat Oncol Biol Phys* 1990;19:535–542.

102. Diehl V, Loeffler M, Pfreundschuh M, et al. Further chemotherapy versus low-dose involved-field radiotherapy as consolidation of complete remission after six cycles of alternating chemotherapy in patients with advance Hodgkin's disease. German Hodgkin's Study Group (GHSG). *Ann Oncol* 1995;6:901–910.

103. Ferme C, Sebban C, Hennequin C, et al. Comparison of chemotherapy to radiotherapy as consolidation of complete or good partial response after six cycles of chemotherapy for patients with advanced Hodgkin's disease: results of the groupe d'etudes des lymphomes de l'Adulte H89 trial. *Blood* 2000;95:2246–2252.

104. Weiner MA, Leventhal B, Brecher ML, et al. Randomized study of intensive MOPP-ABVD with or without low-dose total- nodal radiation therapy in the treatment of stages IIB, IIIA2, IIIB, and IV Hodgkin's disease in pediatric patients: a Pediatric Oncology Group study. *J Clin Oncol* 1997;15:2769–2779.

105. Laskar S, Gupta T, Vimal S, et al. Consolidation radiation after complete remission in Hodgkin's disease following six cycles of doxorubicin, bleomycin, vinblastine, and dacarbazine chemotherapy: is there a need? *J Clin Oncol* 2004;22:62–68.

106. Aleman BM, Raemaekers JM, Tirelli U, et al. Involved-field radiotherapy for advanced Hodgkin's lymphoma. *N Engl J Med* 2003;348:2396–2406.

107. Aleman BMP, Raemaekers JMM, Tomsic R, et al. Involved field radiotherapy for patients in partial remission after chemotherapy for advanced Hodgkin's lymphoma. *Int J Radiat Oncol Biol Phys* 2007;67:19–30.

108. Diehl V, Brillant C, Franklin J, et al. BEACOPP chemotherapy for advanced Hodgkin's disease: results of further analyses of the HD9- and HD12- trials of the German Hodgkin Study Group (GHSG). *Blood* 2004;104:307.

109. Diehl V, Klimm B, Re D. Hodgkin lymphoma: a curable disease: what comes next? *Eur J Haematol Suppl* 2005: 6–13.

110. Vijayakumar S, Myrianthopoulos LC. An updated dose-response analysis in Hodgkin's disease. *Radiother Oncol* 1992;24:1–13.

111. Brincker H, Bentzen SM. A re-analysis of available dose-response and time-dose data in Hodgkin's disease. *Radiother Oncol* 1994;30:227–230.

112. Donaldson SS, Link MP. Combined modality treatment with low-dose radiation and MOPP chemotherapy for children with Hodgkin's disease. *J Clin Oncol* 1987;5:742–749.

113. Maity A, Goldwein JW, Lange B, et al. Comparison of high-dose and low-dose radiation with and without chemotherapy for children with Hodgkin's disease: an analysis of the experience at the Children's Hospital of Philadelphia and the Hospital of the University of Pennsylvania. *J Clin Oncol* 1992;10:929–935.

114. Loeffler M, Diehl V, Pfreundschuh M, et al. Dose-response relationship of complementary radiotherapy following four cycles of combination chemotherapy in intermediate-stage Hodgkin's disease. *J Clin Oncol* 1997;15:2275–2287.

115. Blayney DW, Longo DL, Young RC, et al. Decreasing risk of leukemia with prolonged follow-up after chemotherapy and radiotherapy for Hodgkin's disease. *N Engl J Med* 1987;316:710–714.

116. Andrieu JM, Ifrah N, Payen C, et al. Increased risk of secondary acute non-lymphocytic leukemia after extended-field radiation therapy combined with MOPP chemotherapy for Hodgkin's disease. *J Clin Oncol* 1990;8:1148–1154.

117. van Leeuwen FE, Klokman WJ, Veer MB, et al. Long-term risk of second malignancy in survivors of Hodgkin's disease treated during adolescence or young adulthood. *J Clin Oncol* 2000;18:487–497.

118. Travis LB, Hill D, Dores GM, et al. Cumulative absolute breast cancer risk for young women treated for Hodgkin lymphoma. *J Natl Cancer Inst* 2005;97:1428–1437.

119. Swerdlow AJ, Douglas AJ, Hudson GV, et al. Risk of second primary cancers after Hodgkin's disease by type of treatment: analysis of 2846 patients in the British National Lymphoma Investigation. *BMJ* 1992;304: 1137–1143.

120. Kaldor JM, Day NE, Bell J, et al. Lung cancer following Hodgkin's disease: a case-control study. *Int J Cancer* 1992;52:677–681.

121. Lavey RS, Eby NL, Prosnitz LR. Impact on second malignancy risk of the combined use of radiation and chemotherapy for lymphomas. *Cancer* 1990;66:80–88.

122. Beaty O III, Hudson MM, Greenwald C, et al. Subsequent malignancies in children and adolescents after treatment for Hodgkin's disease. *J Clin Oncol* 1995;13:603–609.

123. Hancock SL, Tucker MA, Hoppe RT. Breast cancer after treatment of Hodgkin's disease. *J Natl Cancer Inst* 1993;85:25–31.

124. Yahalom J, Petrek JA, Biddinger PW, et al. Breast cancer in patients irradiated for Hodgkin's disease: a clinical and pathologic analysis of 45 events in 37 patients. *J Clin Oncol* 1992;10:1674–1681.

125. Salloum E, Doria R, Schubert W, et al. Second solid tumors in patients with Hodgkin's disease cured after radiation or chemotherapy plus adjuvant low-dose radiation. *J Clin Oncol* 1996;14:2435–2443.

126. Bhatia S, Robison LL, Oberlin O, et al. Breast cancer and other second neoplasms after childhood Hodgkin's disease. *N Engl J Med* 1996;334:745–751.

127. Hancock SL, Donaldson SS, Hoppe RT. Cardiac disease following treatment of Hodgkin's disease in children and adolescents. *J Clin Oncol* 1993;11:1208-1215. See comments.

128. Hirsch A, Vander Els N, Straus DJ, et al. Effect of ABVD chemotherapy with and without mantle or mediastinal irradiation on pulmonary function and symptoms in early-stage Hodgkin's disease. *J Clin Oncol* 1996;14:1297–1305.

129. Aleman BMP, Raemaekers JMM, Tirelli U, et al. Involved field radiotherapy for advanced Hodgkin's lymphoma. *N Engl J Med* 2003;348:2396–2406.

130. Duggan D, Petroni G, Johnson J, et al. MOPP/ABV versus ABVD for advanced Hodgkin's disease: preliminary report of CALGB 8952 (with SWOG, ECOG, NCIC). *Proc Am Soc Clin Oncol*1997;16:12a. Abstract 43

131. Hasenclever D, Diehl V. A prognostic score for advanced Hodgkin's disease. International Prognostic Factors Project on Advanced Hodgkin's Disease. *N Engl J Med* 1998;339:1506–1514.

CHAPTER 19 ■ MANAGEMENT OF RECURRENT HODGKIN LYMPHOMA

GEORGE P. CANELLOS AND ANDREAS JOSTING

The problem of relapse of Hodgkin lymphoma following initial therapy can be appreciated from an analysis of large series of patients that include all stages and treatments. Depending on the initial stage and clinical prognostic factors, up to 30% could be expected to relapse following initial induction of remission.[1] Fortunately, second-line (or third-line) therapeutic measures are capable of achieving durable responses and remissions. The biological features of Hodgkin lymphoma that contribute to its sensitivity to chemotherapy/radiation after initial therapy can be retained at the time of relapse, thus allowing for a relatively higher second-line cure rate when compared to most other lymphomas.

Relapse may be defined as the reappearance of disease in sites of prior disease (recurrence) and/or in new sites (extension) after initial therapy and complete response. Progression usually refers to increasing disease after achievement of a minor or no response. An "event" or "failure" refers to the totality of relapse from a complete remission, progression of a partial or minor remission, or death from any cause. Progression of disease refractory to therapy is a failure to achieve any significant response, and represents a rare but significant degree of radiation or drug resistance. Follow-up procedures to detect relapse vary somewhat from institution to institution, but they generally assume a schedule of periodic clinical and radiographic examination every 3 months for the first 2 years, followed by examinations every 4 to 6 months thereafter until annual examinations start after 5 years. Retrospective reviews of follow-up procedures in patients treated for Hodgkin lymphoma with chemotherapy alone[2] and radiation therapy alone[3] reveal that the majority of relapses are detected during physical examination or investigation of symptoms rather than by routine blood tests or radiographic investigations. Depending on stage and risk factor profile, up to 95% of patients with Hodgkin lymphoma at first presentation achieve complete remission or complete remission unconfirmed after the initial standard treatment, including radiotherapy, combination chemotherapy, or combined-modality therapy. Patients who relapse after a first complete remission can achieve a second complete remission with salvage treatment including radiotherapy for localized relapse in previously nonirradiated areas, conventional salvage chemotherapy, or high-dose chemotherapy with stem cell transplantation.

The clinical pattern of relapse can determine the likelihood of success of second-line therapy in achieving a durable second remission. Whenever there is uncertainty, it is useful to document relapse by repeat biopsy. This is especially so in the setting of late relapse, as the risk for other second cancers (non-Hodgkin lymphomas or solid tumors) is present in such patients. Early recurrence from complete remission or progression of a partial remission, especially with persistence of constitutional symptoms or measurable radiographic abnormalities, is most likely to be Hodgkin lymphoma.

In all cases, clinical restaging is recommended at the time of relapse, especially if it may be an asymptomatic localized relapse. Because most patients will receive systemic or combined-modality therapy for relapse, the restaging has more prognostic than therapeutic importance. Late isolated nodal recurrence is associated with a better prognosis than early or disseminated relapse; thus, timing and extent of failure will determine prognosis and the selection of salvage therapy.

The most useful restaging scheme applies the criteria of the Ann Arbor staging system to the extent of disease at the time of relapse and substitutes the letters RS (relapse stage) for CS (clinical stage) or PS (pathologic stage).[4]

It is crucial to define the remission or relapse status, because many salvage treatments are intensive and potentially toxic. Residual abnormalities persisting on CT after treatment of large lymph node masses, especially in the mediastinum, may actually represent a complete remission unconfirmed, with only residual fibrosis and necrosis. Radionuclide scanning with gallium single-photon emission computed tomography (SPECT) or 18-FDG positron emission tomography (PET) has been employed to evaluate residual radiographic abnormalities. Lack of uptake of radionuclide may represent only residual fibrosis/necrosis, and follow-up without therapy is usually recommended. The majority of these radionuclide-negative residual masses do not progress and may continue to regress over long periods of time. Relapse may occur in about 10% to 30% of cases, depending on the initial stage, despite the negative findings on gallium studies following therapy.[5] Persistent avidity for gallium or a more intensely positive PET scan, however, is usually related to residual disease activity.[6] Experienced interpretation of radionuclide scans is crucial, because false-positives can occur with rebound uptake of the isotope in normal thymus gland or with the incidental faint bilateral pulmonary hilar uptake that sometimes follows chemotherapy. In addition, there can be false-positive PET avidity in areas of infection, brown fat, and hyperplastic bone marrow and spleen. Some evidence of minimal PET activity in Hodgkin lymphoma at the completion of therapy can be followed with possible reversion to negativity in a few months. In the PET scan literature, up to 40% of so-called PET- positive findings at the end of therapy do not recur in up to 5 years of follow-up.[7]

RELAPSE FOLLOWING PRIMARY RADIOTHERAPY

In the last 10 to 20 years, primary extended-field or subtotal nodal radiation therapy has included the mantle and peri-aortic and splenic fields unless a prior splenectomy was performed. Relapse within an irradiated nodal site is unusual, ranging from

1.3% to 4.5% over a range of doses from 30 to 45 Gy. However, relapse, if it occurs, will more often be noted in unirradiated contiguous nodes or extranodal sites. Tumor bulk and stage remain the most significant prognostic factors following primary radiation therapy.[8] The relapse rate from primary radiation therapy for stage I–II disease derived from the experience of major radiation therapy centers is in the range of 19% to 32%. Approximately 60% occurred in unirradiated nodal areas and the remainder in extranodal sites such as lung and bone.[9–13]

In recent years, staging laparotomy has been abandoned as a staging approach as most patients now receive combined-modality therapy or, where appropriate, chemotherapy alone. As a result, relapse rates have diminished to the range of 10% to 12% for early stages treated with combined-modality therapy or slightly higher when chemotherapy alone is used. The majority of relapses will recur within 3 years following therapy. Late recurrences are rare but can occur following radiation therapy. One series from the EORTC (European Organization for Research and Treatment of Cancer) demonstrated a 3.5% recurrence rate beyond 5 years.[14]

Durability of remission usually correlates with extent of radiation, and extended-field radiation had a lower recurrence rate than mantle-field radiation alone; however, it did not impact overall survival because of the effectiveness of salvage systemic therapy. The International Database for Hodgkin's Disease is a database with 14,315 patients. They reported that the relapse rate following radiation therapy for clinically and laparotomy-staged patients with localized presentation was 1,154 of 3,750 patients, or 31%, with radiation alone. Combined-modality therapy has cut this in half. Negative prognostic factors tend to diminish when systemic therapy is added in combined-modality therapy. Negative prognostic factors include extent of disease (number of sites) and mediastinal bulk.[15]

Relapse from primary radiation can be salvaged successfully with systemic chemotherapy. In fact, the long-term survival of such patients approaches that achieved with primary systemic therapy of de novo advanced disease. As mentioned above, relapse will more often occur in the nonirradiated sites, and as such could represent tumor that is neither radioresistant nor drug resistant. A selection of series is shown in Table 19.1.[16–20] Negative prognostic factors for a durable secondary chemotherapy-induced remission are age over 50 years, clinical stage at relapse, and early versus late (>4 years) relapse.[21]

The 10-year survival of patients who relapsed from radiation and were treated with combination chemotherapy +/− further radiation from a number of series varied from 57% to 89%, with results improving since the introduction of ABVD.

TABLE 19.1

RESULTS OF SALVAGE CHEMOTHERAPY IN PATIENTS RELAPSING FROM PRIMARY RADIATION THERAPY FOR STAGE I–II HODGKIN LYMPHOMA

Trial site/reference	Patients	Survival
Royal Marsden (UK)[16]	473	63% (10 years)
Peter McCallum (Australia)[17]	70	71% (MOPP chemotherapy, 10 years)
Stanford[18]	99	57% (MOPP, 10 years)
Inst. Cura Tumori (Milan)[19]	63	80% (ABVD, 7 years)
Dana-Farber/Brigham & Women's (Boston)[20]	100	89% (ABVD, 10 years)

In recent years, high-dose therapy with autologous stem cell transplantation has been introduced. In addition, combined-modality therapy has been used for localized relapse. Failure in previously irradiated sites may present a more complicated problem of radiation resistance. In general, failure following irradiation as the sole therapy is a problem of the past, except perhaps for nodular lymphocyte-predominant Hodgkin lymphoma, where radiation therapy still has a major role. Relapse will tend to occur (if it is to occur) earlier in nonirradiated sites.

There is mounting evidence suggesting that radiation therapy routinely used in patients with advanced disease achieving complete remission with chemotherapy does not improve survival.[22,23] Further recent trials in localized nonbulky disease suggest that chemotherapy alone may give equivalent overall survival.[24] The long-term toxicity of radiotherapy to the cardiovascular system and secondary oncogenesis has given pause to the general use of radiation therapy. The salvage results of MOPP versus the now more commonly used regimen, ABVD (doxorubicin, bleomycin, vinblastine, dacarbazine), have been updated by the Dana-Farber/Brigham and Women's Hospital group (formerly the Harvard Joint Center for Radiation Therapy). The 10-year results showed freedom-from-second-relapse and overall survival rates of 70% and 89%. The choice of regimen (MOPP versus ABVD) did not impact outcome. Only age over 50 years was a significant negative factor. Among the factors that influence the success of second-line chemotherapy, nodular-sclerosis histology was a favorable feature. In contrast to the relapse from chemotherapy, the duration of remission following radiation did not influence the outcome of salvage chemotherapy.[20] The tendency to abandon MOPP is understandable given the higher likelihood of secondary myelodysplasia or acute leukemia following alkylating agents. Thus, there may be a new, albeit limited, role for salvage radiation therapy for the fewer than 20% of patients with nonbulky stage I–II disease who relapse only in the original site(s) after treatment with chemotherapy alone. Data from three trials suggest that the majority of these few recurrences will be at the original site of disease and thus potentially salvageable with radiation. Overall then ~80% or more of patients with early favorable Hodgkin lymphoma are likely cured without requiring radiation therapy in their primary treatment.

Patients who present with bulky (>10 cm) mediastinal masses still receive combined modality treatment. Future evaluation with PET may be able to identify patients within this group who might also be spared radiation therapy. Patients with nodular lymphocyte-predominant Hodgkin lymphoma have biological features more typical of a low grade B-cell non-Hodgkin lymphoma. This variant has a very long natural history, with focal relapses and an immunophenotype of the malignant cells that includes a prominence of clonal B-cell markers including CD20 positivity.[25,26] Late isolated relapses can be treated successfully with radiation. Chemotherapy may not be needed and, if needed, the relative durability of remission has not been assessed with adequate numbers of patients to compare ABVD with alkylating agent-containing regimens such as MOPP (nitrogen mustard, vincristine, procarbazine, prednisone). The CD20 positivity contributes to its responsiveness to rituximab, an anti-CD20 monoclonal antibody, as a salvage therapy for more generalized relapse.[27,28]

SALVAGE RADIOTHERAPY FOR PATIENTS WHO RELAPSE AFTER CHEMOTHERAPY

There is an almost anecdotal experience employing radiation therapy as the sole salvage modality for patients in relapse from combination chemotherapy for advanced disease. Since

TABLE 19.2

SALVAGE RADIOTHERAPY ALONE FOLLOWING RELAPSE
FROM CHEMOTHERAPY

Author/reference	Patients	Median follow-up	Freedom from 2nd relapse
Josting (2005)[29]	100	52 months	30% (5 years)
Campbell (2005)[30]	81	16.8 years	33% (10 years)
Uematsu (1993)[31]	14	80 months	36% (7 years)
Brada (1992)[32]	25	60 months	23% (10 years)
Fox (1987)[33]	17	48 months	24% (5 years)

1987, only 260 patients have been reported with a complete remission rate that varied between 45% and 92% and a freedom from second relapse at 5 to 10 years varying from 18% to 46% (Table 19.2).[29–33] The experience would suggest that combined-modality was superior to radiation alone.[31] It is never clear whether selection bias enters into such analyses, but this approach is now rarely used.

In the absence of data derived from randomized trials, nodal or involved-field irradiation is often used in the combined-modality salvage of relapse after chemotherapy in classical Hodgkin lymphoma.

Autologous stem cell support and high-dose combined chemotherapy have been widely used to salvage patients in relapse after systemic or combined-modality therapy. The value of additional radiation therapy in that setting has never been demonstrated in prospective trials. It is frequently added to the program, especially to sites of bulk disease. The implication from retrospective analyses would suggest that involved-field radiation improved the progression-free survival but seemingly did not improve overall survival, except in subgroups of patients.[34] Patients who had not had prior radiation fared somewhat better and had a higher survival rate than those who had prior radiation therapy. Without comparisons matched by prognostic factors, it is difficult to assess the impact of additional radiation. It is noteworthy that, when the data from the Princess Margaret hospital (Toronto) were analyzed for toxicity, there was a high treatment-related mortality (10 patients out of 59, or 17%). The sequence of radiation given prior to the high-dose therapy contributed to the majority of treatment-related deaths (8/10), especially in patients who were irradiated less than 50 days prior to the high-dose therapy.[35]

SALVAGE THERAPY FOR RELAPSED AND REFRACTORY HODGKIN LYMPHOMA FOLLOWING INITIAL SYSTEMIC THERAPY

Prognostic Factors in Relapsed and Refractory Hodgkin Lymphoma

It was first noted in 1979 that the length of remission to first-line chemotherapy had a marked effect on the ability of patients to respond to subsequent salvage chemotherapy.[36] In 1992, the National Cancer institute (NCI) updated their experience with the long-term follow-up of patients who relapsed after polychemotherapy.[37] Derived primarily from investigations involving

failures after MOPP and MOPP variants, the conclusions are thought to be relevant to other chemotherapy programs as well. On this basis, chemotherapy failures can be divided into three subgroups: (a) primary progressive Hodgkin lymphoma, that is, patients who never achieve a complete remission; (b) early relapses within 12 months of complete remission; and (c) late relapses after complete remission lasting longer than 12 months. Using conventional-dose chemotherapy for patients with primary progressive disease, virtually no patient survives more than 8 years. In contrast, the projected 20-year survival rate for patient with early relapse and late relapse was 11% and 22%, respectively.[37]

Primary Progressive Hodgkin Lymphoma

Patients with primary progressive disease (PD), defined as progression during induction treatment or within 90 days after the end of treatment, have a particularly poor prognosis. Conventional salvage regimens have given disappointing results in the vast majority of patients: response to salvage treatment is low and the duration of response is often short. The 8-year overall survival ranges from 0% to 8%.[37,38]

The German Hodgkin Study Group (GHSG) retrospectively analyzed 206 patients with PD to determine outcome after salvage therapy and identify prognostic factors.[39] The 5-year freedom from second failure (FF2F) and overall survival (OS) rates for all patients was 17% and 26%. As reported from transplant centers, the 5-year FF2F and OS for patients treated with HDCT (high dose chemotherapy) plus ASCT (autologous stem-cell support) was 42% and 48%, respectively, but only 33% of all patients received HDCT. The low percentage of patients who received HDCT was due to rapidly fatal disease or life-threatening severe toxicity after salvage therapy. Other reasons not to proceed to HDCT were insufficient stem-cell harvest, poor performance status, and older age. In a multivariate analysis, the Karnofsky performance score at progression ($p < 0.0001$), age over 50 ($p = 0.019$), and attainment of a temporary remission to first-line chemotherapy ($p = 0.0003$) were significant prognostic factors for survival. Patients with none of these risk factors had a 5-year OS of 55% compared with 0% for patients with all three of these unfavorable prognostic factors.

Early and Late Relapsed Hodgkin Lymphoma

The overall prognosis is guarded for patients with advanced disease relapsing after first-line conventional chemotherapy. At present, HDCT followed by ASCT is the treatment of choice for patients with relapsed HD after first-line polychemotherapy. Although the results reported with HDCT in patients with late relapse have been superior to those reported in most series of conventional dose chemotherapy, the use of

HDCT in late relapses had been an area of controversy because patients with late relapse have satisfactory second complete remission rates when treated with conventional chemotherapy with OS ranging from 40% to 55%. However, the HDR-1 trial of the GHSG showed improved FFTF after HDCT compared with conventional chemotherapy also in patients with late relapse.[40]

Many prognostic factors have been described for patients relapsing after first-line chemotherapy. These include age, sex, histology, relapse sites, stage at relapse, bulky disease, B-symptoms, performance status, and extranodal relapse. The impact of these factors is difficult to assess due to confounding factors such as the small number of patients and inclusion of primary progressive Hodgkin lymphoma. In addition, multivariate analyses were not performed systemically.[41–43]

Brice and colleagues performed one of the largest studies evaluating prognostic factors in relapsed Hodgkin lymphoma. Included were 187 patients who relapsed after a first complete remission. At first relapse, treatment was conventional (chemo- and/or radiotherapy) in 44% and HDCT followed by ASCT in 56%. Two prognostic factors were identified by multivariate analysis as correlating with both FF2F and OS. These factors were the initial duration of first remission (<12 months or >12 months; p <0.0001) and stage at relapse (I–II vs. III–IV; p = 0.0013). FF2F was 62% and 32%, respectively; and OS was 87% and 44% according to the presence of 0 or 2 parameters, respectively. Laboratory data were not available in this retrospective analysis.[44]

The GHSG has recently performed a retrospective analysis including a much larger number of relapsed patients (n = 422) than previous reported (Fig. 19.1). The analysis of prognostic factors suggests that the prognosis of a patient with relapsed Hodgkin lymphoma can be estimated according to several factors. The most relevant factors were combined into a prognostic score. This score was calculated on the basis of duration of first remission, stage at relapse, and the presence or absence of anemia at relapse. Early recurrence within 3 to 12 months after the end of primary treatment, relapse stage III or IV, and hemoglobin below 10.5g/dL in female or below 12 g/dL in male patients, contribute to a score with possible values of 0, 1, 2, and 3 in order or worsening prognosis.[45]

This prognostic score allows distinguishing patients with different FF2F and OS. The actuarial 4-year FF2F and OS for patients relapsing after chemotherapy with three unfavorable factors were 17% and 27%, respectively. In contrast, patients with none of the unfavorable factors had FF2F and OS at 4 years of 48% and 83%, respectively. In addition, the prognostic score was also predictive for patients relapsing after radiotherapy, for patients relapsing after chemotherapy who were treated with conventional therapies or with HDCT followed by ASCT, and for patients under 60 years of age and a Karnofsky performance status of 90% or more, being the major candidate groups for dose intensification. The GHSG prognostic factor score uses clinical characteristics that can be easily collected at the time of relapse. It separates groups of patients with substantially different outcomes.

The prognostic factors identified may be useful to tailor the therapy for subgroups of patients, to define homogeneous cohorts for prospective randomized trials, and to identify more precisely patients with poor-risk relapse who should be treated with innovative approaches. Selected salvage regimens published since 1995 are outlined in Table 19.3.

TREATMENT STRATEGIES

The survival of patients treated with conventional chemotherapy after relapse of irradiated early-stage disease is at least equal to that of patients with advanced-stage disease initially treated with chemotherapy. Overall survival (OS) and disease-free survival (DFS) range from 57% to 71%.[46,47] Patients who relapse following radiation therapy alone for localized Hodgkin lymphoma have satisfactory results with combination chemotherapy and are not considered candidates for HDCT and ASCT.

HDCT followed by ASCT has been shown to produce 30% to 65% long-term disease-free survival in selected patients with refractory and relapsed Hodgkin lymphoma.[48–51] In addition, the reduction of early transplant-related mortality from 10% to 25% reported in earlier studies to less than 5% in more recent studies has led to the widespread acceptance of HDCT and ASCT.

Although results of HDCT have generally been better than those observed after conventional-dose salvage therapy, the

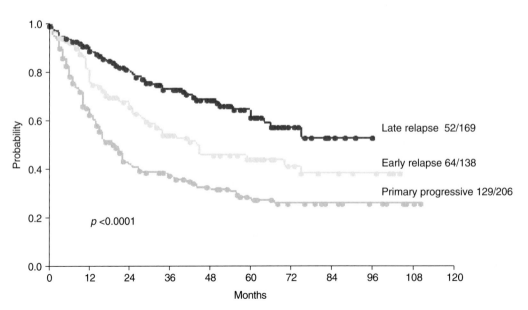

FIGURE 19.1. Actuarial overall survival of patients with primary progressive, early relapsed, or late relapsed Hodgkin lymphoma registered in the GHSG from 1988 to 1999 (n = 513).

TABLE 19.3

SELECTED SALVAGE REGIMENS (PUBLISHED SINCE 1995)

Drug regimen/reference	Dose, route	Schedule
DHAP[70]		
Dexamethasone	40 mg/m² IV	Days 1–4
Cisplatin	100 mg/m² IV continuous infusion	Day 1
Cytarabine	2 g/m² IV over 3 hours q 12 hours	Day 2
G-CSF and cortisosteroid eye drops q 12-17 days		
DEXA-BEAM (German Hodgkin Study Group)[48]		
Dexamethasone	8 mg p.o. q 8 hours	Days 1–10
Carmustine	60 mg/m² IV	Day 2
Etoposide	250 mg/m² IV	Days 4–7
Cytarabine	100 mg/m² IV q 8 hours	Days 4–7
Melphalan	20 mg/m² IV	Day 3
Next cycle given when counts recover		
Mini-BEAM[71]		
BCNU (carmustine)	60 mg/m² IV	Day 1
Etoposide	75 mg/m² IV q. 12 hours	Days 2–5
Cytarabine	100 mg/m² IV q. 12 hours	Days 2–5
Melphalan	30 mg/m² IV × 1	Day 6
Repeated q 4–6 weeks		
ICE[72]		
Ifosfamide	5.0 g/m² continuous infusion 24 hours (equal dose of Mesna)	Day 2
Carboplatin	AUC 5 IV (max 800 mg)	Day 2
Etoposide	100 mg/m² IV	Days 1–3
G-CSF	Usual 2 cycles with a 2-week interval	Days 5–12
GDP (Toronto)[73]		
Gemcitabine	1000 mg/m² IV over 30 min	Days 1, 8
Dexamethoasone	40 mg p.o.	Days 1–4
Cisplatin	75 mg/m²	Days 1, 8
GVD (CALGB)[74]		
Gemcitabine	1000 mg/m²	q 21 days all day 1, 8
Vinorelbine	15 mg/m² IV	
Liposomal doxorubicin	10 mg/m² IV	

validity of these result has been questioned due to the lack of randomized trials. The most compelling evidence for the superiority of HDCT and ASCT in relapsed Hodgkin lymphoma comes from two reports from the British National Lymphoma Investigation (BNLI) and the German Hodgkin Lymphoma Study Group (GHSG) together with the European Group for Blood and Marrow Transplantation (EBMT).

In the BNLI trial, patients with relapsed or refractory Hodgkin lymphoma were treated with a combination of carmustine (BCNU), etoposide, cytarabine, and melphalan at a conventional-dose level (mini-BEAM) or a high-dose level (BEAM) with autologous bone marrow transplantation.[52] The

actuarial 3-year event-free survival (EFS) was significantly better in patients who received high-dose chemotherapy (53% versus 10%). A survival difference has never been demonstrated in this series.

The largest randomized multicenter trial was performed by the GHSG/EBMT to determine the benefit of HDCT in relapsed Hodgkin lymphoma. Patients with relapse after polychemotherapy were randomly assigned between four cycles of Dexa-BEAM (dexamethasone, BCNU, etoposide, ara-C, and melphalan) and two cycles of Dexa-BEAM followed by HDCT (BEAM) and ABMT/PBSCT (peripheral blood stem cell transplant). The final analysis of 144 evaluable patients revealed that among the 117 patients with partial or complete remission after two cycles of chemotherapy, FFTF in the HDCT group was 55% versus 34% for the patients receiving an additional two cycles of chemotherapy. OS was not significantly different.[40]

Sequential High-Dose Chemotherapy

In recent years, sequential high-dose chemotherapy has increasingly been employed in the treatment of solid tumors, hematologic disorders, and lymphoproliferative disorders. Initial results from phase I–II studies indicate that this kind of therapy offers safe and effective treatment.[53–58] In accordance with the Norton-Simon hypothesis,[59] following initial cytoreduction, few non–cross-resistant agents are given at short intervals. In general, PBSCT and the use of growth factors allow the application of the most effective drugs at the highest possible doses at intervals of 1 to 3 weeks. Sequential high-dose chemotherapy thereby enables the highest possible dosing over a minimum period of time (dose intensification).

In 1997, a multicenter phase II trial with a high-dose sequential chemotherapy program and a final myeloablative course was started to evaluate the feasibility and efficacy of this novel regimen in patients with relapsed Hodgkin lymphoma.[60] Eligibility criteria included age 18 to 60 years, histologically proven relapsed or primary progressive Hodgkin lymphoma, second relapse with no prior HDCT, and ECOG performance status of 0 to 1.

The treatment program consists of two cycles of DHAP (dexamethasone, cytosine arabinoside, cisplatin) in the first phase in order to reduce tumor burden before HDCT. Patients with partial or complete remission after two cycles of DHAP receive sequential high-dose chemotherapy consisting of cyclophosphamide 4 g/m^2 IV, methotrexate 8 g/m^2 IV plus vincristine 1.4 mg/m^2 IV and etoposide 2 g/m^2 IV. The final myeloblative course was BEAM (high doses of BCNU, etoposide, cytosine arabinoside, melphalan) followed by PBSCT with at least 2 × 10^6 CD34+ cells/kg.

At the last interim analysis, 102 patients were available for the final evaluation. State of remission was multiple relapse in 10 patients, progressive disease in 16 patients, early relapse in 29 patients, and late relapse in 44 patients. At 18 months of follow-up (range, 3–31 months), results are as follows: response rate after DHAP 87% (23% complete remission, 64% partial remission) and response rate at final evaluation 77% (68% complete remission, 9% partial remission). Toxicity was tolerable with no treatment-related deaths. FFTF and OS for patients with early relapse were 64% and 87% for early relapse; 68% and 81% for late relapse; 30% and 58% for patients with progressive disease, and 55% and 88% for patients with multiple relapse.[60]

In conclusion, sequential administration of high doses of cyclophosphamide, methotrexate, and etoposide is feasible and did not affect the tolerability of final myeloablative BEAM. This new three-phase treatment regimen is well tolerated and feasible in patients with relapsed and primary progressive Hodgkin lymphoma. The preliminary data suggests a high efficacy in relapsed Hodgkin lymphoma patients, warranting further randomized studies.

In January 2001, the GHSG—together with the EORTC, the GEL/TAMO and the EBMT—started a prospective randomized study to compare the effectiveness of a standard HDCT (BEAM) with a sequential HDCT after initial cytoreduction with two cycles of DHAP (HD-R2 protocol, Fig. 19.2). Patients with histologically confirmed early or late relapsed Hodgkin lymphoma, and patients in second relapse with no prior HDCT fulfilling the entry criteria, receive two cycles of dexamethasone, high-dose cytarabine and cisplatin (DHAP) followed by G-CSF (granulocyte colony-stimulating factor).

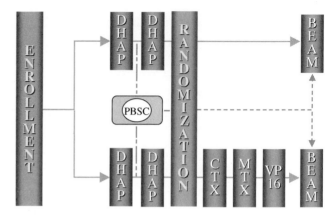

FIGURE 19.2. HDR-2 protocol. A European multicenter study for relapsed Hodgkin lymphoma (GHSG, EORTC, EBMT, GEL/TAMO).

Patients achieving NC, partial remission, or complete remission after DHAP are centrally randomized to receive either BEAM followed by PBSCT (arm A of the study); or high-dose cyclophosphamide plus G-CSF, followed by high-dose methotrexate plus vincristine, followed by high-dose etoposide plus G-CSF, and a final myeloablative course with BEAM (arm B of the study).

Allogeneic Transplantation after Reduced Conditioning

Allogeneic transplantation (alloBMT) has clear advantages compared with autologous transplantation: donor marrow cells uninvolved by malignancy are used, avoiding the risk of infusing occult lymphoma cells, which may contribute to relapse in patients who undergo autologous transplantation. In addition, donor lymphoid cells can potentially mediate a graft-versus-host effect.

Generally, donor availability and age constraints have limited a broader application of alloBMT in Hodgkin lymphoma. Moreover, alloBMT is associated with a high treatment-related mortality rate of up to 75% observed in patients with induction failure, which casts doubt upon the feasibility of this approach in patients with Hodgkin lymphoma.[61–64] In most cases, allogeneic transplantation from HLA-identical siblings is not recommended for patients with Hodgkin lylmphoma. The reduced relapse rate associated with a potential graft-versus-tumor effect is offset by lethal graft-versus-host toxicity.

Nevertheless, patients with induction failure and relapsed patients with additional risk factors have a poor prognosis also after HDCT and ASCT. Therefore, the role of alloBMT should be further evaluated in these patients, taking advantage of new developments like non-myeloablative conditioning regimens and alloPBSCT.

To circumvent the problems inherent to the toxicity and treatment-related mortality associated with allografting, the possibility of achieving engraftment of allogeneic stem cells after immunosuppressive therapy combined with myelosuppressive but non-myeloablative therapy has been assessed. Several groups have recently updated their experience with non-myeloablative conditioning regimens.[65–67]

The EBMT, together with the GEL/TAMO, the EORTC, and the GHSG, activated a multicenter phase II study to evaluate the treatment-related mortality of patients with primary progressive or relapsed Hodgkin lymphoma (early relapse, multiple relapse, and relapse after autologous SCT). Patients with an HLA-compatible sibling donor or an HLA-matched unrelated donor will be treated initially with one or two cycles of DHAP or other salvage protocols to reduce tumor burden before alloPBSCT. PBSC will be collected after G-CSF priming of the donor and reinfused after conditioning with fludarabine and melphalan.

FUTURE DIRECTIONS

Alternative strategies have been developed to improve the outcome of relapsed and resistant Hodgkin lymphoma. These approaches include the development of new cytostatic drugs and biological agents with proven efficacy in preclinical models.

One of the most promising new cytostatic drugs is the new vinca alkaloid, vinorelbine, which has demonstrated activity in Hodgkin lymphoma even in patients pretreated with vincristine or vinblastine.[68] The use of vinorelbine in first- and second-line therapy of Hodgkin lymphoma in order to improve frequency and duration of response is still under investigation. The pyrimidine analogue, gemcitabine, is the only drug currently under investigation that represents a new cytostatic mechanism of action. The "self-potentiating" mechanism of action leads to an enhanced accumulation and prolonged retention of gemcitabine in the malignant cell. The results of gemcitabine in advanced relapsed Hodgkin lymphoma are promising, with an overall response rate of 53% in heavily pretreated patients.[69] It has been combined with other agents in new salvage regimens, as outlined in Table 19.3.[48,71-74]

MAIN PRINCIPLES OF SALVAGE THERAPY FOR PATIENTS WHO HAVE FAILED INITIAL SYSTEMIC THERAPY

1. The majority (80%) of relapses after initial systemic or combined-modality therapy for unfavorable-prognosis (i.e., bulky disease or constitutional symptoms) or advanced-stage Hodgkin lymphoma will occur within 3 years after initial therapy.
2. The majority of these relapses will occur in patients who fail to respond to initial therapy or who have a response duration of less than 12 months. About 25% of relapses will occur beyond 12 months.
3. Residual masses in previous bulky sites of disease may represent only residual necrosis or fibrosis unless radionuclide avidity is clearly demonstrated, there is radiographic progression, or disease is documented by biopsy. Complementary radiation therapy to sites of residual disease in these patients may induce a durable complete response, especially in the setting of initially bulky disease, but the overall impact on survival is nil.
4. Second-line (salvage) systemic therapy is most likely to be successful in patients who relapse after a duration of initial response of more than 12 months whose relapse is confined to limited (specially nodal) sites and who are without constitutional symptoms. The outcome of late progression in an isolated, previously unirradiated nodal site will be better with combined-modality therapy than with chemotherapy or radiation therapy alone.
5. Initial disease progression, failure to respond to initial therapy, and early progression from complete response or partial response merit novel and/or aggressive therapies. Currently this entails high-dose chemotherapy with bone marrow or peripheral stem cell support. The results of the latter approach will also be determined by clinical prognostic factors, such as bulk of residual disease, stage, constitutional symptoms, extranodal disease, and residual sensitivity to cytotoxic drugs.

BIOLOGICAL THERAPY

Biological therapy for relapsed refractory disease employs two general approaches, attacking antigens on the cell surface or directing small molecules against intracellular targets. In the past, the presence of the CD30 antigen was the target of pilot trials of immunotoxins and bispecific monoclonal antibody therapy linking antiCD30 to antiCD16 (Fcγ-receptor III) in order to attract natural killer (NK) cells to the tumor surface.[75] Some minor response was noted; however, patients quickly generated anti-mouse antibodies. The recent availability of humanized mouse monoclonal antiCD30 (SGN-30, Seattle Genetics) and a fully humanized antibody (MDX-060, Medarex) have made further clinical trials possible. However, preliminary experience showed only limited efficacy in relapsed Hodgkin lymphoma but perhaps more consistent activity in CD30-positive anaplastic large-cell lymphoma.[76,77]

The humanized antiCD20 antibody, rituximab, has proven active against the uncommon variant of nodular lymphocyte-predominant Hodgkin lymphoma with rather high initial response rates in this CD20-positive variant.[27,28] In some patients, remission was long-lasting, and the rare CD20- positive classical Hodgkin lymphoma patient may also show response.

Small molecule inhibition of the NFkB proteosome with the drug bortezomid has been attempted in Hodgkin lymphoma. This agent is active in myeloma and mantle-cell lymphoma, but preliminary trials in Hodgkin lymphoma have not been very successful despite the fact that NFkB is upregulated in Hodgkin lymphoma cell lines.

The cellular immunological approach has been limited to the fact that 30% of patients will have Epstein-Barr viral coded antigens, especially LMP1 and LMP2A, on the Hodgkin/Reed-Sternberg cell. The approach has been to generate LMP2A-specific autologous cytotoxic T-cells ex vivo, followed by reinfusion of these activated T-cells. This again has been safe but only marginally active. On the contrary, allogeneic donor leukocyte infusions regardless of EBV status have been administered to patients with progressive disease following allogeneic transplantation. Four of 9 patients responded for a median of 7 months, but graft-versus-host disease developed in 3 patients.[78] Novel therapeutic approaches will follow an expanded knowledge of the molecular events essential to the life of the Reed-Sternberg cell. The precedent has already been set in other hematologic malignancies.

Although some clinical efficacy has been demonstrated in clinical trials with immunotoxins (ITs), none of the currently available ITs seems to be suited for a clinical phase II study.[79,80] Bispecific monoclonal antibodies (BiMoab) such as the recently reported CD30×CD64 BiMoab look more promising with clinical development programs scheduled, including phase III. The use of recombinant DNA technology for site-directed modifications of the IT and the development of humanized IT and BiMoabs might optimize their efficacy. In the future, the hope is to combine standard chemo-/radiotherapy with biological agents for the elimination of residual tumor cells and subsequently more relapse-free long-term survivors.

References

1. Oza AM, Ganesan TS, Leahy M, et al. Patterns of survival in patients with Hodgkin's disease: long follow-up in a single centre. *Ann Oncol* 1993;4:385–392.
2. Radford JA, Eardley A, Woodman C, et al. Follow-up policy after treatment for Hodgkin's disease: too many clinic visits and routine tests? A review of hospital records. *Br Med J* 1997;314:343–346.
3. Torrey MJ, Poen JC, Hoppe RT. Detection of relapse in early-stage Hodgkin's disease. Role of routine follow-up studies. *J Clin Oncol* 1997;15:1123–1130.

4. Josting A. Wolf J, Diehl V. Hodgkin's disease. Prognostic factors and treatment strategies. *Curr Opin Oncol* 2000;12:403–411.

5. Devizzi L, Maffioli L, Bonfante V, et al. Comparison of gallium scan, computed tomography, and magnetic resonance in patients with mediastinal Hodgkin's disease. *Ann Oncol* 1997;8(suppl 1):S53–S56.

6. Jochelson M, Mauch P, Balikian J, et al. The significance of the residual mediastinal mass in treated Hodgkin's disease. *J Clin Oncol* 1985;3: 637–640.

7. Hutchings M, Loft A, Hansen M, et al. FDG-PET after two cycles of chemotherapy predicts treatment failure and progression-free survival in Hodgkin lymphoma. *Blood* 2005;108:52.

8. Spect L. Tumor burden as the main indicator of prognosis in Hodgkin's disease. *Eur J Cancer* 1992;28A;1982–1985.

9. Bessell EM, Moloney AJ, Ellis IO, et al. Prognostic factors affecting disease-free survival in patients with Hodgkin's disease stages IA and IIA treated initially with radiotherapy alone in a single centre during 1973 to 1992. *Radiother Oncol* 1998;49:15–19.

10. Carde P, Burgers JMV, Henry-Amar M, et al. Clinical stages I and II Hodgkin's disease: a specifically tailored therapy according to prognostic factors. *J Clin Oncol* 1988;6:239–252.

11. Mauch P, Tarbell N, Weinstein H, et al. Stage IA and IIA supradiaphragmatic Hodgkin's disease: prognostic factors in surgically staged patients treated with mantle and paraaortic irradiation. *J Clin Oncol* 1988;6: 1576–1583.

12. Gospodarowicz MK, Sutcliffe SB, Bergsagel DE, et al. Radiation therapy in clinical stage I and II Hodgkin's disease. *Eur J Cancer* 1992;28A:1841–1846.

13. Advani RH, Horning SJ. Treatment of early-stage Hodgkin's disease. *Semin Hematol* 1999;36:270–281.

14. Bodis S, Henry-Amar M, Bosq J, et al. Late relapse in early-stage Hodgkin's disease patients enrolled in European Organization for Research and Treatment of Cancer protocols. *J Clin Oncol* 1993;11:225–232.

15. Somers R, Henry-Amar H, Meerwaldt JK, et al, eds. *Treatment strategy in Hodgkin's disease: proceedings of the Paris International Workshop and Symposium held on June 28–30, 1989.* Paris: Les Editions Inserm, John Libby Eurotext; 1990.

16. Horwich A, Spect L, Ashley S. Survival analysis of patients with clinical stages I or II Hodgkin's disease who have relapsed after initial treatment with radiotherapy alone. *Eur J Cancer* 1997;33:848–853.

17. Olver IN, Wolf MM, Cruickshank D, et al. Nitrogen mustard, vincristine, procarbazine, and prenisolone for relapse after radiation in Hodgkin's disease. An analysis of long-term follow-up. *Cancer* 1988;62:233–239.

18. Roach M, Brophy N. Cox R, et al. Prognostic factors for patients relapsing after radiotherapy for early-stage Hodgkin's disease. *J Clin Oncol* 1990;8: 623–629.

19. Santoro A, Viviana S. Villarreal CJR, et al. Salvage chemotherapy in Hodkgin's disease irradiation failures: superiority of doxorubicin-containing regimens over MOPP. *Cancer Treat Rep* 1986;70(3):343–348.

20. Ng AK, Li S, Neuberg D, et al. Comparison of MOPP versus ABVD as salvage therapy in patients who relapse after radiation therapy alone for Hodgkin's disease. *Ann Oncol* 2004;15:270–275.

21. Healy EA, Tarbell NJ, Kalish LA, et al. Prognostic factors for patients with Hodgkin's disease in first relapse. *Cancer* 1993;71:2613–2620.

22. Aleman BMP, Raemaekers JMM, Tirelli U, et al. Involved-field radiotherapy for advanced Hodgkin's lymphoma. *N Engl J Med* 2003;348: 2396–2406.

23. Fermé C, Sebban C, Henniquin C, et al. Comparison of chemotherapy to radiotherapy as consolidation of complete or good partial response after six cycles of chemotherapy for patients with advanced Hodgkn's disease: results of the Groupe d'Etudes des Lymphomes de l'Adulte H89 trial. *Blood* 2000;95:2246–2252.

24. Meyer RM, Gospodarowicz MK, Connors JM, et al. Randomized comparison of ABVD chemotherapy with a strategy that includes radiation therapy in patients with limited-stage Hodgkin's lymphoma: National Cancer Institute of Canada Clinical Trials Group and the Eastern Cooperative Oncology Group. *J Clin Oncol* 2005;23:4634–4642.

25. Wirth A, Yuen K, Barton M, et al. Long-term outcome after radiotherapy alone for lymphocyte-predominant Hodgkin lymphoma. *Cancer* 2005;104: 1221–1229.

26. Nogová L, Reineke T, Eich HT, et al. Extended field radiotherapy, combined modality treatment or involved field radiotherapy for patients with stage IA lymphocyte-predominant Hodgkin's lymphoma: retrospective analysis from the German Hodgkin Study Group (GHSG). *Ann Oncol* 2005;16:1683–1687.

27. Rehwald U, Schulz H, Reiser M, et al. Treatment of relapsed CD20+ Hodgkin lymphoma with the monoclonal antibody rituximab is effective and well tolerated: results of a phase 2 trial of the German Hodgkin Lymphoma Study Group. *Blood* 2003;101:420–424.

28. Ekstrand BC, Lucas JB, Horwitz SM, et al. Rituximab in lymphocyte-predominant Hodgkin disease: results of a phase 2 trial. *Blood* 2003;101: 4285–4289.

29. Josting A, Nogova L, Franklin J, et al. Salvage radiotherapy in patients with relapsed and refractory Hodgkin's lymphoma: a retrospective analysis from the German Hodgkin Lymphoma Study Group. *J Clin Oncol* 23:1522–1529.

30. Campbell B, Wirth A, Milner A, et al. Long-term follow-up of salvage radiotherapy in Hodgkin's lymphoma after chemotherapy failure. *Int J Rad Oncol Biol Phys* 205;63:1538–1545.

31. Uematsu M, Tarbell N, Silver B, et al. Wide-field radiation therapy with or without chemotherapy for patients with Hodgkin disease in relapse after initial combination chemotherapy. *Cancer* 1993;72:207–212.

32. Brada M, Eeles R, Ashley S, et al. Salvage radiotherapy in recurrent Hodgkin's disease. *Ann Oncol* 1992;3:131–135.

33. Fox KA, Lippman SM, Cassady JR, et al. Radiation therapy salvage of Hodgkin's disease following chemotherapy failure. *J Clin Oncol* 1987; 5:38–45.

34. Poen JC, Hoppe RT, Horning SJ. High-dose therapy and autologous bone marrow transplantation for relapsed/refractory Hodgkin's disease: the impact of involved field radiotherapy on patterns of failure and survival. *Int J Rad Oncol Biol Phys* 1996;36:3–12.

35. Tsang RW, Gospodariwicz MK, Sutcliffe SB, et al. Thoracic radiation therapy before autologous bone marrow transplantation in relapsed or refractory Hodgkin's disease. *Eur J Cancer* 1999;35:73–78.

36. Fisher R, De VV, Hubbard S, et al. Prolonged disease-free survival in Hodgkin's disease with MOPP reinduction after first relapse. *Ann Intern Med* 1979;90:761–765.

37. Longo D, Duffey P, Young R, et al. Conventional-dose salvage combination chemotherapy in patients relapsing with Hodgkin's disease after combination chemotherapy: the low probability for cure. *J Clin Oncol* 1992;10:210–218.

38. Bonfante V, Santoro A, Viviani S, et al. Outcome of patient with Hodgkin's disease failing after primary MOPP/ABVD. *J Clin Oncol* 1997;528–534.

39. Josting A, Rueffer U, Franklin J, et al. Prognostic factors and treatment outcome in primary progressive Hodgkin's lymphoma—a report from the German Hodgkin Lymphoma Study Group (GHSG). *Blood* 2000; 96: 1280–1286.

40. Schmitz N, Pfistner B, Sextro M, et al. Aggressive conventional chemotherapy compare with high-dose chemotherapy with autologous haematopoietic stem cell transplantation for relapsed chemosensitive Hodgkin's disease: a randomized trial. *Lancet* 2002;359;2065–2071.

41. Lohri A, Barnett M, Fairey RN, et al. Outcome of treatment of first relapse of Hodgkin's disease after primary chemotherapy: identification of risk factors from the British Columbia experience 1970 to 1988. *Blood* 1991;77: 2292–2298.

42. Ferme C, Bastion Y, Lepage E, et al. The MINE regimen as intensive salvage chemotherapy for relapsed and refractory Hodgkin's disease. *Ann Oncol* 1995;6:543–549.

43. Reece D, Barnett M, Shepherd J, et al. High-dose cyclophosphamide, carmustine (BCNU), and etoposide (VP-16-213) with or without cisplatin (CBV +/− P) and autologous transplantation for patients with Hodgkin's disease who fail to enter a complete remission after combination chemotherapy. *Blood* 1995;86:451–458.

44. Brice P, Bastion Y, Divine M, et al. Analysis of prognostic factors after the first relapse of Hodgkin's disease in 187 patients. *Cancer* 1996;78: 1293–1299.

45. Josting A, Franklin J, May M, et al. A new prognostic score based on treatment outcome of patients with relapsed Hodgkin lymphoma registered in the database of the German Hodgkin Lymphoma Study Group (GHSG). *J Clin Oncol* 2002;20:221–230.

46. Canellos G, Young RC, DeVita VD. Combination chemotherapy for advanced Hodgkin's disease in relapse following extensive radiotherapy. *Clin Pharm Ther* 1972;13:750–758.

47. Santoro A, Viviani S, Villarreal C, et al. Salvage chemotherapy in Hodgkin's disease irradiation failures: superiority of doxorubicin-containing regimens over MOPP. *Cancer Treat Rep*1986;70:343–351.

48. Josting A, Katay I, Rueffer U, et al. Favorable outcome of patient with relapsed or refractory Hodgkin's disease treated with high-dose chemotherapy and stem cell rescue at the time of maximal response to conventional salvage therapy (Dexa-BEAM). *Ann Oncol* 1998;9:289–296.

49. Biermann PJU, Bagin RG, Jagannath S, et al. High dose chemotherapy followed by autologous hematopoietic rescue in Hodgkin's disease: long term follow-up in 128 patients. *Ann Oncol* 1993;4:767–773.

50. Reece DE, Connors JM, Spinelli JJ, et al. Intensive therapy with cyclophosphamide, carmustine, etoposide +/− cisplatin, and autologous bone marrow transplantation for Hodgkin's disease in first relapse after combination chemotherapy. *Blood* 1994;83:1193–1100.

51. Armitage JO, Biermann PJ, Vose JM, et al. Autologous bone marrow transplantation for patients with relapsed Hodgkin's disease. *Am J Med* 1991;91: 605–610.

52. Linch D, Winfield D, Goldstone A, et al. Dose intensification with autologous bone marrow transplantation in relapsed and resistant Hodgkin's disease: results of a BNLI randomized trial. *Lancet* 1993;341:1051–1054.

53. Gianni AM, Siena S, Bregni M, et al. High-dose sequential chemoradiotherapy with peripheral blood progenitor cell support for relapsed or refractory Hodgkin's disease—a 6-year update. *Ann Oncol* 1993;4:889–891.

54. Gianni AM, Bregni M, Siena S. Five-year update of the Milan Cancer Institute randomized trial of high-dose sequential (HDS) vs. MACOP-B therapy for diffuse large-cell lymphomas. *Proc ASCO* 1994;13:373(A 1263).

55. Patrone F, Ballestrero A, Ferrando F, et al. Four-step high-dose sequential chemotherapy with double hematopoietic progenitor-cell rescue for metastatic breast cancer. *J Clin Oncol* 1995;13:840–846.

56. Shea T, Mason JR, Storniolo AM, et al. Sequential cycles of high-dose carboplatin administered with recombinant human granulocyte-makrophase colony-stimulating factor and repeated infusions of autologous peripheral-blood progenitor cells: A novel and effective method for delivering multiple courses of dose-intensive therapy. *J Clin Oncol* 1992;10:464–473.

57. Gianni AM, Taella C, Bregni M, et al. High-dose sequential chemo-radio-therapy, a widely applicable regimen, confers survival benefit to patients with high-risk multiple myeloma. *J Clin Oncol* 1994;12:503–509.

58. Caracciolo D, Gavarotti P, Aglietta M, et al. High-dose sequential chemotherapy with blood and marrow cell autograft as salvage treatment in very poor prognosis, relapsed non-Hodgkin's lymphoma. *Bone Marrow Transplant* 1993;12:621–625.

59. Norton L, Simon R. The Norton-Simon hypothesis revisited. *Cancer Treat Rep* 1986;70:163–169.

60. Josting A, Rudolph C, Mapara M, et al. Cologne high-dose sequential chemotherapy in relapsed and refractory Hodgkin lymphoma—results of a large multi-center study of the German Hodgkin Lymphoma Study Group (GHSG). *Ann Oncol* 2005;16:116–123.

61. Anderson JE, Litzow MR, Appelbaum FR, et al. Allogeneic, syngeneic and autologous marrow transplantation for Hodgkin's disease: the 21-year Seattle experience. *J Clin Oncol* 1993;11:2342–2350.

62. Phillips GP, Reece DE, Barnett MJ, et al. Allogeneic marrow transplantation for refractory Hodgkin's disease. *J Clin Oncol* 1989;7:1039–1045.

63. Jones RJ, Piantadosi S, Mann RB, et al. High-dose cytotoxic therapy and bone marrow transplantation for relapsed Hodgkin's disease. *J Clin Oncol* 1990;8:527–537.

64. Milpied N, Fielding AK, Pearce RM, et al. Allogeneic bone marrow transplantation is not better than autologous transplant for patients with relapsed Hodgkin's disease. *J Clin Oncol* 1996;14:1291–1296.

65. Carella AM, Cavaliere M, Beltrami G, et al. Immunosuppressive nonmyeloablative allografting as salvage therapy in advanced Hodgkin's disease. *Haematologica* 2001;86:1121–1123.

66. Sureda A, Robinson S, De Elvira CR, et al. Allogeneic stem cell transplantation significantly reduces transplant related mortality in comparison with conventional allogeneic transplantation in relapsed or refractory Hodgkin's disease: results of the European Group for Blood and Marrow Transplantation. *Blood* 2003;102 (suppl 1):1461.

67. Schmitz N, Sureda A, Robinson S. Allogeneic transplantation of hematopoietic stem cells after nonmyeloablative conditioning for Hodgkin's disease: indications and results. *Semin Oncol* 2004;31:27–32.

68. Devizzi L, Santoro A, Bonfante V, et al. Vinorelbine: an active drug for the management of patients with heavily pretreated Hodgkin's disease. *Ann Oncol* 1994;5:817–820.

69. Santoro A, Bredenfeld H, Devizzi L, et al. Gemcitabine in the treatment of refractory Hodgkin's disease: results of a multicenter phase II study. *J Clin Oncol* 2000;18:2615–2619.

70. Josting A, Rudolph C, Reiser M, et al. Time-intensified dexamethasone/cisplatin/cytarabine: an effective salvage therapy with low toxicity in patients with relapsed and refractory Hodgkin's disease. *Ann Oncol* 2002;13:1628–1635.

71. Martin A, Fernandez-Jimenez, Caballero MD, et al. Long-term follow-up in patients treated with Mini-BEAM as salvage therapy for relapsed or refractory Hodgkin's disease. *Br J Haematol* 2001;113:161–171.

72. Moskowitz CH, Bertino JR, Glassman JR, et al. Ifosfamide, carboplatin and etoposide: a highly effective cytoreduction and peripheral-blood progenitor-cell mobilization regimen for transplant-eligible patients with non-Hodgkin's lymphoma. *J Clin Oncol* 1999;17:3776–3785.

73. Kuruvilla J, Nagy T, Pintilie M, et al. Similar response rates and superior early progression-free survival with gemcitabine, dexamethaxasone, and cisplatin salvage therapy compared with carmustine, etoposde, cytarabine, and melphalan salvage therapy prior to autologous stem cell transplantation for recurrent or refractory Hodgkin lymphoma. *Cancer* 2006;106:353–360.

74. Bartlett N, Niedzwiecki D, Johnson J, et al. A phase V/II study of gemcitabine vinorelbine and liposomal doxorubicin for relapsed Hodgkin's disease: preliminary results of CALGB 59804. *Proc ASCO* 2003;22:141. Abstract 2275.

75. Hartman F, Renner C, Jung W, et al. Anti-CD16/CD30 bispecific antibody treatment for Hodgkin's disease: role of infusion schedule and costimulation with cytokines. *Clin Cancer Res* 2001;7:1873–1881.

76. Leonard JP, Rosenblatt JD, Bartlett NL, et al. Phase II study of SGN-30 (anti-CD30 monoclonal antibody) in patients with refractory or recurrent Hodgkin's disease. *Blood* 2004;104:721a. Abstract 2635.

77. Ansell SM, Byrd JC, Horwitz SM, et al. Phase I/II, open-label, dose-escalating study of MDX-060 administered weekly for 4 weeks in subjects with refractory/relapsed CD30 positive lymphoma. *Blood* 2004;104:721a. Abstract 2636.

78. Su Z, Peluso MW, Raffegerst SH, et al. The generation of LMP2a-specific cytotoxic T lymphocytes for the treatment of patients with Epstein-Barr virus-positive Hodgkin disease. *Eur J Immunol* 2001;31:947–958.

79. Engert A, Diehl V, Schnell R, et al. A phase I study of an anti-CD25 ricin A chain immunotoxin (RFT5-SMPT-dgA) in patients with refractory Hodgkin's lymphoma. *Blood* 1997;15:403–410.

80. Schnell R, Staak O, Borchmann P, et al. A phase I study with an anti-CD30 ricin A-chain immunotoxin (Ki-4.dgA) in patients with refractory CD30 positive Hodgkin's and-Hodgkin's lymphoma. *Clin Canc Res* 2002;8:1779–1786.

CHAPTER 20 ■ ROLE OF HEMATOPOIETIC STEM-CELL TRANSPLANTATION IN HODGKIN LYMPHOMA

JAMES O. ARMITAGE, ANGELO M. CARELLA, NORBERT SCHMITZ, ARMAND KEATING, AND PHILIP J. BIERMAN

Hodgkin lymphoma is not a common illness, but has had a disproportionate impact on our knowledge of the treatment of malignancies. The principles of staging that were developed for Hodgkin's disease have been applied to other, more common, lymphoid malignancies.[1] Hodgkin's disease was one of the first malignancies for which curative, extended-field radiotherapy was widely applied and was one of the first shown to be curable with combination chemotherapy.[2–4] Thus, it is not surprising that high-dose therapy with autologous bone marrow transplantation was tested in Hodgkin lymphoma early in the development of this procedure.[5–7]

Because patients with Hodgkin lymphoma have a high cure rate when standard therapy is used, most of them will never be candidates for bone marrow transplantation. Unfortunately, not all patients can be cured with standard therapy. Some patients with Hodgkin lymphoma fail to attain an initial remission, and approximately 30% of patients with advanced disease who achieve remission with combination chemotherapy relapse.[8–10]

Most patients who are not cured with radiotherapy for localized Hodgkin lymphoma can be salvaged with subsequent combination chemotherapy.[11–14] However, the outlook for patients who do not achieve remission with combination chemotherapy is poor.[15] Patients who relapse after a complete remission induced by combination chemotherapy can occasionally be cured by second-line chemotherapy regimens.[15–17] The chances for a good outcome are higher in patients who relapse after being in remission for longer periods of time,[15,18,19] but most of these patients still succumb to Hodgkin lymphoma or treatment complications such as myelodysplasia or acute myeloid leukemia. A small proportion of patients with localized relapse after a chemotherapy-induced remission can be cured with salvage radiotherapy or combined-modality therapy.[20–23]

It has been known for many years that some patients who relapse after chemotherapy can be cured with high-dose therapy and autologous hematopoietic stem-cell transplantation (Table 20.1).[24–36] In recent years, the techniques have been greatly improved, prognostic factors have been identified, both allogeneic and autologous transplantation have been tested, and the optimal timing for transplantation has been studied in numerous clinical trials. Although still an expensive procedure, more rapid recovery of hematopiesis with blood-derived hematopoietic stem cells, better use of growth factors and antibiotics, and performance partially or completely as an outpatient have reduced the cost of the procedure.

AUTOLOGOUS HEMATOPOIETIC STEM-CELL TRANSPLANTATION IN HODGKIN LYMPHOMA

Stem-Cell Source

Autologous transplantation involves the replacement of hematopoietic stem cells that have been irreversibly injured by high doses of chemotherapy and/or radiotherapy. This can be accomplished either with bone marrow cells obtained by multiple aspirations from the posterior iliac crest under anesthesia or with blood-derived hematopoietic progenitor cells collected by apheresis. In the early reports of autologous transplantation, bone marrow-derived cells were used.[5–7] However, the use of hematopoietic progenitor cells obtained from the peripheral blood has almost replaced the use of bone marrow, and blood-derived cells may be used exclusively in the future.[37,38] The advantages of using blood-derived cells include the avoidance of general anesthesia and more rapid hematopoietic reconstitution.[39–46] In addition, blood-derived cells can be collected in patients whose pelvic marrow has been damaged by previous radiotherapy or in whom bone marrow metastases are known to be present. However, it is not certain that collections of blood progenitor cells contain fewer tumor cells than would be present in bone marrow.

If blood cells are collected at a time when the marrow is being stimulated by hematopoietic growth factors and/or at the time of hematopoietic recovery from chemotherapy, very few apheresis procedures (occasionally only one) are needed to collect an adequate number of cells (i.e., 2×10^6 CD34+ cells/kg recipient weight).[47] However, this may not be the case with patients who have been extensively pretreated with chemotherapy. Occasionally, adequate numbers of cells cannot be collected from such patients, regardless of the techniques used,[48] although AMD3100 can sometimes allow adequate collection in patients who fail other methods of mobilization.[49]

The relative merits of bone marrow-derived and blood-derived cells have been tested in prospective trials.[42–44,50] Although no differences in therapeutic efficacy were generally observed, more rapid hematopoietic recovery was noted in patients receiving blood-derived cells. There appears to be no difference in the frequency of long-term complications, which might be related more to the high-dose regimen employed than to the rescue product. However, one trial, by the European

TABLE 20.1

COMPARISON OF AUTOLOGOUS HEMATOLPOIETIC STEM-CELL TRANSPLANTATION AND "STANDARD" SALVAGE THERAPY

		Patients		Results	
REFERENCE	TYPE OF STUDY	AUTOBMT	STANDARD	RELAPSE	OS
69	Randomized	20	20	3-year EFS favored autoBMT 53% vs. 10% ($p = 0.025$)	NS
70	Randomized	61	56	39-month EFTF favored autoBMT 55% vs. 34% ($p = 0.019$)	NS
71	Case control	60	103	RFS favored autoBMT 62% vs. 32% ($p < 0.01$)	NS
72	Case control	86	258	Not presented	6-year OS favored autoBMT 38% vs. 29% ($p = 0.058$)

Group for Blood and Marrow Transplantation,[45] found a better 4-year progression-free survival rate in patients who received bone marrow (52% versus 38%; $p = 0.008$) despite the fact that patients who received blood-derived stem cells had a more rapid hematopoietic recovery. Because the results of the European Group for Blood and Marrow Transplantation represented a retrospective, matched-case analysis, they cannot be considered definitive. In two subsequent nonrandomized comparisons there was no disadvange to use of peripheral blood-derived cells.[46,51]

Although it is possible to collect hematopoietic stem cells from patients whose bone marrow is involved by Hodgkin lymphoma, results of transplantation in these patients do not appear to be as good as in patients whose bone marrow shows no evidence of disease. In one trial, the 4-year failure-free survival was 27% for patients without a history of bone marrow involvement, but only 11% in patients with bone marrow involvement at the time cells were collected.[52] This might reflect the inadvertent collection of circulating tumor cells or the effects of an adverse prognostic factor—such as bone marrow involvement by Hodgkin lymphoma. However, bone marrow involvement has not always been found to affect prognosis adversely.[53]

Two studies have found the use of autologous peripheral-blood hematopoietic stem cells to be associated with a higher risk of second malignancy including myelodysplasia/acute myeloid leukemia.[54,55] However, this has not been found in a number of other studies of patients with lymphoma.[46,56,57] Although patients treated for Hodgkin lymphoma are at higher risk for myelodysplasia/acute myeloid leukemia after treatment with alkylating-based regimens, extensive radiotherapy, and multiple treatments after repetitive relapses, it is unclear that the stem-cell source contributes to this risk.

High-Dose Regimens

There is no standard high-dose therapy regimen used for autologous hematopoietic stem-cell transplantation in Hodgkin lymphoma. Unfortunately, there are no comparative trials completed to identify the best of the several regimens that are widely used. Most of the high-dose therapy regimens incorporate various combinations of cyclophosphamide,

carmustine, etoposide, cytarabine, and melphalan. In addition, some investigators have used either total body radiotherapy or more focused radiation as part of their regimen. In centers that prefer to use total body radiotherapy, a history of prior thoracic radiation often makes this impractical because of excess pulmonary toxicity.[58] Radiolabeled antibodies have been tested in Hodgkin lymphoma but are not widely used.[29,59] Some of the most popular high-dose therapy regimens are presented in Table 20.1.

There are wide differences in the dosages of the same drugs used in different high-dose therapy regimens for autologous hematopoietic stem-cell transplantation in Hodgkin lymphoma. For example, using the CBV regimen, the dosage of cyclophosphamide has varied from 4.8 to 7.2 g/m^2, the dosage of carmustine from 300 to 800 mg/m^2, and the dosage of etoposide from 750 to 2,400 mg/m^2.[25,26,31,60] In some cases the drugs are administered in single doses and in others they are administered over several days. Very high doses of carmustine have been problematic and associated with a higher rate of pulmonary toxicity.[61–65]

The effectiveness of the high-dose therapy regimens is related to the amount of disease present at the time they are administered. Patients with the best outlook are those with the least disease at the time of transplantation. For example, one series found a 3-year event-free survival (EFS) of 70% of patients who underwent transplantation with minimal disease, in contrast to a 15% 3-year event-free survival in patients with more bulky lymphoma.[34] Other investigators have had similar results.[20,24,29,30] Patients who have minimal disease at the time of transplantation can have excellent results.[24,66]

Role of Irradiation in High-Dose Therapy Regimens

Radiation therapy is an extremely effective agent in the treatment of lymphoma. When employed as a single agent, radiation therapy is curative for many patients with early-stage Hodgkin lymphoma. Patients who are candidates for high-dose therapy and autologous hematopoietic cell transplantation (HCT) generally have systemic disease; however, locoregional disease may often contribute to relapse in these patients.

Several investigators have analyzed sites of failure after high-dose therapy for relapsed Hodgkin lymphoma. A Vancouver group reported that among 56 transplanted patients, progression or failure occurred in previous sites of disease in 16 of the 17 patients who relapsed.[32] A Seattle report on 127 patients demonstrated that 33 of the 49 patients who relapsed failed exclusively in sites of previous disease.[61]

Investigators from Genoa reported on sites of progression in 50 transplanted patients.[33] Eighty-two percent had progression of disease primarily at initial sites of involvement. Results from Stanford in 100 patients showed that 22 of the 32 patients who relapsed after transplantation relapsed in sites involved immediately prior to transplantation, and an additional three patients relapsed in sites that had been remotely involved.[67] In a similar analysis of patients with Hodgkin lymphoma treated with high-dose chemotherapy at the University of Chicago, 38% of 13 patients who relapsed failed exclusively in sites previously involved, 54% failed in both previously involved and new sites, and only 8% failed exclusively in new sites.[68]

In a collaborative study from St. Bartholomew's and Royal London Hospitals, Queen Mary and Westfield College, Smithfield, London, 100 patients underwent autologous transplantation for relapsed or refractory Hodgkin lymphoma.[69] 81% of the 37 patients who relapsed recurred at previous sites of disease.

Because the reason for failure of the transplant procedure is frequently related to recurrence of lymphoma in the initial sites of involvement, it is easy to understand the rationale for inclusion of locoregional radiation therapy for these salvage programs. If radiation therapy is included, parameters to be addressed include timing (pre- or post-transplant), extent of radiation fields, and dose.

The advantages of using radiation therapy as cytoreductive treatment prior to high-dose therapy are that it can effectively reduce the tumor burden before high-dose treatment, and the risk of interruption or delay of the locoregional radiation therapy is minimal. The primary disadvantages include potential delay of the high-dose therapy and the potential overlapping toxicities of the locoregional irradiation and high-dose therapy, including mucositis and pneumonitis.[70] Cytoreductive radiation treatment may include all sites of relapse, the bulky sites of relapse, sites with an incomplete response, or even more extensive treatment, such as TLI.

Given the logical rationale for locoregional irradiation, it is not surprising that most large published series of high-dose therapy for Hodgkin lymphoma have included locoregional irradiation in at least selected patients. However, there has been wide variation in exactly how to employ it. In some series, radiation is given pretransplant,[31,71,72] although in the majority it is given after transplant.[38,66,73–75] The range of intervals from transplant to irradiation varies from 1 to 4 months.

Often, the fields treated include sites of bulky disease (variably defined) at the time of relapse[31,72,73,76–79] or areas of residual disease after high-dose therapy has been administered.[38,74,78–80] Some have included all sites involved at the time of relapse.[75,80] Others include TLI but with a differential dose, depending upon disease status.[71]

The range of radiation doses employed varies substantially in these series, from 18 to 40 Gy. In general, lower doses are employed in situations where initially nonbulky disease is included in the treatment, or if there has been a complete response to high-dose therapy.

The use of locoregional irradiation in high-dose therapy programs has the potential for altering the patterns of failure and perhaps reducing the risk of failure. For example, in the Stanford series of patients who underwent high-dose therapy for relapse of Hodgkin lymphoma, 49 patients with relapsed stage I–III disease who had involved field irradiation as a component of their salvage treatment had 3-year freedom-from-relapse, survival,

and event-free survival rates of 100%, 85%, and 85%, respectively, compared with only 67%, 60%, and 54% for the 13 patients who received high-dose chemotherapy alone.[67] The difference in freedom from relapse was statistically significant ($p = 0.04$).

In a similar analysis of patients with Hodgkin lymphoma reported from the University of Chicago, the 5-year local control in involved sites was 94% among patients who received irradiation as a component of therapy versus 73% when the sites were not irradiated ($p = 0.008$).[68] At the University of Rochester, the EFS for irradiated patients was 44%, compared to only 28% for patients treated with high-dose chemotherapy alone ($p = 0.03$).[75]

Moskowitz and associates[71] at MSKCC reported the use of more extensive cytoreductive radiation therapy for patients with refractory or relapsed Hodgkin lymphoma. Patients were treated with a second-line chemotherapy program. This was followed by high-dose chemotherapy with a combination of VP16 and CY as preparation for autologous transplantation. Prior to high-dose chemotherapy and peripheral stem-cell transplant, patients who had not received previous irradiation were treated with involved-field irradiation to 18 Gy and TLI to 18 Gy (both with twice-daily fractionation). Patients who had prior irradiation were treated with involved-field irradiation, if organ tolerance would not be exceeded, to a dose of 18 to 36 Gy in 5 to 10 days (twice-daily fractionation), depending on the prior doses received by the involved sites. The EFS rate was 68% and the OS rate was 81% for the 56 patients who underwent transplantation. Only 3 (18%) treatment failures occurred in a site that was irradiated during the salvage program.

There is mounting evidence that locoregional irradiation may be a beneficial component of high-dose therapy programs. As noted, many series reported an improvement in outcome in irradiated patients, although none of the trials was randomized and patients were often selected for radiation because of adverse risk factors such as bulk of disease or incomplete response to systemic therapy. The diversity of ways in which irradiation was incorporated into these studies makes interpretation difficult, making this an area ripe for clinical investigation. Recently, the Australasian Leukemia and Lymphoma Group initiated a clinical trial to test the feasibility of pre- or post-transplant radiation therapy for all patients undergoing high-dose salvage therapy for Hodgkin lymphoma and the non-Hodgkin lymphomas.[81]

The most controversial issue in high-dose therapy regimens in Hodgkin lymphoma has been the timing of involved-field radiotherapy for sites of previous bulky disease. Some investigators believe this should be done before transplantation, while others would reserve it until the patient has recovered from the autologous transplant.[70] What is unclear is which is the best approach—trying to avoid transplant-related toxicity by delaying the radiation or trying to increase the efficacy of the high-dose regimen by using concurrent radiation. Patients with bulky disease might benefit from involved-field radiotherapy administered at some point in their treatment.

COMPARISON OF AUTOLOGOUS HEMATOPOIETIC STEM-CELL TRANSPLANTATION WITH "STANDARD" THERAPY (TABLE 20.1)

A number of phase II clinical trials have reported response rates and failure-free survival curves that appear to be superior to the results of standard salvage therapy.[24,28,31,35,36,74,82] However, the history of oncology is replete with examples of phase II clinical trials that appear to represent a great advance but whose results are not confirmed in prospective randomized trials. The first prospective randomized trial comparing high-dose therapy with bone marrow transplantation versus standard-dose salvage chemotherapy was carried out within the British National Lymphoma Investigation. This study compared high-dose therapy with the BEAM regimen and autotransplantation versus lower doses of the same chemotherapeutic agents.[83] The study was stopped early because of an event-free survival advantage for the high-dose therapy arm. Twenty patients received BEAM and 20 patients received the lower-dose regimen. The event-free survival at 3 years significantly favored the high-dose therapy arm (53% versus 10%; $p = 0.025$). However, the overall survival curves were not different. This might in part be explained by the fact that patients failing in the lower-dose regimen became candidates for transplantation. Although this study shows that high-dose therapy with autotransplantation produces a better response rate than lower doses of the same agents, it does not definitively answer the question of which is the best strategy—early or delayed transplantation.

The German Hodgkin Study Group and the Lymphoma Working Party of the European Group for Blood and Marrow Transplantation carried out a randomized trial comparing chemotherapy-sensitive patients with relapsed Hodgkin lymphoma who were treated with BEAM and autologous hematopoietic stem-cell transplantation or two courses of Dexa-BEAM.[84] The Dexa-BEAM regimen contained dexamethasone plus lower doses of the same agents used in the high-dose regimen. Chemotherapy sensitivity was determined by two cycles of dexa-BEAM. One hundred and sixty-one patients between the ages of 16 and 60 years entered the study. Seventeen patients did not meet study criteria and 81% were chemotherapy sensitive (achieved at least a partial remission with the first two courses of dexa-BEAM). Fifty-six of the chemotherapy-sensitive patients were treated with further dexa-BEAM and 61 patients were randomized to autologous hematopoietic stem-cell transplantation. Five patients randomized to transplantation did not undergo the procedure. At a median follow-up of 39 months, freedom from treatment failure was significantly better for patients in the autologous hematopoietic transplantation arm (55%) than for those in the dexa-BEAM arm (34%) ($p = 0.019$). The significant benefit from transplantation was confined to patients with early and late first relapse. Patients in the study with multiple relapses did not have an advantage in failure-free survival with transplantation. The overall survival did not differ between the two treatments. Recently the 7-year follow-up of this study was reported.

An alternative approach to comparing standard-dose therapy with high-dose therapy is to use matched, historical control patients. One such study was carried out at Stanford University.[85] Sixty patients with relapsed or refractory Hodgkin lymphoma were compared with a matched historical control group that received salvage chemotherapy at standard doses. Survival free from progression of Hodgkin lymphoma was significantly better in the patients who received high-dose therapy and transplantation (62% versus 32%; $p < 0.01$). However, as in the randomized trials, the overall survival did not significantly differ (54% versus 47%).

The Societe Francaise de Greffe de Moelle carried out a case-control study of patients who failed to achieve an initial remission with standard chemotherapy for Hodgkin lymphoma.[86] They compared 86 patients who underwent autologous hematopoietic stem-cell transplantation with 258 matched controls. A variety of transplant-preparative regimens were used and as were a variety of second-line chemotherapy regimens. The 5-year event-free and overall survival for patients undergoing transplantation were 25% and 35%, respectively, and the major factor predicting outcome was whether or not the disease had responded to the last treatment. The 6-year overall survival of patients undergoing autologous hematopoietic stem-cell transplantation was 38% in contrast to 29% of the patients who received salvage therapy at traditional doses ($p = 0.058$).

High-dose therapy and autologous hematopoietic stem-cell transplantation has consistently shown a better response rate and better failure-free survival for patients with relapsed or refractory Hodgkin lymphoma when compared to standard chemotherapy regimens. A lack of difference in overall survival might reflect insuffient follow-up to document a survival advantage, the effect of subsequent transplantation in patients in the standard chemotherapy arms of comparative trials, or conceivably the lack of a sufficient long-term benefit to the high-dose therapy. However, most oncologists have concluded that autologous hematopoietic stem-cell transplantation is a superior treatment for patients with relapsed or refractory Hodgkin lymphoma, and it has becomed the standard therapy in much of the world.

DOES HEMATOPOIETIC STEM-CELL TRANSPLANTATION CURE PATIENTS WITH RELAPSED/REFRACTORY HODGKIN LYMPHOMA?

Because autologous hematopoietic stem-cell transplantation has been performed as a treatment for patients with relapsed or refractory Hodgkin lymphoma for more than 20 years, it is now possible to estimate the durability of remissions induced by this treatment approach. It has become clear that all remissions that last for 5 years or more do not correspond to cure and late relapses sometimes occur.[25] However, the majority of patients who have long remissions never relapse. In 1993, Bierman and colleagues reported long-term follow-up in a series of patients treated at MD Anderson Hospital and the University of Nebraska Medical Center.[25] At the time of the publication some patients had been followed for 10 years and the chance to remain alive and in remission in these patients with very advanced disease was 25%. Some of these patients who were treated at the University of Nebraska Medical Center now continue well for more than 20 years.

Lavoie and associates reported the results in the first 100 patients transplanted in Vancouver, British Columbia.[82] The follow-up of the patients alive ranged from 10 years to over 17 years. Fifty-four percent of patients remained alive and 51% had not progressed. The major cause of death in these patients was recurrent Hodgkin lymphoma (32%) and death from a second malignancy (17%). The latest recurrent Hodgkin lymphoma was seen between 7 and 8 years after transplant.

Akpek and co-workers reported the long-term results of patients undergoing autologous hematopoietic stem-cell transplantation and allogeneic hematopoietic stem-cell transplantation at the Johns Hopkins Oncology Center.[87] The probability of event-free survival at 10 years was 26%, with no difference between those with allogeneic or autologous transplantation. The latest relapse observed was at 10 years in a patient who had undergone autologous hematopoietic stem-cell transplantation.

Josting and associates reported the results of salvage therapy for patients with Hodgkin lymphoma and non-Hodgkin lymphoma who were resistant to their initial treatment.[88] For patients with Hodgkin lymphoma who underwent autologous hematopoietic stem-cell transplantation, 53% with primary refractory disease survived more than 5 years and approximately 20% continued free of disease as long as 8 years.

For some patients, autologous hematopoietic stem-cell transplantation provides the opportunity for cure after failing standard-dose chemotherapy. This appears to be true even for patients who were initially refractory to front-line chemotherapy regimens.

PROGNOSTIC FACTORS WITH AUTOLOGOUS HEMATOPOIETIC STEM-CELL TRANSPLANTATION FOR HODGKIN LYMPHOMA

The same factors that predict outcome for the treatment of Hodgkin lymphoma in other settings also predict the outcome following autologous hematopoietic stem-cell transplantation. This is not surprising, because the anticancer effect is from very intensive use of chemotherapeutic agents and/or radiation. However, several investigators have attempted to develop prognostic models to specifically predict the outcome for patients undergoing autologous hematopoietic stem-cell transplantation for Hodgkin lymphoma (Table 20.2).

Czyz and associates reported a multivariate analysis showing that patients not responding to chemotherapy and having three or more previous chemotherapy regimens had poorer event-free survival and overall survival rates than patients with the opposite characteristics.[89] Sureda and co-workers studied 357 patients undergoing autologous hematopoietic stem-cell transplantation at first relapse and found that a high stage at diagnosis, radiotherapy before coming to transplant, a short first complete remission, and not being in complete remission at the time of the transplant, predicted a poor time to treatment failure.[90] Patients transplanted earlier in the study, those with bulky disease at transplant, those with a short first-remission, those not in remission at the time of transplant, and those with more than one site of extranodal disease had a poorer overall survival.

The International Prognostic Factors project developed a seven-factor system used to predict outcome for primary therapy in the treatment of patients with Hodgkin lymphoma.[91] The seven factors predicting treatment outcome were serum albumin below 4 g/dL, hemoglobin below 10.5 g, male gender, age over 45 years, Ann Arbor Stage IV, white blood cell count above 15×10^9/L, and lymphocyte count below 0.6×10^9/L or 8% of the total white blood cell count. Bierman and colleagues performed a review of 379 patients who underwent autologous hematopoietic stem-cell transplantation between 1984 and 1999 and showed that the same characteristics predicted outcome after autologous hematopoietic stem-cell

transplantation.[92] The 10-year event-free survival rate was 38% for patients with 0 or 1 adverse characteristics, 23% for patients with two or three adverse characteristics, and 7% with patients with four or more adverse characteristics.

Hahn and co-workers described a new prognostic model for event-free survival in patients undergoing autologous or allogeneic hematopoietic stem-cell transplantation.[93] They studied 64 patients undergoing autologous and 18 patients allogeneic transplantation. Significant factors identified included chemotherapy-resistant disease, a low performance status, and more than three chemotherapy regimens. Patients with two or three adverse risk factors had a poorer event-free survival rate at 2 years than those with none or one adverse risk factor (58% versus 11%).

Moskowitz and associates studied 65 consecutive patients with primary refractory or relapsed Hodgkin lymphoma with a two-step protocol involving initial cytoreduction with ifosphomide, carboplatinum, and etoposide, and subsequent autologous hematopoietic stem-cell transplantation following fractionated involved-field radiotherapy, cyclophosphamide, etoposide, and either total lymphoid irradiation or carmustine.[71] Fifty-eight percent of all patients continued free of disease at 43 months at the time of their report. They identified three factors before the initiation of the initial cytoreductive therapy that predicted treatment outcome. These included B-symptoms, extranodal disease, and a complete remission duration of less than one year. Eighty-three percent of patients with none or one adverse risk factor survived free of disease in contrast to only 10% of those with all three adverse risk factors. This study was unique in that it identified factors predicting the outcome in patients at the time of relapse rather than at the time immediately preceding transplantation.

TIMING OF AUTOLOGOUS HEMATOPOIETIC STEM-CELL TRANSPLANTATION IN HODGKIN LYMPHOMA (TABLE 20.3)

Primary Therapy

Bone marrow transplantation has been most effective in a variety of other illnesses when it has been incorporated into the primary treatment of high-risk patients. Transplantation can be reserved for patients who have adverse prognostic factors but achieve an initial remission, or incorporated early into the initial therapy. In non-Hodgkin lymphomas, a significant disease-free survival advantage resulted in some studies when high-risk patients underwent transplantation during their initial remission.

Studies of early transplantation in patients with Hodgkin lymphoma are limited. One series from Italy reported the results

TABLE 20.2

PROGNOSTIC FACTORS FOUND TO BE IMPORTANT IN AUTOLOGUS TRANSPLANTATION IN HODGKIN LYMPHOMA

Chemotherapy resistance

≥3 previous chemotherapy regimens

Brief initial remission

Not in remission at time of transplant

Sites of bulky disease

International Prognostic Factors Score

Performance status

B-symptoms

Extranodal disease

TABLE 20.3

STRATEGIES (TIMING) FOR USE OF BONE MARROW TRANSPLANTATION IN PATIENTS WITH HODGKIN LYMPHOMA

As part of the primary therapy

After failure to achieve an initial remission

After first relapse from chemotherapy-induced complete remission

Second remission

No preceding conventional-dose therapy

After multiple relapses/refractory disease

of high-dose chemotherapy and autologous transplantation in patients with high-risk Hodgkin lymphoma who achieved an initial remission with MOPP/ABVD (mechlorethamine, Oncovin, procarbazine, prednisone/Adriamycin, bleomycin, vinblastine, dacarbazine).[94] In this series, 87% of the patients who underwent transplantation remained in complete remission at 3 years. This was in contrast to the findings in 24 similar patients who could not undergo transplantation in remission. In the latter group, only 33% of the patients continued alive in initial remission.

The European Group for Blood and Marrow Transplantation completed a study in conjunction with the German Hodgkin Study Group comparing 56 patients transplanted in first remission with 168 patients having similar risk factors who underwent standard therapy.[95] Survival free from relapse was improved in patients undergoing early transplantation, but overall survival did not differ.

Federico and associates reported 163 patients who achieved a complete or partial remission after four courses of an anthracycline-containing chemotherapy regimen who were randomly assigned to receive autologous hematopoietic stem-cell transplantation or four more courses of the standard chemotherapy regimen.[96] To enter the study, the patients had to have two of the following adverse prognostic factors: high lactic dehydrogenase level, large mediastinal mass, more than one extranodal site, low hematocrit, and inguinal involvement. The chance to achieve a complete remission (92% versus 89%), remain free of disease for 5 years (75% versus 82%), and remain alive at 5 years (88% versus 88%), did not vary by treatment. The authors concluded that patients responding to the initial four courses of standard-dose chemotherapy have an excellent outcome regardless of the subsequent therapy.

At the present time it is unclear that any group of patients who respond to their initial standard-dose chemotherapy regimen for Hodgkin lymphoma benefit from "adjuvant" autologous hematopoietic stem-cell transplantation. This is in contract to those patients who fail to achieve an initial remission and who are discussed in the next section.

Primary Refractory

One of the most adverse prognostic factors in Hodgkin lymphoma is failure to respond to an initial chemotherapy regimen. Two studies have found a 5-year overall survival rate of 8% and 0% in patients who did not achieve an initial remission with MOPP/ABVD or MOPP, respectively.[15,97] This would seem an obvious setting in which to test the utility of high-dose therapy and autotransplantation to improve treatment outcome.

The North American Autologous Blood and Marrow Transplant Registry reported the results in 122 patients with Hodgkin lymphoma transplanted after they did not achieve an initial complete remission with standard-dose therapy.[98] Fifty percent of the patients achieved a complete remission with the autotransplant and 22% of the patients were refractory to high-dose therapy and progressed. The overall survival at 3 years was 50%, and 38% of patients remained continuously free of disease. The presence of systemic symptoms and a poor performance status were the most adverse risk factors.

The European Group for Blood and Marrow Transplantation reported the results of transplantation in 175 patients with primary refractory Hodgkin lymphoma and found the 5-year progression-free survival rate to be 32%.[99] Interestingly, patients with a longer interval from time of diagnosis of Hodgkin lymphoma to transplant did less well.

Bierman and associates described a 22% 3-year progression-free survival rate in 44% of patients with primary refractory Hodgkin lymphoma.[100] A comparison of matched controls who received further standard therapy after failing an intial

chemotherapy regimen with those who underwent transplant was carried out at Stanford University.[85] Event-free survival at 4 years was 52% for transplantation in contrast to 10% using conventional chemotherapy. However, the overall survival rates did not differ significantly.

All patients who do not achieve complete remission promptly with standard-dose therapy for Hodgkin lymphoma are not equivalent. Unless a careful evaluation is performed, residual masses may be interpreted as evidence of treatment failure when in fact they contain no tumor and the patients might actually be cured. It is also true that patients with chemotherapy-responsive, minimal disease are almost certainly different from those with bulky, progressive disease after the initial treatment regimen. However, it is clear that some patients with Hodgkin lymphoma who fail to achieve an initial complete remission with a high-quality combination chemotherapy regimen can be salvaged by autotransplantation. This is probably the clearest indication for this treatment approach.

After Relapse from Remission

Most patients treated with autologous hematopoietic stem-cell transplantation for Hodgkin lymphoma have been those who relapsed from complete remission. Although patients with more extensive therapy have generally done less well, prolonged failure-free survival has been seen in 40% to 60% of patients transplanted at first treatment failure.

There has been some controversy regarding the timing of high-dose therapy and autologous transplantation for patients who relapse from complete remission. Because patients who have remissions lasting longer than one year can sometimes be cured with further standard therapy,[18,19] the appropriateness of transplantation for such patients has been questioned. However, on prolonged follow-up even patients with long initial remission have a poor ultimate outcome with further standard therapy.[15] Several series have reported excellent results in patients with both a brief and a prolonged initial remission.[31,66]

Transplantation appears to be a superior treatment for patients who have a brief or prolonged initial remission. This is supported by the randomized trial from the German Hodgkin Study Group that showed an advantage in failure-free survival for transplantation over standard therapy for both those with prolonged or brief initial remissions.[84] Some investigators have reported extraordinarily good results in patients with long initial remissions. Reece and associates described a 100% 3-year progression-free survival in such patients,[31] and the Societe Francaise de Greffe de Moelle reported a 93% 4-year survival.[101]

Autologous hematopoietic stem-cell transplantation is regarded by most clinicians as the treatment of choice for patients with relapsed Hodgkin lymphoma. Although there would be almost uniform agreement on this treatment choice for patients with brief initial remission, increasing data support the use of autologous hematopoietic stem-cell transplantation as a salvage therapy for all patients with relapsed Hodgkin lymphoma in whom adequate cells can be collected.

TREATMENT FOR PATIENTS FAILING AUTOLOGOUS HEMATOPOIETIC STEM-CELL TRANSPLANTATION FOR HODGKIN LYMPHOMA

Patients who relapse or progress after autologous hematopoietic stem-cell transplantation for Hodgkin lymphoma generally have a poor outcome. Kewalramani and colleagues reported a median survival in such patients of 26 months.[102] However, some patients can respond to further therapy. Patients who are farther from their autologous transplant are more likely to tolerate further treatment. Some patients, particularly those with late relapse, will tolerate standard combination chemotherapy regimens for Hodgkin lymphoma. In others, particularly those with more extensive previous therapy, new agents such as gemcitabine are sometimes effective. A few patients treated with thalidomide and vinblastine had a marked improvement in B-symptoms.[103]

Younger patients with a compatible donor who fail autologous hematopoietic stem-cell transplantation for Hodgkin lymphoma might be candidates for allogeneic transplantation. The use of non-myeloablative allogeneic transplants has expanded the number of patients who might be candidates. One series reported a 50% 2-year survival using this approach.[104]

ALLOGENEIC HEMATOPOIETIC STEM-CELL TRANSPLANTATION IN HODGKIN LYMPHOMA

Allogeneic bone marrow transplants were first successfully performed in the 1960s.[105–107] Although originally used for leukemia, aplastic anemia, and immunodeficiency states, allogeneic hematopoietic stem-cell transplantation has subsequently been used for a variety of cancers including Hodgkin lymphoma and non-Hodgkin lymphoma. The early results with allogeneic hematopoietic stem-cell transplantation in Hodgkin lymphoma were disappointing because of a high treatment-related mortality rate varying form 31% to 61%.[61,108–110] The explanation for the high treatment-related mortality rate seen in these studies is uncertain, but might include previous thoracic radiotherapy, the selection of very-high-risk patients for allogeneic hematopoietic stem-cell transplantation, and immunodeficiency peculiar to Hodgkin lymphoma leading to infectious complications.

Over the last three decades our understanding of the factors involved in the successful allogeneic hematopoietic stem-cell transplantation have expanded considerably. The techniques of HLA typing have improved and have led to the use of unrelated but matched donors—although HLA-matched siblings still remained preferable. Sources of hematopoietic stem cells for allogeneic transplantation can include those collected from multiple bone marrow aspirations, growth factor-stimulated peripheral blood cell collections, and cord blood. The use of low-dose preparative regimens aimed at immunosuppression rather than tumor ablation has decreased the early mortality rate from the procedure.[104] This technique was developed after it became apparent that much of the anticancer effect from allogeneic hematopoietic stem-cell transplantation was related to destruction of the tumor by the allogeneic lymphocytes. This type of allogeneic hematopoietic stem-cell transplantation has been referred to by various names including reduced intensity, allogeneic hematopoietic stem-cell transplantation, non-myeloablative allogeneic hematopoietic stem-cell transplantation, and mini allogeneic hematopoietic stem-cell transplantation. It must be emphasized that the intensity of the preparative regimen used in non-myeloablative allogeneic hematopoietic stem-cell transplants has varied considerably from those that were only immunosuppressive (e.g., fludarabine and very-low-dose total body radiotherapy) to other regimens that approached traditional myeloablative doses of chemotherapeutic agents.

To obtain the maximum benefit from hematopoietic stem-cell transplantation, and to obtain any benefit from non-myeloablative hematopoietic stem-cell transplantation, it is necessary that there is a graft-versus-Hodgkin lymphoma effect. Several papers dealing with the use of non-myeloablative hematopoietic stem-cell transplantation in patients with Hodgkin lymphoma have argued for such an effect.[111–115] Peggs and associates described the results of reduced-intensity allogeneic hematopoietic stem-cell transplantation in 49 patients with multiply relapsed Hodgkin lymphoma treated in the United Kingdom.[113] Thirty-one patients had HLA-matched related donors and 18 had unrelated donors. The conditioning regimen included fludarabine, melphalan, and alemtuzumab. Patients who had less than a complete response or progression at 3 months could receive donor lymphocyte infusion. All patients in this study engrafted and the 4-year progression-free survival rate was 39%. The 4-year overall survival rate was 56%. Sixteen patients received donor lymphocyte infusion at 3 months because of lack of response or progression and 8 of those patients had a complete response to the donor lymphocyte infusion. The nonrelapsed mortality rate at 2 years was 16%.[113]

Anderlini and co-workers reported 40 patients who received reduced-intensity allogeneic hematopoietic stem-cell transplantation and were treated at the MD Anderson Cancer Center in Houston, Texas.[114] Twenty patients had HLA matched sibling donors and 20 patients unrelated donors. All patients had relapsed and 14 were refractory to previous salvage therapy. The conditioning regimen was either fludarabine, cyclophosphamide, and anti-thymocyte globulin; or fludarabine and melphalan. All patients treated with fludarabine and melphalan had complete response, but that was seen only in 69% of the patients treated with the alternate regimen. The 18-month treatment-related mortality rate was 22%. Fourteen of the 40 patients remained in complete remission at a median follow-up time of 13 months. Patients who received the more myelosuppressive preparative regimen including fludarabine and melphalan had the best outcome (73% versus 39% survival at 18 months).

Although there appears to be a lower treatment-related mortality, it is uncertain that reduced-intensity allogeneic hematopoietic stem-cell transplantation is preferable to full-intensity transplants in patients with Hodgkin lymphoma. Gajewski and associates reported 100 patients with relapsed or refractory Hodgkin lymphoma who underwent a traditional, high-intensity allogeneic hematopoietic stem-cell transplantation.[110] Patients received either a chemotherapy regimen (55%) or a total body irradiation-containing regimen (45%). Patients were treated in the 1980s and early 1990s and reported to the International Bone Marrow Transplant Registry.[110] The treatment-related mortality rate was 61% and the 3-year disease-free survival rate was 15%. Cooney and colleagues reported 10 patients who received allogeneic hematopoietic stem-cell transplantation from HLA-matched siblings (5 patients), partially matched siblings (1), or matched unrelated donors (4).[116] The conditioning regimen was BEAM. None of these patients died in the first 100 days, and 8 of the 10 eventually achieved a complete response. Three patients relapsed and received donor lymphocyte infusions. At 12 months after the allograft, 9 of the 10 patients were alive and 7 in complete remission.

The place of allogeneic hematopoietic stem-cell transplantation for patients with Hodgkin lymphoma remains a point for debate. It appears that there is a graft-versus-Hodgkin lymphoma effect that might be used to advantage. However, the long-term effects of acute and chronic graft-versus-host disease including both mortality and potentially serious morbidity represent a reason for caution in recommending this treatment approach. Patients who fail autologous transplantation can sometimes be rescued with allogeneic hematopoietic stem-cell transplantation. Young, poor-risk patients who have HLA-matched sibling donors might be better candidates for allogeneic hematopoietic stem-cell transplantation than for autologous transplantation.

TANDEM AUTOLOGOUS AND ALLOGENEIC TRANSPLANTATION

Autologous transplantation and myeloablative allografting each offer potential roles in the treatment of Hodgkin lymphoma and non-Hodgkin lymphoma, but each modality has its limitation. High-dose therapy (HDT) followed by ASCT has become the standard therapy for relapsed patients in much of the world. Unfortunately, the relapses following HDT/ASCT remain the most important cause of treatment failure.

Allografting has yielded lower relapse rates compared to autografting in both Hodgkin lymphoma and non-Hodgkin lymphoma, likely due to the graft-versus-lymphoma (GvLy) effect. Overall survival rates after allografting, however, may not be improved because of high mortality risk mediated by combined toxicities of conditioning regimens, immunosuppressive drugs, and GVHD.[61,108,117–120]

Reduced-intensity conditioning for transplant (RICT) is a modification of conventional allografting that aims to exploit GvLy effects while reducing conditioning-related toxicity.[121–130] Because GvLy responses might be insufficient when tumors are bulky and tumor growth is rapid, it was thought that intensive cytoreduction prior to allografting may allow GvLy reaction to be exploited.[131] This tactic could provide the benefit of a conventional allograft but with reduction in the typical acute toxicities and associate mortality of myeloablative therapy; moreover, tandem autografting and RICT might improve outcomes over either approach used alone and over conventional allografting.

The Genoa pioneer study reported 10 patients with Hodgkin lymphoma and 5 with non-Hodgkin lymphoma.[131] The median number of preceding chemotherapy regimens was 2 (range, 1–5). Thirteen of the 15 patients were considered to have poor prognoses due to chemotherapy-refractory disease ($n = 6$), relapse ($n = 8$), or bulky disease at autologous transplantation. BEAM conditioning was used for autologous transplantation. RICT was performed a median of 61 days after autologous transplantation. The allogeneic conditioning consisted of fludarabine and cyclophosphamide with short-course of methotrexate and cyclosporine post-grafting for GVHD prophylaxis. All patients received HLA-identical sibling G-CSF-mobilized peripheral-blood stem-cell (G-PBSC) grafts. At the time of RICT, all patients had disease responses after autologous transplantation with 3 patients achieving complete remissions and the other 12 patients having partial remissions. The toxicity after RICT was mild, because patients did not develop mucositis, severe nausea, or severe neutropenia. Of the 3 patients with complete remissions after autologous transplantation, 1 patient remained in complete remission while 2 patients relapsed; of the relapsed patients, 1 patient achieved a sustained complete remission after additional chemotherapy followed by RICT and remains in complete remission, while the other patient achieved a partial remission after RICT. Nine of 12 patients in partial remission after autologous transplant achieved complete remissions after RICT, while 3 patients had progressive disease. Donor lymphocyte infusions were given to 7 patients, in 2 patients for progressive or persistent disease and in 5 patients for mixed chimerism. At the time of the analysis, 10 patients were alive, while 5 patients died either from progressive disease ($n = 2$), progressive disease and GVHD ($n = 1$), chronic GVHD ($n = 1$), or *Aspergillus* infection ($n = 1$). The severity of GVHD appeared tolerable with only 1 patient dying directly from complications of chronic GVHD. The authors concluded that this approach appeared to be safe and effective for patients with advanced lymphoma.

The same procedure was recently published in 23 patients with advanced lymphoma.[132] Fifteen patients had related donors, 5 patients had unrelated donors, and 3 patients had cord-blood donors. Six patients (26%) remain alive. The 100-day TRM was 9% among all patients and was 0% among matched sibling donors. The conclusion was that the tandem transplant is feasible in advanced lymphoma with low early transplant-related mortality.

In summary, auto-allo transplant is feasible in high-risk Hodgkin lymphoma and non-Hodgkin lymphoma. Future objectives should evaluate this approach in less advanced Hodgkin lymphoma.

LATE EFFECTS OF HEMATOPOIETIC STEM-CELL TRANSPLANTATION IN HODGKIN LYMPHOMA

With standard-dose therapy for Hodgkin lymphoma, it has become apparent that a major problem is late toxicity.[10] This frequently takes the form of second malignancies related to the initial therapy, but other organ injuries, manifested as hypothyroidism, coronary artery disease, and pulmonary disease, can also result. It would be expected that similar effects might be seen in patients undergoing bone marrow transplantation for Hodgkin lymphoma. These patients could exhibit adverse affects of the high-dose therapy regimen, and graft-versus-host disease if an allogeneic transplant was performed, in addition to those incurred during their initial, standard-dose treatment.

In one large study of late effects in patients undergoing autotransplantation for Hodgkin lymphoma or non-Hodgkin lymphoma, most patients were fully functional.[133] However, a number of late toxicities were seen. Hypothyroidism was found in 16% of patients. Sexual dysfunction was surprisingly frequent, being reported by approximately one-third of patients. In 24% of the patients, herpes zoster developed after the transplant. Despite these problems, most patients returned to a normal quality of life and 60% to 80% had returned to work by 1 year post-transplant.[134–136]

The most significant complication of transplantation for lymphoma has been the development of myelodysplasia or acute myeloid leukemia.[55,56,137–139] The actuarial frequency of this event in one series was approximately 10% in patients with Hodgkin lymphoma and did not vary by age.[56] A recent study from the European Group for Blood and Marrow Transplantation suggests that the total amount of therapy, rather than the use of transplantation, is the major factor affecting the incidence of secondary leukemia/myelodysplasia.

CONCLUSIONS

Hematopoietic stem-cell transplantation is an effective therapy in patients with relapsed or refractory Hodgkin lymphoma and can cure some patients unlikely to be cured with other treatments. The technique for performing hematopoietic stem-cell transplantation continues to evolve. Today most patients receive cells collected from the peripheral blood. In combination with hematopoietic growth factors, this has led to rapid return of normal blood cells and has made the procedure safer and possible to carry out as an outpatient. The place of allogeneic hematopoietic stem-cell transplantation remains uncertain, but non-myeloablative allogeneic hematopoietic stem-cell transplantation has a lower-treatment related mortality and has demonstrated the existence of a graft-versus-Hodgkin-lymphoma effect.

Autologous bone marrow or peripheral blood transplantation has become a standard therapy for patients with Hodgkin lymphoma who fail conventional chemotherapy regimens. There is wide agreement that patients who fail to achieve a complete remission or who relapse within 1 year of achieving a complete remission should undergo transplantation. The value of early transplantation in patients who have longer initial remissions remains controversial, but it would be recommended by many oncologists. Transplantation is better when performed early, before patients become refractory to standard-dose therapy. The place of transplantation in the primary therapy of high-risk patients remains an area for study.

References

1. Carbone PP, Kaplan HS, Musshoff K, et al. Report of the Committee on Hodgkin's Disease Staging Classification. *Cancer Res* 1971;31:1860–1861.
2. Peters V. A study in survivals in Hodgkin's disease treated radiologically. *Am J Roentgenol* 1950;63:299–311.
3. Kaplan HS. The radical radiotherapy of regionally localized Hodgkin's disease. *Radiology* 1962;78:553–561.
4. DeVita VT, Jr., Serpick AA, Carbone PP. Combination chemotherapy in the treatment of advanced Hodgkin's disease. *Ann Intern Med* 1970;73:881–895.
5. Carella AM, Santini G, Santoro A, et al. Massive chemotherapy with non-frozen autologous bone marrow transplantation in 13 cases of refractory Hodgkin's disease. *Eur J Cancer Clin Oncol* 1985;21:607–613.
6. Philip T, Dumont J, Teillet F, et al. High dose chemotherapy and autologous bone marrow transplantation in refractory Hodgkin's disease. *Br J Cancer* 1986;53:737–742.
7. Jagannath S, Dicke KA, Armitage JO, et al. High-dose cyclophosphamide, carmustine, and etoposide and autologous bone marrow transplantation for relapsed Hodgkin's disease. *Ann Intern Med* 1986;104:163–168.
8. Urba WJ, Longo DL. Hodgkin's disease. *N Engl J Med* 1992;326:678–687.
9. DeVita VT, Jr., Hubbard SM. Hodgkin's disease. *N Engl J Med* 1993;328:560–565.
10. Rosenberg SA. The management of Hodgkin's disease: half a century of change. The Kaplan Memorial Lecture. *Ann Oncol* 1996;7:555–560.
11. DeVita VT Jr., Simon RM, Hubbard SM, et al. Curability of advanced Hodgkin's disease with chemotherapy. Long-term follow-up of MOPP-treated patients at the National Cancer Institute. *Ann Intern Med* 1980;92:587–595.
12. Olver IN, Wolf MM, Cruickshank D, et al. Nitrogen mustard, vincristine, procarbazine, and prednisolone for relapse after radiation in Hodgkin's disease. An analysis of long-term follow-up. *Cancer* 1988;62:233–239.
13. Vinciguerra V, Propert KJ, Coleman M, et al. Alternating cycles of combination chemotherapy for patients with recurrent Hodgkin's disease following radiotherapy. A prospectively randomized study by the Cancer and Leukemia Group B. *J Clin Oncol* 1986;4:838–846.
14. Cooper MR, Pajak TF, Gottlieb AJ, et al. The effects of prior radiation therapy and age on the frequency and duration of complete remission among various four-drug treatments for advanced Hodgkin's disease. *J Clin Oncol* 1984;2:748–755.
15. Longo DL, Duffey PL, Young RC, et al. Conventional-dose salvage combination chemotherapy in patients relapsing with Hodgkin's disease after combination chemotherapy: the low probability for cure. *J Clin Oncol* 1992;10:210–218.
16. Buzaid AC, Lippman SM, Miller TP. Salvage therapy of advanced Hodgkin's disease. Critical appraisal of curative potential. *Am J Med* 1987;83:523–532.
17. Canellos GP. Is there an effective salvage therapy for advanced Hodgkin's disease? *Ann Oncol* 1991;2(suppl 1):1–7.
18. Fisher RI, DeVita VT, Hubbard SM, et al. Prolonged disease-free survival in Hodgkin's disease with MOPP reinduction after first relapse. *Ann Intern Med* 1979;90:761–763.
19. Viviani S, Santoro A, Negretti E, et al. Salvage chemotherapy in Hodgkin's disease. Results in patients relapsing more than twelve months after first complete remission. *Ann Oncol* 1990;1:123–127.
20. Fox KA, Lippman SM, Cassady JR, et al. Radiation therapy salvage of Hodgkin's disease following chemotherapy failure. *J Clin Oncol* 1987;5:38–45.
21. Mauch P, Tarbell N, Skarin A, et al. Wide-field radiation therapy alone or with chemotherapy for Hodgkin's disease in relapse from combination chemotherapy. *J Clin Oncol* 1987;5:544–549.
22. Roach MIII, Kapp DS, Rosenberg SA, et al. Radiotherapy with curative intent: an option in selected patients relapsing after chemotherapy for advanced Hodgkin's disease. *J Clin Oncol* 1987;5:550–555.
23. Brada M, Eeles R, Ashley S, et al. Salvage radiotherapy in recurrent Hodgkin's disease. *Ann Oncol* 1992;3:131–135.
24. Chopra R, McMillan AK, Linch DC, et al. The place of high-dose BEAM therapy and autologous bone marrow transplantation in poor-risk Hodgkin's disease. A single-center eight-year study of 155 patients. *Blood* 1993;81:1137–1145.
25. Bierman PJ, Bagin RG, Jagannath S, et al. High dose chemotherapy followed by autologous hematopoietic rescue in Hodgkin's disease: long-term follow-up in 128 patients. *Ann Oncol* 1993;4:767–773.
26. Horning SJ, Chao NJ, Negrin RS, et al. High-dose therapy and autologous hematopoietic progenitor cell transplantation for recurrent or refractory Hodgkin's disease: analysis of the Stanford University results and prognostic indices. *Blood* 1997;89:801–813.
27. Wheeler C, Eickhoff C, Elias A, et al. High-dose cyclophosphamide, carmustine, and etoposide with autologous transplantation in Hodgkin's disease: a prognostic model for treatment outcomes. *Biol Blood Marrow Transplant* 1997;3:98–106.
28. Nademanee A, O'Donnell MR, Snyder DS, et al. High-dose chemotherapy with or without total body irradiation followed by autologous bone marrow and/or peripheral blood stem cell transplantation for patients with relapsed and refractory Hodgkin's disease: results in 85 patients with analysis of prognostic factors. *Blood* 1995;85:1381–1390.
29. Crump M, Smith AM, Brandwein J, et al. High-dose etoposide and melphalan, and autologous bone marrow transplantation for patients with advanced Hodgkin's disease: importance of disease status at transplant. *J Clin Oncol* 1993;11:704–711.
30. Burns LJ, Daniels KA, McGlave PB, et al. Autologous stem cell transplantation for refractory and relapsed Hodgkin's disease: factors predictive of prolonged survival. *Bone Marrow Transplant* 1995;16:13–18.
31. Reece DE, Connors JM, Spinelli JJ, et al. Intensive therapy with cyclophosphamide, carmustine, etoposide +/- cisplatin, and autologous bone marrow transplantation for Hodgkin's disease in first relapse after combination chemotherapy. *Blood* 1994;83:1193–1199. See comments.
32. Reece DE, Barnett MJ, Connors JM, et al. Intensive chemotherapy with cyclophosphamide, carmustine, and etoposide followed by autologous bone marrow transplantation for relapsed Hodgkin's disease. *J Clin Oncol* 1991;9:1871–1879.
33. Carella AM, Congiu AM, Gaozza E, et al. High-dose chemotherapy with autologous bone marrow transplantation in 50 advanced resistant Hodgkin's disease patients: an Italian study group report. *J Clin Oncol* 1988;6:1411–1416.
34. Rapoport AP, Rowe JM, Kouides PA, et al. One hundred autotransplants for relapsed or refractory Hodgkin's disease and lymphoma: value of pretransplant disease status for predicting outcome. *J Clin Oncol* 1993;11:2351–2361.
35. Yahalom J, Gulati SC, Toia M, et al. Accelerated hyperfractionated total-lymphoid irradiation, high-dose chemotherapy, and autologous bone marrow transplantation for refractory and relapsing patients with Hodgkin's disease. *J Clin Oncol* 1993;11:1062–1070.
36. Lumley MA, Milligan DW, Knechtli CJ, et al. High lactate dehydrogenase level is associated with an adverse outlook in autografting for Hodgkin's disease. *Bone Marrow Transplant* 1996;17:383–388.
37. Johnston LJ, Horning SJ. Autologous hematopoietic cell transplantation in Hodgkin's disease. *Biol Blood Marrow Transplant* 2000;6:289–300.
38. Argiris A, Seropian S, Cooper DL. High-dose BEAM chemotherapy with autologous peripheral blood progenitor-cell transplantation for unselected patients with primary refractory or relapsed Hodgkin's disease. *Ann Oncol* 2000;11:665–672.
39. Brice P, Marolleau J, Pautier P, et al. High dose chemotherapy and autologous stem cell transplantation for advanced lymphomas: comparison of bone marrow versus peripheral blood stem cell (PBSC) in 147 patients. *Br J Haematol* 1994;87:27.
40. Ager S, Scott MA, Mahendra P, et al. Peripheral blood stem cell transplantation after high-dose therapy in patients with malignant lymphoma: a retrospective comparison with autologous bone marrow transplantation. *Bone Marrow Transplant* 1995;16:79–83.
41. Brunvand MW, Bensinger WI, Soll E, et al. High-dose fractionated total-body irradiation, etoposide and cyclophosphamide for treatment of malignant lymphoma: comparison of autologous bone marrow and peripheral blood stem cells. *Bone Marrow Transplant* 1996;18:131–141.
42. Weisdorf D, Daniels KA, Miller WJ, et al. Bone marrow vs. peripheral blood stem cells for autologous lymphoma transplantation: a prospective randomized trial. *Blood* 1993;82:444a.
43. Schmitz N, Linch DC, Dreger P, et al. Randomised trial of filgrastim-mobilised peripheral blood progenitor cell transplantation versus autologous bone-marrow transplantation in lymphoma patients. *Lancet* 1996;347:353–357. See comments. Published erratum appears in *Lancet* 1996;347: 914.
44. Smith TJ, Hillner BE, Schmitz N, et al. Economic analysis of a randomized clinical trial to compare filgrastim-mobilized peripheral-blood progenitor-cell transplantation and autologous bone marrow transplantation in patients with Hodgkin's and non-Hodgkin's lymphoma. *J Clin Oncol* 1997;15:5–10.
45. Majolino I, Pearce R, Taghipour G, et al. Peripheral-blood stem-cell transplantation versus autologous bone marrow transplantation in Hodgkin's and non-Hodgkin's lymphomas: a new matched-pair analysis of the European Group for Blood and Marrow Transplantation Registry Data. Lymphoma Working Party of the European Group for Blood and Marrow Transplantation. *J Clin Oncol* 1997;15:509–517.
46. Sureda A, Arranz R, Iriondo A, et al. Autologous stem-cell transplantation for Hodgkin's disease: results and prognostic factors in 494 patients from the Grupo Espanol de Linfomas/Transplante Autologo de Medula Osea Spanish Cooperative Group. *J Clin Oncol* 2001;19:1395–1404.

47. Pettengell R, Morgenstern GR, Woll PJ, et al. Peripheral blood progenitor cell transplantation in lymphoma and leukemia using a single apheresis. *Blood* 1993;82:3770–3777.

48. Dreger P, Kloss M, Petersen B, et al. Autologous progenitor cell transplantation: prior exposure to stem cell-toxic drugs determines yield and engraftment of peripheral blood progenitor cell but not of bone marrow grafts. *Blood* 1995;86:3970–3978.

49. Flomenberg N, Devine SM, Dipersio JF, et al. The use of AMD3100 plus G-CSF for autologous hematopoietic progenitor cell mobilization is superior to G-CSF alone. *Blood* 2005;106:1867–1874.

50. Beyer J, Schwella N, Zingsem J, et al. Hematopoietic rescue after high-dose chemotherapy using autologous peripheral-blood progenitor cells or bone marrow: a randomized comparison. *J Clin Oncol* 1995;13:1328–1335.

51. Lieskovsky YE, Donaldson SS, Torres MA, et al. High-dose therapy and autologous hematopoietic stem-cell transplantation for recurrent or refractory pediatric Hodgkin's disease: results and prognostic indices. *J Clin Oncol* 2004;22:4532–4540.

52. Bierman P, Vose J, Anderson J, et al. Comparison of autologous bone marrow transplantation (ABMT) with peripheral stem cell transplantation (PSCT) for patients with Hodgkin's disease. *Blood* 1993;10 (suppl 1):445a.

53. Munker R, Hasenclever D, Brosteanu O, et al. Bone marrow involvement in Hodgkin's disease: an analysis of 135 consecutive cases. German Hodgkin's Lymphoma Study Group. *J Clin Oncol* 1995;13:403–409.

54. Andre M, Henry-Amar M, Blaise D, et al. Treatment-related deaths and second cancer risk after autologous stem-cell transplantation for Hodgkin's disease. *Blood* 1998;92:1933–1940.

55. Miller JS, Arthur DC, Litz CE, et al. Myelodysplastic syndrome after autologous bone marrow transplantation: an additional late complication of curative cancer therapy. *Blood* 1994;83:3780–3786.

56. Darrington DL, Vose JM, Anderson JR, et al. Incidence and characterization of secondary myelodysplastic syndrome and acute myelogenous leukemia following high-dose chemoradiotherapy and autologous stem-cell transplantation for lymphoid malignancies. *J Clin Oncol* 1994;12: 2527–2534.

57. Stone RM, Neuberg D, Soiffer R, et al. Myelodysplastic syndrome as a late complication following autologous bone marrow transplantation for non-Hodgkin's lymphoma. *J Clin Oncol* 1994;12:2535–2542.

58. Phillips GL, Reece DE, Barnett MJ, et al. Allogeneic marrow transplantation for refractory Hodgkin's disease. *J Clin Oncol* 1989;7:1039–1045.

59. Press OW, Eary JF, Appelbaum FR, et al. Radiolabeled-antibody therapy of B-cell lymphoma with autologous bone marrow support. *N Engl J Med* 1993;329:1219–1224. See comments.

60. Spitzer G, Dicke KA, Litam J, et al. High-dose combination chemotherapy with autologous bone marrow transplantation in adult solid tumors. *Cancer* 1980;45:3075–3085.

61. Anderson JE, Litzow MR, Appelbaum FR, et al. Allogeneic, syngeneic, and autologous marrow transplantation for Hodgkin's disease: the 21-year Seattle experience. *J Clin Oncol* 1993;11:2342–2350.

62. Wheeler C, Antin JH, Churchill WH, et al. Cyclophosphamide, carmustine, and etoposide with autologous bone marrow transplantation in refractory Hodgkin's disease and non-Hodgkin's lymphoma: a dose-finding study. *J Clin Oncol* 1990;8:648–656.

63. Weaver CH, Appelbaum FR, Petersen FB, et al. High-dose cyclophosphamide, carmustine, and etoposide followed by autologous bone marrow transplantation in patients with lymphoid malignancies who have received dose-limiting radiation therapy. *J Clin Oncol* 1993;11:1329–1335.

64. Ahmed T, Ciavarella D, Feldman E, et al. High-dose, potentially myeloablative chemotherapy and autologous bone marrow transplantation for patients with advanced Hodgkin's disease. *Leukemia* 1989;3:19–22.

65. Schmitz N, Diehl V. Carmustine and the lungs. *Lancet* 1997;349: 1712–1713.

66. Bierman PJ, Anderson JR, Freeman MB, et al. High-dose chemotherapy followed by autologous hematopoietic rescue for Hodgkin's disease patients following first relapse after chemotherapy. *Ann Oncol* 1996;7:151–156.

67. Poen JC, Hoppe RT, Horning SJ. High-dose therapy and autologous bone marrow transplantation for relapsed/refractory Hodgkin's disease: the impact of involved field radiotherapy on patterns of failure and survival. *Int J Radiat Oncol Biol Phys* 1996;36:3–12.

68. Mundt AJ, Sibley G, Williams S, et al. Patterns of failure following high-dose chemotherapy and autologous bone marrow transplantation with involved field radiotherapy for relapsed/refractory Hodgkin's disease. *Int J Radiat Oncol Biol Phys* 1995;33:261–270.

69. Shamash J, Lee SM, Radford JA, et al. Patterns of relapse and subsequent management following high-dose chemotherapy with autologous haematopoietic support in relapsed or refractory Hodgkin's lymphoma: a two centre study. *Ann Oncol* 2000;11:715–719.

70. Tsang RW, Gospodarowicz MK, Sutcliffe SB, et al. Thoracic radiation therapy before autologous bone marrow transplantation in relapsed or refractory Hodgkin's disease. PMH Lymphoma Group, and the Toronto Autologous BMT Group. *Eur J Cancer* 1999;35:73–78.

71. Moskowitz CH, Nimer SD, Zelenetz AD, et al. A 2-step comprehensive high-dose chemoradiotherapy second-line program for relapsed and refractory Hodgkin disease: analysis by intent to treat and development of a prognostic model. *Blood* 2001;97:616–623.

72. Reece DE, Barnett MJ, Shepherd JD, et al. High-dose cyclophosphamide, carmustine (BCNU), and etoposide (VP16-213) with or without cisplatin (CBV +/− P) and autologous transplantation for patients with Hodgkin's disease who fail to enter a complete remission after combination chemotherapy. *Blood* 1995;86:451–456.

73. Rapoport AP, Meisenberg B, Sarkodee-Adoo C, et al. Autotransplantation for advanced lymphoma and Hodgkin's disease followed by post-transplant rituxan/GM-CSF or radiotherapy and consolidation chemotherapy. *Bone Marrow Transplant* 2002;29:303–312.

74. Ferme C, Mounier N, Divine M, et al. Intensive salvage therapy with high-dose chemotherapy for patients with advanced Hodgkin's disease in relapse or failure after initial chemotherapy: results of the Groupe d'Etudes des Lymphomes de l'Adulte H89 Trial. *J Clin Oncol* 2002;20:467–475.

75. Lancet JE, Rapoport AP, Brasacchio R, et al. Autotransplantation for relapsed or refractory Hodgkin's disease: long-term follow-up and analysis of prognostic factors. *Bone Marrow Transplant* 1998;22:265–271.

76. Philip T, Guglielmi C, Hagenbeek A, et al. Autologous bone marrow transplantation as compared with salvage chemotherapy in relapses of chemotherapy-sensitive non-Hodgkin's lymphoma. *N Engl J Med* 1995; 333:1540–1545. See comments.

77. Perry AR, Peniket AJ, Watts MJ, et al. Peripheral blood stem cell versus autologous bone marrow transplantation for Hodgkin's disease: equivalent survival outcome in a single-centre matched-pair analysis. *Br J Haematol* 1999;105:280–287.

78. Cortelazzo S, Rossi A, Bellavita P, et al. Clinical outcome after autologous transplantation in non-Hodgkin's lymphoma patients with high international prognostic index (IPI). *Ann Oncol* 1999;10:427–432.

79. Gianni AM, Bregni M, Siena S, et al. High-dose chemotherapy and autologous bone marrow transplantation compared with MACOP-B in aggressive B-cell lymphoma. *N Engl J Med* 1997;336:1290–1297. See comments.

80. Rapoport AP, Lifton R, Constine LS, et al. Autotransplantation for relapsed or refractory non-Hodgkin's lymphoma (NHL): long-term follow-up and analysis of prognostic factors. *Bone Marrow Transplant* 1997; 19: 883–890.

81. Wirth A, Prince HM, Wolf MM, et al. Optimal timing to reduce morbidity of involved-field radiotherapy (IFRT) with transplantation for lymphomas: a prospective Australasian leukaemia and lymphoma group study. *Ann Oncol* 2002;13(suppl.2):75. Abstract 249.

82. Lavoie JC, Connors JM, Phillips GL, et al. High-dose chemotherapy and autologous stem cell transplantation for primary refractory or relapsed Hodgkin lymphoma: long-term outcome in the first 100 patients treated in Vancouver. *Blood* 2005;106:1473–1478.

83. Linch DC, Winfield D, Goldstone AH, et al. Dose intensification with autologous bone-marrow transplantation in relapsed and resistant Hodgkin's disease: results of a BNLI randomised trial. *Lancet* 1993;341: 1051–1054.

84. Schmitz N, Pfistner B, Sextro M, et al. Aggressive conventional chemotherapy compared with high-dose chemotherapy with autologous haemopoietic stem-cell transplantation for relapsed chemosensitive Hodgkin's disease: a randomised trial. *Lancet* 2002;359:2065–20.

85. Yuen AR, Rosenberg SA, Hoppe RT, et al. Comparison between conventional salvage therapy and high-dose therapy with autografting for recurrent or refractory Hodgkin's disease. *Blood* 1997;89:814–822.

86. Andre M, Henry-Amar M, Pico JL, et al. Comparison of high-dose therapy and autologous stem-cell transplantation with conventional therapy for Hodgkin's disease induction failure: a case-control study. Societe Francaise de Greffe de Moelle. *J Clin Oncol* 1999;17:222–229.

87. Akpek G, Ambinder RF, Piantadosi S, et al. Long-term results of blood and marrow transplantation for Hodgkin's lymphoma. *J Clin Oncol* 2001;19: 4314–4321.

88. Josting A, Reiser M, Rueffer U, et al. Treatment of primary progressive Hodgkin's and aggressive non-Hodgkin's lymphoma: is there a chance for cure? *J Clin Oncol* 2000;18:332–339.

89. Czyz J, Dziadziuszko R, Knopinska-Postuszuy W, et al. Outcome and prognostic factors in advanced Hodgkin's disease treated with high-dose chemotherapy and autologous stem cell transplantation: a study of 341 patients. *Ann Oncol* 2004;15:1222–1230.

90. Sureda A, Constans M, Iriondo A, et al. Prognostic factors affecting long-term outcome after stem cell transplantation in Hodgkin's lymphoma autografted after a first relapse. *Ann Oncol* 2005;16:625–633.

91. Hasenclever D, Diehl V. A prognostic score for advanced Hodgkin's disease. International Prognostic Factors Project on Advanced Hodgkin's Disease. *N Engl J Med* 1998;339:1506–1514. See comments.

92. Bierman PJ, Lynch JC, Bociek RG, et al. The International Prognostic Factors Project score for advanced Hodgkin's disease is useful for predicting outcome of autologous hematopoietic stem cell transplantation. *Ann Oncol* 2002;13:1370–1377.

93. Hahn T, Benekli M, Wong C, et al. A prognostic model for prolonged event-free survival after autologous or allogeneic blood or marrow transplantation for relapsed and refractory Hodgkin's disease. *Bone Marrow Transplant* 2005;35:557–566.

94. Carella AM, Carlier P, Congiu A, et al. Autologous bone marrow transplantation as adjuvant treatment for high-risk Hodgkin's disease in first complete remission after MOPP/ABVD protocol. *Bone Marrow Transplant* 1991;8:99–103.

95. Schmitz N, Hasenclever D, Brosteanu O, et al. Early high-dose therapy to consolidate patients with high-risk Hodgkin's disease in first complete remission? Results of an EBMT/GHSG matched-pair analysis. *Blood* 1995;10(suppl 1):439a.

96. Federico M, Bellei M, Brice P, et al. High-dose therapy and autologous stem-cell transplantation versus conventional therapy for patients with advanced Hodgkin's lymphoma responding to front-line therapy. *J Clin Oncol* 2003;21:2320–2325.

97. Bonfante V, Santoro A, Viviani S, et al. Outcome of patients with Hodgkin's disease failing after primary MOPP- ABVD. *J Clin Oncol* 1997;15:528–534. See comments.

98. Lazarus HM, Rowlings PA, Zhang MJ, et al. Autotransplants for Hodgkin's disease in patients never achieving remission: a report from the Autologous Blood and Marrow Transplant Registry. *J Clin Oncol* 1999;17:534–545.

99. Sweetenham JW, Taghipour G, Linch DC, et al. Thirty percent of adult patients with primary refractory Hodgkin's disease (HD) are progression free at 5 years after high dose therapy (HDT) and autologous stem cell transplantation (ASCT): data from 290 patients reported to the EBMT. *Blood* 1996;88(suppl 1):486a. Abstract 1932.

100. Bierman PJ, Vose JM, Armitage JO. Autologous transplantation for Hodgkin's disease: coming of age? *Blood* 1994;83:1161–1164.

101. Brice P, Bouabdallah R, Moreau P, et al. Prognostic factors for survival after high-dose therapy and autologous stem cell transplantation for patients with relapsing Hodgkin's disease: analysis of 280 patients from the French registry. Societe Francaise de Greffe de Moelle. *Bone Marrow Transplant* 1997;20:21–26.

102. Kewalramani T, Nimer SD, Zelenetz AD, et al. Progressive disease following autologous transplantation in patients with chemosensitive relapsed or primary refractory Hodgkin's disease or aggressive non-Hodgkin's lymphoma. *Bone Marrow Transplant* 2003;32:673–679.

103. Kuruvilla J, Song KW, Mollee P, et al. A phase II study of thalidomide and vinblastine for palliative patients with Hodgkin's lymphoma. *Hematology* 2006;11:25–29.

104. Robinson SP, Goldstone AH, Mackinnon S, et al. Chemoresistant or aggressive lymphoma predicts for a poor outcome following reduced-intensity allogeneic progenitor cell transplantation: an analysis from the Lymphoma Working Party of the European Group for Blood and Bone Marrow Transplantation. *Blood* 2002;100:4310–4316.

105. Gatti RA, Meuwissen HJ, Allen HD, et al. Immunological reconstitution of sex-linked lymphopenic immunological deficiency. *Lancet* 1968;2:1366–1369.

106. Thomas E, Storb R, Clift RA, et al. Bone-marrow transplantation (first of two parts). *N Engl J Med* 1975;292:832–843.

107. Thomas ED, Storb R, Clift RA, et al. Bone-marrow transplantation (second of two parts). *N Engl J Med* 1975;292:895–902.

108. Milpied N, Fielding AK, Pearce RM, et al. Allogeneic bone marrow transplant is not better than autologous transplant for patients with relapsed Hodgkin's disease. European Group for Blood and Bone Marrow Transplantation. *J Clin Oncol* 1996;14:1291–1296.

109. Jones RJ, Piantadosi S, Mann RB, et al. High-dose cytotoxic therapy and bone marrow transplantation for relapsed Hodgkin's disease. *J Clin Oncol* 1990;8:527–537.

110. Gajewski JL, Phillips GL, Sobocinski KA, et al. Bone marrow transplants from HLA-identical siblings in advanced Hodgkin's disease. *J Clin Oncol* 1996;14:572–578.

111. Porter DL, Stadtmauer EA, Lazarus HM. "GVHD": graft-versus-host disease or graft-versus-Hodgkin's disease? An old acronym with new meaning. *Bone Marrow Transplant* 2003;31:739–746.

112. Grigg A, Ritchie D. Graft-versus-lymphoma effects: clinical review, policy proposals, and immunobiology. *Biol Blood Marrow Transplant* 2004;10:579–590.

113. Peggs KS, Hunter A, Chopra R, et al. Clinical evidence of a graft-versus-Hodgkin's-lymphoma effect after reduced-intensity allogeneic transplantation. *Lancet* 2005;365:1934–1941.

114. Anderlini P, Saliba R, Acholonu S, et al. Reduced-intensity allogeneic stem cell transplantation in relapsed and refractory Hodgkin's disease: low transplant-related mortality and impact of intensity of conditioning regimen. *Bone Marrow Transplant* 2005;35:943–951.

115. Sureda A. Non myeloablative stem cell transplantation for relapsed and resistant Hodgkin's lymphoma. *(EHA Educ Program)* 2005;1:186–191.

116. Cooney JP, Stiff PJ, Toor AA, et al. BEAM allogeneic transplantation for patients with Hodgkin's disease who relapse after autologous transplantation is safe and effective. *Biol Blood Marrow Transplant* 2003;9:177–182.

117. Ratanatharathorn V, Uberti J, Karanes C, et al. Prospective comparative trial of autologous versus allogeneic bone marrow transplantation in patients with non-Hodgkin's lymphoma. *Blood* 1994;84:1050–1055.

118. van Besien KW, Khouri IF, Giralt SA, et al. Allogeneic bone marrow transplantation for refractory and recurrent low-grade lymphoma: the case for aggressive management. *J Clin Oncol* 1995;13:1096–1102.

119. van Besien KW, de Lima M, Giralt SA, et al. Management of lymphoma recurrence after allogeneic transplantation: the relevance of graft-versus-lymphoma effect. *Bone Marrow Transplant* 1997;19:977–982.

120. Peniket AJ, Ruiz de Elvira MC, Taghipour G, et al. An EBMT registry matched study of allogeneic stem cell transplants for lymphoma: allogeneic transplantation is associated with a lower relapse rate but a higher procedure-related mortality rate than autologous transplantation. *Bone Marrow Transplant* 2003;31:667–678.

121. Giralt S, Estey E, Albitar M, et al. Engraftment of allogeneic hematopoietic progenitor cells with purine analog-containing chemotherapy: harnessing graft-versus-leukemia without myeloablative therapy. *Blood* 1997;89:4531–4536.

122. Khouri IF, Keating M, Korbling M, et al. Transplant-lite: induction of graft-versus-malignancy using fludarabine- based nonablative chemotherapy and allogeneic blood progenitor-cell transplantation as treatment for lymphoid malignancies. *J Clin Oncol* 1998;16:2817–2824. See comments.

123. Slavin S, Nagler A, Naparstek E, et al. Nonmyeloablative stem cell transplantation and cell therapy as an alternative to conventional bone marrow transplantation with lethal cytoreduction for the treatment of malignant and nonmalignant hematologic diseases. *Blood* 1998;91:756–763.

124. Sykes M, Preffer F, McAfee S, et al. Mixed lymphohaemopoietic chimerism and graft-versus-lymphoma effects after non-myeloablative therapy and HLA-mismatched bone-marrow transplantation. *Lancet* 1999;353:1755–1759.

125. Childs R, Clave E, Contentin N, et al. Engraftment kinetics after non-myeloablative allogeneic peripheral blood stem cell transplantation: full donor T-cell chimerism precedes alloimmune responses. *Blood* 1999;94:3234–3241.

126. Kottaridis PD, Milligan DW, Chopra R, et al. In vivo CAMPATH-1H prevents graft-versus-host disease following nonmyeloablative stem cell transplantation. *Blood* 2000;96:2419–2425.

127. Khouri IF, Saliba RM, Giralt SA, et al. Nonablative allogeneic hematopoietic transplantation as adoptive immunotherapy for indolent lymphoma: low incidence of toxicity, acute graft-versus-host disease, and treatment-related mortality. *Blood* 2001;98:3595–3599.

128. Alessandrino EP, Bernasconi P, Colombo AA, et al. Thiotepa and fludarabine (TT-FLUDA) as conditioning regimen in poor candidates for conventional allogeneic hemopoietic stem cell transplant. *Ann Hematol* 2001;80:521–524.

129. McSweeney PA, Niederwieser D, Shizuru JA, et al. Hematopoietic cell transplantation in older patients with hematologic malignancies: replacing high-dose cytotoxic therapy with graft-versus-tumor effects. *Blood* 2001;97:3390–3400.

130. Miller KB, Roberts TF, Chan G, et al. A novel reduced intensity regimen for allogeneic hematopoietic stem cell transplantation associated with a reduced incidence of graft-versus-host disease. *Bone Marrow Transplant* 2004;33:881–889.

131. Carella AM, Cavaliere M, Lerma E, et al. Autografting followed by nonmyeloablative immunosuppressive chemotherapy and allogeneic peripheral-blood hematopoietic stem-cell transplantation as treatment of resistant Hodgkin's disease and non-Hodgkin's lymphoma. *J Clin Oncol* 2000;18:3918–3924.

132. Gutman JA, Bearman SI, Nieto Y, et al. Autologous transplantation followed closely by reduced-intensity allogeneic transplantation as consolidative immunotherapy in advanced lymphoma patients: a feasibility study. *Bone Marrow Transplant* 2005;36:443–451.

133. Vose JM, Kennedy BC, Bierman PJ, et al. Long-term sequelae of autologous bone marrow or peripheral stem cell transplantation for lymphoid malignancies. *Cancer* 1992;69:784–789.

134. Chao NJ, Tierney DK, Bloom JR, et al. Dynamic assessment of quality of life after autologous bone marrow transplantation. *Blood* 1992;80:825–830.

135. Bush NE, Haberman M, Donaldson G, et al. Quality of life of 125 adults surviving 6–18 years after bone marrow transplantation. *Soc Sci Med* 1995;40:479–490.

136. Molassiotis A, van den Akker OB, Milligan DW, et al. Quality of life in long-term survivors of marrow transplantation: comparison with a matched group receiving maintenance chemotherapy. *Bone Marrow Transplant* 1996;17:249–258.

137. Traweek ST, Slovak ML, Nademanee AP, et al. Clonal karyotypic hematopoietic cell abnormalities occurring after autologous bone marrow transplantation for Hodgkin's disease and non-Hodgkin's lymphoma. *Blood* 1994;84:957–963.

138. Bhatia S, Ramsay NK, Steinbuch M, et al. Malignant neoplasms following bone marrow transplantation. *Blood* 1996;87:3633–3639.

139. Krishnan A, Bhatia S, Slovak ML, et al. Predictors of therapy-related leukemia and myelodysplasia following autologous transplantation for lymphoma: an assessment of risk factors. *Blood* 2000;95:1588–1593.

CHAPTER 21 ■ PEDIATRIC HODGKIN LYMPHOMA

MELISSA M. HUDSON, DIETER KÖRHOLZ, AND SARAH S. DONALDSON

HISTORICAL ASPECTS OF TREATMENT

Although Hodgkin lymphoma presenting in children is similar to the disease in adults in regard to biology and natural history, some of the features unique to Hodgkin lymphoma in childhood are emphasized in this chapter as a means of augmenting the general discussion of the disease. To appreciate the uniqueness of the disease in children, we must address its historical aspects and treatment. Thirty years ago, pediatric and adult patients with Hodgkin's disease were managed in a similar fashion. Radiation therapy was delivered in high doses and to extended volumes. With radiotherapy alone, during the 1960s and early 1970s, a significant number of patients with Hodgkin's disease were cured. Although the prognosis in children was at first believed to be poorer than in adults, children were later shown to do as well as adults[1] but with a higher risk for the development of late consequences of therapy. The development of the four-drug combination of mechlorethamine (nitrogen mustard), Oncovin (vincristine), procarbazine, and prednisone (MOPP) in the 1960s, and the recognition of the adverse effects of high-dose radiation therapy on musculoskeletal development in survivors, provided the cornerstone for the first investigations of combined-modality therapy in pediatric patients with Hodgkin's disease.[2,3] Pediatric trials implemented in the 1970s modified treatment strategies to address the specific problems of children. They were designed to determine whether multiple cycles of chemotherapy could replace a portion of the needed radiation therapy in laparotomy-staged children with Hodgkin's disease.[4–9] These trials served as the model for institutional and cooperative group investigations of low-dose radiation therapy and chemotherapy in the treatment of pediatric Hodgkin lymphoma.

The development of the four-drug ABVD (Adriamycin [doxorubicin], bleomycin, vinblastine, dacarbazine) regimen and the desire to avoid MOPP-associated sequelae of infertility and secondary leukemia resulted in the use of alternating multiagent chemotherapy regimens.[10,11] The ABVD combination does not cause permanent germ cell dysfunction or an increased risk for leukemogenesis, but does produce a dose-related risk of cardiopulmonary dysfunction.[11] The prototype MOPP/ABVD regimen provided enhanced antineoplastic activity, reduced MOPP-related sequelae because of the limited exposure to alkylating agent chemotherapy, and reduced ABVD-related sequelae because of the limited doses of doxorubicin and bleomycin.[12] This and similar trials of alternating multidrug combinations have shown them to be uniformly efficacious and have led to subsequent pediatric trials in which radiation doses have been further reduced to 15 to 25.5 Gy and volumes reduced to involved fields.[13–19] Monitoring of survivors treated with these regimens thus far indicates a significant reduction in life-threatening toxicity (cardiopulmonary sequelae and secondary malignancies), which has been attributed to the reduced exposure to alkylating drugs, doxorubicin, and bleomycin.[14,15,20]

Until the 1980s, newly diagnosed patients with Hodgkin lymphoma underwent surgical staging with laparotomy and splenectomy to determine the presence and extent of subdiaphragmatic involvement because of the dependence on precise radiation therapy for local disease control. Gradually several factors contributed to the replacement of pathologic staging with clinical staging, including the increased use of systemic therapy in pediatric patients, advances in diagnostic imaging technology to accurately evaluate the retroperitoneal lymph nodes, and the recognition of life-threatening sequelae, including overwhelming bacterial infections in asplenic children. Although precise anatomic staging was required for the design of radiation fields when the treatment plan used radiation therapy alone, histologic confirmation of microscopic abdominal disease became less important when systemic therapy began to be used routinely. Currently, surgical staging is limited to specific nodal sampling in cases with equivocal findings by clinical staging.

By the 1990s, treatment goals in pediatric Hodgkin lymphoma evolved to those of reducing toxicity, while at the same time maintaining the excellent disease-free survival rates in clinically staged children and adolescents and improving the outcome for advanced-stage patients, especially those with extranodal disease. Pediatric trials in the early 1990s established that excellent outcomes could be achieved in favorable early-stage patients treated with fewer than six cycles of multiagent combination chemotherapy and lower radiation doses and volumes. Investigators designed studies to evaluate if patients could be cured with even fewer cycles of nontoxic chemotherapy and to determine in which patients radiotherapy might be safely omitted. In the current century, risk-adapted, response-based treatment approaches are under investigation to identify those patient groups with favorable features and response to therapy who may be candidates for therapy reduction. These trials also aim to better characterize patients at increased risk for treatment failure who might benefit from more aggressive or intensive therapy.

EPIDEMIOLOGY AND PATHOLOGY

The age incidence in Hodgkin lymphoma is bimodal. In industrialized countries, including the United States, the first peak occurs in young adults ages 20 to 30, and the second peak occurs in late adulthood.[21] In developing countries, the first peak is seen before adolescence. Among children less than 15 years of age, the relative risk for Hodgkin lymphoma tends to increase with increasing family size, with a sibship relative risk of 1.28 reported in a Danish study summarizing a population-based database from the Danish Civil Registration system.[22] The trend for birth order was 1.26 among Danish children. Among young adults older than 15 years, the risk for Hodgkin lymphoma decreases with increased sibship size and birth order, with significant differences in the two age groups ($p < 0.05$).

There is a slight overall male predominance in the incidence of Hodgkin lymphoma, which is most marked in the very young children. Hodgkin lymphoma is very rare before the age of 5 years. In children less than 10 years old, the incidence is much higher in boys than in girls, whereas among teenagers, the incidence is approximately equal between the sexes. Table 21.1 summarizes the age and sex distribution of children under 15 years of age in five consecutive German-Austrian pediatric Hodgkin lymphoma studies, confirming the marked sex difference as a function of age.[23]

The etiology of Hodgkin lymphoma remains only partially understood. However, some factors seem to increase the risk of its development. The EBV genome has been found in tumor cells of about one-third of the patients (see Chapter 3).[24] EBV infection seems to be more frequently associated with the development of certain subtypes of Hodgkin lymphoma, namely mixed-cellularity and lymphocyte-depleted subtypes, rather than nodular sclerosis.[25] In young adults, a late infection with mononucleosis is associated with an increased risk of developing EBV-positive Hodgkin lymphoma.[26] Late EBV infection in this group is associated with a higher socioeconomic status, whereas in childhood EBV infection and development of Hodgkin lymphoma is associated with a lower socioeconomic class.[27] Testing for EBV within Reed-Sternberg and Hodgkin cells among children with Hodgkin lymphoma from 10 different countries has shown that EBV strain type 1 is predominant in the United Kingdom, South Africa, Australia, and Greece, whereas EBV type 2 is predominant in Egypt.[28,29] However, as many as 21% of cases show evidence of dual infection, supporting the possibility of an underlying immune deficiency in these cases (see Chapter 3).

Other risk factors for the development of Hodgkin lymphoma include previous infections or medical treatment, genetic predisposition, and environmental factors. In patients with acquired immunodeficiency syndrome, the relative risk of Hodgkin lymphoma is increased ten-fold,[30] whereas a congenital immunodeficiency seems to be associated with a two-fold increased risk.[31] A six-fold increased risk of Hodgkin lymphoma development has been found in patients after allogeneic bone marrow transplantation.[32] In a prospective follow-up of monozygotic twin pairs, the relative risk of Hodgkin lymphoma of the unaffected co-twin was 128, whereas in dizygotic twin pairs no increased risk was found.[33] A strong association of HLA-DPB1-0301 with infectious mononucleosis was detected in patients with EBV-positive Hodgkin lymphoma (odds ratio 17.1), but not in patients with EBV-negative Hodgkin lymphoma (odds ratio 1.24).[34] Finally, recent studies suggest that environmental factors such as traffic-related air pollution[35] or sun-induced vitamin D may affect the development of Hodgkin lymphoma as well its response to treatment.[36]

When the Rye modification of the Lukes and Butler classification of Hodgkin's disease is used, one finds differences in histologic subtypes as a function of age in the pediatric population. The lymphocyte-predominant subtype is seen more commonly in children than adults, the mixed-cellularity subtype is more common in children less than 10 years of age at diagnosis, and the nodular-sclerosing variant is most common in adolescents.[23] Table 21.2 shows the histologic subtypes by age for children less than 15 years old in the German-Austrian DAL-HD-90 study. Historically, the lymphocyte-predominant and nodular-sclerosis subtypes were considered the most favorable, whereas mixed cellularity and lymphocyte depleted were considered less favorable. Today, the lymphocyte-depleted subtype is rarely diagnosed in children from developed countries. With effective combined-modality therapy, as used today, differences in prognosis among histologic subtypes are less apparent.

Hodgkin lymphoma in both adults and children has been rarely associated with a synchronous occurrence with NHL. Molecular studies on the single-cell level reveal that Hodgkin and Reed-Sternberg cells are derived by clonal expansion of germinal center B-cells (see Chapter 5). In one patient who developed a follicular lymphoma 2 years after diagnosis of a Hodgkin lymphoma, molecular single-cell analyses showed that both lymphomas originated from a common precursor.[37] However, recent molecular analysis of such cases reveals that although Hodgkin lymphoma and NHL arise from the same precursor, several different mutations might induce differentiation into HL or NHL cells.[38]

On the other hand, lymphocyte-predominant Hodgkin lymphoma, which is seen with increased frequency in children, has been considered to be a biologically distinct entity in which 90% of children present with an early clinical stage (CS I and II) and have an excellent long-term outcome irrespective of therapy.[39] In the Pediatric Oncology Group experience of 26 cases of stage I–III lymphocyte-predominant Hodgkin lymphoma, the event-free survival after 5 years was 86%.[40] Immunologic evidence now suggests that the nodular variant of lymphocyte-predominant Hodgkin lymphoma is of B-cell origin and behaves in an indolent clinical pattern, with a tendency for late recurrence

TABLE 21.1

AGE AND SEX DISTRIBUTION AMONG 1,025 CHILDREN UNDER 15 YEARS OF AGE ENTERED IN FIVE GERMAN-AUSTRIAN DAL-HD STUDIES 1978–1995

	No. patients	Age		
		<5 years	5 – <10 years	10 – <15 years
Total	1,025	82 (8.0%)	298 (29.1%)	645 (62.9%)
Boys	642	69 (10.8%)	226 (35.5%)	347 (54.0%)
Girls	383	13 (3.4%)	72 (18.8%)	298 (77.8%)
Ratio of boys to girls	1.7:1	5.3:1	3.1:1	1.2:1

From Schellong G. Personal communication. Presented at the Symposium on Childhood Hodgkin's Disease, Istanbul, November 13–15, 1996.

TABLE 21.2

HISTOLOGIC SUBTYPES OF HODGKIN LYMPHOMA AS A FUNCTION OF AGE AMONG CHILDREN LESS THAN 15 YEARS OLD ENTERED INTO THE GERMAN-AUSTRIAN DAL-HD-90 STUDY

	Age	
	<10 years	10 to <15 years
Histologic subtype	No. patients (%)	No. patients (%)
Lymphocyte predominant	13 (8.4)	33 (11.9)
Nodular sclerosis	62 (40.2)	201 (72.3)
Mixed cellularity	77 (50.0)	43 (15.5)
Lymphocyte depleted	1 (0.7)	1 (0.4)
Unknown	1 (0.7)	

From Schellong G. Personal communication. Presented at the Symposium on Childhood Hodgkin's Disease, Istanbul, November 13–15, 1996.

(see Chapter 22).[41] Future recommendations for children with this entity will take into account that lymphocyte-predominant Hodgkin lymphoma seems to be a different entity that behaves differently from classical Hodgkin lymphoma. Thus, following the quite promising results of the French group,[42] several cooperative group studies are evaluating a watch-and-wait strategy for patients after complete resection of involved lymph nodes in order to reduce treatment burden and long-term sequelae.

CLINICAL PRESENTATION AND STAGING

The Ann Arbor staging system, which describes anatomic lymph node regions in Hodgkin's disease, was designed to determine clinical and pathologic extent of disease. The system also provided information about patterns of spread and stage-related prognosis. More recently, however, an appreciation of the importance of tumor size and bulk has led investigators to redefine stages into prognostic groups at variable risk of recurrence as low (early-stage/favorable), intermediate, or high (advanced-stage/unfavorable) risk. When one defines advanced-stage/unfavorable as CS III–IVA or B, as well as CS I–II with large mediastinal disease (more than one-third maximal mediastinal diameter), approximately 66% of clinically staged children are found to have advanced-stage/unfavorable disease, and approximately 33% present with early-stage/favorable disease.[43] When using a three-group risk-adapted system, approximately 40% are low risk, 30% are intermediate risk, and 30% are high risk.[44] At one time, precise staging procedures, including staging laparotomy, were essential to determine appropriate treatment, particularly when radiotherapy alone was used for patients with early-stage disease. However, the risk for serious bacterial infections (bacteremia and meningitis) from encapsulated organisms in asplenic children,[45] the need for prolonged administration of prophylactic antibiotics, and the occurrence of postsurgical complications such as intestinal obstruction, were serious issues in the management of children. The current management approach of chemotherapy-radiotherapy treatment programs has removed the need for the precise anatomic localization of small foci of disease provided by laparotomy staging.

However, in the comparison of treatment results, clinically staged patients cannot be compared directly with the older literature reporting studies that used pathologic staging.

Routine clinical staging for children today includes history and physical examination, with attention to lymph node draining areas including the Waldeyer ring (especially in patients with high cervical nodal disease). Useful and important laboratory studies for the staging and management of disease in children include complete blood count with differential, erythrocyte sedimentation rate or C-reactive protein, serum albumin, and tests of renal and hepatic function, including alkaline phosphatase level and serum lactate dehydrogenase (LDH) level. Important radiographic studies include a chest x-ray (posteroanterior and lateral) to measure the dimensions of mediastinal disease; computed tomography (CT) of the neck, chest, abdomen, and pelvis; and bone-marrow biopsy for all but those children with stage I–IIA disease. [18F]2-fluoro-D-2-deoxyglucose positron emission tomography (PET) is rapidly taking the place of gallium-67 scanning in the staging and follow-up of Hodgkin lymphoma. Data prospectively comparing gallium-67 and PET in children are not yet available. In patients whose mediastinal mass has not completely regressed after therapy, persistent PET or gallium avidity may indicate residual disease.[46,47] The lymphangiogram, once considered the most reliable method to detect retroperitoneal lymph node involvement by Hodgkin lymphoma because of its unique ability to display the internal architecture of lymph nodes,[48] is no longer widely used. A radionuclide bone scan with corresponding plain radiographs, and magnetic resonance imaging (MRI) are useful for the child who presents with bone pain or a serum alkaline phosphatase concentration elevated beyond that expected for age. The MRI may also be useful in the assessment of subdiaphragmatic sites, particularly in the evaluation of fat-encased retroperitoneal lymph nodes.[49]

PROGNOSTIC FACTORS

Improvement in treatment outcomes for children with Hodgkin lymphoma has diminished the importance of prognostic factors. Generally, as therapy improves, prognostic factors change, but remain useful for predicting outcome and defining risk groups. Prognostic factors in pediatric Hodgkin lymphoma comprise patient-related (e.g., age, gender) and tumor-related (e.g., pathologic subtype, disease extent) characteristics. Common prognostic factors described at diagnosis in pediatric trials include gender, histologic subtype, stage, disease bulk (peripheral and mediastinal), number of involved nodal regions, extranodal extension and organ involvement, presence of constitutional symptoms, and laboratory parameters including white blood cell count, lymphocyte count, hemoglobin, albumin, and acute phase reactants. Prognostic factors relevant at relapse comprise intensity of initial chemotherapy, treatment with radiation, response to initial therapy, duration of initial remission, response to salvage therapy, disease stage at relapse, disease bulk at relapse, extranodal relapse, and constitutional symptoms at relapse.

Disease stage represents the most important prognostic variable. Patients with advanced-stage disease, especially stage IV, have an inferior outlook compared to patients with early-stage disease.[50–52] Disease burden is also reflected by the bulk of disease, the number of involved nodal regions, and presence of extranodal extension/involvement. Historically, large mediastinal adenopathy predicted a greater risk for disease recurrence when treated with radiation therapy alone, and also in trials using chemotherapy alone.[51–53] However, effective chemotherapy and escalating radiation doses for patients with bulk or residual post-chemotherapy disease removes the significance of bulk, as demonstrated by the results of the German Austrian multicenter trials.[54]

The presence of constitutional symptoms, likely reflecting cytokine secretion, has been correlated with more biologic aggressiveness and confers a worse prognosis.[17,18,51,52,55] Abnormal hematologic and chemical laboratory parameters including anemia, leukocytosis, lymphopenia, hypoalbuminemia, and elevations of erythrocyte sedimentation rate or C-reactive protein have also been linked to prognosis.[52,55] These abnormalities may indirectly relate to disease burden or biologic activity. Histologic subtype has been less relevant in pediatric studies because of the generally excellent treatment outcomes. However, grade 2 nodular-sclerosing histology has conferred poor outcome in some studies.[56] A recent study of children suggests that EBV infection may predict for an inferior outcome in those with advanced-stage disease or nodular sclerosing.[57]

Early reports of the results of treatment for Hodgkin lymphoma suggested that the youngest patients had the worst prognosis.[58] However, in an analysis of more than 2,200 patients with Hodgkin lymphoma treated and followed at Stanford University during the 30 years between 1961 and 1991, a very young age was shown to be a favorable prognostic factor.[59] Patients less than 10 years of age had a significantly improved freedom from relapse and survival in comparison with adolescents 11 to 16 years of age, and a highly significantly improved outcome compared with patients more than 17 years of age.[59] However, the German-Austrian studies have challenged these observations. From 1978 to 1995, 1,181 children throughout Germany and Austria were treated with uniform combined-modality protocols in five consecutive multicenter studies (DAL-HD-78, HD-82, HD-85, HD-87, HD-90).[17] The disease-free survival rates of children less than 10 years of age ($n = 382$), and of those between 10 and less than 16 years of age ($n = 799$), were nearly identical for the groups considered as a whole and according to stage (Fig. 21.1A).[17] However, the survival was significantly worse in children less than 10 years of age because of the higher rate of fatal infectious episodes among splenectomized children (Fig. 21.1B).[17] In the HD-90 study, splenectomy was omitted. A comparative analysis of children less than 10 years old, between 10 and less than 15 years old, and between 15 and less than 18 years old reveals no significant differences in disease-free survival and survival (Fig. 21.2).[17] These differences are best explained by noting that the HD-90 analysis was limited to patients less than 18 years of age and employed uniform therapy, while the Stanford study evaluated age as a prognostic indicator across pediatric and adult age groups during time periods in which treatment recommendations varied. However, prognostic factors seem to disappear in Hodgkin lymphoma if the patients receive effective treatment.[60] Thus, on one hand, most patients with Hodgkin lymphoma can be cured if treatment is sufficiently intensive, but more intensive treatment is associated with a greater risk of severe long-term sequelae. Therefore, the goal of future trials should shift from prognostic factors to response-based adaptation or factors directly reflecting the biologic nature of the tumor cells.

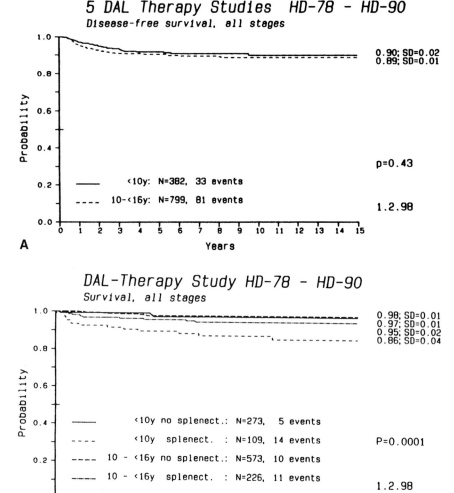

FIGURE 21.1. A: Actuarial disease-free survival by age among children less than 16 years old entered into five consecutive German-Austrian studies. B: Actuarial survival by age and splenectomy among children less than 16 years old entered into five consecutive German-Austrian studies. (From Schellong G, Bramswig JH, Hornig-Franz I. Treatment of children with Hodgkin lymphoma. Results of the German Pediatric Oncology Group. *Ann Oncol* 1992;3:S73, with permission from Harcourt Brace.)

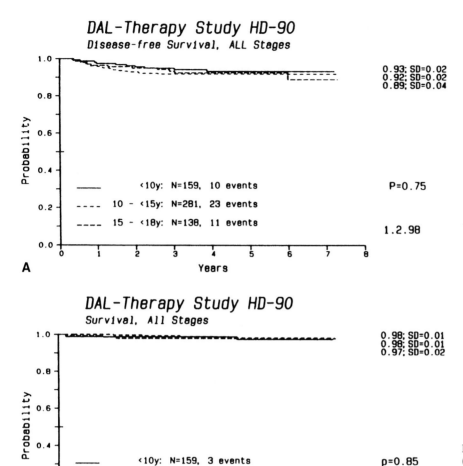

FIGURE 21.2. Actuarial disease-free survival (A) and survival by age group (B) among children less than 18 years old in the German-Austrian DAL-HD-90 study. (From Schellong G, Bramswig JH, Hornig-Franz I. Treatment of children with Hodgkin lymphoma. Results of the German Pediatric Oncology Group. *Ann Oncol* 1992;3:S73, with permission from Harcourt Brace.)

Response to primary therapy is also an important prognostic indicator. In preliminary study results of a randomized controlled trial of risk-adapted combined modality therapy, Nachman and associates[51] did not find a significant survival advantage for patients receiving additional involved-field radiotherapy after complete response to chemotherapy defined by gallium scintigraphy. However, patients randomized to treatment with chemotherapy alone after achieving a complete response to chemotherapy experienced a significantly greater risk of relapse that prompted early closure of the trial. This difference was observed at all treatment strata, but was most marked in patients with advanced and extranodal disease. Dörffel and associates[44] demonstrated that in early-stage Hodgkin lymphoma in children, radiotherapy could be omitted without affecting event-free survival (EFS) when patients were in complete remission defined by cross-sectional imaging. However, in patients with intermediate or advanced stages, EFS rates dropped by about 10% in the group of patients who did not receive radiotherapy. In the future, early response to treatment might become a more reliable tool for treatment stratification, especially when PET is included in the diagnostic program.[61,62] In this regard, Kostakoglu and co-workers[62] demonstrated a significantly better outcome in patients with Hodgkin lymphoma who had a negative PET scan after one cycle of chemotherapy compared to patients with a positive PET scan. As with non-Hodgkin lymphoma (NHL), biologic studies such as gene expression profiling may also help

distinguish molecular subtypes of Hodgkin lymphoma with favorable or poor response to treatment. Devilard and associates[63] found an over-expression of pro-apoptotic genes and down-regulation of tumor-suppressor genes in tumor cells of good responders and up-regulation of genes involved in angiogenesis or cell proliferation in poor responders.

In contrast to newly diagnosed patients with Hodgkin lymphoma, treatment stratification based on response criteria in relapsed patients has not been as well established. For patients treated with high-dose chemotherapy and subsequent autologous hematopoietic cell transplantation, response to salvage treatment appears to be an important factor for treatment stratification. To date, several small cohort studies have reported that a positive PET scan prior to high-dose chemotherapy predicts a poor outcome.[64,65] Other factors have been used for treatment stratification in children with relapsed Hodgkin lymphoma including length of initial remission, primary treatment, and presence of mediastinal or extranodal disease.[66–68]

AGE-RELATED TOXICITY OF TREATMENT

An appreciation of the late effects of the disease and its treatment has become possible with improvements in long-term survival of children and adolescents with Hodgkin lymphoma.

Because children have such a high likelihood of cure, and because they then have many years of life after Hodgkin lymphoma, much attention has been paid to potential late effects among this young age group. However, some of the serious sequelae of treatment are most pronounced in the youngest of patients, in whom growth and development are particularly active when therapy is administered.[69] In addition, cardiac toxicity appears to be age-related, with younger patients at highest risk,[70] and risk continues to evolve as the treated patients age. In this section, we discuss age-related toxicity, which has a significant impact on children and adolescents with Hodgkin lymphoma. The definition of a "pediatric" age group largely depends on treatment-related toxicity. An upper age limit of less than 16 years is appropriate for those with immature skeletal growth. An upper age limit of 18 to 21 years is appropriate when treatment protocols focus on reducing overall therapy and minimizing late organ toxicity. Avoidance of the toxicities mentioned here has become the focus of current protocol therapies. Thus, it is important to realize that current therapy is directed toward avoiding the toxicities observed after treatment programs given several decades ago.

Infertility

Both chemotherapy and radiotherapy can cause testicular and ovarian dysfunction by disrupting the production of testicular and ovarian hormones and damaging the germ cells.[71-80] Exposure of radiation to the testes or ovaries may affect gonadal function by direct or scattered gonadal radiation.[79,81] In addition, testicular and ovarian function can be damaged from exposure to the drugs mechlorethamine, procarbazine, chlorambucil, and cyclophosphamide, all frequently used in the treatment of Hodgkin lymphoma.[72,77,82] Testicular dysfunction has been studied in boys receiving chemotherapy with or without pelvic irradiation for Hodgkin lymphoma.[71,72,74,76,77,83] Cytotoxic drugs, especially the alkylating agents, have been incriminated in the damage to the male gonadal tissue. A complete germinal aplasia occurs following MOPP chemotherapy with azoospermia in at least 80% to 90% of males receiving six to eight cycles of MOPP chemotherapy.[71,78,82] Recovery of spermatogenesis is rare, but has been reported in boys 10 to 15 years after documented azoospermia following six cycles of MOPP,[77] and in adult males following two to three cycles of MOPP chemotherapy.[84] The ChlVPP regimen (chlorambucil, vinblastine, procarbazine, and prednisolone) was developed in an attempt to reduce this chemotherapy-related toxicity; however, testicular function is also severely impaired with this therapy with azoospermia reported in 80% to 90% of males.[73,76] Thus, the ChlVPP and MOPP regimens have similar detrimental effects on germinal epithelial function.

A dose-related incidence of testicular dysfunction is also seen in boys treated with OPPA or OPPA/COPP chemotherapy (Oncovin [vincristine], prednisone, procarbazine, Adriamycin [doxorubicin], cyclophosphamide) with increased FSH levels following 2 cycles of OPPA, 2 OPPA/2 COPP, and 2 OPPA/4–6 COPP at a frequency of 28.9%, 45.5%, and 62.5%, respectively.[72] Pubertal development and testosterone levels are normal, although elevated basal and stimulated luteinizing hormone levels in 24% and 87.8% of boys indicate subclinical Leydig cell damage. It is unknown if this Leydig cell failure resulting in low testosterone values will be permanent.

Testicular function was studied in boys treated with OPA/COMP chemotherapy (Oncovin [vincristine], prednisone, Adriamycin [doxorubicin], cyclophosphamide, methotrexate).[85] Procarbazine, a major gonadotoxic agent, was omitted from OPPA in the German-Austrian HD-85 protocol and replaced by methotrexate in COMP, yielding normal gonadal function in

16 patients treated with two cycles of OPA and in 9 patients treated with two cycles of OPA and two or four cycles of COMP chemotherapy. These data suggest that the dose-dependent testicular damage observed in the OPPA/COPP study resulted from the gonadotoxic agent procarbazine.[85]

Anthracycline-based therapeutic regimens such as ABVD are associated with a lower incidence of testicular damage, with documented azoospermia in only 36% of males treated with ABVD.[71,78] The azoospermia is transitory, and full recovery of spermatogenesis is expected following therapy. Similar results were reported in a study with VEEP chemotherapy (vincristine, epirubicin, etoposide, and prednisolone) where sperm counts were normal in 23 of 25 adult males (93%), and two additional men fathered children 2 and 14 months after the final cycle of VEEP.[86] The German investigators reported normal testicular function in 27 boys with stage I–IIA Hodgkin lymphoma treated with two courses of OEPA (Oncovin [vincristine], etoposide, prednisone, and Adriamycin [doxorubicin]).[83] However, basal FSH levels were outside normal range when the boys received two cycles of OEPA in combination with two or four cycles of COPP (37.5% and 36.4%, respectively). Thus, the combination containing cyclophosphamide and procarbazine is highly gonadotoxic. This toxicity is thought to be a consequence of the effects of procarbazine, although an additional effect of etoposide and cyclophosphamide could not be excluded. Notably, testicular function appears to be retained among adult men with Hodgkin lymphoma treated with the Stanford V protocol (doxorubicin, vinblastine, mechlorethamine, vincristine, bleomycin, etoposide, and prednisone). Thirty-four adult men have fathered normal children following 8 to 12 weeks of Stanford V chemotherapy.[87] Aggressive testicular shielding should be used when administering pelvic irradiation, although this is technically difficult in prepubertal boys. With adequate testicular shielding, high-dose pelvic radiation may be associated with a transient oligospermia or azoospermia but with recovery of function.[88] Although germinal epithelial dysfunction is much more frequently observed than Leydig cell failure, careful long-term evaluation is important so that testosterone replacement therapy can be initiated if Leydig cell failure is documented. Because many male survivors of childhood Hodgkin lymphoma will be infertile after presently available chemotherapy regimens, alternative treatment strategies should be developed to reduce the unacceptably high rates of azoospermia. In addition, cryopreservation of semen should be considered for adolescent boys who face the risk of sterility.[89]

In female patients, the gonadal toxicity of chemotherapy used in the treatment of Hodgkin lymphoma is age-dependent and affects young girls to a lesser extent than adult women receiving similar treatment.[73,75,76,80] Fertility is usually not permanently impaired in prepubertal and pubertal girls treated with chemotherapy alone; those treated prior to the age of 20 to 30 have a high likelihood of retaining or resuming regular ovarian function after a short period of amenorrhea.[75-77,79] In an individual patient with primary or secondary ovarian failure, hormonal replacement therapy is recommended to allow normal pubertal and sexual development and to prevent osteoporosis. Of note, young women who have received alkylator-based chemotherapy such as MOPP, despite return of normal menstrual function, may experience an earlier-than-expected menopause.

Females with Hodgkin lymphoma receiving pelvic nodal irradiation may experience ovarian dysfunction. Direct ovarian radiation in doses of 20 to 35 Gy cause ovarian failure. However, radiation to fields excluding the pelvic lymph nodes does not alter normal menstrual function or cause premature menopause.[90] Oophoropexy can be performed to reduce the dose delivered to the ovaries and preserve fertility. Normal offspring have been produced in women after midline oophoropexy.[91,92] Oophoropexy can be successfully achieved by laparoscopic surgery. Several studies documenting the outcome of pregnancies among cancer survivors, including those previously treated for Hodgkin lymphoma, show no increase in congenital abnormalities in the offspring.[77,92,93]

Thyroid Dysfunction

Thyroid sequelae including hypothyroidism, hyperthyroidism, and benign and malignant thyroid nodules may be seen following treatment among long-term survivors of Hodgkin lymphoma. The multi-institutional retrospective Childhood Cancer Survivor Study (CCSS) reported thyroid abnormalities in 34% of 1,791 5-year survivors of childhood Hodgkin lymphoma treated between 1970 and 1986.[94] Table 21.3 shows the incidence of thyroid abnormalities when compared with sibling controls. Hypothyroidism, defined as chemical or compensated, presents as an elevation of thyroid-stimulating hormone (TSH) in the presence of a normal thyroxine (T4) level. Risk factors for hypothyroidism include a young age at the time of treatment and a high radiation dose to the thyroid gland. Stanford investigators noted while only 17% of children receiving a radiation dose below 26 Gy developed thyroid abnormalities, 78% of those receiving 26 Gy or greater did so.[95] The CCSS observed a dose-related risk for an underactive thyroid with children receiving more than 45 Gy showing a relative risk (RR) of 10.7 (95% CI, 4.7–30.6), those receiving 35 to 44.9 Gy having a RR of 5.5 (CI 2.5–15.3), and those receiving less than 35 Gy with an RR of 3.8 (CI 1.7–10.8). Additional risk factors for an underactive thyroid included time since diagnosis of Hodgkin lymphoma (RR 2.1 [CI 1.7–2.6]); female gender (RR 1.7 [CI 1.4–2.1]); and age at diagnosis above 15 years (RR 1.5 [CI 1.2–1.9]).[94]

Thyroid nodules appear late in the follow-up, with a mean of 14 years. Females have an RR of 4.0 (CI 2.5–6.7) of developing a thyroid nodule. Of all thyroid nodules, fewer than 10% represent thyroid cancer, representing an RR of 18.3 (CI 11.4–27.6) compared to SEER data. Approximately 75% exhibit papillary histology whereas 25% are follicular cancers.[94] Palpable thyroid nodules should be biopsied and monitored periodically by ultrasound.[96]

Follow-up surveillance with annual TSH and T4 levels are recommended for all children undergoing neck irradiation. TSH

elevation signals impending gland failure and may be a carcinogenic stimulus; thus thyroid hormone replacement therapy is recommended. Periodic withdrawal of hormone therapy in asymptomatic patients permits assessment of gland recovery, because as many as 36% of children with biochemically compensated hypothyroidism (elevated TSH in presence of normal free T4) show spontaneous improvement.[95]

Growth, Height, and Musculoskeletal Effects

Information available concerning the effects of treatment on growth patterns and ultimate adult height among children with Hodgkin lymphoma reveal that chronologic age and growth potential at the time of treatment; technical factors including radiation dose, beam energy, and homogeneity; and treatment volume influence musculoskeletal growth and development.[97,98] High doses of radiation delivered to the axial skeleton can cause disproportionate growth.[99] The changes are most marked for children receiving radiation doses in excess of 35 Gy, before the age of 6 years, or during the pubertal growth spurt. Adult height has been measured in 124 children treated for Hodgkin lymphoma with high or low doses of radiation.[98] The relative loss of height based on pretreatment height measurements was 7.7% or 13 cm, when radiation doses greater than 33 Gy were administered to the entire spine to prepubertal children (Fig. 21.3). No disproportionate height was noted comparing standing height with sitting height. A smaller and clinically insignificant impairment of growth was seen in pubertal and postpubertal patients given high-dose, large-volume treatment, and no clinically significant impairment was noted in children receiving lower doses of radiation.[97,98] Thus, current treatment using radiation in doses of 25 Gy or less is recommended to avoid clinically significant growth retardation.

Other side effects of radiation therapy that are difficult to measure quantitatively are narrowing of the thoracic apex, intraclavicular narrowing with symmetric shortening of the clavicles, and atrophy of the soft tissues of the neck. These changes are commonly observed in patients treated many years ago with radiation doses and techniques considered standard at that time. They are particularly prominent in young patients treated with high-dose and large-volume irradiation (Fig. 21.4). More subtle changes in clavicular growth may develop in children treated with contemporary low-dose,

TABLE 21.3

INCIDENCE OF THYROID ABNORMALITIES IN 5-YEAR SURVIVORS OF HODGKIN LYMPHOMA IN CHILDHOOD

Abnormality	% of total	Rate/1000 person-years	Relative risk (95% CI)
Hypothyroidism	28	9.6	17.1 (12.5–24.2)
≥45 Gy			10.7 (4.7–30.6)
35–44.9 Gy			5.5 (4.7–15.3)
<35 Gy			3.8 (1.7–10.8)
Hyperthyroidism	5	1.6	8.0 (4.6–15.1)
≥35 Gy			2.2 (1.2–4.7)
Thyroid nodules	9	2.9	27.0 (13.6–63.9)
≥25 Gy			2.9 (1.4–6.9)

Adapted from Sklar C, Whitton J, Mertens A, et al. Abnormalities of the thyroid in survivors of Hodgkin's disease: data from the Childhood Cancer Survivor Study. *J Clin Endocrinol Metab* 2000;85:3227–3232, with permission.

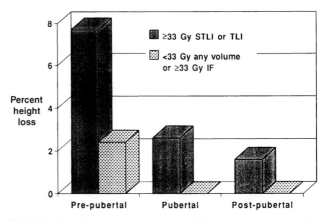

FIGURE 21.3. Height impairment in children from Stanford with Hodgkin lymphoma as a function of pubertal status at the time of treatment and the intensity of treatment administered. (From Willman KY, Cox SR, Donaldson SS. Radiation induced height impairment in pediatric Hodgkin lymphoma. *Int J Radiat Oncol Biol Phys* 1993;28:85, with permission from Elsevier Science.)

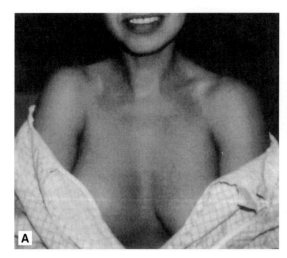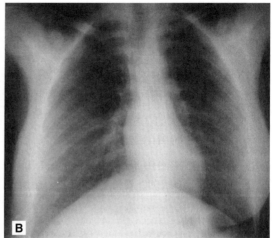

FIGURE 21.4. Clinical (**A**) and radiographic (**B**) 25-year follow-up demonstrating narrowing of the thoracic apex, symmetric shortening of the clavicles, and atrophy of the neck tissues in a woman treated with 40 Gy of total-lymphoid irradiation at age 5. (From Donaldson SS. Effects of irradiation on skeletal growth and development. In: Green DM, D'Angio GJ, eds. *Late effects of treatment for childhood cancer*. New York: Wiley-Liss; 1992: 63, with permission of Wiley-Liss.)

involved-field radiation.[100] Rare late musculoskeletal sequelae include retroperitoneal fibrosis and brachial plexopathy.[101,102] Avascular necrosis is another complication of corticosteroid therapy, although high-dose radiation may also be a contributing factor.[103,104] The current treatment regimens with lower doses and smaller volumes of radiation are designed to lessen and/or eliminate altogether the marked changes seen in young patients treated in the past with high-dose radiation.

Cardiovascular Sequelae

Both radiation therapy and chemotherapy used in the treatment of Hodgkin lymphoma may have toxic effects on the heart and blood vessels, although symptomatic sequelae are uncommon (Table 21.4; see also Chapter 25). External-beam irradiation may affect any of the cardiovascular tissues with the frequency of radiation-related injury related to the total and fractional doses, volume, and specific region of the heart treated, and the relative weighting of the radiation portals.[105] Higher rates of pericardial and coronary artery disease have been observed in patients irradiated by techniques considered unacceptable by contemporary radiation oncologists. Clinically apparent cardiac disease occurs infrequently in survivors of Hodgkin lymphoma treated during childhood or adolescence with modern radiation therapy techniques.[106–108] However, abnormalities of screening echocardiograms observed in some pediatric cohorts emphasize the importance of longitudinal follow-up to determine the incidence of clinically significant pericardial disease and myocardial dysfunction as this group ages.[106,108–110]

The clinical manifestations of radiation-related cardiovascular injury include pericarditis, cardiomyopathy, coronary artery disease with myocardial infarction, conduction system disease, valvular disease, and peripheral vascular disease. Pericardial injury from radiation may present as acute pericarditis during mediastinal radiation, delayed acute pericarditis, chronic pericardial effusions, or chronic constrictive pericarditis.[105] Survivors of Hodgkin lymphoma treated with mediastinal radiation therapy in childhood are also at risk for premature coronary artery disease and acute myocardial infarction.[111–113] Younger age at diagnosis, higher radiation dose, and traditional coronary artery risk factors increase the

risk.[105,114] The potential contribution of chemotherapy to radiation-related cardiac injury is not well established, as combined-modality treatment plans now prescribe lower doses and volumes of mediastinal radiation and protective cardiac shielding. Finally, radiation injury to the cardiovascular microcirculation has been implicated in other sequelae involving the myocardium, conducting system, valves, and peripheral blood vessels that have not been well studied in pediatric cohorts.

Cardiac dysfunction in survivors of Hodgkin lymphoma treated with chemotherapy is most commonly related to anthracycline chemotherapy, particularly with doxorubicin.[115] Clinical manifestations of cardiac injury observed after doxorubicin therapy range from minor rhythm disturbances to

TABLE 21.4

CARDIOPULMONARY COMPLICATIONS AFTER TREATMENT FOR HODGKIN LYMPHOMA

Cardiovascular sequelae
Cardiomyopathy with congestive heart failure
Acute pericarditis
Pericardial effusion
Chronic constrictive pericarditis
Coronary artery disease with myocardial infarction
Conducting system abnormalities (e.g., complete heart or bundle branch block, ventricular arrhythmia)
Valvular dysfunction
Peripheral vascular disease
Pulmonary sequelae
Radiation pneumonitis
Pulmonary fibrosis
Spontaneous pneumothorax
Veno-occlusive disease

life-threatening congestive heart failure. Acute toxicities observed during doxorubicin infusions are relatively common and include sinus and supraventricular tachycardias and premature ventricular complexes. More serious arrhythmias uncommonly occur, including complete heart block, ventricular tachycardia, and sudden death, which have no relationship to the development of chronic cardiomyopathy. Late-onset anthracycline-induced cardiomyopathy may present as congestive heart failure, conduction abnormalities, and ventricular dysrhythmia.[106,116] Chronic toxic effects of anthracycline are manifested as a rapidly progressive biventricular congestive heart failure that is associated with a 50% to 60% early mortality rate. Factors reported to precipitate late cardiac decompensation are childbirth,[117,118] viral infections,[119] isometric exercise,[116] and alcohol and cocaine ingestion.[116]

Several clinical parameters have been associated with an increased risk for doxorubicin-induced cardiomyopathy. The incidence of congestive heart failure begins to increase logarithmically when cumulative doses of doxorubicin exceed 550 mg/m^2.[120] Children show a high frequency of abnormalities of afterload and contractility at lower cumulative doses of anthracyclines in follow-up of long-term survivors.[121] Concomitant treatment exposures (e.g., mediastinal radiation therapy and other chemotherapeutic agents, including cyclophosphamide, ifosfamide, actinomycin D, mitomycin C, and dacarbazine) may intensify the cardiotoxic effects of anthracyclines and lower the threshold cumulative dose to approximately 350 to 400 mg/m^2.[115]

Other chemotherapeutic agents implicated in the development of cardiovascular complications in patients with Hodgkin lymphoma include the vinca alkaloids and alkylating agents. Raynaud syndrome is an uncommon toxicity caused by irreversible microvascular injury in patients treated with the combination of vinblastine and bleomycin.[122] Rarely, myocardial infarctions in patients with Hodgkin's disease have been attributed to vinca alkaloid therapy. Proposed mechanisms for this complication include ischemia resulting from coronary artery spasm or hypercoagulability. Adverse effects of cyclophosphamide on the myocardium are observed primarily when high cumulative doses are administered in the setting of high-dose preparatory regimens for hematopoietic cell transplantation in adults.[123,124] There are no studies of cyclophosphamide-related cardiac sequelae unique to the pediatric population, and so age-related toxicity remains unclear. Conventional doses of cyclophosphamide are generally well tolerated but may exacerbate anthracycline- or radiation-induced cardiac injury.

Pulmonary Sequelae

Several acute and chronic pulmonary complications have been reported following therapy for Hodgkin lymphoma, including radiation pneumonitis, pulmonary fibrosis, spontaneous pneumothorax, and veno-occlusive disease of the lung, although symptomatic sequelae are uncommon among pediatric patients (Table 21.4; see also Chapter 26). Many early studies describing pulmonary sequelae after Hodgkin therapy reflect toxicity caused by treatment practices that have been significantly modified as a result of greater appreciation of late effects and advances in radiation technology. Recent studies of pediatric patients with Hodgkin lymphoma indicate a significant incidence of asymptomatic pulmonary dysfunction after treatment with combined-modality regimens that include radiation therapy and ABVD.[14,15,125] Sequential evaluations after completion of therapy show improvement in pulmonary function in some pediatric cohorts.[126] However, the impact of residual subclinical pulmonary injury remains to be determined as this population ages.

Radiation pneumonitis and pulmonary fibrosis are the most frequent pulmonary complications observed following mantle irradiation. The degree of pulmonary injury from irradiation is related to the total radiation dose, daily fraction size, and treatment volume.[127,128] Mediastinal radiation therapy unavoidably results in irradiation of nearby pulmonary tissues, which can be substantial if extensive nodal involvement is present. Signs and symptoms of radiation pneumonitis develop in up to 20% of patients who receive mantle irradiation. The majority of these patients are asymptomatic, and only 25% require treatment. The use of lung blocks and the administration of chemotherapy in patients with bulky mediastinal disease have reduced the incidence of symptomatic pulmonary dysfunction to less than 5%. Minor restrictive ventilatory defects (reduction in vital capacity and total lung compliance) observed after mediastinal irradiation are increased in patients treated with combined-modality regimens that include ABVD chemotherapy.[126]

Less commonly reported complications after Hodgkin lymphoma include spontaneous pneumothorax and pulmonary veno-occlusive disease. An increased frequency of spontaneous pneumothorax has been observed in patients receiving standard-dose mantle irradiation for Hodgkin lymphoma.[129,130] This complication tends to recur and is seen most commonly in patients with radiographic evidence of pulmonary fibrosis. Reexpansion is often spontaneous, but occasionally tube thoracostomy or rarely pleurectomy is necessary. Pulmonary veno-occlusive disease has been rarely reported in patients with Hodgkin lymphoma.[131]

Second Malignant Tumors

The development of a second malignancy is a serious late treatment complication that occurs among survivors of Hodgkin lymphoma (see Chapter 24). The risk for this complication is multifactorial with potential contributions by hormonal, genetic, behavioral, and treatment factors. Knowledge of tumor suppressor genes such as Rb and p53 and of molecular genetic factors has greatly augmented our understanding of carcinogenesis. However, among survivors of Hodgkin lymphoma, the associations with prior treatment have been given more attention than have the genetic influences that predispose to a second malignancy. In addition, Hodgkin lymphoma is known to be accompanied by defective cellular immunity, which may leave a patient at risk for the development of other malignancies. Finally, in assessing the severity and impact of a second cancer in survivors of Hodgkin lymphoma, it is important to consider all causes of mortality in children and adolescents in whom Hodgkin lymphoma has been previously diagnosed. In the Stanford experience of 694 children and teenagers followed for up to 31 years after treatment for Hodgkin lymphoma and analyzed for causes of death, recurrent Hodgkin lymphoma accounted for more than half of all deaths, accidents or other causes for one-fourth, and secondary cancers for one-fifth.[132]

In the early 1970s, we learned that MOPP and similar derivative alkylating agent chemotherapy produce an excess risk of acute myeloid leukemia (s-AML) and myelodysplasia (MDS) in both adults and children.[133–135] The main risk factor for these leukemias is the cumulative dose and specific type of alkylating agent, as some agents are more leukemogenic than others. The Late Effects Study Group (LESG) reported a standardized incidence ratio (SIR; the ratio of observed to expected cases, or relative risk) for any leukemia of 78.8 (95% CI, 56.6–123.2) and a SIR for s-AML/MDS of 321.3 (95% CI, 207.5–467.1) in children less than 16 years of age treated with chemotherapy.[136] The SIR was reduced to 122 (95% CI, 36–254) with lower cumulative doses of alkylating agents and the omission of mechlorethamine in the German-Austrian OPPA (or OPA)/COPP (or COMP) studies of pediatric Hodgkin lymphoma.[20] The use of ABVD in lieu of MOPP greatly reduced the risk of s-AML and MDS.[137] Treatment with epipodophyllotoxins and nitrosoureas also produce an excess risk of s-AML.[138] Acute lymphoblastic leukemia and chronic myelogenous leukemia have been reported in patients with Hodgkin lymphoma, but their incidence does not exceed that expected on the basis of chance. The s-AML/MDS risk following radiation alone (zero probability in the LESG experience). The highest risk for s-AML/MDS is within the first 5 years of follow-up; it is extraordinarily rare after 10 years of follow-up.[139] The risk for s-AML as a function of prior splenectomy or splenic radiotherapy varies. Although the Institut Gustave-Roussy investigators found an increased relative risk for leukemia following splenectomy (RR, 2.54; $p = 0.018$) and prior splenic irradiation (RR, 3.67; $p = 0.003$) among adults with Hodgkin lymphoma,[140] other large series have not confirmed an increased leukemia incidence following splenectomy among children (see Chapter 24 for further details).[136]

The risk for NHL is also increased following treatment, with a SIR of 11.7 (95% CI, 4.7–24.2) in the most recent update of the LESG[139] and a SIR of 15 (95% CI, 4.9–35) in the five Nordic country experience (Denmark, Finland, Iceland, Norway, and Sweden).[141] This risk may be related to overall immunosuppression associated with the disease and its treatment. Several authors have reported that when the risks for s-AML and NHL are combined, they appear more commonly in adolescents than in children under 10 years of age.[142]

Long-term follow-up of cohorts of pediatric Hodgkin survivors indicate an increasing occurrence of radiation-associated solid tumors. The latency period for the development of a solid tumor is considerably longer than that for the development of leukemia, with solid tumors appearing more than 10 years after treatment; the incidence rises with increasing length of follow-up.[132,139] Figure 21.5 reveals the cumulative incidence of all second malignancies, solid tumors, and secondary leukemia in 1,380 patients with Hodgkin lymphoma in the Late Effects Study Group.[139] The 15-year cumulative probability of solid tumor induction in the original LESG experience following specific treatments was 3.3% (CI, 2.9–3.7) for radiation; 2.9% (CI, 2.3–3.5) for chemotherapy, and 4.6% (CI, 4.4–4.8) for radiation plus chemotherapy.[136] In the recent update of the LESG, the 20-year cumulative incidence of any second malignancy and a solid malignancy after Hodgkin lymphoma was 10.6% and 7.3%, respectively.[139] In this report, the SIR of a solid tumor that arises after treatment for Hodgkin lymphoma was 18.5 (95% CI, 15.2–22.3). The most common solid tumors involved the breast (SIR, 56.7; CI, 40.5–77.3), thyroid (SIR, 36.4; CI, 21.9–56.8), bone (SIR, 37.1; CI, 15.9–73.1), and colorectum (SIR, 36.4; CI, 15.7–71.8) (Table 21.5). Non-melanomatous skin cancers, including basal cell carcinomas, are also common.[143] Many secondary solid tumors can be effectively treated, although previous treatment for Hodgkin lymphoma may limit therapeutic options in some cases.

Much attention has been given to the increasing awareness of the significant risk for breast cancer after treatment for Hodgkin lymphoma. Although early reports showed only a modestly increased risk among women treated with radiation and MOPP chemotherapy, the dramatic increase in risk became apparent when patients were followed longer than 15 years after Hodgkin lymphoma therapy.[144] The relative risk for the development of invasive breast cancer among Hodgkin lymphoma survivors was 4.1 (95% CI, 2.5–5.7) in 885 women (ages 4 to 81 years; mean, 28 years) from Stanford followed for an average of 10 years, or 8,832 person-years of observation.[144] The risk was highest for those who received irradiation before the age of 15 years: the relative risk was 136

(95% CI, 34–37.1) and the absolute risk was 38.4. The relative risk declines with age, but remains elevated in female patients under 30 years of age at the time of irradiation. No increased risk was detected for women older than 30 years at the time of treatment. Similarly, the absolute risk is elevated in these groups until age 30 (Table 21.6).[144] In a follow-up analysis of 694 children with Hodgkin lymphoma, the relative risk for breast cancer was 26.2, with 3,741 person-years at risk. All cases were in female patients; no male breast cancers have been reported.[132] A recent CCSS investigation reported a SIR of 26.3 (95% CI 20.2–33.7) for breast cancer in children treated with chest irradiation for Hodgkin lymphoma; pediatric Hodgkin lymphoma survivors in this cohort who did not receive chest irradiation did not have an elevated risk of breast cancer ($p < 0.001$).[145] This relative risk is similar to other studies of Hodgkin lymphoma where the reported SIR for secondary breast cancer is in the range of 15 to 30.[136,141,146–148]

Factors reported to influence breast cancer risk include age at treatment, radiation dose, and alkylating agent chemotherapy. A high dose of radiation is a risk factor, with most breast cancers arising after 40 to 46 Gy of mantle irradiation, although some reported cases also received 12 to 16 Gy of lung irradiation on the side of the breast cancer.[144] However, a breast radiation dose of 4 Gy or more was associated with a 3.2-fold (95% CI, 1.4–8.2) increased risk in a matched case control study of patients with Hodgkin lymphoma treated at age 30 years or younger who survived for 1 or more years.[149] The risk increased to 8-fold (95% CI, 2.6–26.9) with a radiation dose of more than 40 Gy ($p < 0.001$ for trend). These authors showed that the risk of breast cancer is reduced with ovarian damage from alkylating-agent chemotherapy or pelvic radiation, suggesting that hormonal stimulation appears important for the development of radiation-induced breast cancer.[149] This may explain the observation of increased incidence of breast cancer among adolescent girls treated with radiation,[136,141,150,151] suggesting an unusual sensitivity to pubertal hormones.[152] Others have suggested that patients with Hodgkin lymphoma appear to have a specific susceptibility to the development of excess breast cancers not completely explained by chemotherapy and breast radiation.[153] The impact of genetics on breast cancer (patients receiving combined-modality treatment may carry the BRCA1 or BRCA2 gene) has not yet been evaluated. It is important to investigate the genetic impact as there appears to be an association of breast cancer among girls who have not received breast radiation, but who have a family history of sarcoma suggesting a hereditary cancer predisposition, such as in the Li-Fraumeni syndrome.[145]

Treatment for second solid tumors, particularly breast cancer, must be individualized. However, most oncologists today recommend mastectomy as opposed to breast-conserving therapy with lumpectomy and breast irradiation for a patient previously irradiated for Hodgkin lymphoma. Oncologists must continuously educate their patients on their specific risks. A prospective cohort study of 90 female long-term survivors of Hodgkin lymphoma who received chest irradiation demonstrated that women are often unaware of their increased risk of breast cancer. Thirty-five of 87 (40%) of surveyed women felt they had an equal or lower risk than other women of the same age, and only 41 of 87 (47%) reported having a mammogram within 24 months.[154] For patients with a familial or genetic predisposition of breast cancer, MRI appears more sensitive than mammography in detecting breast tumors, but may be associated with a higher false-positive rate.[155,156] Early detection is particularly important in young female survivors of Hodgkin lymphoma, as breast cancer at a young age is known to have aggressive biologic features.[157] Sex is a factor influencing the risk for a second cancer; female patients have a hazard ratio of 1.8 in comparison with male patients, explained by their

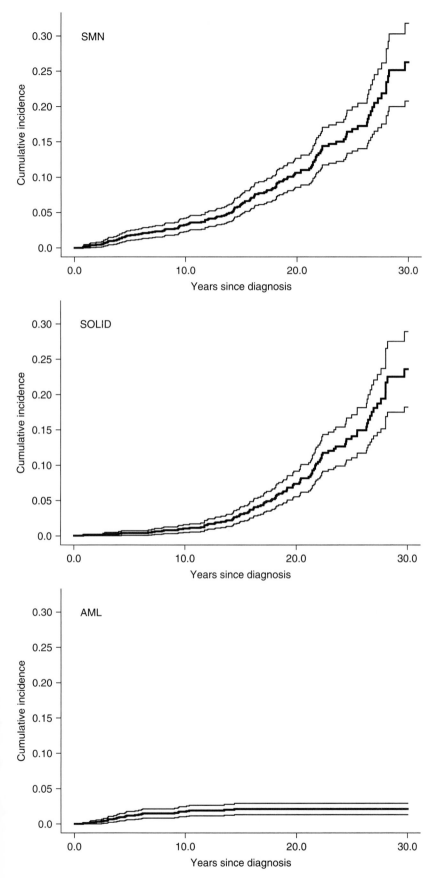

FIGURE 21.5. Cumulative incidence (*middle line*) of all second malignancies (**A**), solid tumors (**B**), and secondary leukemia (**C**) in 1,380 patient with Hodgkin lymphoma in Late Effects Study Group with 95% CI (*upper and lower curves*). (From Bhatia S, Yasui Y, Robison LL, et al. High risk of subsequent neoplasms continues with extended follow-up of childhood Hodgkin's disease: report from the Late Effects Study Group. *J Clin Oncol* 2003;21:4386–4394.)

TABLE 21.5

OBSERVED AND EXPECTED RATE OF SUBSEQUENT MALIGNANCIES IN LESG, ACCORDING TO CANCER DIAGNOSIS

Cancer diagnosis	No. observed/ expected cases	Standardized incidence ratio with 95% CI	Absolute rate per 10^3 person-years	20-year cumulative incidence, %, with 95% CI	30-year cumulative incidence, %, with 95% CI
All cancers[a,b]	143/7.8	18.5 (15.6–21.7)	6.5	10.6 (8.6–12.7)	26.3 (20.8–31.8)
Leukemia[b]	27/0.2	174.8 (115.1–254.3)	1.3	2.1 (1.3–2.9)	2.1 (1.3–2.9)
Non-Hodgkin's lymphoma	7/0.6	11.7 (4.7–24.2)	0.3	1.5 (0.1–1.1)	1.5 (0–3.3)
Solid tumors[c]	109/5.9	18.5 (15.2–22.3)	5.1	7.3 (5.5–9.1)	23.5 (18.2–28.9)
Breast, all[d]	40/0.7	56.7 (40.5–77.3)	1.9	2.0 (1.0–2.9)	7.2 (3.7–10.6)
Breast, females[d]	39/0.7	55.5 (39.5–75.9)	5.3	5.6 (2.8–8.3)	16.9 (9.4–24.5)
Thyroid	19/0.5	36.4 (21.9–56.8)	0.9	1.9 (0.9–2.8)	4.4 (1.3–7.8)
Bone	8/0.2	37.1 (15.9–73.1)	0.4	0.5 (0.1–0.9)	0.8 (0.1–0.4)
Colorectal	8/0.2	36.4 (915.7–71.8)	0.4	0.4 (0–0.8)	2.4 (0.1–4.7)
Gastric	3/0.1	63.9 (12.9–186.9)	0.2	0.3 (0–0.7)	0.6 (0–1.2)
Lung	4/0.2	27.3 (7.4–69.9)	0.2	0.1 (0–0.3)	2.1 (0–4.4)

[a]Excludes non-melanoma skin cancers, including squamous cell cancer ($n = 1$), basal cell cancer ($n = 24$); meningioma ($n = 1$); breast cancer (ductal carcinoma in situ; $n = 2$); benign tumors ($n = 40$); and patients with missing information ($n = 1$).
[b]Date of birth not available for one patient.
[c]Excludes lymphatic ($n = 7$) and hematopoietic tumors ($n = 27$), benign tumors ($n = 40$), and patients with missing information ($n = 1$).
[d]Excludes ductal carcinoma in situ; $n = 2$.
From Bhatia S, Yasui Y, Robison LL, et al. High risk of subsequent neoplasms continues with extended follow-up of childhood Hodgkin's disease: report from the Late Effects Study Group. *J Clin Oncol* 2003;21:4386–4394, with permission.

increased incidence of breast cancer. However, the strongest predictor for development of a second malignancy is relapse of Hodgkin lymphoma, for which the hazard ratio is 2.6 ($p <0.001$).[132] Additionally, exposure to chemotherapeutic regimens containing alkylating agents correlates with the development of leukemia, with a hazard ratio of 10.7 ($p = .03$).

The numerous investigations regarding treatment-related sequelae serve as a guide to the management of children in whom Hodgkin lymphoma has been newly diagnosed. Thus, new protocols must be designed with the following goals kept in mind:

1. Initial treatment should be administered with a curative intent in order to minimize the likelihood of relapse of disease and the aggressive salvage therapy that is mandated by relapse.
2. High doses of irradiation, particularly to the axilla and mediastinum, should be avoided in women younger than 30 years at the time of treatment. Current protocols for pediatric Hodgkin lymphoma in which low-dose involved-field radiotherapy and chemotherapy are used meet this goal.

TABLE 21.6

BREAST CANCER RISK AFTER TREATMENT OF HODGKIN LYMPHOMA

Group	No. at risk	Person-years at risk	Observed/expected events	Relative risk[a] (95% CI)	Absolute Risk[b]
All patients	885	8,759	25/6.13	4.1 (2.5–5.7)	21.5
Age (years)					
<15	76	776	3/0.02	136 (34–371)	38.4
15–19	156	1696	3/0.16	19 (4.7–51)	16.7
20–24	180	1807	9/0.47	19 (9.3–35)	47.2
25–29	173	1853	7/0.96	7.3 (3.2–14)	32.6
30–39	177	1651	1/1.75	0.6 (0.0–2.8)	—
40–49	51	502	1/1.08	0.9 (0.0–4.6)	—
≥50	72	474	1/1.69	0.6 (0.0–2.9)	—

[a]Relative risk calculated as ratio of observed to expected events, with 95% confidence intervals (CI).
[b]Absolute risk expressed as excess numbers of cases per 10,000 person-years.
From Hancock SL, Tucker MA, Hoppe RT. Breast cancer after treatment of Hodgkin's disease. *J Natl Cancer Inst* 1993;85:25, with permission.

Risk-based guidelines for follow-up of patients treated for Hodgkin lymphoma have been organized by the Children's Oncology Group.[158] The recommendations vary based on specific treatment exposures, but include the following evaluations for most children treated with contemporary combined-modality therapy:

1. A follow-up evaluation should be performed annually by a health care provider who is knowledgeable about the survivor's treatment and its associated health risks.

2. The complete blood count should be monitored for at least 10 years after administration of alkylating agent or epipodophyllotoxin chemotherapy to evaluate for leukemia and myelodysplastic syndrome.

3. A thorough physical examination should be performed annually with a particular focus on clinical history and physical findings that could represent manifestations of late treatment toxicity. This examination should include inspection of skin lesions and soft tissues in radiation treatment fields, palpation of the thyroid gland of patients treated with cervical radiation, and cardiopulmonary assessment in patients treated with anthracycline chemotherapy, bleomycin, or chest radiation.

4. Heightened breast cancer surveillance should be undertaken in any woman who was 30 years or younger when treated with thoracic radiation. Specific recommendations include monthly breast self-examination beginning at puberty; annual clinician breast exam until age 25 years, then every 6 months; and yearly mammography, beginning 8 years after radiation or at age 25 years, whichever comes last.

5. Cardiovascular function assessment should be performed on a periodic basis with the specific frequency based on age at treatment, cumulative dose of anthracycline therapy, and thoracic radiation dose.

6. Pulmonary function should be evaluated at baseline for patients treated with bleomycin or thoracic radiation, and repeated as clinically indicated.

7. Specific signs or symptoms in a patient previously treated for Hodgkin lymphoma that could possibly suggest a new primary tumor (i.e., bone pain, dysphagia, cough, pigmented skin lesion) should be promptly evaluated.

8. Survivors should be educated about risk factors for treatment-related morbidity, methods of risk reduction, and the value of physical and screening examinations.

9. Specific attention should be paid to the risks for overwhelming sepsis in patients who have had splenectomy or splenic irradiation and appropriate immunization programs should be completed.

More detailed information about risk-based assessments in pediatric Hodgkin survivors is summarized at http://www.survivorshipguidelines.org.

CURRENT TRIALS

In the 1970s, several pediatric institutions and cooperative groups initiated clinical trials evaluating combined-modality therapy for pediatric patients with Hodgkin lymphoma. Late sequelae of treatment, identified during long-term follow-up of survivors of childhood disease, guided the development of protocol therapy. The desire to avoid treatment-related toxicity observed in long-term survivors of Hodgkin lymphoma continues to influence protocol development. Trials of risk-adapted, response-based therapy with restricted doses of anthracyclines, bleomycin, and alkylating agents are underway aiming to reduce the burden of treatment by decreasing or completely omitting radiotherapy. Recent study results demonstrate that

patients with favorable presentations of localized disease are excellent candidates for therapy reduction. However, some modifications of therapy for patients with unfavorable and advanced disease produce inferior disease control.[43,159-163] In addition, two large cooperative trials reported an EFS advantage for patients treated with combined-modality therapy including low-dose, radiation consolidation, although survival was unaffected due to effective retrieval therapy.[44,51] These results underscore the need for caution with which investigators must proceed when attempting to reduce late effects of treatment. Tables 21.7 and 21.8, which summarize the results of selected series of combined-modality trials, provide specific details of the evolution of pediatric Hodgkin therapy.

Chemotherapy Alone Versus Combined-Modality Therapy

Several investigators have demonstrated disease-free survival rates in children with Hodgkin lymphoma treated with chemotherapy alone that are comparable with those observed after combined-modality therapy (Table 21.9). Chemotherapy-alone protocols have several advantages: (a) single-modality treatment with chemotherapy can be used in developing countries, where radiation equipment and trained personnel may be lacking; (b) precise surgical or clinical staging, which may be difficult to accomplish in some centers, is not needed; and (c) long-term growth and neoplastic complications associated with radiation therapy are avoided with chemotherapy alone. The potential disadvantages of chemotherapy-alone regimens include (a) higher exposure to alkylating drugs (compared with exposures in combined-modality regimens) and (b) increased morbidity from myelosuppression, gonadal injury, and secondary leukemia.

Evaluation of the efficacy of chemotherapy-only treatment regimens has been difficult because most reports describe outcome after nonrandom treatment assignments in small clinically staged cohorts. In addition, several trials specifically exclude patients with unfavorable risk features based on bulk and number of involved nodal sites. Early trials reported satisfactory outcomes in children treated with MOPP and similar therapies containing alkylating agents.[164-168] Acute hematologic and infectious toxicity was acceptable and manageable in centers with limited resources. As anticipated, the limited reports describing long-term gonadal toxicity indicated a high incidence of irreversible sterility and possibly germinal epithelial damage in boys treated with six or more cycles of combination chemotherapy containing alkylating agents, regardless of their pubertal status.[169] Long-term toxicity has not been thoroughly evaluated, and it may be underestimated because of the difficulty or unwillingness of patients to return for follow-up evaluations after completion of therapy.

Later chemotherapy-only trials in pediatric patients with Hodgkin lymphoma sought to improve cure rates and reduce treatment sequelae related to alkylating agent chemotherapy by using alternating non–cross-resistant regimens (MOPP/ABVD, COPP/ABV hybrid, CVPP/EBO [cyclophosphamide, vinblastine, procarbazine, prednisone/Epirubicin, bleomycin, vincristine (Oncovin)])[162,170-172] or by using combinations without alkylating agents, such as ABVD or EVAP/ABV (etoposide, vinblastine, cytosine arabinoside, cis-platinum, doxorubicin, bleomycin, and vincristine).[159,173] Most of these trials comprised small cohorts of clinically staged patients with early-stage Hodgkin lymphoma; some trials specifically excluded patients with "bulky" disease. Results indicate that treatment with six cycles of alternating chemotherapy programs can produce disease-free survival rates comparable in short-term follow-up with those achieved with combined-modality regimens of

TABLE 21.7

EUROPEAN-SOUTH AMERICAN COMBINED-MODALITY TRIALS IN PEDIATRIC HODGKIN LYMPHOMA

Institution or group (Ref.)	Stage	Chemotherapy	Radiation therapy	No. patients	Outcome (years)			
					EFS (%)	DFS (%)	FFS (%)	Survival (%)
Institut Gustave-Roussy[8]	All stages	6 MOPP	40 Gy, IF	40	86 (15)			93 (15)
		3 MOPP	40 Gy, IF	20				
SFOP MDH-82[16]	I–IIA	4 ABVD	20–40 Gy, IF	79		90 (6)		
	I–IIA	2 MOPP/2 ABVD	20–40 Gy, IF	67		87 (6)		
	I–IIB	3 MOPP/3 ABVD	20–40 Gy, EF	31				92 (6)
	III	3 MOPP/3 ABVD	20–40 Gy, EF	40		82 (6)		
	IV	3 MOPP/3 ABVD	20–40 Gy, EF	21		62 (6)		
SFOP MDH-90[55]	I–II, good responders	4 VBVP	20 Gy, IF	171		91 (5)		97.5 (5)
	I–II, poor responders	4 VBVP + 1–2 OPPA	20 Gy, IF	27		78 (5)		
Germany-Austria HD-82[9]	IA/B, IIA	2 OPPA	35 Gy, IF	100	98 (9)			100 (9)
	IIB–IIIA	2 OPPA/2 COPP	30 Gy, IF	53	94 (9)			96 (9)
	IIIB, IV	2 OPPA/4 COPP	25 Gy, IF	50	86 (9)			85 (9)
HD-85[9]	IA/B, IIA	2 OPA	35 Gy, IF	53	85 (6)			98 (6)
	IIB–IIIA	2 OPA/2 COMP	30 Gy, IF	21	55 (6)			95 (6)
	IIIB, IV	2 OPA/4 COMP	25 Gy, IF	24	49 (6)			100 (6)
HD-90[17]	IA/B, IIA	2 OEPA/2 OPPA	25 Gy, IF	274	93/96 (5)			100/100 (5)
	IIB–IIIA	2 OEPA/2 OPPA + 2 COPP	25 Gy, IF	123	90/96 (5)			100/97 (5)
	IIIB, IV	2 OEPA/2 OPPA + 4 COPP	20 Gy, IF	178	83/91 (5)			98/89 (5)
HD-95[44]	I–IIA	2 OEPA/2 OPPA	20–35 Gy, IF	281	94 (5)			
	II$_E$A, IIB, IIIA	2 OEPA/2 OPPA + 2 COPP	20–35 Gy, IF	212	92 (5)			
	II$_E$B, III$_E$A/B, IIIB, IVA/B	2 OEPA/2 OPPA + 4 COPP	20–35 Gy, IF	265	90 (5)			
AEIOP MH-83[18]	IA	3 ABVD	20–40 Gy, IF	83			95 (7)	
	IIA (M/T <0.33)	3 ABVD	20–40 Gy, R					
	IIA (M/T ≥0.33)	3 MOPP/3 ABVD	20–40 Gy, R	132			81 (7)	86 (7)
	IIIA	3 MOPP/3 ABVD	20–40 Gy, EF					
	IIIB-IV	5 MOPP/5 ABVD	20–40 Gy, EF				60 (7)	
	III	6–10 ChlVPP	35 Gy, IF	80			73 (10)	84 (10)
	IV	6–10 ChlVPP	35 Gy, IF	27			38 (10)	71 (10)
Royal Marsden[165]	I–III	8 VEEP	30–35, IF	46			82 (5)	93 (5)
Argentina[177]	I–IV	6 CVPP	30–40 Gy, IF	43	87 (5)			
	Intermediate prognostic group[a]	6 AOPE	30–40 Gy, IF	21	67 (5)			
	Unfavorable	CCOPP/CAPTe	30–40 Gy, IF	24	83 (5)			

[a]Intermediate prognostic group determined on the basis of age, symptoms, stage, and number of nodal regions.
EFS, event-free survival; DFS, disease-free survival; FFP, freedom from progression; MOPP, Mustargen, Oncovin, procarbazine, prednisone; ABVD, Adriamycin, bleomycin, vinblastine, dacarbazine; OPPA, Oncovin, prednisone, procarbazine, Adriamycin; CAPTe, cyclophosphamide, Adriamycin, prednisone, teniposide; COPP, cyclophosphamide, Oncovin, procarbazine, prednisone; CCOPP, CCNU, vincristine, procarbazine, prednisone; COMP, cyclophosphamide, Oncovin, methotrexate, prednisone; OEPA, Oncovin, etoposide, prednisone, Adriamycin; ChlVPP, chlorambucil, vinblastine, procarbazine, prednisolone; OPA, Oncovin, prednisone, Adriamycin; CVPP, cyclophosphamide, vincristine, prednisone, procarbazine; AOPE, Adriamycin, Oncovin, prednisone, etopside; IF, involved field; EF, extended field; R, regional; MMR, mediastinal mass rates; M/T, mediastinal mass/thorax rates; VBVP, vinblastine, bleomycin, etoposide, prednisone; VEEP, vincristine, etoposide, epirubicin, prednisolone.

TABLE 21.8

NORTH AMERICAN COMBINED-MODALITY TRIALS IN PEDIATRIC HODGKIN LYMPHOMA

Institution or group (ref.)	Stage	Chemotherapy	Radiation therapy	No. patients	EFS (%)	DFS (%)	RFS (%)	Survival (%)
Stanford[4]	PS I–II	6 MOPP	15–25 Gy, IF	27			96 (5)	100 (5)
	PS III–IV	6 MOPP	15–25 Gy, IF	28			84 (5)	78 (5)
Stanford[15]	CS/PS I–III	3 MOPP/ 3 ABVD	15–25 Gy, IF	44	100 (10)			100 (10)
	CS/PS IV	3 MOPP/ 3 ABVD	15–25 Gy, IF	13	69 (10)			85 (10)
St. Jude[14]	CS I–IIB	4–5 COP(P)/ 3–4 ABVD	20 Gy, IF	28		96 (5)		96 (5)
	CS III–IV	4–5 COP(P)/ 3–4 ABVD	20 Gy, IF	57		93 (5)		93 (5)
Stanford, St. Jude, Dana Farber Consortium[184]	CSI/II, no bulk	4 VAMP	15–25.5 Gy, IF	110	93 (5)			99 (5)
Stanford, St. Jude, Dana Farber Consortium[43]	CS I/II, bulky CS III/IV	6 VEPA	15–25.5 Gy, IF	56	68 (5)			82 (5)
Stanford, St. Jude, Dana Farber Consortium[163]	CS IA/IIB, bulky CS IIB	3 VAMP/ 3 COP	15–25.5 Gy, IF	77	83 (6)			93 (6)
	CS III, IV	3 VAMP/ 3 COP	15–25.5 Gy, IF	82	68 (6)			93 (6)
Intergroup Hodgkin's[5]	PS I–II	6 MOPP	≥35 Gy	97			95 (5)	90 (5)
Pediatric Oncology Group[19]	CS/PS IIB, IIIA$_2$, IIIB, IV	4 MOPP/ 4 ABVD	21 Gy, TLI	62	77 (3)			91 (3)
Pediatric Oncology Group[178]	CS/PS IIB, IIIA$_2$, IIIB, IV	4 MOPP/ 4 ABVD	21 Gy, EF	80	80 (5)			87 (5)
Children's Cancer Group[13]	PS III–IV	12 ABVD	21 Gy, R	64	87 (3)			89 (3)
Children's Cancer Group[178]	PS III/IV	6 ABVD	21 Gy, EF	54	87 (4)			90 (4)
Children's Cancer Group[51]	CS IA/B, IIA without adverse features[a]	4 COPP/ABV	21 Gy, IF	294	97 (3)			100 (3)
	CS I/II with adverse features,[a] CS IIB, CS III	6 COPP/ABV	21 Gy, IF	394	87 (3)			95 (3)
	CS IV	COPP/ABV + CHOP + Ara-C/VP-16	21 Gy, IF	141	90 (3)			100 (3)

[a]Adverse features defined as hilar adenopathy, involvement of more than 4 nodal regions, mediastinal tumor ≥33% of chest diameter, node or nodal aggregate >10 cm.
CS, clinical stage; PS, pathologic stage; MOPP, Mustargen, Oncovin, procarbazine, prednisone; ABVD, Adriamycin, bleomycin, vinblastine, dacarbazine; CHOP, cyclophosphamide, doxorubicin, Oncovin, prednisone; COP(P), cyclophosphamide, Oncovin, procarbazine, prednisone; IF, involved field; EF, extended field; EFS, event-free survival; DFS, disease-free survival; R, regional, RFS, relapse-free survival; TLI, total lymphoid irradiation.

TABLE 21.9

TREATMENT RESULTS IN PEDIATRIC HODGKIN LYMPHOMA WITH CHEMOTHERAPY ALONE

Institution or group (ref.)	Stage	Chemotherapy	No. patients	Outcome (years)			
				EFS (%)	DFS (%)	RFS (%)	Survival (%)
Pediatric Oncology Group[178]	CS IIB, IIA2, IIIB, IV	4 MOPP/4 ABVD	81	79 (5)			96 (5)
Children's Cancer Group[180]	PS III/IV	6 MOPP/6 ABVD	57	77 (4)			84 (4)
Children's Cancer Group[51]	CS IA/B, IIA (without adverse features)[a]	4 COPP/ABV	106	91 (3)			100 (3)
	CS I/II with adverse features,[a] CS IIB, CS III	6 COPP/ABV	394	83 (3)			100 (3)
	CS IV	COPP/ABV + CHOP + Ara-C/VP-16	141	81 (3)			94 (3)
German Multicenter HD-95[44]	CS II$_E$A, III$_E$A/B, IIIB, IVA/B	2 OPPA/OEPA + 4 COPP	57	80 (5)			90 (5)
U.K. Children's Cancer Study Group[166]	CS IV	6–8 ChlVPP	67	55 (5)			81 (5)
Australia/ New Zealand[168]	CS I–IIB	6–8 MOPP or 6 ChlVPP	38			92 (4)	94 (4)
Australia/ New Zealand[175]	CS IA–IVA	3 EVAP/ABV	25			60 (3.5)	100 (3.5)
Australia/ New Zealand[162]	CS I–IV	5–6 VEEP	53	78 (5)			92 (5)
Nicaragua[172]	I, IIA	6 COPP	14	100 (3)			100 (3)
	CS IIIB, IV	8–10 COPP-ABV	23	75 (3)			
The Netherlands[174]	CS I–IV (<4 cm node)	6 MOPP	21	91 (5)			100 (5)
	CS I–IV	6 ABVD	17	70 (5)			94 (5)
	CS 1–IV	3 MOPP/3 ABVD	21	91 (5)			91 (5)
Madras, India[173]	CS IIB–IVB	6 COPP/ABV	43	90 (5)			
Argentina[176]	CS IA, IIA	3 CVPP	10	86 (6.7)			
	CS IB, IIB	6 CVPP	16	87 (6.7)			
Costa Rica[164]	CS IA–IIIA	6 CVPP	52			90 (5)	100 (5)
	CS IIIB, IV	6 CVPP/6 EBO	24			60 (5)	81 (5)
Uganda[170]	CS I–IIIA	6 MOPP	38		75 (5)		
	CS IIIB–IV	6 MOPP	10		60 (5)		

[a]Adverse features defined as hilar adenopathy, involvement of more than 4 nodal regions, mediastinal tumor ≥33% of chest diameter, node or nodal aggregate >10 cm.
EFS, event-free survival; DFS, disease-free survival; RFS, relapse-free survival; CS, clinical stage; PS, pathologic stage; POG, Pediatric Oncology Group; MOPP, Mustargen, Oncovin, procarbazine, prednisone; ABVD, Adriamycin, bleomycin, vinblastine, dacarbazine; COPP, cyclophosphamide, Oncovin, procarbazine, prednisone; CVPP, cyclophosphamide, vincristine, procarbazine, prednisone; EBO, Epirubicine, bleomycin, Oncovin; EVAP, etoposide, vinblastine, cytosine arabinoside, cis-platium; ChlVPP, vinblastine, procarbazine, prednisone; OPPA, Oncovin, prednisone, procarbazine, Adriamycin; OEPA, Oncovin, etoposide, prednisone, Adriamycin; ChlVPP, chlorambucil, vinblastine, procarbazine, prednisolone; OPA, Oncovin, prednisone, Adriamycin; CVPP, cyclophosphamide, vincristine, prednisone, procarbazine; VEEP, vincristine, etoposide, epirubicin, prednisolone.

fewer than six cycles of chemotherapy plus low-dose, involved-field radiation. Acute toxicity related to these regimens appears to be acceptable; however, follow-up is not available to evaluate long-term morbidity.

There are few randomized trials comparing chemotherapy alone with combined-modality treatment in children. The Grupo Argentino de Tratamiento de Leucemia Aguda (GATLA) compared chemotherapy with CVPP alone (CVPP is a modification of MOPP in which cyclophosphamide and vinblastine are substituted for the mechlorethamine and vincristine of MOPP) versus CVPP plus involved-field radiotherapy (30–40 Gy) in patients with CS I–IV. In patients with stage I and II disease, CVPP alone produced event-free survival and overall survival rates similar to those produced by CVPP plus radiotherapy. However, patients with stage I and II disease and unfavorable characteristics (more than two nodal areas, lymph nodes larger than 5 cm, or bulky mediastinal disease) treated with CVPP plus radiotherapy had a superior disease-free survival and overall survival than did similar patients treated with CVPP alone. Also, among patients with CS III and IV, the combined-modality (CVPP plus radiotherapy) group had better disease-free survival rates than did the group treated with CVPP alone.[174] In a second GATLA study, a prognostic index was designed that took into account the number of involved nodes, systemic symptoms, and the presence of bulky mediastinal disease at the time of diagnosis. In the favorable group, patients were randomized to receive three or six cycles of CVPP without radiotherapy. Study results demonstrated that three cycles of CVPP without radiotherapy are equally as effective as six cycles in the favorable-risk group.[175]

North American pediatric cooperative group randomized trials also organized longitudinal trials comparing treatment with combined-modality therapy to chemotherapy alone. The Pediatric Oncology Group investigated combined-modality therapy versus MOPP/ABVD chemotherapy alone in advanced-stage pediatric Hodgkin lymphoma.[176] Of 161 patients in remission after completion of eight cycles of alternating MOPP/ABVD, 81 were randomized to observation and 80 to receive low-dose total-nodal or subtotal-nodal radiation therapy. Event-free survival and overall survival (based on treatment intent) were not significantly improved by the addition of low-dose radiation therapy. However, analysis based on treatment actually delivered indicated an event-free survival advantage for patients who received combined-modality therapy.[177] Similarly, Children's Cancer Group investigators tested combined-modality therapy consisting of ABVD for six cycles plus 21 Gy of irradiation to involved, extended, or total-lymphoid fields (depending on stage) versus 12 months of alternating MOPP/ABVD in laparotomy-staged children with stage III or IV Hodgkin lymphoma. At four years, there was no statistically significant difference in event-free survival or survival between the two groups; however, the children randomized to ABVD and radiotherapy had a four-year event-free survival of 87%, compared with 77% for those receiving chemotherapy only.[178] The pattern of relapse was predominantly nodal and was heavily biased toward sites of prior involvement, whether nodal or extranodal. The children randomized to ABVD and radiotherapy had a four-year survival of 90%, compared with 84% for patients randomized to chemotherapy alone.[178]

These POG and CCG results, and the inferior disease control observed in a small group of advanced-stage patients treated with ABVD alone,[159] suggest that combined-modality therapy given according to protocol may effect an improved outcome. By contrast, a study by Kelly and co-workers[179] investigated if early response could be enhanced by using an induction therapy with four cycles of dose-intensive BEACOPP. Rapid responders, defined by greater than 70% reduction in disease burden, received gender-specific consolidation therapy (COPP/ABV in females and ABVD in males) in an effort to reduce the risk of gender-associated toxicities. Early results demonstrate feasibility and efficacy of this approach, but median follow-up of the cohort is very short. If results are maintained with subsequent follow-up, this study will support the concept proposed by Loeffler and associates[180] that at an effective dose level of chemotherapy, additional radiotherapy will not improve treatment results.

Children's Cancer Group investigators reported the early results of a randomized controlled trial comparing survival outcomes in children treated with COPP/ABV hybrid chemotherapy alone to those treated with COPP/ABV hybrid chemotherapy plus low-dose, involved-field radiation.[51] Treatment assignment was based on clinical features including the presence of B-symptoms, hilar adenopathy, mediastinal and peripheral lymph node bulk, and the number of involved nodal regions. Patients achieving a complete response to chemotherapy (defined as more than 70% tumor regression

and a negative gallium scan in previously gallium-positive areas) were eligible for randomization to receive low-dose, involved-field radiation or no further therapy. A significantly greater number of relapses among patients treated with chemotherapy alone resulted in early closure of the study. The difference in 3-year event-free survival was most marked for patients with stage IV disease who had a 90% event-free survival if randomized to receive combined-modality therapy with involved-field radiation compared to 81% in those randomized to receive chemotherapy alone. Estimates for overall survival are not different between the randomized groups due to successful salvage therapy after relapse, but follow-up of the cohort is early. German and Austrian investigators also implemented a longitudinal (GPOH-HD-95) trial testing individualization of therapy based on disease characteristics, gender, and response to chemotherapy. Patients with a complete response to chemotherapy as defined by longitudinal imaging did not receive radiotherapy. The 5-year EFS rates for early-stage disease was 97% for patients achieving a complete remission with chemotherapy and 94% for those who did not achieve a complete remission with chemotherapy and underwent subsequent radiotherapy. However, the 5-year EFS was significantly lower in patients with intermediate- and advanced-stage disease treated with chemotherapy alone (91%) compared to those treated with combined-modality therapy (79%).[44] Overall survival rates did not differ, indicating that patients who fail can attain a second remission following retrieval therapy. Notably, previous studies of long-term survivors indicate that treatment for relapse increases the risk of second malignancies and early mortality, underscoring the importance of assigning the most effective, as well as least toxic, therapy at disease presentation.[132,181]

The debate continues as to whether the best course of action is to err on the side of overtreatment to optimize disease response to primary therapy, or whether to let patients who require more intensive therapy, particularly radiation, declare themselves by poor response to, or failure to, primary therapy. Most investigators agree that the potential benefits of radiation therapy in improving disease control outweigh the potential adverse sequelae in patients with (a) bulky mediastinal lymphadenopathy occupying more than 33% of the thoracic cavity, (b) advanced-stage disease in whom combination chemotherapy has resulted in only a partial response, and (c) refractory or progressive disease. In the absence of these clinical features, multiple studies have indicated that an equivalent proportion of children with Hodgkin lymphoma can be cured with aggressive combination chemotherapy or less intensive chemotherapy plus irradiation. The risk for late sequelae of chemotherapy, such as infertility, secondary leukemia, and cardiopulmonary dysfunction, as well as the increased risk for disease recurrence, must be balanced against the risk for sequelae of radiation, particularly the development of subsequent malignancies.

Risk-Adapted Therapy

Risk-adapted trials generally assign treatment based on clinical presentations defined as low, intermediate, or high risk. Unfortunately, risk categorizations vary per trial, making direct comparison of treatment outcomes difficult. A low-risk clinical presentation is defined by most trials as localized (stage I–II) nodal involvement in the absence of B-symptoms and lymph node bulk. Bulky mediastinal lymphadenopathy is designated when the ratio of the maximum measurement of the mediastinal lymph nodes to intrathoracic cavity on upright chest radiograph is 33% or more. Some studies also consider lymph node bulk outside the mediastinum in the risk assessment; this designation has ranged across studies from 4 cm to 10 cm. Likewise, the number of nodal sites considered as low risk varies, but generally is defined as fewer than 3 or 4 involved nodal regions.

The standard treatment approach for patients with low-risk presentations of Hodgkin lymphoma involves two to four cycles of chemotherapy with or without low-dose, involved-field radiation. Most multiagent regimens used for low-risk patients include little or no alkylating-agent chemotherapy.[44,51,55,182] Pediatric investigators from Stanford, Dana Farber, and St. Jude observed excellent outcomes using four cycles of vinblastine, doxorubicin, methotrexate, and prednisone (VAMP) and low-dose, involved-field radiation therapy. Five-year event-free survival and overall survival for low-risk patients treated with combined-modality therapy including the VAMP regimen were 93% and 99%, respectively.[175] Incorporation of etoposide in other regimens permits a lower cumulative dose of anthracycline or alkylating-agent chemotherapy; the disadvantage of this approach is the rare complication of secondary acute myeloid leukemia (s-AML).[44,55,56,183] French investigators reported a 5-year event-free survival of 91.5% in favorable-risk patients who achieved a good response following four cycles of the VBVP regimen (vinblastine, bleomycin, etoposide, and prednisone) followed by 20 Gy to involved-fields.[55] The German-Austrian group also reported that disease-free survival could be maintained with a potential for less gonadal toxicity in male patients by substituting etoposide for procarbazine in the vincristine, prednisone, procarbazine, and doxorubicin (OPPA) regimen.[44,56] Similarly, Pediatric Oncology Group investigators observed excellent outcomes in children with early-stage Hodgkin lymphoma treated with combined-modality therapy consisting of four courses of doxorubicin, bleomycin, vincristine, and etoposide (DBVE) followed by 25.5-Gy involved-field irradiation. At a median follow-up of 8.4 years, the 6-year overall and event-free survival rates for patients treated with combined-modality therapy with DBVE were 98% and 91%, respectively.[183] Thus far, the cumulative dose of etoposide in these trials has been associated with only a rare case of s-AML. Therefore, the benefits of reduced gonadal and cardiac toxicity appear to outweigh the risk of leukemogenesis with the restricted use of etoposide in regimens for low-risk Hodgkin lymphoma.

Several recent and ongoing trials aim to eliminate radiation therapy for low-risk patients with favorable responses to chemotherapy. Children's Cancer Group investigators reported a significantly higher 3-year event-free survival in patients who received 21-Gy involved-field radiation consolidation (97%), compared to those who were treated with four cycles of COPP/ABV chemotherapy alone (91%).[51] However, early treatment results in the group randomized to chemotherapy alone suggest that many patients with low-risk disease can be cured using this approach. The most recent German multicenter trial also demonstrated that outcome was not compromised by omitting involved-field radiation in low-risk patients who achieved a complete response following treatment with two cycles of OPPA or OEPA chemotherapy.[44] Preliminary studies indicate that local control is not compromised by reducing involved-field radiation dose to 15 Gy in patients who achieve an early complete response to VAMP chemotherapy.[184] Their ongoing consortium trial is investigating whether radiation can be eliminated for this favorable group.

The intermediate-risk group is characterized by patients with stage I/II disease who have one or more unfavorable features, and sometimes patients with stage IIIA disease. Patients with intermediate-risk disease have been treated similarly to those with advanced (stage III/IV) disease in some risk-adapted pediatric trials, or assigned a therapy that is intermediate in intensity in others. The criterion for unfavorable disease features has not been consistent across trials and may include the presence of B-symptoms; lymph node bulk; hilar lymph involvement; involvement of 3, 4, or more lymph node regions; and extranodal extension to contiguous structures. A high-risk presentation includes patients with advanced stage IIIB or IVA/B. This risk designation earns patients the most dose-intensive chemotherapy assignment therapy, which in most cases includes low-dose, involved-field radiation consolidation.

Chemotherapy used for intermediate- and high-risk Hodgkin lymphoma usually includes derivatives combinations of MOPP and ABVD. COPP has largely replaced MOPP in pediatric trials because cyclophosphamide is less myelosuppressive and leukemogenic than mechlorethamine.[20] Etoposide has been incorporated in regimens for intermediate- and high-risk Hodgkin lymphoma with the goal of improving antitumor activity and reducing cumulative doses of alkylating and anthracycline chemotherapy. However, substitution of non–alkylating- agent chemotherapy like methotrexate or etoposide as an alternative to alkylating-agent chemotherapy is associated with inferior event-free survival among patients with high-risk clinical presentations.[43,161,163]

The standard treatment approach prescribes a non–cross-resistant chemotherapy combination on a twice-monthly schedule for a total of 6 months. Low-dose (15.0- to 25.5-Gy), involved-field radiation therapy may be delivered between treatment cycles or, more commonly, following completion of chemotherapy to consolidate remission. An alternative approach uses dose-intensive multiagent chemotherapy administered at weekly intervals for a period of 3 to 5 months, during which myelosuppressive agents are alternated with non-myelosuppressive agents. The abbreviated therapy duration provides the advantage of increased dose-intensity, reduced therapy duration, and decreased cumulative chemotherapy doses, which should theoretically reduce the potential for the development of chemotherapy resistance and treatment toxicity. Most pediatric trials consolidate with low-dose, involved-field radiation to sites of bulky or residual disease. Notably, the German HD-90 study demonstrated loss of prognostic significance of bulky disease and number of involved nodal regions using a risk-adapted chemotherapy assignment and a response-based escalation of radiation dose in cases of insufficient remission following chemotherapy.[54]

SALVAGE THERAPY

In children, because the likelihood of cure with initial treatment programs is high, the experience with salvage therapy programs is limited.[66–68,185,186] Little has been published specifically addressing the salvage approach for patients treated with contemporary risk-adapted therapy.[68] Localized nodal relapse of minimal tumor burden is more amenable to salvage treatment than is extensive, widespread relapse. Disease that progresses during initial treatment and early relapse (within 1 year) after initial therapy are associated with a poorer outcome than is late relapse occurring many months or years after initial treatment. Patients with multiple relapses after one or more conventional chemotherapy regimens also have a poor outcome.

Starting in 1986, the German-Austrian Pediatric Hodgkin Lymphoma Study Group performed a prospective study of salvage therapy for children with first relapse or early progression.[68] This salvage study used ifosfamide, etoposide, and prednisone (IEP) along with ABVD, COPP, CEP (CCNU, etoposide, prednimustine), and additional radiotherapy as standard treatment. The disease-free survival (DFS) and overall survival rates after 10 years were 62% and 75%. A multivariant risk factor analysis revealed that time between end of primary treatment and diagnosis of relapse is the most important factor determining outcome of the patients: the DFS rate of patients with progression was 41%, whereas in patients with late relapse it was 86%. The second significant risk factor was primary treatment group. In general, patients with a primary diagnosis of early-stage Hodgkin lymphoma had a better prognosis than patients with intermediate or advanced stages. Thus, there is a potential for cure of Hodgkin lymphoma after relapse, but the likelihood of cure depends on several factors, including the nature of the initial therapy.

There is emerging experience with autologous bone-marrow or stem-cell transplantation in children.[66,67,185,186] The European Bone Marrow Transplant Group Lymphoma Registry reported outcomes for pediatric patients undergoing autologous bone marrow transplantation similar to those for adults, but cautioned about the necessity of monitoring such patients for late treatment sequelae.[186] Subsequent pediatric trials indicate reveal progression-free survival rates of approximately 50% after myeloablative chemotherapy with autologous bone-marrow or peripheral stem-cell transplantation. Predictors of favorable outcome have varied across studies and include extranodal disease at first relapse, disease sensitivity at time of transplant, presence of mediastinal mass at time of transplant, length of initial remission, and primary induction failure.[66–68,186] Allogeneic bone-marrow transplantation has also been used for relapsed Hodgkin lymphoma. Despite its association with a lower relapse rate (felt to be related to a "graft-versus-lymphoma" effect), the high rate of treatment-associated mortality after allogeneic transplantation results in event-free survival rates similar to those seen in patients treated with autologous transplantation.

QUALITY-OF-LIFE ISSUES

Among long-term survivors of pediatric Hodgkin lymphoma, quality-of-life issues have been addressed only in general terms in studies that include the entire population of Hodgkin lymphoma survivors and thus focus on adult issues, or they have been included in reports of cancers in childhood in general and have not focused specifically on pediatric Hodgkin lymphoma (see Chapter 27). Many definitions of quality of life have been offered. Among cancer patients, quality of life has been defined as a personal sense of well-being encompassing physical, psychological, social, and spiritual domains.[187] Changes in one of these four domains may influence one's perception in another domain. Furthermore, quality of life is best defined from the patient's own perspective.[188] Thus, among children with Hodgkin lymphoma, the opinion of a parent or family member is not as useful as the individual patient's personal perception about health status and/or nonmedical aspects of life. Such patients have almost without exception reached adulthood by the time long-term quality-of-life issues are investigated, which further explains the paucity of reports related specifically to quality of life among pediatric long-term survivors.

As goals of management of cancer patients include cure as well as restoration of function, a qualitative and quantitative measurement of functional status frequently used in the evaluation of adult patients is the Karnofsky Performance Status (KPS) scale.[189] This scale was not developed for use in children, but has been adapted for assessment of children.[190] However, the KPS scale is not entirely appropriate for children, as it measures one's ability to care for oneself, the degree of assistance needed, and the ability to conduct normal activities. In pediatric oncology, the Lansky Play Performance Scale for Children is considered more suitable, as it quantifies the degree to which cancer disrupts a child's play.[191] However, as pediatric Hodgkin lymphoma may affect an age range from early childhood through adolescence to young adulthood, neither of these measurements of functional status is adequate

for the entire population of interest. Both scales focus on short-term assessment, most appropriate while a patient is undergoing treatment; neither was designed to address the long-term issues associated with a highly curable disease such as Hodgkin lymphoma.[190]

Quality of life in patients with Hodgkin lymphoma is often divided into two components: quality of life during treatment and that after treatment.[192–194] Issues most commonly addressed are shown in Table 21.10. These concerns are enormous for anyone in whom Hodgkin lymphoma has been diagnosed and treated during childhood because of the number of years of potential long-term survival. During a course of treatment, concerns most disruptive to a child often include alopecia, whereas a parent may be most concerned about nutrition. Prolonged acute morbidity, such as the nausea and vomiting that may be seen with repeated cycles of chemotherapy, may cause a teenager to resist or refuse potentially life-saving therapy.

Changes in body image and loss of self-esteem occur in nearly one-half (49%) of patients from 1 to 21 years after treatment for Hodgkin lymphoma (median, 9 years).[195,196] Loss of body image correlates with symptoms of depression and stage of disease. The perception of change in body image may correlate directly with physical alterations attributed to treatment administered during childhood, particularly impairment of musculoskeletal growth and development.

Although such impairment is often difficult to quantify, it is common for male survivors to attempt body-building to augment the atrophy and muscular wasting that may follow high-dose irradiation when administered in the prepubertal years. Other physical complaints reported among pediatric survivors of Hodgkin lymphoma include disfigurement (30%), neurologic problems (30%), dyspnea (15%), and easy fatigability (5%).[193] With modern treatment approaches, including newer radiation techniques, lower radiation doses to more restricted fields, and less toxic chemotherapy agents, these problems will likely be less severe for those more recently treated.

Sexual problems have been reported in 22% to 37% of survivors of Hodgkin lymphoma.[196,197] The issues relate to problems of future longevity, possible sterility, and reproductive

TABLE 21.10

LONG-TERM EFFECTS ON QUALITY OF LIFE AFTER TREATMENT FOR HODGKIN LYMPHOMA IN CHILDHOOD

MEDICAL ISSUES
Nausea and vomiting
Second malignancy
Reproductive problems
Cognitive impairment
Organ dysfunction
  Thyroid
  Cardiac
  Pulmonary
  Musculoskeletal

PSYCHOSOCIAL ISSUES
Marital
Sexual
Work-related
Insurance
Socioeconomic

PSYCHOLOGICAL ISSUES

dysfunction, whether they were treated when children or adults. However, this concern is of particular relevance to adolescents and/or young adults, who face developmental aspects of intimacy and child-rearing. No differences in psychosocial adaptation or function have been seen among survivors of Hodgkin lymphoma treated with MOPP, ABVD, or MOPP alternating with ABVD, although the ABVD combination is reported to have fewer adverse effects on male fertility.[197]

As a rule, survivors of Hodgkin lymphoma are less likely to marry than persons without a prior diagnosis of cancer, and if they do marry, they tend to do so at a later age. A higher rate of divorce among male survivors has been reported in comparison with age- and race-specific statistics for the United States (23% versus 5.4%; $p = 0.002$).[195] On the other hand, other investigators have found that survivors of Hodgkin lymphoma have closer marital relationships, with increased support and communication during and after the illness.[198] Education and employment issues require long-term adjustments following therapy. In one review, 17% of children dropped out of school, citing cancer therapy as a reason.[193] In another report, 42% of employed survivors of Hodgkin lymphoma cited problems in the workplace.[195] The perception of job discrimination as a result of having had Hodgkin lymphoma has been reported in 11% of patients, with assertions of job discrimination.[199] Overall, 36% of survivors of Hodgkin lymphoma perceive negative social and economic effects related to employment, income, and education.[199]

Discrimination in the military has also been reported for both young patients and adults. When discrimination is not reported, it is generally because of failure to reveal a cancer history on an application form. Today, Department of Defense Directive 6130, from March 31, 1986, "Physical Standards for Enlistment, Appointment, and Induction," makes it possible for survivors of childhood cancer to serve in the armed forces, military reserves, and Reserved Officers Training Corps. By this directive, persons with a history of childhood cancer who have not received therapy for 5 years and are free of cancer will be considered fit for acceptance into the armed forces on a case-by-case basis.[200]

Survivors of Hodgkin lymphoma continue to report difficulties in obtaining insurance because their risk for dying of Hodgkin lymphoma or of treatment-related causes is higher than that of the normal population. Health insurance was denied to 22% of patients in one study, and 15% had no health insurance in another.[199,201] Health coverage concerns may affect vocational advancement, as some survivors feel they cannot accept a better position for fear of losing group health coverage. In North Carolina, survivors of childhood cancer were found to be more likely to be denied health insurance than their siblings, with an odds ratio of 15.1. In addition, the health insurance policies of these persons excluded care for preexisting medical conditions more often than did those of their siblings, with an odds ratio of 5.5. The cancer survivors reported problems in obtaining health insurance more frequently than did their siblings, with an odds ratio of 22.8.[202] Similarly, life insurance may be denied outright, or survivors may have to purchase policies with restrictive clauses. Life insurance problems are reported in 11% to 31% of disease-free survivors of Hodgkin lymphoma.[195,197] Terms of insurance policies and contracts are constantly changing. Cancer survivors who have problems with insurance should seek help from hospital insurance departments, local independent insurance agents, state insurance commission offices, patient support groups, and community agencies. Pediatric protocol therapy, coordinated by the cooperative clinical trials groups, has evolved as the standard of care for children with cancer. This standard has resulted in the development of safe and effective therapy for the majority of

children with malignancies. Denial of payment still can be expected for investigational or experimental (phase I) therapy. However, Childhood Cooperative Group phase II and III clinical trials should be routinely reimbursed.[200] Patients are encouraged to appeal claims denied for treatment prescribed by a therapeutic trial.

The significance of quality-of-life effects among survivors of childhood Hodgkin lymphoma is probably underestimated, as only recently has research funding become available to study these important issues. Although some investigators report that survivors of Hodgkin lymphoma seem to have learned to cope with problems related to their disease and treatment,[203] others caution that the impact of the disease and treatment can still be felt 10 to 18 years after treatment.[204]

Continued attention to these important issues is essential if the stigmata and sequelae suffered by survivors of Hodgkin lymphoma are to be reversed.

Children in whom Hodgkin lymphoma is diagnosed require continuous follow-up and assessment throughout their lives. During the childhood years, they should be managed by a multidisciplinary team concerned with the disease and its late effects. The issue arises regarding who should provide follow-up when a child reaches adulthood. Ideally, such persons will be followed by an internist or family practice physician for general medical concerns, and by a multidisciplinary oncology team concerned with late effects. With this dual management approach, long-term survivors have the greatest likelihood of having all late effects recognized and optimally managed.

THE FUTURE

Although efficacy in terms of event-free survival is typically estimated within 5 years of study entry, treatment-related morbidity and its affect on mortality require many more years to accurately assess. Today, many investigators of pediatric Hodgkin lymphoma still favor using combined-modality therapy for most children, as this approach offers the possibility of clinical staging, lower doses, smaller volumes of radiation, and fewer cycles of less toxic chemotherapy in comparison with single-modality therapy. However, despite the fact that recent investigations suggest that combined-modality therapy offers the highest probability of EFS for the majority children, the optimal treatment approach for an individual patient may vary. Host factors such as age and gender are routinely considered in regards to enhanced risks for specific treatment toxicities like musculoskeletal growth impairment, cardiopulmonary dysfunction, infertility, and second malignancy. The presence of constitutional symptoms, extranodal disease, tumor bulk, and number of involved nodal sites are among the cancer-related factors that are considered in the balance to determine the most effective and least toxic treatment approach.

Treatment programs in the new millennium still emphasize chemotherapy regimens that limit the cumulative doses of alkylating agents, anthracyclines, and bleomycin, with or without low-dose, involved-field radiation therapy to reduce the frequency and severity of treatment sequelae. Dose-intensive regimens are currently under study by pediatric groups with the goal of increasing anti-tumor effect and limiting cumulative doses of potentially toxic agents. When delivered over a short duration, dose-intensive regimens offer the potential to minimize cumulative doses and thus long-term toxicity. However, acute toxicity, especially myelosuppression and neuropathy, may be greater than that observed following conventional chemotherapy administered on a twice-monthly schedule. The OPPA/COPP combination featured in the German multicenter studies was one of the first dose-intensive regimens used in pediatric combined-modality trials.[9] Contemporary trials are attempting to emulate this success using regimens with lower doses of alkylating agents. The current Children's Oncology Group's intermediate-risk trial features a dose/time-intensive approach with ABVE-PC as the backbone therapy that eliminates procarbazine and restricts doxorubicin and etoposide doses. Similarly, pediatric Hodgkin consortium investigators from St. Jude, Stanford, and Boston are testing Stanford V and response-based (15–25.5 Gy), involved-field radiation therapy for children and adolescents with advanced and unfavorable disease.

Several contemporary trials are exploring early response as assessed by PET-CT imaging as a surrogate of long-term outcome to guide the need for therapy escalation or reduction.[61,62,205] In low-risk Hodgkin lymphoma, European and North American investigators are testing the prognostic accuracy of early resolution of FDG avidity as a guide to de-escalate therapy by omission of involved-field radiation. The long-term goal is to reduce the burden of therapy by using a treatment approach that adapts the type and intensity of initial chemotherapy to prognostic characteristics of the disease and unique risks of gender-related toxicity, and bases the indication for radiation on response to primary chemotherapy.

So far lymphocyte-predominant Hodgkin lymphoma has been treated according to protocols for classical Hodgkin lymphoma. However, the pathology and epidemiology of the disease suggest that lymphocyte-predominant Hodgkin lymphoma is a unique B-cell malignancy that (a) affects mainly boys, (b) presents as localized disease, (c) has a propensity for late relapse, and (d) is highly salvageable at relapse (see Chapter 22). Thus, ongoing trials for the treatment of early-stage lymphocyte-predominant Hodgkin lymphoma aim to postpone therapy in patients who present with localized and completely resected disease. This approach is supported by some European and North American investigators who have observed prolonged complete remission after complete resection of involved lymph nodes in patients with lymphocyte-predominant disease.[42,44,206] Thus, future trials for patients with lymphocyte-predominant Hodgkin lymphoma will be designed independent of protocols for patients with classical Hodgkin lymphoma.

The improvement of treatment efficacy for patients with high-risk disease remains challenging. More aggressive treatment approaches are clearly needed for some patients with advanced-stage disease; however, identification of patients at risk for treatment failure remains difficult. Prognostic data currently available have failed to distinguish a specific group of patients who would clearly benefit from early intensification of treatment.[207] The excellent cure rates accomplished with contemporary conventional regimens has limited the use of more intensive therapies, such as hematopoietic stem-cell transplantation, to the setting of salvage therapy. Identification of biologic factors that correlate with tumor response and host predisposition to treatment toxicity will be critical to more accurately guide risk-adapted therapeutic recommendations and improve outcome in high-risk patients.

Contemporary treatment planning for pediatric patients with Hodgkin lymphoma involves a multidisciplinary approach from the time of diagnosis. Factors that should be considered when therapy is designed include the age and physical maturity of the patient, disease stage and bulk, and potential treatment sequelae. Recommended therapy should provide the best opportunity for long-term disease-free survival with the lowest risk for severe treatment toxicity. In particular, efforts should be made to reduce or eliminate treatment exposures that increase the risk for serious treatment sequelae and so influence early mortality. With this approach, investigators have pioneered the effort to provide safe and effective treatment for pediatric patients with Hodgkin lymphoma and other childhood cancers.

References

1. Teillet F, Schweisguth O. Hodgkin's disease in children. Notes on diagnosis and prognosis based on experiences with 72 cases in children. Clin Pediatr (Phila) 1969;8:698–704.
2. Devita VT, Jr., Serpick AA, Carbone PP. Combination chemotherapy in the treatment of advanced Hodgkin's disease. Ann Intern Med 1970;73:881–895.
3. Donaldson SS. Pediatric Hodgkin's disease—focus on the future. In: Van Eys J, Sullivan M, eds. Status of the curability of childhood cancers., New York: Raven Press; 1980:235.
4. Donaldson SS, Link MP. Combined modality treatment with low-dose radiation and MOPP chemotherapy for children with Hodgkin's disease. J Clin Oncol 1987;5:742–749.
5. Gehan EA, Sullivan MP, Fuller LM, et al. The intergroup Hodgkin's disease in children. A study of stages I and II. Cancer 1990;65:1429–1437.
6. Jenkin D, Chan H, Freedman M, et al. Hodgkin's disease in children: treatment results with MOPP and low-dose, extended-field irradiation. Cancer Treat Rep 1982;66:949–959.
7. Maity A, Goldwein JW, Lange B, et al. Comparison of high-dose and low-dose radiation with and without chemotherapy for children with Hodgkin's disease: an analysis of the experience at the Children's Hospital of Philadelphia and the Hospital of the University of Pennsylvania. J Clin Oncol 1992;10:929–935.
8. Oberlin O, Boilletot A, Leverger G, et al. Clinical staging, primary chemotherapy, and involved field radiotherapy in childhood Hodgkin's disease. Eur Paediatr Haematol Oncol 1985;2:65–70.
9. Schellong G, Bramswig JH, Hornig-Franz I. Treatment of children with Hodgkin's disease—results of the German Pediatric Oncology Group. Ann Oncol 1992;3(suppl 4):73–76.
10. Klimo P, Connors JM. MOPP/ABV hybrid program: combination chemotherapy based on early introduction of seven effective drugs for advanced Hodgkin's disease. J Clin Oncol 1985;3:1174–1182.
11. Santoro A, Bonadonna G, Bonfante V, et al. Alternating drug combinations in the treatment of advanced Hodgkin's disease. N Engl J Med 1982;306:770–775.
12. Santoro A, Bonadonna G, Valagussa P, et al. Long-term results of combined chemotherapy-radiotherapy approach in Hodgkin's disease: superiority of ABVD plus radiotherapy versus MOPP plus radiotherapy. J Clin Oncol 1987;5:27–37.
13. Fryer CJ, Hutchinson RJ, Krailo M, et al. Efficacy and toxicity of 12 courses of ABVD chemotherapy followed by low-dose regional radiation in advanced Hodgkin's disease in children: a report from the Children's Cancer Study Group. J Clin Oncol 1990;8:1971–1980.
14. Hudson MM, Greenwald C, Thompson E, et al. Efficacy and toxicity of multiagent chemotherapy and low-dose involved-field radiotherapy in children and adolescents with Hodgkin's disease. J Clin Oncol 1993;11:100–108.
15. Hunger SP, Link MP, Donaldson SS. ABVD/MOPP and low-dose involved-field radiotherapy in pediatric Hodgkin's disease: the Stanford experience. J Clin Oncol 1994;12:2160–2166.
16. Oberlin O, Leverger G, Pacquement H, et al. Low-dose radiation therapy and reduced chemotherapy in childhood Hodgkin's disease: the experience of the French Society of Pediatric Oncology. J Clin Oncol 1992;10:1602–1608.
17. Schellong G. Treatment of children and adolescents with Hodgkin's disease: the experience of the German-Austrian Paediatric Study Group. Baillieres Clin Haematol 1996;9:619–634.
18. Vecchi V, Pileri S, Burnelli R, et al. Treatment of pediatric Hodgkin disease tailored to stage, mediastinal mass, and age. An Italian (AIEOP) multicenter study on 215 patients. Cancer 1993;72:2049–2057.
19. Weiner MA, Leventhal BG, Marcus R, et al. Intensive chemotherapy and low-dose radiotherapy for the treatment of advanced-stage Hodgkin's disease in pediatric patients: a Pediatric Oncology Group study. J Clin Oncol 1991;9:1591–1598.
20. Schellong G, Riepenhausen M, Creutzig U, et al. Low risk of secondary leukemias after chemotherapy without mechlorethamine in childhood Hodgkin's disease. German-Austrian Pediatric Hodgkin's Disease Group. J Clin Oncol 1997;15:2247–2253.
21. Grufferman S, Delzell E. Epidemiology of Hodgkin's disease. Epidemiol Rev 1984;6:76–106.
22. Westergaard T, Melbye M, Pedersen JB, et al. Birth order, sibship size and risk of Hodgkin's disease in children and young adults: a population-based study of 31 million person-years. Int J Cancer 1997;72:977–981.
23. Schellong G. Presented at the symposium on childhood Hodgkin's disease. XXIX Meeting of the International Society of Pediatric Oncology, Istanbul, Turkey. September, 1997.
24. Flavell KJ, Murray PG. Hodgkin's disease and the Epstein-Barr virus. Mol Pathol 2000;53:262–269.
25. Glaser SL, Lin RJ, Stewart SL, et al. Epstein-Barr virus-associated Hodgkin's disease: epidemiologic characteristics in international data. Int J Cancer 1997;70:375–382.
26. Alexander FE, Lawrence DJ, Freeland J, et al. An epidemiologic study of index and family infectious mononucleosis and adult Hodgkin's disease (HD): evidence for a specific association with EBV+ve HD in young adults. Int J Cancer 2003;107:298–302.

27. Gutensohn N, Cole P. Childhood social environment and Hodgkin's disease. *N Engl J Med* 1981;304:135–140.

28. Weinreb M, Day PJ, Niggli F, et al. The consistent association between Epstein-Barr virus and Hodgkin's disease in children in Kenya. *Blood* 1996;87:3828–3836.

29. Weinreb M, Day PJ, Niggli F, et al. The role of Epstein-Barr virus in Hodgkin's disease from different geographical areas. *Arch Dis Child* 1996;74:27–31.

30. Goedert JJ. The epidemiology of acquired immunodeficiency syndrome malignancies. *Semin Oncol* 2000;27:390–401.

31. Filipovich AH, Mathur A, Kamat D, et al. Primary immunodeficiencies: genetic risk factors for lymphoma. *Cancer Res* 1992;52:5465s–5467s.

32. Rowlings PA, Curtis RE, Passweg JR, et al. Increased incidence of Hodgkin's disease after allogeneic bone marrow transplantation. *J Clin Oncol* 1999;17:3122–3127.

33. Mack TM, Cozen W, Shibata DK, et al. Concordance for Hodgkin's disease in identical twins suggesting genetic susceptibility to the young-adult form of the disease. *N Engl J Med* 1995;332:413–418.

34. Alexander FE, Jarrett RF, Cartwright RA, et al. Epstein-Barr virus and HLA-DPB1-* 0301 in young adult Hodgkin's disease: evidence for inherited susceptibility to Epstein-Barr virus in cases that are EBV(+ve). *Cancer Epidemiol Biomarkers Prev* 2001;10:705–709.

35. Raaschou-Nielsen O, Hertel O, Thomsen BL, et al. Traffic-related air pollution at the place of residence and risk of cancer among children. *Ugeskr Laeger* 2002;164:2283–2287.

36. Porojnicu AC, Robsahm TE, Ree AH, et al. Season of diagnosis is a prognostic factor in Hodgkin's lymphoma: a possible role of sun-induced vitamin D. *Br J Cancer* 2005;93:571–574.

37. Marafioti T, Hummel M, Foss HD, et al. Hodgkin and reed-sternberg cells represent an expansion of a single clone originating from a germinal center B-cell with functional immunoglobulin gene rearrangements but defective immunoglobulin transcription. *Blood* 2000; 95:1443–1450.

38. Rosenquist R, Menestrina F, Lestani M, et al. Indications for peripheral light-chain revision and somatic hypermutation without a functional B-cell receptor in precursors of a composite diffuse large B-cell and Hodgkin's lymphoma. *Lab Invest* 2004;84:253–262.

39. Sandoval C, Venkateswaran L, Billups C, et al. Lymphocyte-predominant Hodgkin disease in children. *J Pediatr Hematol Oncol* 2002;24: 269–273.

40. Karayalcin G, Behm FG, Gieser PW, et al. Lymphocyte predominant Hodgkin disease: clinico-pathologic features and results of treatment – the Pediatric Oncology Group experience. *Med Pediatr Oncol* 1997;29: 519–525.

41. Regula DP, Jr., Hoppe RT, Weiss LM. Nodular and diffuse types of lymphocyte predominance Hodgkin's disease. *N Engl J Med* 1988;318: 214–219.

42. Pellegrino B, Terrier-Lacombe MJ, Oberlin O, et al. Lymphocyte-predominant Hodgkin's lymphoma in children: therapeutic abstention after initial lymph node resection—a study of the French Society of Pediatric Oncology. *J Clin Oncol* 2003;21:2948–2952.

43. Friedmann AM, Hudson MM, Weinstein HJ, et al. Treatment of unfavorable childhood Hodgkin's disease with VEPA and low-dose, involved-field radiation. *J Clin Oncol* 2002;20:3088–3094.

44. Dorffel W, Luders H, Ruhl U, et al. Preliminary results of the multicenter trial GPOH-HD 95 for the treatment of Hodgkin's disease in children and adolescents: analysis and outlook. *Klin Padiatr* 2003;215:139–145.

45. Donaldson SS, Glatstein E, Vosti KL. Bacterial infections in pediatric Hodgkin's disease: relationship to radiotherapy, chemotherapy and splenectomy. *Cancer* 1978;41:1949–1958.

46. Jerusalem G, Beguin Y, Fassotte MF, et al. Whole-body positron emission tomography using 18F-fluorodeoxyglucose for posttreatment evaluation in Hodgkin's disease and non-Hodgkin's lymphoma has higher diagnostic and prognostic value than classical computed tomography scan imaging. *Blood* 1999;94:429–433.

47. Weiner M, Leventhal B, Cantor A, et al. Gallium-67 scans as an adjunct to computed tomography scans for the assessment of a residual mediastinal mass in pediatric patients with Hodgkin's disease. A Pediatric Oncology Group study. *Cancer* 1991;68:2478–2480.

48. Baker LL, Parker BR, Donaldson SS, et al. Staging of Hodgkin disease in children: comparison of CT and lymphography with laparotomy. *AJR Am J Roentgenol* 1990;154:1251–1255.

49. Hanna SL, Fletcher BD, Boulden TF, et al. MR imaging of infradiaphragmatic lymphadenopathy in children and adolescents with Hodgkin disease: comparison with lymphography and CT. *J Magn Reson Imaging* 1993;3: 461–470.

50. Bader SB, Weinstein H, Mauch P, et al. Pediatric stage IV Hodgkin disease. Long-term survival. *Cancer* 1993;72:249–255.

51. Nachman JB, Sposto R, Herzog P, et al. Randomized comparison of low-dose involved-field radiotherapy and no radiotherapy for children with Hodgkin's disease who achieve a complete response to chemotherapy. *J Clin Oncol* 2002;20:3765–3771.

52. Smith RS, Chen Q, Hudson MM, et al. Prognostic factors for children with Hodgkin's disease treated with combined-modality therapy. *J Clin Oncol* 2003;21:2026–2033.

53. Mauch P, Tarbell N, Weinstein H, et al. Stage IA and IIA supradiaphragmatic Hodgkin's disease: prognostic factors in surgically staged patients treated with mantle and paraaortic irradiation. *J Clin Oncol* 1988;6: 1576–1583.

54. Dieckmann K, Potter R, Hofmann J, et al. Does bulky disease at diagnosis influence outcome in childhood Hodgkin's disease and require higher radiation doses? Results from the German-Austrian pediatric multicenter trial DAL-HD-90. *Int J Radiat Oncol Biol Phys* 2003;56:644–652.

55. Landman-Parker J, Pacquement H, Leblanc T, et al. Localized childhood Hodgkin's disease: response-adapted chemotherapy with etoposide, bleomycin, vinblastine, and prednisone before low-dose radiation therapy-results of the French Society of Pediatric Oncology study MDH90. *J Clin Oncol* 2000;18:1500–1507.

56. Schellong G. The balance between cure and late effects in childhood Hodgkin's lymphoma: the experience of the German-Austrian Study-Group since 1978. *Ann Oncol* 1996;7(suppl 4):67–72.

57. Claviez A, Tiemann M, Luders H, et al. Impact of latent Epstein-Barr virus infection on outcome in children and adolescents with Hodgkin's lymphoma. *J Clin Oncol* 2005;23:4048–4056.

58. Schellong G, Hornig-Franz I, Rath B, et al. Reducing radiation dosage to 20–30 Gy in combined chemo-/radiotherapy of Hodgkin's disease in childhood. A report of the cooperative DAL-HD-87 therapy study. *Klin Padiatr* 1994;206:253–262.

59. Cleary SF, Link MP, Donaldson SS. Hodgkin's disease in the very young. *Int J Radiat Oncol Biol Phys* 1994;28:77–83.

60. Hasenclever D. The disappearance of prognostic factors in Hodgkin's disease. *Ann Oncol* 2002;13(suppl 1):75–78.

61. Carde P, Koscielny S, Franklin J, et al. Early response to chemotherapy: a surrogate for final outcome of Hodgkin's disease patients that should influence initial treatment length and intensity? *Ann Oncol* 2002;13(suppl 1): 86–91.

62. Kostakoglu L, Coleman M, Leonard JP, et al. PET predicts prognosis after 1 cycle of chemotherapy in aggressive lymphoma and Hodgkin's disease. *J Nucl Med* 2002;43:1018–1027.

63. Devilard E, Bertucci F, Trempat P, et al. Gene expression profiling defines molecular subtypes of classical Hodgkin's disease. *Oncogene* 2002;21: 3095–3102.

64. Becherer A, Jaeger U, Szabo M, et al. Prognostic value of FDG-PET in malignant lymphoma. *Q J Nucl Med* 2003;47:14–21.

65. Filmont JE, Czernin J, Yap C, et al. Value of F-18 fluorodeoxyglucose positron emission tomography for predicting the clinical outcome of patients with aggressive lymphoma prior to and after autologous stem-cell transplantation. *Chest* 2003;124:608–613.

66. Baker KS, Gordon BG, Gross TG, et al. Autologous hematopoietic stem-cell transplantation for relapsed or refractory Hodgkin's disease in children and adolescents. *J Clin Oncol* 1999;17:825–831.

67. Lieskovsky YE, Donaldson SS, Torres MA, et al. High-dose therapy and autologous hematopoietic stem-cell transplantation for recurrent or refractory pediatric Hodgkin's disease: results and prognostic indices. *J Clin Oncol* 2004;22:4532–4540.

68. Schellong G, Dorffel W, Claviez A, et al. Salvage therapy of progressive and recurrent Hodgkin's disease: results from a multicenter study of the pediatric DAL/GPOH-HD study group. *J Clin Oncol* 2005;23:6181–6189.

69. Donaldson SS, Kaplan HS. Complications of treatment of Hodgkin's disease in children. *Cancer Treat Rep* 1982;66:977–989.

70. Hancock SL, Tucker MA, Hoppe RT. Factors affecting late mortality from heart disease after treatment of Hodgkin's disease. *JAMA* 1993;270: 1949–1955.

71. Anselmo AP, Cartoni C, Bellantuono P, et al. Risk of infertility in patients with Hodgkin's disease treated with ABVD vs MOPP vs ABVD/MOPP. *Haematologica* 1990;75:155–158.

72. Bramswig JH, Heimes U, Heiermann E, et al. The effects of different cumulative doses of chemotherapy on testicular function. Results in 75 patients treated for Hodgkin's disease during childhood or adolescence. *Cancer* 1990;65:1298–1302.

73. Clark ST, Radford JA, Crowther D, et al. Gonadal function following chemotherapy for Hodgkin's disease: a comparative study of MVPP and a seven-drug hybrid regimen. *J Clin Oncol* 1995;13:134–139.

74. Green DM, Brecher ML, Lindsay AN, et al. Gonadal function in pediatric patients following treatment for Hodgkin disease. *Med Pediatr Oncol* 1981;9:235–244.

75. Horning SJ, Hoppe RT, Kaplan HS, et al. Female reproductive potential after treatment for Hodgkin's disease. *N Engl J Med* 1981;304: 1377–1382.

76. Mackie EJ, Radford M, Shalet SM. Gonadal function following chemotherapy for childhood Hodgkin's disease. *Med Pediatr Oncol* 1996;27:74–78.

77. Ortin TT, Shostak CA, Donaldson SS. Gonadal status and reproductive function following treatment for Hodgkin's disease in childhood: the Stanford experience. *Int J Radiat Oncol Biol Phys* 1990;19:873–880.

78. Viviani S, Santoro A, Ragni G, et al. Gonadal toxicity after combination chemotherapy for Hodgkin's disease. Comparative results of MOPP vs ABVD. *Eur J Cancer Clin Oncol* 1985;21:601–605.

79. Wallace WH, Shalet SM, Hendry JH, et al. Ovarian failure following abdominal irradiation in childhood: the radiosensitivity of the human oocyte. *Br J Radiol* 1989;62:995–998.

80. Whitehead E, Shalet SM, Blackledge G, et al. The effect of combination chemotherapy on ovarian function in women treated for Hodgkin's disease. *Cancer* 1983;52:988–993.

81. Hamre MR, Robison LL, Nesbit ME, et al. Effects of radiation on ovarian function in long-term survivors of childhood acute lymphoblastic leukemia: a report from the Childrens Cancer Study Group. *J Clin Oncol* 1987;5: 1759–1765.

82. Sherins RJ, Olweny CL, Ziegler JL. Gynecomastia and gonadal dysfunction in adolescent boys treated with combination chemotherapy for Hodgkin's disease. *N Engl J Med* 1978;299:12–16.

83. Gerres L, Bramswig JH, Schlegel W, et al. The effects of etoposide on testicular function in boys treated for Hodgkin's disease. *Cancer* 1998;83: 2217–2222.

84. da Cunha MF, Meistrich ML, Fuller LM, et al. Recovery of spermatogenesis after treatment for Hodgkin's disease: limiting dose of MOPP chemotherapy. *J Clin Oncol* 1984;2:571–577.

85. Hassel JU, Bramswig JH, Schlegel W, et al. Testicular function after OPA/COMP chemotherapy without procarbazine in boys with Hodgkin's disease. Results in 25 patients of the DAL-HD-85 study. *Klin Padiatr* 1991;203:268–272.

86. Hill M, Milan S, Cunningham D, et al. Evaluation of the efficacy of the VEEP regimen in adult Hodgkin's disease with assessment of gonadal and cardiac toxicity. *J Clin Oncol* 1995;13:387–395.

87. Horning SJ, Williams J, Bartlett NL, et al. Assessment of the stanford V regimen and consolidative radiotherapy for bulky and advanced Hodgkin's disease: Eastern Cooperative Oncology Group pilot study E1492. *J Clin Oncol* 2000;18:972–980.

88. Pedrick TJ, Hoppe RT. Recovery of spermatogenesis following pelvic irradiation for Hodgkin's disease. *Int J Radiat Oncol Biol Phys* 1986;12: 117–121.

89. Kliesch S, Behre HM, Jurgens H, et al. Cryopreservation of semen from adolescent patients with malignancies. *Med Pediatr Oncol* 1996;26:20–27.

90. Madsen BL, Giudice L, Donaldson SS. Radiation-induced premature menopause: a misconception. *Int J Radiat Oncol Biol Phys* 1995;32: 1461–1464.

91. Hadar H, Loven D, Herskovitz P, et al. An evaluation of lateral and medial transposition of the ovaries out of radiation fields. *Cancer* 1994;74: 774–779.

92. Le Floch O, Donaldson SS, Kaplan HS. Pregnancy following oophoropexy and total nodal irradiation in women with Hodgkin's disease. *Cancer* 1976;38:2263–2268.

93. Holmes GE, Holmes FF. Pregnancy outcome of patients treated for Hodgkin's disease: a controlled study. *Cancer* 1978;41:1317–1322.

94. Sklar C, Whitton J, Mertens A, et al. Abnormalities of the thyroid in survivors of Hodgkin's disease: data from the Childhood Cancer Survivor Study. *J Clin Endocrinol Metab* 2000;85:3227–3232.

95. Constine LS, Donaldson SS, McDougall IR, et al. Thyroid dysfunction after radiotherapy in children with Hodgkin's disease. *Cancer* 1984;53:878–883.

96. Metzger ML, Howard SC, Hudson MM, et al. Natural history of thyroid nodules in survivors of pediatric Hodgkin lymphoma. *Pediatr Blood Cancer* 2006;46:314–319.

97. Papadakis V, Tan C, Heller G, et al. Growth and final height after treatment for childhood Hodgkin disease. *J Pediatr Hematol Oncol* 1996;18: 272–276.

98. Willman KY, Cox RS, Donaldson SS. Radiation induced height impairment in pediatric Hodgkin's disease. *Int J Radiat Oncol Biol Phys* 1994;28: 85–92.

99. Probert JC, Parker BR. The effects of radiation therapy on bone growth. *Radiology* 1975;114:155–162.

100. Merchant TE, Nguyen L, Nguyen D, et al. Differential attenuation of clavicle growth after asymmetric mantle radiotherapy. *Int J Radiat Oncol Biol Phys* 2004;59:556–561.

101. Chao N, Levine J, Horning SJ. Retroperitoneal fibrosis following treatment for Hodgkin's disease. *J Clin Oncol* 1987;5:231–232.

102. Hancock SL, Hoppe RT. Long-term complications of treatment and causes of mortality after Hodgkin's disease. *Semin Radiat Oncol* 1996;6:225–242.

103. Prosnitz LR, Lawson JP, Friedlaender GE, et al. Avascular necrosis of bone in Hodgkin's disease patients treated with combined modality therapy. *Cancer* 1981;47:2793–2797.

104. Rossleigh MA, Smith J, Straus DJ, et al. Osteonecrosis in patients with malignant lymphoma. A review of 31 cases. *Cancer* 1986;58:1112–1116.

105. Adams MJ, Lipshultz SE, Schwartz C, et al. Radiation-associated cardiovascular disease: manifestations and management. *Semin Radiat Oncol* 2003;13:346–356.

106. Adams MJ, Lipsitz SR, Colan SD, et al. Cardiovascular status in long-term survivors of Hodgkin's disease treated with chest radiotherapy. *J Clin Oncol* 2004;22:3139–3148.

107. Green DM, Gingell RL, Pearce J, et al. The effect of mediastinal irradiation on cardiac function of patients treated during childhood and adolescence for Hodgkin's disease. *J Clin Oncol* 1987;5:239–245.

108. Kadota RP, Burgert EO Jr., Driscoll DJ, et al. Cardiopulmonary function in long-term survivors of childhood Hodgkin's lymphoma: a pilot study. *Mayo Clin Proc* 1988;63:362–367.

109. Brosius FC III, Waller BF, Roberts WC. Radiation heart disease. Analysis of 16 young (aged 15 to 33 years) necropsy patients who received over 3,500 rads to the heart. *Am J Med* 1981;70:519–530.

110. Iarussi D, Pisacane C, Indolfi P, et al. Evaluation of left ventricular function in long-term survivors of childhood Hodgkin disease. *Pediatr Blood Cancer* 2005;45:700–705.

111. Cohen SI, Bharati S, Glass J, et al. Radiotherapy as a cause of complete atrioventricular block in Hodgkin's disease. An electrophysiological-pathological correlation. *Arch Intern Med* 1981;141:676–679.

112. Hancock SL, Donaldson SS, Hoppe RT. Cardiac disease following treatment of Hodgkin's disease in children and adolescents. *J Clin Oncol* 1993;11:1208–1215.

113. Scholz KH, Herrmann C, Tebbe U, et al. Myocardial infarction in young patients with Hodgkin's disease–potential pathogenic role of radiotherapy, chemotherapy, and splenectomy. *Clin Investig* 1993;71:57–64.

114. Hull MC, Morris CG, Pepine CJ, et al. Valvular dysfunction and carotid, subclavian, and coronary artery disease in survivors of hodgkin lymphoma treated with radiation therapy. *JAMA* 2003;290:2831–2837.

115. Adams MJ, Lipshultz SE. Pathophysiology of anthracycline- and radiation-associated cardiomyopathies: implications for screening and prevention. *Pediatr Blood Cancer* 2005;44:600–606.

116. Steinherz LJ, Steinherz PG, Tan CT, et al. Cardiac toxicity 4 to 20 years after completing anthracycline therapy. *JAMA* 1991;266:1672–1677.

117. Freter CE, Lee TC, Billingham ME, et al. Doxorubicin cardiac toxicity manifesting seven years after treatment. Case report and review. *Am J Med* 1986;80:483–485.

118. Goorin AM, Borow KM, Goldman A, et al. Congestive heart failure due to adriamycin cardiotoxicity: its natural history in children. *Cancer* 1981;47: 2810–2816.

119. Ali MK, Ewer MS, Gibbs HR, et al. Late doxorubicin-associated cardiotoxicity in children. The possible role of intercurrent viral infection. *Cancer* 1994;74:182–188.

120. Von Hoff DD, Layard MW, Basa P, et al. Risk factors for doxorubicin-induced congestive heart failure. *Ann Intern Med* 1979;91:710–717.

121. Lipshultz SE, Frassica JJ, Orav EJ. Cardiovascular abnormalities in infants prenatally exposed to cocaine. *J Pediatr* 1991;118:44–51.

122. Doll DC, Ringenberg QS, Yarbro JW. Vascular toxicity associated with antineoplastic agents. *J Clin Oncol* 1986;4:1405–1417.

123. Mills BA, Roberts RW. Cyclophosphamide-induced cardiomyopathy: a report of two cases and review of the English literature. *Cancer* 1979;43: 2223–2226.

124. O'Connell TX, Berenbaum MC. Cardiac and pulmonary effects of high doses of cyclophosphamide and isophosphamide. *Cancer Res* 1974;34: 1586–1591.

125. Bossi G, Cerveri I, Volpini E, et al. Long-term pulmonary sequelae after treatment of childhood Hodgkin's disease. *Ann Oncol* 1997;8(suppl 1): 19–24.

126. Marina NM, Greenwald CA, Fairclough DL, et al. Serial pulmonary function studies in children treated for newly diagnosed Hodgkin's disease with mantle radiotherapy plus cycles of cyclophosphamide, vincristine, and procarbazine alternating with cycles of doxorubicin, bleomycin, vinblastine, and dacarbazine. *Cancer* 1995;75:1706–1711.

127. Dubray B, Henry-Amar M, Meerwaldt JH, et al. Radiation-induced lung damage after thoracic irradiation for Hodgkin's disease: the role of fractionation. *Radiother Oncol* 1995;36:211–217.

128. Kaplan HS, Stewart JR. Complications of intensive megavoltage radiotherapy for Hodgkin's disease. *Natl Cancer Inst Monogr* 1973;36:439–444.

129. Libshitz HI, Banner MP. Spontaneous pneumothorax as a complication of radiation therapy to the thorax. *Radiology* 1974;112:199–201.

130. Rowinsky EK, Abeloff MD, Wharam MD. Spontaneous pneumothorax following thoracic irradiation. *Chest* 1985;88:703–708.

131. Polliack A. Late therapy-induced cardiac and pulmonary complications in cured patients with Hodgkin's disease treated with conventional combination chemo-radiotherapy. *Leuk Lymphoma* 1995;15(suppl 1):7–10.

132. Wolden SL, Lamborn KR, Cleary SF, et al. Second cancers following pediatric Hodgkin's disease. *J Clin Oncol* 1998;16:536–544.

133. Kushner BH, Zauber A, Tan CT. Second malignancies after childhood Hodgkin's disease. The Memorial Sloan-Kettering Cancer Center experience. *Cancer* 1988;62:1364–1370.

134. Meadows AT, Baum E, Fossati-Bellani F, et al. Second malignant neoplasms in children: an update from the Late Effects Study Group. *J Clin Oncol* 1985;3:532–538.

135. Meadows AT, Obringer AC, Marrero O, et al. Second malignant neoplasms following childhood Hodgkin's disease: treatment and splenectomy as risk factors. *Med Pediatr Oncol* 1989;17:477–484.

136. Bhatia S, Robison LL, Oberlin O, et al. Breast cancer and other second neoplasms after childhood Hodgkin's disease. *N Engl J Med* 1996;334: 745–751.

137. Cimino G, Papa G, Tura S, et al. Second primary cancer following Hodgkin's disease: updated results of an Italian multicentric study. *J Clin Oncol* 1991;9:432–437.

138. van Leeuwen FE, Chorus AM, van den Belt-Dusebout AW, et al. Leukemia risk following Hodgkin's disease: relation to cumulative dose of alkylating agents, treatment with teniposide combinations, number of episodes of chemotherapy, and bone marrow damage. *J Clin Oncol* 1994;12: 1063–1073.

139. Bhatia S, Yasui Y, Robison LL, et al. High risk of subsequent neoplasms continues with extended follow-up of childhood Hodgkin's disease: report from the Late Effects Study Group. *J Clin Oncol* 2003;21:4386–4394.

140. Dietrich PY, Henry-Amar M, Cosset JM, et al. Second primary cancers in patients continuously disease-free from Hodgkin's disease: a protective role for the spleen? *Blood* 1994;84:1209–1215.

141. Sankila R, Garwicz S, Olsen JH, et al. Risk of subsequent malignant neoplasms among 1,641 Hodgkin's disease patients diagnosed in childhood and adolescence: a population-based cohort study in the five Nordic countries. Association of the Nordic Cancer Registries and the Nordic Society of Pediatric Hematology and Oncology. *J Clin Oncol* 1996;14: 1442–1446.

142. Beaty OIII, Hudson MM, Greenwald C, et al. Subsequent malignancies in children and adolescents after treatment for Hodgkin's disease. *J Clin Oncol* 1995;13:603–609.

143. Perkins JL, Liu Y, Mitby PA, et al. Nonmelanoma skin cancer in survivors of childhood and adolescent cancer: a report from the childhood cancer survivor study. *J Clin Oncol* 2005;23:3733–3741.

144. Hancock SL, Tucker MA, Hoppe RT. Breast cancer after treatment of Hodgkin's disease. *J Natl Cancer Inst* 1993;85:25–31.

145. Kenney LB, Yasui Y, Inskip PD, et al. Breast cancer after childhood cancer: a report from the Childhood Cancer Survivor study. *Ann Intern Med* 2004;141:590–597.

146. Metayer C, Lynch CF, Clarke EA, et al. Second cancers among long-term survivors of Hodgkin's disease diagnosed in childhood and adolescence. *J Clin Oncol* 2000;18:2435–2443.

147. Swerdlow AJ, Barber JA, Hudson GV, et al. Risk of second malignancy after Hodgkin's disease in a collaborative British cohort: the relation to age at treatment. *J Clin Oncol* 2000;18:498–509.

148. van Leeuwen FE, Klokman WJ, Veer MB, et al. Long-term risk of second malignancy in survivors of Hodgkin's disease treated during adolescence or young adulthood. *J Clin Oncol* 2000;18:487–497.

149. Travis LB, Hill DA, Dores GM, et al. Breast cancer following radiotherapy and chemotherapy among young women with Hodgkin disease. *JAMA* 2003;290:465–475.

150. Mauch PM, Kalish LA, Marcus KC, et al. Second malignancies after treatment for laparotomy staged IA-IIIB Hodgkin's disease: long-term analysis of risk factors and outcome. *Blood* 1996;87:3625–3632.

151. Tarbell NJ, Gelber RD, Weinstein HJ, et al. Sex differences in risk of second malignant tumours after Hodgkin's disease in childhood. *Lancet* 1993;341: 1428–1432.

152. Hamilton AS, Mack TM. Puberty and genetic susceptibility to breast cancer in a case-control study in twins. *N Engl J Med* 2003;348:2313–2322.

153. Guibout C, Adjadj E, Rubino C, et al. Malignant breast tumors after radiotherapy for a first cancer during childhood. *J Clin Oncol* 2005;23:197–204.

154. Diller L, Medeiros Nancarrow C, Shaffer K, et al. Breast cancer screening in women previously treated for Hodgkin's disease: a prospective cohort study. *J Clin Oncol* 2002;20:2085–2091.

155. Kriege M, Brekelmans CT, Boetes C, et al. Efficacy of MRI and mammography for breast-cancer screening in women with a familial or genetic predisposition. *N Engl J Med* 2004;351:427–437.

156. Lehman CD, Blume JD, Weatherall P, et al. Screening women at high risk for breast cancer with mammography and magnetic resonance imaging. *Cancer* 2005;103:1898–1905.

157. Gonzalez-Angulo AM, Broglio K, Kau SW, et al. Women age < or = 35 years with primary breast carcinoma: disease features at presentation. *Cancer* 2005;103:2466–2472.

158. Landier W, Bhatia S, Eshelman DA, et al. Development of risk-based guidelines for pediatric cancer survivors: the Children's Oncology Group long-term follow-up guidelines from the Children's Oncology Group Late Effects Committee and Nursing Discipline. *J Clin Oncol* 2004;22:4979–4990.

159. Behrendt H, Brinkhuis M, Van Leeuwen EF. Treatment of childhood Hodgkin's disease with ABVD without radiotherapy. *Med Pediatr Oncol* 1996;26:244–248.

160. Ekert H, Toogood I, Downie P, et al. High incidence of treatment failure with vincristine, etoposide, epirubicin, and prednisolone chemotherapy with successful salvage in childhood Hodgkin disease. *Med Pediatr Oncol* 1999;32:255–258.

161. Hudson MM, Krasin M, Link MP, et al. Risk-adapted, combined-modality therapy with VAMP/COP and response-based, involved-field radiation for unfavorable pediatric Hodgkin's disease. *J Clin Oncol* 2004;22: 4541–4550.

162. Lobo-Sanahuja F, Garcia I, Barrantes JC, et al. Pediatric Hodgkin's disease in Costa Rica: twelve years' experience of primary treatment by chemotherapy alone, without staging laparotomy. *Med Pediatr Oncol* 1994;22: 398–403.

163. Shankar AG, Ashley S, Atra A, et al. A limited role for VEEP (vincristine, etoposide, epirubicin, prednisolone) chemotherapy in childhood Hodgkin's disease. *Eur J Cancer* 1998;34:2058–2063.

164. Atra A, Higgs E, Capra M, et al. ChlVPP chemotherapy in children with stage IV Hodgkin's disease: results of the UKCCSG HD 8201 and HD 9201 studies. *Br J Haematol* 2002;119:647–651.

165. Behrendt H, Van Bunningen BN, Van Leeuwen EF. Treatment of Hodgkin's disease in children with or without radiotherapy. *Cancer* 1987;59: 1870–1873.

166. Ekert H, Waters KD, Smith PJ, et al. Treatment with MOPP or ChlVPP chemotherapy only for all stages of childhood Hodgkin's disease. *J Clin Oncol* 1988;6:1845–1850.

167. Jacobs P, King HS, Karabus C, et al. Hodgkin's disease in children. A ten-year experience in South Africa. *Cancer* 1984;53:210–213.

168. Olweny CL, Katongole-Mbidde E, Kiire C, et al. Childhood Hodgkin's disease in Uganda: a ten year experience. *Cancer* 1978;42:787–792.

169. Ekert H, Waters KD. Results of treatment of 18 children with Hodgkin disease with MOPP chemotherapy as the only treatment modality. *Med Pediatr Oncol* 1983;11:322–326.

170. Baez F, Ocampo E, Conter V, et al. Treatment of childhood Hodgkin's disease with COPP or COPP-ABV (hybrid) without radiotherapy in Nicaragua. *Ann Oncol* 1997;8:247–250.

171. Sripada PV, Tenali SG, Vasudevan M, et al. Hybrid (COPP/ABV) therapy in childhood Hodgkin's disease: a study of 53 cases during 1989-1993 at the Cancer Institute, Madras. *Pediatr Hematol Oncol* 1995;12:333–341.

172. van den Berg H, Zsiros J, Behrendt H. Treatment of childhood Hodgkin's disease without radiotherapy. *Ann Oncol* 1997;8(suppl 1):15–17.

173. Ekert H, Fok T, Dalla-Pozza L, et al. A pilot study of EVAP/ABV chemotherapy in 25 newly diagnosed children with Hodgkin's disease. *Br J Cancer* 1993;67:159–162.

174. Sackmann-Muriel F, Bonesana AC, Pavlovsky S, et al. Hodgkin's disease in childhood: therapy results in Argentina. *Am J Pediatr Hematol Oncol* 1981;3:247–254.

175. Sackmann-Muriel F, Zubizarreta P, Gallo G, et al. Hodgkin disease in children: results of a prospective randomized trial in a single institution in Argentina. *Med Pediatr Oncol* 1997;29:544–552.

176. Weiner MA, Leventhal B, Brecher ML, et al. Randomized study of intensive MOPP-ABVD with or without low-dose total-nodal radiation therapy in the treatment of stages IIB, IIIA2, IIIB, and IV Hodgkin's disease in pediatric patients: a Pediatric Oncology Group study. *J Clin Oncol* 1997;15: 2769–2779.

177. Marcus RB, Weiner MA, Chauvenet AR. Radiation in pediatric Hodgkin's disease [in reply]. *J Clin Oncol* 1998;16:392.

178. Hutchinson RJ, Fryer CJ, Davis PC, et al. MOPP or radiation in addition to ABVD in the treatment of pathologically staged advanced Hodgkin's disease in children: results of the Children's Cancer Group phase III trial. *J Clin Oncol* 1998;16:897–906.

179. Kelly KM, Hutchinson RJ, Sposto R, et al. Feasibility of upfront dose-intensive chemotherapy in children with advanced-stage Hodgkin's lymphoma: preliminary results from the Children's Cancer Group study CCG-59704. *Ann Oncol* 2002;13(suppl 1):107–111.

180. Loeffler M, Hasenclever D, Diehl V. Model based development of the BEA-COPP regimen for advanced stage Hodgkin's disease. German Hodgkin's Lymphoma Study Group. *Ann Oncol* 1998;9(suppl 5):S73–S78.

181. Hudson MM, Poquette CA, Lee J, et al. Increased mortality after successful treatment for Hodgkin's disease. *J Clin Oncol* 1998;16:3592–3600.

182. Donaldson SS, Hudson MM, Lamborn KR, et al. VAMP and low-dose, involved-field radiation for children and adolescents with favorable, early-stage Hodgkin's disease: results of a prospective clinical trial. *J Clin Oncol* 2002;20:3081–3087.

183. Tebbi CK, Mendenhall N, London WB, et al. Treatment of stage I, IIA, IIIA(1) pediatric Hodgkin disease with doxorubicin, bleomycin, vincristine and etoposide (DBVE) and radiation: a Pediatric Oncology Group (POG) study. *Pediatr Blood Cancer* 2006;46:198–202.

184. Krasin MJ, Rai SN, Kun LE, et al. Patterns of treatment failure in pediatric and young adult patients with Hodgkin's disease: local disease control with combined-modality therapy. *J Clin Oncol* 2005;23:8406–8413.

185. Claviez A, Klingebiel T, Beyer J, et al. Allogeneic peripheral blood stem cell transplantation following fludarabine-based conditioning in six children with advanced Hodgkin's disease. *Ann Hematol* 2004;83: 237–241.

186. Williams CD, Goldstone AH, Pearce R, et al. Autologous bone marrow transplantation for pediatric Hodgkin's disease: a case-matched comparison with adult patients by the European Bone Marrow Transplant Group Lymphoma Registry. *J Clin Oncol* 1993;11:2243–2249.

187. Ferrell BR, Hassey Dow K. Quality of life among long-term cancer survivors. *Oncology (Williston Park)* 1997;11:565. Discussion on p. 572.

188. Gill TM, Feinstein AR. A critical appraisal of the quality of quality-of-life measurements. *JAMA* 1994;272:619–626.

189. Karnofsky DA, Burchenal JH. The clinical evaluation of chemotherapeutic agents in cancer. In: Macleod CM, ed. *Evaluation of chemotherapeutic agents.* New York: Columbia University Press; 1949:191.

190. Jenney ME, Kane RL, Lurie N. Developing a measure of health outcomes in survivors of childhood cancer: a review of the issues. *Med Pediatr Oncol* 1995;24:145–153.

191. Lansky LL, List MA, Lansky SB, et al. Toward the development of a play performance scale for children (PPSC). *Cancer* 1985;56:1837–1840.

192. Hoerni B, Eghbali H. Quality of life during and after treatment of Hodgkin's disease. *Recent Results Cancer Res* 1989;117:257–269.

193. Wasserman AL, Thompson EI, Wilimas JA, et al. The psychological status of survivors of childhood/adolescent Hodgkin's disease. *Am J Dis Child* 1987;141:626–631.

194. Yellen SB, Cella DF, Bonomi A. Quality of life in people with Hodgkin's disease. *Oncology (Williston Park)* 1993;7:41–45. Discussion on p. 46.

195. Fobair P, Hoppe RT, Bloom J, et al. Psychosocial problems among survivors of Hodgkin's disease. *J Clin Oncol* 1986;4:805–814.

196. Bloom JR, Fobair P, Gritz E, et al. Psychosocial outcomes of cancer: a comparative analysis of Hodgkin's disease and testicular cancer. *J Clin Oncol* 1993;11:979–988.

197. Kornblith AB, Anderson J, Cella DF, et al. Comparison of psychosocial adaptation and sexual function of survivors of advanced Hodgkin disease treated by MOPP, ABVD, or MOPP alternating with ABVD. *Cancer* 1992;70:2508–2516.

198. Hannah MT, Gritz ER, Wellisch D, et al. Changes in marital status and sexual functioning in long-term survivors and their spouses: testicular cancer versus Hodgkin's disease. *Psychosocial Oncol* 1992;1:89.

199. Kornblith AB, Anderson J, Cella DF, et al. Hodgkin disease survivors at increased risk for problems in psychosocial adaptation. The Cancer and Leukemia Group B. *Cancer* 1992;70:2214–2224.

200. Monaco GP, Fiduccia D, Smith G. Legal and societal issues facing survivors of childhood cancer. *Pediatr Clin North Am* 1997;44:1043–1058.

201. Hubbard SM, Longo DL. Treatment-related morbidity in patients with lymphoma. *Curr Opin Oncol* 1991;3:852–862.

202. Vann JC, Biddle AK, Daeschner CW, et al. Health insurance access to young adult survivors of childhood cancer in North Carolina. *Med Pediatr Oncol* 1995;25:389–395.

203. Joly F, Henry-Amar M, Arveux P, et al. Late psychosocial sequelae in Hodgkin's disease survivors: a French population-based case-control study. *J Clin Oncol* 1996;14:2444–2453.

204. van Tulder MW, Aaronson NK, Bruning PF. The quality of life of long-term survivors of Hodgkin's disease. *Ann Oncol* 1994;5:153–158.

205. Korholz D, Claviez A, Hasenclever D, et al. The concept of the GPOH-HD 2003 therapy study for pediatric Hodgkin's disease: evolution in the tradition of the DAL/GPOH studies. *Klin Padiatr* 2004;216: 150–156.

206. Murphy SB, Morgan ER, Katzenstein HM, et al. Results of little or no treatment for lymphocyte-predominant Hodgkin disease in children and adolescents. *J Pediatr Hematol Oncol* 2003;25:684–687.

207. Faguet GB. Hodgkin's disease: basing treatment decisions on prognostic factors. *Leuk Lymphoma* 1995;17:223–228.

CHAPTER 22 ■ CLINICAL PRESENTATION AND TREATMENT OF LYMPHOCYTE-PREDOMINANT HODGKIN LYMPHOMA

LUCIA NOGOVÁ, JEREMY FRANKLIN, VOLKER DIEHL, AND ANDREAS ENGERT

Lymphocyte-predominant Hodgkin lymphoma (LPHL) is rare, accounting for about 5% of all Hodgkin lymphoma cases in Western countries.[1] Patients with LPHL usually present with early clinical stage, cervical or inguinal involvement, and few if any adverse prognostic factors. Patients are predominantly male and most frequently in the 25- to 45-year age group. The disease progresses slowly, with fairly frequent relapses, which are rarely fatal.

This chapter describes the clinical characteristics, prognosis, and management of LPHL in comparison to classical Hodgkin lymphoma (cHL) subtypes, with special consideration given to the question of reducing primary treatment for patients with LPHL in early favorable stages.

HISTOLOGY

For more than half a century, efforts have been made to classify Hodgkin lymphoma pathologically. The aim was to establish reproducible and clinically useful categories and to understand better the underlying pathology of the disease. A lucid and comprehensive understanding of LPHL or "nodular paragranuloma" has been hampered by several factors, including the rarity of this diagnosis, with only occasional referrals to major centers. Therefore, published reports included few patients, and histologic subclassifications often diverged substantially, mainly because of ignorance of the origin and nature of the tumor cells. The unique biological and immunologic processes responsible for the cellular architecture of the tumor lesion, the clinical presentation, and the prognosis of this disease were also largely unknown. An indolent form of Hodgkin lymphoma morphologically characterized by a lymphocytic and histiocytic (L&H) background was first distinguished from other types in 1937 with use of the terms "early Hodgkin" and later (1944) "paragranuloma."[2] In 1966 it was renamed Hodgkin lymphoma of the L&H type and subdivided into a nodular and a diffuse form.[3] For practical reasons, these two infrequent subforms were combined at the Rye conference[4] into LPHL. Accordingly, the International Lymphoma Study Group proposed in the Revised European American Lymphoma (REAL) classification[5] to rename it as lymphocyte-predominant Hodgkin lymphoma (LPHL) and separate it from the other Hodgkin lymphoma subtypes as a clinicopathologic entity by subsuming these under the term "classical Hodgkin lymphoma."

Histologically, the nodular pattern of LPHL is characterized by the presence of atypical L&H or "popcorn" cells, embedded in a non-neoplastic nodular background composed mostly of small B-lymphocytes. In the diffuse pattern, the L&H cells are set against a diffuse background of reactive T-cells. L&H cells usually express the B-cell marker CD20 and lack expression of CD15 and CD30, the characteristic markers for cHL.[6] According to the current WHO definition, at least a partial nodular pattern is required for the diagnosis of lymphocyte-predominant Hodgkin lymphoma.[7] A purely diffuse pattern would be classified as a diffuse large B-cell lymphoma or T-cell-rich B-cell lymphoma.[8] The histopathologic pattern of LPHL differs from cHL, in which a few morphologically abnormal mononucleated and multinucleated giant cells, termed Hodgkin and Reed-Sternberg cells, are surrounded by a reactive infiltrate composed of T-cells, histiocytes, eosinophils, and plasma cells.[9]

It has been shown that LPHL and cHL are malignant B-cell lymphomas of germinal-center origin.[10] Furthermore, new published data demonstrate that a number of B-cell signal-transducing molecules are absent or reduced in Reed-Sternberg cells, whereas they are largely preserved in L&H cells and in non-Hodgkin B-cell lymphomas.[11] This may support the idea of distinct oncogenic mechanisms underlying the two forms of Hodgkin lymphoma, that is, cHL and LPHL.

RELATIONSHIP BETWEEN HISTOLOGY AND PROGNOSIS

In 1944, Jackson and Parker found that paragranuloma patients often remained disease-free for many years or had only localized recurrences of the disease showing very little proliferation activity. This contrasted with the short life expectancy of most Hodgkin lymphoma patients. Westling,[12] Harrison,[13] Wright,[14] and others confirmed the features of paragranuloma patients showing good survival, nonprogressive relapses, and transformation to granuloma. However, the results of other investigators cast some doubt on the prognostic value of histopathology. Peters, in 1950,[15] classified 113 patients according to both histologic subtype (a modification of Jackson and Parker's scheme) and extent of disease (using three clinical stages). The results demonstrated that clinical stage is a stronger prognostic factor than histologic subtype, and that within a given clinical stage, prognosis shows little or no dependence on histology. All patients received intensive involved-field or extended-field irradiation; this may well explain the generally good results and the reduced effect of histology on prognosis, which is representative of the trends in later years. Studies based on the Rye classification,[16–20] however, suggested that patients with LPHL had a better prognosis than those with other histologic subtypes.

319

In spite of the diminishing difference in clinical outcome between LPHL and the other forms of cHL, there is mounting evidence by morphologic, immunologic, and molecular-genetic data that nodular LPHL is a distinct disease entity, resembling more closely the indolent follicular non-Hodgkin lymphomas than cHL[21,22] Because LPHL accounts for only about 5% of all Hodgkin lymphoma cases, conclusive studies concerning pathogenetic, morphologic, and clinical aspects are lacking. Therefore in 1994 an international group of clinicians and pathologists under the auspices of the European Task Force on Lymphomas (ETFL) started a multicenter effort to collect pathologic and clinical material from patients primarily diagnosed as having LPHL, in order to better understand this rare disease.[1] The purpose was to investigate the clinical characteristics and course of patients diagnosed with LPHL and lymphocyte-rich classical Hodgkin lymphoma (LRcHL), classified by morphologic and immunophenotypic criteria. The Revised European-American classification of lymphoma neoplasms[5] formed the basis for the histopathologic classification. Clinical data and biopsy material (paraffin blocks) of all available cases diagnosed initially as LPHL (lymphocyte predominant-Rye) were collected from 17 European and American centers. Clinical data were obtained on stage, age, sex, laparotomy, B-symptoms, E-stage, mediastinal tumor, bulky disease, type of organ involvement, survival, relapse, number of relapses, death, causes of death, and therapy. Seven patients who were not treated or had surgery only, and patients younger than 16 years, were excluded from the analysis. Cases were newly classified, without prior knowledge of any corresponding clinical data, by a team of expert pathologists according to a modified REAL classification using morphologic and immunohistochemical criteria. The following categories were used: LPHL (n = 219 cases; 51%), LRcHL (n = 115; 27%), non-Hodgkin lymphoma (n = 12; 3%), cHL (n = 19; 5%), reactive lesions (n = 14; 3%), and technically inadequate sample (n = 47; 11%). Originally, LPHL was subdivided according to lymph node architecture into nodular (n = 189), diffuse (n = 9), and nodular and diffuse (n = 19) cases, but because no significant differences between these categories in clinical characteristics or prognosis were seen, they were pooled for subsequent analysis. For purposes of comparison, data were drawn from all evaluable patients in the multicenter trials of the German Hodgkin Lymphoma Study Group (GHSG) recruiting from 1988 to 1992[23] who were classified by the GHSG pathology panel as having nodular-sclerosis Hodgkin lymphoma or mixed-cellularity Hodgkin lymphoma.[24]

Furthermore, from these ETFL studies a new pathologically defined entity emerged: the lymphocyte-rich classical Hodgkin lymphoma (LRCHL), characterized by Reed-Sternberg cells, which are CD20 negative but CD30 and CD15 positive.

CLINICAL PRESENTATION OF LPHL

Age and Gender

According to the ETFL project results, LPHL has a similar age distribution (median 35 years) to cHL, whereas patients with LRcHL are older on average, with a median age of 43 years. Approximately 70% of LPHL and LRcHL cases were male (Table 22.1). This is similar to mixed-cellularity Hodgkin lymphoma and different from the nearly equal gender balance for nodular-sclerosis Hodgkin lymphoma. The new GHSG analysis comparing 394 patients with LPHL and 7,904 patients with cHL treated in the GHSG trials between 1988 and 2002 showed similar age and gender distribution: the median age was 37 in the LPHL group and 33 years in the cHL group. Patients with LPHL were predominantly males (75%).[25]

Stage and Systemic Symptoms

Table 22.1 shows that both LPHL and LRcHL cases (ETFL project) are mainly patients with early-stage disease: 53% of LPHL and 46% of patients with LRcHL had stage I disease and only 6% of each group had stage IV. This contrasts markedly with cHL. B-symptoms were observed in 10% LPHL, 11% LRcHL, and 42% nodular-sclerosis patients in the German trials.

The newer GHSG analysis demonstrates even higher rates of patients with early-stage LPHL: of 394 patients with LPHL, 63% were in early stage, 16% in intermediate stage, and 21% in advanced stage of disease. Of the 7,904 patients with cHL analyzed, 22% were in early, 39% in intermediate, and 39% in advanced stages, respectively. About 9% of patients with LPHL developed B-symptoms compared to 40% patients with cHL.[25]

In the other published studies, stage I accounted for 34% to 59% and stage IV for 1% to 12%. Thus, the proportion of early stages is consistently higher compared with cHL, and stage IV is much rarer. B-symptoms were present in 6% to 15% of cases. The average distribution of stages was as follows: stage I, 49%; stage II, 24%; stage III, 20%; stage IV, 7%; B-symptoms, 11%.[26-30]

TABLE 22.1

ETFL PROJECT: PATIENT CHARACTERISTICS

	LP (n = 219)	LRc (n = 115)	NS (n = 599)	MC (n = 174)
Age (median)	35 yr[a]	41 yr[a]	28 yr	35 yr
Sex (male)	74%	69%	49%	73%
Stage I	53%	46%	10%	21%
II	28%	24%	47%	32%
III	14%	24%	29%	35%
IV	6%	6%	14%	13%
B-symptoms	10%	11%	42%	35%

[a]For comparability with the GHSG trials, where entry is restricted to patients under 75 years of age, patients 75 or older were excluded in calculating these medians. Unrestricted values are 35 years for LPHL and 43 years for LRcHL.
LP, lymphocyte-predominant Hodgkin lymphoma; LRc, lymphocyte-rich classical Hodgkin lymphoma; NS, nodular sclerosis Hodgkin lymphoma; MC, mixed cellularity Hodgkin lymphoma.

TABLE 22.2

ETFL PROJECT: PATIENT CHARACTERISTICS

Type of involvement	LP (*n* = 219)	LRc (*n* = 115)	NS (*n* = 599)	MC (*n* = 174)
Bulky	13%	11%	54%	40%
Mediastinal	7%	15%	80%	40%
Spleen	8%	15%	10%	22%
Bone marrow	1%	1%	3%	10%
Liver	3%	3%	3%	5%
Lung	1%	4%	10%	1%
Skeletal	1%	0%	6%	3%
Other organ	2%	3%	8%	1%

LPHL, lymphocyte-predominant Hodgkin lymphoma; LRcHL, lymphocyte-rich classical Hodgkin lymphoma; NS, nodular sclerosis Hodgkin lymphoma; MC, mixed cellularity Hodgkin lymphoma.

Organ Involvement and Other Negative Prognostic Factors

Table 22.2 shows that site-specific organ involvement occurred with similar low frequency in LPHL and LRcHL in the ETFL analysis. It is chiefly lung involvement in nodular-sclerosis Hodgkin lymphoma and bone-marrow involvement in mixed-cellularity Hodgkin lymphoma that account for the higher fractions of stage IV cases among the cHL cases. The prognostic factors of bulky disease and mediastinal involvement are both comparatively rare in LPHL and in LRcHL; mediastinal disease occurred in only 7% of LPHL and 15% of LRcHL cases (*p* = 0.04). A small but fairly consistent percentage (1–4%) of patients with liver involvement is described in the other studies for which organ involvement rates are reported. Mediastinal involvement rates between 3% and 15% were found.[26–30]

For a reliable comparison of lymph node involvement between LPHL and other Hodgkin lymphoma subtypes, the analysis by Mauch and co-workers[31] of 719 patients uniformly staged using laparotomy and splenectomy is particularly suitable. Table 22.3 shows the prevalence of involvement of sites of lymphocyte predominance, nodular sclerosis, and mixed cellularity/lymphocyte depletion. LPHL seems to be localized more often in peripheral sites, such as upper neck, epitrochlear, and inguinal nodes. In contrast, central sites such as mediastinum, lung hila, lower neck, and upper abdomen are less frequently involved.

CLINICAL COURSE AND TREATMENT OUTCOME

LPHL in Early Favorable Stages

Clinical course and treatment outcome differ substantially by LPHL stages.[1,25] The ETFL project found differences in clinical outcome between early favorable stages, early unfavorable stages (early stages with risk factors or intermediate stages), and advanced stages.[1] According to this analysis, LPHL early favorable-stage patients can be sufficiently treated with reduced-intensity programs having less severe side effects.

TABLE 22.3

PREVALENCE (%) OF INVOLVEMENT IN NODAL SITES AND SPLEEN ACCORDING TO HISTOLOGIC SUBTYPE[a]

Involved site	LP (*n* = 63)	NS (*n* = 433)	MC/LD (*n* = 223)	*p* value
Upper neck	14	4	4	0.006
Side of neck (L,R)	41, 46	62, 55	53, 60	0.002 (L)
Axilla (L,R)	14, 13	15, 11	14, 16	NS
Mediastinum	8	73	46	<0.0001
Lung hilum (L,R)	5, 3	15, 14	8, 9	0.006
Upper abdomen	5	13	18	0.01
Lower abdomen	8	8	17	0.002
Inguinal (L,R)	10, 10	1, 1	3, 3	0.001

[a]Based on 719 laparotomy-staged patients reported by Mauch and associates.[31]
LP, lymphocyte predominant; NS, nodular sclerosis; MC/LD, mixed cellularity/lymphocyte depletion.

Analyses performed by the European Organization for Research and Treatment of Cancer (EORTC) suggested that the Hodgkin lymphoma-related death rate in patients treated for Hodgkin lymphoma decreases during the years after diagnosis. The overall mortality is higher compared to the general population, largely due to cardiac failures and secondary cancers.[32] Consequently, several new treatment approaches aimed at reducing toxicity were evaluated for patients with early favorable-stage LPHL to avoid side effects of standard treatment. Establishing a standard treatment for LPHL in early favorable stages is difficult due to the low incidence of LPHL and the very few events observed in this entity. As a result, treatment of early favorable LPHL stages is rather heterogeneous, including extended- and involved-field radiation, combined modality treatment, and more recently, monoclonal antibodies.[33–37]

Pediatric study groups reported nonrandomized case studies with small numbers of patients[38,39] suggesting that a watch-and-wait strategy after initial lymph-node resection may be an appropriate treatment. Pellegrino and associates retrospectively analyzed 27 children (median age, 10 years) most of whom had localized LPHL, who received either standard treatment or were not treated beyond initial lymphadenectomy. With a median follow-up of 70 months, overall survival was 100% and overall event-free survival (EFS) was 69%. EFS rates were not significantly different between the two groups. Patients with residual mass after initial surgery had a worse EFS if they did not receive additional treatment. Thus, treatment in these cases reduces the number of relapses but has no impact on overall survival.[38]

An American group of pediatric oncologists reported 15 children and adolescents (median age, 11 years) with localized LPHL. Patients received a selected therapy: those with stage I disease whose were disease-free after excision of the involved lymph node were carefully followed without further treatment. Patients with stage I or II disease who had incomplete resections were treated with brief chemotherapy consisting of vincristine, doxorubicin, cyclophosphamide, and prednisone. All treated patients reached complete remission; one patient in stage II relapsed 6 years after the initial diagnosis.[39]

These retrospective studies on small numbers of pediatric patients indicate promising results for early favorable LPHL. Treatment of this relatively benign malignancy, particularly in pediatric patients, strongly aims at avoiding adverse events such as growth retardation, infertility, hypothyroidism, cardiopulmonary complications, and second malignancies.

Schlembach and colleagues conducted an analysis on 36 patients with LPHL with nonbulky IA or IIA supradiaphragmatic or subdiaphragmatic disease and suggested involved-field or regional radiotherapy alone as an adequate treatment in patients with stage IA disease. The 5-year relapse-free and overall survival rates for the 20 patients with stage IA LPHL after involved-field or regional radiotherapy were 95% and 100%, respectively.[37] However, a larger patient number with longer follow-up will help to clarify the risk of cardiac toxicity, solid tumors, and late relapses that result from involved-field or regional radiotherapy.

Hoskin and associates published an analysis of 603 patients with clinical stage I and II Hodgkin lymphoma treated with radiotherapy alone. Patients with stage IA and IIA were randomized to receive involved-field or extended-field radiotherapy. The treatment failure after 25 years for patients with stage IA and IIA was 44% after extended-field and 54% after involved-field radiation. The incidence of second malignancies was 21% after involved-field and 20% after extended-field treatment. There were no significant differences in the causes of death between the randomized arms. Involved-field radiotherapy for patients with stage IA and IIA Hodgkin lymphoma results in an 11% greater risk of relapse compared with extended-field radiotherapy, but had no impact on overall survival and risk of second malignancy at 25 years. Although these data showed promising results in terms of low late toxicity, the analysis included no separate data on patients with stage IA LPHL.[40]

An Australian group published an analysis of 202 patients with LPHL in Stage I–II who were treated with radiotherapy alone. The treatment included predominantly mantle and inverted-Y field techniques. The overall survival rate at 15 years was 83% and freedom from progression was observed in 82% of the patients. There was no relapse and only 1 patient with non-Hodgkin lymphoma was reported after 15 years. Causes of death at 15 years were LPHL in 3% of patients, non-Hodgkin lymphoma in 2% of patients, in-field malignancy in 2% of patients, in-field cardiac/respiratory causes in 4% of patients, and other causes in 6% of patients. The authors demonstrated that radiotherapy may be curative for patients with stage I–II of LPHL and suggested that limited-field radiotherapy might be used without loss of treatment efficacy in this patient group.[36]

The GHSG reviewed all LPHL cases registered in the GHSG database and compared the different treatment approaches such as extended-field and involved-field radiation as well as combined-modality treatment for patients with stage IA LPHL. A total of 131 patients with LPHL in clinical stage IA without risk factors were analyzed; 45 patients were treated with extended-field radiotherapy, 45 patients had involved-field radiation, and 41 patients received combined-modality treatment. The median follow-up was 78 months in the extended-field group, 40 months after combined-modality treatment, and 17 months after involved-field radiotherapy, respectively. A total of 129 patients achieved complete remission (CR and CRu): 98% after extended-field radiotherapy, 100% after involved-field radiation, and 95% after combined- modality treatment. With a median follow-up of 43 months there were 5% relapses and only 3 patients died. Toxicity of treatment was generally mild, with most events observed after combined-modality treatment. After a median observation of 43 months the FFTF rate was 95% and overall survival (OS) rate 99% for all patients (Fig. 22.1). FFTF rates at 24 months were 100% for extended-field, 92% for involved–field, and 97% for combined-modality treatment (Fig. 22.2). In terms of remission induction, involved-field radiotherapy for stage IA LPHL is as effective as extended-field or combined-modality treatment. However, longer follow-up is needed before final conclusions can be drawn on the optimal therapy.[35] After their H7 trial (1988–1993), the EORTC has also adopted involved-field radiotherapy as standard treatment for stage IA LPHL.[41] Similarly, the guidelines panel of the National Cancer Center Network (NCCN) in the United States recommends local-regional irradiation as the treatment of choice for stage IA LPHL.[42] Thus, involved-field radiotherapy is currently being regarded as standard treatment for patients with stage IA LPHL.

LPHL in Early Unfavorable (Intermediate) and Advanced Stages

Due to the excellent treatment results in early favorable LPHL stages, several more recent analyses focused on outcome differences between LPHL and cHL to determine the suitable treatment for early unfavorable and advanced LPHL stages.[37,43,44]

Primary treatment results in the two major histopathologic groups of the ETFL project were identical, with 96% complete remission for both LPHL and LRcHL, somewhat higher than for the cHL cases of the GHSG (nodular sclerosis, 89%; mixed cellularity, 93%). There were slightly more relapses in the LPHL group (21% versus 17%). Survival and failure-free survival were analyzed using Hodgkin-specific measures

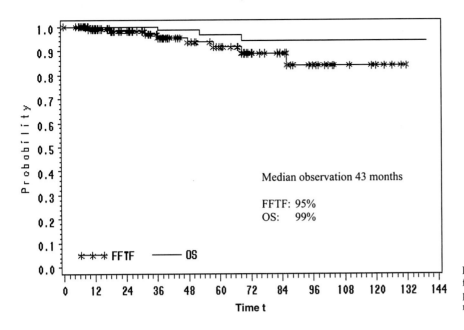

FIGURE 22.1. Freedom from treatment failure (FFTF) and overall survival (OS) for patients with stage IA lymphocyte-predominant Hodgkin lymphoma. Time in months.

because therapy-related or other non-lymphoma deaths were not relevant. Both survival and failure-free survival were significantly worse for those cases originally diagnosed as LPHL that were reclassified as cHL (*n* = 19) or as non-Hodgkin lymphoma (*n* = 12) by the ETFL review panel. It is apparent that the review process separated out a small fraction of cases with poor prognosis that did not belong to the LPHL or LRcHL groups. The LRcHL group is, however, not necessarily representative of cHL in general, because all of these cases had originally been classified as LPHL. Surprisingly, older patients were more frequent in both the cHL and non-Hodgkin lymphoma groups (47% and 58%, respectively, were over 50 years old at diagnosis). The survival and failure-free survival comparison of the ETFL groups of LPHL and LRcHL with cHL cases from the GHSG at 8 years were 95% (survival) and 74% (failure-free survival) for LPHL, and 87% (survival) and 75% (failure-free survival) for LRcHL. Overall survival was 89% for LPHL and 74% for

LRcHL at 8 years. Although survival is slightly worse for LRcHL, this difference was not significant (*p* = 0.067 for survival; *p* = 0.57 for failure-free survival). In addition, there is no difference when compared with the nodular-sclerosis or mixed-cellularity cases of the GHSG database. There is a trend towards better failure-free survival, but even if it is real, it is likely accounted for by the preponderance of early-stage cases in LPHL and LRcHL (Table 22.1). The indolent course with frequent but nonaggressive recurrences has long been regarded as typical of LPHL. The ETFL project results showed a tendency (not statistically significant) to more frequent late relapses and better long-term survival in LPHL compared with LRcHL or cHL. In general, the literature does not substantiate the assertion that patients with LPHL experience a late recurrence (after 10 years or more) more frequently than other Hodgkin lymphoma subtypes; however, long-term follow-up data for LPHL are scant.[1]

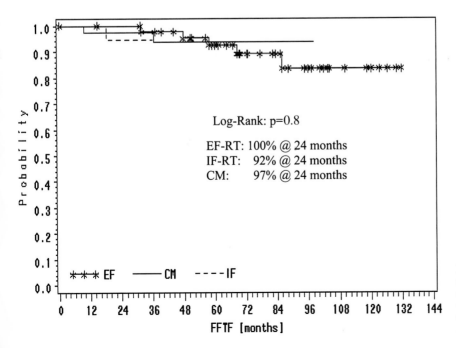

FIGURE 22.2. Freedom from treatment failure (FFTF) according to different treatment strategies for patients with stage IA lymphocyte predominant Hodgkin lymphoma. EF-RT, extended field irradiation; IF-RT, involved field irradiation; CM, combined modality therapy.

The GHSG recently published a new analysis comparing clinical characteristics and treatment outcome of patients with LRcHL with other Hodgkin lymphoma histologic subtypes. From a total of 2,715 patients with biopsy-proven Hodgkin lymphoma treated within the GHSG trials, 4% of patients with LRcHL, 5% with LPHL, 62% with nodular sclerosis, 27% with mixed cellularity, and 1% with lymphocyte depletion were identified. Comparison between LRcHL and LPHL showed that although on the basis of immunology and bio-chemistry LRcHL belongs to cHL, it clinically more closely resembles LPHL. In general there were no major differences in the clinical characteristics of patients with LRcHL and LPHL except for the significantly lower numbers of elevated erythrocyte sedimentation rate and B-symptoms in LPHL. The authors concluded that LRcHL and LPHL are the most curable Hodgkin lymphoma subtypes, with almost all patients responding to therapy and with excellent long-term EFS rates. Primary treatment outcome of LRcHL and LPHL is excellent with 30-month EFS rates of 97% and 94%, respectively without significant difference. The authors explained the differences between the previously published analysis of ETFL project[1] and the recent data by a different mechanism of selection. In the ETFL project, only patients with LRcHL who were previously misclassified as having LRcHL were reviewed.[45]

A French group analysis of 500 patients with Hodgkin lymphoma including 42 LPHL, 144 cHL without mediastinal involvement (MI), and 314 cHL patients with MI showed identical clinical characteristics for patients with LPHL and for patients with cHL without MI. These patient patterns were significantly different from those of patients with cHL with MI. The 15-year Hodgkin lymphoma mortality rates were similarly low in patients with LPHL and patients with cHL without MI. The study suggests that LPHL and patients with cHL without MI have a similar prognosis after a brief anthracycline-based chemotherapy followed by extended-field radiation.[44]

The GHSG recently retrospectively analyzed 8,298 patients with Hodgkin lymphoma treated on the GHSG trials: 394 patients with LPHL and 7,904 patients with cHL. A total of 91% of LPHL patients versus 86% of patients with cHL in early stage, 86% versus 83% in intermediate stage, and 79% versus 75% in advanced stage reached CR/CRu (Table 22.4). Some 0.3% patients with LPHL developed progressive disease compared to 3.7% of patients with cHL. The relapse rate of patients with LPHL was very similar to patients with cHL (8.1% versus 7.9%). There were 2.5% secondary malignancies in LPHL and 3.7% in cHL, and 4.3% LPHL and 8.8% patients with cHL died (Table 22.5). The FFTF rates for LPHL and patients with cHL at a median observation of 41 or 48 months were 92% and 84%, respectively. The OS for LPHL and patients with cHL was 96% and 92%, respectively. There was no difference in treatment outcome in terms of CR/CRu, progressive disease, and mortality between LPHL and cHL. Surprisingly there were also no differences in patients with relapses.[25]

It seems almost impossible to conduct randomized trials for patients with LPHL to compare stage-adapted treatment schedules due to the very low incidence and few events. The published data show that the treatment outcome of LPHL early unfavorable and advanced stages is not different from those of cHL. A future effort should be given to the identification of prognostic risk factors in these two LPHL stage groups. The current recommendation is to treat early unfavorable and advanced stages of LPHL according to the treatment protocols for cHL.

Role of Monoclonal Antibodies in LPHL

Therapy with monoclonal antibodies would be an option associated with lower treatment-related toxicity and very few if any late adverse effects. The GHSG conducted a phase-II trial to evaluate the chimeric monoclonal antibody rituximab in patients with relapsed or refractory LPHL.[33] Fourteen adults with CD20+ Hodgkin lymphoma at a median of 9 years after initial diagnosis received rituximab at standard doses once weekly for 4 weeks. The overall response was 86% with 20+ month duration of response.

The Stanford group published their results on 22 adult patients with either untreated or previously treated LPHL who received rituximab also at standard doses.[34] The overall response rate in this study was 100%. However, with a short median follow-up of 13 months, 9 patients had relapsed. Rituximab appeared to be less effective in patients with larger lymph nodes, stage III or IV disease, and more than 2 involved nodal regions. Both the GHSG study and this trial showed little toxicity and good feasibility, and suggest that rituximab might become a new treatment option for patients with CD20+ Hodgkin lymphoma. Another possible option would be to combine rituximab with cytotoxic drugs or radiotherapy in CD20+ Hodgkin lymphoma.

Prognosis after Relapse

In the ETFL study, most recurrences (76%) after an initial diagnosis of LPHL were confirmed as LPHL. However, 14% could not be clearly identified as Hodgkin lymphoma and 10% were classified as other Hodgkin lymphoma. In contrast,

TABLE 22.5

TREATMENT OUTCOME OF PATIENTS WITH LPHL AND CHL IN THE GHSG STUDIES

	LPHL (n = 394)	cHL (n = 7904)
Progress (%)	0.3	3.7
Relapse (%)	8.1	7.9
Secondary malignancies(%)	2.5	3.7
Death (%)	4.3	8.8

TABLE 22.4

TREATMENT OUTCOME (CR/CRu) OF PATIENTS WITH LPHL AND cHL IN THE GHSG STUDIES

Histology	Early stage (%)	Intermediate stage (%)	Advanced stage (%)	Total (%)
LPHL (n = 394)	91	86	79	88
cHL (n = 7904)	86	83	75	81

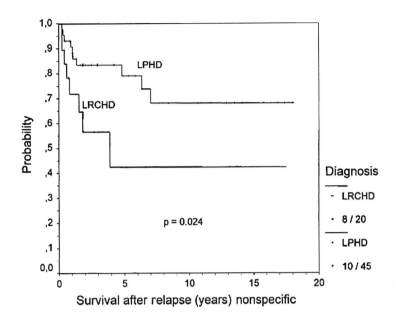

FIGURE 22.3. Survival after relapse (nonspecific) for lymphocyte-predominant Hodgkin lymphoma (LPHD) and lymphocyte-rich Hodgkin lymphoma (LRCHD).

more than half of the first recurrences after LRcHL were diagnosed as classical or unclassifiable Hodgkin lymphoma. Patients with LRcHL had a worse prognosis than patients with LPHL after relapse ($p = 0.024$) (Fig. 22.3). Further analysis revealed that this difference could partly be explained by the older average age of patients with LRcHL. Nevertheless, subgroup analysis of patients younger than 45 years also revealed a favorable prognosis after relapse for patients with LPHL (Fig. 22.4). Patients with LPHL also showed a tendency to more favorable survival after relapse compared with patients with cHL ($p = 0.050$). This, however, should be interpreted with caution because the patients with LPHL more often had early stage at first diagnosis and usually received less intensive first-line therapy.

Multiple relapses were observed in 12 of 45 relapsing patients (27%) in the LPHL group. There was only one multiple relapse in 19 patients (5%) with initial LRcHL ($p = 0.044$). Information on the sequence of relapse diagnoses was very incomplete but suggested that transformation to cHL is rare.

Surprisingly, the recent GHSG analysis showed no differences in terms of relapses between patients with LPHL or cHL

treated in three GHSG study generations. The relapse rate of LPHL was very similar to patients with cHL (8.1% versus 7.9%). However, further analyses are needed to better define an exact ratio of relapses between LPHL and patients with cHL.[25]

Nodular and Diffuse LPHL: Clinical Differences

Nodular LPHL is considered by many investigators to be a distinct entity within the spectrum of Hodgkin lymphoma, with a better prognosis than cHL. There are conflicting data, however, about the nature and prognosis of the diffuse and mixed variants of LPHL.

As mentioned earlier, in the ETFL project data no significant prognostic differences were observed between cases with nodular, diffuse, and nodular-plus-diffuse architecture. Neither were any differences in patient or disease characteristics visible. However, because there were only 9 purely diffuse cases (4%), the project data are inconclusive on these points.

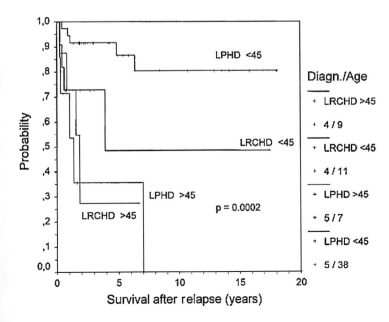

FIGURE 22.4. ETFL project. Survival after relapse of patients with lymphocyte-predominant Hodgkin lymphoma (LPHD), and lymphocyte-rich classical Hodgkin lymphoma (LRCHD) subdivided according to age above or below 45 years.

The study from Crennan and associates also revealed no prognostic differences between nodular and diffuse LPHL.[26] Others observed better but non significant relapse-free survival for diffuse cases ($p = 0.06$) without any sign of survival differences.[29]

Difficulties can occur in the differential diagnosis between diffuse LPHL and both LRcHL and T-cell–rich B-cell lymphoma.[46–48] The inclusion of a few borderline cases in the diffuse LPHL samples could explain the apparently worse prognosis in some reports. Moreover, the small proportion of diffuse cases diagnosed in the ETFL study, which had shrunk as further efforts were made to detect nodularity, casts doubt on the clinical relevance of this subdivision. In addition, these findigs underscore the need for a standardized expert review on histology for LPHL and related cases.

Relationship to Other Lymph Node Disorders Secondary to Non-Hodgkin Lymphoma After LPHL

The enhanced number of cases of non-Hodgkin lymphoma after primary LPHL has an impact on (a) choice of monitoring strategy after primary treatment and diagnostic measures in the event of a malignancy, (b) choice of primary treatment to destroy a potential concomitant non-Hodgkin lymphoma, and (c) choice of primary treatment to avoid treatment-related non-Hodgkin lymphoma. In the ETFL project, complete data on occurrence of second malignancies after LPHL were not collected, but all deaths from a second malignancy were recorded (Table 22.6). There were two fatal non-Hodgkin lymphomas following LPHL ($n = 219$) and two following LRcHL ($n = 115$). Median follow-up was 6.8 years for LPHL and 8.2 years for LRcHL. Four additional nonfatal occurrences of secondary

non-Hodgkin lymphoma were documented, 2 directly following primary LPHL and 2 after one or more relapses of LPHL, giving a total of at least 6 non-Hodgkin lymphomas after 219 cases of primary LPHL (2.9%).

These rates can be compared with those for Hodgkin lymphoma as a whole from the International Database on Hodgkin Disease (IDHD).[49] Of 12,411 patients with Hodgkin lymphoma, 106 developed a secondary non-Hodgkin lymphoma (0.9%), and the cumulative incidence rate for non-Hodgkin lymphoma was estimated as 1.0% after 10 years. A significantly higher risk for secondary non-Hodgkin lymphoma, increased by a factor 1.8, was found for patients with LPHL compared to nodular sclerosis and mixed cellularity ($p < 0.01$). On the basis of this evidence, an approximately two- to threefold higher rate of secondary non-Hodgkin lymphoma following LPHL compared with cHL is likely. In the IDHD analysis, combined-modality therapy was associated with an increased risk for developing non-Hodgkin lymphoma in univariate analysis but not in multivariate analysis.

Retrospective evaluation of data from patients with LPHL who developed a non-Hodgkin lymphoma indicates an aggressive clinical course with poor survival. Huang and co-workers retrospectively analyzed 21 patients with diffuse large B-cell lymphoma arising either concurrently with or subsequent to a diagnosis of LPHL. The median OS and FFS for the entire group were only 35 and 11 months, respectively. The predicted 5-year OS and FFS were 31 and 18%. Although the median survival was poor for the whole group, patients who achieved a complete remission with aggressive combination chemotherapy had a favorable outcome regardless of risk factors. Regimens for classical Hodgkin lymphoma appeared to be ineffective.[50]

In summary, there is evidence that non-Hodgkin lymphomas are more common following LPHL than other cHL subtypes. Treatment seems to play little role in causing secondary non-Hodgkin lymphoma.

TABLE 22.6

ETFL PROJECT: FATAL SECONDARY MALIGNANCIES

Diagnosis	Cause of death	Age at death (years)	Primary therapy	HL relapse
LPHL	Leukemia/MDS	77	CMT	No
LPHL	Leukemia/MDS	62	RT	Yes
LPHL	Leukemia/MDS	66	RT	No
LPHL	Leukemia/MDS	34	CT	Yes
LPHL	Leukemia/MDS	75	RT	No
LPHL	NHL	57	CT	No
LPHL	NHL	51	RT	No
LPHL	Solid tumor	67	RT	No
LPHL	Solid tumor	79	CT	Yes
LPHL	Solid tumor	83	RT	No
LRcHL	Leukemia/MDS	36	CMT	No
LRcHL	NHL	72	CT	No
LRcHL	NHL	45	RT	Yes
LRcHL	Solid tumor	82	RT	No

LPHL, lymphocyte-predominant Hodgkin lymphoma; MDS, myelodysplastic syndrome; CMT, combined modality treatment; RT, radiotherapy; CT, chemotherapy alone; NHL, non-Hodgkin lymphoma; LRcHL lymphocyte-rich classical Hodgkin lymphoma.

CONCLUSIONS

LPHL is typically diagnosed in male patients with a median age of 35 years presenting as early-stage disease without systemic symptoms or other adverse prognostic factors. These clinical features distinguish LPHL from cHL, which more often presents in advanced stage and with more adverse prognostic factors.

Historically, patients with LPHL in earlier stages had a better prognosis compared to patients with cHL. However, modern protocol treatment resulted in the disappearance of this difference. When patients of the same stage are compared, no significant differences in survival or failure-free survival were seen for LPHL as compared to cHL cases in the GHSG database. Patients with LPHL tend to relapse more frequently and late relapses are more common. However, their overall prognosis is better.

There is no conclusive evidence for clinical or prognostic differences between the nodular, diffuse, or mixed forms of LPHL. Studies differ widely in the proportion of diffuse cases; in the ETFL cohort only 4% of LPHL cases were purely diffuse. This division does not seem to be clinically relevant.

Secondary low-grade non-Hodgkin lymphomas occur more frequently after LPHL than after cHL. They seem to be disease related rather than treatment induced.

The resemblance of LPHL to nonmalignant disorders, with favorable clinical presentation and good survival rates even after relapse, suggests that the optimal primary treatment strategy might be less intensive than for cHL. Late toxicities, which contribute considerably to overall mortality, could thus be reduced. The long survival of selected patients with early favorable-stage LPHL who have had no treatment beyond lymph node excision could favor a watch-and-wait strategy, although only after rigorous staging. New experimental therapy techniques such as immunotherapy might also be suitable. These possibilities must first be tested in a large-scale prospective study.

The GHSG, EORTC, and NCCN recommend involved-field radiotherapy as a standard treatment for LPHL in early favorable stages. For early unfavorable stages and advanced stages, no differences in treatment outcome were found between LPHL and cHL. These stages should be treated according to standard Hodgkin lymphoma treatment guidelines.

References

1. Diehl V, Sextro M, Franklin J, et al. Clinical presentation, course, and prognostic factors in lymphocyte-predominant Hodgkin's disease and lymphocyte-rich classical Hodgkin's disease: report from the European Task Force on Lymphoma Project on Lymphocyte-Predominant Hodgkin's Disease. *J Clin Oncol* 1999;17:776–783.
2. Jackson H, Parker F. Hodgkin's disease II. Pathology. *N Engl J Med* 1944;231.
3. Lukes RJ, Butler JJ. The pathology and nomenclature of Hodgkin's disease. *Cancer Res* 1966;26:1063–1083.
4. Lukes RJB, Hicks EB. Natural history of Hodgkin's disease as related to its pathologic picture. *Cancer* 1966;19.
5. Harris NL, Jaffe ES, Stein H, et al. A revised European-American classification of lymphoid neoplasms: a proposal from the International Lymphoma Study Group. *Blood* 1994;84:1361–1392.
6. Anagnostopoulos I, Hansmann ML, Franssila K, et al. European Task Force on Lymphoma project on lymphocyte predominance Hodgkin disease: histologic and immunohistologic analysis of submitted cases reveals 2 types of Hodgkin disease with a nodular growth pattern and abundant lymphocytes. *Blood* 2000;96:1889–1899.
7. Jaffe E, Harris NL, Stein H, et al. *Pathology and Genetics of tumours of haematopoietic and lymphoid tissues.* Lyon, France: IARC Press; 2001: 241–243.
8. Nicholas DS, Harris S, Wright DH. Lymphocyte predominance Hodgkin's disease—an immunohistochemical study. *Histopathology* 1990;16: 157–165.
9. Thomas RK, Re D, Wolf J, et al. Part I: Hodgkin's lymphoma—molecular biology of Hodgkin and Reed-Sternberg cells. *Lancet Oncol* 2004;5:11–18.
10. Braeuninger S, Kueppers R, Strickler JG, et al. Hodgkin and Reed-Sternberg cells in lymphocyte predominance Hodgkin disease represent clonal populations of germinal center-derived tumor cells. *Proc Natl Acad Sci USA* 1997;94:9337–9342.
11. Marafioti T, Pozzobon M, Hansmann ML, et al. Expression of intracellular signaling molecules in classical and lymphocyte predominance Hodgkin disease. *Blood* 2004;103:188–193.
12. Westling P. Studies of the prognosis in Hodgkin's disease. *Acta Radiol* 1965; 245(suppl):5.
13. Harrison CV. Benign Hodgkin's disease (Hodgkin's paragranuloma). *J Pathol Bacteriol* 1952;64:513–518.
14. Wright CJE. The "benign" form of Hodgkin's disease (Hodgkin's paragranuloma). *J Pathol Bacteriol* 1960;80:157–171.
15. Peters MV. A study of survivals in Hodgkin's disease treated radiologically. *Am J Roentgenol* 1950;63:299–311.
16. Franssila KO, Heiskala MK, Heiskala HJ: Epidemiology and histopathology of Hodgkin's disease in Finland. *Cancer* 39:1280–1288,1977
17. Keller AR, Kaplan HS, Lukes RJ, et al. Correlation of histopathology with other prognostic indicators in Hodgkin's disease. *Cancer* 1968;22:487–499.
18. Landsberg T, Larsson LE. Hodgkin's disease retrospective clinico-pathologic study in 149 patients. *Acta Radiol Ther Phys Biol* 1969;8:390–414.
19. Gough J. Hodgkin's disease: a correlation of histopathology with survival. *Int J Cancer* 1970;5:273–281.
20. Kaplan HS. Hodgkin's disease and other malignant lymphomas: advances and prospects. G.H.A. Clowes Memorial Lecture. *Cancer Res* 1976;36:3863–3878.
21. Regula DP Jr, Hoppe RT, Weiss LM. Nodular and diffuse types of lymphocyte predominance Hodgkin's disease. *N Engl J Med* 1988;318:214–219.
22. Jaffe ES, Zarate-Osorno A, Medeiros LJ. The interrelationship of Hodgkin's disease and non-Hodgkin's lymphomas—lessons learned from composite and sequential malignancies. *Semin Diagn Pathol* 1992;9:297–303.
23. Loeffler M, Pfreundschuh M, Ruhl U, et al. Risk factor adapted treatment of Hodgkin's lymphoma: strategies and perspectives. *Recent Results Cancer Res* 1989;117:142–162.
24. Georgii A, Fischer R, Hubner K, et al. Classification of Hodgkin's disease biopsies by a panel of four histopathologists. Report of 1,140 patients from the German National Trial. *Leuk Lymphoma* 1993;9:365–370.
25. Nogova L, Reineke T, Josting A, et al. Lymphocyte-predominant and classical Hodgkin's lymphoma—comparison of outcomes. *Eur J Haematol* 2005(suppl):106–110.
26. Crennan E, D'Costa I, Liew KH, et al. Lymphocyte predominant Hodgkin's disease: a clinicopathologic comparative study of histologic and immunophenotypic subtypes. *Int J Radiat Oncol Biol Phys* 1995;31:333–337.
27. Pappa VI, Norton AJ, Gupta RK, et al. Nodular type of lymphocyte predominant Hodgkin's disease. A clinical study of 50 cases. *Ann Oncol* 1995;6:559–565.
28. von Wasielewski R, Werner M, Fischer R, et al. Lymphocyte-predominant Hodgkin's disease. An immunohistochemical analysis of 208 reviewed Hodgkin's disease cases from the German Hodgkin Study Group. *Am J Pathol* 1997;150:793–803.
29. Bodis S, Kraus MD, Pinkus G, et al. Clinical presentation and outcome in lymphocyte-predominant Hodgkin's disease. *J Clin Oncol* 1997;15:3060–3066.
30. Orlandi E, Lazzarino M, Brusamolino E, et al. Nodular lymphocyte predominance Hodgkin's disease: long-term observation reveals a continuous pattern of recurrence. *Leuk Lymphoma* 1997;26:359–368.
31. Mauch PM, Kalish LA, Kadin M, et al. Patterns of presentation of Hodgkin disease. Implications for etiology and pathogenesis. *Cancer* 1993;71:2062–2071.
32. Cosset JM, Henry-Amar M, Meerwaldt JH. Long-term toxicity of early stages of Hodgkin's disease therapy: the EORTC experience. EORTC Lymphoma Cooperative Group. *Ann Oncol* 1991;2(suppl 2):77–82.
33. Rehwald U, Schulz H, Reiser M, et al. Treatment of relapsed CD20+ Hodgkin lymphoma with the monoclonal antibody rituximab is effective and well tolerated: results of a phase 2 trial of the German Hodgkin Lymphoma Study Group. *Blood* 2003;101:420–424.
34. Ekstrand BC, Lucas JB, Horwitz SM, et al. Rituximab in lymphocyte-predominant Hodgkin disease: results of a phase 2 trial. *Blood* 2003;101:4285–4289.
35. Nogova L, Reineke T, Eich HT, et al. Extended field radiotherapy, combined modality treatment or involved field radiotherapy for patients with stage IA lymphocyte-predominant Hodgkin's lymphoma: a retrospective analysis from the German Hodgkin Study Group (GHSG). *Ann Oncol* 2005; 16:1683–1687.
36. Wirth A, Yuen K, Barton M, et al. Long-term outcome after radiotherapy alone for lymphocyte-predominant Hodgkin lymphoma: a retrospective multicenter study of the Australasian Radiation Oncology Lymphoma Group. *Cancer* 2005;104:1221–1229.
37. Schlembach PJ, Wilder RB, Jones D, et al. Radiotherapy alone for lymphocyte-predominant Hodgkin's disease. *Cancer J* 2002;8:377–383.
38. Pellegrino B, Terrier-Lacombe MJ, Oberlin O, et al: Lymphocyte-predominant Hodgkin's lymphoma in children: therapeutic abstention after initial lymph node resection—a Study of the French Society of Pediatric Oncology. *J Clin Oncol* 2003;21:2948–2952.
39. Murphy SB, Morgan ER, Katzenstein HM, et al. Results of little or no treatment for lymphocyte-predominant Hodgkin disease in children and adolescents. *J Pediatr Hematol Oncol* 2003;25:684–687.
40. Hoskin PJ, Smith P, Maughan TS, et al. Long-term results of a randomised trial of involved field radiotherapy vs extended field radiotherapy in stage I and II Hodgkin lymphoma. *Clin Oncol (R Coll Radiol)* 2005;17:47–53.

41. Raemaekers J, Kluin-Nelemans H, Teodorovic I, et al. The achievements of the EORTC Lymphoma Group. European Organisation for Research and Treatment of Cancer. *Eur J Cancer* 2002;38(suppl 4):S107–S113.

42. Hoppe RT, Advani RH, Bierman PJ, et al. Hodgkin disease/lymphoma. Clinical practice guidelines in oncology. *J Natl Compr Canc Netw* 2006;4:210–230.

43. Wilder RB, Schlembach PJ, Jones D, et al: European Organization for Research and Treatment of Cancer and Groupe d'Etude des Lymphomes de l'Adulte very favorable and favorable, lymphocyte-predominant Hodgkin disease. *Cancer* 94:1731–1738, 2002

44. Feugier P, Labouyrie E, Djeridane M, et al. Comparison of initial characteristics and long-term outcome of patients with lymphocyte-predominant Hodgkin lymphoma and classical Hodgkin lymphoma at clinical stages IA and IIA prospectively treated by brief anthracycline-based chemotherapies plus extended high-dose irradiation. *Blood* 2004;104:2675–2681.

45. Shimabukuro-Vornhagen A, Haverkamp H, Engert A, et al. Lymphocyte-rich classical Hodgkin's lymphoma: clinical presentation and treatment outcome in 100 patients treated within German Hodgkin's Study Group trials. *J Clin Oncol* 2005;23:5739–5745.

46. Poppema S. Lymphocyte-predominance Hodgkin's disease. *Int Rev Exp Pathol* 1992;33:53–79.

47. Hansmann ML, Stein H, Dallenbach F, et al. Diffuse lymphocyte-predominant Hodgkin's disease (diffuse paragranuloma). A variant of the B-cell-derived nodular type. *Am J Pathol* 1991;138:29–36.

48. Schmidt U, Metz KA, Leder LD. T-cell-rich B-cell lymphoma and lymphocyte-predominant Hodgkin's disease: two closely related entities? *Br J Haematol* 1995;90:398–403.

49. Henry-Amar M. Second cancer after the treatment for Hodgkin's disease: a report from the International Database on Hodgkin's Disease. *Ann Oncol* 1992;3(suppl 4):117–128.

50. Huang JZ, Weisenburger DD, Vose JM, et al. Diffuse large B-cell lymphoma arising in nodular lymphocyte predominant Hodgkin lymphoma: a report of 21 cases from the Nebraska Lymphoma Study Group. *Leuk Lymphoma* 2004;45:1551–1557.

LATE EFFECTS

CHAPTER 23 ■ LIFE EXPECTANCY IN HODGKIN LYMPHOMA

ANDREA K. NG, PETER M. MAUCH, AND RICHARD T. HOPPE

Hodgkin lymphoma is a highly curable form of malignancy that mostly affects young adults. Currently, over three-quarters of patients presenting with Hodgkin lymphoma will be cured, and the chance of cure among early-stage, favorable-prognosis Hodgkin lymphoma is over 90%. As the number of survivors of Hodgkin lymphoma increases and as they are followed over a longer period of time, however, it is becoming evident that their average survival does not revert completely to that of the age-matched general population.[1-9] The excessive mortality that patients face after they are cured of their Hodgkin lymphoma is largely a result of the long-term effects from management of their disease. A number of investigators have independently demonstrated that although cumulative Hodgkin lymphoma-specific mortality levels off over time, intercurrent deaths continue to rise with time, and with long enough follow-up, combinations of treatment-related mortality including second malignancies, cardiac diseases, and infections exceed mortality from Hodgkin lymphoma.[2,5,6,8,9]

Detailed knowledge and comprehensive understanding of the timing and distribution of mortality causes among survivors of Hodgkin lymphoma are crucial for physicians involved in their follow-up care. It may also help clarify the expectations on the overall prognosis of the affected patients and their families. The identification of factors that influence the long-term survival of patients with Hodgkin lymphoma may facilitate development of strategies that can help to prolong their life expectancy, as well as improve their quality of life. Potential approaches include modifying initial treatment to minimize acute and late toxicity, implementing risk reduction, prevention, and screening programs targeted at specific late effects.

In this chapter, we will summarize the data on the major causes of excessive deaths over time in patients who had been treated for Hodgkin lymphoma, factors that affect Hodgkin lymphoma-specific mortality, intercurrent mortality, and overall mortality. In addition, based on available information, we will propose ways that may improve the overall survival of patients successfully treated for Hodgkin lymphoma, and minimize the long-term sequelae associated with their diagnosis and treatment.

LONG-TERM RELATIVE CAUSES OF MORTALITY AFTER TREATMENT OF HODGKIN LYMPHOMA

A number of studies have evaluated the long-term outcomes of patients who have survived Hodgkin lymphoma.[1-14] Provencio and associates compared the long-term mortality of 477 patients with Hodgkin lymphoma with the general population.[15] At a median follow-up time of 8 years, the overall relative survival estimates, at 5, 10, and 15 years were 0.82, 0.73, and 0.71, respectively, suggesting that survival continued to be compromised long after the initial diagnosis. In this study, however, the causes of mortality were not reported. A limited number of studies are available that comprehensively evaluated the relative causes of mortality after Hodgkin lymphoma therapy. The distribution of the causes of mortality is highly dependent on the length of follow-up of the individual studies. Studies with inadequate follow-up time will only capture short-term causes of mortality such as deaths as a result of refractory or relapsing disease, and deaths related to immediate treatment toxicity. In order to capture events with protracted latency and to have a more accurate sense of the delayed causes of death, an adequate follow-up period is essential.

Table 23.1 summarizes the results of studies that reported causes of mortality among patients treated for Hodgkin lymphoma.[2-4,7-9,13] It is difficult to directly compare the results of these studies, as the follow-up times, initial stage distribution, types of treatment, and grouping of mortality causes vary from study to study. Also, different investigators may define "intercurrent" and "treatment-related" deaths differently. For instance, in the study by the International Database on Hodgkin's Disease, intercurrent deaths included deaths from cardiac causes or infections but did not include deaths from second malignancies.[2] Nevertheless, it is apparent that in studies with relatively short follow-up, Hodgkin lymphoma death has by far the greatest impact on mortality,[1,2,4] but for studies with longer follow-up time,[6-9] other causes of death, especially second malignancies and cardiac toxicities, increasingly contribute to the overall mortality.

Three of the studies were of adequate duration to include the period of time when deaths from Hodgkin lymphoma begin to be exceeded by deaths from other causes.[7-9] In the most recent update from the Netherlands Cancer Institute, examining long-term causes of death in patients treated for Hodgkin lymphoma at age 40 or younger, mortality from causes other than Hodgkin lymphoma surpassed that from Hodgkin lymphoma at 23 years (Fig. 23.1).[9] Data from the Harvard Joint Center for Radiation Therapy showed that deaths from second malignancies and cardiac toxicities combined exceeded deaths from Hodgkin lymphoma after 15 years of follow-up.[8] At 20 years after treatment, deaths from second cancers had the greatest impact on mortality (Fig. 23.2). Data from Stanford University revealed that the curves for the actuarial probability of death due to Hodgkin lymphoma and death due to other causes (including cardiovascular, secondary cancer, infection, pulmonary, gastrointestinal, accident/suicide, and unknown causes) intersect at 15 years after treatment.[7] The risk of dying from Hodgkin lymphoma beyond 15 years

TABLE 23.1

LONG-TERM CAUSES OF DEATH IN HODGKIN LYMPHOMA

Institution	Sample size	% Stages I–II	Mean or median follow-up	Number dead at follow-up	Distribution of mortality
IDHD[2]	14,225	63.6%	87.6 mo (mean)	4,139	Hodgkin lymphoma 67.1% Acute treatment-related 5.6% SM 10% Other intercurrent 13.9% (including cardiac, infections) Unspecified 3.4%
EORTC[3]	1,660	100%	Not stated	320	Hodgkin lymphoma 52.8% Acute treatment-related 8.1% SM 14.4% Cardiac 7.5% Intercurrent death 10% Unspecified 7.2%
BNLI[4]	1,057	Not stated	80 months (median)	43[a]	SM 30.2% Cardiac 14.0% Infection 30.2% Accident/suicide 7.0% Other 18.6%
Stanford[7]	2,498	59%	Not stated	754	Hodgkin lymphoma 44% Other cancers 21% Cardiovascular 16% Pulmonary 7% Infection 4% Accidental 2% Hematologic 1% Gastrointestinal 1% Other, multiple 2% Unknown 3%
Specht et al[13,b]	3,888	Majority	Not stated	360[a]	SST 26% SL 3.9% NHL 2.8% Cardiac 33.0% Pulmonary/iatrogenic 6.1% Infection 8.6% Other known cause 4.7% Unknown causes 11.7%
Harvard[8]	1,080	100%	12 years (median)	161	Hodgkin lymphoma 37% SM 37% Cardiac 11% Infection 4% Pulmonary 3% Miscellaneous 8%
The Netherlands Cancer Institute[9]	1,261	57%	17.8 years	113	Hodgkin lymphoma 54.5% Acute treatment-related 2.1% SM 21.7% Cardiac 9.4% Pulmonary 1.7% Infection 1.7% Others 8.9%

[a]Cause of death excluded Hodgkin lymphoma.
[b]Meta-analysis of 23 randomized trials for patients with early-stage disease.
NHL, non-Hodgkin lymphoma; IDHD, International Database on Hodgkin Disease; SM, second malignancy; EORTC, European Organization for Research and Treatment of Cancer; BNLI, British National Lymphoma Investigation; SM, second malignancy; SST, secondary solid tumors; SL, secondary leukemia; NHL, non-Hodgkin lymphoma.

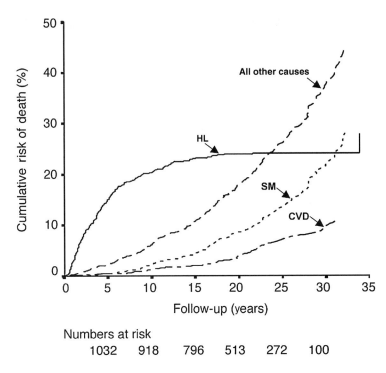

Numbers at risk
1032   918   796   513   272   100

FIGURE 23.1. Data from the Netherlands Cancer Institute on causes of mortality over time. (Adapted from Aleman BM, van den Belt-Dusebout AW, Klokman WJ, et al. Long-term cause-specific mortality of patients treated for Hodgkin's disease. *J Clin Oncol* 2003;21:3431–3439, Fig. 1, p. 3233, with permission.)

only rose slightly, while the risk of death from other causes increased sharply after 15 years (Fig. 23.3).

Limited data are also available addressing the issue of competing mortality and long-term causes of death in patients with childhood Hodgkin lymphoma. In a study from St. Jude Children's Research Hospital on 387 patients treated for pediatric Hodgkin lymphoma, with a median follow-up time of 15 years, the 20-year cumulative incidence of death from Hodgkin lymphoma was 9.8% while that from second malignancy was 4.3%.[16] Similar to studies on the adult population, Hodgkin lymphoma mortality plateaus after 15 years, while mortality from other causes continued to increase with time. In this study, despite the relatively long follow-up time, Hodgkin lymphoma was the leading cause of death, accounting for 51% of all deaths. Long-term follow-up studies of children differ from those of adults, however, particularly when assessing risk of adult-onset disease, and it is important to take attained age into account in addition to follow-up length when assessing specific late complications.[17]

It is clear that patients who enjoy long-term survival after treatment for Hodgkin lymphoma continue to face a markedly increased mortality risk. As illustrated by data from Harvard,[8] the absolute excess risk for all causes of deaths continued to increase at more than 15 years after initial diagnosis when patients are no longer at risk for death from Hodgkin lymphoma (Table 23.2). Absolute excess risk can be calculated as follows, expressed as absolute excess risk per 10,000 person-years:

$$\frac{(observed\ events - expected\ events)}{number\ of\ person\ years\ of\ follow-up} \times 10,000$$

The persistently increased risk of death emphasizes the importance of life-long follow-up care. Additional time is need to determine whether the excessive mortality in these patients will plateau or continue to rise, and when, if ever, their overall survival rate will return to that of the general population. In the following sections, we will describe each of the major causes of death in patients treated for Hodgkin lymphoma, their relative impact on overall mortality over time, and potential ways to minimize these fatal events.

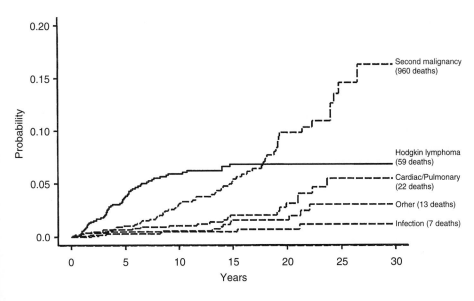

FIGURE 23.2. Data from Harvard on causes of mortality over time. (Adapted from Ng AK, Bernardo MP, Weller E, et al. Long-term survival and competing causes of death in patients with early-stage Hodgkin's disease treated at age 50 or younger. *J Clin Oncol* 2002;20:2101–2108, Fig. 2, p. 2106, with permission.)

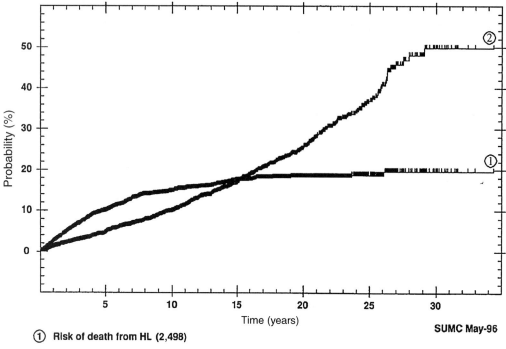

① **Risk of death from HL (2,498)**

② **Risk of death from other causes (2,498)**

FIGURE 23.3. Data from Stanford on causes of mortality over time. (Adapted from Hoppe RT. Hodgkin's disease: complications of therapy and excess mortality. *Ann Oncol* 1997;8(suppl 1): S115—S118, Fig. 1, p. S116, with permission.)

HODGKIN LYMPHOMA MORTALITY

Host- and Disease-Related Factors

The majority of the studies reporting on competing mortality over time in patients with Hodgkin lymphoma found that deaths due to Hodgkin lymphoma were largely limited to the first 10 to 15 years after treatment.[7–9,14] Hodgkin lymphoma-specific mortality is most closely related to the likelihood of refractory or relapsed disease. A number of factors have been identified as predictive of Hodgkin lymphoma relapse, most of which were based on patients treated with radiation therapy alone. These include age, disease stage, number of sites of disease, size of disease (large mediastinal adenopathy), constitutional symptoms, and extranodal disease (see Chapter 12).[18–23] Cooperative groups have used varying combinations of these factors, which largely reflect disease burden, potential for dissemination of disease, and the ability of the patient to tolerate treatment, to separate patients with early-stage disease into favorable- versus unfavorable-prognosis groups (see Chapters 16 and 17).[24–27]

In a study from Harvard Joint Center for Radiation Therapy on 1,080 patients with early-stage Hodgkin lymphoma, the competing causes of death were analyzed separately for patients with favorable and unfavorable prognosis (defined as presence

TABLE 23.2

DATA FROM HARVARD SHOWING COMPETING MORTALITY OVER TIME IN PATIENTS WITH STAGE I—II HODGKIN LYMPHOMA

Time interval (yr)	AR—all causes (per 10,000 PY)	RR—all causes[a]	No. dead of HL	Deaths excluding Hodgkin lymphoma		
				Dead	RR[a]	AR
All Pts	104.2	6.4 (5.5, 7.4)	60	101	4.0 (3.3, 4.9)	58.2
0–5	116.7	9.9 (7.7, 12.7)	38	25	3.9 (2.6, 5.7)	38.4
5–10	89.3	6.2 (4.3, 8.4)	17	21	3.5 (2.1, 5.2)	41.7
10–15	87.3	4.8 (3.2, 6.9)	5	22	4.0 (2.5, 5.8)	66.9
15–20	99.5	4.3 (2.6, 6.8)	0	18	4.3 (2.6, 6.8)	99.5
20+	157.5	4.9 (2.7, 8.1)	0	15	4.9 (2.8, 8.1)	157.5

[a]Numbers in parenthesis indicate the 95% confidence interval.
RR, relative risk; AR, absolute excess risk; HL, Hodgkin lymphoma; PY, person-years.

TABLE 23.3

DATA FROM HARVARD SHOWING COMPETING MORTALITY OVER TIME IN PATIENTS WITH STAGE I–II HODGKIN LYMPHOMA, ACCORDING TO PROGNOSTIC GROUPS

Time interval (PY)	AR—all causes (per 10,000 PY)	RR—all causes[a]	No. dead of HL	Deaths excluding Hodgkin lymphoma		
				Dead	RR[a]	AR
Favorable Prognosis Pts (n = 660)	78.0	4.9 (3.9, 6.1)	24	56	3.4 (2.6, 4.5)	48.6
0–5 (3,010)	56.3	5.2 (3.2, 7.8)	10	11	2.7 (1.4, 4.8)	23.1
5–10 (2,254)	80.2	5.6 (3.5, 8.2)	11	11	2.8 (1.4, 5.0)	31.3
10–15 (1,554)	79.3	4.3 (2.5, 7.1)	3	13	3.5 (1.9, 6.0)	60.0
15–20 (870)	83.9	3.7 (1.8, 6.8)	0	10	3.7 (1.8, 6.8)	83.9
20+ (472)	191.9	5.7 (2.8, 10.1)	0	11	5.6 (2.8, 10.1)	191.9
Unfavorable Prognosis Pts (n = 420)	148.0	9.1 (7.3, 11.3)	36	45	5.1 (3.6, 6.6)	74.1
0–5 (1,842)	215.5	18.2 (13.0, 24.1)	28	14	6.1 (3.3, 10.2)	63.5
5–10 (1,323)	104.8	7.5 (4.3, 12.2)	6	10	4.7 (2.2, 8.6)	59.4
10–15 (901)	101.2	5.8 (2.9, 10.4)	2	9	4.8 (2.2, 9.1)	79.0
15–20 (520)	125.7	5.4 (2.3, 10.7)	0	8	5.4 (2.3, 10.7)	125.7
20+ (287)	100.8	3.6 (1.0, 9.2)	0	4	3.6 (1.0, 9.2)	100.8

[a]Number in parenthesis indicate the 95% confidence interval.
RR, relative risk; AR, absolute excess risk; PY, person-years.

of B-symptoms, large mediastinal adenopathy, and 4 or more sites of disease).[8] The results are summarized in Table 23.3. Among patients with favorable-prognosis disease, 24 of the 80 deaths were due to Hodgkin lymphoma (30%), while among patients with unfavorable-prognosis disease, 36 of the 81 deaths were from Hodgkin lymphoma (44%). This was despite the fact that patients with unfavorable-prognosis disease were more likely to have received combined modality therapy compared with the favorable-prognosis group (64% versus 14%). In addition, a distinctive pattern of excess mortality over time was observed between the two groups of patients. In patients with favorable-prognosis disease, the absolute excess risk of mortality from all causes increased with time, predominantly from causes other than Hodgkin lymphoma, as patients were further out from initial diagnosis and treatment. In contrast, in the unfavorable-prognosis group, the absolute excess risk of mortality from all causes was the greatest in the first 5 years, and this was predominantly due to Hodgkin lymphoma deaths. The findings suggest that additional efforts are needed to limit long-term treatment-related mortality in patients with favorable-prognosis disease, while the priority in the management of patients with unfavorable-prognosis disease, including patients with advanced-stage disease, should continue to be optimizing disease control.

For patients with advanced-stage disease, a seven-factor prognostic scoring system was developed by the International Prognostic Factors Project that predicted 5-year rates of freedom from progression.[28] These included hypoalbuminemia, anemia, male sex, age of 45 years or older, stage IV disease, leukocytosis, and lymphocytopenia. The freedom-from-progression of disease at 5 years in patients with 0, 1, 2, 3, 4, and 5 or more number of factors was 84%, 77%, 67%, 60%, 51%, and 42%, respectively. The identification of these factors that significantly predicted for the likelihood of relapse had

important implications on selecting high-risk patients for more aggressive up-front treatment and for patient selection and stratifications as part of clinical trials. Of note, these factors were also found to independently predict for overall survival, although deaths specifically due to Hodgkin lymphoma were not separately reported.

Treatment-Related Factors

In addition to host- and disease-related factors, treatment-related factors have also been shown to affect relapse-free survival. Among patients with early-stage Hodgkin lymphoma, several trials comparing radiation therapy alone versus combined-modality therapy have shown a significantly higher relapse rate with radiation therapy alone,[29–31] although in most of these trials, the difference in relapse-free survival did not translate into a survival difference, due to the excellent salvage rate associated with radiation therapy alone and the potentially higher treatment-related morbidity and mortality with combined-modality therapy. This subject matter is well-illustrated by results of the meta-analysis by Specht and associates on early-stage Hodgkin lymphoma.[13] The authors found that the addition of chemotherapy to radiation therapy in stage I–II Hodgkin lymphoma halved the relapse rate, leading to a higher Hodgkin lymphoma-specific survival of borderline significance ($p = 0.07$) in the combined-modality therapy arm. However, they observed a 9% increase in the odds of death from known causes other than Hodgkin lymphoma in the combined-modality therapy group, and 11% if unknown causes are included with the deaths from other causes. Even though the elevated mortality from other causes was not statistically significant in the combined-modality therapy group, it was sufficient to counterbalance the borderline significantly higher Hodgkin lymphoma-specific survival in patients who received combined-modality therapy, such that no overall survival differences were observed between radiation therapy alone versus combined modality therapy.

However, there are data to suggest that a large enough difference in treatment efficacy may translate into significant differences in survival outcome. One example is the preliminary results of the United Kingdom Lymphoma Group LY-07 Trial,[32] comparing 4 weeks of vincristine, doxorubicin, prednisolone, etoposide, cyclophosphamide, and bleomycin (VAPEC-B) plus involved-field radiation therapy versus mantle radiation therapy alone in clinical stage I–II patients with favorable-prognosis disease. At a median follow-up time of 51 months, the 5-year relapse-free survival of the mantle radiation therapy alone arm was 70%, which was significantly lower than that of the combined-modality therapy arm of 87% ($p = 0.002$). A significant difference in overall survival between the two arms was also observed (92% versus 98%, $p = 0.036$). Although Hodgkin lymphoma-specific mortality was not separately reported, the difference in overall survival was likely mostly driven by Hodgkin lymphoma-specific mortality, as there were 5 Hodgkin lymphoma deaths in the mantle alone arm versus no Hodgkin lymphoma deaths in the combined-modality therapy arm.

For patients with unfavorable-prognosis and/or advanced-stage Hodgkin lymphoma, trials comparing different systemic regimens have shown differences in relapse-free survival rates. The superiority of the adriamycin, bleomycin, vinblastine, dacarbazine (ABVD) regimen over mechlorethamine, vincristine, procarbazine, and prednisone (MOPP) was demonstrated by the CALGB trial showing a significant failure-free survival benefit with the ABVD-based regimens in patients with advanced-stage disease.[33] In the most recent update, with a median follow-up of 14 years,[34] the significant difference in failure-free survival persisted, but there continued to be no overall survival differences, likely due to successful salvage in the inferior chemotherapy arm. However, in trials with treatment arms that are associated with markedly different disease control rates, significant survival differences can be seen. The German Hodgkin Study Group (GHSG) HD9 trial compared cyclophosphamide, vincristine, procarbazine, prednisone, adriamycin, bleomycin, vinblastine, and dacarbazine (COPP-ABVD),[35] a combination of bleomycin, etoposide, doxorubicin, cyclophosphamide, vincristine, procarbazine, and prednisone

(BEACOPP) in standard doses, and BEACOPP in increased doses in patients stage IIB or advanced-stage Hodgkin lymphoma. The 5-year freedom-from-treatment failure of the three arms were 69%, 76%, and 87% ($p < 0.001$), significantly favoring the increased-dose BEACOPP arm. Despite the higher treatment toxicity and secondary acute leukemia risk in the increased-dose BEACOPP arm, this more intensive chemotherapy arm was associated with a significant survival benefit when compared with the COPP-ABVD arm (91% versus 83%, $p = 0.002$). The findings suggest that with a sufficiently large difference in disease control rates between two treatment regimens, the excess of Hodgkin lymphoma deaths from refractory or recurrent disease overpowers lower treatment-related mortality associated with the less aggressive treatment approach.

Minimizing Hodgkin Lymphoma Mortality: Clinical Implications

The dilemma confronting physicians in deciding on the optimal management approach for patients with Hodgkin lymphoma is to balance between the goals of maximizing Hodgkin lymphoma-specific survival by comprehensive staging and adequate treatment, while reducing the long-term mortality from treatment-related causes. Although reducing treatment to limit toxicity is an important goal, there are scenarios in which the reduced treatment-related mortality may not be enough to offset the Hodgkin lymphoma deaths when clearly inadequate treatments are used. Treatment programs that involve use of less than standard therapy should therefore only be used in the setting of a clinical trial, in which patients can be closely monitored for potential excessive relapses.

Intercurrent Mortality

Unlike Hodgkin lymphoma-specific deaths, which tend to take place in the initial part of the follow-up period and have been relatively well documented, other causes of death in survivors of Hodgkin lymphoma occur later and their effect on long-term survival is still being defined. Of particular concern is the evidence of the rising risk of death from other causes with increasing follow-up time. As illustrated in Table 23.4, data from Stanford, Harvard, and the Netherlands Cancer

TABLE 23.4

DATA FROM STANFORD, HARVARD, AND THE NETHERLANDS CANCER INSTITUTE SHOWING ABSOLUTE EXCESS RISK[a] OF DEATH FROM CAUSES OTHER THAN HODGKIN LYMPHOMA ACCORDING TO FOLLOW-UP INTERVAL

Follow-up interval (yr)	Stanford				Harvard	Netherlands Cancer Institute[b]
	Stage I–II (1962–1980)	Stage I–II (1980–1996)	Stage III–IV (1962–1980)	Stage III–IV (1980–1996)	Stage I–II, age <50 (1969–1997)	All Stages, age <41 (1965–1987)
0–5	45	17	130	70	38.4	45
5–10	84	16	132	72	41.7	74
10–15	106	44	158	219	66.9	76
15–20	156	—	222	—	99.5	150
≥20	296	—	383	—	157.5	175
>30	—	—	—	—	—	275

[a]Expressed as per 10,000 person-years.
[b]Estimated from graph.

TABLE 23.5

DATA FROM STANFORD AND HARVARD SHOWING RELATIVE AND ABSOLUTE EXCESS RISKS OF SECOND MALIGNANCY AND CARDIAC DEATHS IN HODGKIN LYMPHOMA SURVIVORS

	Stanford	Harvard
O/E number of second malignancy deaths	104/16.6	59/5.3
RR of second malignancy death	6.3	11.2
AR of second malignancy death (/10,000 person-years)	43.5	41.2
O/E number of cardiac deaths	88/28.8	17/5.2
RR of cardiac death	3.1	3.2
AR of cardiac death (/10,000 person-years)	28	9.0

O/E, observed to expected; RR, relative risk; AR, absolute excess risk.

Institute showed increasing absolute excess risk of death from causes other than Hodgkin lymphoma at increasing follow-up interval.[7–9]

The two major causes of deaths other than Hodgkin lymphoma in the long-term survivors are second malignancies and cardiac diseases. Table 23.5 shows the results from Stanford and Harvard on the relative risk and absolute excess risk of death from these causes.[7,8] The other main causes of deaths in survivors of Hodgkin lymphoma include infection and pulmonary toxicities.

SECOND MALIGNANCIES

Development of second malignancies is a long-term complication that has received increasing attention since the early 1970s, and has been a growing contribution to the long-term mortality of patients treated for Hodgkin lymphoma (see Chapter 24). The elevated risk for second tumors in patients with Hodgkin lymphoma has been attributed to several factors, including direct leukemogenic or carcinogenic effects of the treatments, an impaired immune system related to treatments or the disease itself, and underlying genetic susceptibility to environmental carcinogens. Second malignancies after Hodgkin lymphoma can be divided into three main categories: leukemia, non-Hodgkin lymphoma, and solid tumors. The relative impact of each type of second malignancy on overall mortality depends on the timing and frequency of its occurrence and the survival outcome after its development.

Leukemia

Impact of Secondary Leukemia on Overall Survival

The prognosis of leukemia after Hodgkin lymphoma is extremely poor, and is almost uniformly fatal. The median survival is typically less than 6 months.[36,37] Recent data suggested that aggressive treatment of the secondary leukemia with high-dose therapy and allogeneic stem-cell transplantation may not provide a survival benefit over conventional-dose palliative chemotherapy or no therapy.[37] Despite the poor survival outcome, leukemia accounts for less than 5% of all mortality in patients with Hodgkin lymphoma,[9,13] due to the relative rarity of leukemia among survivors of Hodgkin lymphoma, with an estimated long-term cumulative risk of only 1 to 4%.[37–39] The risk is even lower in the modern era with the replacement of the MOPP regimen by ABVD, as alkylating agent-based chemotherapy is the key contributor to leukemia after Hodgkin lymphoma treatment.

Factors Associated with Risks of Secondary Leukemia

Exposure to alkylating-agent chemotherapy has clearly been identified by a number of series as the main culprit for secondary acute nonlymphocytic leukemia, the predominant form of leukemia after Hodgkin lymphoma.[37,40–44] The most comprehensive study on leukemia risk following Hodgkin lymphoma treatment with respect to chemotherapy history is a case-control study by van Leeuwen and colleagues from the Netherlands Cancer Institute.[41] Detailed information was obtained for 44 cases of leukemia and compared against 124 matched controls. The cumulative dose of mechlorethamine was identified as the most important factor in determining leukemia risk. A significantly elevated risk was particularly seen for patients who received a cumulative dose of greater than 110 mg. A study from the same group reported that leukemia risk in patients treated with chemotherapy prior to 1980, compared with patients treated after 1980, was approximately three-fold higher.[45] Patients treated in the earlier period received predominantly MOPP chemotherapy, while the more recently treated patients received mainly alternating MOPP/ABVD, in which the total dose of alkylating chemotherapy agents is lower. The results again demonstrated the association between mechlorethamine-based chemotherapy and secondary leukemia.

A French study compared the 15-year risk of secondary leukemia in 869 patients with Hodgkin lymphoma treated with either MOPP or ABVD chemotherapy. A total of 11 cases of acute nonlymphoblastic leukemia (ANLL) and 2 cases of acute lymphoblastic leukemia (ALL) were observed.[46] The 15-year actuarial risk of ANLL was 3.4% after MOPP chemotherapy and 0.7% after ABVD chemotherapy. This study with long-term results confirmed the lower risk of leukemia in patients treated with the ABVD regimen.

In recent years, alternative chemotherapy regimens have been developed in an attempt to improve the cure rate of patients with advanced Hodgkin lymphoma. Stanford V is a 12-week, 7-drug regimen (mechlorethamine, doxorubicin, vinblastine, vincristine, bleomycin, etoposide, and prednisone) that contains lower cumulative doses of mechlorethamine, Adriamycin, and bleomycin than MOPP and ABVD, respectively, and with the addition of radiation therapy to 36 Gy for patients with initial disease of 5 cm or larger. Thus far, this regimen does not appear to be associated with an increased leukemia risk.[47] The dose-escalated BEACOPP regimen, developed by the GHSG, has been shown to have significantly better treatment outcome than conventional-dose chemotherapy in patients with advanced Hodgkin lymphoma.[35] However, it is associated with a 2.9% actuarial risk of secondary leukemia at 5 years, and additional follow-up time is needed to determine the long-term leukemia risk with the use of this regimen.

High-dose therapy with autologous hematopoietic stem-cell transplantation is increasingly used as a potentially curative treatment strategy for patients with relapsed or refractory Hodgkin lymphoma after conventional chemotherapy. Several studies have shown that this approach may be associated with an increased risk of secondary myelodysplastic syndrome/acute myeloid leukemia (MDS/AML).[48-52] Factors including the extent of pretransplant therapy, types of conditioning regimen, use of peripheral blood stem cells, and older age at transplantation have been implicated in contributing to the risk.[48-50,52]

Investigators have also explored the relationship between radiation therapy and subsequent leukemia risk. Several studies found leukemia risk after radiotherapy alone for Hodgkin lymphoma to be negligible.[39,53-57] Whether radiation therapy adds to the leukemia risk of chemotherapy is controversial, and the results vary from study to study. In one large case-control study from a collaborative study group,[40] 163 cases of leukemia following treatment for Hodgkin lymphoma were reviewed. The results demonstrated that when the number of cycles of chemotherapy was held constant, addition of radiotherapy did not increase the risk of leukemia above that produced by the use of chemotherapy alone. On the other hand, in a study by Delwail and co-workers among patients who received MOPP chemotherapy, patients who received extended-field radiation therapy had an actuarial risk of secondary leukemia of 13.9%, versus 2.4% among patients treated with limited-field radiation therapy.[46] The extent of radiation therapy, however, did not have an impact on the leukemia risk in the group of patients treated with ABVD chemotherapy.

The association between splenectomy and increased risk for secondary leukemia was first reported by van Leeuwen and associates in 1987.[58] Their findings were confirmed by a number of subsequent studies, some of which controlled for the amount of chemotherapy received,[40,58-60] while others have not been able to come to the same conclusion.[53,61,62] Similar elevated risk has not been observed in patients who were splenectomized for other reasons (e.g., trauma),[63] implying that cancer risk after a splenectomy may be influenced by a patient's baseline immune status.

Minimizing Secondary Leukemia Mortality: Clinical Implications

Given the overwhelming evidence of the association between high doses of alkylating agents and leukemia risk, the most effective way to minimize leukemia deaths is to limit the dose of alkylating agents. Although MOPP is no longer used as part of initial treatment for Hodgkin lymphoma, it is sometimes used in the salvage setting. Also, some of the newer chemotherapy regimens do contain alkylating agents, and longer follow-up time is needed to determine the true magnitude of the leukemia risk. Available data suggest that the risk of secondary leukemia risk may be especially increased in patients who are receiving both extended-field radiation therapy and alkylating agent-based chemotherapy. Efforts should therefore be made to avoid large-field radiation therapy in patients who are treated with some of the newer regimens that contain high doses of alkylating agents.[35] As high-dose therapy with autologous stem-cell transplantation is increasingly used for patients with refractory or relapse disease after chemotherapy, ways to decrease the risk of secondary MDS/AML include avoiding the use of total body irradiation, and by substituting cytostatic drugs that do not have leukemic potential for alkylating agents and topoisomerase II inhibitors in the preparative regimens.

Non-Hodgkin Lymphoma

Impact of Non-Hodgkin Lymphoma on Overall Survival

The long-term cumulative risk of non-Hodgkin lymphoma after Hodgkin lymphoma ranges from 1% to 6%, and its reported absolute excess risk ranges from 2.5 to 14/10,000 person-years.[36,38,39,64] The risk of non-Hodgkin lymphoma is slightly lower than the risk of secondary leukemia, and the associated prognosis is better than that for patients with leukemia. Its contribution to the overall mortality of survivors of Hodgkin lymphoma is estimated to be less than 5%.[9,12,13] The German Hodgkin Study Group reviewed 51 cases of secondary non-Hodgkin lymphoma after Hodgkin lymphoma, and found diffuse large-B cell lymphoma to be the most common histology, accounting for 78% of the cases.[64]

The survival outcomes of non-Hodgkin lymphoma after Hodgkin lymphoma are comparable to those observed in stage III or IV aggressive primary non-Hodgkin lymphoma, in which the 5-year overall survival rates range between 30% and 40%.[55,59,64,65] In one study, the treatment outcome of non-Hodgkin lymphoma that developed after Hodgkin lymphoma was found to be significantly worse in those with a shorter time from initial Hodgkin lymphoma therapy.[64] This may be due to either a more aggressive composite lymphoma that was not detected at the initial Hodgkin lymphoma diagnosis, or compromised treatment of the non-Hodgkin lymphoma due to the recent Hodgkin lymphoma therapy. In that study, the authors also showed that better treatment outcome was achieved when patients received doxorubicin-based chemotherapy.

Factors Associated with Risks of Non-Hodgkin Lymphoma

The risk of developing non-Hodgkin lymphoma after Hodgkin lymphoma appears to be relatively independent of the time from completion of treatment, or type of initial treatment received.[39,55,62,64] Results from several larger series suggested that there may be an elevated risk after more extensive treatment.[45,59] Other factors that have been associated with increased risk for non-Hodgkin lymphoma include older age at diagnosis[66] and lymphocyte-predominant histology.[59,67] Overall, however, there appears to be a lack of consistent pattern on risk factors for subsequent development of non-Hodgkin lymphoma. It may partly reflect pathologic misclassification in some of the studies, or differences in diagnostic criteria for Hodgkin lymphoma and non-Hodgkin lymphoma. Development of non-Hodgkin lymphoma after Hodgkin lymphoma treatments may be multifactorial. It may be directly treatment-induced, or it could be part of the natural course of Hodgkin lymphoma, especially for the lymphocyte predominant subtype.[68,69] The excessive risk could also be a result of the immunosuppressed status of patients with Hodgkin lymphoma, similar to the increased non-Hodgkin lymphoma risk in other groups of immunocompromised patients such as transplant patients or patients infected with the human immunodeficiency virus.[70]

Minimizing Non-Hodgkin Lymphoma Mortality: Clinical Implications

The possible association between treatment extent and non-Hodgkin lymphoma risk suggested by some of the larger series stresses the importance of tailored treatment and minimizing overtreatment for patients with Hodgkin lymphoma. In addition, careful pathologic review by an expert hematopathologist at the time of initial Hodgkin lymphoma diagnosis, as well as in cases of suspected disease recurrence versus subsequent non-Hodgkin lymphoma, are crucial in ensuring delivery of proper therapy. Approximately 70% to 80% of cases of non-Hodgkin lymphoma after Hodgkin lymphoma are of aggressive histology, and aggressive treatment should be pursued in these patients, as the disease is curable in up to one-half of the cases.[64] Such treatment, however, may not be warranted in patients who develop indolent lymphoma.

Solid Tumors

Impact of Solid Tumors on Overall Survival

In contrast to leukemia, which rarely occurs beyond 10 to 15 years after therapy for Hodgkin lymphoma, the risk of developing solid tumor continues to increase beyond 15 years. In some series with long enough follow-up time, solid tumors have constituted over three-quarters of all cases of second malignancies.[36,38,39,71,72] In a study on competing mortality by Aleman and co-workers,[9] solid tumors accounted for 10% of all deaths in patients treated for Hodgkin lymphoma. Important determining factors of the survival outcome in these patients included the specific types of solid tumors that developed and the stage of the solid tumor at diagnosis.

Breast cancer is one of the most common solid tumors after Hodgkin lymphoma in most series, and it appears to be associated with a reasonable prognosis. In a study from the Memorial Sloan Kettering Cancer Center, the 6-year disease-free survival rates for node-negative and node-positive breast cancers after Hodgkin lymphoma were 85% and 33%,[73] respectively, and were noted to be similar to the survival outcome of patients presenting with primary breast cancers. Wolden and associates from Stanford reported on results of 71 cases of breast cancer after Hodgkin lymphoma,[74] and found the 10-year disease-specific survival for patients with in situ disease, stage I, stage II, stage III, and stage IV disease to be 100%, 88%, 55%, 60%, and 9%, respectively. These results were also comparable to those reported in the general population. Lung cancer is another of the most common solid tumors observed after Hodgkin lymphoma. Compared with breast cancer, however, it is associated with a considerably worse prognosis. Laurie and associates reported on the clinical course of 19 patients who developed lung cancer after Hodgkin lymphoma.[75] The median survival was 5.1 months for the entire cohort, and the 14 patients who had unresectable disease all died of their lung cancer at a median time of 3 months. Das and colleagues evaluated the treatment outcome of 33 patients with lung cancer after Hodgkin lymphoma and found a median survival of 9 months.[76] Because of the significantly worse survival outcome associated with lung cancer, it has a much greater impact on the overall survival of patients with a history of Hodgkin lymphoma. In the study by Aleman and associates,[9] lung cancer was responsible for 4.3% of all deaths, while breast cancer only accounted for 0.9% of all deaths in patients treated for Hodgkin lymphoma.

Solid tumors are a late-developing complication that will play an increasing part in negatively affecting the survival of patients who have been successfully treated for Hodgkin lymphoma. Understanding the pattern of and factors that influence their development may help in finding ways to diminish their risks, or to improve their survival outcomes (e.g., through prevention and/or early detection and treatment).

Factors Associated with Risks of Solid Tumor after Treatment for Hodgkin Lymphoma

Radiation Treatment Field. Data from retrospective studies showed that the majority of solid cancers arise within or in close vicinity to the previous radiation therapy treatment fields, suggesting that smaller field size may be associated with a lower solid tumor risk. However, because of the long latency to solid tumor development, it can be difficult to reliably determine the location of the cancer with respect to the initial treatment fields. Several studies have found a significant correlation between the initial Hodgkin lymphoma radiation treatment field size and the subsequent risk of solid tumor development. Biti and associates of the University of Florence found that the 15-year cumulative probability of developing a solid tumor was 5.1% among patients treated with involved-field/mantle radiation therapy, compared with 11.6% among patients treated with subtotal or total nodal irradiation.[77] Results from the International Database for Hodgkin's Disease showed a 1.84-fold higher risk of solid tumor in patients who received subtotal or total nodal irradiation compared with local radiation therapy.[59] Other studies, however, were only able to detect a nonsignificant trend of an association between the radiation treatment field extent and the solid tumor risk.[44,78] These studies are largely retrospective and are thus limited by the differences in follow-up time of patients treated with extended- versus limited-field radiation therapy. The best data on the issue of the relationship between radiation field size and second malignancy risk will therefore need to come from long-term results of prospective randomized trials that include different radiation therapy fields in the treatment arms. In the German Hodgkin Study Group HD 8 trial comparing chemotherapy followed by extended-field versus involved-field radiation therapy,[79] there was a trend of a lower risk of second malignancy in the involved-field radiation therapy arm (4.6% versus 2.8%), which was not statistically significant ($p = 0.191$). However, the follow-up time was only 54 months, and additional time is needed to determine the solid tumor risks of the two arms.

Radiation Dose. Several case-control studies carefully looked at the dose–response relationship in the development of breast cancer and lung cancer.[80–83] The radiation dose at the site of the second tumor was estimated in the case patients and was compared to the dose to a comparable location in the control subjects. These studies all showed a significant trend of increasing risk of tumor development with increasing radiation dose. Van Leeuwen and colleagues reported on 30 cases of lung cancer following Hodgkin lymphoma and 62 matched controls,[80] and found that patients in whom the radiation dose to a specific part of the lung was 9 Gy or more have a 9.6-fold increased risk of lung cancer compared to those who received a dose of less than 1 Gy. In another case-control study by Travis et al,[82,84] evaluating 222 cases of lung cancer and 444 matched controls, a radiation dose of 5 Gy or higher to a specific location in the lung was associated with a six-fold risk of lung cancer compared to a dose of less than 5 Gy. The same group also evaluated risk factors for breast cancer after Hodgkin lymphoma in 105 cases of breast cancer and 266 matched controls.[83,85] Using a dose of under 4 Gy as reference, a radiation dose of more than 40 Gy to a specific location to the breast was associated with an eight-fold risk of breast cancer. In a separate case-control study on breast cancer after Hodgkin lymphoma, van Leeuwen and associates found that patients who received 38.5 Gy or more had a relative risk of 4.5 when compared to patients who received less than 4Gy.[81] A linear dose–response relationship may not be the case for all solid tumors. In one study on childhood cancer survivors, the risk of thyroid cancer increased with radiation doses up to

20–29 Gy, but the risk fell after 30 Gy.[86] However, when specifically looking at survivors of Hodgkin lymphoma, a dose–response relationship could not be established because of the small number of cases in the low-dose strata.

Chemotherapy. The contribution of chemotherapy alone to the risk of solid tumor is more difficult to ascertain because in the majority of the available studies, the number of patients treated with chemotherapy alone was too low to allow for any meaningful conclusions. However, in the cohort of patients from the British National Lymphoma Investigation group, 31% of the population was treated with chemotherapy alone, with predominantly alkylating agent-based chemotherapy.[39] In their retrospective cohort study on 5,519 patients, the relative risks of developing a lung cancer after radiation therapy alone or chemotherapy alone were both significantly increased at 2.9 (95% C.I. 1.9–4.1) and 3.3 (95% C.I. 2.2–4.7), respectively. A nested case-control study on lung cancer after Hodgkin lymphoma was subsequently published by the same group, comparing 88 cases of lung cancer with 176 matched controls.[87] Compared with patients who were never exposed to mechlorethamine, those who were ever treated with mechlorethamine were at a significantly higher risk of developing a lung cancer (RR = 1.69, 95% C.I. 1.01–2.86). In the case-control study by Travis and co-workers on lung cancer after Hodgkin lymphoma,[82] among patients who received less than 5 Gy of radiation therapy, those who were treated with alkylating-agent chemotherapy had a four-fold risk of lung cancer compared with patients who did not receive alkylating agents.

Two case-control studies on breast cancer after Hodgkin lymphoma, however, showed a significantly decreased risk of breast cancer after alkylating chemotherapy exposure.[81,83] The relationship was dose related, with decreasing breast cancer risk with increasing number of cycles of chemotherapy. Both studies also showed that the risk of breast cancer was significantly reduced in women who had premature menopause. The study by van Leeuwen and associates further showed that the younger the age at menopause, the lower was the risk of breast cancer.[81] The protective effect of chemotherapy-induced premature menopause against subsequent breast cancer development may have implications on recommendations on use of hormone replacement therapy, and on the role of chemopreventive agents in female survivors of Hodgkin lymphoma.

Age. Reports on the relationship between age at diagnosis and treatment of Hodgkin lymphoma and overall risk of solid tumors are conflicting.[38,39,71] This may be due to differences in the type of second tumor and the age group of the patient population under consideration, and the methods of risk estimation. One consistent finding, however, is the increased risk of breast cancer for females treated for Hodgkin lymphoma at a young age.[38,39,71] The cut-off age ranges from 25 to 35, beyond which the risk of breast cancer appeared to be no longer significantly increased.

Gender. Tarbell and associates at Harvard were the first to report a female predominance among patients with solid tumors.[88] A review of a larger pediatric patient population at St. Jude confirmed that second malignancies were more common in female patients, even when those with breast cancer were excluded.[16,89] The Late Effect Study Group found, on multivariate analysis, that female sex was an independent predictor for secondary solid tumors, with a relative risk of 2.9 (95% C.I of 1.5–5.4).[61]

Patient Habits: Tobacco Use. The contribution of tobacco use to the risk of lung cancer in survivors of Hodgkin lymphoma has been addressed by several case-control studies.[82,84,87,90] In a study by van Leeuwen and associates[90] in which the smoking history was known in 90% of the patient population, the authors found that patients who smoked more

than 10 pack-years after Hodgkin lymphoma were at a six-fold increased risk for lung cancer compared to those with a less than 1 pack-year history of smoking. The multiplicative effect between smoking and Hodgkin therapy exposure is well-demonstrated in a study by Travis and co-workers.[82,84] Compared to survivors who were exposed to less than 5 Gy of radiation therapy, never received alkylating-agent chemotherapy, and who were light smokers or nonsmokers, patients who received both radiation therapy and alkylating agents were at a seven-fold increased risk of lung cancer. However, for patients who were exposed to radiation therapy, alkylating agents, and also had a more than 10 pack-year history of smoking, their risk of lung cancer was 49 times higher than patients who had none of the exposures.

Predisposing Genetic Factors. Studies addressing potential underlying molecular mutations that may contribute to the risk of second malignancy after Hodgkin lymphoma have largely been negative. However, there is indirect evidence suggesting that genetic factors may play a role in the second malignancy risk. In a report from Stanford, among the 6 patients who developed malignant melanoma, 5 had precursor nevi in the specimen upon pathology review, or had clinical characteristics of dysplastic nevus syndrome.[55] It was hypothesized that immune deficits in patients with Hodgkin lymphoma, when exacerbated by their treatment, may allow the transformation of precursor nevi to cutaneous melanoma, similar to that observed in renal transplant patients. The authors also observed that these patients appeared to have unusual responses to radiation therapy, with significant atrophy, neurologic deficits, pulmonary fibrosis, and retroperitoneal fibrosis, raising the possibility of an inherently increased tissue sensitivity to ionizing radiation.

In a recent case-control study by Hill and associates among women without a family history of breast cancer and/or ovarian cancer, exposure to radiation doses of 5 Gy or higher was associated with a 5.8-fold risk of breast cancer development compared to those who were exposed to less than 5 Gy.[91] Interestingly, among women with a family history of breast cancer and/or ovarian cancer, a significant dose–response relationship was not observed, and the relative risk of breast cancer was 0.8 in those who received the higher doses of radiation therapy. These results suggest that exposure to radiation therapy is unlikely to be associated with a larger increase in breast cancer risk among women with a positive family history. It was hypothesized that in women with a family history and who may be mutation carriers, unrepaired damaged cells might undergo cell death rather than serve as cancer-initiating cells when exposed to therapeutic doses of radiation.

Minimizing Solid Tumor Mortality: Clinical Implications

Hodgkin Lymphoma Treatment Reduction. Results of retrospective cohort studies and case-control studies described above indicate that the risk of solid tumor after Hodgkin lymphoma therapy is related to the cumulative treatment exposure, with some of the studies suggesting that smaller radiation field size and lower radiation dose may be associated with lower risk of specific types of cancer. A number of ongoing multi-institutional randomized trials are investigating different ways to reduce treatment for Hodgkin lymphoma, especially among patients with early-stage, favorable-prognosis disease.[92,93] Treatment arms include use of abbreviated chemotherapy, reduced radiation field size, and reduced radiation dose. Trials have also been conducted that test the elimination of radiation therapy in early-stage patients, although in two of the trials, the chemotherapy alone arms were closed due to high relapse rates.[92,94] Due to the long latency to solid tumor development, at least 10 to 15 year follow-up data will be needed to determine whether the treatment reductions will translate into lower risk of solid tumors.

Early Detection of Solid Tumors. Early detection through screening tests has been shown to improve the stage-distribution or even reduce mortality in a number of cancer types in the normal population. However, there is a paucity of data establishing the effectiveness of solid tumor screening strategies in survivors of Hodgkin lymphoma. One needs to be cautious in extrapolating data on cancer screening in the general population to survivors of Hodgkin lymphoma for a number of reasons. The clinical nature of tumors that develop after Hodgkin lymphoma therapy may be different from that of de novo cancers. In addition, prior radiation exposure may cause soft-tissue changes that may influence the results of radiographic screening studies. Finally, survivors of Hodgkin lymphoma face other competing mortality that may affect their benefit from early cancer detection.

Diller and colleagues conducted a prospective cohort study on 90 female survivors of Hodgkin lymphoma, evaluating the utility of mammographic screening and assessing patient awareness of breast cancer risk.[95] A total of 12 breast cancers were found during the study period, all of which were less than 2 cm in size and were detectable on mammograms. In addition, it was found that 40% of women were unaware of their increased risk of breast cancer, although women who had received information from an oncologist were more likely to correctly assess their risk than women who received information from other sources. Results of this study showed that screening mammography can detect small breast cancers in this group of relatively young patients, and the results also highlight the importance of patient education regarding their breast cancer risks. Given the high risk of breast cancer after Hodgkin lymphoma therapy, our current recommendation is yearly screening mammography beginning 8 years after mediastinal radiation therapy, or when the patient reaches 40, whichever comes first.

Recent data showed that breast MRI is significantly more effective than mammography in detecting breast cancer in carriers of *BRCA-1* or *BRCA-2*, or in women with traditional breast cancer risk factors.[96,97] However, the role of breast MRI as a breast cancer screening tool has not been studied in female survivors of Hodgkin lymphoma. These patients have a similar level of risk of breast cancer as carriers of *BRCA-1* and *BRCA-2*. Survivors of Hodgkin lymphoma also tend to be young with denser breasts, and therefore may share the same limitations as *BRCA-1* and *BRCA-2* carriers in their breast cancer detection rate by mammography. Therefore, there may be a role for breast MRI screening in women who have undergone chest irradiation for Hodgkin lymphoma at a young age.

The National Cancer Institute conducted a randomized lung cancer screening trial (http://www.cancer.gov/nlst) comparing annual low-dose chest computed tomography versus annual chest x-ray in high-risk patients based on their smoking history. The study is now closed to recruitment and data analysis is underway. Whether lung cancer screening may be of benefit to survivors of Hodgkin lymphoma is unclear, but their high lung cancer risk may justify its implementation, particularly among smokers, given the known multiplicative effect of tobacco use and prior Hodgkin lymphoma therapy on lung cancer risk. Das and associates preformed a cost-effective analysis on annual low-dose chest CT in survivors of Hodgkin lymphoma starting at 5 years out from treatment.[98] The incremental cost-effective ratio of annual screening for smokers was $35,000 per quality-adjusted life year saved, which was well within the range of other well-established cancer screening tests.

Risk Reduction and Prevention. Prevention strategies may have an important impact on specific subtypes of second malignancy after Hodgkin lymphoma. Examples of the more obvious risk-reduction strategies include smoking cessation programs and counseling on sun-safety practice, which can be incorporated into the follow-up plan of patients.

The role of chemoprevention in these patients is less clear. Tamoxifen has been shown to reduce breast cancer incidence by 30% to 40% in at-risk, but otherwise healthy women in large phase III trials.[99] It is unknown whether similar results will be achieved in survivors of Hodgkin lymphoma. The substantial impact of hormonal exposure on breast cancer risk demonstrated in the case-control studies on breast cancer after Hodgkin lymphoma support the potential value of selective estrogen receptor modulators for breast cancer prevention in these patients. However, barriers that need to be taken into consideration include costs, side effects, and the teratogenic effects of the medications, limiting the use to only women who have completed child-bearing. A feasibility study was conducted at the Dana-Farber Cancer Institute on the use of tamoxifen as chemoprevention in young women who received mantle irradiation for Hodgkin lymphoma.[100] A disappointingly low enrollment rate of only 11.5% in this pilot study led to the conclusion that a randomized trial addressing this question is unlikely to be feasible. Concerns with side effects of tamoxifen were one of the most frequently quoted reasons for opting out of the study. Allen and co-workers constructed a decision-analytic model on 5 years of tamoxifen as chemoprevention in female survivors of Hodgkin lymphoma.[101] Assuming a 10-year duration protective effect of tamoxifen, the incremental cost-effectiveness ratio was under $50,000 per quality-adjusted life-year saved if tamoxifen were to start 10 years after radiation therapy, and the use of tamoxifen was cost-saving if its use were to start 15 years after radiation therapy.

CARDIAC MORTALITY

Impact of Cardiac Diseases on Overall Mortality

After Hodgkin lymphoma and second malignancies, cardiovascular disease is the third most common cause of death following treatment for Hodgkin lymphoma, contributing to approximately 10% to 15% of all causes of mortality.[3,4,7–9,13] Most of the studies showed that the excess risk of cardiac mortality increases with increasing follow-up time, and remains elevated beyond 20 to 25 years after Hodgkin lymphoma therapy. A wide spectrum of cardiac complications after Hodgkin lymphoma treatments has been observed, including pericarditis, pancarditis, pericardial effusions, pericardial fibrosis, congestive heart failure, valvular defects, conduction defects, and coronary artery disease (see Chapter 25).[102–105] The most common fatal cardiovascular complication after Hodgkin lymphoma therapy, however, is acute myocardial infarction secondary to coronary artery disease. At Stanford University, results on 2,232 patients treated for Hodgkin lymphoma were reported, in which 88 patients died of cardiac diseases.[106] Over 60% of the cardiac deaths were from acute myocardial infarction. The absolute excess risk for acute myocardial infarction deaths increased from 6.4 to 70.6/10,000 person-years, and the relative risk increased from 2.0 to 5.6, within 5 years of Hodgkin lymphoma diagnosis and at greater than 20 years from diagnosis, respectively.

Factors Associated with Cardiac Morbidity and Mortality after Hodgkin lymphoma Therapy

Mediastinal Radiation Therapy

A number of studies have documented an association between mediastinal irradiation and risk of fatal cardiovascular complications. Boivin and associates reported results on 957 patients treated for Hodgkin lymphoma, and found that the standardized mortality ratio of death from coronary artery disease was significantly elevated at 2.1 (95% C.I. of 1 to 3.9, $p < 0.05$) in patients who have received mediastinal radiation therapy, while the risk was not increased in patients who were not irradiated.[107] In a collaborative study from 11 cancer treatment centers that included 4,665 patients with Hodgkin lymphoma, a significantly elevated relative risk of 2.56 of death from myocardial infarction (C.I. of 1.11 to 5.93) was observed after mediastinal irradiation, but not after chemotherapy.[108] Cosset and associates found that among 499 patients who received mantle-field irradiation, there was a 3.9% cumulative incidence at 10 years of acute myocardial infarction, but in 138 patients who did not receive mediastinal irradiation, no acute myocardial infarctions were observed.[109] In the Stanford series, among the 171 patients who received no mediastinal irradiation or less than 30 Gy to the mediastinum, no significantly increased risk of heart disease death was observed.[106] In their pediatric and adolescent population, 85% of the acute myocardial infarction deaths occurred in patients who had received mediastinal doses of 36 Gy or more.[102]

At Stanford, cardiac and subcarinal blocking was introduced in 1972, resulting in a decline in relative risk for non-myocardial infarction cardiac death from 5.3 to 1.4 in subsequent years.[106] However, the implementation of the blocking did not affect the risk of death from acute myocardial infarction, likely because the blocks did not shield the proximal coronary arteries, where the Hodgkin lymphoma was primarily located.

Treatment techniques used in the earlier years with 60-cobalt or orthovoltage equipment, anterior field weighting, daily fractions larger than 2 Gy treatment to one field per day, and lack of cardiac blocking, all resulted in higher cardiac doses or dose inhomogeneity. In the multi-institutional study by Boivin and co-workers, the relative risk for fatal myocardial infarction after mediastinal irradiation was associated with the time period of Hodgkin lymphoma therapy.[108] Patients treated from 1940 to 1966, which is during the era when orthovoltage irradiation and anterior or predominantly anterior techniques were employed, had a higher relative risk of acute myocardial infarction death than patients treated from 1967 to 1985 (6.33 versus 1.97), although the difference did not achieve statistical significance. At the University of Rochester, cardiac evaluations were performed on 50 patients with Hodgkin lymphoma treated predominantly with modern techniques using megavoltage radiation therapy, subcarinal blocking, and dose fraction under 2 Gy, and 86% of the patients were treated with equally weighted parallel opposed AP-PA mantle fields daily.[110] The estimated mean central cardiac dose was 35 Gy in 1.5 to 2.0 Gy fractions. With an average follow-up of 13.5 years, other than some modest abnormalities in a minority of patients, most had ejection fraction and myocardial perfusion that were within normal limits, suggesting intact cardiac function in most patients irradiated for Hodgkin lymphoma using modern techniques.

Anthracyclines

The doses of anthracyclines used in Hodgkin lymphoma therapy as part of the ABVD regimen are typically limited (50 mg/m² per cycle, usual 300 to 400 mg/m² total dose).

However, even at relatively low cumulative doses, it can contribute to late cardiac toxicity and cardiac deaths. In a prospective study conducted by Aviles and associates, 476 patients with stage III–IV Hodgkin lymphoma were randomized to receive six cycles of ABVD, EBVD (epirubicin instead of doxorubicin), and MBVD (mitoxantrone instead of doxorubicin).[111] At a median follow-up time of 11.5 years, among the 191 patients randomized to receive six cycles of ABVD (cumulative dose of doxorubicin of 400 mg/m²), clinical cardiac events were observed in 9% and cardiac mortality was observed in 7% of patients. Compared with the age- and gender-matched normal population, the relative risk of cardiac mortality was 46.4 (95% C.I., 39.8–89.4) and the absolute excess risk was 39/10,000 person-years. In this study, radiation therapy was not given as part of the initial Hodgkin lymphoma therapy, and the cardiac toxicity can therefore be more directly attributed to the use of anthracyclines.

Traditional Cardiac Risk Factors

Risk factors for coronary heart disease that have been identified in the normal population include hypertension, hypercholesterolemia, diabetes, smoking, family history, low physical activity, and obesity. There have been emerging data on the relative contributions of these traditional cardiac risk factors to cardiac complications in survivors of Hodgkin lymphoma. In a study by Glanzmann and associates on survivors of Hodgkin lymphoma, the relative risk of ischemic cardiac disease patients with known cardiac risk factors was significantly elevated at 2.36, compared to a relative risk of 0.96 for those without cardiac risk factors.[112] In a study from the University of Florida on cardiac disease after Hodgkin lymphoma, hypertension and hypercholesterolemia were significantly associated with the risk of coronary artery disease, and all patients who developed coronary artery disease had at least one traditional cardiac risk factor.[105] Strasser and associates conducted a case-control study evaluating cardiac complications after Hodgkin lymphoma, and found that independent risk factors for the development of cardiac events included family history of premature cardiac disease, hypertension, and hypercholesterolemia.[113]

Minimizing Cardiac Mortality: Clinical Implications

Hodgkin Lymphoma Treatment Reduction

Improvements in radiation therapy techniques over the last few decades have reduced the risk of cardiac complications and mortality by reducing the dose to the heart and the volume of heart irradiated. These include use of equal daily doses from anterior and posterior fields, daily fraction sizes of 2 Gy or less, extended source-to-skin distances, megavoltage equipment, and routine use of cardiac blocks. The use of three-dimensional treatment planning and the further dose reduction and radiation field size reduction being investigated in ongoing trials may further reduce the risk of cardiac complications. Trials are currently ongoing investigating the use of more limited radiation treatment fields, lower radiation therapy doses, reduced number of cycles of chemotherapy, and use of modified chemotherapy regimens with lower cumulative anthracycline doses.[92,93,114] However, the major challenge that remains from the radiation therapy perspective is the proximity of anterior mediastinal adenopathy to the proximal coronary arteries. Long-term results from these trials will provide information on whether these treatment modifications will lead to reduced cardiac morbidity and mortality.

Early Detection

Subclinical cardiac abnormalities may precede clinical symptoms by years or decades, and the dysfunction can progress over time. By the time survivors of Hodgkin lymphoma present with clinically apparent or symptomatic cardiac disease, irreparable damage may have already been done. Early detection through cardiac screening tests may allow intervention before the disease becomes debilitating, irreversible or fatal. Appropriate interventions based on the screening results may include pharmacological interventions, endocarditis prophylaxis, angioplasty, coronary artery bypass graft, valve replacement, or pacemaker placement. In a study from Stanford University, 294 asymptomatic survivors of Hodgkin lymphoma were prospectively screened with electrocardiogram and echocardiogram.[103] Significant valve disease was detected in 29% of the patients. The valvular abnormality was detected by auscultation in only 6.3% of the cases. In addition, it was noted that valvular disease, regional wall-motion abnormality, and pericardial disease increased with increasing follow-up time.

At this time, the types of screening tests to be performed, timing in relationship to initial Hodgkin lymphoma treatment, frequency, and target population are unresolved issues that need to be addressed. Novel serum markers including C-reactive protein, a biomarker of generalized inflammation associated with atherosclerosis; brain neutriotide protein, a biomarker of left ventricular dysfunction associated with congestive heart failure; and homocysteine, a marker for accelerated atherosclerosis, may also have a role in future cardiac screening protocols in these patients.

Risk Reduction and Prevention

Modification of some of the cardiac risk factors, including blood pressure control with antihypertensives and use of cholesterol-lowering agents, has been shown to effectively reduce cardiac mortality in the general population. Because of the relative young age of most survivors of Hodgkin lymphoma and the general lack of awareness of their increased cardiac risks, they may not be as aggressively screened for and be treated for cardiac risk factors as older patients or other high-risk patients. Prompt recognition and intervention for treatable cardiac risk factors are important first steps in preventing cardiovascular disease. Other interventions to be considered, depending on the risk profile of patients, include an exercise program, dietary modifications, a weight reduction program, and counseling for smoking cessation.

INFECTION

The contribution of infectious complications to the overall mortality of patients treated for Hodgkin lymphoma varies according to the era in which the patients were treated and the length of follow-up time. In most of the recent series, infection accounts for less than 5% of all deaths.[7–9] The most serious and life-threatening infection is overwhelming sepsis, seen predominantly in post-splenectomy patients, with a crude overall incidence estimated to be 2% to 3%.[115–117] In addition to the high associated mortality rate of up to 66%, the clinical course is rapid, and death can ensue within hours of onset of the infection. Although most of these highly fatal bacterial sepses occur around or shortly after treatment, fatal overwhelming sepsis has been described up to 47 years after a splenectomy.[115]

Survivors of Hodgkin lymphoma are at increased infectious risks due to underlying immunologic defects associated with Hodgkin lymphoma, as well as various diagnostic and therapeutic interventions, including chemotherapy, radiation therapy, splenectomy, or splenic irradiation. A number of changes in the management of patients with Hodgkin lymphoma, however, have resulted in a decline in infectious mortality after Hodgkin lymphoma therapy. These include use of less myelosuppressive chemotherapeutic agents, availability of more effective supportive care in patients with myelosuppression or acute infections, decreased performance of staging laparotomy and splenectomy, routine vaccination administration in asplenic patients,[118,119] and the increased awareness of the danger of overwhelming sepsis and importance of prompt antibiotic therapy. At Stanford, the crude incidence of fatal infection among patients treated for Hodgkin lymphoma who were disease-free at the time of death decreased from 0.96% during the period from 1962 to 1980 to 0.38% during the period from 1980 to 1996.[120]

PULMONARY MORTALITY

Pulmonary toxicities after Hodgkin lymphoma treatment are well-documented, ranging from acute interstitial pneumonitis to chronic lung injury such as pulmonary fibrosis and recurrent pleural effusions.[121–129] Specific combination chemotherapy regimens have also been shown to be associated with increased lung toxicity, including the vinblastine, bleomycin, and methotrexate (VBM) regimen,[130,131] and regimens that contain both bleomycin and gemcitabine.[132,133] The addition of mediastinal irradiation appears to further exacerbate the pulmonary toxicity associated with bleomycin.[123,126,134,135] In a study from the National Cancer Institute, 80 patients with Hodgkin lymphoma presenting with large mediastinal disease were treated with MOPP alternated with ABVD chemotherapy, followed by mantle radiation therapy.[135] The radiation fields were shaped to conform to the pre-chemotherapy tumor volume. Treatment-related pneumonitis developed in 16% and some pulmonary reaction was noted in 21% of patients. One 51-year-old patient died of treatment-related pneumonitis. In the EORTC H6U trial, 2 patients in the ABVD and radiotherapy arm died from lung toxicity.[134] Both cases were in patients with bulky mediastinal disease, and one of the patients received a daily fraction size of 2.5 Gy. Efforts to limit the extent of the radiation field by inclusion of only the post-chemotherapy volume and the use of fraction sizes of 2 Gy or less can help reduce the risk of pulmonary complications. Regimens have been developed that contain a lower cumulative dose of bleomycin. Trials are also ongoing investigating the use of a reduced number of cycles of ABVD chemotherapy, or elimination of the bleomycin from the treatment program; and the use of lower doses of radiation therapy, which may further reduce the risk of pulmonary toxicity.

There is evidence that older patients may be more prone to pulmonary toxicity and mortality. In a CALGB study, Canellos and associates reported fatal lung toxicity in 3 patients, aged 42, 69, and 72, among the 115 advanced-stage patients treated with ABVD.[33] In a retrospective study from Harvard on 175 Hodgkin lymphoma patients treated with ABVD with or without radiation therapy, 5 patients died of pulmonary toxicity, with 3 of the 5 patients being age 60 or older.[136] In a recent study from the Mayo clinic on 141 patients with Hodgkin lymphoma treated with bleomycin-containing regimens, 18% of patients developed bleomycin lung toxicity, which was associated with a 24% mortality rate. The risk of pulmonary mortality was 28% in patients 40 or more years of age versus 7% in patients age under 40 ($p = 0.006$).[137] Therefore, careful monitoring of pulmonary function during treatment, especially in older patients, is important, and there should be a low threshold to discontinue the bleomycin when there are signs or symptoms of lung compromise.

CONCLUSIONS

The life expectancy of patients diagnosed with Hodgkin lymphoma has improved significantly over the last several decades, largely due to improvements in staging and treatments over the years. Given the already high cure rate of Hodgkin lymphoma, the greatest potential to further improve the survival of patients affected by the disease is through reducing excess mortality from late complications of treatment. This can be accomplished by continued efforts in exploring treatment reduction without compromising cure in newly diagnosed patients, and in survivors of Hodgkin lymphoma; and by continued careful documentation of the broad range of late effects over time in order to fully appreciate the scope of the problems faced by these patients. The types of screening tests, preventative measures, and interventions; their timing in relation to initial Hodgkin lymphoma therapy; the optimal target population; and the effectiveness of these follow-up programs, need to be explored. Education of both patients and primary care physicians, who often are the main health care professionals following the patients years after their cure, about the various types of late complications and management approaches, will also be crucial for successful long-term follow-up care of these patients.

References

1. van Rijswijk R, Verbeek J, Haanen C, et al. Major complications and causes of death in patients treated for Hodgkin's disease. *J Clin Oncol* 1987;5:1624–1633.
2. Henry-Amar M, Somers R. Survival outcome after Hodgkin's disease: a report from the International Data Base on Hodgkin's Disease. *Semin Oncol* 1990;17:758–768.
3. Cosset J, Henry-Amar M, Meerwaldt J. Long-term toxicity of early stage of Hodgkin's disease therapy: the EORTC experience. *Ann Oncol* 1991;2(suppl 2):77–82.
4. VanghanHudson B, VanghanHudson G, Linch D, et al. Late mortality in young British National Lymphoma Investigation patients cured of Hodgkin's disease. *Ann Oncol* 1994;5:565–566.
5. Mauch P, Kalish L, Marcus K, et al. Long-term survival in Hodgkin's disease: relative impact of mortality, secondary tumor, infection and cardiovascular disease. *Cancer J Sci Am* 1995;1:33–42.
6. Hancock S, Hoppe R. Long-term complications of treatment and causes of mortality after Hodgkin's disease. *Semin Radiat Oncol* 1996;6:225–242.
7. Hoppe R. Hodgkin's disease. Complications of therapy and excess mortality. *Ann Oncol* 1997;8(suppl 1):S115–S118.
8. Ng AK, Bernardo MP, Weller E, et al. Long-term survival and competing causes of death in patients with early-stage Hodgkin's disease treated at age 50 or younger. *J Clin Oncol* 2002;20:2101–2108.
9. Aleman BM, van den Belt-Dusebout AW, Klokman WJ, et al. Long-term cause-specific mortality of patients treated for Hodgkin's disease. *J Clin Oncol* 2003;21:3431–3439.
10. Hancock S, Hoppe R, Horning S, et al. Intercurrent death after Hodgkin's disease treated with radiotherapy and adjuvant MOPP trials. *Ann Intern Med* 1988;109:183–189.
11. Vlachake M, Ha C, Hagemeister F, et al. Long-term outcome of treatment for Ann Arbor stage I Hodgkin's disease: patterns of failure, late toxicity and second malignancies. *Int J Radiat Oncol Biol Phys* 1997;39:609–616.
12. Loeffler M, Brosteanu O, Hasenclever D, et al. Meta-analysis of chemotherapy versus combined modality therapy trials in Hodgkin's disease. *J Clin Oncol* 1998;16:818–829.
13. Specht L, Gray K, Clarke M, et al. Influence of more extensive radiotherapy and adjuvant chemotherapy on long-term outcome of early-stage Hodgkin's disease: a metaanalysis of 23 randomized trials involving 3,888 patients. *J Clin Oncol* 1998;16:830–843.
14. Hodgson DC, Zhang-Salomons J, Rothwell D, et al. Evolution of treatment for Hodgkin's disease: a population-based study of radiation therapy use and outcome. *Clin Oncol (R Coll Radiol)* 2003;15:255–263.
15. Provencio M, Garcia-Lopez FJ, Bonilla F, et al. Comparison of the long-term mortality in Hodgkin's disease patients with that of the general population. *Ann Oncol* 1999;10:1199–1205.
16. Hudson MM, Poquette CA, Lee J, et al. Increased mortality after successful treatment for Hodgkin's disease. *J Clin Oncol* 1998;16:3592–3600.
17. Yasui Y, Liu Y, Neglia JP, et al. A methodological issue in the analysis of second-primary cancer incidence in long-term survivors of childhood cancers. *Am J Epidemiol* 2003;158:1108–1113.
18. Hoppe R, Coleman C, Cox R, et al. The management of stage I-II Hodgkin's disease with irradiation alone or combined modality therapy: the Stanford experience. *Blood* 1982;59:455–465.
19. Crnkovich M, Leopold K, Hoppe R, et al. Stage I to IIB Hodgkin's disease: the combined experience at Stanford University and the Joint Center for Radiation Therapy. *J Clin Oncol* 1987;5:1041–1049.
20. Specht L, Nordentoft A, Cold S, et al. Tumor burden as the most important prognostic factors in early stage Hodgkin's disease. Relations to other prognostic factors in early-stage Hodgkin's disease and implications for choice of treatment. *Cancer* 1988;61:1719–1727.
21. Mauch P, Tarbell N, Weinstein H, et al. Stage IA and IIA supradiaphragmatic Hodgkin's disease: prognostic factors in surgically staged patients treated with mantle and paraaortic irradiation. *J Clin Oncol* 1988;6:1576–1583.
22. Gospodarowicz M, Sutcliffe S, Clark R, et al. Analysis of supradiaphragmatic clinical stages I and II Hodgkin's disease treated with radiation alone. *Int J Radiat Oncol Biol Phys* 1992;22:859–865.
23. Henry-Amar M, Tirelli U, Dupoy N. Age less than 50 versus greater than 50 years as a prognostic factor in 1624 patients with stage I-II Hodgkin's disease entered in EORTC clinical trials since 1964. *Ann Oncol* 1990;1(suppl):3. Abstract.
24. Cosset JM, Henry-Amar M, Meerwaldt JH, et al. The EORTC trials for limited stage Hodgkin's disease. The EORTC Lymphoma Cooperative Group. *Eur J Cancer* 1992;28A:1847–1850.
25. Sieber M, Engert A, Diehl V. Treatment of Hodgkin's disease: results and current concepts of the German Hodgkin's Lymphoma Study Group. *Ann Oncol* 2000;11(suppl 1):81–85.
26. Meyer RM, Gospodarowicz MK, Connors JM, et al. Randomized comparison of ABVD chemotherapy with a strategy that includes radiation therapy in patients with limited-stage Hodgkin's lymphoma: National Cancer Institute of Canada Clinical Trials Group and the Eastern Cooperative Oncology Group. *J Clin Oncol* 2005;23:4634–4642.
27. Gisselbrecht C, Mounier N, Andre M, et al. How to define intermediate stage in Hodgkin's lymphoma? *Eur J Haematol* 2005;75, suppl 66:111–114.
28. Hasenclever D, Diehl V. A prognostic score for advanced Hodgkin's disease. International Prognostic Factors Project on Advanced Hodgkin's Disease. *N Engl J Med* 1998;339:1506–1514.
29. Hagenbeek A, Eghbali H, Fermé C, et al. Three cycles of MOPP/ABV hybrid and involved-field irradiation is more effective than subtotal nodal irradiation in favorable supradiaphragmatic clinical stages I–II Hodgkin's disease: preliminary results of the EORTC-GELA H8-F randomized trial in 543 patients. *Blood* 2000;96:576a.
30. Press OW, LeBlanc M, Lichter AS, et al. Phase III randomized intergroup trial of subtotal lymphoid irradiation versus doxorubicin, vinblastine, and subtotal lymphoid irradiation for stage IA to IIA Hodgkin's disease. *J Clin Oncol* 2001;19:4238–4244.
31. Sieber M, Franklin J, Tesch H, et al. Two cycles ABVD plus extended field radiotherapy is superior to radiotherapy alone in early stage Hodgkin's disease: results of the German Hodgkin's Lymphoma Study Group (GHSG) trial HD7. *Blood* 2002;100:A341.
32. Radford JA, Williams MV, Hancock BW, et al. Minimal initial chemotherapy plus involved field radiotherapy (RT) vs. mantle field RT for clinical stage IA/IIA supradiaphragmatic Hodgkin's disease (HD). Results of the UK Lymphoma Group LY07 trial. *Eur J Haematol* 2004;73:E08a.
33. Canellos G, Anderson J, Propert K, et al. Chemotherapy of advanced Hodgkin's disease with MOPP, ABVD or MOPP alternating with ABVD. *N Engl J Med* 1992;327:1478–1484.
34. Canellos GP, Niedzwiecki D. Long-term follow-up of Hodgkin's disease trial. *N Engl J Med* 2002;346:1417–1418.
35. Diehl V, Franklin J, Pfreundschuh M, et al. Standard and increased-dose BEACOPP chemotherapy compared with COPP-ABVD for advanced Hodgkin's disease. *N Engl J Med* 2003;348:2386–2395.
36. Ng AK, Bernardo MV, Weller E, et al. Second malignancy after Hodgkin disease treated with radiation therapy with or without chemotherapy: long-term risks and risk factors. *Blood* 2002;100:1989–1996.
37. Josting A, Wiedenmann S, Franklin J, et al. Secondary myeloid leukemia and myelodysplastic syndromes in patients treated for Hodgkin's disease: a report from the German Hodgkin's Lymphoma Study Group. *J Clin Oncol* 2003;21:3440–3446.
38. van Leeuwen FE, Klokman WJ, Veer MB, et al. Long-term risk of second malignancy in survivors of Hodgkin's disease treated during adolescence or young adulthood. *J Clin Oncol* 2000;18:487–497.
39. Swerdlow AJ, Barber JA, Hudson GV, et al. Risk of second malignancy after Hodgkin's disease in a collaborative British cohort: the relation to age at treatment. *J Clin Oncol* 2000;18:498–509.
40. Kaldor J, Day N, Clarke E, et al. Leukemia following Hodgkin's disease. *N Engl J Med* 1990;322:7–13.
41. van Leeuwen F, Chorus A, vandenBelt-Dusebout A, et al. Leukemia risk following Hodgkin's diseae: relation to cumalative dose of alkylating agents, treatment wtih teniposide combinations, number of episodes of chemotherapy, and bone marrow damage. *J Clin Oncol* 1994;12:1063–1073.
42. Tucker M, Meadows A, Boice J, et al. Leukemia after therapy with alkylating agents for childhood cancer. *J Natl Cancer Inst* 1987;78:459–464.
43. Swerdlow A, Barber J, Horwich A, et al. Second malignancy in patients with Hodgkin's disease treated at the Royal Marsden Hospital. *Br J Cancer* 1997;75:116–123.

44. Chronowski GM, Wilder RB, Levy LB, et al. Second malignancies after chemotherapy and radiotherapy for Hodgkin disease. *Am J Clin Oncol* 2004;27:73–80.

45. vanLeeuwen F, Klokman W, Hagenbeek A, et al. Second cancer risk following Hodgkin's disease: a 20-year follow-up study. *J Clin Oncol* 1994;12:312–325.

46. Delwail V, Jais JP, Colonna P, et al. Fifteen-year secondary leukaemia risk observed in 761 patients with Hodgkin's disease prospectively treated by MOPP or ABVD chemotherapy plus high-dose irradiation. *Br J Haematol* 2002;118:189–194.

47. Horning SJ, Hoppe RT, Breslin S, et al. Stanford V and radiotherapy for locally extensive and advanced Hodgkin's disease: mature results of a prospective clinical trial. *J Clin Oncol* 2002;20:630–637.

48. Pedersen-Bjergaard J, Andersen MK, Christiansen DH. Therapy-related acute myeloid leukemia and myelodysplasia after high-dose chemotherapy and autologous stem cell transplantation. *Blood* 2000;95:3273–3279.

49. Krishnan A, Bhatia S, Slovak ML, et al. Predictors of therapy-related leukemia and myelodysplasia following autologous transplantation for lymphoma: an assessment of risk factors. *Blood* 2000;95:1588–1593.

50. Metayer C, Curtis RE, Vose J, et al. Myelodysplastic syndrome and acute myeloid leukemia after autotransplantation for lymphoma: a multicenter case-control study. *Blood* 2003;101:2015–2023.

51. Bhatia R, Van Heijzen K, Palmer A, et al. Longitudinal assessment of hematopoietic abnormalities after autologous hematopoietic cell transplantation for lymphoma. *J Clin Oncol* 2005;23:6699–6711.

52. Lavoie JC, Connors JM, Phillips GL, et al. High-dose chemotherapy and autologous stem cell transplantation for primary refractory or relapsed Hodgkin lymphoma: long-term outcome in the first 100 patients treated in Vancouver. *Blood* 2005;106:1473–1478.

53. Andrieu J, Ifrah N, Payen C, et al. Increased risk of secondary acute non-lymphocytic leukemia after extended-field radiation therapy combined with MOPP chemotherapy for Hodgkin's disease. *J Clin Oncol* 1990;8:1148–1154.

54. Valagussa P, Santoro A, Fossati-Bellani F, et al. Second acute leukemia and other malignancies following treatment for Hodgkin's disease. *J Clin Oncol* 1986;4:830–837.

55. Tucker M, Coleman C, Cox R, et al. Risk of second cancers after treatment for Hodgkin's disease. *N Engl J Med* 1988;318:76–81.

56. Pedersen-Bjergaard J, Specht L, Lansen S, et al. Risk of therapy-related leukaemia and pre-leudaemia after Hodgkin's disease. Relation to age, cumulative dose of alkylating agents and time from chemtherapy. *Lancet* 1987;2:83–88.

57. Coleman M, Easton D, Horwich A, et al. Second malignancies and Hodgkin's disease—-the Royal Marsden Hospital experience. *Radiother Oncol* 1988;11:229–238.

58. van Leeuwen F, Somers R, Hart A. Splenectomy in Hodgkin's disease and second leukaemias. *Lancet* 1987;2:210–211. Letter.

59. Henry-Amar M. Second cancer after the treatment for Hodgkin's disease: a report from the International Data Base Hodgkin's Disease. *Ann Oncol* 1992;3(suppl 4):117–128.

60. Tura S, Fiacchini M, Zinzani P, et al. Splenectomy and the increased risk of secondary acute leukemia in Hodgkin's disease. *J Clin Oncol* 1993;11:925–930.

61. Bhatia S, Robison L, Oberlin O, et al. Breast cancer and other second neoplasms after childhood Hodgkin's disease. *N Engl J Med* 1996;334:745–751.

62. Abrahamsen J, Andersen A, Hannisdal E, et al. Second malignancies after treatment of Hodgkin's disease: the influence of treatment, follow-up time, and age. *J Clin Oncol* 1993;11:255–261.

63. Robinette C, Fraumeni J. Splenectomy and subsequent mortality in veterans of the 1939–45 war. *Lancet* 1977;2:127–129.

64. Rueffer U, Josting A, Franklin J, et al. Non-Hodgkin's lymphoma after primary Hodgkin's disease in the German Hodgkin's Lymphoma Study Group: incidence, treatment, and prognosis. *J Clin Oncol* 2001;19:2026–2032.

65. Fisher R, Gaynor E, Dahlberg S, et al. Comparison of a standard regimen (CHOP) with 3 intensive chemotherapy regimen for advanced non-Hodgkin's lymphoma. *N Engl J Med* 1993;328:1002–1006.

66. Mauch P, Kalish L, Marcus K, et al. Second malignancies after treatment for laparotomy-staged IA-IIIB Hodgkin's disease: long-term analysis of risk factors and outcome. *Blood* 1996;87:3625–3632.

67. Swerdlow A, Douglas A, VaughanHudson G, et al. Risk of second primary cancer after Hodgkin's disease in patients in the British National Lymphoma Investigation: relationships to host factors, histology and stage of Hodgkin's disease, and splenectomy. *Br J Cancer* 1993;68:1006–1011.

68. Rudiger T, Gascoyne RD, Jaffe ES, et al. Workshop on the relationship between nodular lymphocyte predominant Hodgkin's lymphoma and T cell/histiocyte-rich B cell lymphoma. *Ann Oncol* 2002;13(suppl 1):44–51.

69. Huang JZ, Weisenburger DD, Vose JM, et al. Diffuse large B-cell lymphoma arising in nodular lymphocyte predominant Hodgkin lymphoma: a report of 21 cases from the Nebraska Lymphoma Study Group. *Leuk Lymphoma* 2004;45:1551–1557.

70. Penn I. Cancers complicating organ transplantation. *N Engl J Med* 1990; 323:1767–1769.

71. Dores GM, Metayer C, Curtis RE, et al. Second malignant neoplasms among long-term survivors of Hodgkin's disease: a population-based evaluation over 25 years. *J Clin Oncol* 2002;20:3484–3494.

72. Cellai E, Magrini SM, Masala G, et al. The risk of second malignant tumors and its consequences for the overall survival of Hodgkin's disease patients and for the choice of their treatment at presentation: analysis of a series of 1524 cases consecutively treated at the Florence University Hospital. *Int J Radiat Oncol Biol Phys* 2001;49:1327–1337.

73. Yahalom J, Petrek J, Biddinger P, et al. Breast cancer in patients irradiated for Hodgkin's disease: a clinical and pathological analysis of 45 events in 37 patients. *J Clin Oncol* 1992;10:1674–1681.

74. Wolden SL, Hancock SL, Carlson RW, et al. Management of breast cancer after Hodgkin's disease. *J Clin Oncol* 2000;18:765–772.

75. Laurie SA, Kris MG, Portlock CS, et al. The clinical course of nonsmall cell lung carcinoma in survivors of Hodgkin disease. *Cancer* 2002;95:119–126.

76. Das P, Ng AK, Stevenson MA, et al. Clinical course of thoracic cancers in Hodgkin's disease survivors. *Ann Oncol* 2005;16:793–797.

77. Biti G, Cellai E, Magrini S, et al. Second solid tumors and leukemia after treatment for Hodgkin's disease: an analysis of 1121 patients from a single institution. *Int J Radiat Oncol Biol Phys* 1994;29:25–31.

78. Dietrich P, Henry-Amar M, Cosset J, et al. Second primary cancers in patients continuously disease-free from Hodgkin's disease: a protective role for the spleen? *Blood* 1994;84:1209–1215.

79. Engert A, Schiller P, Josting A, et al. Involved-field radiotherapy is equally effective and less toxic compared with extended-field radiotherapy after four cycles of chemotherapy in patients with early-stage unfavorable Hodgkin's lymphoma: results of the HD8 trial of the German Hodgkin's Lymphoma Study Group. *J Clin Oncol* 2003;21:3601–3608.

80. VanLeeuwen F, Klokman W, Stovall M, et al. Roles of radiotherapy and smoking in lung cancer following Hodgkin's disease. *J Natl Cancer Inst* 1995;87:1530–1537.

81. van Leeuwen FE, Klokman WJ, Stovall M, et al. Roles of radiation dose, chemotherapy, and hormonal factors in breast cancer following Hodgkin's disease. *J Natl Cancer Inst* 2003;95:971–980.

82. Travis LB, Gospodarowicz M, Curtis RE, et al. Lung cancer following chemotherapy and radiotherapy for Hodgkin's disease. *J Natl Cancer Inst* 2002;94:182–192.

83. Travis LB, Hill DA, Dores GM, et al. Breast cancer following radiotherapy and chemotherapy among young women with Hodgkin disease. *JAMA* 2003;290:465–475.

84. Travis LB, Gilbert E. Lung cancer after Hodgkin lymphoma: the roles of chemotherapy, radiotherapy and tobacco use. *Radiat Res* 2005;163:695–696.

85. Travis LB, Hill D, Dores GM, et al. Cumulative absolute breast cancer risk for young women treated for Hodgkin lymphoma. *J Natl Cancer Inst* 2005;97:1428–1437.

86. Sigurdson AJ, Ronckers CM, Mertens AC, et al. Primary thyroid cancer after a first tumour in childhood (the Childhood Cancer Survivor Study): a nested case-control study. *Lancet* 2005;365:2014–2023.

87. Swerdlow AJ, Schoemaker MJ, Allerton R, et al. Lung cancer after Hodgkin's disease: a nested case-control study of the relation to treatment. *J Clin Oncol* 2001;19:1610–1618.

88. Tarbell N, Gelber R, Weinstein H, et al. Sex differences in risk of second malignant tumors after Hodgkin's disease in childhood. *Lancet* 1993;341:1428–1432.

89. Beaty III O, Hudson M, Greenwald C, et al. Subsequent malignancies in children and adolescents after treatment for Hodgkin's disease. *J Clin Oncol* 1995;13:603–609.

90. van Leeuwen F, Somers R, Taal B, et al. Increased risk of lung cancer, non-Hodgkin's lymphoma, and leukemia following Hodgkin's disease. *J Clin Oncol* 1989;7:1046–1058.

91. Hill DA, Gilbert E, Dores GM, et al. Breast cancer risk following radiotherapy for Hodgkin lymphoma: modification by other risk factors. *Blood* 2005;106:3358–3365.

92. Noordijk E, Thomas J, Fermé C, et al. First results of the EORTC-GELA H9 randomized trials: the H9-F trial (comparing 3 radiation dose levels) and H9-U trial (comparing 3 chemotherapy schemes) in patients with favorable or unfavorable early stage Hodgkin's lymphoma (HL). *ASCO Annual Meeting Proceedings* 2005;23:561s.

93. Eich H, Mueller R, Engert A, et al. Comparison of 30 Gy versus 20 Gy involved field radiotherapy after two versus four cycles ABVD in early stage Hodgkin's lymphoma: interim analysis of the German Hodgkin Study Group trial HD10. *Int J Radiat Oncol Biol Phys* 2005;63(suppl 1):S1–S2.

94. Nachman JB, Sposto R, Herzog P, et al. Randomized comparison of low-dose involved-field radiotherapy and no radiotherapy for children with Hodgkin's disease who achieve a complete response to chemotherapy. *J Clin Oncol* 2002;20:3765–3771.

95. Diller L, Medeiros Nancarrow C, Shaffer K, et al. Breast cancer screening in women previously treated for Hodgkin's disease: a prospective cohort study. *J Clin Oncol* 2002;20:2085–2091.

96. Warner E, Plewes DB, Hill KA, et al. Surveillance of BRCA1 and BRCA2 mutation carriers with magnetic resonance imaging, ultrasound, mammography, and clinical breast examination. *JAMA* 2004;292:1317–1325.

97. Kriege M, Brekelmans CT, Boetes C, et al. Efficacy of MRI and mammography for breast-cancer screening in women with a familial or genetic predisposition. *N Engl J Med* 2004;351:427–437.

98. Das P, Ng A, Earle C, et al. Decision analysis on computed tomography screening for lung cancer in Hodgkin's disease survivors. *Ann Oncol* 2006;17:785–793.

99. Gasco M, Argusti A, Bonanni B, et al. SERMs in chemoprevention of breast cancer. *Eur J Cancer* 2005;41:1980–1989.
100. Garber J, Ng A, Mauch P, et al. A feasibility study of tamoxifen chemoprevention in Hodgkin's disease (HD) survivors. Frontiers in Cancer Prevention Research Conference; 2002. Abstract.
101. Allen M, Ng A, Mauch P, et al. A decision and cost-effectiveness analysis on tamoxifen as chemoprevention for breast cancer in young women treated with radiation therapy for Hodgkin's disease. *Int J Radiat Oncol Biol Phys* 2002;54(supp 1):103.
102. Hancock S, Donaldson S, Hoppe R. Cardiac disease following treatment of Hodgkin's disease in children and adolescents. *J Clin Oncol* 1993;11:1208–1215.
103. Heidenreich PA, Hancock SL, Lee BK, et al. Asymptomatic cardiac disease following mediastinal irradiation. *J Am Coll Cardiol* 2003;42:743–749.
104. Adams MJ, Lipsitz SR, Colan SD, et al. Cardiovascular status in long-term survivors of Hodgkin's disease treated with chest radiotherapy. *J Clin Oncol* 2004;22:3139–3148.
105. Hull MC, Morris CG, Pepine CJ, et al. Valvular dysfunction and carotid, subclavian, and coronary artery disease in survivors of Hodgkin lymphoma treated with radiation therapy. *JAMA* 2003;290:2831–2837.
106. Hancock S, Tucker M, Hoppe R. Factors affecting late mortality from heart disease after treatment of Hodgkin's disease. *JAMA* 1993;270:1949–1955.
107. Boivin J, Hutchison G. Coronary heart disease mortality after irradiation for Hodgkin's disease. *Cancer* 1982;49:2470–2475.
108. Boivin J, Hutchison G, Lubin J, et al. Coronary artery disease mortality in patients treated for Hodgkin's disease. *Cancer* 1992;69:1241–1247.
109. Cosset J, Henry-Amar M, Pallae-Cosset B, et al. Pericarditis and myocardial infarctions after Hodgkin's disease therapy. *Int J Radiat Oncol Biol Phys* 1991;21:447–449.
110. Constine L, Schwartz R, Savage D, et al. Cardiac function, perfusion and morbidity in irradiated long-term survivors of Hodgkin's disease. *Int J Radiat Oncol Biol Phys* 1997;39:897–906.
111. Aviles A, Neri N, Nambo JM, et al. Late cardiac toxicity secondary to treatment in Hodgkin's disease. A study comparing doxorubicin, epirubicin and mitoxantrone in combined therapy. *Leuk Lymphoma* 2005;46:1023–1028.
112. Glanzmann C, Huguenin P, Lutolf UM, et al. Cardiac lesions after mediastinal irradiation for Hodgkin's disease. *Radiother Oncol* 1994;30:43–54.
113. Strasser JF, Li S, Neuberg D, et al. Late cardiac toxicity after mediastinal radiation therapy for Hodgkin's disease. *Int J Radiat Oncol Biol Phys* 2004;60:S217.
114. Horning S, Hoppe R, Advani R, et al. Efficacy and late effects of Stanford V chemotherapy and radiotherapy in untreated Hodgkin's disease: mature data in early and advanced stage patients. *Blood* 2004;104:308. Abstract.
115. Waldron D, Harding B, Duigran J. Overwhelming infection occurring in the immediate post-splenectomy period. *Br J Clin Pract* 1989;43:421–422.
116. Frezzato M, Castaman G, Rodeghiero F. Fulminant sepsis in adults splenectomized for Hodgkin's disease. *Haematologica* 1993;78(suppl 2):73–33.
117. Jockovich M, Mendenhall NP, Sombeck MD, et al. Long-term complications of laparotomy in Hodgkin's disease. *Ann Surg* 1994;219:615–624.
118. Molrine DC, George S, Tarbell N, et al. Antibody responses to polysaccharide and polysaccharide-conjugate vaccines after treatment of Hodgkin disease. *Ann Intern Med* 1995;123:828–834.
119. Chan C, Molrine D, George S, et al. Pneumococcal conjugate vaccine primes for antibody response to polysaccharide pneumococcal vaccine following treatment of Hodgkin's disease. *J Infect Dis* 1996;173:256–258.
120. Hancock S, Hoppe R. Long-term complications of treatment and cancer mortality after Hodgkin's disease. *Semin Radiat Oncol* 1996;6:225–242.
121. Brice P, Tredaniel J, Monsuez JJ, et al. Cardiopulmonary toxicity after three courses of ABVD and mediastinal irradiation in favorable Hodgkin's disease. *Ann Oncol* 1991;2(suppl 2):73–76.
122. Allavena C, Conroy T, Aletti P, et al. Late cardiopulmonary toxicity after treatment for Hodgkin's disease. *Br J Cancer* 1992;65:908–912.
123. Hirsch A, Vander Els N, Straus DJ, et al. Effect of ABVD chemotherapy with and without mantle or mediastinal irradiation on pulmonary function and symptoms in early-stage Hodgkin's disease. *J Clin Oncol* 1996;14:1297–1305.
124. Villani F, Viviani S, Bonfante V, et al. Late pulmonary effects in favorable stage I and IIA Hodgkin's disease treated with radiotherapy alone. *Am J Clin Oncol* 2000;23:18–21.
125. Brockstein BE, Smiley C, Al-Sadir J, et al. Cardiac and pulmonary toxicity in patients undergoing high-dose chemotherapy for lymphoma and breast cancer: prognostic factors. *Bone Marrow Transplant* 2000;25:885–894.
126. Horning S, Adhikari A, Rizk N, et al. Effects of treatment for Hodgkin's disease on pulmonary function: results of a prospective study. *J Clin Oncol* 1994;2:297–305.
127. Lund M, Kongerud J, Nome O, et al. Lung function impairment in long-term survivors of Hodgkin's disease. *Ann Oncol* 1995;6:495–501.
128. Morrone N, GanaeSilvaVolope V, Dourado A, et al. Bilateral pleural effusion due to mediastinal fibrosis induced by radiotherapy. *Chest* 1993;4:1276–1278.
129. Rodriguez-Garcia J, Fraile G, Moreno M, et al. Recurrent massive pleural effusions as a late complication of radiotherapy in Hodgkin's disease. *Chest* 1991;4:1165–1166.
130. Horning SJ, Hoppe RT, Mason J, et al. Stanford-Kaiser Permanente G1 study for clinical stage I to IIA Hodgkin's disease: subtotal lymphoid irradiation versus vinblastine, methotrexate, and bleomycin chemotherapy and regional irradiation. *J Clin Oncol* 1997;15:1736–1744.
131. Moody AM, Pratt J, Hudson GV, et al. British National Lymphoma Investigation: pilot studies of neoadjuvant chemotherapy in clinical stage Ia and IIa Hodgkin's disease. *Clin Oncol (R Coll Radiol)* 2001;13:262–268.
132. Friedberg JW, Neuberg D, Kim H, et al. Gemcitabine added to doxorubicin, bleomycin, and vinblastine for the treatment of de novo Hodgkin disease: unacceptable acute pulmonary toxicity. *Cancer* 2003;98:978–982.
133. Bredenfeld H, Franklin J, Nogova L, et al. Severe pulmonary toxicity in patients with advanced-stage Hodgkin's disease treated with a modified bleomycin, doxorubicin, cyclophosphamide, vincristine, procarbazine, prednisone, and gemcitabine (BEACOPP) regimen is probably related to the combination of gemcitabine and bleomycin: a report of the German Hodgkin's Lymphoma Study Group. *J Clin Oncol* 2004;22:2424–2429.
134. Carde P, Hagmbeek A, Hayat M, et al. Clinical staging versus laparotomy and combined modality with MOPP versus ABVD in early-stage Hodgkin's disease: the H6 twin randomized trials for the European Organization for Research and Treatment of Cancer Lymphoma Cooperative Group. *J Clin Oncol* 1993;11:2258–2272.
135. Longo D, Glatstein E, Duffey P, et al. Alternating MOPP and ABVD chemotherapy plus mantle-field radiation therapy in patients with massive mediastinal Hodgkin's disease. *J Clin Oncol* 1997;15:3338–3346.
136. Ng AK, Bernardo MV, Silver B, et al. Mid- and post-ABVD gallium scanning predicts for recurrence in early-stage Hodgkin's disease. *Int J Radiat Oncol Biol Phys* 2005;61:175–184.
137. Martin WG, Ristow KM, Habermann TM, et al. Bleomycin pulmonary toxicity has a negative impact on the outcome of patients with Hodgkin's lymphoma. *J Clin Oncol* 2005;23:7614–7620.

CHAPTER 24 ■ SECOND CANCERS AFTER TREATMENT OF HODGKIN LYMPHOMA

FLORA E. VAN LEEUWEN, ANTHONY J. SWERDLOW, AND LOIS B. TRAVIS

Now that the majority of patients with Hodgkin lymphoma have such a favorable prognosis, it has become increasingly important to evaluate the long-term complications of treatment. Paradoxically, research conducted over the last three decades has clearly demonstrated that some treatments used to control cancer have the potential to induce new (second) primary malignancies. Of all late complications of treatment, second malignancies are generally considered to be the most serious, because they cause not only substantial morbidity but also considerable mortality. For example, among long-term survivors of Hodgkin lymphoma, second cancer deaths have been reported to be the largest contributor to the substantial excess mortality that these patients experience.[1-3] Increased risk of second cancers has been observed after both radiotherapy and chemotherapy.

In any discussion of treatment-related second malignancies, it is of primary importance to remember that not all second cancers are caused by treatment. The occurrence of two primary malignancies in the same individual may have several causes. It may represent a chance occurrence (in which case the two cancers developed as a result of unrelated factors); it may result from host susceptibility factors (e.g., genetic predisposition or immunodeficiency); it may be linked to carcinogenic influences in common; or it may represent an effect of treatment for the first tumor or an effect of, or evolution of, the primary tumor.[4,5] In view of the high prevalence of cancer in the general population and the increasing incidence of most cancers with age, background etiologic factors other than treatment are likely to be responsible for a substantial proportion of second cancers especially in older populations. Therefore, whenever a clinical impression arises that a specific combination of two distrinct primary malignancies occurs more frequently than expected, comparison with cancer risk in the general population is imperative. If a second malignancy has been demonstrated to occur in excess, the contributions of other risk factors and the role of host susceptibility factors need to be ruled out convincingly before the risk increase can be attributed to treatment. The evaluation of the carcinogenic effects of therapy is further complicated by the fact that therapeutic agents are frequently given in combination. Appropriate epidemiologic and statistical methods are required to quantify the excess risk and to unravel treatment factors responsible for it.

Whenever one is interpreting results of second cancer studies, it must be kept in mind that the problem of treatment-induced malignancies has arisen by virtue of the successes of cancer treatment. As more becomes known about the effects of various treatment factors on second cancer risk, therapies may be modified to decrease second cancer risk while maintaining equal levels of therapeutic effectiveness.

This chapter addresses major aspects of second malignancy risk following treatment for Hodgkin lymphoma. After a brief overview of the carcinogenic effects of radiation therapy and chemotherapy, we first discuss the methods used for assessing second cancer risk. Subsequently, a review is given of the risks of leukemia, non-Hodgkin lymphoma (NHL), and selected solid tumors in patients treated for Hodgkin lymphoma. Emphasis is on large studies that were published recently. Clinical implications of the most important findings are discussed, and, finally, we suggest some directions for future research.

CARCINOGENIC PROPERTIES OF RADIATION AND CYTOTOXIC DRUGS

Radiation

There is abundant literature demonstrating the carcinogenic potential of ionizing radiation. The ability of radiation to induce malignancies, particularly squamous cell carcinomas of the skin, sarcomas, and leukemia, was already recognized more than a half century ago.[6-8] Several comprehensive reviews of the carcinogenic effects of radiation have been published.[9-11] Most knowledge about radiation effects in humans has derived from epidemiologic studies of the atomic bomb survivors in Japan,[12-14] occupationally irradiated workers,[15,16] patients exposed to large amounts of diagnostic radiation,[15,16] and patients treated with radiation for malignant[17-22] and nonmalignant diseases.[23,24] Almost all types of cancer can be caused by exposure to ionizing radiation, with the probable exception of chronic lymphocytic leukemia.[12,12,25,26] Certain sites, such as the thyroid, the female breast, and bone marrow, appear to be more radiosensitive than others.[11]

The excess risk of leukemia attributable to radiation is observed within a few years of exposure, with a peak after 5 to 9 years, and declines slowly thereafter.[12,17,24,26,27] Increased risks of solid tumors have been shown to take much longer to emerge. Although increased risks have been reported in the 5- to 9-year period following irradiation,[24,28-32] most solid tumors do not occur in excess until 10 years after radiation exposure, and for some cancers (e.g., breast and bladder), excess risks seem to emerge only 15 years or even longer following irradiation. After a minimum induction period of 5 to 10 years, solid tumor risk appears to follow a time-response model consistent with a multiplicative relationship with the underlying incidence in the population; that is, risk after exposure is proportional to the background incidence of cancer over time.[26,33] It is not known at the present time whether the relative risk remains elevated throughout life. Studies in the atomic bomb survivors[13] and in women treated for benign gynecologic disorders[34] have shown that the excess relative risk per Gray tends to be fairly stable over time for at least 30 years following radiation. However, an update of the mortality experience of ankylosing spondylitis patients showed that, 25 years after irradiation, risk had decreased for a number of malignancies, particularly lung cancer.[24] In the few studies of second cancer risk in which the time course beyond 25 years from first treatment was evaluated, the relative risk (RR) of solid tumor development remained increased at the same level[35] or tended to decrease in very long-term survivors.[29,36–38] The most recent cancer incidence report on the Japanese atomic bomb survivors, with 42 years of follow-up, indicated that the excess relative risk decreased with time for the younger age-at-exposure groups, and remained virtually constant for the older cohorts.[13] Cancer incidence data from the atomic bomb survivors and five other groups exposed to radiation have been analyzed to address specifically the evolution of risk with increasing time since exposure in childhood.[39] Ten to 15 years after radiation exposure, the relative risk of solid tumors decreased with increasing follow-up time (5.7–6.1 % per year). The excess absolute risk, however, significantly increased with time since exposure.[39]

An important part of our knowledge of radiation carcinogenesis derives from populations exposed to relatively low levels of radiation, such as the atomic bomb survivors. Extrapolation of radiation effects from low doses to the high dose ranges used therapeutically cannot be done with certainty[10] because of the possibility of cell killing at high doses (see below). Therefore, recent studies of second cancer risk have focused on the shape of the radiation dose–response curve in the high-dose range.

For leukemia, data from most low-dose studies are compatible with a linear dose–response trend in risk for doses below 1.5 to 2 Gy.[12,17,25] There is consistent evidence that the excess risk of leukemia per unit radiation dose to the active bone marrow is much higher at low doses than at the high doses administered for the treatment of malignant disease.[11,17,25] This phenomenon has been attributed to cell killing or inactivation of potentially leukemic cells at the higher radiation doses.[17,27] Many studies in cancer patients have shown that high radiation doses to limited fields, such as commonly used in the treatment of Hodgkin lymphoma, confer very little or no increased risk of leukemia.[40–43] In contrast, a significant risk of leukemia (6%) has been observed in patients with NHL receiving total-body irradiation with low doses of radiation to large volumes of bone marrow.[44,45] Both in the atomic bomb survivors and in patients who received radiotherapy for cervical cancer, leukemia risk appeared to increase with increasing average dose to the bone marrow until about 4 Gy, above which leukemia risk was progressively reduced with increasing dose.[10,17,46] However, a study of leukemia risk in survivors of uterine cancer showed little evidence for such a clear downturn in risk.[25] More research is needed to investigate how dose fractionation and proportion of total bone marrow irradiated affect leukemia risk.

With regard to solid tumors, studies in populations exposed to relatively low levels of radiation have convincingly shown that the risk increases linearly with radiation dose in the lower dose ranges (up to about 5 Gy).[10,33] The excess absolute rates of breast cancer for a specified dose were found to be remarkably similar across studies in the Japanese atomic bomb survivors and in medically irradiated populations in the United States.[33,47] Recently, two studies have examined whether a linear dose–response extends to the higher dose ranges used therapeutically.[21,22] They evaluated mantle-field irradiation given for Hodgkin lymphoma, which results in a large dose gradient across the breast (i.e., 3–42 Gy at a midline dose of 40 Gy). Both studies showed increasing risk of breast cancer over this entire dose range, with eight-fold increased risk for the highest dose category (median dose 42 Gy) compared with the lowest one (<4 Gy). However, the slope of the dose–response curve appeared to be less steep than observed in studies in the low-dose range.[33] A recent comparison of relative and absolute excess risks in eight irradiated cohorts showed that breast cancer

risk was increased to a lesser extent after low-dose-rate protracted exposures compared with acute and fractionated high-dose-rate exposures.[33]

The risk of lung cancer also rises with increasing radiation dose in the lower dose range[13,24] as well as in the high-dose range (see also Table 24.6).[21,48] A leveling of risk at doses of 10 Gy or more has been observed for radiation-induced thyroid cancer.[49,50] However, even at thyroid doses up to 60 Gy, the risk of thyroid cancer did not decrease in one study.[49] A recent case-control study of thyroid cancer in the Childhood Cancer Survivor Study cohort showed that risk increased with radiation doses up to 20 to 29 Gy (RR, 9.8; 95% confidence interval [CI], 3.2–34.8).[51] At doses greater than 30 Gy, the risk appeared to decrease, although numbers were rather small to draw definitive conclusions. The reduction in radiation dose–response at high doses is consistent with a cell-killing effect. For bone sarcoma, two studies in survivors of childhood cancer[20,52] show no evidence of increased risk for doses less than 10 Gy to the site of the bone tumor. Beyond 10 Gy, risk for bone sarcoma rose sharply with increasing dose, reaching over 90-fold at doses of 30 to 50 Gy.[52]

Young age at radiation exposure has been found to be a strong risk factor for the development of most radiation-associated solid cancers in relative risk terms.[10,13,15,26,29–31,38,50,53] For example, in atomic bomb survivors who were less than 10 years old at the time of bombing, the excess relative risk of breast cancer per Gray was five times that of women who were over 40 years old when exposed.[14] Irradiation may thus affect cells of the mammary ducts before full organ development begins. A strong trend of increasing breast cancer relative risk with decreasing age at exposure was also observed in patients irradiated for Hodgkin lymphoma.[29,30,38,54] Significantly greater RRs with younger age at radiation exposure have been reported for lung cancer,[29,30] thyroid cancer,[13,29] bone sarcoma,[29,31,53] and gastrointestinal cancer.[29,30,38] After radiation in childhood, the excess relative risk per Gy for thyroid cancer (RR, 7.7; 95% CI, 2.1–28.7) is higher than for any other solid malignancy.[13]

Issues that need to be clarified by further research include the duration of radiation-induced cancer risk, the effects of dose fractionation and, importantly, the interaction of radiotherapy with environmental carcinogens (e.g., smoking, hormonal factors, chemotherapy, and the role of gene–environment and gene–gene interactions).[55] Because the mechanisms underlying the carcinogenic effects of radiation are still poorly understood, research should also focus on the identification of specific (somatic) gene alterations associated with the development of radiation-induced cancer.[56,57] The mutational spectrum of the p53 tumor suppressor gene in radiation-induced lung cancer may differ from that observed in smoking-related lung cancer.[58–60] Further, microsatellite alterations, which indicate widespread genomic instability, occur with greater frequency in lung and breast cancers after Hodgkin lymphoma than in sporadic cancers.[61] Increasing evidence suggests that genetic factors contribute to the development of radiation-induced cancers. This is perhaps best demonstrated in survivors of hereditary retinoblastoma who harbor a heterozygous germline mutation in the RB1 tumor-suppressor gene, and who have a much greater risk of developing osteosarcomas within the radiation field than children irradiated for nonhereditary retinoblastoma.[62] In addition, two studies showed that patients with a positive family history of cancer are more likely to develop radiation-associated second malignancies,[63,64] and BRCA1/2 mutation carriers were recently shown to have an increased risk of breast cancer following diagnostic radiation exposures at young ages.[65] In view of the postulated radiation sensitivity of heterozygous carriers of the mutated ataxia-telangiectasia (ATM) gene, it has been speculated that AT heterozygotes (approximately 1.0% of the population) may have an increased risk of radiation-induced cancer, specifically breast cancer.[66,67] In two studies, however, no ATM mutations were found in a total of

56 women who had developed breast cancer after radiation therapy for Hodgkin lymphoma.[64,68] Further studies should focus on the identification of other genes that may influence susceptibility to the DNA-damaging effects of radiation.[55] Such research will provide more insight into the mechanisms underlying radiation carcinogenesis and will also be of clinical benefit in minimizing radiation exposure to the most susceptible subgroups.

Chemotherapy

The carcinogenic potential of chemotherapy was recognized much later than that of ionizing radiation. This obviously has to do with the fact that chemotherapeutic agents were not introduced in cancer treatment until the late 1940s,[69] and modern multiagent combination chemotherapy, which is now known to have the strongest carcinogenic potential, was not used until the 1960s. Until the introduction of combination chemotherapy, patients treated with antineoplastic agents rarely lived long enough for an increased risk of second malignancies to become manifest. A review of the literature indicates that, generally, it takes 5 to 20 years from the introduction of a drug into clinical practice before a carcinogenic effect of the agent becomes evident.[69-71] Evidence of the carcinogenicity of chemotherapeutic agents has not only come from clinical observations but also, to a great extent, from in vivo and in vitro laboratory studies. Pioneering work in this field was conducted before clinical studies had shown increased risk of second malignancies following chemotherapy.[72-74]

The predominant malignancy associated with chemotherapy is acute myeloid leukemia (AML). The leukemogenicity of chemotherapy in man was first discovered in patients treated for multiple myeloma, following the introduction of melphalan and other alkylating agens in 1962. The first report suggesting a role of alkylating agents was published in 1970,[75] and the association was confirmed in a number of subsequent studies.[76,77] MOPP combination chemotherapy for Hodgkin lymphoma (consisting of mechlorethamine, vincristine, procarbazine, and prednisone) was introduced in 1967 and its leukemogenic potential became evident in the 1970s.[78-80] Large elevated risks of AML have subsequently been demonstrated following combination-alkylating agent chemotherapy for many other malignancies.[81,82]

Chemotherapy is far more potent than radiation therapy in inducing leukemia. In recent years it has become evident that there are at least two different syndromes of treatment-related leukemia: "classic" alkylating agent–induced AML and AML related to the topoisomerase II inhibitors.[83-85]

Alkylating agents with known leukemogenic effects in humans are mechlorethamine, chlorambucil, cyclophosphamide, melphalan, semustine, lomustine, carmustine, prednimustine, busulfan, and dihydroxybusulfan.[81,84] The relative leukemogenicity of these drugs is not completely known, and studies in this field are surrounded by methodologic problems. First, chemotherapeutic drugs are commonly given in combination, which renders it difficult to disentangle their effects. Second, the leukemogenic potency of drugs can be compared in different ways: in terms of absolute (cumulative) drug dose (in grams, or grams/m²) or in terms of units of equal therapeutic or clinical effect.[40,86] Convincing evidence has accumulated that, with both definitions, cyclophosphamide is substantially less leukemogenic than melphalan, mechlorethamine, chlorambucil, lomustine, and thiotepa.[40,41,43,87-91] There is general agreement that cumulative cyclophosphamide doses below 20 g do not confer an appreciable increase of leukemia risk.[43,89,91] Only a few studies have compared the leukemogenic potency of alkylating agents other than cyclophosphamide.[90,91]

There is abundant evidence that the risk of alkylating agent–related AML rises with increasing cumulative dose. Most studies that attempted to disentangle the effects of cumulative dose, duration of use, and dose intensity, reported that cumulative dose appeared to be the strongest determinant of risk.[43,91]

The relative risk of alkylating agent–related leukemia (compared with the general population) begins to increase 2 years after start of chemotherapy, peaks in the 5- to 10-year follow-up period, and decreases afterwards.[32,40,41,92] Even in large patient series, the number of patients has been too small to determine whether 15 to 20 years post-treatment the risk of leukemia returns to the background level of the population.[32,93] More than 50% of leukemias following alkylating-agent therapy present initially as myelodysplasia (MDS), whereas de novo AML is preceded by MDS much less frequently.[32,81] Most cases of myelodysplastic syndrome progress to AML within a year.[32,81,94] Cytogenetic studies of alkylating agent–related AML/MDS have shown unbalanced chromosome aberrations, primarily with loss of whole chromosomes 5 and/or 7 or various parts of the long arms of these chromosomes.[94,95] Morphologically, alkylating agent–related AML is most commonly of French-American-British (FAB) subtypes M1 and M2, but all subtypes except M3 have been observed.[81]

The International Agency for Research on Cancer (IARC) recently concluded that the epipodophyllotoxins etoposide and teniposide are probably carcinogenic to humans.[96] As compared with "classical" alkylating agent–induced AML, epipodophyllotoxin-related AML has a shorter induction period (median 2 to 3 years following treatment), and generally lacks a preceding myelodysplastic phase. Further, this type of AML appears to be characterized by balanced translocations involving chromosome bands 11q23 and 21q22. These chromosome aberrations are more frequently associated with the development of acute monoblastic or myelomonocytic leukemia (M4 or M5 according to the FAB criteria).[84,97,98] Evidence has accumulated that the anthracyclines doxorubicin and 4-epidoxorubicin, which are intercalating topoisomerase II inhibitors, may induce a similar type of AML as the one related to epipodophyllotoxin treatment.[40,99,100] It is unclear whether epipodophyllotoxin-related AML has a better prognosis than "classic" alkylating agent-related AML, which is notoriously resistant to anti-leukemic treatment.[95,101]

Just as the pharmacology of effective cancer chemotherapy is impacted by pharmacokinetics and pharmacodynamics, these influences likely contribute to the development of AML. The possible role of polymorphisms in drug-metabolizing genes, including the cytochrome P-450 enzymes, glutathione S-transferases, and arylamine N-acetyltransferases in chemotherapy-related leukemias, has been reviewed.[102] The U.S. Children's Oncology Group is currently conducting a study of polymorphisms in drug-metabolizing enzymes and indicators of genotoxicity to possibly identify patients treated for Hodgkin lymphoma who are at increased risk of therapy-associated complications, including second cancer.[103] Other factors in the development of chemotherapy-related leukemias may include interindividual differences in repair of DNA damage,[104,105] germ-line mutations in tumor-suppressor genes,[102,106] administration of concomitant medications, and interpatient variation in renal and hepatic function. Yeoh and associates[107] suggested that gene expression profiling of pediatric ALL might indicate which patients are at increased risk of secondary AML, independent of treatment. Clarification of the interrelationships between various factors are critical to a better understanding of individual susceptibility to AML. Because cancer patients frequently receive large doses of cytotoxic drugs, interindividual differences in drug absorption, distribution, metabolism, and excretion are accentuated. Until these influences and their interrelationships are better understood, empiric end-points, such as the development of acute hematopoetic toxicity following chemotherapy, might be explored for their value as possible surrogate markers of AML risk.[91] Whether chemoprotectants such as amifostine (WR-2721), which ameliorates the myelosuppressive effects of alkylating agents,[108] might possibly contribute to decreased risks of second leukemias, should be examined.

Many chemotherapeutic agents are known mutagens and animal carcinogens,[109] and the induction period of solid tumors may be longer than the observation period available in published research. Thus, the question of whether the increased risks of leukemia after chemotherapy may be later followed by excess solid tumors is important. To date, the causal link between cyclophosphamide and bladder cancer represents one of the few established relationships between a specific cytostatic drug and a solid tumor.[110,111] Risk of bladder cancer rises significantly with increasing cumulative dose of cyclophosphamide, with 15-fold excess risk among patients receiving doses of 50 g or more. Similarly, increasing cumulative doses of mechlorethamine or procarbazine given to treat Hodgkin lymphoma have been strongly associated with increasing lung cancer risk when evaluated separately (p trend for dose for each <0.001),[19] consistent with the ability of these drugs to induce lung tumors in laboratory animals.[109] Moreover, mechlorethamine is similar in chemical structure to sulfur mustard, an established human lung carcinogen when inhaled.[112] Elevated risks of bone sarcomas[20,52] have also been observed after alkylating-agent chemotherapy, although the responsible cytostatic agents have not been clearly identified. Prolonged follow-up studies are warranted to determine whether specific agents affect solid tumor risk, and if so, whether they add to or multiply radiation-associated risks.

METHODS OF ASSESSING SECOND CANCER RISK

The *cohort study* and the *nested case-control study* are the epidemiologic study designs generally used in second cancer research.[113] Case reports have an important role in the early recognition of potential associations between different malignancies.[75,77] However, because of lack of information on the underlying population at risk, case reports are not useful in quantifying risks.

In a cohort study of second cancer risk, a large group of patients (the cohort) with a specified first malignancy is followed up for a number of years to determine the incidence of second (and subsequent) malignancies. In nearly all studies of second cancer risk, the cohorts have been defined retrospectively from existing data sources. Useful sources for the identification of such cohorts are population-based cancer registries, hospital-based tumor registries, or clinical trial databases (see below). Because most cohort studies of second cancer risk have been conducted retrospectively, follow-up of all patients in such studies is completed up to some point in the recent past. In order to evaluate whether second cancer risk in the cohort is increased compared with cancer risk in the general population, the observed number of second cancers in the cohort is compared with the number expected on the basis of cancer incidence rates in the general population. This can be done in a so-called "person-years" type of analysis. In this approach, adjustment is made for the distribution of the cohort according to age, sex, and calendar period, while the observation period of individual patients (person-years at risk) is also taken into account. The expected site-specific numbers of second primary cancers in the cohort are derived by multiplying the person-years by age-, sex-, and calendar period–specific incidence rates of cancers of all selected sites from a population-based cancer registry. Ideally, the cancer incidence rates used to calculate the expected numbers are derived from the same source population as that from which the cohort has been drawn. The *relative risk* (RR) of developing a second cancer is estimated by the ratio of the observed number of second cancer cases in the cohort to the number expected. In epidemiologic terminology, the observed-to-expected ratio is often called the standardized incidence ratio

(SIR). For cancer deaths, the equivalent measure is the standardized mortality ratio (SMR), in which observed second malignancy deaths are compared with expected numbers of deaths.

A disadvantage of the person-years method as applied in its simplest form is that it assumes the risk of second cancer development to be constant over time; that is, it assumes the second cancer experience of 1,000 patients followed for 1 year to be comparable to that of 100 patients followed for 10 years. When this assumption is inappropriate (as with treatment-related cancers developing after an induction period), it is more informative to calculate RRs within specified post-treatment intervals (usually 5-year periods).[114,115] Such a procedure highlights situations in which an inadequate number of patients are followed for a sufficient amount of time to evaluate the long-term carcinogenic risks of treatment.

When the observed-to-expected ratio is increased, the question arises whether the risk increase is caused by the treatment. This can be evaluated by comparing RRs between treatment groups, preferably with a reference group of patients not treated with radiation therapy or chemotherapy. Such a comparison group is available when second cancer risk is examined in patients with breast or testicular cancer but, unfortunately, not for patients with Hodgkin lymphoma. When the observation period (or survival rate) differs between treatments, their overall observed-to-expected ratios cannot be validly compared. In such cases, treatment-specific RRs must be calculated by interval after start of therapy. To allow valid comparisons between treatments it is also possible, in Poisson regression analysis, to adjust treatment-specific observed-to-expected ratios for differences in age at treatment and time since treatment (see below). However, when too few patients are left for observation in one treatment group beyond a particular duration of follow-up, comparisons of second cancer risk between treatments are not appropriate beyond that observation period. A temporal trend of excess second cancer risk may in itself provide an important initial clue to treatment-related causes; for example, the risk of solid malignancy following radiation therapy for Hodgkin lymphoma generally increases with time since exposure.

Second cancer risk in the cohort (and in different treatment groups) can also be expressed by the *cumulative* (actuarial estimated) risk,[116] which gives the proportion of patients expected to develop a second malignancy by time t (e.g., 5 years from diagnosis) if they do not die before then. When the cohort's death rate from causes other than second malignancy is high, the assumptions underlying the actuarial method may not be valid. This particularly concerns the assumption that, in patients who died due to other causes, second malignancy risk would have followed the temporal pattern observed in those who survived. In such cases actuarial risk tends to overestimate the true risk and competing-risk techniques should be used to estimate cumulative risk.[117–120] In comparing estimates of cumulative risk across studies, it is important to keep in mind that this measure of risk depends very strongly on the age distribution of a specific cohort; because of the low background incidence of cancer at young ages, cohorts of Hodgkin lymphoma patients that include patients treated as children will report much lower cumulative risks than cohorts including adults only. Furthermore, cumulative risks for different treatments will only be comparable if the treatment groups have a similar age distribution, and if they do not there will be a bias toward lower apparent risks in whichever treatment group is youngest. Most studies reporting cumulative risks make no comparison with cancer risk in the general population, yet population-expected cumulative risks over time can be easily calculated on the basis of cancer incidence rates from a population-based registry.[121]

Because certain treatment-related cancers are rare in the general population (e.g., leukemia, sarcoma), a high RR (compared to the population) may still translate into a rather low cumulative risk. *Absolute excess risk* (AER), which estimates the excess number of second malignancies occurring per 10,000 patients per year (beyond those expected from rates in the general population), perhaps best reflects the second cancer burden in a cohort. This risk measure is also the most appropriate one to judge which second malignancies contribute most to the excess risk. The calculation of observed-to-expected ratios on the basis of person-years analysis, and the calculation of cumulative risks using life-table analysis, involve rather simple statistical methods, which have a strong intuitive appeal. Besides these elementary methods, statistical modeling with Cox proportional hazards model and Poisson regression techniques is increasingly being used to refine the quantification of second cancer risk (e.g., by estimating dose– and time–response relationships) and to examine the interplay between treatment variables and other factors.[122,123]

Each of the data sources that are commonly used to constitute cohorts has specific advantages and disadvantages. Population-based cancer registries have large numbers of patients available, which allows the detection of even small excess risks of second cancers.[4,124,125] An additional advantage is that the observed and expected numbers of cancers come from the same reference population. Disadvantages include limited availability of treatment data, underreporting of second cancers[4,41,126] (in particular hematologic malignancies), and inconsistent diagnostic criteria for second cancers. Population-based registries differ greatly in these aspects and hence in their usefulness for second cancer studies. If treatment data are not available, it is impossible to know whether excess risk for a second malignancy is related to treatment or to shared etiology with the first cancer. Underreporting of second cancers clearly leads to an underestimation of second cancer risk. Far higher risks of second leukemia following Hodgkin lymphoma have been found in hospital series[31,32] than in population-based studies.[41,125] Part of this difference, however, may be attributable to the more intensive treatments administered in large treatment centers.[41] Despite their disadvantages, population-based registries are well suited to evaluate broadly which second cancers occur in excess following a wide spectrum of different first primary malignancies. They are also a valuable starting point for case-control studies that evaluate treatment effects in detail (see below).

A major advantage of clinical trial databases is that detailed treatment data on all patients are available. Comparison of second cancer risk between the treatment arms of the trial controls for any intrinsic risk for a second malignancy associated with the first cancer. However, a limitation of most trials is the small number of patients involved. Although this problem can be overcome by combining data from a number of trials, multicenter trial series pose other problems, such as difficulties in accessing medical records and histologic slides of patients in multiple centers. Further, the main end-points of interest in most clinical trials are treatment response and survival, and many trials do not routinely collect information on second malignancies or on full systematic long-term follow-up, so that follow-up data to a fixed end date may be very incomplete (and biased). Ideally, routine reporting and assessment of second malignancy risk should become an integral part of clinical trial research.[55,127]

Many large cancer treatment centers maintain registries of all admitted patients. Most of these registries have been in existence for decades and collect extensive data on treatment and follow-up. They share the advantages of clinical trial databases without having their disadvantages. Investigators using hospital tumor registries have ready access to the medical records; often a review of the histologic slides of the first and the second malignancy can also be arranged easily, or is conducted routinely. An additional advantage is that, compared with trial data, hospital registries provide a wider range of treatments and dose levels, which may yield important information on drug and radiation carcinogenesis. Most studies of second cancer risk following Hodgkin lymphoma have been based on hospital registries.[31,32,78,128–130]

The cohort study is not an efficient study design for examining detailed treatment factors (e.g., cumulative dose of alkylating agents) in relation to second cancer risk. In order to yield stable estimates of second cancer risk, cohorts need to be large, rendering the collection of detailed treatment data time-consuming and costly. In such cases, to assess treatment-related risks without the practical difficulty of gathering detailed treatment data for many hundreds or thousands of patients, a "nested" case-control study within an existing cohort is the preferred approach. The case group consists of all patients identified with the second cancer of interest, and the controls are a random sample of all patients in the cohort who did not develop the cancer concerned, although they experienced the same amount of follow-up time. To achieve maximum statistical power, most case-control studies of second cancer risk use a design in which more than one control is individually matched to each second cancer "case." Matching factors employed in most studies include sex, year of birth, and year at diagnosis of the first primary cancer. The most important criterion for control selection is that each control must have survived, without developing the second cancer of interest, for at least as long as the interval between the diagnosis of the first and the second malignancy of the corresponding case. Even if the control group is three times as large as the case group, detailed treatment data need be collected for only a small proportion of the total cohort. In each case-control study it is critical to the validity of the study results that the controls are truly representative of all patients who did not develop the second cancer of interest. For example, biased results may be obtained when controls with untraceable records are replaced by controls with traceable records.

In the analysis of a case-control study of second cancer risk, treatment factors are compared between cases and controls. Treatments that have been administered more often, for a longer duration, or with a higher dose to the case group than to the controls are associated with increased risk of developing the second malignancy of interest. It is important to understand that in a nested case-control study, the risk associated with specific treatments is estimated relative to the risk in patients receiving other treatment and *not* relative to the risk in the general population. The cumulative risk of developing a second malignancy cannot be derived using data from a case-control study alone. Estimates of the AERs associated with specific treatments can be derived, however, if the case-control study follows a cohort analysis in which observed-to-expected ratios were calculated for broad treatment groups. Although case-control methodology has only come into widespread use for the investigation of second cancer risk in recent decades,[44,131] several landmark studies have already demonstrated its strengths.[17,19–22,40–43,111,132]

INCIDENCE AND RISK FACTORS OF SELECTED SECOND CANCERS

Overall Risk of Leukemia, Non-Hodgkin Lymphoma (NHL), and Solid Malignancy

Since the first reports in the early 1970s noting an of increased second cancer risk in patients treated for Hodgkin's disease,[79,80,133] many treatment centers have reported on second cancer risk. An excess of AML in chemotherapy-treated patients and an increased risk of solid tumors in radiation-treated patients have been consistently noted. For 11 large cohort studies published since 1990, the overall RRs of selected second malignancies compared with the general population are given in Tables 24.1 (predominantly adults) and Table 24.2 (children).

TABLE 24.1

RELATIVE RISKS OF SECOND MALIGNANCY FOR SELECTED SITES IN RECENT LARGE[a] COHORT STUDIES OF PATIENTS WITH HODGKIN LYMPHOMA; PREDOMINANTLY ADULTS

Site	Henry-Amar[92] • International • N = 12,411[b] • Ages ≥15 • Med. fup ~7 yrs • Yrs of dx 1960–87 ♂ RR(n)	♀ RR(n)	Boivin[138] • U.S. and Canada • N = 10,472[b] • All ages • Med. fup 7.1 yrs • Yrs of dx 1940–87 RR(n)	van Leeuwen[32] • Netherlands • N = 1,939[b] • All ages • Med. fup 9.2 yrs • Yrs of dx 1966–86 RR(n)	Swerdlow[30] • Britain • N = 5,519[b] • All ages • Med. fup 8.5 yrs • Yrs of dx 1963–93 RR(n)	van Leeuwen[38] • Netherlands • N = 1,253[b] • Ages <40 • Med. fup 14.1 yrs • Yrs of dx 1966–86 RR(n)	Dores[29] • International • N = 32,591[b] • All ages • Med. fup <10 yrs • Yrs of dx 1935–94 RR(n)	Foss Abrahamsen[164] • Norway • N = 1,024[b] • All ages • Med. fup 14 yrs • Yrs of dx 1968–85 RR(n)	Ng[54] • U.S. • N = 1,319[b] • All ages • Med. fup 12 yrs • Yrs of dx 1969–97 RR(n)
Stomach	1.7 (14)	0.8 (2)	d	1.6 (4)	2.2c (13)	10.9c (7)	1.9c (80)	4.4c (12)	d
Colon	1.9c (18)	0.9 (5)	d	2.5 (8)	2.3c (18)	2.8 (3)	1.6c (129)	1.9 (9)	d
Pancreas	1.7 (6)	0.9 (1)	d	d	1.0c (3)	d	1.5c (40)	1.3 (2)	d
Lung	2.2c (68)	4.6c (27)	d	3.7c (31)	3.4c (78)	7.0c (13)	2.9c (377)	5.1c (26)	4.9c (22)
Bone	6.2c (4)	6.5 (2)	d	–(0)	10.7c (4)	d	3.8c (9)	d	d
Soft tissue	2.8 (3)	1.6 (1)	d	8.8c (3)	3.9c (3)	12.1c (3)	5.1c (32)	d	d
Bone and soft tissue	d	d	12.0c (24)	d		d		d	26.6c (11)
Melanoma	1.9 (7)	1.2 (4)	2.2c (15)	4.9c (5)	2.3 (6)	5.5c (7)	1.7c (52)	2.8c (8)	3.3c (7)
Female breast	d	1.5c (39)	1.4 (39)	1.3 (8)	1.4 (19)	5.2c (27)	2.0c (234)	3.8c (23)	6.7c (39)
Cervix	d	1.4 (9)	d	5.9c (4)	2.1 (7)	d	2.0c (37)	1.5 (2)	d
Bladder	0.44 (4)	1.8 (3)	d	2.0 (4)	0.8 (5)	d	1.4c (66)	d	d
Prostate	0.47 (5)		d	1.5 (3)	0.8 (4)	d	1.0 (98)	1.7 (10)	d
Thyroid	5.1c (5)	1.5 (3)	4.5c (13)	–(0)	7.6c (5)	15.2c (4)	4.1c (47)	d	5.6c (5)
NHL	35.6c (79)	24.2c (27)	5.6c (35)	20.6c (23)	14.0c (50)	21.5c (16)	5.5c (162)	24.2c (31)	16.5c (24)
Leukemia	28.6 (102)	25.7c (56)	23.9c (122)	34.7c (31)	14.6c (45)	37.5c (18)	9.9c (249)	13.0c (14)	82.5c (23)
All solid	d	d	d	2.4 (93)	2.2c (227)	6.1c (106)	2.0c (1726)	d	3.5c (131)
All sites	3.0c (410)	2.6c (221)	2.7c (521)	3.5c,e (146)	2.9c (322)	7.0 (137)	2.3c (2153)	3.5c (194)	4.6c (181)

[a] Only includes studies with ≥100 second malignancies; for cohorts included in several reports, only the paper with the longest follow-up is included.

[b] Number of patients with Hodgkin lymphoma included in the study.

[c] Significantly elevated ($p < 0.05$).

[d] Data not published.

[e] Excluding nonmelanoma skin cancers.

NHL, non-Hodgkin lymphoma; Med. fup, median follow up; Yrs of dx, years of diagnosis; ♂, male; ♀, female; RR, relative risk; n, number of second malignacies.

TABLE 24.2

RELATIVE RISKS OF SECOND MALIGNANCY OF SELECTED SITES IN RECENT LARGE[a] COHORT STUDIES OF PATIENTS WITH HODGKIN LYMPHOMA; *CHILDREN AND ADOLESCENTS*

Site	Sankila[141] • Nordic countries • N = 1,641[b] • Ages ≤20 • Med. fup 10 yrs • Yrs of dx 1940–1991 RR(n)	Metayer[37] • International • N = 5,925[b] • Ages ≤20 • Med. fup 10.5 yrs • Yrs of dx 1935–1994 RR(n)	Bhatia[35] • U.S. • N = 1,380[b] • Ages ≤16 • Med. fup 17 yrs • Yrs of dx 1955–1986 RR(n)
Stomach	– (0)	13.8[c] (5)	63.9[c] (3)
Colon	3.6 (1)	4.7[c] (4)	36.4[c] (8)[d]
Pancreas	–[e]	10.8[c] (2)	–[e]
Lung	– (0)	5.1[c] (6)	27.3[c] (4)
Bone	–[e]	9.7[c] (5)	37.1[c] (8)
Soft tissue	–[e]	15.1[c] (9)	–[e]
Bone and soft tissue	10.0[c] (3)	–[e]	–[e]
Melanoma	2.7 (2)	1.9 (5)	–[e]
Female breast	17.0[c] (16)	14.1[c] (52)	55.5[c] (39)
Cervix	– (0)	6.1[c] (10)	–[e]
Bladder	–[e]	4.3 (2)	–[e]
Prostate	–[e]	–[e]	–[e]
Thyroid	33.0[c] (9)	13.7[c] (22)	36.4[c] (19)
NHL	15.0[c] (5)	6.9[c] (10)	11.7[c] (7)
Leukemia	17.0[c] (7)	20.9[c] (28)	174.8[c] (27)
All solid	–[e]	7.0[c] (157)	18.5[c] (109)
All sites	7.7[f] (62)	7.7[c] (195)	18.5[c] (143)

[a]Only includes studies with ≥100 second malignancies; for cohorts included in several reports, only the paper with the longest follow-up is included.
[b]Number of patients Hodgkin lymphoma included in the study.
[c]Significantly elevated *(p <0.05)*.
[d]Colorectal.
[e]Data not published.
[f]Partially includes nonmelanoma skin cancers.
NHL, non-Hodgkin lymphoma; Med. fup, median follow up; Yrs of dx, years of diagnosis; RR, relative risk; n, number of second malignancies.

The largest RR (10- to 15-fold) is observed for all leukemia taken together (with even greater risk for AML (22-fold)), followed by a 6- to 14-fold increased risk for NHL, and 4- to 10-fold excesses for connective tissue, bone, and thyroid cancer. Moderately increased risks (2- to 4-fold) are observed for a number of solid tumors, such as cancers of the lung, stomach, esophagus, colon, breast, mouth and pharynx, cervix, and melanoma. Because leukemia and NHL are diseases with a low incidence in the general population, even a high RR compared with the population may translate into a low cumulative (actu-

arial) risk, as well as a low AER. As shown in Figure 24.1,[38] for the entire follow-up period, the cumulative risk of solid tumors far exceeds that of leukemia or NHL. AER is the best measure to judge which subsequent tumors contribute most to the second cancer burden. Table 24.3 gives AERs from the two largest studies in Table 24.1, showing that, compared with the general population, patients treated for Hodgkin lymphoma experience an excess of about 45 malignancies per 10,000 person-years of observation. Solid tumors account for the majority of excess cancers (approximately 30 per 10,000 patients per year), with

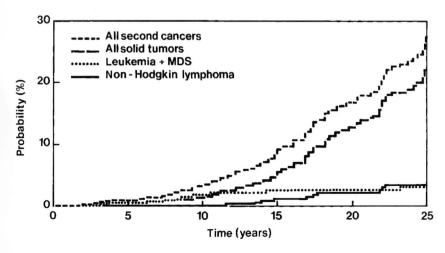

FIGURE 24.1. Cumulative risk of second cancers after Hodgkin lymphoma. (Adapted with permission from van Leeuwen FE, Klokman WJ, van't Veer MB, et al. Long-term risk of second malignancy in survivors of Hodgkin's disease treated during adolescence or young adulthood. *J Clin Oncol* 2000;18:487–497.)

TABLE 24.3

RELATIVE RISK AND ABSOLUTE EXCESS RISK OF SECOND MALIGNANCIES AFTER HODGKIN LYMPHOMA: RESULTS FROM TWO LARGE RECENT STUDIES

| Site or type | Dores[29]
• International
• N = 32,591[a]
• All ages
• Med. fup <10 yrs
• Yrs of dx 1935–1994 | | | | Swerdlow[30]
• Britain
• N = 5,519[a]
• All ages
• Med. fup 8.5 yrs
• Yrs of dx 1963–1993 | | | |
	Observed cases	Relative risk[b] (O/E cases)	95% CI	AER[c] (per 10,000 patients/year)	Observed cases	Relative risk[b] (O/E cases)	95% CI	AER[c] (per 10,000 patients/year)
All malignancies	2,153	2.3	2.2–2.4	47.2	322	2.9	2.6–3.2	44.5
Leukemia	249	9.9	8.7–11.2	8.8	45	14.6	10.7–19.2	8.9
NHL	162	5.5	4.7–6.4	5.2	50	14.0	10.5–18.3	9.9
Solid tumors	1,726	2.0	1.9–2.0	33.1	227	2.2	1.9–2.5	25.7
Tongue, mouth, pharynx	75	3.3	2.6–4.1	2.1	6	2.8	1.1–5.8	0.8
Esophagus	29	2.8	1.8–4.0	0.7	5	2.0	0.7–4.3	0.5
Stomach	80	1.9	1.5–2.4	1.5	13	2.2	1.2–3.6	1.5
Colon	129	1.6	1.4–1.9	2.0	18	2.3	1.4–3.6	2.2
Rectum	52	1.2	0.9–1.6	0.4	7	1.3	0.5–2.5	0.3
Pancreas	40	1.5	1.1–2.0	0.5	3	1.0	0.2–2.6	0
Lung	377	2.9	2.6–3.2	9.7	8	3.4	2.7–4.2	11.7
Female breast	234	2.0	1.8–2.3	10.5	19	1.4	0.9–2.1	3.1
Uterine cervix	37	2.0	1.4–2.7	1.6	7	2.1	0.9–4.1	0.8
Prostate	98	1.0	0.8–1.2	-0.1	4	0.8	0.2–1.7	-0.3
Bladder	66	1.4	1.1–1.8	0.8	5	0.8	0.3–1.8	-0.2
Central nervous system	36	1.5	1.1–2.1	0.5	7	2.5	1.1–4.8	0.9
Thyroid	47	4.1	3.0–5.5	1.4	5	7.6	2.7–16.4	0.9
Bone	9	3.8	1.7–7.2	0.3	4	10.7	3.3–24.8	0.8
Connective tissue	32	5.1	3.5–7.2	1.0	3	3.9	1.0–10.1	0.5
Melanoma	52	1.7	1.3–2.3	0.9	6	2.3	0.9–4.6	0.7

NHL, non-Hodgkin lymphoma; Med. fup, median follow up; Yrs of dx, years of diagnosis; 95% CI, 95% confidence interval.
[a]Number of patients with Hodgkin lymphoma included in the study.
[b]Observed cases/expected cases; expected numbers based on age-, gender-, and calendar-period specific cancer incidence in the population.
[c]AER, absolute excess risk = excess number of cases (observed minus expected) per 10,000 patients per year.

lung cancer contributing 10 to 12 excess cases per 10,000 person-years. Leukemia and NHL each account for about 8 to 9 cases per 10,000 person-years. These figures, however, depend on the age distribution of the particular cohort.

Temporal Trends for Leukemia, NHL, and Solid Malignancy

Temporal patterns of increased second malignancy risk vary by tumor site, as is illustrated in Table 24.4. In most studies, increased leukemia risk is observed as early as 2 to 4 years following initiation of chemotherapy, with peak occurrence between 5 and 9 years and decreasing risks thereafter.[29,30,32,35,38,41,134] In studies with large numbers of long-term survivors, significantly increased RRs are still observed for 15 years after first treatment.[29,30,32,35,38,54,93] The RR of NHL is already greatly increased in the first 5 years after treatment (Table 24.4). In some studies, the risk remains rather constant over time,[29,54,134] whereas others report that risk increases with time since treatment.[31,32] The RR of solid tumors is minimally elevated in the 1 to 4 year follow-up period, and increases steadily with increasing follow-up time from 5 years since first treatment (Table 24.4).[29–32,38,54,92,134] For some tumor sites

(breast, thyroid, esophagus), the excess risk does not become apparent until after 10 or even 15 years of observation. In studies that include data on 20-year survivors, the RR of solid tumors continued to increase through the 15- to 20-year follow-up period.[29,30,32,35,38,54,92,135,136] Four recent studies reported on the time course of risk 20 or more years after treatment.[29,35,38,54] In an international population-based study by Dores and associates,[29] a downturn in the RR for all solid tumors combined was observed after 25 years of follow-up, with RRs of 3.0 and 1.8 among patients in the 20- to 24-year interval and 25-year survivors, respectively (Table 24.4). A Dutch study in patients diagnosed with Hodgkin lymphoma before age 40 reported a RR for solid tumors of 5.3 among 25-year survivors, compared with a RR of 8.8 in the 20- to 24-year interval. This suggests that the RR may decrease in very long-term survivors. However, Ng and co-workers[54] reported an increasing RR of solid malignancy throughout follow-up, and Bhatia and co-workers[35] found in survivors of pediatric Hodgkin lymphoma a rathers 20- to 24-fold increased risk from 15 to over 30 years after diagnosis.

Because the RRs of leukemia, NHL and solid tumors all show distinctive patterns with time since first treatment, the AERs in long-term survivors differ greatly from those observed in the entire patient population. Table 24.4 clearly shows that the AERs of solid malignancies increase at a much

TABLE 24.4

RELATIVE RISKS AND ABSOLUTE EXCESS RISKS OF SECOND CANCERS AFTER HODGKIN LYMPHOMA, ACCORDING TO TIME SINCE DIAGNOSIS[a]

	Time since diagnosis				
	1–9 years	10–14 years	15–19 years	20–24 years	≥25 years
Number of patients entering interval	32,591	11,326	6,195	2,861	1,111
All solid tumors					
O/E (95% CI)	1.6 (1.5–1.7)	2.4 (2.2–2.7)	2.5 (2.2–2.8)	3.0 (2.5–3.5)	1.8 (1.4–2.3)
AER	19.2	50.2	63.5	109.6	62.4
Lung cancer					
O/E (95% CI)	2.7 (2.4–3.1)	3.4 (2.7–4.3)	2.9 (2.1–4.0)	4.6 (3.2–6.5)	0.8 (0.3–1.9)
AER	8.1	12.2	11.6	27.7	-2.4
Female breast cancer					
O/E (95% CI)	1.2 (1.0–1.5)	2.7 (2.1–3.5)	3.8 (2.9–4.9)	3.0 (1.9–4.5)	3.3 (2.0–5.2)
AER	1.7	19.4	40.1	36.0	52.6
Stomach cancer					
O/E (95% CI)	1.3 (0.9–1.8)	3.7 (2.4–5.5)	2.6 (1.2–4.8)	3.2 (1.3–6.6)	2.1 (0.6–5.4)
AER	0.5	4.1	2.8	5.2	4.0
NHL					
O/E (95% CI)	4.9 (3.9–6.0)	8.2 (6.0–11.0)	4.7 (2.6–7.8)	5.7 (2.6–10.8)	4.4 (1.4–10.3)
AER	4.1	9.0	5.3	8.0	7.4
AML					
O/E (95% CI)	27.7 (23.3–32.7)	17.2 (10.9–25.8)	2.6 (0.3–9.4)	10.1 (2.7–25.9)	0 (0.0–11.5)
AER	7.7	5.1	0.6	3.9	-0.6

[a]Adapted from results by Dores GM, Metayer C, Curtis RE, et al. Second malignant neoplasms among long-term survivors of Hodgkin's disease: a population-based evaluation over 25 years. *J Clin Oncol* 2002;20:3484–3494.
O/E, observed/expected; 95% CI, 95% confidence interval; NHL, non-Hodgkin lymphoma; AML, acute myeloid leukemia; AER, absolute excess risk = excess number of cases per 10,000 patients per year.

steeper rate than the RRs, related to the fact that, with longer follow-up, patients grow older and their background rate of cancer rises strongly. Consequently, the AER amounts to about 100 excess cancer cases per 10,000 20-year survivors per year, as compared to 45/10,000 per year in all patients. Based on estimates from the study by Dores and associates,[29] solid cancers contribute by far the most to the AER in 20-year survivors, with 92 excess cases per 10,000 patients per year, followed by NHL (8/10,000/year) and AML (2/10,000/year). In females, breast cancer accounts for most of the AER of solid tumors in 20-year survivors (42/10,000/year) (Table 24.3).[29] Lung cancer accounts for 17 excess cases per 10,000 patients per year in 20-year survivors of both sexes combined. Below, we describe in more detail the magnitude of the risk increases for leukemia, NHL, and selected solid tumors. In addition, we discuss treatment and other factors associated with the excess risk.

Risk of Leukemia

The risk of secondary leukemias following Hodgkin lymphoma has been actively studied since the early 1970s. Leukemia was the first malignancy for which elevated risk after treatment for Hodgkin lymphoma was systematically noticed, probably because of the relatively short latency period, the rarity of acute leukemia in the general population, and the large RR. Most large treatment centers have reported their experience with second leukemias. Overall, risks compared with the general population have been reported to be

10- to over 80-fold increased (Tables 24.1 and 24.2). Nearly all studies show that the RR of leukemia is higher than that of NHL and much greater than that of solid tumors overall (Tables 24.1 and 24.2). Because the background risk of leukemia in the population is low, however, this strongly increased RR translates into a relatively low cumulative risk, ranging between 1.4% and 4.1% at 15 years.[30–32,35,38,92,137] Overall, AER has varied between 9 and 30 excess cases per 10,000 patients per year (Table 24.3).[29,30,93]

Although the RRs of leukemia are greatly elevated, leukemia is a rare outcome, and any one series has limited ability to examine all of the suspected cofactors in the development of leukemia. This review focuses primarily on the current questions that are being addressed in large studies. The major areas of active research include the relationship with specific treatments, the variation in risk by age at treatment for Hodgkin lymphoma, the association with splenectomy, and the time period after which excess risk levels off.

Most leukemias that occur after Hodgkin lymphoma are AML related to alkylating-agent exposure.[31,41,91,92,134,138] The actuarial risks at 15 years vary substantially with treatment categories, from 0% to 0.6% among those receiving only radiation therapy to as high as 16.5% at 15 years in chemotherapy-treated groups.[31,32,137,139,140] The RRs of leukemia associated with specific treatment categories also vary widely, depending on the referent category and considered subtypes. The RRs in chemotherapy-treated patients tend to be over 20-fold increased in cohort analyses that use population-based comparisons of all leukemia risks, over 50-fold increased with population-based estimates of AML risks, and less in case-control analyses, where the referent category usually consisted of patients treated with radiation therapy alone.[31,32,41,91,129,140–142]

Radiotherapy alone is associated with a small, or no, increased risk of leukemia compared to the risk in the general population,[30,31,38,91,92] while alkylating-agent chemotherapy is linked with greatly elevated risk. Several studies have compared the leukemogenicity of different chemotherapy regimens. Where exposure has been quantified, risk appears to be most related to total dose of alkylating agents or nitrosoureas.[41,42,91,129,140] Risk of AML rises sharply with an increasing number of MOPP (mechlorethamine, vincristine, procarbazine, prednisone) (or MOPP-like) cycles.[41,91] The risk associated with 10 to 12 MOPP cycles appears to be approximately three to five times higher than the risk following 6 MOPP cycles.[41,91] Total dose of alkylators and nitrosoureas is likely the explanation of the reports of higher risk associated with salvage chemotherapy or maintenance chemotherapy,[91,92,143] but there is evidence that retreatment may be a factor in risk.[91,134,140,144] Among those treated with variations of MOPP that substitute chlorambucil for mechlorethamine, the risks appear similar, but with melphalan or cyclophosphamide in place of mechlorethamine, the risks are lower.[31,91,129,138,145] Mechlorethamine and procarbazine are usually given in combination, so it is difficult to disentangle the effects of each. One study, in which the cumulative doses of individual cytostatic drugs were available, and in which mechlorethamine and procarbazine doses were not highly correlated, showed that mechlorethamine rather than procarbazine had the strongest effect on leukemia risk.[91] Since the 1980s, MOPP-only chemotherapy has been gradually replaced by ABV(D) (doxorubicin, bleomycin, vinblastine and dacarbazine)-containing regimens in many centers. There are only a few reports of AML occurrence following ABV(D) alone. Patients treated with ABVD in the Milan Cancer Institute, where this regimen was designed, were shown to have a significantly lower risk of AML than MOPP-treated patients (15-year cumulative risks of 0.7% and 9.5%, respectively).[137] Another study showed that patients treated with MOPP/ABV(D)-containing regimens in the 1980s had substantially lower risk of AML/MDS than patients treated in the 1970s with MOPP alone (10-year cumulative risks of 2.1% and 6.4%, respectively, $p = 0.07$).[32] The German-Austrian Pediatric Hodgkin's Disease Group observed a low risk of AML (1.1% at 15 years) following regimens that contained relatively low doses of procarbazine, doxorubicin and cyclophosphamide, without mechlorethamine.[146] A recent international collaborative study showed that the AER of AML declined significantly after 1984, from 7.0 to 4.2 per 10,000 patients per year in those diagnosed before age 35 years, and from 16.4 to 9.9 per 10,000 patient-years in those diagnosed at 35 years or after.[93]

There is, however, concern about the role of anthracyclines and epipodophyllotoxins (both of which are topoisomerase II inhibitors) in the risk of leukemia. Limited evidence suggests that doxorubicin in combination with higher doses of alkylating agents and/or epipodophyllotoxins may have a synergistic effect on the risk of AML. Recent analyses of the German Hodgkin Lymphoma Study Group also show low risks of AML after COPP-ABVD (mechlorethamine replaced by cyclophosphamide) and standard BEACOPP (bleomycin, etoposide, doxorubicin combined with COPP), while substantially increased risk of AML was observed for the escalated BEACOPP regimen (actuarial risk at 5 years of 2.5%).[147,148]

An important question is whether radiation therapy adds to the leukemia risk associated with chemotherapy. Evidence that combined-modality treatment results in greater risk than chemotherapy alone is provided by several reports,[92,137,149] whereas other large series indicate that the risk of AML after combined treatment is comparable to that after chemotherapy alone.[30–32,35,41,91,138,140] These inconsistent results may be due partly to differences in treatment regimens between studies, but also to lack of adjustment for type and amount of chemotherapy in some reports. The interaction between radiation therapy and chemotherapy could be evaluated most rigorously in the large case-control study by Kaldor and associates,[41] which included 163 cases of leukemia following Hodgkin lymphoma. When examining the combined effects of radiation dose to the active bone marrow and number of mechlorethamine-procarbazine containing cycles, it was found that for each category of radiation dose (<10, 10–20, >20 Gy to the marrow), leukemia risk clearly increased with the number of chemotherapy cycles. In contrast, among patients with a given number of chemotherapy cycles, risk of leukemia did not consistently increase with higher radiation dose. Taken together, the preponderance of available data does not support the hypothesis that the combination of chemotherapy and radiation therapy confers a higher risk of leukemia than chemotherapy alone.

Therapeutic intensification with autologous stem-cell transplantation (ASCT) is increasingly being used for patients with relapsing lymphoma. Relatively high actuarial risks (4–15% at 5 years) of AML and myelodysplasia have been observed after ASCT for Hodgkin lymphoma. Evidence suggests that much of the risk is related to intensive pretransplant chemotherapy.[150–154] Forrest and colleagues recently compared the risk of AML/MDS in 202 patients who had undergone ASCT to 1530 patients who underwent conventional therapy for Hodgkin lymphoma.[155] The 15-year cumulative incidence of developing AML/MDS was 1.1% (95% CI, 0.6–1.8) for those treated with conventional therapy alone, and 3.6% (95% CI, 0.9–9.6) for those undergoing ASCT ($p = 0.22$). In multivariate analysis, leukemia risk was also not influenced by ASCT.[155]

The influence of host-related factors such as age on leukemia risk in survivors of Hodgkin lymphoma treatment has been examined in a number of studies and was recently reviewed elsewhere.[156] The reported higher *cumulative* risk of AML in older Hodgkin lymphoma patients compared with younger ones just reflects the higher baseline incidence of the disease in older persons. In the few studies that have analyzed RR of leukemia by age, based on comparisons to general population expectations, no differences between age groups were observed,[31,38,157] or the RR of AML was even significantly greater at younger ages than at older (Table 24.5).[29,30,41] A large international collaborative study recently showed that the AER of AML was significantly greater in patients diagnosed with Hodgkin lymphoma at age 35 years and older than in those diagnosed before age 35,[93] likely related to the larger background incidence of AML at older ages.

The role of splenectomy in the etiology of treatment-related leukemia remains somewhat controversial. Since the initial report of an association in 1987,[158] most large groups have evaluated their data. The most recent update of the Dutch data reveals a persistent three-fold risk associated with splenectomy, controlled for type and dose of chemotherapy.[91] In this group of patients, there was no increased risk of leukemia in those who received splenic irradiation and therefore had functional hyposplenism. The effect of splenectomy has also been found by independent groups,[41,92,137,138,159,160] most of which demonstrate risks that are about doubled. In a large meta-analysis, however, splenectomy was not a significant risk factor for leukemia.[92] Other separate groups with smaller numbers have also not found splenectomy to be a risk factor.[140,145,146,149] The biological plausibility of the relationship is not completely clear. An alteration in immune status by splenectomy has been postulated.[158]

The risk of AML in relation to treatment-associated acute and chronic bone marrow toxicity has been examined in only

TABLE 24.5

RELATIVE RISKS OF VARIOUS SECOND MALIGNANCIES, ACCORDING TO AGE AT DIAGNOSIS OF HODGKIN LYMPHOMA[a]

Age at diagnosis	All second cancers	All solid cancers	Female breast	Lung	GI tract	NHL	AML
			Dores et al. (International, 2002) O/E				
<21 yrs	7.7[b]	7.0[b]	14.2[b]	5.5[b]	10.0[b]	6.9[b]	39.2[b]
21–30 yrs	4.3[b]	3.6[b]	3.7[b]	5.4[b]	3.9[b]	7.5[b]	31.7[b]
31–40 yrs	2.7[b]	2.1[b]	1.2	4.0[b]	2.1[b]	8.7[b]	35.7[b]
41–50 yrs	2.5[b]	2.1[b]	1.7[b]	3.5	2.3[b]	5.3[b]	28.6[b]
51–60 yrs	2.0[b]	1.8[b]	1.0	3.4[b]	1.6[b]	4.3[b]	21.2[b]
≥61 yrs	1.3[b]	1.2[b]	1.1	1.5[b]	1.0	3.8[b]	5.9[b]
			Swerdlow et al. (U.K., 2000) O/E				
<15 yrs	26.1[b]	—	7.7[b,c]	24.1[b]	9.1[b,c]	33.3[b]	0
15–24 yrs	7.0[b]	—		15.3[b]		8.0[b]	53.6[b]
25–34 yrs	4.1[b]	—	0.8[b,d]	6.4[b]	2.8[b,d]	9.4[b]	26.3[b]
35–44 yrs	3.0[b]	—		5.3[b]		15.7[b]	22.4[b]
45–54 yrs	2.6[b]	—	0.8	4.1[b]	1.8	11.9[b]	17.2[b]
≥55 yrs	1.9[b]	—	1.1	2.2[b]	1.6[b]	18.7[b]	10.5[b]

[a]Adapted from results by Dores GM, Metayer C, Curtis RE, et al. Second malignant neoplasms among long-term survivors of Hodgkin's disease: a population-based evaluation over 25 years. *J Clin Oncol* 2002;20:3484–3494; and Swerdlow AJ, Barber JA, Hudson GV, et al. Risk of second malignancy after Hodgkin's disease in a collaborative British cohort: the relation to age at treatment. *J Clin Oncol* 2000;18:498–509.
[b]$p < 0.05$.
[c]Joint category age at diagnosis <15 and 15–24.
[d]Joint category age at diagnosis 25–44.
O/E, observed/expected; NHL, non-Hodgkin lymphoma; AML, acute myeloid leukemia.

two studies to date.[91] Significantly increased risks of leukemia were found among patients who developed thrombocytopenia, either in response to initial therapy or during follow-up. After adjustment for type and amount of chemotherapy, patients who showed a ≥70% decrease in platelet counts after initial treatment had an approximately five-fold higher risk of developing leukemia than patients who showed a decrease of 50% or less.[91] Severe acute thrombocytopenia may indicate greater bioavailability of cytotoxic drugs, which would likely contribute to the development of leukemia. In support of these findings, a study of leukemia risk after autologous bone-marrow transplantation found that low platelet counts at the time of transplant were predictive for MDS/AML development in NHL patients who had received intensive pretransplant chemotherapy.[161]

Risk of Non-Hodgkin Lymphoma

The first observation of NHL in patients previously treated for Hodgkin's disease dates back to the early 1970s[162] and was soon followed by other case reports. However, Krikorian and associates were the first to demonstrate a clearly elevated cumulative risk, which amounted to 4.4% at 10 years in patients given both irradiation and chemotherapy.[163] Subsequently, other investigators confirmed that patients with Hodgkin lymphoma are at increased risk of developing NHL.[29–32,35,38,54,92,134,164] In most studies, the person-year analysis shows that, compared with the risk in the general population, the RR for NHL, ranges between 6 and 36 (Tables 24.1 and 24.2). Because the background risk of NHL in the

general population is low, this fairly high RR translates into a relatively low cumulative risk, ranging between 2% and 4% at 20 years[30,38,165] in the larger studies. AER in these studies has varied between 5 and 10 excess NHL cases per 10,000 patients per year (Table 24.3).[29,30]

The causes of the excess risk are not well understood. Because increased risks of NHL occur in immunosuppressed patients, such as transplant recipients,[166] and because Hodgkin lymphoma may be accompanied by immunosuppression,[167] several investigators have argued that the elevated risk of NHL may be attributed to Hodgkin lymphoma itself rather than to its treatment. This view is supported by several studies in which risk did not vary appreciably between treatments.[30,31,157] However, in other studies, the risk of NHL was found to be lowest among patients treated with radiation therapy alone, and highest among patients who received intensive combined-modality treatment, both initially and for relapse.[32,92,163,165,168] The inconsistent results regarding the relation to treatment may be partly attributed to diagnostic misclassification, that is, misdiagnosis of the primary tumor as Hodgkin lymphoma when it represented NHL according to modern lymphoma classification schemes.[165] Rueffer and colleagues[165] reported that an expert panel of pathologists reviewing the histology of 4,104 patients with Hodgkin lymphoma (German Hodgkin Lymphoma Study Group) rejected 114 cases (2.1%) initially diagnosed as Hodgdkin lymphoma and rediagnosed them as primary NHL. In only very few studies were diagnostic pathology slides of the second NHL and original Hodgkin lymphoma reviewed in order to avoid such misclassification.[32,134,165]

The majority of cases of second NHL diagnosed after Hodgkin lymphoma are intermediate or aggressive lymphomas of B-cell immunophenotype.[165,169,170] Second NHL more often arises in extranodal sites (compared with primary NHL)[171]; in two series, extranodal involvement was observed in 61%[165] and 79% of cases.[170]

Some evidence indicates that transformation to NHL may be part of the natural history of the lymphocyte-predominant subtype of Hodgkin lymphoma,[171,172] a hypothesis that would explain the association between lymphocyte-predominant Hodgkin lymphoma and NHL risk observed in the International Database on Hodgkin's disease and the British National Lymphoma Investigation.[173] Other investigators argued that the clinical, histologic, and immunophenotypic findings of NHL in these patients were analogous to those of NHL arising in immunosuppressed patients, suggesting that immunodeficiency plays a role in the pathogenesis of second NHL in patients treated for Hodgkin lymphoma.[170] It may be that more than one of the above mechanisms operates in the development of NHL following treatment for Hodgkin lymphoma. Although transformation to NHL may be part of the natural history of some types of Hodgkin lymphoma, the role of intensive combined-modality treatment and its associated immunosuppression should be explored further. In such future studies it is desirable that all slides of the second NHL and the original Hodgkin lymphoma diagnosis are reviewed by an expert pathologist.

Risk of Solid Cancers

Despite the large RRs of leukemia and NHL in the early years after treatment of Hodgkin lymphoma, most of the long-term excess risk of second malignancies derives from solid cancers (Table 24.3). In recent studies with 15 years or more of follow-up, 65% to 75% of second malignancies have been solid cancers (Tables 24.1 and 24.2).[29,30,35,37,38,54] Large cohort studies of patients with Hodgkin lymphoma have consistently shown raised risks of lung cancer, breast cancer, gastrointestinal cancers considered in aggregate, malignant melanoma (although sometimes not significantly), bone and soft tissue cancers, and thyroid cancer (Tables 24.1 and 24.2).[29,30,32,35,37,38,54,138,164] In the largest studies there were also significantly elevated risks of cancers of the mouth, tongue and pharynx, salivary gland, esophagus, stomach, small intestine, colon, pancreas, cervix, and bladder.[29,30] The risk of solid tumor development depends greatly on age at treatment, follow-up interval, and therapy given for Hodgkin lymphoma.

The RR for solid cancer overall, compared to general population expectations, is about 2.0 to 4.5 in long-term follow-up of studies of predominantly adult patients (Table 24.1),[29,30,38,54] but much larger, 8 to 18.5, in children (Table 24.2).[35,37] This latter finding reflects a general trend toward greater RRs of solid cancer at younger ages rather than a dichotomy between children and adults (Table 24.5).[29,30,38] The AER of solid cancer in adults[29,30,38,54] or children[35,37] with Hodgkin lymphoma has ranged from 25 to 60 excess cases per 10,000 Hodgkin lymphoma patients per year in large and recent studies (Table 24.3). The variation in AERs with age is less clear than the pattern for RRs: in one large study the absolute risks slightly increased with age, from age 15 onwards,[30] but in another they decreased.[29]

Results of studies have been inconsistent with regard to whether solid cancer risks might differ by gender. The RR of solid tumors was slightly greater for women in two large studies of (predominantly) adult patients,[29,30] due largely to breast cancer excesses, and was also greater for women in a large study of patients treated in childhood.[37] AERs of solid cancers after treatment of adult Hodgkin lymphoma have been found to be substantially greater in women[29] or to be similar between the sexes.[30]

Unlike the pattern for leukemia, solid-tumor RRs do not reach a peak in the early years after first treatment for Hodgkin lymphoma, but rather continue to rise for at least 25 years (Table 24.4).[29,30,35,37,38,54,164] Typically, the risk is raised little if at all in the first 5 years but substantially, severalfold, raised thereafter. In studies in children, however, increased risks have also been reported in the first 5 of first 10 years after treatment.[35,37] It should be noted that the large RRs at young ages, when background (general population) cancer rates are low, equate with relatively low absolute risks of cancer. However, if the same magnitude of RR persists as the patients grow older, then very large absolute risks of second malignancy will occur (Table 24.4).

The late manifestation of the strongly increased RRs of solid tumors in patients treated for Hodgkin lymphoma at a young age might point to a prolonged induction period, but it may also be due to this young patient group reaching an age at which solid tumor incidence begins to rise in the general population. Only three recent studies distinguished the separate contributions of age at first treatment and attained age.[29,37,38] Solid tumor risk was greatest among patients treated at a young (≤20 years) age, but the greatest RR emerged *before* the patients attained the age range at which solid tumors normally occur. Among patients first treated at age 20 or younger in the largest study to date, the RR of developing a solid tumor at ages 40 to 59 was significantly lower than the RR of solid tumor development before age 40 (RR 2.3 versus 10.5).[29,37] It is notable that a similar finding has been reported with regard to breast cancer risk among atomic bomb survivors in Japan.[174]

The risk of solid cancer overall, and of several specific solid malignancies (see below), is raised after radiation therapy, due to the carcinogenic effects of ionizing radiation.[10] The sites for which excess solid cancers have been reported in survivors of Hodgkin lymphoma treatment (e.g., lung, breast, gastrointestinal tract, thyroid, bone, connective tissue) are those for which elevated risks have also been described in other radiation-exposed cohorts.[175–177] Excesses of melanoma, however, are more likely to be related to immunosuppression accompanying Hodgkin lymphoma or its treatment, because elevated risks appear as early as in the 1- to 4-year follow-up interval.[30,178] Emergence of increased risk of cervical cancer 10 years after diagnosis of Hodgkin lymphoma may also be related to defects in cellular immunity that may facilitate the progression of human papillomavirus-related neoplasia.[37]

In recent years evidence has emerged that chemotherapy can also increase the risk of specific solid malignancies, in particular lung cancer (see below).[19,22,30,138,178,179] Although increased risks of lung cancer (compared with the general population) after chemotherapy alone were found in a few studies,[30,180] most investigations have not observed elevated risks of solid malignancy following chemotherapy alone.[31,32,38,92,140] However, the expected number of solid tumors 10 or more years after chemotherapy alone was less than two in nearly all negative studies, rendering it impossible to exclude a moderate increase in risk. If chemotherapy affects solid-tumor risk, one would expect that patients receiving combined-modality treatment would have a greater RR than patients treated solely with radiotherapy. Only one study to date has reported a significantly greater risk for solid cancers overall following chemotherapy and radiotherapy compared with irradiation alone,[157] whereas no such difference has been found in the majority of investigations.[31,32,92,134,140,181] However, for the gastrointestinal tract[30,38,136] and lung,[19,179] larger risks were observed after combined-modality treatment than after irradiation alone.

The inconsistent results reported with regard to the influence of chemotherapy on solid-tumor risk may be partly related to the fact that most studies considered all solid tumors combined, whereas chemotherapy may differentially affect the risk of tumors at disparate sites. One study demonstrated that the addition of salvage chemotherapy to initial radiotherapy, as compared to radiation therapy alone, did not influence the risk of solid cancers overall, but significantly increased the risk of solid tumors other than breast cancer (RR of 9.4 versus 4.7 for initial irradiation alone).[38] Conversely, patients who received salvage chemotherapy were found to experience significantly lower risks of breast cancer than patients treated with radiation therapy alone (RRs of 2.8 and 7.6, respectively) (see below).[38]

Next we discuss risk factors for lung and breast cancer, the two sites accounting for the largest absolute excess of solid malignancy after Hodgkin lymphoma.

Lung Cancer

In several large cohort studies with 15 or more years of follow-up, the site accounting for the largest absolute excess of solid malignancy after Hodgkin lymphoma is the lung (Table 24.3).[29,30] In Britain, over a quarter of all excess malignancies were lung cancers.[30] However, in other studies only 10% to 15% of excess second malignancies were lung cancers, and breast was the most common site.[38,54] An excellent review of risk factors for lung cancer after Hodgkin lymphoma has recently been published.[182] The risk of lung cancer after Hodgkin lymphoma depends on time since treatment, age at treatment, treatments administered for Hodgkin lymphoma, and smoking.

The RR of lung cancer is slightly if at all raised in the initial 5 years after first treatment, with larger RRs, usually around 5 or greater, thereafter until at least 25 years.[19,29,30,38,54,164] RRs of lung cancer are greater for patients treated at young than at older ages.[19,30,38,54,164] Dores and colleagues[29] reported that the RR of lung cancer decreased from a 5.5-fold increase (compared to the general population) for patients diagnosed

before age 21 to a 1.5-fold excess for patients diagnosed at age 61 or above. In the U.K. study[30] the RRs for lung cancer decreased from 20-fold among those diagnosed before age 25 to a 2.2-fold excess for patients diagnosed at age 55 or above (Table 24.5).

Risk of lung cancer is substantially raised in Hodgkin lymphoma patients treated with radiation therapy (with or without chemotherapy).[19,30,32,38,164,182] The first study investigating the effect of radiation dose estimated the dose to the lobe of the lung in which lung cancer occurred, and found a strong dose–response relationship between radiation dose and risk of lung cancer. There was a RR of 9.6 for a dose of 9 Gy or more compared to less than 1 Gy, although with a possible downturn in risk for doses of 15 Gy or greater.[183] Risk after Hodgkin lymphoma was not related to number of courses of radiation therapy.[183]

A recent much larger international collaborative case-control study also examined lung cancer risk in relation to the radiation dose to the specific location in the lung in which cancer later developed.[19] This study included 222 lung cancer patients and 444 matched controls (patients with Hodgkin lymphoma in whom lung cancer had not been diagnosed).[19,48] Case patients developed lung cancer after an average of 10.8 years. The risk increased with increasing radiation dose to the area of the lung in which cancer later developed (p for trend <0.001; see also Table 24.6). The risk estimates for the highest dose categories of 30.0 to 39.9 Gy and 40 or more Gy compared to no radiation therapy were 8.5 (95% CI, 3.3–24) and 6.3 (95% CI, 2.2–19), respectively, suggesting that the risk might level off at very high doses.[48] The linear model provided a good fit to the area: neither the addition of a dose-squared term nor adding a term to reflect a decline in risk due to cell killing significantly improved the fit of the linear model (p >0.5 in both cases).[48] Two studies addressed the modifying effects of the patient's smoking habits on radiation therapy-associated risks. In the Dutch study, the increase in risk of lung cancer with increasing radiation dose was significantly

TABLE 24.6

RELATIVE RISKS OF BREAST AND LUNG CANCERS AFTER HODGKIN LYMPHOMA, ACCORDING TO RADIATION DOSE TO AFFECTED SITE IN BREAST/LUNG AND NUMBER OF CYCLES OF ALKYLATING CHEMOTHERAPY

Lung cancer[a]				Breast cancer[b]			
Radiation dose to affected site in lung (Gy)	Cases/controls	Relative risk	95% CI	Radiation dose to affected site in breast (Gy)	Cases/controls	Relative risk	95% CI
0	43/87	1.0	(Referent)	0–3.9	15/76	1.0	(Referent)
>0–4.9	27/84	1.6	0.5–5.2	4.0–6.9	13/30	1.8	0.7–4.5
5–14.9	14/18	4.2	0.7–21	7.0–23.1	16/30	4.1	1.4–12.3
15.0–29.9	14/22	2.7	0.2–15	23.2–27.9	9/30	2.0	0.7–5.9
30.0–39.9	60/102	8.5	3.3–24	28.0–37.1	20/31	6.8	2.3–22.3
≥40.0	31/45	6.3	2.2–19	37.2–40.4	12/31	4.0	1.3–13.4
				40.5–61.3	17/29	8.0	2.6–26.4
No. of cycles of alkylating agents				No. of cycles of alkylating agents			
0	74/188	1.0	(Referent)	0	68/132	1.0	(Referent)
1–4	22/44	4.0	1.3–12.5	1–4	10/20	0.7	0.3–1.7
5–8	58/89	6.2	2.6–17.1	5–8	17/55	0.6	0.3–1.1
≥9	28/29	13.0	4.3–45	≥9	4/29	0.2	0.1–0.7

[a]Adapted with permission from results by Gilbert ES, Stovall M, Gospodarowicz M, et al. Lung cancer after treatment for Hodgkin's disease: focus on radiation effects. *Radiat Res* 2003;159:161–173.
[b]Adapted with permission from results by Travis LB, Hill DA, Dores GM, et al. Breast cancer following radiotherapy and chemotherapy among young women with Hodgkin's disease. *JAMA* 2003;290:465–475.

TABLE 24.7

RISK OF LUNG CANCER IN PATIENTS WITH HODGKIN LYMPHOMA ACCORDING TO TYPE OF TREATMENT AND SMOKING HISTORY[a]

Treatment for Hodgkin lymphoma		RR (95% CI) by smoking category (no. of case patients; control patients)[b]	
Radiation ≥5 Gy	Alkylating agents	Nonsmoker, light, other[c]	Moderate-heavy[d]
No	No	1.0[e] (11 case patients; 76 control patients)	6.0 (1.9 to 20.4) p = 0.002 (10 case patients; 22 control patients)
Yes	No	7.2 (2.9 to 21.2) p <0.001 (33 case patients; 73 control patients)	20.2 (6.8 to 68) p <0.001 (20 case patients; 17 control patients)
No	Yes	4.3 (1.8 to 11.7) p <0.001 (40 case patients; 105 control patients)	16.8 (6.2 to 53) p <.001 (33 case patients; 30 control patients)
Yes	Yes	7.2 (2.8 to 21.6) p <0.001 (28 case patients; 60 control patients)	49.1 (15.1 to 187) p <0.001 (24 case patients; 10 control patients)

[a]Adapted with permission from Travis LB, Gospodarowicz M, Curtis RE, et al. Lung cancer following chemotherapy and radiotherapy for Hodgkin's disease. *J Natl Cancer Inst* 2002;94:182–192.
[b]Represents estimated tobacco smoking habit 5 years before diagnosis date of lung cancer and corresponding date in control patients, with the use of information recorded up to 1 year before these dates.
[c]This group includes nonsmokers, light current cigarette smokers (less than one pack per day), former cigarette smokers, smokers of cigar and pipes only, and patients for whom tobacco smoking habit was not stated.
[d]Moderate (one to two packs per day) and heavy (two or more packs per day) current cigarette smokers.
[e]Reference group.
RR, relative risk; 95% CI, 95% confidence interval.

greater among patients who smoked after diagnosis of Hodgkin lymphoma than among those who refrained from smoking.[183] Thus, there was evidence for a more than multiplicative relation between smoking-related and radiation-related risks (i.e., the RR for smoking plus radiation therapy was greater than would be obtained by multiplying the separate RRs for these exposures). Travis and collaborators[19,48] observed that the increased RRs from smoking appeared to multiply the elevated risks from radiation (Table 24.7). Both studies imply that there are large AERs for lung cancer among irradiated patients who smoke.

An important question is whether chemotherapy for Hodgkin lymphoma can also cause lung cancer. Several recent studies have indeed observed that chemotherapy significantly increased the risk of lung cancer.[19,30,134,182,184] The British National Lymphoma Investigation cohort study of 5,519 patients[30] showed a significantly elevated risk of lung cancer following chemotherapy alone, with the RR (3.3; 95% CI, 2.2–4.7) compared to the general population being of similar magnitude to that observed in patients treated with either radiation therapy (RR = 2.9; 95% CI, 1.9–4.1) or combined-modality treatment (RR = 4.3; 95% CI, 2.9–6.2). Two large, recent case-control studies have investigated the separate and joint roles of chemotherapy, radiation, and smoking in detail.[19,179] In both reports, there was a clear trend of increasing lung cancer risk with greater number of cycles of alkylating chemotherapy (p trend <0.001; Table 24.6[19]) or MOPP-chemotherapy (p trend = 0.07[179]). In the study by Travis and colleagues,[19] data were also collected on cumulative dose of individual cytotoxic drugs. As reviewed earlier, among

patients treated with MOPP, increasing total dose of mechlorethamine or procarbazine was strongly associated with increasing lung cancer risk when evaluated separately (p trend for dose for each <0.001).[19] In the same international collaboration,[19] in which also individual radiation dosimetry was performed, risk of lung cancer after treatment with alkylating agents and radiation together was as expected if individual excess RRs were summed: RRs of 4.2 (95% CI, 2.1–8.8) were observed for patients given alkylating agents alone, 5.9 (95% CI, 2.7–13.5) for patients treated with radiation therapy alone (>5 Gy), and 8.0 (95% CI, 3.6–18.5) for those who received combined-modality treatment, compared with the reference group of patients who received no alkylating agents and had a radiation dose of 5 Gy or less.[19] As was observed for the joint effects of smoking and radiation therapy, the risks from smoking appeared to at least multiply risks from alkylating chemotherapy.[19]

Smoking remains the major cause of lung cancer in patients treated for Hodgkin lymphoma, as is evident from the observation that only 7 out of 222 cases included in the study by Travis and associates[19] occurred in patients who had never smoked. Further, it was estimated that 9.6% of all lung cancers were due to treatment, 24% were due to smoking, but 63% were due to treatment and smoking in combination; the remainder (3%) represented tumors in which neither smoking nor treatment played a role.

In summary, both supradiaphragmatic radiation therapy and chemotherapy contribute to the elevated risk of lung cancer after Hodgkin lymphoma. In addition, the above data suggest that patients with Hodgkin lymphoma who smoke will have a considerably greater risk of lung cancer after chest radiation therapy and/or chemotherapy than those who do not smoke, and this is in accord with experience in other radiation-exposed groups.[10] As a consequence, smokers who have received chest radiation therapy should be particularly strongly advised to refrain from smoking. The evidence implicating specific chemotherapeutic agents as carcinogenic to the lung is less clear. It is not yet known whether modern chemotherapy regimens other than MOPP also increase the risk of lung cancer. The role of lung cancer screening in patients treated for Hodgkin lymphoma has not yet been assessed, but an international study is planned to study the efficacy of screening with low-dose spiral CT.[182]

Breast Cancer

The strongly elevated risk of breast cancer following radiotherapy for Hodgkin lymphoma has become a major concern for female survivors.[29,38,53,185–188] In several recent studies breast cancer contributes most to the AER of second malignancy in female Hodgkin lymphoma survivors.[3,35,38,189] Several review articles have addressed the magnitude of the risk of breast cancer after Hodgkin lymphoma and risk factors for its development.[190–192] The risk of breast cancer after Hodgkin lymphoma greatly depends on age at treatment, time since treatment, therapies given for Hodgkin lymphoma, and hormonal factors.

The overall RR of breast cancer in women treated for Hodgkin lymphoma has been only modestly raised in studies that inclued all age groups—about 1.5 to 2.2 in most investigations (Table 24.1).[29,30,32,92,125,138,193] Larger RRs (4- to 7-fold) were observed in studies with predominantly young adults, or a large proportion of long-term survivors.[3,38,135,164] AERs for all ages have been around 2 to 10 per 10,000 Hodgkin lymphoma patients per year (Table 24.3),[29,30,32] again with a greater risk (20 to 30 per 10,000 per year) in recent studies with predominantly young adults and/or a large proportion of long-term survivors.[3,38,164] Breast cancer clearly is the most frequent long-term malignant complication of radiation therapy in women with Hodgkin lymphoma treated under about age 25. The RR of breast cancer after treatment at ages under 16 has ranged from 17 to 458,[141,142] with most studies showing RRs around 50 to 100.[3,35,38,135,194–197] Several studies covering the whole age range have shown that the RR of developing breast cancer increases dramatically with younger age at first irradiation (or start of treatment) (Table 24.5).[3,29,30,38,164,194] A strong trend of increasing RR of breast cancer with decreasing age at exposure has also been observed in other radiation-exposed cohorts.[14,198–200] In a Dutch study, 15-year Hodgkin lymphoma survivors who had radiation treatment before 20 years of age had an 18-fold increased risk of breast cancer, compared to the general population of the same age; women irradiated at ages 20 to 29 had a six-fold increased risk; and a small, nonsignificant increase was observed for women irradiated at ages 30 or older (RR, 1.7).[38] Similar trends, with even larger RRs, have been reported from Stanford University[135] and Harvard-affiliated hospitals.[3] Most studies show that breast cancer risk is not elevated compared with the general population in women treated after age 30 (Table 24.5),[29,30] but others report doubled risk[3,164]

Studies have differed as to whether the steep increase in RR of breast cancer with decreasing age at treatment extends into childhood. It has been hypothesized that the risk increase might be most pronounced after treatment at ages 10 to 16 years, assuming that the increased breast tissue proliferation during puberty might be associated with a greater sensitivity to develop radiation-induced breast cancer.[37,187,198,201] However, two recent studies with sufficient follow-up reported that, for

women treated before age 20, the RR compared with age-matched peers from the general population did not consistently vary by age at treatment.[33,195] It is important to note here that consequently, prepubertal radiation exposure increases the RR to the same extent as exposure during puberty. In the atomic bomb survivors and other radiation-exposed cohorts, the RR also did not vary by exposure age for ages under 20.[202] In most studies the AER of breast cancer is also highest after treatment before age 20,[29,38,54] but shows little variation between exposure at ages 20 to 35.

The huge variation across studies in estimated risk of breast cancer, especially in young patients, is not surprising in view of the large differences between series in important variables such as the proportion of patients irradiated, duration of follow-up and completeness of follow-up. Generally, surveys with more complete follow-up have found lower RRs of breast cancer[29,30,38,141,197] than those in which completeness of follow-up was less satisfactory or not addressed.[140,157,194] Incomplete follow-up may lead to overestimation of second malignancy risk if patients who remain well lose contact with clinical follow-up, while those with second cancer come to attention because of this. The very high *actuarial* risks reported in two U.S. studies (34% at 25 years after first treatment for women treated at ages under 20,[194] and 35% at 40 years of age for those treated under age 16[140]) may be exaggerated estimates, not only because of losses to follow-up, but also because the actuarial method is less appropriate when including events that occur at follow-up intervals later than those at which data for most of the patients were censored.[185] In a Dutch study, with (nearly) complete follow-up, the 25-year actuarial risk of breast cancer amounted to 16%, both for women first treated before age 20 and at ages 20 to 30.[38] The recent study by Bhatia and colleagues from the U.S. Late Effects Study Group[35] extended the follow-up of the earlier study on this cohort of pediatric Hodgkin lymphoma survivors[140] and calculated cumulative incidence of breast cancer using competing risk methods.[120] The cumulative incidence of breast cancer as a function of age of the female cohort of Hodgkin lymphoma survivors who received mantle radiation was 13.9% at age 40 years and reached 20.1% (95% CI, 11.1–29.0) at age 45 years, which was much lower than the estimate of 35% at age 40 years in the previous study from the same group (Fig. 24.2).[140] Subsequently, Bhatia and colleagues in their recent paper conducted sensitivity analyses, based on the assumption that patients lost to follow-up are alive and did not develop breast cancer. With this conservative assumption, the overall SIR for breast cancer decreased from 55.5 (95% CI, 39.5–75.9) to 21.7 (95% CI, 15.4–29.6). The true risk is expected to be somewhere in between these values.[35] Kenney and colleagues[195] recently reported quite similar risk estimates, that is, a cumulative incidence of 12.9% (95% CI, 9.3–16.5) at age 40 in the U.S. Childhood Cancer Survivor Study.

Travis and collaborators[203] recently estimated treatment-specific cumulative absolute risks of breast cancer for young women treated for Hodgkin lymphoma. For a survivor who was treated at age 25 with a chest radiation dose of at least 40 Gy without alkylating agents, the cumulative absolute risks of breast cancer by age 35, 45, and 55 years were 1.4% (95% CI, 0.9–2.1), 11.1% (95% CI, 7.4–16.3), and 29.0% (95% CI, 20.2–40.1), respectively.[203]

The raised risk of breast cancer develops late, and is typically observed from 15 or more years after first treatment (Table 24.4).[29,30,38,54,164] In patients treated as children, however, large and highly significant risks have been seen earlier, after 5 years[196] or 10 years,[141] or even in the first 5 years after treatment[35]; some of these early excesses may reflect the effect of screening or the operation of underlying genetic factors.

The main cause of the high risk of breast cancer after Hodgkin lymphoma is mantle radiation therapy. There are few stable estimates of the RR for this treatment compared

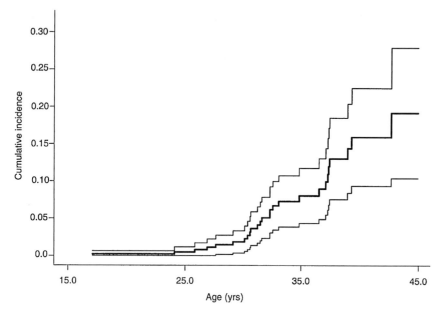

FIGURE 24.2. Cumulative incidence *(middle line)* of breast cancer as a function of age of a cohort of female survivors of Hodgkin lymphoma, with 95% CIs (upper and lower curves). (Adapted from Bhatia S, Yasui Y, Robison LL, et al. High risk of subsequent neoplasms continues with extended follow-up of childhood Hodgkin's disease: report from the Late Effects Study Group. *J Clin Oncol* 2003; 21:4386–4394.)

with other treatments, because in many cohort studies 80% to over 90% of patients received supradiaphragmatic radiation therapy[35,38,54,164] and in other cohort studies treatment data were not available.[29] In the British cohort reported by Swerdlow and colleagues, a large proportion of patients had been treated with chemotherapy alone, and the risk of breast cancer was increased only after radiation therapy without chemotherapy.[30] In women treated at ages younger than 25 years, the risk of breast cancer was 14.4-fold (95% CI, 5.7–29.3) increased after radiation therapy alone, which was significantly greater than the RR of 4.6 among those treated with mixed modalities; no breast cancers occurred in women trated solely with chemotherapy. Among women treated before age 45, these RRs were 3.4 (95% CI, 1.6–6.3), 0.7 (95% CI, 0.1–2.6), and 0.7 (95% CI, 0.02–3.7), respectively.

The strong trend in breast cancer risk by time since treatment is also strongly suggestive of a radiogenic effect. Furthermore, in several cohort studies almost all cases of breast cancer after Hodgkin lymphoma have been in or at the margin of the radiation field: for instance, 16 of 16 cases,[141] 22 of 26,[135] and all of 42 cases[35] in three publications. In the large, population-based study by Travis and colleagues,[21] 49% of 105 breast cancers occurred in the unblocked chest treatment field, 24% under the lung blocks, 15% at the blocked edge, 8% in the field edge, and 3% out-of-beam, with relative location not known for one patient. In studies of the relation of risk to dose of radiation therapy, all but two of 25 cases reported by Hancock and associates had received a mantle dose of 40 Gy or greater,[135] whereas Bhatia and associates found a significant dose–response relationship for patients treated in childhood, with a RR of 23.7 for more than 40 Gy compared to 5.9 for dose of 20 to 40 Gy.[140]

From studies examining other radiation exposures, it is well established that, in the low-dose range, breast-cancer risk increases linearly with radiation dose.[33,200] In discussing the possibility of dose reductions in mantle radiation therapy, an important question therefore is whether linear dose–response extends to the high-dose range used for Hodgkin lymphoma treatment.

Recently, two case-control studies investigated the independent and joint effects of radiation therapy dose to the affected area in the breast and chemotherapy.[21,22] The Dutch study included 48 patients who developed breast cancer 5 or more years after treatment for Hodgkin lymphoma and 175 matched controls. All women had been treated for Hodgkin lymphoma

at age 40 years or younger. The radiation dose to the area of the breast where the patient's tumor had developed was estimated for each case-control set, based on simulation films of the original Hodgkin lymphoma radiotherapy and mammograms indicating the position of the breast tumor. The risk of breast cancer increased significantly with increasing radiation dose *(p* trend = 0.01), with a RR of 5.2 (95% CI, 1.3–1.0) for patients who received 38.5 Gy or more, as compared to those who received less than 4 Gy. Patients who received chemotherapy and radiation therapy had significantly decreased risk as compared to those treated with radiation alone (RR = 0.39; *p* = 0.005). For patients who never received chemotherapy, the risk of breast cancer increased more strongly with increasing radiation dose (RR = 12.7 for patients receiving 38.5 Gy or more) than among patients also treated with chemotherapy. The substantial risk reduction associated with chemotherapy was attributable to its effect on menopausal age. Reaching menopause before age 36 (25% of the controls) was associated with a strongly reduced risk of breast cancer (RR = 0.06; 95% CI, 0.01–0.45). These results indicate that ovarian hormones are probably a crucial factor to promote tumorgenesis once radiation has produced an initiating event.[22]

Travis and associates investigated the roles of radiation and chemotherapy dose in a large international collaborative case-control study[21] of women treated for Hodgkin lymphoma at age 30 years or less. The study included 105 patients with Hodgkin lymphoma and 266 matched controls in whom breast cancer had not developed (38% of cases were also included in the Dutch report[22]). Median time to breast cancer in the case patients was 18 years. Risk of breast cancer increased with increasing radiation therapy dose to the location in which the subsequent tumor developed, with an 8.0-fold (95% CI, 2.6–26.4) increased risk for doses of 41 to 61 Gy, compared to doses below 4 Gy (*p* for trend <0.001) (Table 24.6). Risk of breast cancer decreased with increasing number of alkylating agent cycles (*p* = 0.003 for trend); the RR associated with nine or more cycles of alkylating chemotherapy compared to no alkylating chemotherapy was 0.2 (95% CI, 0.1–0.7) (Table 24.6). A 60% decrease in breast cancer risk was observed among women who received 5 Gy or more to the ovaries, compared to those who received lower doses. As in the Dutch study, women who became menopausal before age 40 experienced significant reductions in breast cancer risk. Remarkably, the relation between alkylating agent treatment and breast cancer risk differed between North America and European centers. Within Europe, significant reductions in risk were observed (for six cycles: RR = 0.33; 95% CI, 0.15–0.65), while in North America the RR associated with six cycles of alkylating agent therapy was close to unity (RR = 0.97; 95% CI, 0.41–2.0).

It is likely that the reduction in risk in European Hodgkin lymphoma survivors, but not in North American women, is related to the much higher prevalence of hormone therapy in North America compared to Europe. Hormone replacement therapy (HRT) is an established risk factor for breast cancer[204,205] and may counteract the protective effect of chemotherapy. In the international study information on HRT use was not available.[21] In the Dutch case-control study, information on reproductive risk factors was obtained from the women themselves and it appeared indeed that the prevalence of HRT use was very low: 78% never used HRT and 10% had used HRT for less than 3 years.[22]

In summary, mantle radiation therapy at young ages is associated with a very high risk of breast cancer after 15 years and later, and this hazard needs to be borne in mind both when selecting treatment for girls and young women with Hodgkin lymphoma and when following patients treated in this way. Reductions of radiation dose and field size (replacement of mantle radiation therapy by involved-field/involved-node irradiation) in current treatment protocols are expected to result in lower breast cancer risk. Gonadotoxic chemotherapy such as the MOPP regimen appears to reduce the increased risk of breast cancer from radiation therapy through the induction of premature menopause. The use of hormone replacement therapy may negate this favorable effect of chemotherapy, but direct information about this is lacking. It has not been examined whether modern, less gonadotoxic chemotherapy, such as ABVD, affects breast cancer risk.

SURVIVAL AFTER SECOND CANCER DIAGNOSIS

Despite a multitude of reports on the magnitude of second cancer risk in patients treated for Hodgkin lymphoma, few studies have examined survival after such a diagnosis. Van Leeuwen and colleagues reported that, in their cohort of 1,253 patients treated for Hodgkin lymphoma 74 (51%) of the 145 patients who developed a second malignancy died of this disease (median follow-up 3.5 yrs).[38] Second cancer deaths represented 16% of all deaths in that cohort; the 25-year actuarial risk of death was 24.2% for Hodgkin lymphoma and 13.5% for second malignancy.[1] In a more recently treated series from several Harvard-affiliated hospitals, mortality from Hodgkin lymphoma was lower and the 20-year cumulative mortality rates (accounting for competing risks) were 8% for Hodgkin lymphoma and 9.8% (95% CI, 7.0–12.6) for second malignancy.[3] As noted earlier, however, such rates are highly dependent on the age distribution of the particular cohort. Van Leeuwen and associates[38] determined the impact of second malignancies on overall survival. Assuming that deaths from second cancer had not occurred (by censoring), it was calculated that the proportion of surviving patients at 25 years increased by 8%, from 55% to 63%.

Ng and colleagues recently presented survival data by second tumor site in a cohort of 1,319 Hodgkin lymphoma patients in whom 181 second malignancies were observed.[54] The median follow-up time after diagnosis of a second malignancy was 3 years. The 5-year overall survival rate after second malignancy was 38.1%, and the median survival time was 3 years for all second tumor sites combined. Survival following development of acute leukemia was poor, with a 5-year overall

survival estimate of only 4.9%, and a median survival time of 0.4 years. Seventeen of the 23 patients who developed acute leukemia died within 1 year of diagnosis. The 5-year overall survival rates after diagnosis of second malignancy for patients who developed solid tumors and non-Hodgkin lymphoma were 42.1% and 49.6%, respectively. The corresponding median survival times were 4.3 years and 2.4 years, respectively. The survival curves after the development of any second malignancy are shown in Figure 24.2, and survival curves after the development of solid tumors, leukemia, and non-Hodgkin lymphoma are shown in Figure 24.3. Among the solid tumors, prognosis was the poorest in patients who developed lung cancer, with a median survival time of only 1 year. The 5-year survival estimate after development of a gastrointestinal cancer was 12.4% (median survival time, 1.9 years). In patients who developed breast cancer, the 5-year overall survival estimate was more favorable (76.1%), and the median survival time had not yet been reached. The survival outcome by type of second malignancy is summarized in Table 24.8.

A number of studies have reported on survival after a diagnosis of selected second malignancies. With regard to secondary AML or MDS after treatment for Hodgkin lymphoma, the literature consistently shows an extremely poor prognosis, worse than for de novo leukemia. In series reported in the 1980s, reviewed in the previous edition of this book, the outcome of therapy-related AML/MDS was nearly always fatal.[156,206] In one survey, more promising results were reported with the use of bone-marrow transplantation in patients with secondary AML/MDS, with a 27% disease-free survival at 5 years.[207] However, these results require some caution in interpretation in that they were based on a very small patient group; the vast majority was subjected to allogeneic transplantation. Another recent series from the German Hodgkin Lymphoma Study Group showed no apparent survival benefit from allogeneic stem-cell transplantation.[148] A special concern in this heavily pretreated patient population is the risk of regimen-related toxicity; other problems include infection, graft-versus-host disease, and leukemia recurrence.

With regard to NHL after treatment for Hodgkin lymphoma, the German Hodgkin Lymphoma Study Group recently showed that the prognosis seems worse than reported for primary NHL.[165] It must be noted, however, that a direct comparison with de novo NHL patients was not made. Rueffer and coworkers examined survival of 51 cases of secondary NHL from a clinical trial database of 5,406 Hodgkin lymphoma patients. Five NHL patients had no further therapy because of rapidly progressive disease. For the remaining patients, the overall response rate was 43% (36% complete response and 7% partial response). The actuarial 2-year freedom from treatment failure and overall survival for all patients were 24% and 30%, respectively; and for patients with diffuse large-cell lymphoma, they were 28% and 35%, respectively. For the 21 NHL patients with diffuse large-cell lymphoma treated with a doxorubicin-containing regimen, overall survival at 2 years was 50% and 2-year freedom from treatment failure was 54%.[165] Time of occurrence of secondary NHL after first diagnosis of Hodgkin lymphoma and variables employed in the age-adjusted International Prognostic Index significantly influenced treatment outcome. Survival was significantly worse for patients who developed NHL within a year from the Hodgkin lymphoma diagnosis. Patients with T-cell lymphoma had a poor outcome, with 6 of 7 patients dying between 3 and 28 months after diagnosis. Patients belonging to the high/high-intermediate risk group or low/low-intermediate risk group had a 2-year freedom from treatment failure of less than 10% and 40% respectively. Thus, patients with secondary NHL and favorable prognostic features can often be cured with multiagent chemotherapy regimens, but this is not true for those with unfavorable subtypes.

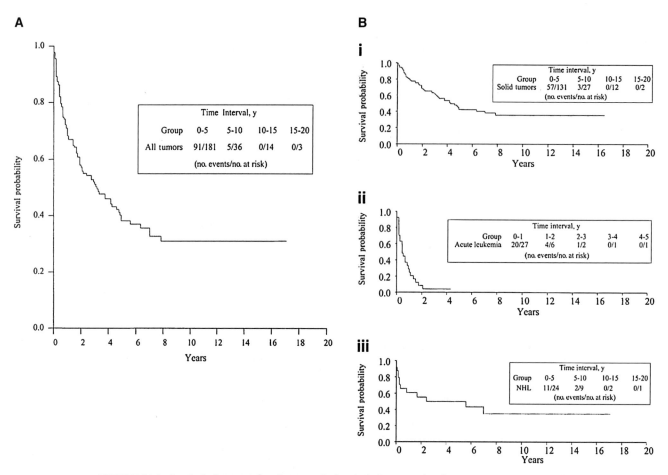

FIGURE 24.3. Survival after second malignancy. **A:** Survival after second malignancy in patients treated for Hodgkin lymphoma. **B:** Survival after solid tumors (**i**), acute leukemia (**ii**), and non-Hodgkin lymphoma (**iii**) in patients treated for Hodgkin lymphoma. (Adapted with permission from Ng AK, Bernardo MV, Weller E, et al. Second malignancy after Hodgkin disease treated with radiation therapy with or without chemotherapy: long-term risks and risk factors. *Blood* 2002;100:1989–1996.)

TABLE 24.8

SURVIVAL OUTCOME AFTER DIAGNOSIS OF SELECTED SECOND MALIGNANCIES[a]

Second malignancy	N	5-year survival estimate (%)	95% CI	Median survival, years
All sites	181	38.1	(29.7–46.5)	3.2
Acute leukemia	23	4.9	(0.0–14.2)	0.4
NHL	24	49.6	(28.0–71.2)	2.4
Solid tumors	131	42.1	31.6–52.5)	4.3
Breast	39	76.1	(57.4–94.8)	Not yet reached
Lung	22	0.0	—	1.0
Gastrointestinal	24	12.4	(0–28.1)	1.9
Sarcoma	11	14.4	(0–40.2)	4.3
Genitourinary	11	81.8	(59.0–100.0)	Not yet reached
Head and neck	7	38.1	(0–77.2)	2.9
Melanoma	7	80.0	(44.9–100)	Not yet reached
Thyroid	5	100.0	—	Not yet reached
Gynecological	4	50.0	(1.0–99.0)	1.4

[a]Adapted with permission from Ng AK, Bernardo MV, Weller E, et al. Second malignancy after Hodgkin disease treated with radiation therapy with or without chemotherapy: long-term risks and risk factors. *Blood* 2002;100:1989–1996.
95% CI, 95% confidence interval; N, number of selected second malignancies; NHL, non-Hodgkin lymphoma.

With regard to lung cancer after treatment for Hodgkin lymphoma, there are again no studies directly comparing the prognosis with that of de novo lung tumors. Laurie and colleagues[208] observed a median survival of 3 months for 14 patients with inoperable disease treated in one center. The results were worse than expected for patients with inoperable disease treated with modern chemotherapy and radiation therapy. Behringer and colleagues reported that 21 of 30 patients in their series had died by 21 months after diagnosis of lung cancer.[209] Neither study reported stage-specific data. It seems that lung cancer after treatment for Hodgkin lymphoma carries a similarly poor or even worse prognosis as compared with de novo lung cancer.[54,182] Previous treatment for Hodgkin lymphoma may compromise the ability to deliver appropriate treatment for secondary lung cancer.

With regard to breast cancer after Hodgkin lymphoma treatment, several studies have described clinicopathologic characteristics[188,210–212] and some have compared survival with that reported for sporadic breast cancers.[188,212] Yahalom and co-workers reported on characteristics of 45 breast cancers occurring in 37 patients diagnosed at the Memorial Sloan-Kettering Cancer Center in New York.[212] Compared with patients with primary breast cancer, women who developed a second breast cancer after Hodgkin lymphoma were more likely to be young, to develop bilateral disease (8 of 37; 4 had synchronous bilateral tumors), and to have breast tumors that involved the medial half of the breast. By contrast, no significant differences in nuclear and histologic grade, lymphocytic reaction, and lymphatic invasion were detected between second and first primary tumors. Apparently, all patients received locoregional treatment only, and prognosis strongly depended on the axillary nodal status (positive in 31% of patients). The 6-year disease-free survival rates were 85% for patients with node-negative tumors and 33% for patients with axillary involvement. According to the authors, these survival rates were similar to those of patients with primary breast cancer seen at the same cancer center.

Cutuli and colleagues reported on 76 breast cancers in 63 women treated for Hodgkin lymphoma between 1941 and 1988.[210] The cancers included 10 ductal carcinomas in situ and 2 fibrosarcomas. The median age at diagnosis of the first breast cancer was 42 years. An unusually high rate of bilateral tumors was observed (21%). TNM classification showed 13% T0 (ductal carcinoma in situ), 26% T1, 29% T2, 11% T3, and 9% T4 tumors. Among 50 axillary dissections for invasive carcinomas, histologic involvement was found in 31 cases (62%). Forty-five tumors were treated by mastectomy, without ($n = 35$) or with ($n = 10$) radiation therapy, whereas 27 tumors had lumpectomy, without ($n = 7$) or with radiation therapy ($n = 20$). After a median follow-up of 40 months, 7 patients (11%) had developed isolated local recurrence, 20 patients (32%) had developed metastases (all died), 38 were in complete remission, and 5 died of intercurrent disease. The 5-year disease-specific survival rate was 61%. The 5-year disease-specific survival rate for pN0, pN1–3, and pN ≥3 groups were 91%, 66%, and 0%, respectively ($p < 0.0001$) and 100%, 88%, 64%, and 23% for the T0, T1, T2, and T3/T4 groups, respectively.

Wolden and colleagues reported on clinicopathological characteristics and survival of 71 cases of breast cancer in 65 women treated for Hodgkin lymphoma at Stanford University.[188] The median age at diagnosis of breast cancer was 43 years. Only 10% of patients developed bilateral breast cancer. Sixty-three percent of cancers were detected by self-examination, 30% by mammography, and 7% by physician examination. Thirteen percent of breast cancers were noninvasive; 85% of all invasive cancers were ductal carcinomas, similar to the prevalence of this histology in the general population. Twenty-two percent were medially located,

and 83% of all cancers were developed within or at the margin of a prior radiotherapy field. TNM classification showed 63% T1 tumors, 27% T2, and 9% T3/T4. Axillary lymph nodes involvement was present in 27% of patients. The stage distribution was significantly more favorable in patients diagnosed after 1990, when more intensive screening among women treated for Hodgkin lymphoma was introduced. Both the stage distribution and other clinicopathologic features (63% positive estrogen receptors) were similar to reported figures for the general breast cancer population. Ninety-five percent of invasive cancers were managed by mastectomy, because of prior radiation for Hodgkin lymphoma. Of the two women who underwent lumpectomy with breast irradiation, one developed tissue necrosis in the region overlapping with the previous mantle field. Adjuvant systemic therapy (48% of patients) was well tolerated, doxorubicin was infrequently used because of concern about prior cardiotoxic treatments for Hodgkin lymphoma. The 5-year disease-specific survival was 88% for stage I, 55% for stage II, and 60% for stage III, similar to rates reported for the general breast cancer population.[188] Although none of the above studies directly compared the clinicopathologic characteristics and prognosis of breast cancers after Hodgkin lymphoma with a series of age-matched first primary breast cancers, it seems that, except for a greater risk of bilaterality and medial location, the features of breast cancer after Hodgkin lymphoma are quite similar to those of sporadic breast cancer.

Most authors advise mastectomy for women with breast cancer after irradiation for Hodgkin lymphoma. However, Deutsch and colleagues recently showed, based on 12 cases, that breast-conserving surgery followed by breast irradiation is possible.[213] With modern low-dose involved-field radiation therapy for Hodgkin lymphoma and accurate records of doses and fields of exposure, conservative management of subsequent breast cancers is theoretically possible if the estimated cumulative dose is acceptable.[192]

CLINICAL IMPLICATIONS

The occurrence of treatment-related cancers is a major problem in survivors of Hodgkin lymphoma. Therefore, the results discussed in this chapter have multiple clinical implications. First, increased knowledge of treatment factors responsible for the occurrence of second cancers is of crucial importance for the development of new treatment strategies. Clinical research should focus on the development of therapeutic regimens with lesser carcinogenic potential, without compromising the excellent cure rates that have been achieved. Despite the strongly increased risks observed for several cancer sites, the issue of treatment-induced second cancers must always be viewed in relation to the dramatic increase in survival rates of patients with Hodgkin lymphoma since intensive radio- and chemotherapy were introduced. When a specific treatment is the optimal means by which to cure the patient, the treatment should obviously not be abandoned because of its carcinogenic effects. The short- and long-term risks of second malignancy (and other complications) that are associated with alternative treatment regimens should be weighed carefully against the therapeutic benefits of the treatments. The arbitrary alteration of a therapy successful against a particular malignancy in order to mitigate second cancer risk is unwarranted. Hence, changes in therapy to reduce the risk of late complications should be made only in the context of carefully designed clinical trials that can evaluate whether the overall efficacy of treatment is maintained. Conversely, trials of new treatments need to be accompanied by long-term assessment of the extent of second cancer and other late adverse effects. The replacement of MOPP chemotherapy with the far less leukemogenic ABV-based regimens introduced in the 1980s has shown that it is indeed possible to reduce second cancer risk while maintaining equal levels of therapeutic effectiveness. It is to be expected that the reduction of dose and fields of irradiation, as applied in several recent Hodgkin lymphoma trials, will result in a lower risk of solid tumors.[189]

Knowledge of risk factors for second malignancy has also made it possible to identify patient groups at high risk of developing second cancers as a result of treatments that they have received in the past. Whenever effective screening methods are available, these should be considered for the patients' follow-up program to improve their survival from a second primary malignancy. In some cases, preventive strategies (e.g., smoking cessation) may substantially reduce the risk of developing a treatment-related cancer.

Patients with Hodgkin lymphoma who have been disease-free for more than 5 years are often told that they are cured; as a result, they are sometimes discharged from further routine follow-up by their treating physicians. Yet paradoxically, after 5 years, the risk of developing a solid cancer increases rapidly. Treating physicians, family physicians, and also the patients themselves must be made aware of the high risk of second malignancy. This may constitute a strong argument in favor of long-term or even lifelong medical surveillance. The risk of a particular second malignancy depends on the treatment administered for Hodgkin lymphoma but also on various patient characteristics, such as age and sex. This implies that advice to the patient, and additional screening methods during follow-up, may need to vary among different patient groups.

In all patients with Hodgkin lymphoma, special attention should be given throughout follow-up to new clinical signs or symptoms of lymphoma. The greatly increased risk of NHL demonstrates the importance of performing biopsies to discriminate between recurrent Hodgkin lymphoma and NHL. Because smokers experience a significantly greater risk of lung cancer in relation to radiotherapy than nonsmokers, physicians should make a special effort to dissuade Hodgkin lymphoma patients from smoking even before treatment starts, and also in the course of follow-up. If this is successful, the excess risk of lung cancer following Hodgkin lymphoma may decrease substantially in the future. The usefulness of screening for lung cancer in survivors of Hodgkin lymphoma is questionable. Therefore, results of research on the efficacy of screening with spiral CT in Hodgkin lymphoma survivors should be awaited before such screening is introduced into clinical practice.[182] Women treated with mantle-field irradiation before age 35 are at greatly increased risk of breast cancer. The importance of regular breast examinations should be explained to them. From about 8 years after irradiation (but not before age 25), there is a strong argument that the follow-up program for these women should include yearly breast palpation and breast imaging. Because mammography is known to be less sensitive in young women, due to the density of the breast tissue and because of the particular undesirability or radiation doses to the young breast, breast magnetic resonance imaging (MRI) rather than mammography should be considered at younger ages. Recent studies comparing the screening efficacy of contrast-enhanced breast MRI screening and mammography show that breast MRI has a greater sensitivity in young women at high risk of breast cancer.[214] The diagnostic process of the breast tumors in two Hodgkin lymphoma series illustrates that routine mammography alone has only limited value in this young patient group.[32,135] However, two other series showed that 90% or more of breast cancer cases after Hodgkin lymphoma were evident on mammogram.[215,216] With respect to other second malignancies, physicians should also be alert to the higher risk of gastrointestinal cancers in patients treated with para-aortic and pelvic radia-

tion fields. Thorough examination of gastrointestinal complaints is indicated.

In regard to the clinical implications of the findings discussed in this chapter, it is important to keep in mind that, over the past decades, there has been a continuous evolution of new therapies aimed at increasing treatment efficacy and/or, more recently, decreasing the risk of acute and late complications. Thus, the results presented in this chapter reflect the risks associated with treatments used 5 to 20 years ago. This is not a fault resulting from defective research, but rather a logical inevitability: one cannot, by definition, know what will happen several years after an exposure that has been introduced only a few years ago. This fact, which is inherent to the study of late effects, implies that the risks observed in published studies cannot always be extrapolated directly to patient populations currently being treated. Whereas some treatments have changed little, there has been a general tendency in radiotherapy to restrict radiation therapy to involved nodes, thus minimizing radiation dose to surrounding normal tissues and, recently, also to decrease the tumor dose. With regard to chemotherapy, the total dose of alkylating agents has been reduced while new cytostatic agents have been introduced, the long-term effects of which are not yet known (e.g., the epipodophyllotoxins). In most cases it is very difficult, if not impossible, to predict the effect of these treatment alterations on second cancer risk, in particular since it has become clear that both chemotherapy and radiation therapy can affect solid malignancy risk. It is only through large, well-designed, and long-term follow-up studies that the effects of such new treatments on second-cancer risk can be evaluated.

DIRECTIONS FOR FUTURE RESEARCH

In this final section we give some directions for future research with respect to second-cancer risk following Hodgkin lymphoma.

First, more data are needed with regard to the evolution of second cancer risk over prolonged follow-up periods. The risks of developing second malignancies more than 25 years following treatment of Hodgkin lymphoma are not known. It is not clear whether the radiation-related increased RRs of solid tumors observed in the 10- to 25-year follow-up interval will remain elevated with more prolonged follow-up or will decrease at some point in time. This question is of great importance in view of the fact that, even with constant RRs over time, the aging of a cohort of survivors of Hodgkin lymphoma treatment with more prolonged follow-up will result in greatly increased AERs of second malignancy. In view of existing data showing that the risk of most solid tumors increases with decreasing age at first treatment, it is important to carefully consider age at treatment in future studies.

Another question of major importance is which chemotherapy regimens (and specific agents) contribute to the increased risk of solid tumors. So far it has only been shown that MOPP chemotherapy increases the risk of lung cancer. Therefore, large and long-term follow-up studies are needed to examine whether other chemotherapy regimens, possibly in interaction with radiotherapy, affect the risk of specific solid tumors. Effects of chemotherapy on solid-cancer risk are likely to be site-specific as well as agent-specific, so there is a need for detailed (case-control) studies of the risk of selected solid tumors in relation to the cumulative dose of various cytostatic drugs.

Furthermore, little is known so far about possible interaction between treatment effects (radiotherapy, chemotherapy) on the one hand and environmental carcinogens (e.g., smoking) or hormonal risk factors on the other. For example, it is of great interest to further examine whether reproductive risk factors and hormone treatment following chemotherapy-induced premature menopause affect radiation-related breast cancer in young female survivors of Hodgkin lymphoma.

Genetic susceptibility likely also plays a role in the pathogenesis of treatment-related second malignancies. An intriguing research question regarding genetic predisposition relates to the assumed greater radiation sensitivity of p53 mutation carriers, carriers of the BRCA1/2 genes, and heterozygous carriers of the mutated ataxia telangiectasia gene. Future studies should aim to examine whether carriers of mutations in these and other genes have an increased risk of radiation-induced cancer, specifically breast cancer. Because the mechanisms underlying the carcinogenic effects of radiation are still poorly understood, research should also focus on the identification of specific (somatic) gene alterations associated with the development of radiation-induced cancer.[56,57] Recent studies have suggested that the mutational spectrum of the p53 tumor suppressor gene in radiation-induced lung cancer may differ from that observed in smoking-related lung cancer.[58–60] Also, preliminary data using comparative genomic hybridization techniques show that breast cancers following radiation for Hodgkin lymphoma are characterized by a distinct molecular profile, compared to sporadic breast cancers from age-matched women.[217] With the rapid advances in molecular biology, our understanding of radiation carcinogenesis at the molecular level is likely to increase significantly in the years to come.[55] New cohorts should be assembled to evaluate the extent of second-cancer risk (leukemia, NHL, solid tumors) associated with treatments introduced in the 1990s (in particular, new chemotherapy regimens). It is only through future long-term follow-up studies that the late effects of such treatments can be evaluated.

Finally, it is of great importance to evaluate the benefits as well as possible adverse effects of screening and lifelong medical surveillance in survivors of Hodgkin lymphoma.

Although knowledge about the carcinogenic effects of Hodgkin lymphoma treatments has increased substantially over the last decade, it is clear that many important questions remain to be answered. The long induction period of many carcinogenic agents, including radiation, as well as the continuous evolution of new therapies necessitate the evaluation of the risk of second malignancy for many years to come. Proper and innovative epidemiologic methods, preferably incorporating biological measurements, are needed to quantify the risk, to identify treatment factors responsible for such risk, and to shed light on the mechanisms of therapy-induced carcinogenesis.

References

1. Aleman BM, van den Belt-Dusebout AW, Klokman WJ, et al. Long-term cause-specific mortality of patients treated for Hodgkin's disease. *J Clin Oncol* 2003 Sep 15;21(18):3431–9.
2. Aviles A, Neri N, Cuadra I, et al. Second lethal events associated with treatment for Hodgkin's disease: a review of 2980 patients treated in a single Mexican institute. *Leuk Lymphoma* 2000;39:311–319.
3. Ng AK, Bernardo MP, Weller E, et al. Long-term survival and competing causes of death in patients with early- stage Hodgkin's disease treated at age 50 or younger. *J Clin Oncol* 2002;20:2101–2108.
4. Boice JD, Jr., Storm HH, Curtis RE, et al. Introduction to the study of multiple primary cancers. *Natl Cancer Inst Monogr* 1985;68:3–9.
5. Travis LB. Therapy-associated solid tumors. *Acta Oncol* 2002;41:323–333.
6. Court-Brown WM, Doll R. *Leukaemia and aplastic anaemia in patients irradiated for ankylosing spondylitis.* London: Her Majesty's Stationary Office; 1957.
7. Martland HS. The occurrence of malignancy in radioactive persons: a general review of data gathered in the study of the radium dial painters, with special reference to the occurrence of osteogenic sarcoma and the interrelationship of certain blood diseases. *Am J Cancer* 1931;15:2435–2516.
8. Upton AC. Physical carcinogenesis: radiation, history and sources. In: Becker FF, ed. *Cancer: a comprehensive treatise.*New York: Plenum Press; 1975:387–404.
9. Inskip PD. Second cancers following radiotherapy. In: Neugut AI, Meadows AT, Robinson, eds. *Multiple primary cancers: incidence, etiology, diagnosis and prevention.* Baltimore: Williams & Wilkins; 1999:91–135.
10. National Research Council.Committee to Assess Health Risks from Exposure to Low Levels of Ionizing Radiation. *Health risks from exposure to low levels of ionizing radiation: BEIR VII phase 2.* Washington, DC: National Academies Press; 2006.
11. Boice JD. Ionizing radiation. In: Schottenfeld DS, Fraumeni JF Jr., eds. *Cancer epidemiology and prevention*, 3rd ed. New York: Oxford University Press. 2006;259–293.
12. Preston DL, Kusumi S, Tomonaga M, et al. Cancer incidence in atomic bomb survivors. Part III. Leukemia, lymphoma and multiple myeloma, 1950–1987. *Radiat Res* 1994;137:S68–S97. Erratum appears in *Radiat Res* 1994;139:129.
13. Thompson DE, Mabuchi K, Ron E, et al. Cancer incidence in atomic bomb survivors. Part II: solid tumors, 1958–1987. *Radiat Res* 1994;137(suppl 2):S17–S67.
14. Tokunaga M, Land CE, Tokuoka S, et al. Incidence of female breast cancer among atomic bomb survivors, 1950-1985. *Radiat Res* 1994;138:209–223.
15. Smith PG, Doll R. Mortality from cancer and all causes among British radiologists. *Br J Radiol* 1981;54:187–194.
16. Wang JX, Inskip PD, Boice JD Jr., et al. Cancer incidence among medical diagnostic x-ray workers in China, 1950 to 1985. *Int J Cancer* 1990;45:889–895.
17. Boice JD, Jr., Blettner M, Kleinerman RA, et al. Radiation dose and leukemia risk in patients treated for cancer of the cervix. *J Natl Cancer Inst* 1987;79:1295–1311.
18. Hancock SL, Tucker MA, Hoppe RT. Breast cancer after treatment of Hodgkin's disease. *J Natl Cancer Inst* 1993;85:25–31.
19. Travis LB, Gospodarowicz M, Curtis RE, et al. Lung cancer following chemotherapy and radiotherapy for Hodgkin's disease. *J Natl Cancer Inst* 2002;94:182–192.
20. Tucker MA, D'Angio GJ, Boice JD Jr., et al. Bone sarcomas linked to radiotherapy and chemotherapy in children. *N Engl J Med* 1987;317:588–593.
21. Travis LB, Hill DA, Dores GM, et al. Breast cancer following radiotherapy and chemotherapy among young women with Hodgkin's disease. *JAMA* 2003;290:465–475.
22. van Leeuwen FE, Klokman WJ, Stovall M, et al. Roles of radiation dose, chemotherapy, and hormonal factors in breast cancer following Hodgkin's disease. *J Natl Cancer Inst* 2003;95:971–929.
23. Lundell M, Mattsson A, Karlsson P, et al. Breast cancer risk after radiotherapy in infancy: a pooled analysis of two Swedish cohorts of 17,202 infants. *Radiat Res* 1999;151:626–632.
24. Weiss HA, Darby SC, Doll R. Cancer mortality following x-ray treatment for ankylosing spondylitis. *Int J Cancer* 1994;59:327–338.
25. Curtis RE, Boice JD Jr., Stovall M, et al. Relationship of leukemia risk to radiation dose following cancer of the uterine corpus. *J Natl Cancer Inst* 1994;86:1315–1324.
26. United Nations Scientific Committee on the Effects of Atomic Radiation (UNSCEAR). UNSCEAR 2000 report to General Assembly, with scientific annexes, sources and effects of ionizing radiation. New York: United Nations; 2000.
27. Boice JD Jr. Carcinogenesis— synopsis of human experience with external exposure in medicine. *Health Phys* 1988;55:621–630. Review.
28. Boice JD Jr., Engholm G, Kleinerman RA, et al. Radiation dose and second cancer risk in patients treated for cancer of the cervix. *Radiat Res* 1988;116:3–55.
29. Dores GM, Metayer C, Curtis RE, et al. Second malignant neoplasms among long-term survivors of Hodgkin's disease: a population-based evaluation over 25 years. *J Clin Oncol* 2002;20:3484–3494.
30. Swerdlow AJ, Barber JA, Hudson GV, et al. Risk of second malignancy after Hodgkin's disease in a collaborative British cohort: the relation to age at treatment. *J Clin Oncol* 2000;18:498–509.
31. Tucker MA, Coleman CN, Cox RS, et al. Risk of second cancers after treatment for Hodgkin's disease. *N Engl J Med* 1988;318:76–81.
32. van Leeuwen FE, Klokman WJ, Hagenbeek A, et al. Second cancer risk following Hodgkin's disease: a 20-year follow- up study. *J Clin Oncol* 1994;12:312–325.
33. Preston DL, Mattsson A, Holmberg E, et al. Radiation effects on breast cancer risk: a pooled analysis of eight cohorts. *Radiat Res* 2002;158:220–235.
34. Inskip PD, Monson RR, Wagoner JK, et al. Cancer mortality following radium treatment for uterine bleeding. *Radiat Res* 1990;123:331–344. Erratum appears in *Radiat Res* 1991;128:326.
35. Bhatia S, Yasui Y, Robison LL, et al. High risk of subsequent neoplasms continues with extended follow-up of childhood Hodgkin's disease: report from the Late Effects Study Group. *J Clin Oncol* 2003;21:4386–4394.
36. de Vathaire F, Hawkins M, Campbell S, et al. Second malignant neoplasms after a first cancer in childhood: temporal pattern of risk according to type of treatment. *Br J Cancer* 1999;79:1884–1893.
37. Metayer C, Lynch CF, Clarke EA, et al. Second cancers among long-term survivors of Hodgkin's disease diagnosed in childhood and adolescence. *J Clin Oncol* 2000;18:2435–2443.
38. van Leeuwen FE, Klokman WJ, van't Veer MB, et al. Long-term risk of second malignancy in survivors of Hodgkin's disease treated during adolescence or young adulthood. *J Clin Oncol* 2000;18:487–497.

39. Little MP, de Vathaire F, Charles MW, et al. Variations with time and age in the risks of solid cancer incidence after radiation exposure in childhood. *Stat Med* 1998;17:1341–1355.
40. Kaldor JM, Day NE, Pettersson F, et al. Leukemia following chemotherapy for ovarian cancer. *N Engl J Med* 1990;322:1–6. See comments.
41. Kaldor JM, Day NE, Clarke EA, et al. Leukemia following Hodgkin's disease. *N Engl J Med* 1990;322:7–13. See comments.
42. Tucker MA, Meadows AT, Boice JD Jr., et al. Leukemia after therapy with alkylating agents for childhood cancer. *J Natl Cancer Inst* 1987;78:459–464.
43. Curtis RE, Boice JD Jr., Stovall M, et al. Risk of leukemia after chemotherapy and radiation treatment for breast cancer. *N Engl J Med* 1992;326:1745–1751. See comments.
44. Greene MH, Young RC, Merrill JM, et al. Evidence of a treatment dose response in acute nonlymphocytic leukemias which occur after therapy of non-Hodgkin's lymphoma. *Cancer Res* 1983;43:1891–1898.
45. Travis LB, Weeks J, Curtis RE, et al. Leukemia following low-dose total body irradiation and chemotherapy for non-Hodgkin's lymphoma. *J Clin Oncol* 1996;14:565–571.
46. Shimizu Y, Kato H, Schull WJ. Studies of the mortality of A-bomb survivors. 9. Mortality, 1950–1985: Part 2. Cancer mortality based on the recently revised doses (DS86). *Radiat Res* 1990;121:120–141.
47. Little MP, Boice JD Jr. Comparison of breast cancer incidence in the Massachusetts tuberculosis fluoroscopy cohort and in the Japanese atomic bomb survivors. *Radiat Res* 1999;151:218–224.
48. Gilbert ES, Stovall M, Gospodarowicz M, et al. Lung cancer after treatment for Hodgkin's disease: focus on radiation effects. *Radiat Res* 2003;159:161–173.
49. Tucker MA, Jones PH, Boice JD Jr., et al. Therapeutic radiation at a young age is linked to secondary thyroid cancer. The Late Effects Study Group. *Cancer Res* 1991;51:2885–2888.
50. Ron E, Lubin JH, Shore RE, et al. Thyroid cancer after exposure to external radiation: a pooled analysis of seven studies. *Radiat Res* 1995;141:259–277.
51. Sigurdson AJ, Ronckers CM, Mertens AC, et al. Primary thyroid cancer after a first tumour in childhood (the childhood cancer survivor study): a nested case-control study. *Lancet* 2005;365:2014–2023.
52. Hawkins MM, Wilson LM, Burton HS, et al. Radiotherapy, alkylating agents, and risk of bone cancer after childhood cancer. *J Natl Cancer Inst* 1996;88:270–278.
53. Neglia JP, Friedman DL, Yasui Y, et al. Second malignant neoplasms in five-year survivors of childhood cancer: childhood cancer survivor study. *J Natl Cancer Inst* 2001;93:618–629.
54. Ng AK, Bernardo MV, Weller E, et al. Second malignancy after Hodgkin disease treated with radiation therapy with or without chemotherapy: long-term risks and risk factors. *Blood* 2002;100:1989–1996.
55. Travis LB, Rabkin CS, Brown LM, et al. Cancer survivorship—genetic susceptibility and second primary cancers: research strategies and recommendations. *J Natl Cancer Inst* 2006;98: 15–25.
56. Sankaranarayanan K, Chakraborty R. Cancer predisposition, radiosensitivity and the risk of radiation-induced cancers. I. Background. *Radiat Res* 1995;143:121–143. Review.
57. Greenblatt MS, Bennett WP, Hollstein M, et al. Mutations in the p53 tumor suppressor gene: clues to cancer etiology and molecular pathogenesis. *Cancer Res* 1994;54:4855–4878. Review.
58. De Bendetti VMG, Travis LB, Welsh JA. P53 mutations in lung cancer following radiation therapy for Hodgkin's disease. *Cancer Epidemiol Biomarkers Prev* 1996;5:93.
59. Vahakangas KH, Samet JM, Metcalf RA, et al. Mutations of p53 and ras genes in radon-associated lung cancer from uranium miners. *Lancet* 1992;339:576–580.
60. Taylor JA, Watson MA, Devereux TR, et al. p53 mutation hotspot in radon-associated lung cancer. *Lancet* 1994;343:86–87. See comments.
61. Behrens C, Travis LB, Wistuba II, et al. Molecular changes in second primary lung and breast cancers after therapy for Hodgkin's disease. *Cancer Epidemiol Biomarkers Prev* 2000;9:1027–1035.
62. Wong FL, Boice JD Jr., Abramson DH, et al. Cancer incidence after retinoblastoma. Radiation dose and sarcoma risk. *JAMA* 1997;278:1262–1267. See comments.
63. Kony SJ, de Vathaire F, Chompret A, et al. Radiation and genetic factors in the risk of second malignant neoplasms after a first cancer in childhood. *Lancet* 1997;350:91–95. See comments.
64. Nichols KE, Levitz S, Shannon KE, et al. Heterozygous germline ATM mutations do not contribute to radiation-associated malignancies after Hodgkin's disease. *J Clin Oncol* 1999;17:1259.
65. Andrieu N, Easton DF, Chang-Claude J, et al. Effect of chest x-rays on the risk of breast cancer among BRCA 1/2 mutation carriers in the international BRCA1/2 carrier cohort study: a report from EMBRACE, GENEPSO, GEO-HEBON, and IBCCS Collaborators' group. *Jour Clini Oncol.* 2006; 24:3361–3366.
66. Easton DF. Cancer risks in A-T heterozygotes. *Int J Radiat Biol* 1994;66:S177–S182. Review.
67. Swift M, Morrell D, Massey RB, et al. Incidence of cancer in 161 families affected by ataxia- telangiectasia. *N Engl J Med* 1991;325:1831–1836.
68. Broeks A, Russell NS, Floore AN, et al. Increased risk of breast cancer following irradiation for Hodgkin's disease is not a result of ATM germline mutations. *Int J Radiat Biol* 2000;76:693–698.
69. Rieche K. Carcinogenicity of antineoplastic agents in man. *Cancer Treat Rev* 1984;11:39–67. Review.
70. Sieber SM, Adamson RH. Toxicity of antineoplastic agents in man, chromosomal aberrations antifertility effects, congenital malformations, and carcinogenic potential. *Adv Cancer Res* 1975;22:57–155.
71. Stolley PD, Hibberd PL. Drugs. In: Schottenfeld D, Fraumeni JF, eds. *Cancer epidemiology and prevention*. Philadelphia: WB Saunders; 1982:304–317.
72. Haddow A, Harris R, Kon GAR. The growth-inhibitory and carcinogenic properties of 4-Aminostilbene and derivatives. *Philos Trans R Soc* 1948; 241(series A):247.
73. Schmähl D, Thomas C, Auer R. *Iatrogenic carcinogenesis*. Berlin: Springer Verlag; 1977.
74. Shimkin B, Weisburger JH, Weisburger EK. Bioassay of 29 alkylating chemicals by the pulmonary-tumor response in strain A mice. *J Natl Cancer Inst* 1966;36:915–923.
75. Kyle RA, Pierre RV, Bayrd ED. Multiple myeloma and acute myelomonocytic leukemia. *N Engl J Med* 1970;283:1121–1125.
76. Bergsagel DE, Bailey AJ, Langley GR, et al. The chemotherapy on plasma-cell myeloma and the incidence of acute leukemia. *N Engl J Med* 1979;301:743–748.
77. Rosner F, Grunwald H. Multiple myeloma terminating in acute leukemia. Report of 12 cases and review of the literature. *Am J Med* 1974;57:927–939. Review.
78. Coleman CN, Williams CJ, Flint A, et al. Hematologic neoplasia in patients treated for Hodgkin's disease. *N Engl J Med* 1977;297:1249–1252.
79. Canellos GP, Arseneau JC, Straus VT, et al. Second malignancies complicating Hodgkin's disease in remission. *Lancet* 1975;1:947–949.
80. Bonadonna G, De Lena M, Banfi A, et al. Secondary neoplasms in malignant lymphomas after intensive therapy. *N Engl J Med* 1973;288: 1242–1243.
81. Levine EG, Bloomfield CD. Leukemias and myelodysplastic syndromes secondary to drug, radiation, and environmental exposure. *Semin Oncol* 1992;19:47–84. Review.
82. van Leeuwen FE, Travis LB. Second cancers. In: DeVita VT Jr., Hellman S, Rosenberg SA, eds. *Cancer principles and practice of oncology*. 7th ed. Philadelphia: Lippincott Williams & Wilkins; 2005:2575–2602.
83. Pedersen-Bjergaard J, Philip P, Larsen SO, et al. Therapy-related myelodysplasia and acute myeloid leukemia. Cytogenetic characteristics of 115 consecutive cases and risk in seven cohorts of patients treated intensively for malignant diseases in the Copenhagen series. *Leukemia* 1993;7:1975–1986.
84. Pedersen-Bjergaard J, Rowley JD. The balanced and the unbalanced chromosome aberrations of acute myeloid leukemia may develop in different ways and may contribute differently to malignant transformation. *Blood* 1994;83:2780–2786. Review.
85. Smith MA, Rubinstein L, Ungerleider RS. Therapy-related acute myeloid leukemia following treatment with epipodophyllotoxins: estimating the risks. *Med Pediatr Oncol* 1994;23:86–98. Review.
86. Kaldor JM, Day NE, Hemminki K. Quantifying the carcinogenicity of antineoplastic drugs. *Eur J Cancer Clin Oncol* 1988;24:703–711.
87. Cuzick J, Erskine S, Edelman D, et al. A comparison of the incidence of the myelodysplastic syndrome and acute myeloid leukaemia following melphalan and cyclophosphamide treatment for myelomatosis. A report to the Medical Research Council's working party on leukaemia in adults. *Br J Cancer* 1987;55:523–529.
88. Greene MH, Harris EL, Gershenson DM, et al. Melphalan may be a more potent leukemogen than cyclophosphamide. *Ann Intern Med* 1986;105:360–367.
89. Travis LB, Curtis RE, Stovall M, et al. Risk of leukemia following treatment for non-Hodgkin's lymphoma. *J Natl Cancer Inst* 1994;86:1450–1457.
90. Travis LB, Holowaty EJ, Bergfeldt K, et al. Risk of leukemia after platinum-based chemotherapy for ovarian cancer. *N Engl J Med* 1999;340:351–357.
91. van Leeuwen FE, Chorus AM, van den Belt-Dusebout AW, et al. Leukemia risk following Hodgkin's disease: relation to cumulative dose of alkylating agents, treatment with teniposide combinations, number of episodes of chemotherapy, and bone marrow damage. *J Clin Oncol* 1994;12:1063–1073.
92. Henry-Amar M. Second cancer after the treatment for Hodgkin's disease: a report from the International Database on Hodgkin's Disease. *Ann Oncol* 1992;3(suppl 4):117–128.
93. Schonfeld SJ, Gilbert ES, Dores GM, et al. Acute myeloid leukemia following Hodgkin lymphoma: a population-based study of 35,511 patients. *J Natl Cancer Inst* 2006;98:215–218.
94. Michels SD, McKenna RW, Arthur DC, et al. Therapy-related acute myeloid leukemia and myelodysplastic syndrome: a clinical and morphologic study of 65 cases. *Blood* 1985;65:1364–1372.
95. Pedersen-Bjergaard J, Philip P, Larsen SO, et al. Chromosome aberrations and prognostic factors in therapy-related myelodysplasia and acute non-lymphocytic leukemia. *Blood* 1990;76:1083–1091.
96. IARC. Some antiviral and antineoplastic drugs, and other pharmaceutical agents. *IARC Monogr Eval Carcinog Risk Chem Hum* 2000;76:177.
97. Pedersen-Bjergaard J, Philip P. Balanced translocations involving chromosome bands 11q23 and 21q22 are highly characteristic of myelodysplasia and leukemia following therapy with cytostatic agents targeting at DNA-topoisomerase II. *Blood* 1991;78:1147–1148. Letter.
98. Rubin CM, Arthur DC, Woods WG, et al. Therapy-related myelodysplastic syndrome and acute myeloid leukemia in children: correlation between chromosomal abnormalities and prior therapy. *Blood* 1991;78:2982–2988.

99. Sandoval C, Pui CH, Bowman LC, et al. Secondary acute myeloid leukemia in children previously treated with alkylating agents, intercalating topoisomerase II inhibitors, and irradiation. *J Clin Oncol* 1993;11:1039–1045.

100. Pedersen-Bjergaard J, Sigsgaard TC, Nielsen D, et al. Acute monocytic or myelomonocytic leukemia with balanced chromosome translocations to band 11q23 after therapy with 4-epi- doxorubicin and cisplatin or cyclophosphamide for breast cancer. *J Clin Oncol* 1992;10:1444–1451. See comments.

101. Neugut AI, Robinson E, Nieves J, et al. Poor survival of treatment-related acute nonlymphocytic leukemia. *JAMA* 1990;264:1006–1008.

102. Felix CA. Chemotherapy-related second cancers. In: Neugut AI, Meadows AT, Robinson E, eds. *Multiple primary cancers.* Philadelphia: Lippincott Williams & Wilkins; 1999:137–164.

103. Kelly KM, Perentesis JP. Polymorphisms of drug metabolizing enzymes and markers of genotoxicity to identify patients with Hodgkin's lymphoma at risk of treatment-related complications. *Ann Oncol* 2002;13(suppl 1):34–39.

104. Ben-Yehuda D, Krichevsky S, Caspi O, et al. Microsatellite instability and p53 mutations in therapy-related leukemia suggest mutator phenotype. *Blood* 1996;88:4296–4303.

105. Zhu YM, Das-Gupta EP, Russell NH. Microsatellite instability and p53 mutations are associated with abnormal expression of the MSH2 gene in adult acute leukemia. *Blood* 1999;94:733–740.

106. Smith MA, McCaffrey RP, Karp JE. The secondary leukemias: challenges and research directions. *J Natl Cancer Inst* 1996;88:407–418. Review.

107. Yeoh EJ, Ross ME, Shurtleff SA, et al. Classification, subtype discovery, and prediction of outcome in pediatric acute lymphoblastic leukemia by gene expression profiling. *Cancer Cell* 2002;1:133–143.

108. Alberts DS. Protection by amifostine of cyclophosphamide-induced myelosuppression. *Semin Oncol* 1999;26(suppl 7):37–40. Review.

109. Overall evaluations of carcinogenicity: an updating of IARC monographs volumes 1 to 42. *IARC Monogr Eval Carcinog Risks Hum Suppl* 1987;7:1–440.

110. Kaldor JM, Day NE, Kittelmann B, et al. Bladder tumours following chemotherapy and radiotherapy for ovarian cancer: a case-control study. *Int J Cancer* 1995;63:1–6.

111. Travis LB, Curtis RE, Glimelius B, et al. Bladder and kidney cancer following cyclophosphamide therapy for non-Hodgkin's lymphoma. *J Natl Cancer Inst* 1995;87:524–530.

112. Blair A, Kazerouni N. Reactive chemicals and cancer. *Cancer Causes Control* 1997;8:473–490.

113. Kaldor JM, Day NE, Shiboski S. Epidemiological studies of anticancer drug carcinogenicity. *IARC Sci Publ* 1986;78:189–201.

114. Makuch R, Simon R. Recommendations for the analysis of the effect of treatment on the development of second malignancies. *Cancer* 1979;44:250–253.

115. Schoenberg BS, Myers MH. Statistical methods for studying multiple primary malignant neoplasms. *Cancer* 1977;40:1892–1898.

116. Kaplan EL, Meier P. Non-parametric estimation from incomplete observations. *J Am Stat Assoc* 1958;53:457–481.

117. Darrington DL, Vose JM, Anderson JR, et al. Incidence and characterization of secondary myelodysplastic syndrome and acute myelogenous leukemia following high-dose chemoradiotherapy and autologous stem-cell transplantation for lymphoid malignancies. *J Clin Oncol* 1994;12: 2527–2534.

118. Mauch PM, Kalish LA, Marcus KC, et al. Long-term survival in Hodgkin's disease: relative impact of mortality, second tumors, infection, and cardiovascular disease. *Cancer J Sci Am* 1995;1:33–42.

119. Pepe MS, Mori M. Kaplan-Meier, marginal or conditional probability curves in summarizing competing risks failure time data? *Stat Med* 1993;12:737–751.

120. Gooley TA, Leisenring W, Crowley J, et al. Estimation of failure probabilities in the presence of competing risks: new representations of old estimators. *Stat Med* 1999;18:695–706.

121. Travis LB, Curtis RE, Glimelius B, et al. Second cancers among long-term survivors of non-Hodgkin's lymphoma. *J Natl Cancer Inst* 1993;85:1932–1937.

122. Breslow NE, Day NE. *Statistical methods in cancer research.* Volume II. *The design and analysis of cohort studies.* Interrnational Society for Research on Cancer (Lyon, FR) IARC Sci Publ; 1987.

123. Cox DR. Regression models and life-tables. *J R Stat Soc B* 1972;334:187–202.

124. Boice JD, Jr., Day NE, Andersen A, et al. Second cancers following radiation treatment for cervical cancer. An international collaboration among cancer registries. *J Natl Cancer Inst* 1985;74:955–975.

125. Kaldor JM, Day NE, Band P, et al. Second malignancies following testicular cancer, ovarian cancer and Hodgkin's disease: an international collaborative study among cancer registries. *Int J Cancer* 1987;39:571–585.

126. Storm HH, Prener A. Second cancer following lymphatic and hematopoietic cancers in Denmark, 1943–80. *Natl Cancer Inst Monogr* 1985;68:389–409.

127. Greene MH. Is cisplatin a human carcinogen?. *J Natl Cancer Inst* 1992;84:306–312.

128. Dietrich PY, Henry-Amar M, Cosset JM, et al. Second primary cancers in patients continuously disease-free from Hodgkin's disease: a protective role for the spleen? *Blood* 1994;84:1209–1215.

129. Swerdlow AJ, Barber JA, Horwich A, et al. Second malignancy in patients with Hodgkin's disease treated at the Royal Marsden Hospital. *Br J Cancer* 1997;75:116–123.

130. Valagussa P, Santoro A, Fossati-Bellani F, et al. Second acute leukemia and other malignancies following treatment for Hodgkin's disease. *J Clin Oncol* 1986;4:830–837.

131. Ewertz M, Machado SG, Boice JD, Jr., et al. Endometrial cancer following treatment for breast cancer: a case-control study in Denmark. *Br J Cancer* 1984;50:687–692.

132. Boice JD, Jr., Harvey EB, Blettner M, et al. Cancer in the contralateral breast after radiotherapy for breast cancer. *N Engl J Med* 1992;326:781–785.

133. Arseneau JC, Sponzo RW, Levin DL, et al. Nonlymphomatous malignant tumors complicating Hodgkin's disease. Possible association with intensive therapy. *N Engl J Med* 1972;287:1119–122.

134. Swerdlow AJ, Douglas AJ, Hudson GV, et al. Risk of second primary cancers after Hodgkin's disease by type of treatment: analysis of 2846 patients in the British National Lymphoma Investigation. *BMJ* 1992;304:1137–1143.

135. Hancock SL, Tucker MA, Hoppe RT. Breast cancer after treatment of Hodgkin's disease. *J Natl Cancer Inst* 1993;85:25–31.

136. Birdwell SH, Hancock SL, Varghese A, et al. Gastrointestinal cancer after treatment of Hodgkin's disease. *Int J Radiat Oncol Biol Phys* 1997;37:67–73.

137. Valagussa PA, Bonadonna G. Carcinogenic effects of cancer treatment. In: Peckham M, Pinedo H, Veronesi U, eds. *Oxford textbook of oncology.* Oxford: Oxford University Press; 1995:2348.

138. Boivin JF, Hutchison GB, Zauber AG, et al. Incidence of second cancers in patients treated for Hodgkin's disease. *J Natl Cancer Inst* 1995;87:732–741. See comments.

139. Henry-Amar M, Dietrich PY. Acute leukemia after the treatment of Hodgkin's disease. *Hematol Oncol Clin North Am* 1993;7:369–387. Review.

140. Bhatia S, Robison LL, Oberlin O, et al. Breast cancer and other second neoplasms after childhood Hodgkin's disease. *N Engl J Med* 1996;334:745–751.

141. Sankila R, Garwicz S, Olsen JH, et al. Risk of subsequent malignant neoplasms among 1,641 Hodgkin's disease patients diagnosed in childhood and adolescence: a population-based cohort study in the five Nordic countries. Association of the Nordic Cancer Registries and the Nordic Society of Pediatric Hematology and Oncology. *J Clin Oncol* 1996;14:1442–1446.

142. Mauch PM, Kalish LA, Marcus KC, et al. Second malignancies after treatment for laparotomy staged IA-IIIB Hodgkin's disease: long-term analysis of risk factors and outcome. *Blood* 1996;87:3625–3632.

143. Cimino G, Papa G, Tura S, et al. Second primary cancer following Hodgkin's disease: updated results of an Italian multicentric study. *J Clin Oncol* 1991;9:432–437.

144. Devereux S, Selassie TG, Vaughan Hudson G, et al. Leukaemia complicating treatment for Hodgkin's disease: the experience of the British National Lymphoma Investigation. *BMJ* 1990;301:1077–1080.

145. Abrahamsen JF, Andersen A, Hannisdal E, et al. Second malignancies after treatment of Hodgkin's disease: the influence of treatment, follow-up time, and age. *J Clin Oncol* 1993;11:255–261. See comments.

146. Schellong G, Riepenhausen M, Creutzig U, et al. Low risk of secondary leukemias after chemotherapy without mechlorethamine in childhood Hodgkin's disease. German-Austrian Pediatric Hodgkin's Disease Group. *J Clin Oncol* 1997;15:2247–2253.

147. Diehl V, Franklin J, Pfreundschuh M, et al. Standard and increased-dose BEACOPP chemotherapy compared with COPP-ABVD for advanced Hodgkin's disease. *N Engl J Med* 2003;348:2386–2395.

148. Josting A, Wiedenmann S, Franklin J, et al. Secondary myeloid leukemia and myelodysplastic syndromes in patients treated for Hodgkin's disease: a report from the German Hodgkin's Lymphoma Study Group. *J Clin Oncol* 2003;21:3440–3446.

149. Andrieu JM, Ifrah N, Payen C, et al. Increased risk of secondary acute nonlymphocytic leukemia after extended-field radiation therapy combined with MOPP chemotherapy for Hodgkin's disease. *J Clin Oncol* 1990;8:1148–1154. Review. See comments.

150. Abruzzese E, Radford JE, Miller JS, et al. Detection of abnormal pretransplant clones in progenitor cells of patients who developed myelodysplasia after autologous transplantation. *Blood* 1999;94:1814–1819.

151. Andre M, Henry-Amar M, Blaise D, et al. Treatment-related deaths and second cancer risk after autologous stem-cell transplantation for Hodgkin's disease. *Blood* 1998;92:1933–1940.

152. Park S, Brice P, Noguerra ME, et al. Myelodysplasias and leukemias after autologous stem cell transplantation for lymphoid malignancies. *Bone Marrow Transplant* 2000;26:321–326.

153. Traweek ST, Slovak ML, Nademanee AP, et al. Myelodysplasia and acute myeloid leukemia occurring after autologous bone marrow transplantation for lymphoma. *Leuk Lymphoma* 1996;20:365–372. Review.

154. Pedersen-Bjergaard J, Pedersen M, Myhre J, et al. High risk of therapy-related leukemia after BEAM chemotherapy and autologous stem cell transplantation for previously treated lymphomas is mainly related to primary chemotherapy and not to the BEAM-transplantation procedure. *Leukemia* 1997;11:1654–1660.

155. Forrest DL, Hogge DE, Nevill TJ, et al. High-dose therapy and autologous hematopoietic stem-cell transplantation does not increase the risk of second neoplasms for patients with Hodgkin's lymphoma: a comparison of conventional therapy alone versus conventional therapy followed by autologous hematopoietic stem-cell transplantation. *J Clin Oncol* 2005;23:7994–8002.

156. van Leeuwen FE, Swerdlow AJ, Valagussa P, et al. Second cancers after treatment of Hodgkin's disease. In: Mauch PM, Armitage JO, Diehl V, et al., eds. *Hodgkin's disease*. Philadelphia: Lippincott Williams & Wilkins; 1999:607–632.

157. Mauch PM, Kalish LA, KC, et al. Second malignancies after treatment for laparotomy staged IA- IIIB Hodgkin's disease: long-term analysis of risk factors and outcome. *Blood* 1996;87:3625–3632.

158. van Leeuwen FE, Somers R, Hart AA. Splenectomy in Hodgkin's disease and second leukaemias. *Lancet* 1987;2:210–211. Letter.

159. Meadows AT, Obringer AC, Marrero O, et al. Second malignant neoplasms following childhood Hodgkin's disease: treatment and splenectomy as risk factors. *Med Pediatr Oncol* 1989;17:477–484.

160. Tura S, Fiacchini M, Zinzani PL, et al. Splenectomy and the increasing risk of secondary acute leukemia in Hodgkin's disease. *J Clin Oncol* 1993;11: 925–930.

161. Stone RM, Neuberg D, Soiffer R, et al. Myelodysplastic syndrome as a late complication following autologous bone marrow transplantation for non-Hodgkin's lymphoma. *J Clin Oncol* 1994;12:2535–2542.

162. Burns CP, Stjernholm RL, Kellermeyer RW. Hodgkin's disease terminating in acute lymphosarcoma cell leukemia. A metabolic study. *Cancer* 1971;27:806–811.

163. Krikorian JG, Burke JS, Rosenberg SA, et al. Occurrence of non-Hodgkin's lymphoma after therapy for Hodgkin's disease. *N Engl J Med* 1979;300: 452–458.

164. Foss Abrahamsen A, Andersen A, Nome O, et al. Long-term risk of second malignancy after treatment of Hodgkin's disease: the influence of treatment, age and follow-up time. *Ann Oncol* 2002;13:1786–1791.

165. Rueffer U, Josting A, Franklin J, et al. Non-Hodgkin's lymphoma after primary Hodgkin's disease in the German Hodgkin's Lymphoma Study Group: incidence, treatment, and prognosis. *J Clin Oncol* 2001;19:2026–2032.

166. Penn I. Cancers complicating organ transplantation. *N Engl J Med* 1990;323:1767–1769. Editorial, comment.

167. van Rijswijk RE, Sybesma JP, Kater L. A prospective study of the changes in immune status following radiotherapy for Hodgkin's disease. *Cancer* 1984;53:62–69.

168. Prosper F, Robledo C, Cuesta B, et al. Incidence of non-Hodgkin's lymphoma in patients treated for Hodgkin's disease. *Leuk Lymphoma* 1994;12:457–462.

169. Amini RM, Enblad G, Sundstrom C, et al. Patients suffering from both Hodgkin's disease and non-Hodgkin's lymphoma: a clinico-pathological and immuno-histochemical population-based study of 32 patients. *Int J Cancer* 1997;71:510–516.

170. Zarate-Osorno A, Medeiros LJ, Longo DL, et al. Non-Hodgkin's lymphomas arising in patients successfully treated for Hodgkin's disease. A clinical, histologic, and immunophenotypic study of 14 cases. *Am J Surg Pathol* 1992;16:885–895.

171. Bennett MH, MacLennan KA, Vaughan Hudson G, et al. Non-Hodgkin's lymphoma arising in patients treated for Hodgkin's disease in the BNLI: a 20-year experience. British National Lymphoma Investigation. *Ann Oncol* 1991;2(suppl 2):83–92.

172. Kim H, Zelman RJ, Fox MA, et al. Pathology Panel for Lymphoma Clinical Studies: a comprehensive analysis of cases accumulated since its inception. *J Natl Cancer Inst* 1982;68:43–67.

173. Swerdlow AJ, Douglas AJ, Vaughan Hudson G, et al. Risk of second primary cancer after Hodgkin's disease in patients in the British National Lymphoma Investigation: relationships to host factors, histology and stage of Hodgkin's disease, and splenectomy. *Br J Cancer* 1993;68:1006–1011.

174. Land CE. Studies of cancer and radiation dose among atomic bomb survivors. The example of breast cancer. *JAMA* 1995;274:402–407. See comments.

175. Boice JD, Jr., Land CE, Preston DL. Ionizing radiation. In: Schottenfeld D, Fraumeni JF Jr., eds. *Cancer epidemiology and prevention*. 2nd ed. New York: Oxford University Press; 1996:319–354.

176. Miller AB, Howe GR, Sherman GJ, et al. Mortality from breast cancer after irradiation during fluoroscopic examinations in patients being treated for tuberculosis. *N Engl J Med* 1989;321:1285–1289.

177. United Nations Scientific Committee on the Effects of Atomic Radiation. *Sources and effects of ionizing radiation: UNSCEAR 1994 report to the general assembly with scientific annexes*. New York: United Nations; 1994.

178. Tucker MA, Misfeldt D, Coleman CN, et al. Cutaneous malignant melanoma after Hodgkin's disease. *Ann Intern Med* 1985;102:37–41.

179. Swerdlow AJ, Schoemaker MJ, Allerton R, et al. Lung cancer after Hodgkin's disease: a nested case-control study of the relation to treatment. *J Clin Oncol* 2001;19:1610–1618.

180. Travis LB, Curtis RE, Bennett WP, et al. Lung cancer after Hodgkin's disease. *J Natl Cancer Inst* 1995;87:1324–1327.

181. Hancock SL, Hoppe RT. Long-term complications of treatment and causes of mortality after Hodgkin's disease. *Semin Radiat Oncol* 1996;6: 225–242.

182. Lorigan P, Radford J, Howell A, et al. Lung cancer after treatment for Hodgkin's lymphoma: a systematic review. *Lancet Oncol* 2005;6:773–779.

183. van Leeuwen FE, Klokman WJ, Stovall M, et al. Roles of radiotherapy and smoking in lung cancer following Hodgkin's disease. *J Natl Cancer Inst* 1995;87:1530–1537.

184. Kaldor JM, Day NE, Bell J, et al. Lung cancer following Hodgkin's disease: a case-control study. *Int J Cancer* 1992;52:677–681.

185. Donaldson SS, Hancock SL. Second cancers after Hodgkin's disease in childhood *N Engl J Med* 1996;334:792–794. Editorial. See comments.

186. Wolf J, Schellong G, Diehl V. Breast cancer following treatment of Hodgkin's disease—more reasons for less radiotherapy? *Eur J Cancer* 1997;33:2293–2294. Editorial.

187. Goss PE, Sierra S. Current perspectives on radiation-induced breast cancer. *J Clin Oncol* 1998;16:338–347. Review. See comments.

188. Wolden SL, Hancock SL, Carlson RW, et al. Management of breast cancer after Hodgkin's disease. *J Clin Oncol* 2000;18:765–772.

189. Yahalom J. Breast cancer after Hodgkin disease: hope for a safer cure. *JAMA* 2003;290:529–531.

190. Clemons M, Loijens L, Goss P. Breast cancer risk following irradiation for Hodgkin's disease. *Cancer Treat Rev* 2000;26:291–302.

191. Horwich A, Swerdlow AJ. Second primary breast cancer after Hodgkin's disease. *Br J Cancer* 2004;90:294–298.

192. Deniz K, O'Mahony S, Ross G, et al. Breast cancer in women after treatment for Hodgkin's disease. *Lancet Oncol* 2003;4:207–214.

193. Travis LB, Curtis RE, Boice JD Jr. Late effects of treatment for childhood Hodgkin's disease. *N Engl J Med* 1996;335:352–353. Letter.

194. Aisenberg AC, Finkelstein DM, Doppke KP, et al. High risk of breast carcinoma after irradiation of young women with Hodgkin's disease. *Cancer* 1997;79:1203–1210.

195. Kenney LB, Yasui Y, Inskip PD, et al. Breast cancer after childhood cancer: a report from the Childhood Cancer Survivor Study. *Ann Intern Med* 2004;141:590–597.

196. Travis LB, Curtis RE, Boice JD Jr. Late effects of treatment for childhood Hodgkin's disease. *N Engl J Med* 1996;335:352–353.

197. Wolden SL, Lamborn KR, Cleary SF, et al. Second cancers following pediatric Hodgkin's disease. *J Clin Oncol* 1998;16:536–544. See comments.

198. Boice JD Jr., Preston D, Davis FG, et al. Frequent chest x-ray fluoroscopy and breast cancer incidence among tuberculosis patients in Massachusetts. *Radiat Res* 1991;125:214–222.

199. Hildreth NG, Shore RE, Dvoretsky PM. The risk of breast cancer after irradiation of the thymus in infancy. *N Engl J Med* 1989;321:1281–1284.

200. Ronckers CM, Erdmann CA, Land CE. Radiation and breast cancer: a review of current evidence. *Breast Cancer Res* 2005;7:21–32.

201. Boice JD Jr. Radiation and breast carcinogenesis. *Med Pediatr Oncol* 2001;36:508–513.

202. Land CE, Tokunaga M, Koyama K, et al. Incidence of female breast cancer among atomic bomb survivors, Hiroshima and Nagasaki, 1950–1990. *Radiat Res* 2003;160:707–717.

203. Travis LB, Hill D, Dores GM, et al. Cumulative absolute breast cancer risk for young women treated for Hodgkin lymphoma. *J Natl Cancer Inst* 2005;97:1428–1437.

204. Beral V. Breast cancer and hormone-replacement therapy in the Million Women Study. *Lancet* 2003;362:419–427. Erratum in Lancet 2003; 362:1160.

205. Collaborative Group on Hormonal Factors in Breast Cancer. Breast cancer and hormone replacement therapy: collaborative reanalysis of data from 51 epidemiological studies of 52,705 women with breast cancer and 108,411 women without breast cancer. *Lancet* 1997;350:1047–1059.

206. Hoyle CF, de Bastos M, Wheatley K, et al. AML associated with previous cytotoxic therapy, MDS or myeloproliferative disorders: results from the MRC's 9th AML trial. *Br J Haematol* 1989;72:45–53.

207. Longmore G, Guinan EC, Weinstein HJ, et al. Bone marrow transplantation for myelodysplasia and secondary acute nonlymphoblastic leukemia. *J Clin Oncol* 1990;8:1707–1714.

208. Laurie SA, Kris MG, Portlock CS, et al. The clinical course of nonsmall cell lung carcinoma in survivors of Hodgkin disease. *Cancer* 2002;95:119–126.

209. Behringer K, Josting A, Schiller P, et al. Solid tumors in patients treated for Hodgkin's disease: a report from the German Hodgkin Lymphoma Study Group. *Ann Oncol* 2004;15:1079–1085.

210. Cutuli B, Dhermain F, Borel C, et al. Breast cancer in patients treated for Hodgkin's disease: clinical and pathological analysis of 76 cases in 63 patients. *Eur J Cancer* 1997;33:2315–2320.

211. Gervais-Fagnou DD, Girouard C, Laperriere N, et al. Breast cancer in women following supradiaphragmatic irradiation for Hodgkin's disease. *Oncology* 1999;57:224–231.

212. Yahalom J, Petrek JA, Biddinger PW, et al. Breast cancer in patients irradiated for Hodgkin's disease: a clinical and pathologic analysis of 45 events in 37 patients. *J Clin Oncol* 1992;10:1674–1681. See comments.

213. Deutsch M, Gerszten K, Bloomer WD, et al. Lumpectomy and breast irradiation for breast cancer arising after previous radiotherapy for Hodgkin's disease or lymphoma. *Am J Clin Oncol* 2001;24:33–34.

214. Kriege M, Brekelmans CT, Boetes C, et al. Efficacy of MRI and mammography for breast-cancer screening in women with a familial or genetic predisposition. *N Engl J Med* 2004;351:427–437.

215. Dershaw DD, Yahalom J, Petrek JA. Breast carcinoma in women previously treated for Hodgkin disease: mammographic evaluation. *Radiology* 1992;184:421–423.

216. Diller L, Medeiros Nancarrow C, Shaffer K, et al. Breast cancer screening in women previously treated for Hodgkin's disease: a prospective cohort study. *J Clin Oncol* 2002;20:2085–2091.

217. Broeks A, Russell NH, van Leeuwen FE, et al. Breast tumors induced by high dose radiation display similar genetic profiles. *Breast Cancer Res* 2005;7(suppl 2):S43.

CHAPTER 25 ■ CARDIOVASCULAR LATE EFFECTS AFTER TREATMENT OF HODGKIN LYMPHOMA

STEVEN L. HANCOCK

Cardiovascular diseases are more prevalent and develop earlier in life in survivors of Hodgkin lymphoma than in the general population, and have been the most common cause of excess morbidity and mortality other than malignant neoplasms. Most severe, early cardiovascular reactions to treatment, such as acute radiation pericarditis, myocarditis, pancarditis, and acute heart failure associated with anthracyclines, have become rare events due to current therapies that have reduced the volume and dose of irradiation to the heart and limited anthracycline exposure. However, late cardiovascular complications of therapy remain a significant concern and challenge for the management of treated individuals. Identified problems include premature coronary artery disease with manifestations that range from silent ischemia to acute myocardial infarction and sudden cardiac death. Cardiac irradiation may lead to decreased left ventricular mass, delayed restrictive cardiomyopathy with signs of diastolic dysfunction, and associated symptoms of fatigue and impaired exercise tolerance. Delayed restrictive or constrictive pericarditis, and pancarditis with both pericardial and myocardial fibrosis, can lead to pleural effusions and subsequent signs and symptoms of biventricular failure. Mediastinal irradiation has increased risks for valvular heart disease, abnormalities of the cardiac conduction system, and arrhythmia. Delayed onset of left ventricular failure from cardiomyopathy has been reported sporadically after anthracycline-based chemotherapy regimens. However, the incidence of late anthracycline toxicity in treated populations of large size is yet to be clearly defined. Peripheral vascular stenosis and stroke have been observed in several treated populations.

Studies of mortality rates in several populations of Hodgkin lymphoma survivors with prolonged follow-up suggest the magnitude of these risks. Death was attributed to cardiovascular disease in 16% of 754 deaths among 2,498 patients treated for Hodgkin lymphoma at Stanford between 1960 and 1995[1] and in 13.7% of 124 deaths among 794 patients treated at the Joint Center for Radiation Therapy between 1969 and 1995.[2] Among patients treated for early stages of Hodgkin lymphoma on European Organization for the Research and Treatment of Cancer (EORTC) and British National Lymphoma Investigation (BNLI) protocols, 7% and 14% of deaths were attributed to myocardial infarction.[3,4] Among 258 patients treated in the Netherlands between 1965 and 1980, 4.7% died of ischemic heart disease—a rate that was 5.3 times the rate observed in the general Dutch population.[5] There is some evidence that improvements in therapy have decreased these risks among more recently treated patients. Among patients treated for stage I or II Hodgkin lymphoma at Stanford, the incidence of cardiovascular death

within 15 years of treatment decreased from 5.4% for those treated between 1962 and 1980 to 0.8% for those treated from 1980 to 1996.[6]

HISTORICAL ASPECTS AND TREATMENT FACTORS AFFECTING RISK

During the era when supervoltage and megavoltage therapeutic radiation sources were first applied to the treatment of Hodgkin lymphoma, the heart was generally believed to be relatively resistant to radiation injury. Occasional case reports suggested potential risks of acute electrocardiographic changes, arrhythmia, fibrosis of the myocardium and/or pericardium, and acute myocardial infarction. In the late 1960s and early 1970s, systematic studies of patients who had been treated with mediastinal irradiation for Hodgkin lymphoma documented a more serious pattern of risk, as reviewed by Stewart and Fajardo.[7] In 1967, Cohn and associates[8] reported a series of 21 cases of radiation-induced heart disease evaluated at Stanford, 11 of whom were treated for Hodgkin lymphoma using the mantle technique described by Kaplan.[9] These cases presaged the findings of larger, population-based studies during the subsequent three decades, documenting risks of acute pericarditis, chronic constrictive pericarditis, valvular heart disease, and premature coronary artery disease.

Most of the early studies focused on radiation carditis, a mixture of clinical entities that spanned the spectrum of acute pericarditis, post-irradiation pericardial effusion, chronic pericarditis with constriction, and direct myocardial injury. Myocardial fibrosis was initially inferred from the observation that 5 of 10 patients with severe late constrictive pericarditis did not derive clinical benefit from surgical pericardiectomy.[10] Autopsies from such patients demonstrated diffuse pericardial, endocardial, and myocardial fibrosis. Observation of these clinical syndromes led to a series of pathologic and experimental studies characterizing the response of the parietal and visceral pericardium, myocardium, and endocardium to ionizing radiation.[10–14] Direct valvular injury was sporadically reported in autopsy series of children[15] and young adults[16] but was not a feature of cardiac injury by irradiation in experimental systems. Similarly, premature coronary artery disease, although clinically suspected on the basis of sporadic case reports of acute myocardial infarction in younger patients, was not a common feature noted in early pathologic or experimental studies of radiation-induced heart disease.

The role of radiation as an etiologic factor in valvular or coronary artery diseases was doubted by experts as late as 1984.[14]

Studies of patients treated for Hodgkin lymphoma with mantle-field irradiation at Stanford and the University of California provided the first indication of a dose-response for radiation pericarditis or myocardial injury.[12] Most of the patients irradiated for Hodgkin lymphoma before 1971 had at least 60% of the cardiac volume included in the mediastinal portion of a mantle field. A dose of 40 Gy in 20 fractions over a treatment period of 4 weeks appeared to approximate the threshold for pericardial injury. No cases of pericarditis were observed after doses below 36 Gy. The risk was 2% with doses in the range of 36 to 40 Gy and 6% with doses of 40 to 48 Gy, which were the doses most often used for treatment of mediastinal Hodgkin lymphoma. Risks rose rapidly with the use of higher radiation doses—particularly among those patients who received more than one course of mediastinal irradiation for recurrent disease. A much higher incidence of constrictive pericarditis and myocardial injury was reported from centers that had emphasized dose delivery through an anterior mediastinal field alone or had used anteriorly weighted 60-Co fields rather than equally weighted anterior and posterior fields generated by linear accelerators.[16,17] Based on these studies, it appeared that high dose per fraction was an important factor contributing to the risk of pericardial and myocardial injury.[17,18] The use of subcarinal blocking was instituted at Stanford in 1971 and served to limit the radiation exposure of most of the myocardium to 30 to 35 Gy. This decreased the incidence of early pericardial injury to 2.5% from a 7% incidence observed with partial left ventricular shielding or a 20% incidence observed when radiation fields encompassed the entire heart.[19] A study of cases of constrictive pericarditis that required surgery at Stanford suggested that such blocking techniques may have increased the latent interval between irradiation and the development of constriction without affecting the incidence of the problem.[20] Patients who underwent pericardiectomy between 1970 and 1980 were usually irradiated before the routine use of subcarinal blocking and underwent surgery an average of 4.75 years after irradiation; those who underwent pericardiectomy between 1980 and 1985 usually had subcarinal blocking and underwent surgery an average of 11 years after irradiation. The authors of this study noted that no patients irradiated after 1980 at Stanford had required pericardiectomy. The survival impact of limiting cardiac radiation dose was verified in a subsequent study from Stanford. The relative risk of death from cardiac diseases other than acute myocardial infarction decreased from 5.1 to 1.7 (not significantly increased) in association with the use of left ventricular and subcarinal blocking during mediastinal irradiation.[21] The increased use of initial chemotherapy for patients who present with bulky mediastinal masses of Hodgkin lymphoma has also improved cardiac protection for many patients by reducing the volume of heart that is incidentally irradiated in order to encompass lymphadenopathy. These combined-modality programs also eliminated the need to use low-dose irradiation of the entire cardiac silhouette to treat cardiophrenic angle or juxtadiaphragmatic lymph nodes, which were relatively common sites for recurrence of mediastinal Hodgkin lymphoma when these nodal regions were initially untreated.[22] The routine use of such strategies to limit the dose and volume of cardiac irradiation has virtually eliminated the complications of constrictive pericarditis and pancarditis from the management of patients treated for Hodgkin lymphoma.

The first suggestions of an association between mediastinal irradiation for Hodgkin lymphoma and premature coronary artery disease were reports of acute myocardial infarction deaths in a 19-year-old man 4 years after mediastinal irradiation and a 15-year-old boy 16 months after mantle irradiation.[8,23] Autopsy findings in the younger patient showed diffuse, severe intimal proliferation and atheromatous change in the proximal coronary arteries with no significant atherosclerosis apparent in other, unirradiated vessels. In the late 1970s, Kopelson and Herwig[24] reported 10 patients who developed angina pectoris, acute myocardial infarction, or sudden death from acute myocardial infarction before 40 years of age after receiving mediastinal irradiation for Hodgkin lymphoma. Pohjola-Sintonen and co-workers[25] reported severe coronary artery disease arising in 2 males at 12 and 31 years of age following treatment for Hodgkin lymphoma 7 and 10 years earlier. Both were treated with anterior radiation fields alone to estimated epicardial doses of 40 and 52 Gy.

In the first population-based study, Boivin et al.[26] evaluated coronary heart disease mortality among 957 patients treated for Hodgkin lymphoma between 1942 and 1975 at either the Harvard Joint Center for Radiation Therapy or the Massachusetts General Hospital. They observed a higher annual probability of death from coronary disease among patients who had received mediastinal irradiation in comparison to those who received no cardiac irradiation. However, the relative risk for death from coronary artery disease in this population was 1.5, which was not significantly elevated. A subsequent analysis of 590 patients treated at the Joint Center for Radiation Therapy between 1969 and 1980 reported 13 deaths from acute myocardial infarction (only one of which occurred before 40 years of age) and a significantly elevated relative risk (RR) of myocardial infarction death of 6.7 (95% confidence interval [CI], 2.91–13.3).[27]

Among patients with early stages of Hodgkin lymphoma entered in EORTC trials, acute myocardial infarction was the second most common cause of intercurrent death. The standardized mortality ratio (SMR) for the risk of death from acute myocardial infarction was significantly increased for those treated either before or after 40 years of age (SMR, 14.9 [95% CI, 5.5–32.3] versus SMR, 6.6 [95% CI, 3.3–11.9]), respectively.[3] Cosset and associates[28] reported a 3.9% 10-year cumulative incidence rate of acute myocardial infarction after Hodgkin lymphoma treatment at Institut Gustave-Roussy; 13 acute myocardial infarctions occurred among 499 patients who received mediastinal irradiation for Hodgkin lymphoma. There were no myocardial infarctions in the 138 patients whose treatments did not include mediastinal irradiation.

Investigators from the British National Lymphoma Investigation reported that 14% of 43 deaths were attributed to myocardial infarction among 1,043 patients cured of Hodgkin lymphoma after treatment before 30 years of age.[4]

In a case-cohort study that compiled records of 4,665 patients treated for Hodgkin lymphoma at 11 American and Canadian centers, Boivin et al. reported an age-adjusted relative risk of acute myocardial infarction death of 2.56 (95% CI, 1.11–5.93) after treatments that included mediastinal irradiation and 0.97 (95% CI, 0.53–1.77) after chemotherapy.[26] The risk of death from myocardial infarction appeared to be higher among those irradiated after 60 years of age and lower among those treated before 40 years of age. The risk for death from myocardial infarction was significantly increased within 5 years of treatment and appeared to remain elevated with more prolonged follow-up.

Among 2,232 patients treated for Hodgkin lymphoma at Stanford between 1960 and 1991, 55 deaths were attributed to acute myocardial infarction, representing a relative risk or standardized mortality ratio of 3.2 (95% CI, 2.3–4.0) and an absolute risk of 17.8 excess deaths per 10,000 person-years of observation after therapy.[21] The risk of myocardial infarction death tended to be higher among patients treated with radiation alone (RR, 4.1 [95% CI, 2.8–5.5]) than among those who received both chemotherapy and mediastinal irradiation (RR, 2.7 [95% CI, 1.5–3.8]). The risk of death from myocardial infarction was not significantly increased for those who received no mediastinal irradiation (RR, 1.7 [95% CI, 0.7–3.5]) or for those who received mediastinal irradiation in doses less

TABLE 25.1

EFFECT OF AGE AT IRRADIATION ON RISK OF DEATH FROM
ACUTE MYOCARDIAL INFARCTION (AMI) AFTER TREATMENT
OF HODGKIN LYMPHOMA

Age at irradiation (years)	Observed/expected events	Relative risk (RR)[a]	95% confidence intervals	Absolute risk (AR)[a,b]
Less than 10	0/0.002	—	—	—
10 through 19	6/0.13	44.7	18.0–93.0	12.4
20 through 29	8/1.1	7.3	3.4–13.8	9.0
30 through 39	14/2.7	5.1	2.9–7.4	27.4
40 through 49	9/3.0	3.0	1.4–5.5	43.6
50 or more	12/6.8	1.8	1.0–3.0	—

[a]χ for trend in AMI-RR: $p < 0.0001$; χ for trend in AMI-AR: 2.6, $p = 0.01$.
[b]Absolute risk is expressed as excess cases per 10,000 person-years.
Adapted with permission from Hancock SL, Tucker MA, Hoppe RT. Factors affecting late mortality from heart disease after treatment of Hodgkin's disease. *JAMA* 1993;270:1949–1955.

than 30 Gy (RR, 4.2 [95% CI, 0.7–13.8]). The introduction of routine left ventricular and subcarinal blocking in 1971 had a modest impact upon the risk of death from acute myocardial infarction (RR before 1972: 3.7 [95% CI, 2.3–5.1] and RR after 1972: 3.4 [95% CI, 2.0–4.8]). For most patients who received mediastinal irradiation, the proximal coronary arteries were likely to be located within the unblocked portion of the radiation field, adjacent to mediastinal lymphadenopathy.

In contrast to the study by Boivin et al., the study from Stanford showed that treatment at a young age conferred a higher relative risk of acute myocardial infarction death than treatment at an older age. The risk of infarction death decreased significantly with advancing age at irradiation and was not significantly increased among patients irradiated at 50 years of age or older. The relative risk decreased from 44.7 for those irradiated at 10 to 19 years of age to 1.8 for those irradiated at 50 years of age or older (Table 25.1). However, the annualized, absolute risk of death from myocardial infarction after exposure tended to increase with increasing age at irradiation from 12.4 excess cases per 10,000 person-years of observation for those treated between 10 and 19 years of age to 43.6 excess cases for those irradiated between 40 and 49 years of age.

In the Stanford experience, the risk of death from acute myocardial infarction was significantly increased within 5 years of irradiation with 12 events (twice the number expected) and an absolute risk of 6.4 excess events per 10,000 person-years of follow-up. Both the relative risk and the absolute risk after exposure increased significantly with more prolonged follow-up, reaching a relative risk of 5.6 and an absolute risk of 70.6 extra deaths per 10,000 person-years of observation among patients whose follow-up exceeded 20 years (Table 25.2). This trend to increased risk at more prolonged latency may have been confounded by variations in radiation technique, because patients treated in the earlier eras generally received less cardiac blocking, higher daily fraction size, higher total doses, and higher epicardial daily doses due to treatment of anterior and posterior fields on alternate days.

Acute myocardial infarction death tended to occur at a younger age than is common. The relative risk was 52.4 for patients younger than 30 years of age; it declined progressively to 2.2 for those between 50 and 59 years of age, and was not significantly increased for those 60 years of age or older (Table 25.3). There was no association between chemotherapy exposure and an increased risk of death due to premature coronary artery disease. Cardiac risk factors were not clearly documented among these patients, although the prevalence of cigarette smoking in the Stanford population appeared to be significantly lower than expected in the general population.

The association of increased myocardial infarction risk with high-dose mediastinal irradiation at a young age was underscored by another study that focused on 635 patients treated for Hodgkin lymphoma before 21 years of age at

TABLE 25.2

LATENCY OF RISK FOR DEATH FROM ACUTE MYOCARDIAL INFARCTION (AMI)
AFTER TREATMENT OF HODGKIN LYMPHOMA

Years after initial Hodgkin lymphoma Tx	Observed/expected events	Relative risk[a]	95% confidence intervals	Absolute risk[a,b]
0 through 4	12/6.0	2.0	1.1–3.3	6.4
5 through 9	17/4.7	3.6	2.2–4.5	20.1
10 through 14	11/3.7	3.0	1.6–5.2	20.5
15 through 19	11/2.2	5.0	2.6–8.7	54.2
Over 20	4/0.7	5.6	1.8–13.6	70.6

[a]χ for trend in relative risk of AMI death: 2.3, $p = 0.02$; χ for trend in absolute risk of AMI death: 3.8, $p = 0.0002$.
[b]Absolute risk is expressed as excess cases per 10,000 person-years.
Adapted with permission from Hancock SL, Tucker MA, Hoppe RT. Factors affecting late mortality from heart disease after treatment of Hodgkin's disease. *JAMA* 1993;270:1949–1955.

TABLE 25.3

RISK FOR DEATH FROM ACUTE MYOCARDIAL INFARCTION AFTER TREATMENT OF HODGKIN LYMPHOMA ACCORDING TO AGE AT DEATH

Years of age at death from AMI	Observed/expected events	Relative risk	95% confidence intervals	Absolute risk[a]
Under 30	1/0.19	52.4	0.0–259	—
30 through 39	7/0.37	18.8	8.2–37.2	9.0
40 through 49	14/2.0	7.0	4.0–10.0	21.4
50 through 59	12/2.7	4.5	2.4–7.5	39.0
60 through 69	11/5.0	2.2	1.2–3.8	52.7
70 or more	10/6.2	1.6	0.8–2.9	—

[a]Absolute risk is expressed as excess cases per 10,000 person-years.
Adapted with permission from Hancock SL, Tucker MA, Hoppe RT. Factors affecting late mortality from heart disease after treatment of Hodgkin's disease. *JAMA* 1993;270:1949–1955.

Stanford.[29] Seven patients died of myocardial infarction, with a standardized mortality ratio of 41.5 (95% CI, 18.1–82.1). Three young patients sustained nonfatal myocardial infarctions, and three others required revascularization procedures for severe coronary artery disease. Among these younger patients, all coronary events arose from 6 to 20 years after mediastinal radiation doses that ranged from 42 to 45 Gy.

The effect of radiation dose in determining the subsequent risk for premature coronary disease is uncertain. Brierley and associates[30] summarized cardiac morbidity observed after treatment of Hodgkin lymphoma in 611 patients at Princess Margaret Hospital, where most patients received mediastinal radiation doses of 35 Gy in 20 fractions. The actuarial incidence of heart disease at 15 years was 10% for those whose mediastinum was irradiated and 12% for those who received no mediastinal irradiation. Mediastinal irradiation was not identified as a significant risk factor for cardiac disease. The relative risk of death from myocardial infarction was estimated at 1.55 (95% CI, 0.71–2.95).

Glanzmann and colleagues[31] reported a relative risk of acute myocardial infarction death of 4.2 (95% CI, 1.8–8.3) and a relative risk of either sudden death or myocardial infarction death of 6.7 (95% CI, 3.5–11.2) among 352 patients treated at University Hospital, Zurich, 93% of whom received 30 to 42 Gy with dose per fraction ranging from 1.3 to 2.1 Gy. The excess risk for coronary mortality appeared to be confined to males and was higher after treatment with chemotherapy and irradiation (RR, 10 [95% CI, 4.3–19.7]) than with irradiation alone (RR, 5 [95% CI, 1.6–11.7]). Excess coronary artery disease mortality was observed despite lower mediastinal irradiation doses than were implicated in the Stanford experience. However, fatal or nonfatal coronary artery disease events were largely confined to individuals with known coronary risk factors of smoking, hypertension, obesity, or hypercholesterolemia. No adverse cardiac event had occurred among the 74 patients who lacked identifiable risk factors and had received no chemotherapy. Nine of the 13 patients who had sudden death or a fatal myocardial infarction and 2 of 3 patients who sustained nonfatal myocardial infarctions had no antecedent angina pectoris or other cardiac symptoms in this series. This absence of prodromal symptoms was also common in the Stanford experience[21,29] and has led to assessment of strategies for screening populations at potential risk at both institutions, as discussed below.

Conventional risk factors for coronary artery disease appeared to be prevalent co-factors for coronary risk in several other studies. King and associates reported a relative risk of 2.8 for death from myocardial infarction among 326 patients treated to an average mediastinal dose of 44 Gy at the University of Rochester.[32] Conventional coronary risk factors were prevalent among the deceased, including smoking (72%), hypercholesterolemia (78%), obesity (61%), hypertension (33%), and family history (28%). Among 404 patients treated with radiation for Hodgkin lymphoma at the University of Florida, at least one conventional coronary risk factor was identified in all of the 32 cases who developed symptomatic coronary artery disease after a median mid-mediastinal radiation dose of 36 Gy.[33] In a long-term follow-up analysis of 258 patients treated for Hodgkin lymphoma in the Netherlands, Reinders and associates found a standardized mortality ratio of 5.3 for deaths from ischemic heart disease and a relative risk for 2.7 for hospitalization for ischemic heart conditions.[5] In this population the risk appeared higher among those irradiated at or above 30 years of age. However, the risk for coronary events or hospitalization became significantly increased within 5 through 9 years after treatment. The mean dose to the inferior mediastinum was 37.2 Gy at a dose rate of 1.64 Gy per fraction. The authors found no difference in the risk of an ischemic cardiac event when both fields were irradiated each day instead of treating anterior and posterior fields on alternate days. Specific data on conventional coronary risk factors except for gender were not available in this study.

Unusual valvular injury attributed to irradiation was reported in two autopsy studies of children and young adults treated with mediastinal irradiation, and mitral insufficiency was reported in early analyses from Stanford.[7,15,16] Nonetheless, appreciation of the contribution of mediastinal irradiation for Hodgkin lymphoma to the risk of valvular heart disease has been a relatively recent finding. Most of the evidence for valvular disease derives from echocardiographic studies of Hodgkin lymphoma survivors. Mitral or aortic valve thickening was found in 27% of 41 Hodgkin lymphoma or mediastinal seminoma survivors studied in the early-1980s by Perrault and co-workers[34] and in 2 of 28 Hodgkin lymphoma patients studied by Pohjola-Sintonen and associates.[25] Valvular insufficiency was the most common finding in echocardiographic studies of 25 young-adult Hodgkin lymphoma patients, with tricuspid regurgitation identified in 22, mitral regurgitation in 9, and aortic regurgitation in one. Studies of cardiopulmonary function in 116 Norwegians treated for Hodgkin lymphoma with mediastinal irradiation with or without chemotherapy identified cardiopulmonary dysfunction in 75% of females and 41% of males.[35] On echocardiographic studies, 15% of these patients had aortic regurgitation, 7% had mitral regurgitation, and 2% had both aortic and mitral regurgitation that exceeded grade 1 severity.[36] None of 40 control subjects had valvular regurgitation that exceeded grade 1 in severity. Valvular dysfunction affected 46% of the women and 16% of the men in this study, and female gender appeared to be an independent risk factor for valvular injury or symptomatic cardiopulmonary dysfunction in this population.

Female gender was not identified as a specific risk factor for cardiac dysfunction or valvular heart disease among 144 patients studied by Glanzmann and associates after mediastinal irradiation that generally ranged from 30 to 42 Gy for Hodgkin lymphoma.[31] Only 3 patients had symptomatic valvular heart disease. However, the authors found abnormal valvular thickening in 29% of patients, with a cumulative incidence that rose from 8% after 10 years to 66% among patients treated more than 25 years before the study. Glanzmann and associates also found support for increased valvular abnormality with more prolonged follow-up through repeated echocardiography of 74 patients 1 to 6 years after an initial study that occurred more than 10 years after therapy; 8% of the subjects whose valves were normal developed signs of thickening, and 37% of the subjects with thickening had progression of valvular abnormality on subsequent study.

Although most of the valvular abnormalities identified by echocardiographic screening after mediastinal irradiation for Hodgkin lymphoma have not been associated with clinical symptoms, valvular heart disease has contributed to excess morbidity and mortality. Among 635 patients treated for Hodgkin lymphoma before 21 years of age at Stanford, 3 expired of complications related to valvular heart disease and 3 had undergone surgical replacement of damaged valves.[29] Four of 1,597 patients treated at Stanford at 21 years of age or older died of valvular heart disease or complications related to valve replacement.[21] Clinically significant valvular heart disease developed at a median of 22 years after Hodgkin lymphoma treatment at the University of Florida, affecting 25 of the 415 patients studied.[33] The median mid-mediastinal radiation dose was reported to be 37 Gy for those affected, compared to 33 Gy for those unaffected. The risk for requiring valve surgery was 8.42 relative to expected rates in the general population estimated from National Hospital Discharge Survey data.

RADIATION FACTORS ASSOCIATED WITH CARDIAC TOXICITY

The risks of acute radiation pericarditis and delayed constrictive pericarditis after irradiation for Hodgkin lymphoma have been clearly associated with the volume of the heart irradiated and the dose of radiation received. Stewart and co-workers have estimated that the threshold for significant pericardial injury is 40 Gy if more than 60% of the heart is included in the radiation field and 55 to 60 Gy if less than 15% of the cardiac volume is irradiated.[12,37] The risk of pericarditis rises steeply with doses above 40 Gy when subcarinal blocking is not employed. Among patients treated with doses approximating 44 Gy, early pericarditis affected 20% of patients treated to 60% or more of the heart in the absence of blocking, 7% in whom blocks shielded the left ventricle, and 2.5% who had both left ventricular shielding and placement of a subcarinal block to limit ventricular exposure to 30 Gy.[19] Late constrictive pericarditis has been exceedingly rare among patients treated with mediastinal doses of 44 Gy or less when exposure of the entire cardiac silhouette has been limited to 15 to 25 Gy and subcarinal blocking has been added between 25 and 35 Gy. Among patients treated at Stanford, the risk of death from cardiac diseases other than acute myocardial infarction has not been significantly increased among patients treated since the introduction of subcarinal blocking in 1971 or among cohorts who received mediastinal irradiation doses of 30 Gy or less.[21]

Because the risk of premature coronary disease has varied with treatment technique, use of chemotherapy, age at treatment, duration of observation, and prevalence of conventional coronary risk factors, it is difficult to draw firm conclusions about the relationships between radiation dose, volume of the heart irradiated, and coronary-artery disease risk. Investigators at Princess Margaret Hospital have reported no significant increase in the risk of acute myocardial infarction death among 611 patients with stage I or II Hodgkin lymphoma, 246 of whom received mantle irradiation to a usual dose of 35 Gy using a fraction size of 1.75 Gy.[30] Among patients treated in Zurich, Glanzmann and associates observed a very high relative risk of acute myocardial infarction or sudden death of 8.6 (CI, 4.5–15.3) in men who received approximately 40 Gy in 1.5- to 1.8-Gy fractions but observed no excess risk among women who had received similar treatment (RR, 1.72 [CI, 0.04–9.6]).[31] They also found that the risk for fatal or nonfatal ischemic coronary events appeared to be confined to those who had known risk factors for coronary artery disease, including smoking, hypertension, diabetes, obesity, or hypercholesterolemia (RR, 2.36 [CI, 1.42–3.68] with risk factors versus 0.96 [CI, 0.20–2.77] with no known risk factors). The prevalence of known coronary risk factors was unknown in the population of patients irradiated at Stanford, where the usual mediastinal dose was 44 Gy administered in 1.8- to 2.2-Gy fractions.[21] The relative risk of myocardial infarction death was significantly increased among women in this population (RR 2.6 [CI, 1.2–5.0]), suggesting some potential difference in risk associated with dose when compared with the Zurich experience. Dose effect remained unclear in the overall Stanford experience, because the relative risks were similar with or without subcarinal blocking (RR 3.4 [CI, 2.0–4.5] versus RR 3.7 [CI, 2.3–5.1]) or with mediastinal doses above or below 30 Gy (RR, 3.5 [CI, 2.5–4.5] versus 4.2 [CI, 0.7–13.8]). Cosset and colleagues were also unable to demonstrate a relationship between total dose or fraction size and the risk of acute myocardial infarction death in a comparison of 499 patients who had received mediastinal irradiation for Hodgkin lymphoma in comparison with 138 patients who were not irradiated.[28] Reinders and co-workers reported a standardized mortality ratio of 5.3 for death from ischemic heart disease for patients irradiated to mean total dose of 37.2 Gy at a fraction size of 1.64 Gy.[5] They concluded that "data in the literature suggest 30 Gy to be a relatively safe dose with respect to the potential development of (serious) cardiac complications."

The relationship between radiation dose, cardiac volume, and the subsequent development of valvular heart disease has also been difficult to discern due to the relatively small number of events, prolonged latency for the development of clinically apparent valvular disease, and evolving radiation techniques. Glanzmann and associates[31] evaluated the latency of valvular abnormality after radiation by means of echocardiographic studies that were performed in 144 patients treated with mediastinal irradiation for Hodgkin lymphoma in Zurich between 1964 and 1994. Forty-two patients (29%) had aortic or mitral valvular thickening apparent on cardiac echogram, 4 of whom had grade 3 lesions. The cumulative incidence of valvular thickening 10 years after irradiation was 8% but rose to 45% at 20 years with grade 3 changes in 4.1%. Among patients who had repeat echocardiography from 1 to 6 years after an initial study, 8% of patients with normal heart valves at their initial study developed valvular thickening and 37% of those with abnormal valves showed progression of valvular abnormality.

Two hundred and ninety-four asymptomatic Hodgkin lymphoma survivors were studied with transthoracic echocardiography at Stanford an average of 15 ± 7 years after a mean mediastinal radiation dose of 43 Gy.[38] Valvular disease was several-fold increased in comparison with age and gender-adjusted rates reported from the Framingham population. Prolonged latency was a significant factor in the appreciation of valvular disease. Aortic regurgitation, for example, was observed in 60% of individuals studied more than 20 years after irradiation, versus 4% for those studied within 10 years of treatment. Valvular thickening was also dependent upon the time since therapy. Aortic thickening was observed in 13%

of patients within 10 years of treatment and 61% of those studied more than 20 years after treatment.

Adams and co-workers[39] also identified a high prevalence of valvular disease among 48 survivors of Hodgkin lymphoma without symptoms of cardiac disease studied by transthoracic echo an average of 14.3 years after mediastinal irradiation at young age (median radiation dose: 40 Gy; median age at treatment 16.5 years). They found significant increases in the incidence of mitral regurgitation (21 observed versus 9.7 expected) and aortic regurgitation (19 observed versus 0.0 expected).

IMPACT OF CHEMOTHERAPY

At present, studies in populations treated for Hodgkin lymphoma have shown variable associations between chemotherapy exposure in combined-modality regimens and subsequent risks for cardiac disease. The relative risk of death from acute myocardial infarction in the Stanford population was slightly lower among patients treated with mediastinal irradiation and MOP(P) (mechlorethamine, Oncovin [vincristine], and procarbazine, given with or without prednisone) than with irradiation alone (RR, 2.8 [CI, 1.6–4.0] versus RR, 3.8 [CI, 2.0–5.1]).[21] Factors that may have contributed to this reduced risk included the use of lower average mediastinal radiation doses and a somewhat shorter follow-up duration for the cohort of patients treated with combined therapy. The mean mediastinal dose was 43.3 Gy for radiation alone versus 40.7 Gy for combined therapy, and the median follow-up was 9.1 years after radiation alone versus 8.1 years with combined treatment. Among patients treated in Zurich, the relative risk of acute myocardial infarction or sudden death was somewhat higher after combined therapy than after radiation alone (RR, 10 [CI, 4.3–19.7] versus RR, 5 [CI, 1.6–11.7]).[31]

The increasing use of anthracycline-based chemotherapy regimens such as ABVD (Adriamycin [doxorubicin], bleomycin, vinblastine, and dacarbazine) raises concern about late cardiac toxicity after the treatment of Hodgkin lymphoma. Studies using clinical and morphologic end-points have shown that mediastinal irradiation potentiates cardiac toxicity from anthracyclines. Using light and electron microscopic techniques Billingham and associates[40] developed a system for grading myofibrillary loss in endomyocardial biopsies obtained during cardiac catheterizations and found that histologic findings preceded and correlated with the risk of congestive cardiomyopathy. Billingham and associates[41] found that patients who had received cardiac irradiation had greater myocyte degeneration and an increased incidence of congestive heart failure than patients who received comparable doses of Adriamycin without irradiation. They also found evidence for doxorubicin recall of acute radiation injury, noting capillary endothelial cell damage typical of acute radiation injury in a patient who received doxorubicin 10.5 years after irradiation.

Late cardiac decompensation after anthracycline therapy has been better documented among individuals treated for Hodgkin lymphoma during childhood than among adults. Steinherz and associates[42] identified 15 patients among a screened population of 300 who developed abnormalities of cardiac conduction, dysrhythmia, or congestive failure between 6 and 19 years after exposure to daunorubicin or doxorubicin in doses ranging from 285 to 870 mg per square meter of body surface area. Some patients who had no early evidence of cardiac injury developed acute cardiac decompensation more than 10 years after anthracycline exposure. Although stresses unique to adolescent development may have played a role in these occasional episodes of cardiac decompensation after anthracycline exposure, there is little published data regarding cardiac function beyond the first decade in individuals who received anthracycline therapy during early adulthood.

Several groups have used echocardiography and radionuclide imaging techniques to assess the contribution of doxorubicin to

cardiac dysfunction in Hodgkin lymphoma survivors. LaMonte and colleagues[43] concluded that significant abnormalities were likely to be low, reporting normal resting and exercise function in 15 of 19 patients treated with the MOPP/ABVD regimen and varying doses of radiation to the mediastinum. Two patients had decreased left ventricular ejection fraction at rest, and two others had a diminished left ventricular response to exercise. Similarly, Allavena and co-workers[44] found signs of diminished left ventricular function in only 6% of Hodgkin lymphoma patients and could not differentiate between treatment with radiation alone or combined with MOPP or MOPP/ABVD. Among 40 patients screened with echocardiography after three cycles of ABVD and mediastinal irradiation to doses of 40 to 45 Gy, 38 had a normal left ventricular ejection fraction and 2 had borderline low values of 50%.[45]

Functional impairment associated with combined irradiation and anthracycline-containing regimens for Hodgkin lymphoma may be greater when administered during childhood. Pihkala and associates[46] reported abnormally low left ventricular ejection fraction for 50% of children who had received both doxorubicin and mediastinal irradiation (to a median dose of 24 Gy with a range from 11 to 51 Gy) compared with 8% of children who had received mediastinal irradiation alone to a median dose of 40 Gy. Careful analyses of late intercurrent morbidity and mortality in large populations of Hodgkin lymphoma patients treated with anthracycline-based regimens such as ABVD with and without irradiation are clearly needed to confirm the lack of cardiac decompensation more than a decade beyond these therapies.

Only 4 of the 48 patients with Hodgkin lymphoma studied by Adams and associates[39] at a median of 14.3 years after treatment had anthracycline exposure. However, they reported an association with aortic insufficiency ($p = 0.0025$), impaired left ventricular function (lower LV fractional shortening and higher LV wall stress on echocardiography), and higher average 24-hour heart rate on Holter monitor than in patients who had no anthracycline exposure.

Although long-term studies assessing the risk of late chronic heart failure after anthracycline-based chemotherapy regimens for Hodgkin lymphoma are lacking, Moser and associates observed a significant elevation of this risk in Dutch and Belgian patients treated on EORTC trials for high grade non-Hodgkin lymphoma with doxorubicin-based regimens when compared to the general Dutch population.[47] When analysis was confined to patients who received no secondary treatment regimens, the standardized incidence ratio for developing chronic heart failure was 3.1 after chemotherapy alone, 3.6 after chemotherapy and irradiation, 7.1 after chemotherapy and hematopoietic progenitor cell transplantation, and 12.5 after chemotherapy, irradiation, and transplantation. Although more than half of the patients treated for non-Hodgkin lymphoma also received mediastinal irradiation at doses of 30 Gy after complete response to chemotherapy or 40 Gy after partial response, the risk of acute myocardial infarction and coronary artery disease was equivalent to that observed in the general Dutch population. Whether the risk of developing chronic heart failure varies with the age at anthracycline exposure is uncertain. This may be a factor in the limited report of this problem in populations treated for Hodgkin lymphoma at a younger age than patients with non-Hodgkin lymphomas.

VASCULAR COMPLICATIONS

Elerding and associates[48] analyzed pooled retrospective data on 910 patients from M. D. Anderson Cancer Center who had received irradiation to the neck, including 247 patients treated for Hodgkin lymphoma, 119 patients treated for non-Hodgkin lymphoma, and 537 patients with squamous cell carcinomas of the head and neck. They reported a 6.9% incidence of cerebrovascular accidents over a 9-year period of observation. By their estimates the relative risk of stroke was nearly twice that expected in a general population, but this increase was not statistically significant ($p = 0.39$). These events occurred an average of 9 years after irradiation at an average of 64 years of age. The incidence of stroke among the patients treated for Hodgkin lymphoma was not specified. However, Elerding and associates also prospectively studied 77 patients more than 5 years after treatment radiation fields that included the neck for Hodgkin lymphoma with carotid phonoangiograms and ocular plethysmography. Seventeen patients (22%) had abnormal phonoangiogram studies, suggesting turbulent flow in the carotid system. Four others had audible bruits on auscultation and were excluded from the phonoangiogram study because turbulence may have originated in the innominate or subclavian systems. Twelve of the patients studied (16%) had abnormal ocular plethysmography, suggesting significant impairment of blood flow through the carotid system due to stenosis. The patients treated for Hodgkin lymphoma who developed apparent vascular stenosis averaged 38 years of age at the time of these studies.

Recently, Hull and associates identified noncoronary vascular events in 30 of 404 patients treated for Hodgkin lymphoma at the University of Florida.[33] The events included stroke in 10, transient ischemic attacks in 7, carotid artery stenosis in 14, and subclavian artery stenosis in 7 patients. Stroke and transient ischemic events tended to affect individuals treated at an older age and at a relatively short interval after therapy. These events developed at a median interval of 5.6 years after radiation exposure at a median age of 51 years. Carotid or subclavian stenosis more often developed at prolonged intervals after irradiation at a younger age. The median interval from Hodgkin lymphoma treatment to diagnosis of stenosis was 21 years after treatment at a median age of 20 years. Risk factors associated with peripheral vascular disease, hypertension, and diabetes mellitus were more prevalent among the older individuals who experienced stroke or transient ischemic attacks than among those who developed carotid or subclavian stenosis.

A similar, age-related pattern was also observed among 21 patients who developed vascular stenosis after irradiation for Hodgkin lymphoma, non-Hodgkin lymphoma, or seminoma at Stanford.[49] In 9 of the cases noncoronary vascular diseases were diagnosed at a median interval of 9.1 years after treatment at a median of 61 years of age. For these patients the relationship between therapy and risk seemed uncertain. However, 12 patients developed major arterial stenoses in irradiated regions at an unusually young age, suggesting a role of irradiation in the pathogenesis of the disorder. Those events developed at a median interval of 16.9 years after radiation exposure at a median of 33 years of age.

Studies from the Childhood Cancer Survival Group have shown a strong association between mantle radiation exposure before 21 years of age (median dose, 40 Gy) and increased risk of late-occurring stroke.[50] Compared with siblings, the relative risk for stroke among Hodgkin lymphoma survivors was 4.32 (95% CI, 2.01–9.29) and was 5.62 among those patients who received mantle irradiation. The median interval from diagnosis of Hodgkin lymphoma to stroke was 17.5 years, and the median age at the time of stroke was 33 years (range, 21 to 45 years). Late vascular stenosis appears to be a sporadic event that has affected a minority of patients after treatment for Hodgkin lymphoma. However, there are no published studies in which substantial populations of patients have been systematically screened for occult vascular stenosis. Because age, race, and gender-specific general population incidence rates for these vascular diseases are not available, the magnitude of excess risk associated with Hodgkin lymphoma therapy has not been well quantified. New less-invasive vascular imaging, such as CT angiography or magnetic resonance angiography, seem particularly useful in evaluating patients with potential vascular stenosis after irradiation (Figs. 25.1 and 25.2).

Venous thrombotic disease that primarily involves the axillary-subclavian venous system has also been reported during chemotherapy or combined-modality therapy of Hodgkin lymphoma.[51,52] The risk for these episodes has been primarily attributed to the desiccant action of some chemotherapy agents or the presence of indwelling infusion catheters, and appears to be unrelated to Hodgkin lymphoma activity.

A number of studies have documented abnormalities of the cardiac conduction system after mediastinal irradiation for Hodgkin lymphoma.[13,16,25,53–55] Bundle branch block on electrocardiogram has been attributed to ventricular injury affecting the Purkinje branches from high radiation dose to the epicardium.[37] Patients with bundle branch block patterns

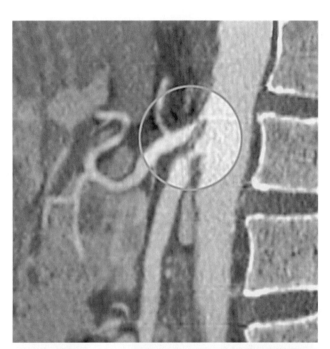

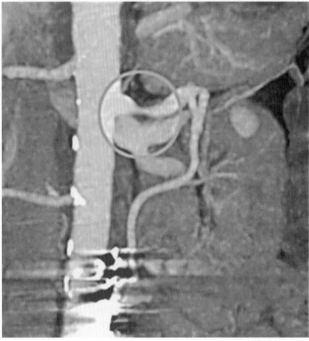

FIGURE 25.1. A: 3D reconstruction of a CT scan demonstrating stenosis at the origin of the celiac artery and superior mesenteric artery in a 55-year-old man with malabsorption and postprandial pain 32.8 years after para-aortic irradiation to 44Gy. B: 3D reconstructed CT scan of the same patient showing narrowing at the origin of the left renal artery.

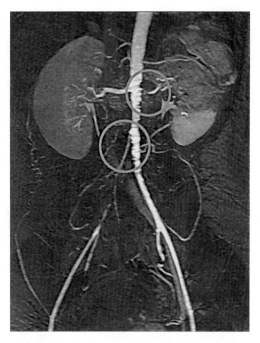

FIGURE 25.2. Magnetic resonance angiogram (MRA) showing diffuse disease involving the abdominal aorta, left renal artery, and right common iliac artery in a 42-year-old woman treated with 40 Gy total lymphoid irradiation at the age of 5 for stage III-B NSHL. Note the decreased perfusion of the mid and superior poles of the left kidney as a result of high-grade stenosis of the main left renal artery and occlusion of the proximal right common iliac artery with collaterals supplying the more distal iliac arteries.

or prolonged PR interval on electrocardiography may develop atrioventricular block and require implantation of a permanent pacemaker.

The prevalence of arrhythmia and cardiac conduction defects after Hodgkin lymphoma therapy varies widely by report and very likely depends upon radiation dose to the epicardium, interval after treatment, and upon the electrocardiographer's threshold for defining abnormality. Watchie and colleagues[56] reported a high prevalence of conduction abnormalities, including bundle branch block, among 40 patients who underwent resting and exercise testing an average of 5 years after extended-field irradiation or combined-modality therapy for extensive, intrathoracic Hodgkin lymphoma. Subjects were selected for study because their initial extent of disease involvement and treatment were likely to represent the "maximum degree of dysfunction" after Hodgkin lymphoma therapy. Despite the relatively early interval to testing, 17.5% of the subjects had significant conduction defects and 35% had abnormalities of borderline significance. Adams and associates[39] identified conduction defects in 75% of 48 patients treated for Hodgkin lymphoma who were subjected to extensive screening. The subjects were treated before 25 years of age and studied at a median interval of 14.3 years after treatment (median treatment age 16.5 years and median mediastinal radiation dose 40 Gy). In contrast, Heidenreich and colleagues reported that resting electrocardiography was rarely abnormal in 294 asymptomatic patients screened an average of 15 years after a mean mediastinal radiation dose of 43.5 Gy. The prevalence of various electrocardiographic conduction abnormalities was similar to general population rates reported from the Framingham Heart Study.[38] However, signs of left ventricular hypertrophy, right bundle branch block, and Q-wave abnormalities were noted to increase with increasing time after irradiation. These specific abnormalities became more common than expected in the general population.

Heidenreich and co-workers[38] also observed an increase in resting heart rate with increasing periods of time after treatment (70 ± 13 beats per minute within 10 years, 74 ± 12 beats per minute from 11 to 20 years, 81 ± 10 beats per minute more than 20 years after treatment). Among 47 patients studied by Adams and associates,[39] 9 (19%) had sinus tachycardia with a resting heart rate that exceeded 100 beats per minute. Holter monitor studies showed that 62% of their subjects had persistent tachycardia or a monotonous heart rate without normal physiologic variability over the course of 24 hours. Their findings suggested a high prevalence of autonomic dysfunction after mantle irradiation. The authors correlated self-reported symptoms from a quality-of-life questionnaire and observed an association between increased resting heart rate and difficulties in completing vigorous or moderate activities. Some have questioned whether persistent sinus tachycardia at rates exceeding 100 beats per minute in some patients after mediastinal irradiation may represent functional denervation of the heart and may indicate a consequent inability to perceive angina pectoris. Similar phenomena have been documented among individuals after cardiac transplantation or associated with the autonomic dysfunction of severe diabetes mellitus.[57–59]

CLINICAL PRESENTATIONS

Acute pericarditis may develop during or after mediastinal irradiation for Hodgkin lymphoma and is clinically similar to viral or idiopathic pericarditis.[19,37] It is usually transient and self-limited. Patients report chest pains that are often pleuritic in character and may be affected by position. Auscultation may reveal a pericardial friction rub, and chest roentgenogram may or may not show an enlarged, globular cardiac silhouette. The electrocardiogram may show low voltage, when significant effusions are present, diffuse ST-segment elevation across the precordium in the early phase, and diffuse T-wave inversion during later stages. Acute pericarditis is generally treated with nonsteroidal antiinflammatory agents, unless symptoms are severe and persistent. Corticosteroids may be useful for refractory episodes, but symptomatic episodes of pericarditis may recur during steroid withdrawal and may result in steroid dependency. Cardiac tamponade may develop during the course of acute pericarditis with effusion, and should be suspected when dyspnea is reported. Clinical signs include neck vein elevation and a paradoxical pulse.

Echocardiography is useful in establishing the diagnosis. Pericardiocentesis may eliminate tamponade. However, thoracoscopic procedures or open pericardiectomy may be required when symptomatic pericardial effusion and constrictive pericarditis coexist. One episode of myocardial infarction without clinically significant coronary occlusion after irradiation for Hodgkin lymphoma was reported to arise due to vasospasm apparently induced by acute pericarditis.[60] Pericardial effusion may present as an increased heart size on routine follow-up chest radiograph in the absence of symptoms. Most such effusions resolve without intervention, although many patients are treated with nonsteroidal anti-inflammatory agents. Tamponade is rare. Some small effusions may persist in an apparently benign form and have been observed as late findings on echocardiographic studies of asymptomatic patients. Pericarditis, pericardial effusion, and pneumonitis have also developed at prolonged intervals after irradiation following abrupt withdrawal of corticosteroid medications.[29,61] Exposure to some chemotherapeutic agents, such as gemcitabine, can also induce pericarditis as a "recall" reaction after prior mediastinal irradiation.[62]

Constrictive pericarditis may present insidiously with exertional dyspnea and pleural effusions or may present with signs of biventricular failure with exertional dyspnea, peripheral edema, hepatomegaly, and tamponade (Fig. 25.1).[7,21,28,29,37]

Pericardial effusion may or may not be present on echocardiographic evaluation. Ventricular size and wall motion are usually normal on echogram. Echocardiography, CT, or MRI scans of the thorax may feature prominent pericardial thickening to support this diagnosis. Cardiac catheterization is usually necessary to document equalization of diastolic filling pressures in the left and right ventricles. Treatment requires surgical pericardiectomy, but this has been associated with increased morbidity and a 21% mortality rate in irradiated patients, presumably due to coexisting myocardial, pulmonary, and pleural fibrosis in many patients.[20]

The strategies used to decrease radiation dose and volume during mediastinal irradiation for Hodgkin lymphoma appear to have substantially reduced the incidence of constrictive pericarditis and should reduce surgical risks for the rare individual who may develop this complication.

Among the clinical sequelae of mediastinal irradiation, coronary artery disease has been particularly difficult to diagnose before cardiac injury from acute myocardial infarction or sudden death. In part, this may be attributable to cardiac symptoms that arise at an earlier age than is typical for coronary artery disease. However, many patients appear to have had no symptoms before a catastrophic event. Among 55 deaths attributed to myocardial infarction in patients treated for Hodgkin lymphoma at Stanford, 38 patients had no prior history of heart disease or record of symptoms suggesting angina pectoris.[21] Similarly, 9 of 13 acute myocardial infarction deaths or sudden deaths reported in Hodgkin lymphoma survivors from Zurich occurred in individuals who had no history of cardiac disease or angina pectoris.[31] Two of these patients had normal electrocardiography, echocardiography, and myocardial perfusion scintigraphy within 6 months of death. Significant ischemia may be clinically silent, may produce unusual manifestations, such as exertional dyspnea, and may be associated with coronary ostial stenosis induced by radiation.[57]

Although the valvular heart disease that arises after irradiation may be identified by cardiac auscultation during routine follow-up of treated patients, Heidenreich and colleagues have advocated transthoracic echocardiography for individuals who are more than 10 years after mediastinal irradiation.[38] Among 294 asymptomatic patients who had been treated for Hodgkin lymphoma, clinically significant valvular dysfunction and thickening increased with the interval after exposure and appeared to be independent of attained age. Among those tested, 29% had indications for endocarditis prophylaxis, including the majority of patients tested more than 20 years after treatment. Cardiac auscultation findings were frequently misleading. An isolated systolic murmur was the most common auscultatory finding in Hodgkin lymphoma survivors who had evidence of aortic regurgitation identified on echocardiography.[63] The rate of progression of established valvular heart disease after irradiation is not clearly appreciated. For this reason, cardiac murmurs suggesting mitral or aortic valvular disease should be evaluated by echocardiography and patients with more than minimal amounts of valvular insufficiency should have regular cardiologic follow-up with annual or biennial echocardiography to judge the need for and appropriate timing of valvular surgery.

Chronic pleural effusions may be a late development after high-dose mediastinal irradiation for Hodgkin lymphoma and present a difficult diagnostic and therapeutic dilemma.[37] Evaluation generally requires thoracentesis to evaluate potential malignant or infectious causes, assessment of thyroid and pulmonary function, thoracic CT scanning, and biopsy of pulmonary or pleural lesions that may be suspicious for malignancy. This often yields no adequate pulmonary or pleural pathology that is sufficient to explain persistent or recurrent effusion. Thorough cardiac evaluation should be performed including electrocardiography, echocardiography, and consideration of cardiac catheterization with coronary angiography to ensure the absence of pericardial constriction or potentially correctable left ventricular dysfunction, such as silent ischemia. Often, the etiology of such effusions remains obscure. These effusions may persist and vary in volume over many years and have generally been attributed to sclerosis of mediastinal lymphatics.

CARDIAC FUNCTIONAL EVALUATION AND SCREENING

Studies that have aimed to quantify the extent of cardiopulmonary dysfunction in survivors of Hodgkin lymphoma through various combinations of rest and exercise echocardiography and radionuclide scintigraphy scanning have reached variable conclusions. Watchie and associates[56] reported results of cardiac and pulmonary exercise testing for 57 patients an average of 5 years after treatment. Forty subjects had extensive thoracic irradiation with or without chemotherapy for extensive intrathoracic Hodgkin lymphoma. The authors concluded that symptomatic cardiopulmonary dysfunction was quite rare, with only one patient complaining of limitation. In contrast, Lund and co-workers[36] reported a high rate of cardiopulmonary dysfunction and disability among 116 patients treated for Hodgkin lymphoma in Norway and tested 5 to 14 years later. Signs of cardiac or pulmonary dysfunction affected 75% of women and 41% of the men who underwent echocardiography, exercise testing, and pulmonary function testing; 27% of those patients who had signs of diminished function on both cardiac and pulmonary testing reported disability, as did 4% of those with less impairment on testing. In a smaller series decreased left ventricular ejection fraction was found to correlate with irradiation techniques that encompassed the entire heart but was not observed in patients who had some portion of the heart shielded during irradiation for Hodgkin lymphoma.[64] None of the 16 patients studied in this series had symptomatic impairment. A high rate of cardiopulmonary dysfunction was also documented in a small series of patients treated with mantle-field irradiation during childhood.[65]

Exercise echocardiography and radionuclide perfusion imaging have been used to screen Hodgkin lymphoma survivors for occult coronary artery disease or silent ischemia. In two early studies comparing resting and exercise thallium-201 single photon emission tomographic scans after irradiation for Hodgkin lymphoma, 61% and 84% of the patients had abnormal distribution of thallium uptake.[66,67] Coronary arteriography was not performed to confirm coronary obstruction. However, Maunoury and associates[66] reported that the patterns of the perfusion defects observed after irradiation were not typical for an obstruction in a single major coronary artery and attributed exercise-induced defects to small coronary vessel disease and fixed perfusion deficits to myocardial fibrosis. Functional testing has been reported for 144 patients treated for Hodgkin lymphoma in Zurich.[31] Resting ECG was normal in 88%. During exercise testing the ECG became abnormal in 8% of patients, with 4% having unequivocal signs of myocardial ischemia and 3% showing ascending patterns of ST segment depression suspicious for ischemia. One hundred of these patients underwent myocardial perfusion scintigraphy with technetium-99m–methoxy-isobutyl-isonitril (99mTc-MIBI): 4 patients had abnormalities suggesting ischemia, 3 were considered equivocal for ischemia, and 93 were normal. The report of this study did not specify whether these electrocardiographic or nuclear perfusion abnormalities suggesting ischemia were confirmed on subsequent arteriography.

Constine and associates reported results of equilibrium radionuclide angiocardiography and resting and stress electrocardiography and perfusion imaging in 50 asymptomatic patients an average of 9.1 years after Hodgkin lymphoma therapy.[68] Subjects had a mean treatment age of 26 years and had received a mean central cardiac radiation dose of 35 Gy. Measures of ventricular function (left ventricular ejection fraction, mean peak filling rate, and end-diastolic volumes) were generally normal. Two of 38 patients had signs of exercise-induced ischemia on perfusion scintigraphy but did not undergo arteriography to confirm the presence of coronary disease.

At Stanford 294 asymptomatic patients were studied with stress imaging studies an average of 15 years after Hodgkin lymphoma treatments that included a mean mediastinal irradiation dose of 43.5 Gy.[69] Stress-induced wall-motion abnormality suggesting ischemia was identified in 5% of subjects through comparison of resting and exercise echocardiograms. Myocardial perfusion imaging with MIBI showed stress-induced perfusion defects in 11% of the subjects. Follow-up coronary arteriography in the 14% of patients who had abnormal screening studies showed that 55% of them had stenosis affecting at least one coronary artery that exceeded 50%. The prevalence of coronary stenosis greater than 50% was 7.5%, and 2.7% had severe coronary stenosis affecting three vessels or the left main coronary disease that was clinically unsuspected. Screening led to bypass graft surgery in 7 patients. Conventional coronary risk factors, such as older age, smoking, hypertension, dyslipidemia, and diabetes, were not prevalent in the screened population and were not predictive of coronary risk. Although exercise testing with ventricular imaging by echocardiography and radionuclide perfusion imaging identified individuals at risk for acute myocardial infarction or sudden death, a significant percentage of the screened population developed symptomatic coronary artery disease, suggesting either a high rate of progression of coronary stenosis or the need for more sensitive and specific screening tests. Doppler echocardiography showed evidence of abnormal diastolic function in 40 of 282 patients studied at Stanford.[70] Diastolic dysfunction was mild in 9% and moderate in 5% of those tested. Signs of exercise-induced ischemia were more common in patients who had diastolic dysfunction than in those with normal diastolic function (23% versus 11%). Cardiac event-free survival was significantly impaired among the 40 patients with diastolic dysfunction compared with the 242 patients who had normal diastolic function. The prevalence of diastolic dysfunction and follow-up cardiac events as a function of age is summarized in Table 25.4.

Echocardiography also showed evidence of decreasing left ventricular mass and left ventricular ejection fraction as a function of time since irradiation. These findings were more common in patients after irradiation for Hodgkin lymphoma than in general population rates reported from screening in the Framingham Heart Study.[38]

In their study of echocardiography and exercise stress testing in 48 Hodgkin lymphoma survivors treated at young age, Adams and associates also reported a high prevalence of impaired left ventricular fractional shortening, decreased left ventricular mass, and diastolic changes suggestive of restrictive cardiomyopathy.[39] The authors observed a correlation between signs of diastolic dysfunction on echocardiography and physical limitations and symptoms reported by the participants on a questionnaire instrument. The authors found a high prevalence of restrictive cardiomyopathy, valvular abnormalities, conduction defects, autonomic dysfunction, and significantly reduced peak oxygen consumption during exercise. They advocated multimodality screening for these problems even among patients treated with modern radiotherapy protocols, and advised repeated evaluations due to the apparent progression of cardiac dysfunction with increasing time after treatment.

The optimum time to screen for ischemia or other signs of cardiac dysfunction is yet to be determined. In the Stanford study, the yield of screening for signs of exercise-induced ischemia increased when 10 years had elapsed since mediastinal irradiation. However, the risk for death from acute myocardial infarction was significantly increased within 10 years of radiation in the era of treatment when mediastinal doses averaged 44 Gy. Glanzmann and colleagues[31] have advocated exercise myocardial perfusion imaging at 5-year intervals after therapy.

Thus far, screening for coronary artery disease and other forms of post-irradiation cardiac dysfunction have primarily relied upon changes in ventricular function or perfusion induced by exercise. New cardiac imaging techniques with CT angiography and magnetic resonance angiography may offer more direct approaches to defining proximal coronary artery stenosis. Radiation-associated changes on cardiac magnetic resonance imaging in one patient are shown in Figure 25.3.

TABLE 25.4

DIASTOLIC DYSFUNCTION, AGE, AND CARDIAC EVENT RISK IN SURVIVORS OF HODGKIN LYMPHOMA

Doppler finding	n (%)	Number with cardiac events (% of n)
20–39 y		
Normal	107 (94)	3 (3)
Mild diastolic dysfunction	0	0
Moderate diastolic dysfunction	7 (6)	2 (29)
40–49 y		
Normal	99 (87)	7 (6)
Mild diastolic dysfunction	10 (9)	1 (10)
Moderate diastolic dysfunction	5 (4)	1 (20)
≥50 y		
Normal	36 (67)	4 (11)
Mild diastolic dysfunction	16 (30)	4 (25)
Moderate diastolic dysfunction	2 (4)	1 (50)

Adapted with permisssion from Constine LS, Schwartz RG, Savage DE, et al. Cardiac function, perfusion, and morbidity in irradiated long-term survivors of Hodgkin's disease. *Int J Radiat Oncol Biol Phys* 1997;39:897–906.

MINIMIZING CARDIOVASCULAR RISKS

Newer treatment approaches for Hodgkin lymphoma have attempted to limit the total radiation dose and radiation dose per fraction through treatment limited to involved fields after chemotherapy regimens that substitute for the prophylactic nodal irradiation. The long-term impact of mediastinal irradiation at reduced doses remains to be determined. Patients who have already received mediastinal irradiation should have periodic assessment of known cardiac risk factors and optimal medical management to minimize risk. This is underscored by the association of known cardiac risk factors with markedly increased risk for acute myocardial infarction death despite apparently moderate cardiac doses and dose rate in the University Hospital, Zurich study[31] and the recent study of Dutch and Belgian patients with Hodgkin lymphoma.[5] Efforts should aim at cessation of cigarette smoking and optimal management of lipids, glucose intolerance, and hypertension. Physicians who follow patients after treatment for Hodgkin lymphoma must recall that coronary artery disease may develop at unusually young age and may be manifested by

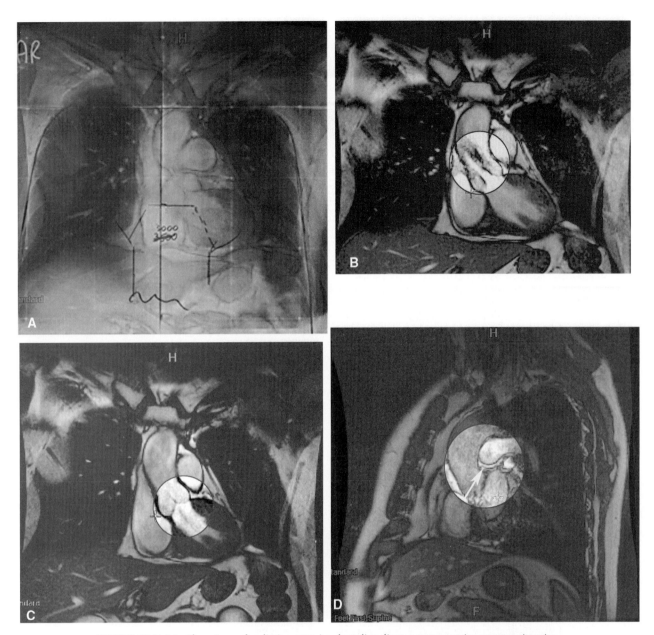

FIGURE 25.3. Manifestations of radiation-associated cardiac disease on magnetic resonance imaging. A: Anterior mantle field planning radiogram from 1980 superimposed on coronal MRI of the heart obtained in 2005. The inferior cardiac structures are shifted cephalad compared with the cardiac silhouette from the planning radiogram. This is possibly due to a combination of volume loss in irradiated lung tissue and interval weight gain. A subcarinal block was added to the mediastinal portion of the radiation field at a dose of 30 Gy. The aortic valve is located immediately cephalad to the subcarinal block in the mediastinal region irradiated to 44 Gy. B: Coronal MRI of the heart in the same patient obtained during systole showing a jet of turbulence from aortic stenosis. C: Coronal MRI of the heart in the same patient obtained during diastole showing a jet of turbulence from aortic regurgitation. D: Oblique images of the heart showing mild to moderate narrowing of the proximal segment of the left main coronary artery.

unusual symptoms, such as exertional dyspnea, asthma-like symptoms, dyspepsia, or exertional fatigue. Unusual symptoms such as these should prompt stress testing and consideration of coronary arteriography, because current exercise tests have a significant and poorly defined false-negative rate. For asymptomatic patients previously exposed to mediastinal irradiation doses of 35 Gy or more, periodic screening for ventricular dysfunction and inducible coronary ischemia with ventricular imaging studies at rest and after peak exercise may decrease the observed risk for acute myocardial infarction and sudden cardiac death. Further research is needed to determine if screening and intervention prolongs survival and to determine the optimal timing for initial and subsequent studies.

References

1. Hoppe RT. Hodgkin's disease: complications of therapy and excess mortality. *Ann Oncol* 1997;8(suppl 1):115–118.
2. Mauch PM, Kalish LA, Marcus KC, et al. Long-term survival in Hodgkin's disease. *Cancer J Sci Am* 1995;1:33.
3. Henry-Amar M, Hayat M, Meerwaldt JH, et al. Causes of death after therapy for early stage Hodgkin's disease entered on EORTC protocols. EORTC Lymphoma Cooperative Group. *Int J Radiat Oncol Biol Phys* 1990;19:1155–1157.
4. Vaughan Hudson B, Vaughan Hudson G, Linch DC, et al. Late mortality in young BNLI patients cured of Hodgkin's disease. *Ann Oncol* 1994;5(suppl 2):65–66.
5. Reinders JG, Heijmen BJ, Olofsen-van Acht MJ, et al. Ischemic heart disease after mantlefield irradiation for Hodgkin's disease in long-term follow-up. *Radiother Oncol* 1999;51:35–42.

6. Hancock SL, Hoppe RT. Long-term complications of treatment and causes of mortality after Hodgkin's disease. *Semin Radiat Oncol* 1996;6:225–242.
7. Stewart JR, Fajardo LF. Radiation-induced heart disease. Clinical and experimental aspects. *Radiol Clin North Am* 1971;9:511–531.
8. Cohn KE, Stewart JR, Fajardo LF, et al. Heart disease following radiation. *Medicine (Baltimore)* 1967;46:281–298.
9. Kaplan HS. The role of intensive radiotherapy in the management of Hodgkin's disease. *Cancer* 1966;19:356.
10. Fajardo LF, Stewart JR. Experimental radiation-induced heart disease. I. Light microscopic studies. *Am J Pathol* 1970;59:299–316.
11. Fajardo LF, Stewart JR. Capillary injury preceding radiation-induced myocardial fibrosis. *Radiology* 1971;101:429–433.
12. Stewart JR, Fajardo LF. Dose response in human and experimental radiation-induced heart disease. Application of the nominal standard dose (NSD) concept. *Radiology* 1971;99:403–408.
13. Rubin E, Camara J, Grayzel DM, et al. Radiation-induced cardiac fibrosis. *Am J Med* 1963;34:71–75.
14. Stewart JR, Fajardo LF. Radiation-induced heart disease: an update. *Prog Cardiovasc Dis* 1984;27:173–194.
15. Greenwood RD, Rosenthal A, Cassady R, et al. Constrictive pericarditis in childhood due to mediastinal irradiation. *Circulation* 1974;50:1033–1039.
16. Broesius FC, Walller BF, Roberts WG. Radiation heart disease: analysis of 16 young (aged 15 to 33 years) necropsy patients who received over 3500 rads to the heart. *Am J Med* 1981;70:519–530.
17. Byhardt R, Brace K, Ruckdeschel J, et al. Dose and treatment factors in radiation-related pericardial effusion associated with the mantle technique for Hodgkin's disease. *Cancer* 1975;35:795–802.
18. Morton DL, Glancy DL, Joseph WL, et al. Management of patients with radiation-induced pericarditis with effusion: a note on the development of aortic regurgitation in two of them. *Chest* 1973;64:291–297.
19. Carmel RJ, Kaplan HS. Mantle irradiation in Hodgkin's disease. An analysis of technique, tumor eradication, and complications. *Cancer* 1976;37:2813–2825.
20. Cameron J, Oesterle SN, Baldwin JC, et al. The etiologic spectrum of constrictive pericarditis. *Am Heart J* 1987;113:354–360.
21. Hancock SL, Tucker MA, Hoppe RT. Factors affecting late mortality from heart disease after treatment of Hodgkin's disease. *JAMA* 1993;270:1949–1955.
22. Blank N, Castellino RA. The intrathoracic manifestations of the malignant lymphomas and the leukemias. *Semin Roentgenol* 1980;15:227–245.
23. Prentice RT. Myocardial infarction following radiation. *Lancet* 1965;10:388.
24. Kopelson G, Herwig KJ. The etiologies of coronary artery disease in cancer patients. *Int J Radiat Oncol Biol Phys* 1978;4:895–906.
25. Pohjola-Sintonen S, Totterman KJ, Salmo M, et al. Late cardiac effects of mediastinal radiotherapy in patients with Hodgkin's disease. *Cancer* 1987;60:31–37.
26. Boivin JF, Hutchinson GB, Lubin JH, et al. Coronary artery disease mortality in patients treated for Hodgkin's disease. *Cancer* 1992;69:1241–1247.
27. Tarbell NJ, Thompson L, Mauch P. Thoracic irradiation in Hodgkin's disease: disease control and long-term complications. *Int J Radiat Oncol Biol Phys* 1990;18:275–281.
28. Cosset JM, Henry-Amar M, Pellae-Cosset B, et al. Pericarditis and myocardial infarctions after Hodgkin's disease therapy. *Int J Radiat Oncol Biol Phys* 1991;21:447–449.
29. Hancock SL, Donaldson SS, Hoppe RT. Cardiac disease following treatment of Hodgkin's disease in children and adolescents. *J Clin Oncol* 1993;11:1208–1215. See comments.
30. Brierley JD, Rathmell AJ, Gospodarowicz MK, et al. Late effects of treatment for early-stage Hodgkin's disease. *Br J Cancer* 1998;77:1300–1310.
31. Glanzmann C, Kaufmann P, Jenni R, et al. Cardiac risk after mediastinal irradiation for Hodgkin's disease. *Radiother Oncol* 1998;46:51–62.
32. King V, Constine LS, Clark D, et al. Symptomatic coronary artery disease after mantle irradiation for Hodgkin's disease. *Int J Radiat Oncol Biol Phys* 1996;36:881–889.
33. Hull MC, Morris CG, Pepine CJ, et al. Valvular dysfunction and carotid, subclavian, and coronary artery disease in survivors of hodgkin lymphoma treated with radiation therapy. *JAMA* 2003;290:2831–2837.
34. Perrault DJ, Levy M, Herman JD, et al. Echocardiographic abnormalities following cardiac radiation. *J Clin Oncol* 1985;3:546–551.
35. Lund MB, Kongerud J, Boe J, et al. Cardiopulmonary sequelae after treatment for Hodgkin's disease: increased risk in females? *Ann Oncol* 1996;7:257–264.
36. Lund MB, Ihlen H, Voss BM, et al. Increased risk of heart valve regurgitation after mediastinal radiation for Hodgkin's disease: an echocardiographic study. *Heart* 1996;75:591–595.
37. Stewart JR, Hancock EW, Hancock SL. Radiation injury to the heart: risk factors, diagnosis, prevention and treatment. In: Meyer JL, ed. *Radiation injury. Advances in management and prevention.* Vol 32. Basel: Karger; 1999:71–84.
38. Heidenreich PA, Hancock SL, Lee BK, et al. Asymptomatic cardiac disease following mediastinal irradiation. *J Am Coll Cardiol* 2003;42:743–749.
39. Adams MJ, Lipsitz SR, Colan SD, et al. Cardiovascular status in long-term survivors of Hodgkin's disease treated with chest radiotherapy. *J Clin Oncol* 2004;22:3139–3148.
40. Billingham ME, Bristow MR, Glatstein E, et al. Adriamycin cardiotoxicity: endomyocardial biopsy evidence of enhancement by irradiation. *Am J Surg Pathol* 1977;1:17–23.
41. Billingham ME, Mason JW, Bristow MR, et al. Anthracycline cardiomyopathy monitored by morphologic changes. *Cancer Treat Rep* 1978;62:865–872.
42. Steinherz LJ, Steinherz PG, Tan C. Cardiac failure and dysrhythmias 6-19 years after anthracycline therapy: a series of 15 patients. *Med Pediatr Oncol* 1995;24:352–361.
43. LaMonte CS, Yeh SD, Straus DJ. Long-term follow-up of cardiac function in patients with Hodgkin's disease treated with mediastinal irradiation and combination chemotherapy including doxorubicin. *Cancer Treat Rep* 1986;70:439–444.
44. Allavena C, Conroy T, Aletti P, et al. Late cardiopulmonary toxicity after treatment for Hodgkin's disease. *Br J Cancer* 1992;65:908–912.
45. Brice P, Tredaniel J, Monsuez JJ, et al. Cardiopulmonary toxicity after three courses of ABVD and mediastinal irradiation in favorable Hodgkin's disease. *Ann Oncol* 1991;2(suppl 2):73–76.
46. Pihkala J, Saarinen UM, Lundstrom U, et al. Myocardial function in children and adolescents after therapy with anthracyclines and chest irradiation. *Eur J Cancer* 1996;32A:97–103.
47. Moser EC, Noordijk EM, van Leeuwen FE, et al. Long-term risk of cardiovascular disease after treatment for aggressive non-Hodgkin lymphoma. *Blood* 2006;107:29122919.
48. Elerding SC, Fernandez RN, Grotta JC, et al. Carotid artery disease following external cervical irradiation. *Ann Surg* 1981;194:609–615.
49. Patel DA, Kochanski J, Suen AW, et al. Clinical manifestations of noncoronary atherosclerotic vascular disease after moderate dose irradiation. *Cancer* 2006;106:718–725.
50. Bowers DC, McNeil DE, Liu Y, et al. Stroke as a late treatment effect of Hodgkin's Disease: a report from the Childhood Cancer Survivor Study. *J Clin Oncol* 2005;23:6508–6515.
51. Seifter EJ, Young RC, Longo DL. Deep venous thrombosis during therapy for Hodgkin's disease. *Cancer Treat Rep* 1985;69:1011–1013.
52. Schreiber DP, Kapp DS. Axillary-subclavian vein thrombosis following combination chemotherapy and radiation therapy in lymphoma. *Int J Radiat Oncol Biol Phys* 1986;12:391–395.
53. Totterman KJ, Pesonen E, Siltanen P. Radiation-related chronic heart disease. *Chest* 1983;83:875–878.
54. Slama MS, Le Guludec D, Sebag C, et al. Complete atrioventricular block following mediastinal irradiation: a report of six cases. *Pacing Clin Electrophysiol* 1991;14:1112–1118.
55. Cohen SI, Bharati S, Glass J, et al. Radiotherapy as a cause of complete atrioventricular block in Hodgkin's disease. An electrophysiological-pathological correlation. *Arch Intern Med* 1981;141:676–679.
56. Watchie J, Coleman CN, Raffin TA, et al. Minimal long-term cardiopulmonary dysfunction following treatment for Hodgkin's disease. *Int J Radiat Oncol Biol Phys* 1987;13:517–524.
57. Aronow H, Kim M, Rubenfire M. Silent ischemic cardiomyopathy and left coronary ostial stenosis secondary to radiation therapy. *Clin Cardiol* 1996;19:260–262.
58. O'Sullivan JJ, Conroy RM, MacDonald K, et al. Silent ischaemia in diabetic men with autonomic neuropathy. *Br Heart J* 1991;66:313–315.
59. Bertolet BD, Belardinelli L, Hill JA. Absence of adenosine-induced chest pain after total cardiac afferent denervation. *Am J Cardiol* 1993;72:483–484.
60. Yahalom J, Hasin Y, Fuks Z. Acute myocardial infarction with normal coronary arteriogram after mantle field radiation therapy for Hodgkin's disease. *Cancer* 1983;52:637–641.
61. Castellino RA, Glatstein E, Turbow MM, et al. Latent radiation injury of lungs or heart activated by steroid withdrawal. *Ann Intern Med* 1974;80: 593–599.
62. Vogl DT, Glatstein E, Carver JR, et al. Gemcitabine-induced pericardial effusion and tamponade after unblocked cardiac irradiation. *Leuk Lymphoma* 2005;46:1313–1320.
63. Heidenreich PA, Schnittger I, Hancock SL, et al. A systolic murmur is a common presentation of aortic regurgitation detected by echocardiography. *Clin Cardiol* 2004;27:502–506.
64. Savage DE, Constine LS, Schwartz RG, et al. Radiation effects on left ventricular function and myocardial perfusion in long term survivors of Hodgkin's disease. *Int J Radiat Oncol Biol Phys* 1990;19:721–727.
65. Kadota RP, Burgert EO, Jr., Driscoll DJ, et al. Cardiopulmonary function in long-term survivors of childhood Hodgkin's lymphoma: a pilot study. *Mayo Clin Proc* 1988;63:362–367.
66. Maunoury C, Pierga JY, Valette H, et al. Myocardial perfusion damage after mediastinal irradiation for Hodgkin's disease: a thallium-201 single photon emission tomography study. *Eur J Nucl Med* 1992;19:871–873.
67. Gustavsson A, Eskilsson J, Landberg T, et al. Late cardiac effects after mantle radiotherapy in patients with Hodgkin's disease. *Ann Oncol* 1990;1: 355–363.
68. Constine LS, Schwartz RG, Savage DE, et al. Cardiac function, perfusion, and morbidity in irradiated long-term survivors of Hodgkin's disease. *Int J Radiat Oncol Biol Phys* 1997;39:897–906.
69. Heidenreich PA, Schnittger I, Strauss HW, et al. Screening for coronary artery disease after mediastinal irradiation for Hodgkin's disease. *J Clin Oncol* 2007:32–42.
70. Heidenreich PA, Hancock SL, Vagelos RH, et al. Diastolic dysfunction after mediastinal irradiation. *Am Heart J* 2005;150:977–982.

CHAPTER 26 ■ OTHER COMPLICATIONS OF THE TREATMENT OF HODGKIN LYMPHOMA

JULIE M. VOSE, LOUIS S. CONSTINE, AND SIMON B. SUTCLIFFE

Late complications of treatment are generally of two types: treatment-induced tissue or organ dysfunction, and mutagenic consequences of cytotoxic therapies. The differential diagnosis of symptomatology acquired after therapy must always include recurrent primary tumor (Hodgkin lymphoma), development of a new primary tumor (second malignancy), late effects of prior therapy, or other disease processes. Late complications can be a function of surgery, radiation, chemotherapy, the disease itself, or a combination of the etiologies. The damage that is caused by disease or its treatment includes vascular interruption, slowed tissue repair, altered metabolism or clearance of drugs, and genetic alterations. The long-term complications that may occur as a consequence of these therapies are outlined in this chapter.

ENDOCRINE

Thyroid

A spectrum of clinically significant thyroid abnormalities may occur in patients treated for Hodgkin lymphoma. Primary hypothyroidism is most frequent, but Graves disease, autoimmune thyroiditis, euthyroid Graves ophthalmopathy, benign cysts and nodules, and papillary or follicular thyroid cancers occur with a defined frequency.[1,2] Among 1,787 patients treated for Hodgkin lymphoma at Stanford University, the 20-year actuarial risk for the development of any thyroid abnormality was 50%.[2] Direct radiation exposure to the thyroid gland, incidental to cervical radiation therapy, is the predominant therapeutic insult.

Hypothyroidism

Primary hypothyroidism is a frequent consequence of supraclavicular or cervical irradiation. Subclinical hypothyroidism is defined as an elevation of the basal thyroid-stimulating hormone (TSH) level and an increased TSH response to thyrotropin-releasing hormone (TRH) provocation, but with normal serum triiodothyronine (T3)/thyroxine (T4) levels and no clinical symptoms of hypothyroidism. Clinical hypothyroidism is defined as the clinical symptoms of hypothyroidism associated with an elevation in basal TSH levels, increased TSH response to TRH, and depressed serum levels of T4 or T3. The legion of symptoms includes cold intolerance, constipation, inordinate weight gain, dry skin, brittle hair, menorrhagia or spotting, muscle cramps or generalized muscle weakness, and slowed mentation. Signs include a round puffy face, slow speech, hoarseness, hypokinesia, delayed relaxation of deep tendon reflexes, periorbital or peripheral edema, and pleural or pericardial effusions.[3] The incidence of hypothyroidism following therapeutic irradiation for Hodgkin lymphoma varies in different reports depending on radiation dose and technique, patient age, interval to and type of laboratory testing (e.g., T4, T3, free T4, TSH), and the thoroughness of the history and physical examination. Consequently, if an elevated serum TSH concentration is the determinant, then 4% to 79% of patients become affected.[4,5] A study by Hancock and associates[2] of 1,677 patients with Hodgkin lymphoma irradiated to the thyroid showed that the actuarial risk at 26 years for overt or subclinical hypothyroidism was 47%. Although the peak incidence occurred at 2 to 3 years, and half the risk was manifested within 5 years, some patients developed hypothyroidism as long as 20 years after therapy.

Radiation dose is the most relevant parameter in predicting the likelihood of hypothyroidism. Radiation technique determines dose deposition, including the use of differential anterior versus posterior field weighting and cervical or specific thyroid blocks.[6] An increasing incidence of hypothyroidism above threshold doses of 20 to 30 Gy has been reported.[4,5] Constine and associates[5] noted thyroid abnormalities in 4 of 24 children (17%) who received mantle irradiation of 26 Gy or less, and in 74 of 95 children (78%) who received greater than 26 Gy; the relationship of basal TSH to radiation dose was significant ($p <0.001$). In a report by Bhatia and associates,[4] the relative risk of hypothyroidism increased by 1.02/Gy, ($p <0.001$) (Fig. 26.1). Other factors may affect risk for radiation-induced hypothyroidism. Prior to age 16 years, radiation therapy dose was the predominant determinant of risk, whereas female gender and chemotherapy were additional risk factors in older patients.[2,4,5] The influence of chemotherapy on the development of thyroid dysfunction appears to be negligible.[4,5]

Hyperthyroidism

Thyrotoxicosis may occur following mantle or cervical irradiation for Hodgkin lymphoma. Hancock and colleagues[2] report that approximately 2% of patients ($n = 34$) developed Graves disease. Almost all had a diffuse goiter, high free thyroxine (FT4), low TSH, and increased thyroid uptake of radioiodine. Half of these patients developed infiltrative ophthalmopathy, as did an additional 4 patients who did not have overt hyperthyroidism. The relative risk for Graves disease was 7.2 to 20.4. Six patients developed silent thyroiditis characterized by transient mild symptoms of thyrotoxicosis, an increased serum FT4 and low TSH, no thyroid enlargement or tenderness, and low thyroid uptake of radioiodine.[7] All of

383

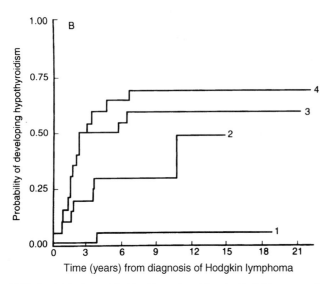

FIGURE 26.1. Actuarial risk of hypothyroidism in 89 children treated for Hodgkin lymphoma. Curve 1 represents the risk in 13 children who did not undergo irradiation to the thyroid, curve 2 the risk in 10 children who received less than 30 Gy, curve 3 the risk in 26 children who received between 30 and 45 Gy, and curve 4 the risk in 40 children who received greater than 45 Gy ($p = 0.002$). (Reprinted with permission from Bhatia S, Ramsay N, Bantle J, et al. Thyroid abnormalities after therapy for Hodgkin's disease in childhood. *Oncologist* 1996;1:62.)

these patients subsequently developed hypothyroidism. The mechanism of Graves disease is an autoimmune dysregulation of unknown etiology.

Thyroid Enlargement, Benign and Malignant Nodules

An excess frequency of benign and malignant thyroid nodules occurs following radiation therapy for Hodgkin lymphoma. This risk appears to vary according to age at treatment, which may also reflect the known association of radiation dose and induced thyroid cancers. In a report by Boivin and co-workers[8] of 10,472 patients with Hodgkin lymphoma, the relative risk was 4.5 (95% confidence interval [CI], 2.4–7.7) overall, and 1.3 (95% CI, 0.3–6.1) after radiation therapy. Children appear to be at greater risk. In a report on 1,380 children with Hodgkin lymphoma from the Late Effects Study Group, the relative risk was 32.7 (95% CI, 15.3–55.3).[4]

Ovary

Radiation and chemotherapy for Hodgkin lymphoma can cause transient or permanent effects on reproductive capacity, endocrine integrity, and sexual function. The concerns of survivors range from their functional status to consequences on the health of their offspring. The complexity of defining these sequelae stems from the differential dose-dependent effects caused by different chemotherapy agents, radiation therapy, and their combination. Injury to the ovaries can cause both sterilization and suppressed hormone production because of the relationship of the latter to the presence of ova and maturation of the primary follicle.[9]

Depending on the radiation dose, fertility may be transiently preserved due to survival of relatively radioresistant follicles in the late stages of development. Conversely, sterility may be transient due to survival of primordial follicles, although the duration of subsequent fertility may be shortened due to reduction of the total number of follicles or acceleration in the rate of follicular atresia. These observations may explain why girls treated prior to puberty, who have a greater complement of ova than do older women, are more likely to retain ovarian function after radiation therapy.

The dose of radiation that will ablate ovarian function depends on the patient's age and whether the dose is fractionated. Data from Ash[10] summarized the effect of fractionated radiation therapy on ovarian function in women of reproductive age (Table 26.1). Doses of 12 to 15 Gy in women 40 years of age or younger induced menopause, whereas women older than 40 years became menopausal after 4 to 7 Gy. Permanent sterility occurred in up to 60% of females 15 to 40 years of age who received 5 to 6 Gy to the ovaries. After single fractions, temporary sterility can occur with ovarian doses of 1.7 to 6.4 Gy, and permanent sterility after 3.2 to 10 Gy.[11] Wallace and colleagues[12] reviewed data to estimate a median lethal dose (LD_{50}) of 6 Gy for the oocyte.

If pelvic irradiation is a potential component of therapy, the ovaries should be relocated in order to effectively shield them. An oophoropexy may be performed by open procedure or laparoscopically. Typically, the ovaries are moved to a midline position in front of or behind the uterus. Alternately, they may be moved laterally to the iliac wings or paracolic gutter, or even heterotopically autotransplanted into a remote location (e.g., the arm).[13]

TABLE 26.1

EFFECT OF FRACTIONATED IRRADIATION ON OVARIAN FUNCTION IN WOMEN OF REPRODUCTIVE AGE

Minimum ovarian dose (Gy)[a]	Effect
0.6	No deleterious effect
1.5	No deleterious effect in most young women; some risk of sterilization especially in women age >40 years
2.5–5.0	Variable: age 15–40 years, 30–40% sterilized permanently; age >40 years, >90% sterilized permanently
5–8	Variable: age 15–40 years, 50–70% sterilized permanently, temporary amenorrhea in some of remainder; age >40 years, >90% sterilized permanently
>8	100% permanently sterilized

[a]No attempt has been made to allow for variation in mode of fractionation.
Modified from Ash P. The influence of radiation on fertility in man. *Br J Radiol* 1980;53:271, with permission.

Several chemotherapeutic agents used to treat Hodgkin lymphoma are capable of causing ovarian dysfunction, including cyclophosphamide and mechlorethamine.[9,14] The age of the patient, the dose of chemotherapy, and the combined use of irradiation are all relevant to the potential for ovarian injury. For example, prepubertal girls are apparently more resistant to large cumulative doses of cyclophosphamide than are adults. In a report by Horning and associates[15] of patients treated with MOP(P) (mechlorethamine, Oncovin [vincristine], procarbazine, and prednisone) or PAVe (procarbazine, Alkeran [L-phenylalanine mustard], and vinblastine),[15] 75% of women younger than 20 years maintained menses while only 30% of women 30 years or older continued to menstruate. In those patients who also received pelvic irradiation, 28% had irregular menses and 52% had amenorrhea (Table 26.2). Among the women treated with chemotherapy alone, 10 pregnancies occurred in 8 women, resulting in 6 normal births, 1 premature birth, and 3 therapeutic abortions. Among those receiving combined radiation and chemotherapy, 7 pregnancies occurred among 5 women, resulting in 6 normal births and 1 premature birth. More complex chemotherapy regimens are also associated with secondary amenorrhea. In a study of 405 patients treated with combination chemotherapy for advanced-stage Hodgkin lymphoma in the German Hodgkin Lymphoma Study Group, 51.4% of pateints receiving eight cycles of dose-escalated BEACOPP had continuous amenorrhea.[16] Amenorrhea was significantly more frequent after dose-excalated BEACOPP compared with ABVD or standard BEACOPP (p = 0.007). Amenorrhea was more pronouced in women with advanced—stage Hodgkin lymphoma (p <0.0001), women older than 30 years at treatment (p = 0.0065), and in women who did not take oral contraceptives during chemotherapy (p = 0.0002). However, long-term follow-up of patients treated with the Stanford V regimen has documented little impact on menstrual function and 72 conceptions out of 256 patients.[17]

Strategies for protecting the ovaries from chemotherapy-induced damage have been suggested. Administration of hormones to suppress ovarian function during chemotherapy might increase its resistance. Autotransplanting the ovary to a remote site, such as the arm, and then using a tourniquet to decrease the exposure to chemotherapy has also been suggested. A report of using orthotopic reimplantation of cryopreserved ovarian cortical strips after high-dose treatment for Hodgkin lymphoma has been published.[18] This report demonstrated a temporary increase in estradiol that was associated with one menstrual period. However, the effect was lost by 9 months later, with a return to amenorrhea. Other options include the use of donor eggs for use in patients with iatrogenic amenorrhea. With the use of oocyte donation , in vitro fertilization, and estradiol and progesterone administration, several successful pregancies have been reported.[19]

TABLE 26.2

FREQUENCY OF AMENORRHEA FOLLOWING TREATMENT WITH COMBINATION CHEMOTHERAPY

Regimen	Patient age	Frequency of amenorrhea (no. patients)
MVPP	All ages	63% (20/32)
	<30 years	52% (17/33)
	30–51 years	86% (31/36)
MOPP		
Full course	All ages	39% (17/44)
Full course	<30 years	11% (4/36)
Full course	30–45 years	56% (10/18)
3 cycles	16–30 years	3% (1/31)
3 cycles	31–45 years	61% (11/18)
ChlVPP	All ages	19% (6/32)
ChlVPP/EAV	All ages	80% (16/20)
COPP/ABVD		
4 cycles	<40 years	55%
BEACOPP base	<40 years	32%
BEACOPP esc		
8 cycles	<40 years	67%

M(O/V)PP, mechlorethamine, (vincristine/vinblastine), procarbazine, prednisone; ChlVPP, chlorambucil, vincristine, prednisone, procarbazine; EAV, etoposide, Adriamycin, vincristine; COPP, cyclophosphamide, vincristine, procarbazine, prednisone; ABVD, doxorubicin, bleomycin, vinblastine, dacarbazine; BEACOPP, bleomycin, etoposide, doxorubicin, cyclophosphamide, vinvristine, procarbazine, and prednisone. (16) From Behringer K, Breuer K, Reineke T, et al. Secondary amenorrhea after Hodgkin's lymphoma is influenced by age at treatment, stage of disease, chemotherapy regimen, and the use of oral contraceptives during therapy: a report from the German Hodgkin's Lymphoma Study Group. *J Clin Oncol* 2005;23:7555–7564.

Testes

The testes can be exposed to radiation directly, by scatter, or by transmission through shielding blocks. Because the spermatogonia are exquisitely sensitive to radiation, even small doses can produce measurable damage. Depression of sperm counts is discernible at doses as low as 0.15 Gy. This decrease in sperm counts may evolve over 3 to 6 weeks following irradiation, and, depending on the dose, recovery may take 1 to 3 years. Complete sterilization may occur with fractionated irradiation to a dose of 1 to 2 Gy, though some patients will recover.[20] Spermatocytes generally fail to complete maturation division at doses of 2 to 3 Gy and are visibly damaged after 4 to 6 Gy with resulting azoospermia. At the highest doses, permanent sterility is frequent. At lower doses this reduced sperm count is seen 60 to 80 days after exposure, which is the time that maturation would otherwise be complete.[21] Multiple small fractions of radiation are more toxic to spermatogenesis than are large, single fractions. This reverse fractionation effect is due to the extreme radiosensitivity of the testicular germinal epithelium, the small number of stem cells, and rapid cell turnover.[20,21] In contrast to the extreme radiosensitivity of the germinal epithelium, Leydig cell function is more resistant, and consequently testosterone production is generally normal below radiation doses of 10 to 20 Gy.[22]

In a report from Stanford, 83% of men treated with pelvic irradiation using testicular shielding were oligospermic or azoospermic when tested within 18 months of therapy, but only 12% remained azoospermic when tested more than 26 months after therapy.[23] The testes of young children may be more difficult to protect from irradiation due to technical difficulty in shielding the prepubertal testes. Stanford investigators assessed gonadal function in 20 boys treated for Hodgkin lymphoma, 8 with radiation therapy alone.[24] Four of the boys, irradiated at 13 to 15 years of age and receiving pelvic doses of 0, 40, 44, and 44 Gy, respectively, have fathered children 3 to 19 years after radiation therapy. Three had azoospermia 10 to 15 years after irradiation, and one other boy had testicular atrophy at biopsy 1 year after irradiation. Five additional boys had received chemotherapy and 20 to 44 Gy of pelvic irradiation at 8 to 15 years of age. Four were azoospermic 3 to 10 years later, and one had fathered a child.

The testicular germinal epithelium is susceptible to damage produced by several chemotherapeutic agents used in the

treatment of Hodgkin lymphoma including cyclophosphamide, mechlorethamine, and procarbazine. The effects are
almost certainly dose related where data are available for this
assessment.[25] For example, azoospermia is consistently
induced with a cumulative dose of 18 g of cyclophosphamide
in men, and this effect is commonly permanent. When MOPP
chemotherapy is used, six or more cycles will sterilize 90% of
males, whereas three or fewer cycles will cause oligospermia
in 25%.[26,27] Reports are variable on the recovery of sperm
numbers, with ranges from 0% to 50% (usually 10–25%),
and latent intervals up to 10 years (usually 2–5 years).[26,28]
ABVD (Adriamycin, bleomycin, vinblastine, and dacarbazine)
appears to spare fertility, although transient azoospermia is
reported in up to 50% of patients.[29] A recent report from
M. D. Anderson Cancer Center also documents rapid recovery (3–4 months) of spermatogenesis after three cycles of
NOVP (Novantrone, Oncovin, vinblastine, and prednisone)
chemotherapy.[30]

Prepubertal patients may have a slightly decreased sensitivity to chemotherapy-induced gonadal toxicity compared with
adults, but irreversible azoospermia can still occur after the
use of alkylating agents. In a report by Sherins and associates[31]
of 13 pubertal boys treated with MOPP, 9 (69%) demonstrated gynecomastia and had evidence of germinal aplasia on
testicular biopsy.

Current efforts to protect patients from chemotherapy or
radiation-induced damage to spermatogenesis involve eliminating those agents known to damage spermatogenesis, and
optimizing testicular shielding from irradiation. Work in an
animal model demonstrates that pretreatment with testosterone and estradiol, which reversibly inhibits the completion
of spermatogenesis, protects spermatogonial stem cells from
procarbazine and radiation.[32] However, complete data are not
yet available in clinical trials, with some trials demonstrating
no protective effects.

BONE AND SOFT TISSUE

Detrimental effects of treatment for Hodgkin lymphoma on
bone and soft tissue are most problematic in children (see
Chapter 21), and predominantly result from radiation therapy. These effects are rarely seen in adults. The pathophysiology of radiation injury to growing bone is probably attributable
to damage to the chondroblasts.[33] Essentially the predominant
effect on long bones is shortening, and on flat bones it is
hypoplasia.

The crucial factors that determine outcome include the following: (a) the radiation total and fractional dose (as well as
energy, beam type); (b) which bone(s), epiphyseal plate(s), and
muscles are encompassed; (c) patient age and genetic constitu-
tion (including growth potential); and (d) other components
of therapy (steroids, chemotherapeutic agents).[33,34] The greatest retardation of spinal growth occurred in children irradiated during the periods of most active growth (under 6 years
of age and during puberty) and at doses greater than 35 Gy.[31]
Patients receiving less than 33 Gy demonstrated significant
impairment in standing and sitting height for the prepubertal
age group only (Fig. 26.2).[35]

Bone Damage

Although scoliosis and kyphosis may result from spinal or
flank irradiation, children treated for Hodgkin lymphoma are
uncommonly affected due to the relative symmetry of the radiation fields and the low doses currently used. Slipped femoral
capital epiphysis is a clinically significant adverse effect
observed in patients following irradiation of the femoral

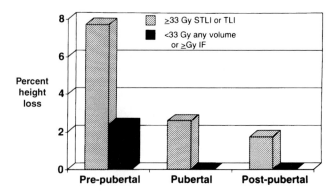

FIGURE 26.2. Relative height impairment for six groups according to
age at treatment and radiation dose/volume. (Reprinted with permission from Willman K, Cox R, Donaldson S. Radiation induced height
impairment in pediatric Hodgkin's disease. *Int J Radiat Oncol Biol
Phys* 1994;28:85.)

head.[36] There is a threshold dose of 25 Gy for this complication. It occurred in about half the children irradiated at less
than 4 years of age (7 of 15), as compared to only 1 of 21 children 5 to 15 years old. The mechanism of femoral capital epiphyseal plate slippage is postulated to be a radiation-induced
delay in maturation of the epiphyseal plate with disruption of
normal calcification and bone matrix deposition.

Avascular necrosis of the femoral or humeral heads can
occur 2 to 3 years following irradiation, but most commonly
occurs in the setting of combined-modality therapy.[37] The
etiology of this complication is unclear but may be related to
the combined use of steroids and irradiation or corticosteroids alone. Libshitz and Edeikin[38] reported necrosis in 16
of 44 children receiving 30 to 60 Gy to the femoral heads;
this was bilateral in 4 of 5 children treated to both hips. This
debilitating injury is fortunately rare when the femoral and
humeral heads are shielded and/or when lower radiation
doses are used.[33]

A variety of other uncommon skeletal abnormalities can be
seen after irradiation for Hodgkin lymphoma in young children,
including sternal deformity (hypoplasia, asymmetry, pectus exca-
vatum, pectus carinatum), clavicular shortening, hypoplasia of
the iliac bones or lower ribs, cartilaginous exostoses, osteochon-
dromata, and hypoplasia of the mandible.[39] A common effect of
chemotherapy is skeletal demineralization (osteoporosis) leading
to fractures following use of corticosteroids.

The most common chronic radiation effect on muscle is
hypoplasia. The muscles treated are smaller, although the
effects on strength are not pronounced. Thus the effect is more
cosmetic than functional. However, marked fibrosis can occur,
which produces stiffness, a decrease in range of motion of a
joint, and even pain. The frequency and severity of hypoplasia,
as previously stated, essentially depends on the age, developmental status, sex, and growth potential of the patient. In
young children, radiation doses of 15 to 25 Gy can cause varying degrees of hypoplasia. This is most evident in the neck and
upper thorax.[36] Certainly, doses of 35 to 45 Gy will impair
muscle development in adolescent patients. Rare individuals
who have been treated more than once with cumulative doses
of greater than 50 Gy will demonstrate significant fibrosis.[40]

Soft Tissue

In the growing breast, the most sensitive structure is the breast
bud. Doses of as little as 10 Gy to the breast bud will cause the
breast to be hypoplastic; doses above 20 Gy may ablate development altogether.[41] Doses of 20 Gy or more to other areas of
the breast will impair development in those areas. Even low

doses of radiation during puberty may impair subsequent lactation.[41]

Damage to developing teeth causes cosmetic and functional difficulties throughout life. The age of the child at the time of therapy, the radiation dose, and the use of chemotherapy determine the consequences. The defects that occur are most pronounced in children treated before age 6 and can include malocclusion, enamel hypoplasia, hypodontia, microdontia, enamel opacities, altered root development, shortening of premolar roots, and thinning of the roots with constriction.[42] However, Hodgkin lymphoma is rare in patients younger than 6 years of age.

Another long-term complication affecting soft tissue is retroperitoneal fibrosis. This is a problem in the retroperitoneal area that can cause ureteral obstruction and occurs typicall 8 to 15 years after the treament. This complication is usally associated with higher doses of radiation to the retroperitoneal area.[43]

Salivary Glands

Radiation injury to the major salivary glands (parotid, submandibular, sublingual) is associated primarily with an increased risk for caries, alterations in taste, and discomfort due to mouth dryness. Salivary gland irradiation causes a qualitative and quantitative change in salivary flow. Chemotherapy may also independently diminish salivary function, though its effects are less severe and transient.[44] However, anthracycline use may exacerbate radiation effects.

Salivary gland damage may be evident after 20 Gy of fractionated irradiation. Salivary flow rate drops rapidly during a course of fractionated irradiation. Postradiotherapy xerostomia is irreversible if all major salivary glands are treated with doses of 50 to 60 Gy, which almost never occurs in the treatment of Hodgkin lymphoma. Excellent oral hygiene and attentive dental care are the keys to dealing with the effect of irradiation on teeth and salivation. Prior to radiation and chemotherapy, a dental evaluation is indicated. As possible, foci of infection, loose exfoliating primary teeth and orthodontic appliances should be removed. The daily use of topical fluoride can dramatically reduce the frequency of radiation caries in the treated patient. Xerostomia is palliatively treated with saliva substitutes and sialagogues. Recent data support the efficacy of pilocarpine in improving saliva production and relieving symptoms of xerostomia, with minor risks that are predominantly limited to sweating.

Gastrointestinal Tract

The most systematic examination of late gastrointestinal tract complications following treatment for Hodgkin lymphoma is from the European Organization for the Research and Treatment of Cancer (EORTC) H2 and H5 trials conducted between 1972 and 1981.[45] These trials enrolled patients with clinical stage (CS) I and II Hodgkin lymphoma, registered all data including the type of complication prospectively, and comprised treatment groups with or without laparotomy, receiving radiation to mantle and paraaortic ± splenic fields according to three fractionation regimens. The report documented 36 late radiation injuries in 516 patients on the H2 and H5 protocols who received infradiaphragmatic irradiation—25 with ulcers of stomach or duodenum, 2 with severe gastritis, 6 with small-bowel obstruction or perforation, and 3 with both an ulcer and bowel obstruction. The complication rate was 2.7% in the non-laparotomy cohort and 11.5% in the laparotomy group. The highest risk of complications was in patients who had a laparotomy and subdiaphragmatic irradiation with 3.3-Gy fractions.

The median time to bowel injury from initiation of therapy was 14 months (3–92 months) for ulcers and gastritis, and 18 months (5–115 months) for small-bowel lesions.

In current practice, several factors would predict that gastrointestinal morbidity would be less prevalent than in the report from the EORTC.[45] These include the abandonment of laparotomy as a staging technique; the established use of contemporary techniques to optimize dose, fractionation, and dosimetry; and the increasing use of combined-modality approaches that limit the necessity for abdominal irradiation encompassing structures other than limited axial nodal regions.

Esophageal strictures can occur in patients who have received chest irradiation, or more commonly combined-modality therapy. In a report from Mahboubi and Silber,[46] esopageal strictures were found 1 to 10 years after therapy in 5 of 18 lymphoma patients who had a history of esophagitis. Three of the 5 patients had received doses greater than 40 Gy. This complication can also occur quite late, with reports up to 14 to 30 years after the therapy.[47]

Irradiation of the liver beyond tolerance levels results in sclerosis and thrombosis of small hepatic veins; sinusoidal and hepatic congestion; centrilobular necrosis and subsequent fibrosis; and a resultant shrunken liver demonstrating severe vascular damage, liver cell atrophy, lobular collapse, and periportal vein and bile duct fibrosis. Clinically, early radiation injury may be manifest as abnormal liver function tests, hepatomegaly, radionuclide imaging abnormalities (absence of Kupffer cell uptake of radionuclide within the irradiated area), and ascites. In the absence of other predisposing factors, radiation tolerance of the whole liver is considered to be approximately 25 to 30 Gy using conventional fractionation techniques. Transient abnormalities of liver function and imaging tests have been reported in the majority of patients receiving 20 Gy to the whole liver plus 40 Gy to the left lobe for stage III Hodgkin lymphoma despite the absence of clinical symptomatology.[48]

A wide variety of chemotherapeutic agents used in Hodgkin lymphoma may have hepatic effects. Transient elevation of alkaline phosphatase and transaminases were reported in approximately 20% of patients treated with MOPP.[49] Dimethyltriazeno imidazole carboxamide (dacarbazine or DTIC) commonly causes mild biochemical hepatic dysfunction at doses employed in the ABVD regimen,[50] procarbazine has been associated with granulomatous hepatitis,[51] and corticosteroids have a recognized association with acute pancreatitis and avascular necrosis of the femoral head.[52] Despite these associations, clinically relevant chemotherapy-related hepatotoxicity is remarkably uncommon in the absence of other predisposing factors.

Late Treatment Injury to the Urinary Tract

The radiation tolerance of the kidney has been well established, with a maximum tolerable dose limit of 20 Gy for whole-kidney irradiation.[53] In current practice, the configuration of abdominal radiation fields for the treatment of known or suspected Hodgkin lymphoma may comprise the midline upper abdominal nodes, the pelvic nodes, and spleen. Coverage of the spleen necessitates the irradiation of the upper third to half of the left kidney to full tumor dose.[54] Such irradiation has not resulted in elevations of serum blood urea nitrogen or creatinine, or in hypertension. Appropriately executed therapy using accepted radiation techniques and established chemotherapy regimens usually do not result in clinically apparent long-term renal dysfunction.

Conventionally applied pelvic radiation fields for Hodgkin lymphoma do not necessitate inclusion of substantial portions of bladder within the tumor volume. In current practice, bulky pelvic disease usually is managed with a combined-modality approach resulting in a more limited radiation volume. Partial bladder irradiation to 35 to 40 Gy and whole-bladder scatter doses from pelvic irradiation fields do not result in clinical late bladder injury or dysfunction.

Bladder toxicity from cyclophosphamide is well recognized, both as fibrosis following cumulative long-term exposure[55] and as hemorrhagic cystitis following cyclophosphamide in various chemotherapy schedules or, more significantly, in combination with radiation therapy.[56] Appropriate hydration to prevent accumulation of toxic metabolites of cyclophosphamide within the bladder is the established procedure to avoid acute cystitis risk and subsequent progression to bladder fibrosis and the development of bladder carcinoma.[57]

Late Treatment Injury to the Skin

The skin response to radiation is predictable, dose dependent, and characterized by an acute reaction during and shortly after the course of treatment. Chronic radiation injury may occur many months to years after radiation and may occur as a direct consequence of the acute reaction or may develop without antecedent clinically apparent damage. Chronic injury is manifest as thin, atrophic, telangiectatic skin with variable pigmentation (both hyper- and hypopigmentation). Erosion and ulceration may occur, wound healing is poor and infection common, and the predisposition to the development of cutaneous malignancies of various histologic types is well recognized.[58]

Chronic skin injury is usually seen in two circumstances. First is the use of radical irradiation where the full tumor dose is required either in the skin (cutaneous and/or subcutaneous tumor) or where the tumor volume of interest necessitates incorporation of the skin within the high-dose volume (subcutaneous lymph nodes, cutaneous lymphatic involvement, etc.). The other is the use of beam energies (orthovoltage or low-energy beam) or treatment techniques (e.g., inappropriate dosimetry, skin-applied bolus for missing tissue correction) that result in deposition of full dose in the skin and subcutaneous tissues and an inappropriate ratio of skin dose to tumor dose. In current practice, late skin injury is rarely, if ever, seen, given appropriate consideration of tumor dose (30–40 Gy), fractionation (1.5–2 Gy per day), treatment of all fields daily, selection of appropriate beam energy to achieve skin sparing, and use of the technique to establish uniformity of dose within the volume of interest with remotely applied compensation or attenuation for missing tissue contour correction.

Alopecia within the radiation field is universal with fractionated doses to 35 to 40 Gy despite the use of skin-sparing techniques. Facial, scalp, and body hair epilates during radiation therapy and starts to regrow 3 months after completion of therapy. Similarly, radiation effects on sweat glands recover, although increased dryness of the skin may be a long-term effect. The use of combined-modality therapy with conventional radiation dose (35–40 Gy) and, more specifically, the ABVD regimen may result in enhanced acute skin reaction, and more variable recovery of body hair and sweat gland function.

Cutaneous hyperpigmentation commonly follows acute radiation reactions but usually resolves with natural desquamation over a period of weeks. Hyperpigmentation is frequently seen with bleomycin administration,[59] often at sites of skin trauma (e.g., excoriations associated with pruritus, trauma, pressure). Doxorubicin is also associated with hyperpigmentation, particularly of skin creases, palms and soles, face, oral mucosa, and tongue. Nail changes are not uncommon, consisting of darkening of the nail bed (bleomycin and doxorubicin); dystrophic change (bleomycin); and pigmented, hypopigmented, and/or transverse depressions of the nail occurring with successive courses of chemotherapy.

Radiation recall reactions are induced by administration of chemotherapy (certain drugs) or corticosteroids. They manifest themselves as a radiation effect (skin erythema or pneumonitis within the radiation field) and occur with or after the administration of the chemotherapy. These reactions may not have occurred previously or may have been seen with the radiation. Increased radiosensitivity of skin is associated with doxorubicin and bleomycin, and increased photosensitivity with dacarbazine and vinblastine. This may enhance the acute skin reaction during radiation therapy and delay recovery following radiation. Radiation recall reaction is also seen with doxorubicin and may occur when doxorubicin-based therapy is administered weeks to months following radiation and with each course of chemotherapy. Gemcitabine has also been associated with radiation recall dermatitis in patients receiving salvage chemotherapy for Hodgkin lymphoma.[60]

Late Treatment Effects on the Immune System

Even before any treatment is administered to patients diagnosed with Hodgkin lymphoma, an immunodeficiency state is often present. Patients with Hodgkin lymphoma often exhibit lymphocytopenia, which is mainly ascribed to a reduction of CD4+ T-cells. Blood lymphocytes of untreated Hodgkin patients are poorly activated by mitogens and antigens, which preferentially stimulate T-cells.[61,62] Furthermore, the proliferative response of T-lymphocytes cultured with autologous non–T-lymphocytes is usually impaired or absent.[63] Although lymphocytopenia is present in all clinical stages, it tends to be more pronounced in patients with advanced disease.[61,64] Few studies have included patients who were tested both before and after treatment for Hodgkin lymphoma. In a relatively large study of patients retested 2 to 56 months following termination of radiotherapy for Hodgkin lymphoma, the responses to concanavalin A (ConA) and PPD, but not to pokeweed mitogen (PWM), were significantly reduced shortly after total nodal irradiation. The mitogen response did not increase with time after treatment; however, it did with PPD stimulation.[65] Following cytotoxic chemotherapy, a moderate to severe T-cell depletion is also observed. In a prospective study by Van Rijswik and associates,[66] 20 previously untreated patients with stage III and IV Hodgkin lymphoma were evaluated before modified MOPP therapy, after three courses, and within 3 months of the completion of six cycles. There was no change in the B-cells; however, T-lymphocytopenia was observed 2 years or more after cytotoxic drug therapy.

Deficiencies in the humoral immune system in patients with untreated Hodgkin lymphoma are minimal. Antibody titers that develop after immunization with pneumococcal polysaccharide vaccine in patients with untreated Hodgkin lymphoma are normal.[67] Radiotherapy and cytotoxic drug therapy may suppress a subsequent antibody response. Suppression was most pronounced following total-nodal irradiation plus cytotoxic drug therapy.[67] The antibody response recovered with time after therapy and became normal in several patients after 3 years.[68] Following curative radiotherapy and cytotoxic drug therapy, serum immunoglobulin IgG, IgA, and IgE concentrations are slightly decreased.[69] The reduction of serum IgM in patients who achieve a complete remission may be more pronounced. Splenectomy may partly contribute to the decline in serum IgM concentrations. Treated and potentially cured patients with Hodgkin lymphoma often have reduced serum IgM levels and a poor antibody response after immunization with microbial antigens.

Splenectomy was used in the past as a routine diagnostic and staging procedure in patients with Hodgkin lymphoma to assess the extent of abdominal disease. Splenectomy, however, may be associated with acute and late surgical complications and an increased risk of septicemia as a result of encapsulated bacteria, predominantly pneumococci.[70] With splenectomy, 20% to 25% of the phagocytic cell mass of the body is removed, leading to a diminished capacity for clearing circulating bacteria.[71] Removal of the spleen may also result in persistent blood-cell abnormalities. Neutrophilia, lymphocytosis, eosinophilia, and thrombocytosis are regular findings after splenectomy, but cell counts tend to return closer to normal over weeks to months.[72] Splenectomy causes a relative increase in lymphocyte counts (both T- and B-cell), which can be observed in patients in long-term remission. However, reduced IgM levels, and possibly impaired B-cell response, contribute to the persistent lifelong threat of overwhelming postsplenectomy infections in splenectomized patients who have been treated for Hodgkin lymphoma.

Due to the immunodeficiencies outlined above, patients with Hodgkin lymphoma are at increased risk for infections that depend on an intact cell-mediated immune capability for control. Infections seen with increased frequency in patients with Hodgkin lymphoma include varicella zoster, fungi, toxoplasmosis, listeriosis, and pneumocystis.[73,74] Long-term survivors are also at increased risk for bacterial infections. Among identifiable factors predisposing patients to infection are advanced age, advanced disease, and prior extensive radiotherapy and cytotoxic drug therapy.[75] *Streptococcus pneumoniae* is the most common and serious infection seen. Removal of the spleen predisposes patients to developing septicemia, which is caused predominantly by pneumococci, although *Haemophilus influenzae*, *Escherichia coli*, and *Staphylococcus aureus* may be isolated. Patients who are to have a splenectomy should be vaccinated for *S. pneumoniae* prior to the procedure to help to prevent infection with encapsulated organisms. In addition, all patients with Hodgkin lymphoma should be cautioned regarding their increased risk of bacterial sepsis and opportunistic infections. Patients who have undergone splenic irradiation may be at similar risk and should also be immunized prior to irradiation and every 5 to 7 years in follow-up.

Late Hematologic Complications

A number of chronic effects of Hodgkin lymphoma and its therapy on hematopoietic tissues can be demonstrated in long-term survivors of the disease. A decrease in the reserve of hematopoietic tissue can be evident in patients treated with chemotherapeutic agents such as alkylating agents and/or irradiation. This may be manifested only as slight cytopenias during times of normal health; however, under stress, such as a severe infection, an impaired response may be present due to the lack of a normal reserve capacity.

Although impaired immunocompetence is a feature present in most patients with Hodgkin lymphoma, evidence of immune activation is present as well. These alterations suggest that imbalances in cell populations, particularly of T-cells, result in both compromised immunity and, at the same time, hyperreactivity. Autoantibodies directed against red blood cells, platelets, neutrophils, and lymphocytes are common in patients with Hodgkin lymphoma and can lead to immunohemolytic anemia, immune thrombocytopenic purpura, autoimmune neutropenia, and lymphopenia. These immune phenomena can predate the diagnosis of Hodgkin lymphoma and sometimes are a sign of relapse.

All chemotherapy agents used in the treatment of Hodgkin lymphoma affect hematopoietic cell proliferation. The inhibition of hematopoiesis is a reflection of a decline in DNA synthesis, most often by alkylation of nucleic acids, as well as mitotic inhibition. Because the stem-cell population is predominantly

noncycling, antimetabolites, generally cycle-specific, are less likely to result in stem-cell depletion than alkylating agents. Chronic myelosuppressive effects of agents administered to patients with Hodgkin lymphoma appear more profound on occasion and may be demonstrated up to 2 years after the initial administration.[76] There may also be effects on the marrow stromal elements, which could cause problems with bone marrow reserve for possible future autologous hematopoietic stem cell transplantation.

Radiation induces both stromal and stem cell compartment injury.[77] Fibrosis in the bone marrow may be seen after radiation-induced injury and may effect long-term hematopoiesis.[78,79] The combination of damage induced by chemotherapy and radiation therapy can be additive or synergistic, with resultant prolonged cytopenias that are never corrected to normal levels. These effects can also lead to reduced marrow reserve and problems with adequate collections for hematopoietic stem-cell transplantation.

Patients have reduced marrow reserve after autologous bone-marrow transplantation, which limits subsequent treatment with combination chemotherapy or large-field irradiation. This limit in marrow reserve is due to prior chemotherapy and transplantation of limited numbers of hematopoietic stem cells. Caution should be exercised in using myelosuppressive drugs after autologous bone-marrow transplantation.

Numerous compounds have been recognized as lymphoma- or leukemia-inducing agents such as procarbazine, nitrosoureas, and alkylating agents (see Chapter 24).[80,81] Chemical carcinogenesis results from a multistep process of initiation and promotion. The development of secondary myelodysplasia may have a prolonged natural history with or without progression to acute leukemia, or alternatively the development of acute leukemia can appear to be very abrupt. Early in the course of dysmyelopoietic states, a blunted response to hematopoietic stress during infection may signal the appearance of the syndrome. As more severe changes progress, various degrees of pancytopenia my be present.[82] Laboratory evaluation of dysmyelopoiesis also can identify abnormalities of red-cell morphology, nucleated red blood cell forms, megaloblastoid cells, pseudo—Pleger-Huet neutrophils, immature white blood cells, monocytosis, dysmyelopoietic megakarocytic progenitors, and Auer rods.

Cytogenetic abnormalities are common, particularly involvement of chromosomes 5, 7, and 17.[83] Karyotypic evolution and the presence of complex cytogenetic abnormalities are indications of a leukemic evolution.[83] A report from Stanford University analyzed the survival of 690 patients with Hodgkin lymphoma beginning 1 year after the initial diagnosis. The actuarial risks of developing acute leukemia at 5 and 7 years were 1.5% and 2%, respectively.[84] These figures are similar to other studies, with the cumulative risks of acute myelogenous leukemia development of 3% to 5.5% at 5 years and 8% to 10% at 10 years.[85,86] The highest risk of development occurs at 6 to 7 years, with the critical window of 2 to 12 years. Chemotherapy and combined-modality therapy approaches appear to be the major risk factors for leukemia. The use of nitrosourea-containing combinations has been found to be a significant risk as compared to ABVD as frontline therapy.[87] Treatment of secondary leukemias can often be difficult due to relative chemotherapy insensitivity and complex cytogenetic abnormalities. The goal of treatment of secondary leukemias in young patients otherwise cured of Hodgkin lymphoma should be eradication, and an aggressive approach with induction, consolidation, and high-dose therapy and transplantation when indicated should be planned.

Patients treated for Hodgkin lymphoma are also at increased risk for the development of non-Hodgkin lymphoma.[88] The etiology of lymphomas observed after treatment of Hodgkin lymphoma is not known, although several explanations are possible. The profound immunosuppression of Hodgkin lymphoma, both de novo and treatment related, may allow oncogenic viruses to proliferate and produce lymphomas. The appearance of non-Hodgkin lymphomas may also represent a spectrum of the natural history of the disease. Patients who develop non-Hodgkin lymphomas have an excellent chance of long-term survival and should be treated aggressively in hopes of eradicating the lymphoma.

Genomic instability induced by chemotherapy or radiation has been demonstrated in long-term survivors of treatment for Hodgkin lymphoma. In a study of 49 patients with Hodgkin lymphoma, chromosomes were checked prior to therapy and at several time-points following therapy. A greater frequency of spontaneous cytogenetic abnormalities was observed in untreated patients with Hodgkin's disease compared to the general population. Following chemotherapy and radiation, the chromosomal abnormalities increased; however, some went away over time.[89] Studies with longer follow-up of patients who are in remission have also demonstrated that the mean frequency and patterns of both spontaneous and induced aberrations in remision pateints were significantly different in long-term follow analysis—up to 31 years in remission.[90]

Late Neurologic Compications of Therapy for Hodgkin Lymphoma

Radiation therapy is associated with toxicity to normal tissue, which is unavoidably included in the port of treatment. This damage can result from either direct damage to the nerve tissue or indirect damage to supporting tissues, such as the arterial supply. Radiation disorders of the spinal cord are occasionally seen in patients with Hodgkin lymphoma because the spinal cord is unavoidably included in the radiation field of many patients. Two types of radiation-induced myelopathy have been reported. The first occurs within a few months of treatment and is manifested by the complaint of an electric shock—like sensation below the neck, precipitated by neck flexion (Lhermitte sign).[91] The sensation is not accompanied by neurologic signs and is self-limiting. This syndrome probably represents reversible demyelination of sensory fibers in the cervical spinal cord. Chronic progressive radiation myelopathy is a disabling disorder most commonly reported after mantle and para-aortic irradiation due to an overdose at the match line.[92] The onset is insidious, with an initial slow progression and then often stabilization. Symptoms of chronic progressive radiation myelopathy include paresthesias, weakness, and bowel/bladder dysfunction. The signs are frequently of hemicord dysfunction (Brown-Séquard syndrome) or transverse myelopathy. The disorder may end in death or severe disability.

Peripheral nerves can also be adversely affected by radiation therapy. Areas adjacent to the spinal cord are most commonly affected. The brachial plexus is frequently in the portals of radiation for cervical, supraclavicular, and axillary lymph nodes as well as the apex of the lung. Brachial plexopathy usually begins with paresthesias or dysesthesias of the arm or hand, which is followed by weakness. Pain is usually not an early complaint and may not occur during the course of the disease. The onset is insidious and usually slowly progressive. In general, the dose of radiation to the brachial plexus that causes nerve injury is greater than 60 Gy.[93] Because Hodgkin patients usually receive 35 to 40 Gy, this complication is unusual except in cases of retreatment. The differential diagnosis of brachial plexopathy includes tumor as well as other benign causes, such as inflammatory plexopathy. A tumor often presents initially with pain, followed by neurologic disability and sometimes Horner syndrome as well. Brachial plexus neuropathies can also occur on viral illnesses or related to a reaction to vaccination on rare occasions.

Several of the chemotherapeutic agents used to treat Hodgkin lymphoma can also cause neurotoxicity alone or in combination with radiation therapy. The most common agents used in Hodgkin lymphoma that have been associated with neurotoxicity are the vinca alkyloids such as vincristine and vinblastine. Neurotoxicity is caused by destruction of neurotubules and is the dose-limiting factor of these agents.[94] Vincristine produces a peripheral neuropathy in patients treated with repeated doses.[95] This neuropathy is usually manifested by paresthesias initially, depression of the ankle jerk reflex, and eventually areflexia.[96] Sensation deficits are usually mild and typically partially or completely reversible once the treatment has been discontinued.[97] Distal weakness may occur, usually after sensory complaints are prominent. The motor deficits may show little improvement and the patient may have chronic neuropathic disability. Vinblastine can cause similar neurotoxicity but it is often milder in nature than that of vincristine.

Paraneoplastic syndromes have also occasionally been associated with Hodgkin lymphoma (see Chapter 28). These disorders can either precede the diagnosis or occur when the tumor is quiescent. Occasional reports of syndromes such as the myasthenic syndrome as seen with small-cell cancer of the lung, the POEMS (polyneuropathy, organomegaly, endocrinopathy, M protein, skin changes) syndrome with osteosclerotic myeloma,[98] and subacute cerebellar degeneration as seen in cancer of the ovary[99] have been reported. Most of these syndromes do not respond to treatment. Several of them are self-limited or respond to treatment of the primary tumor.[100]

Corticocerebellar degeneration is a purely degenerative process largely confined to the cerebellar cortex. Patients with Hodgkin lymphoma who have this disorder, but have no inflammation, have also been described. This diagnosis has preceded the diagnosis of Hodgkin lymphoma in some patients by as much as 8 years. Most patients develop a pancerebellar deficit acutely or subacutely. Most patients are significantly disabled, having severe truncal and limb ataxia, and sometimes also having nystagmus, myoclonus, and mental symptoms. The pathologic hallmark is the loss of neurons in the Purkinje cell layer—the loss occurs evenly throughout the cerebellum.

Late Pulmonary Effects

Patients with Hodgkin lymphoma often have disease in the chest, which can cause direct damage to the pulmonary tissue due to direct invasion. In addition, some of the treatment modalites used, such as radiation therapy to the mediastinal structures, and chemotherapy with potential lung toxicity such as bleomycin, may cause additional damage to the lung parenchyma. Studies of long-term survivors of therapy for Hodgkin lymphoma has demonstrated pulmonary dysfunction in 10% to 20% of patients.[101,102] Mediastinal fibrosis has been associated with radiation therapy alone as well as combined-modality therapy.[103] Suggested risk factors for the development of bleomycin-induced lung toxicity include age, bleomycin dose, renal insufficiency, radiation therapy to the chest, underlying lung disease, smoking history, and the use of granulocyte-stimulating factor support.[104] A large study of 951 patients who received therapy for lymphoma demonstrated that pulmonary toxicity was associated with smoking, radiation therapy to the mediastinum, bleomycin use, hypertension, and receiving salvage chemotherpy.[105] Another recent study evaluated 141 patients treated with a bleomycin-containing regimen.[106] In this study, bleomycin pulmonary toxicity was observed in 18% of the patients. Age over 40 years, ABVD as initial therapy, and the use of G-CSF were associated with an increased risk for the development of bleomycin induced lung toxicity. The 5-year overall survival in patients without bleomycin-induced lung toxicity was 90% and the survival with the lung toxicity was 63% ($p = 0.001$). The mortality rate was 4.2% in patients without lung toxicity and 24% in patients with the pulmonary syndrome. Newer chemotherapy agents have been substituted to attempt to decrease toxicity; however, to date this has not met with too much success. One example is the substitution of gemcitabine for etoposide in the BEACOPP regimen. Bredenfeld and associates[107] evaluated 27 patients with the substitution of gemcitabine for etoposide in the BEACOPP regimen. In this study, out of the first 14 pateints, 8 developed significant pulmonary toxicity and the addition was discontinued. It appeared that the addition of gemcitabine to bleomycin significantly increased the pulmonary complications. To minimize pulmonary toxicity, limiting the amount of chest irradiation, careful monitoring of diffusion capacity during bleomycin therapy, management of hypertension, and eliminating smoking for the patient would help to reduce this risk.

References

1. Hancock S, McDougall I, Constine L. Thyroid abnormalities after therapeutic external radiation. *Int J Radiat Oncol Biol Phys* 1995;31:1165.
2. Hancock S, Cox R, McDougall I. Thyroid diseases after treatment of Hodgkin disease. *N Engl J Med* 1991;325:599.
3. McDougall IR. *Thyroid disease in clinical practice.* London: Chapman & Hall Medical; 1992:304.
4. Bhatia S, Ramsay N, Bantle J, Mertens A, Robson L. Thyroid abnormalities after therapy for Hodgkin's disease in childhood. *Oncologist* 1996;1:62.
5. Constine LS, Donaldson SS, McDougall IR, et al. Thyroid dysfunction after radiotherapy in children with Hodgkin's disease. *Cancer* 1984;53:878.
6. Marcial-Vega VA, Order SE, Lastner G, et al. Prevention of hypothyroidism related to mantle irradiation for Hodgkin's disease: preoperative photon study. *Int J Radiat Oncol Biol Phys* 1990;18:613.
7. Petersen M, Keeling CA, McDougall IR. Hyperthyroidism with low radioiodine uptake after head and neck irradiation for Hodgkin's disease. *J Nucl Med* 1989;30:255.
8. Boivin J, Hutchison G, Zauber A, et al. Incidence of second cancers in patients treated for Hodgkin's disease. *J Natl Cancer Inst* 1995;87:732.
9. Green DM. Fertility and pregnancy outcome after treatment for cancer in childhood or adolescence. *Oncologist* 1997;2:171.
10. Ash P. The influence of radiation on fertility in man. *Br J Radiol* 1980;53:271.
11. Lushbaugh CC, Casarett GW. The effects of gonadal irradiation in clinical radiation therapy: a review. *Cancer* 1976;37:1111.
12. Wallace WHB, Shalet SM, Hendry JH, et al. Ovarian failure following abdominal irradiation in childhood: the radiosensitivity of the human oocyte. *Br J Radiol* 1989;62:995.
13. Leporrier M, vonTheobald P, Roffe J, Muller G. A new technique to protect ovarian function before pelvic irradiation: heterotopic ovarian autotransplantation. *Cancer* 1987;60:2201.
14. Mackie E, Radford M, Shalet S. Gonadal function following chemotherapy for childhood Hodgkin's disease. *Med Pediatr Oncol* 1996;27:24.
15. Horning WJ, Hoppe RT, Kaplan HS, et al. Female reproductive potential after treatment for Hodgkin's disease. *N Engl J Med* 1981;304:1377.
16. Behringer K, Breuer K, Reineke T, et al. Secondary amenorrhea after Hodgkin's lymphoma is influenced by age at treatment, stage of disease, chemotherapy regimen, and the use of oral contraceptives during therapy: a report from the German Hodgkin's Lymphoma Study Group. *J Clin Oncol* 2005;23:7555–7564.
17. Horning SJ, Hoppe RT, Advani R, et al. Efficacy and late effects of Stanford V chemotherapy and radiotherapy in untreated Hodgkin's disease: mature data in early and advanced stage patients. *Blood* 2004;104:308a.
18. Radford JA, Lieberman BA, Brison DR, et al. Orthotopic reimplantation of cryopreserved ovarian cortical strips after high-dose chemotherapy for Hodgkin's lymphoma. *Lancet* 2001;357:1172–1175.
19. Anselmo PA, Cavalieri E. Aragona C, et al. Successful pregnancies following an egg donation program in women with previously treated Hodgkin's disease. *Haematologica* 2001;86:624–628.
20. Griffin JE, Wilson JD. Disorders of the testes and the male reproductive tract. In: Wilson JD, Foster DW, eds. *Williams' textbook of endocrinology.* Philadelphia: WB Saunders; 1992:799.
21. Heller GC. Effects on the germinal epithelium of radiobiological factors in manned space flight. In: Langham WH, ed. *NRC publication 1487.* Washington, DC: National Academy of Sciences, National Research Council; 1967:124.
22. Izard M. Leydig cell function and radiation: a review of the literature. *Radiother Oncol* 1995;34:1.
23. Pedrick TJ, Hoppe RT. Recovery of spermatogenesis following pelvic irradiation for Hodgkin's disease. *Int J Radiat Oncol Biol Phys* 1986;12:117.
24. Sy Ortin TT, Shastak CA, Donaldson SS. Gonadal status and reproductive function following treatment for Hodgkin's disease in childhood: the Stanford experience. *Int J Rad Oncol Biol Phys* 1990;19:873.
25. Sanders JE. Effects of bone marrow transplantation on reproductive function. In: Green DM, D'Angio GJ, eds. *Late effects of treatment for childhood cancer.* New York: Wiley-Liss, 1992:95.
26. da Cunha M, Meistrich M, Fuller L, et al. Recovery of spermatogenesis after treatment for Hodgkin's disease: limiting dose of MOPP chemotherapy. *J Clin Oncol* 1984;2:571.
27. Braumswig J, Heimes U, Heiermann E, et al. The effects of different cumulative doses of chemotherapy on testicular function. Results in 75 patients treated for Hodgkin's disease during childhood or adolescence. *Cancer* 1990;65:1298.
28. Heikens J, Behrendt H, Adriaanse R, Berghout A. Irreversible gonadal damage in male survivors of pediatric Hodgkin's disease. *Cancer* 1996;78:2020.
29. Kulkarni S, Sastry P, Saikia T, et al. Gonadal function following ABVD therapy for Hodgkin's disease. *Am J Clin Oncol* 1997;20:354.
30. Meistrich M, Wilson G, Mathur K, et al. Rapid recovery of spermatogenesis after mitoxantrone, vincristine, vinblastine, and prednisone chemotherapy for Hodgkin's disease. *J Clin Oncol* 1997;15:3488.
31. Sherins RJ, Olweny CLM, Ziegler JL. Gynecomastia and gonadal dysfunction in adolescent boys treated with combination chemotherapy for Hodgkin's disease. *N Engl J Med* 1978;299:12.
32. Kurdoglu B, Wilson G, Parchuri N, et al. Protection from radiation-induced damage to spermatogenesis by hormone treatment. *Radiat Res* 1994;139:97.
33. Dawson WB. Growth impairment following radiotherapy in childhood. *Clin Radiol* 1968;19:241.
34. Eifel P, Donaldson S, Thomas P. Response of growing bone to irradiation: a proposed late effects scoring system. *Int J Radiat Oncol Biol Phys* 1995;31:1301.
35. Willman K, Cox R, Donaldson S. Radiation induced height impairment in pediatric Hodgkin's disease. *Int J Radiat Oncol Biol Phys* 1994;28:85.
36. Chapman JA, Deakin DP, Green JH. Slipped upper femoral epiphysis after radiotherapy. *J Bone Joint Surg* 1980;62B:337.
37. Prosnitz LR, Lawson JP, Friedlaender GE, et al. Avascular necrosis of bone in Hodgkin's disease patients with combined modality therapy. *Cancer* 1981;47:2793.
38. Libshitz A, Edeikin BS. Radiotherapy changes of the pediatric hip. *AJR* 1981;137:585.
39. Rutherford H, Dodd GD. Complications of radiation therapy; growing bone. *Semin Roentgenol* 1974;9:15.
40. Gillette E, Mahler P, Powers B, Gillette S, Vujaskovic Z. Late radiation injury to muscle and peripheral nerve. *Int J Radiat Oncol Biol Phys* 1995;31:1309.
41. Rosenfield N, Haller J, Berdon W. Failure of development of the growing breast after radiation therapy. *Pediatr Radiol* 1989;19:124.
42. Maguire A, Craft A, Evans R, et al. The long-term effects of treatment on the dental condition of children surviving malignant disease. *Cancer* 1987;60:2570.
43. Chao N, Levin J, Horning SJ. Retroperitoneal fibrosis following treatment for Hodgkin's disease. *JCL* 1987;5:231–232.
44. Schubert M, Izutsu K. Iatrogenic causes of salivary gland dysfunction. *J Dent Res* 1987;66:680.
45. Cosset J-M, Henry-Amar M, Burgers JMV, et al. Late radiation injuries of the gastrointestinal tract in the H2 and H5 EORTC Hodgkin's disease trials: emphasis on the role of exploratory laparotomy and fractionation. *Radiother Oncol* 1988;13:61.
46. Mahboubi S, Silber JH. Radiation-induced esophageal strictures in children with cancer. *Eur Radiol* 1997;7:119–122.
47. Kaplinsky C, Kornreich L, Tiomny E, et al. Esophageal obstruction 14 years after treatment for Hodgkin's disease. *Cancer* 1991;68:903–905.
48. Poussin-Rosillo H, Nisee LZ, D Angio GJ. Hepatic radiation tolerance in Hodgkin's disease patients. *Radiology* 1976;121:461.
49. DeVita VT, Serpick AA, Carbone PP. Combination chemotherapy in the treatment of advanced Hodgkin's disease. *Ann Intern Med* 1970;73:881.
50. Johnson RO, Metter G, Wilson W, et al. Phase I evaluation of DTIC (NSC-45388) and other studies in malignant melanoma in the Central Oncology Group. *Cancer Treat Rep* 1976;60:183.
51. Stolinsky DC, Solomon J, Pugh RP, et al. Clinical experience with procarbazine in Hodgkin's disease, reticulum cell sarcoma, and lymphosarcoma. *Cancer* 1979;26:984.
52. Nakashima Y, Howard JM. Drug induced acute pancreatitis. *Surg Obstet Gynecol* 1977;145:105.
53. Kunkler PB, Farr FR, Luxton RW. The limit of renal tolerance to x-rays. *Br J Radiol* 1952;25:190.
54. Koster A, Kimmig B, Müller-Schmipfle, et al. MR tomographie und MR angiographic—eine neue methode zur bestrahlungs-planung abdomineller grossfelder. *Strahlenther Onkol* 1992;168:230.
55. Johnson WW, Meadows DC. Urinary-bladder fibrosis and telangiectasia associated with long term cyclophosphamide therapy. *N Engl J Med* 1977;284:290.
56. Jayalkshamma B, Pinkel D. Urinary bladder toxicity following pelvic irradiation and simultaneous cyclophosphamide therapy. *Cancer* 1976;28:701.
57. Pathak AB, Advani SH, Gopal R, et al. Urinary bladder cancer following cyclophosphamide therapy for Hodgkin's disease. *Leuk Lymphoma* 1992;8:503.
58. Tranenkle HL. Late radiation injury and cutaneous neoplasms. In: Helm F, ed. *Cancer dermatology.* Philadelphia: Lea & Febiger; 1979:99.

59. Yagoda A, Mukherji B, Young C, et al. Bleomycin, an antitumour antibiotic. Clinical experience in 274 patients. *Ann Intern Med* 1972;77:861.
60. Marisavljevic D, Ristic B, Hajder J, et al. Gemcitiabine induced radiation recall dermatitis in a patient with resistant Hodgkin lymphoma. *Am J Hematol* 2005;80:91.
61. Holm G, Mellstedt H, Bjorkholm M, et al. Lymphocyte abnormalities in untreated patients with Hodgkin's disease. *Cancer* 1976;37:751.
62. Case DC, Hansen JA, Corrales E, et al. Comparison of multiple in vivo and in vitro parameters in untreated patients with Hodgkin's disease. *Cancer* 1976;38:1807.
63. Begemann M, Claas G, Falke H. Impaired autologous mixed lymphocyte reactivity in Hodgkin's disease. *Klin Wochenschr* 1982;60:19.
64. Wedelin C, Bjorkholm M, Johansson B, et al. Clinical and laboratory findings in untreated patients with Hodgkin's disease with special reference to age. *Med Oncol Tumor Pharmacother* 1984;1:33.
65. Bjorkholm M, Wedelin C, Holm G, et al. Longitudinal studies of blood lymphocyte capacity in Hodgkin's disease. *Cancer* 1981;48:2010.
66. Van Rijswijk REN, Sybesm JPHB, Kater L. A prospective study of the changes in the immune status before, during, and after multiple-agent chemotherapy for Hodgkin's disease. *Cancer* 1983;51:637.
67. Levine AM, Overturf GD, Field RF, et al. Use and efficacy of pneumococcal vaccine in patients with Hodgkin's disease. *Blood* 1979;54:1171.
68. Minor DR, Schiffman G, McIntosh LS. Response of patients with Hodgkin's disease to pneumococcal vaccine. *Ann Intern Med* 1979;90:887.
69. Amlot PL, Green L. Serum immunoglobulins G, A, M, D, and E concentration in lymphomas. *Cancer* 1979;40:371.
70. Singer DB. Postsplenectomy sepsis. In: Rosenberg HS, Bolands RP, eds. *Perspectives on pediatric pathology.* Chicago: Year Book Medical; 1973:185.
71. Schulkind ML, Ellis EF, Smith RT. Effect of antibody upon clearance of I-125-labelled pneumococci by the spleen and liver. *Pediatr Res* 1967;1:178.
72. Lipson RL, Bayrd ED, Watkins CH. The postsplenectomy blood picture. *Am J Clin Pathol* 1959;32:526.
73. Goffinet DR, Glatstein EJ, Merigan TC. Herpes zoster-varicella infections and lymphoma. *Ann Intern Med* 1972;76:235.
74. Ruskin J, Remington JS. *Pneumocystis carinii* infection in the immunosuppressed host. *Antimicrob Agents Chemother* 1967;7:70.
75. Notter D, Grossman Z, Rosenberg SA, et al. Infections in patients with Hodgkin's disease: a clinical study of 300 consecutive adult patients. *Rev Infect Dis* 1980;2:761.
76. Botnick LE, Hannon EC, Hellman S. Multisystem stem cell failure after apparent recovery from alkylating agents. *Cancer Res* 1978;38:1942.
77. Nelson DF, Chaffey JT, Hellman S. Late effects of x-irradiation on the ability of mouse bone marrow to support hematopoiesis. *Int J Radiat Oncol Biol Phys* 1977;2:39.
78. Knospe WA, Blom J, Crosby WH. Regeneration of locally irradiated bone marrow—I. Dose dependent long term changes in the rat, with particular emphasis upon vascular and stromal reaction. *Blood* 1966;28:398.
79. Slanina J, Musshoff K, Rahner T, Stiasny R. Long-term side effects in irradiated patients with Hodgkin's disease. *Int J Radiat Oncol Biol Phys* 1977;2:1.
80. Dexter TM, Schofield R, Lajtha LG, Moore M. Studies on the mechanism of chemical leukaemogenesis. *Br J Cancer* 1974;30:325.
81. O'Gara RW, Adamson RH, Kelly MG, Dalgaard DW. Neoplasms of the hematopoietic system in nonhuman primates: report of one spontaneous tumor and two leukemias induced by procarbazine. *J Natl Cancer Inst* 1971;46:1121.
82. Weiden PL, Lerner KG, Gerdes A, et al. Pancytopenia and leukemia in Hodgkin's disease: report of three cases. *Blood* 1973;42:571.
83. Anderson RL, Bagby GC, Richert-Boe K, et al. Therapy-related preleukemic syndrome. *Cancer* 1981;47:1867.
84. Coleman CN, Williams CJ, Flint A, et al. Hematologic neoplasia in patients treated for Hodgkin's disease. *N Engl J Med* 1977;297:1249.
85. Pedersen-Bjergaard J, Larsen SO. Incidence of acute nonlymphocytic leukemia, preleukemia, and acute myeloproliferative syndrome up to 10 years after treatment of Hodgkin's disease. *N Engl J Med* 1982; 307:965.
86. Blayney DW, Longo DL, Young RC, et al. Decreasing risk of leukemia with prolonged follow-up after chemotherapy and radiotherapy for Hodgkin's disease. *N Engl J Med* 1987;316:710.
87. Yahalom J, Voss R, Leizerowitz R, et al. Secondary leukemia following treatment of Hodgkin's disease: ultra structural and cytogenetic data in two cases with a review of the literature. *Am J Clin Pathol* 80: 1983;231.
88. Razis DV, Diamond HD, Craver LF. Hodgkin's disease associated with other malignant tumors and certain non-neoplastic diseases. *Am J Med Sci* 1959;238:327.
89. M'kacher R, Girinsky T, Koscielny S, et al. Baseline and treatment–induced chromosomal abnormalities in peripheral blood lymphocytes of Hodgkin's lymphoma patients. *Int J Radiat Oncol Biol Phys* 2003;57:321–326.
90. Ryabchenko N, Nasovova V, Antoschina M, et al. *Int J Radiat Biol* 2003;79:251–257.
91. Carmel RJ, Kaplan HS. Mantle irradiation in Hodgkin's disease. *Cancer* 1976;37:2813.
92. Reagan TJ, Thomas JE, Colby MY Jr. Chronic progressive radiation myelopathy: its clinical aspects and differential diagnosis. *JAMA* 1968;203:128.
93. Kori SH, Foley KM, Posner JB. Brachial plexus lesions in patients with cancer:100 cases. *Neurology* 1981;31:45.
94. Jellinger K. Pathologic effects of chemotherapy. In: Walker MD, ed. *Oncology of the nervous system.* Amsterdam: Martinus Nijhoff; 1983:416.
95. Young DF, Posner JB. Nervous system toxicity of chemotherapy agents. In: Vinken PJ, Bruyn GW, eds. *Handbook of clinical neurology,* vol. 39. Amsterdam: North-Holland; 1980:126.
96. Casey EB, Jellife AM, LeQuesne PM, et al. Vincristine neuropathy: clinical and electrophysiological observations. *Brain* 1973;96:69.
97. Sandler SG, Tobin W, Henderson ES. Vincristine-induced neuropathy: a clinical study of fifty leukemic patients. *Neurology* 1969;19:367.
98. Kelly JJ, Kyle RA, Miles JM, et al. Osteosclerotic myeloma and peripheral neuropathy. *Neurology* 1983;33:202.
99. Greenlee JE, Brashear HR. Antibodies to cerebellar Purkinje cells in patients with paraneoplastic cerebellar degeneration and ovarian carcinoma. *Ann Neurol* 1983;14:609.
100. Carr I. The Ophelia syndrome: memory loss in Hodgkin's disease. *Lancet* 1982;1:844.
101. Robinson LL, Green DM, Hudson M, et al. Long-term outcomes of adult survivors of childhood cancer. *Cancer* 2005;104:2557–2564.
102. Camus P, Costabel U. Drug-induced respiratory disease in patients with hematological diseases. *Semin Respir Crit Care Med* 2005;26:458–481.
103. Brusamolino E, Lazzarino M, Orlandi E, et al: Early-stage Hodgkin's disease: Long-term results with radiotherapy alone or combined radiotherapy and chemotherapy. *Ann Oncol* 1994;5:S101–S106.
104. Sleijfer S. Bleomycin induced pneumonitis. *Chest* 2001;120:617–624.
105. Moser EC, Noordijk EM, Carde P, et al. Late non-neoplastic events in patients with aggressive non-Hodgkin's lymphoma in four randomized European Organisation for Research and Treatment of Cancer Trials. *Clin Lymphoma Myeloma* 2005;6:122–130.
106. Martin WG, Ristow KM, Habermann TM, et al. Bleomycin pulmonary toxicity has a negative impact on the outcome of patinets with Hodgkin's lymphoma. *J Clin Oncol* 2005;23:7614–7620.
107. Bredenfeld H, Franklin J, Nogova L, et al. Severe pulmonary toxicity in patients with advanced stage Hodgkin's disease treated with a modified beomycin, doxorubicin, cyclophosphamide, vincristine, procarbazine, prednisone, and gemcitabein combination of gemcitabine and bleomycin: A report of the German Hodgkin's lymphoma Study Group. *JCO* 2004;22:2424–2429.

CHAPTER 27 ■ ASSESSING THE QUALITY OF LIFE IN PATIENTS WITH HODGKIN LYMPHOMA: INSTRUMENTS AND CLINICAL TRIALS

HENNING FLECHTNER, MICHEL HENRY-AMAR, PATRICIA FOBAIR, FLORENCE JOLY, AND JENS-ULRICH RUEFFER

HISTORY AND BACKGROUND

In 1948, the World Health Organization (WHO) offered a redefinition of health as a state of complete physical, mental, and social well-being and not merely the absence of disease or infirmity.[1] In the same year, Karnofsky and Burchenal proposed a rating scale designed to help physicians assess the effects of treatment by comparing patients' performance before and after therapeutic intervention.[2] In 1960, the term *quality of life* was used by the U.S. Presidential Commission on National Goals. In 1964, these goals were used to stimulate programs that would examine the quality and needs of individual lives, and develop programs to improve quality of life.[3] By 1977, "quality of life" became a key word for the retrieval of journal articles in the United States National Library of Medicine. Since the mid-1980s, there have been hundreds of articles per year referring to "quality of life and cancer," and the number has constantly risen since to well over 1,500 papers in 2005. In 1989, the U.S. Congress passed the Outcomes Assessment Research Act to create the Agency for Health Care Policy and Research, whose task it is to measure functional status, well-being, and satisfaction with care along with other end-points to evaluate policies that affect patient outcomes.[1] Very recently, *patient-reported outcome [PRO]* became the widely accepted notion for any health-status measurement that comes directly from the patient. The FDA *Guidance for Industry* about PRO measures states that "in clinical trials, a PRO instrument can be used to measure the impact of an intervention on one or more aspects of patients' health status, hereafter referred to as PRO concepts, ranging from the purely symptomatic [response of a headache] to more complex concepts [e.g., ability to carry out activities of daily living], to extremely complex concepts such as quality of life, which is widely understood to be a multi-domain concept with physical, psychological, and social components," thereby placing quality of life under the evolving umbrella of PRO concepts.[4]

Background

Quality of life includes psychological and social functioning as well as physical functioning, and incorporates positive as well as negative aspects of disease or infirmity and it can be viewed as a metaphor for the physical, psychological, and social health of patients after treatment for cancer. Health-related quality of life can be defined as the value assigned for the duration of life as modified by social opportunities, perceptions, functional states, and impairments that are influenced by disease or treatment.[5]

Qualitative and Quantitative Measurements

The patient's qualitative perspective or subjective view is a major component of the quality-of-life concept.[6] However, quality of life is also a quantifiable, multidimensional concept, encompassing perceptions of both positive and negative aspects produced by a disease or its treatment. It is the multidimensionality of life that provides the various domains or dimensions to be evaluated using quantitative methods. These domains include physical, functional, emotional or psychological, social, and spiritual well-being.[7,8]

Dimensions of Quality of Life

Physical well-being includes symptoms of the disease, side effects of treatment, and acute or chronic limitations in physical activity, self-care, mobility, sleep, body image, energy, and fatigue.[6,7] These may occur acutely as a result of the disease or treatment, and long-term as part of the recovery process. A review of the literature on late effects and psychosocial recovery after cancer suggests that physical adjustment after treatment is associated with the stage of the disease and the extent of treatment required.[9]

Functional well-being includes the ability to perform both work and leisure activities. An earlier analysis found that survivors of Hodgkin lymphoma had more difficulties in completing work tasks than a comparison group of patients treated for testicular cancer.[10] Using a measure of physical performance at work and at leisure, it was found that compromised physical performance was more likely to be observed in leisure activities than in work-related activities.[11,12]

Psychological or emotional well-being includes both positive and negative aspects. It is estimated that some degree of emotional distress may occur in more than 40% of patients during the course of their illness.[1] Main aspects include anxiety and depression as well as mechanisms to cope with the potential stressful and traumatic events that may occur in the course of a cancer experience. It is very important to know about the emotional state of a patient, and in studies of survivors of Hodgkin lymphoma at Stanford University in 1986, around

20% of patients reported elevated levels of depression and distress an average of 9 years following treatment.[13]

Social well-being includes perceived social support, functional family support, ability to engage in leisure activities and work, and financial success. Cella[6] also suggests that measures of intimacy and sexuality be added to the assessment of social well-being. Patients with poor support systems have been found to be more depressed, vulnerable, angry and unsettled, and more likely to reject overtures from others.[14] Positive associations between the emotional support patients received and their social well-being are established and it was also found that successful social integration led to lower levels of depression.[15]

Hannah and associates[16] found that survivors of Hodgkin lymphoma often reported difficulties in communication in the marital relationship; these difficulties in part were founded on a fear of recurrence or death and the avoidance of talking about problems. In their study, 41% of men with Hodgkin lymphoma reported problems with sexual frequency 3 years after treatment.

Spiritual well-being includes the sense of purpose and meaning in life, and emphasis on religious issues and values.[17] This important domain has been noted but not frequently studied, and only recently have validated instruments been developed. In the Stanford series of survivors of Hodgkin lymphoma, 44% of patients reported that they changed their view of life, 23% found that their self-esteem increased, 22% found that the importance of relationships increased, and 11% found that there were no benefits.[13] Coping with the disease and its treatment were the toughest problem for 60% of survivors of Hodgkin lymphoma, while 40% reported that family and career problems provided greater challenges to them than the cancer. The greatest source of social support came from family and friends (56%), and faith in religion, self-belief, and treatment (44%).

Why Should the Quality of Life of Cancer Patients be Assessed?

The concern about the late effects of the disease and treatment (including quality of life) for survivors of cancer provides the impetus to more formally study these issues. Health practitioners and providers will increasingly seek qualitative and quantitative data to support their choices in treatment based on differing concerns for mortality, morbidity, and quality of life. For example, patients with Hodgkin lymphoma now enjoy increased survival due to improvements in treatment,[18] and many are young and have many potentially productive years after completion of treatment. Clinical trials that may not demonstrate differences in survival or event-free survival may allow recommendations for less toxic treatment based on quality-of-life measurements, which might allow increased productivity at work and improved functioning outside of work. Thus, studies that lead to reducing late effects and psychosocial burdens among survivors of Hodgkin lymphoma will continue to provide benefit to patients as survival and freedom from recurrence continue to improve. A recent international expert meeting sponsored by the Rockefeller Foundation was held in Bellagio, Italy to devise strategies "reducing mortality and improving the quality of life of long-term survivors of Hodgkin lymphoma."[19]

QUALITY-OF-LIFE ASSESSMENT IN HODGKIN LYMPHOMA

For many years the focus among health professionals was in improving treatment and reducing mortality among patients with Hodgkin lymphoma. As the major efforts have been directed toward increasing cure and minimizing late effects, it is understandable that quality-of-life assessment has had less effect on the treatment of Hodgkin lymphoma than on the treatment of other malignancies such as lung or breast cancer.[20,21] Major developments in quality-of-life assessment have been accomplished in palliative treatment, where there has been concern about the value of treatment to patients.[22] To date, most studies on quality of life have been conducted in patients with lung and breast cancer, two of the most common cancers.[23,24]

The majority of the quality-of-life instruments developed in the early 1980s were directed at assessing the short-term effects of disease and treatment, including the acute side effects of chemotherapy and radiotherapy (e.g., nausea and vomiting, hair loss). Most of the quality-of-life assessments measured the general and physical condition of the patient. Measurements included assessment of pain, gastrointestinal problems (diarrhea, constipation), and sleep disturbance, among other more psychological issues.[25] Patients were typically in their 50s, 60s, or older, and thus the studies provided an assessment of quality of life for an aging individual having to cope with a life-threatening illness. There were few studies that focused on younger patients and their quality of life after returning to their jobs, new marriages, and families. Large differences exist between pediatric and adult oncology in the development of quality-of-life instruments.[26] Assessment of quality of life in pediatric and young-adult oncology patients has mainly focused on cure and the psychosocial consequences after inducing complete remission.[27] Cross-sectional studies were employed rather than longitudinal trials due to limitations in resources and measurements.[26] Many of these measurements were lengthy, time-consuming, and unsuitable for longitudinal follow-up studies. Studies investigating the late effects and sequelae in Hodgkin lymphoma used instruments from a variety of research fields including data on socioeconomic status and occupational situation,[13,28-31] while disease-specific instruments were developed for many of the more common adult cancers. As a consequence, there are no quality-of-life instruments ready for use in Hodgkin lymphoma. In contrast there are a number of well-established, internationally validated instruments for quality-of-life assessment that focus on acute effects of treatment and shorter periods of follow-up in the palliative treatment of patients.[32,33] From the beginning, these instruments were developed for longitudinal studies, using repeated measurements in clinical trials.[34,35] There still is a need for quality-of-life instruments that inquire about the needs of surviving patients after active treatment and recovery have taken place.[36] To further enhance the effectiveness of treatment and reduce as much as possible the acute and late side effects, more information is needed about how patients cope with the illness and late effects of treatment and whether they are able to return to normal life. This makes prospective longitudinal approaches desirable, that is, data taken on quality of life during and following treatment. To obtain information from the patient's point of view, instruments are needed to address the relevant issues from the beginning of therapy to 10 and 15 years later.[37]

METHODS AND INSTRUMENTS

The main constructs of assessing the quality of life of a patient do not aim at fixed definitions of quality of life but consider the important influences on a patient's quality of life.[25,38] The two major sources that influence quality of life are the disease itself and the treatment administered. This has led to a change over the years from the notion of quality of life as a broader concept to the more restricted notion of health-related quality of life.[33] Three broad domains of quality of life—physical, psychoemotional, and social—are defined by the WHO. Although these domains are widely accepted internationally, major problems remain as to how to arrive at valid, reliable, and meaningful data reflecting the influence of illness and treatment.[39]

Two approaches are available. The first has an expert rater do the assessment, such as the physician or health professional; examples are the Karnofsky Performance Scale, used in the assessment of the physical effects of the disease and treatment,[2,20] and the Spitzer Index, which assesses five dimensions of quality of life.[40] The second approach has patients rating their own experience and quality of life; this subjective information can be collected through interviews, questionnaires, or a combination of the two.

Interviews

The interview approach is useful in informing the research team about important issues with which patients cope. Interviews can improve the reliability of data when patients are disadvantaged by age, language, or disease process. They can be time-consuming and expensive, as it requires personnel skilled in interviewing. Interview methods vary from face-to-face, psychologically oriented interviews lasting a couple of hours, to structured telephone interviews lasting a few minutes.[41,42] One format involves a highly structured approach that holds the interviewer tightly to the questionnaire, and at the other extreme are open, exploratory interviews that refrain from restricting the patient's answer. Telephone interviews are sometimes used to supplement data not collected, or to complete partial answers on forms.[41]

Questionnaires

The most established method of assessing quality of life is the use of self-administered questionnaires. Over the last 2 to 3 decades, a number of questionnaires have been developed for assessment of quality of life. In general, most instruments measure either generic health-related quality of life or cancer-specific quality of life. Basic principles have been established internationally on how to construct quality-of-life instruments and how to validate them. Most instruments approach quality of life as a multidimensional construct by employing multi-item scales and single items for the different domains of quality of life. For the generic health-related quality-of-life instrument, there is wide agreement that at least the domains of physical, emotional, and social functioning as well as global assessments of health and well-being should be assessed. This is also true for the more specific cancer-oriented instruments where these domains constitute the core of what is assessed and are complemented by other domains more specifically pertaining to cancer (assessment of the side effects of treatment and symptoms of the disease). Recent developments make use of a modular approach by which the main domains are covered by a core instrument, and other domains, dealing with tumor or treatment-specific phenomena, are available as add-on modules.[25,34]

A time-frame has to be given to the patient from whom an assessment is requested. Apart from the diary-type instruments, where patients are asked to assess their quality of life daily or weekly on different items, the time-frames most often given are 1 and 2 weeks. Usually four- to seven-point scales are used to obtain severity ratings. Widely used are Likert-type scales and the scaling technique of summated scales. Each item has equal weight within the scale and the grading of the item uses equal intervals. Equal weighting is, in principle, questionable, but sufficient data from many sources are available to show that this kind of scaling exhibits the necessary robustness. Although other scoring techniques have been scientifically explored, the standard procedure for the scoring of scales uses unweighted summed scores of the contributing items. Other instruments use the visual or linear analog type of scales where only the ends of the poles are defined and the distance between them (usually 10 cm) is held constant. The patient marks a cross on the line where appropriate or at given linear intervals.[23] Most questionnaires generate scale scores and single-item scores, usually transformed uniformly on a 0 to 100 (worst to best) scale like the European Organization for the Research and Treatment of Cancer Quality-of-Life Core Questionnaire (EORTC QLQ-C30).[35] The psychometric properties of the instrument are of utmost importance. Validity, reliability, and responsiveness to change over time are anchor points and have to be investigated and proven.[43]

Validity

Aspects of validity include face validity, content validity, criterion-related validity, construct validity, and discriminant and predictive validity. Discriminant and predictive validity are of particular clinical relevance and importance because they refer to the properties of an instrument that can distinguish between groups of patients and predict outcome, which is the main interest of quality-of-life research in the clinical trials.[22]

Reliability

The usual test-retest reliability and inter-rater reliability are not so important for quality-of-life assessment because inter-rater reliability is not applicable to self-reports (exceptions are instruments such as the Spitzer Index, which uses rater assessments), and test-retest is in many situations difficult to perform because of the natural changes that occur in the treatment and disease process. Because quality-of-life measures usually do not aim at addressing trait variables, stability over time should only be expected for shorter periods of time (days). As a third measure, the internal consistency (Cronbach's alpha) of scales is often used, and values above 0.7 are regarded as sufficient for conducting group comparisons.[44]

Responsiveness Over Time

Responsiveness refers to sensitivity to change and to the clinical significance of observed changes in health status or quality of life over time.[45] Investigation of responsiveness will become more important because for most quality-of-life questionnaires there are no normative or reference data available, and an increasing amount of reported data needs interpretation frames for controls for determining the clinical value of the observed changes.[46]

Cross-Cultural Validation

Cross-cultural validation is needed today due to increasing international collaboration. Most of the major questionnaires have either gone from national development to international field testing procedures or from the start have undergone international testing.[47] Guidelines for translation (forward-backward procedures) and adaptation to language (e.g., in some languages male, female, and mixed gender forms of the questionnaires are necessary) have been developed and are standardized.[48]

Instruments

The general disadvantage of all available standard instruments is the lack of a Hodgkin lymphoma-specific module. The wide range of key interval times (treatment period, follow-up, long-term surveillance) is not adequately covered by existing instruments. Most published trials in Hodgkin lymphoma that address late effects and quality of life use different instruments (mainly questionnaires, but also mixed questionnaire-interview approaches) that focus on psychological outcome including mood, depression, psychosocial adaptation, and psychiatric symptoms.[49] Besides this complex of psychological outcomes, the socioeconomic impact of the disease is also evaluated, for example, living circumstances, occupational situation, leisure activities, family life, and drinking and smoking habits.[50–54] Infertility and sexual problems as a consequence of treatment have received particular attention.[55] As outlined above, these assessment instruments were derived from the general assessment of late effects from a variety of research fields and illnesses. Only recently have explicit quality-of-life measures, such as the EORTC QLQ-C30, been included in cross-sectional studies.[31,37,53]

Few published reports have addressed both late effects and longitudinal quality-of-life assessment. For quality-of-life assessment, a variety of instruments have been tested (validated) that can distinguish between generic health outcome measures. They include the Nottingham Health Profile (NHP),[56] Sickness Impact Profile (SIP),[57] Medical Outcome Study Short Form 36 (MOS SF-36),[58] EuroQoL,[59] World Health Organization Quality-of-Life WHOQOL,[60] Dartmouth COOP Function Charts,[61] and cancer-specific questionnaires such as the EORTC QLQ-C30/36,[35] Functional Assessment of Cancer Therapy (FACT, or the newer version, FACIT),[62] Functional Living Index: Cancer (FLIC),[63] Spitzer Index,[40] Cancer Rehabilitation Evaluation System (CARES),[64,65] and the Rotterdam Symptom Checklist.[66] All newer instruments use patient self-assessment of the perceived quality of life. Apart from the broader and general domains of quality of life, there is agreement about the necessity of assessing specific disease- and treatment-related problems (e.g., body image, sexuality, fatigue, spirituality, and gender issues, as well as issues pertaining to very old or very young patients). To accomplish this, a number of groups follow the modular approach in the development of questionnaires (FACT-G and the QLQ-C30 represent core instruments) and supplement the core instrument by specific tumor- or treatment-related modules.[35,67]

One of the difficulties in designing Hodgkin lymphoma-specific modules is that, unlike other cancers, the particular problems are not easily identified. Apart from problems of sexuality and fertility, many side effects of radiation therapy (xerostomia) and chemotherapy (alopecia and peripheral neuropathy) are only temporary.

Fatigue

A frequently reported problem after treatment for Hodgkin lymphoma is fatigue.[68] Although certainly not restricted to or in any way pathognomonic of Hodgkin lymphoma, fatigue seems to occur in a high proportion of patients successfully treated for Hodgkin lymphoma.[69–72] Over the last 5 years, there has been increased research on assessment of fatigue, and instruments are now available to measure the different aspects of this symptom.[73,74] As with quality of life in general, current opinion perceives fatigue as a combined construct with a number of dimensions. One dimension refers to physical and mental fatigue in accordance with what would be seen after intensive exercise or work. Other aspects include motivation, activity, and cognition, and the connection with mood states such as depression.[74] Interestingly, the available data suggest that a great proportion of the fatigue reported by patients is not due primarily to physical condition. Particularly in surviving patients after Hodgkin lymphoma or breast cancer, high levels of fatigue occur with normal levels of physical functioning.[71,75]

An example of an instrument that assesses fatigue is the Multidimensional Fatigue Inventory (MFI-20), which uses 20 items on five subscales.[73] Other questionnaires or modules for the assessment of fatigue are also available.[69,74]

The European Approach

Because no Hodgkin- or lymphoma-specific module for the assessment of quality of life and fatigue was available, the EORTC Lymphoma Group (EORTC LG) together with the French Groupe D'Etude des Lymphomes de L'Adulte (GELA) and the German Hodgkin Study Group (GHSG), and in close liaison and collaboration with the EORTC Quality of Life Group (EORTC QLG), devised an alternative way to measure quality of life and fatigue in patients with Hodgkin lymphoma.[37] The main elements of the EORTC QLQ C30 core instrument were supplemented by already-existing instruments or modules addressing in particular the dimensions of fatigue, sexuality, and fear of childlessness, and, as single questions, the special side effects of chemotherapy and radiotherapy.

The first use of this EORTC H8 Quality of Life (QL) questionnaire, developed for repeated measurement and extensively tested within the trial groups, has yielded promising results concerning psychometrics, applicability, and appropriateness of content. The H8-QL questionnaire is to date available in 10 European languages and is complemented by the Life Situation Questionnaire (LSQ), developed originally in Caen (France). The LSQ is currently available in French, German, and English and is being prepared for further international evaluation. It addresses the following areas: general living circumstances (e.g., housing), work history and current occupational status, marital status and family relationships, health records, family medical history, current health status, leisure activities, and economic and insurance problems related to Hodgkin lymphoma.[37,53]

Children and Adolescents

Only recently there has been progress in the development of instruments to measure quality of life and late effects in pediatric oncology.[76] Quality-of-life assessment in children must address normal developmental issues in such areas as peer relations, school, family, and play, which differ from the topics addressed in adult instruments. Questionnaires must also be suitably administered. In children under the age of 10 or 11, self-reporting is neither reliable nor feasible; proxy ratings by the parents or caregivers are necessary. A number of proxy and self-rating tools are already available from child psychology and psychiatry but no established and tested instruments exist for quality-of-life research in children and adolescents with Hodgkin lymphoma.[77,78]

Elderly

As with the quality-of-life assessment in pediatric oncology, only in the last few years have the problems of elderly patients been noticed.[79] Quality-of-life assessment in elderly patients must address the aspects of daily living and the adjustment to physical and mental disabilities. Questionnaires must be suitably devised and administered and the patients may need assistance in filling out the forms. For a subgroup of patients, self-reporting is no longer reliable or feasible; proxy ratings by caregivers are necessary. Some proxy and self-rating tools are meanwhile available from geriatrics but no validated instruments exist for quality-of-life research in elderly patients with Hodgkin lymphoma.[80]

Quality-Adjusted Life Years (QALYs)

The concept of QALYs[81,82] adjusts survival time (months/years) by a factor derived from quality-of-life measures, integrating quantity and quality of survival into one measurement. The use of QALYs allows integrating quality-of-life data into standard survival data (curves) to facilitate clinical decision making. Despite the attractiveness of this concept, a number of problems have arisen. One problem concerns calculated comparisons, because by this method, for example, one year with a 100% quality of life equals 10 years with a 10% quality of life. Obviously, a number of assumptions have to be made in comparing time and the quality of life. A second problem is related to the generation of adjustment factors and the time interval to which they are assigned. One of the assumptions is that time intervals with constant quality of life can be identified and that the corresponding adjustment factor (ranging from 0 to 1) can be measured accurately. Even if time intervals can be identified with a sufficient reliability to obtain quality-of-life indicators, it is still uncertain which quality-of-life domains are the most relevant for generating adjustment factors. In attempting to address some of these problems, different approaches have been taken to define time intervals and to generate quality-of-life adjustment factors for them.[83]

One of the more advanced methods is known as Time Without Symptoms and Toxicity (TWiST), or more recently Q-TWiST, which applies a patient-derived qualifying component to the adjustment process.[84,85] The patients who have primarily been studied with TWiST (e.g., breast cancer patients) had cancers with different pattern of outcomes and side effects than patients with Hodgkin lymphoma (in which there is a high probability of long-term survival, and late complications of treatment are extremely important). Years after treatment, normal life events can be as influential as the prior life-threatening illness. To make valid judgments, normal populations must be included to control for these variables. Thus, QALYs concepts rarely have been employed in Hodgkin lymphoma, but there are studies that have applied the methodology to cost-effectiveness analyses.[86] Furthermore, mixed-effects models making use of Q-TWiST approaches may prove useful in longitudinal quality-of-life studies with incomplete data sets as, one study suggests, also for Hodgkin lymphoma.[85]

USE OF QUALITY-OF-LIFE DATA

There are three general uses for quality-of-life measures to assist professionals in predicting patient outcomes and in planning patient-care programs: (a) to evaluate the extent of change in the quality of life of an individual or group across time or as an end-point in evaluating treatment outcome; (b) to predict outcome, prognosis, patient survival, or response to future treatment; and (c) to assess rehabilitation needs, and determine problem areas and coping patterns among various patient subgroups.[87–90]

Quality of Life as an Independent Variable

Quality-of-life measures can be used as either independent or dependent variables. In effectiveness of treatment studies, quality of life is used as an independent variable. In Example 1, quality of life after an intervention in patients versus controls is the independent variable, while survival time, or time to recurrence, is the dependent variable. Spiegel and associates[89] used quality-of-life measures among breast cancer patients randomized to treatment or controls. In an analysis of survival time (the dependent measure), they found that those patients in the group with intervention enjoyed a survival benefit of 18 months compared to patients in the control group.

Example 1: Effectiveness of Treatment Studies

$$= \frac{QL + Treatment\ versus\ Controls}{Survival\ Time,\ Time\ to\ Recurrence}$$

Rehabilitation studies provide a second example of quality of life used as an independent variable. In Example 2, quality-of-life measures are combined with medical variables to form the independent variable, with the dependent variable being a predictor such as depression or anxiety. Rehabilitation studies provide an example of data from quality-of-life measures that might be grouped as both independent and dependent variables.[90]

Example 2: Rehabilitation Studies

$$= \frac{Quality\ of\ Life + Medical\ Variables}{Patient\ Depression/QL\ Measures}$$

Using data from a cross-sectional group of Hodgkin patients, Fobair and colleagues[13] examined how return of energy and severity of treatment were predicted by depression scores at follow-up. Although the intent of the study was to describe the patients' problems, there was interest in using the results to inform the support services of the patient-care problems. In this analysis of data from 403 patients treated for Hodgkin lymphoma, the independent variables were energy loss, physical functioning, medical condition, stage of disease and type of treatment, and age at treatment. The dependent variable was the depression score on the CES-D.

Quality of Life as a Dependent Variable

Quality-of-life scores are used as the dependent or outcome measure in clinical trials (Example 3) comparing two treatments of similar biological effectiveness, to determine which treatment had the least emotional, social, or physical dysfunctioning.

Example 3: Comparison of Treatment Studies

$$= \frac{Treatment\ 1\ versus\ Treatment\ 2}{Quality-of-Life\ Scores}$$

In psychosocial studies, quality-of-life scores are used as dependent measures when data on the effectiveness of one or more interventions versus controls is analyzed for outcome. In medical outcome studies, quality of life can be viewed as being "as important as the conventional outcomes of survival and toxicity of therapy." Coates and Gebski[91] found that quality-of-life scores provided an independent predictor of survival duration for cancer patients when assessing the impact of the disease and its treatment.

The clinical applications of quality-of-life data benefit both the analysis of clinical trials and clinical practice. When used as an independent or predictive variable, quality-of-life data guide clinical decisions based on the effectiveness of treatment and assist in the early detection of morbidity. Used as a dependent measure, in the comparison of different treatments, quality of life helps to determine patient preferences among treatment choices in a systematic and quantifiable manner, and has prognostic value in predicting survival among patients treated for advanced disease "as patients perceive disease progression before it is clinically evident."[92]

APPLYING QUALITY-OF-LIFE INSTRUMENTS TO PATIENTS

There are three main reasons why investigators might measure quality of life: (a) to assess need for rehabilitation resources, (b) to use information as a predictor of outcome or prognosis, and (c) to have an end-point in evaluating treatment outcome. An overview of the main characteristics and instruments used in the most recent published quality-of-life studies in Hodgkin lymphoma are listed in Table 27.1. Results from these 38

TABLE 27.1

QUALITY-OF-LIFE STUDIES IN HODGKIN LYMPHOMA (N = 38)

Author	Study type, population	Survey modality	Instruments used	FU (yrs)	PR (%)	Areas explored
Hoerni et al. 1986[93] (n = 150)	Cross-sectional study Adult survivors of HL	SAQ	NV	2–7	—	Quality of life Information
Cella & Tross 1986[94] (n = 60)	Cross-sectional study Adults with HL compared with 20 healthy men	SAQ Interview	BSI DSFI subscales) IES RSES DAQ GAS	0.5–10	—	Psychosocial adaptation Emotion Sexuality Body image
Fobair et al. 1986[13] (n = 403)	Cross-sectional study Adults with HL	SAQ Interview	CES-D POMS	9 (1–21)	95	Psychosocial adaptation Sense of well-being Family relationship Employment
Wasserman et al. 1987[95] (n = 40)	Cross sectional study Children with HL	Interview	NV	7–19	—	Physical sequelae Social difficulties Experience of having a cancer
Devlen et al. 1987[96] (n = 120)	Prospective study Adults with HL and lymphoma	Interview	NV (treatment toxicity) Wechsler memory test	—	95	Toxicity of treatment Psychiatric morbidity Social morbidity
Bloom et al. 1989[12] (n = 85)	Cross-sectional study Adults with HL compared with adults with testicular cancer	SAQ Interview	POMS Social Support Scale SAS	3	—	Social morbidity Employment
Carpenter et al. 1989[97] (n = 43)	Cross-sectional study Adult survivors of HL	Interview	PAIS BDS (subscales) DSFI STAI	4–7 (0.5–13)	—	Psychosocial status Anxiety Sexuality
Hannah et al. 1992[16] (n = 24)	Cross-sectional study Adults with HL and their spouses compared with 34 adults with testicular cancer and their spouses	Interview	FES	—	—	Marital functioning Sexual functioning
Kornblith et al. 1992[98] (n = 93)	Cross-sectional study Adult survivors of HL	Interview	PAIS BSI POMS IES	2.2 (1–5)	76	Psychological, sexual, familial and vocational functioning
Kornblith et al. 1992[51] (n = 273)	Cross-sectional study Adult survivors of HL	Interview	PAIS BSI POMS IES DSF (subscales)	6.3 (1–20)	91	Psychosocial adaptation Sexuality Employment
Harrer et al. 1993[50] (n = 61)	Cross-sectional study Adult survivors of HL	Interview	FKV 102 FLZ	5 (1–16)	88	Coping strategies Life satisfaction
Bloom et al. 1993[10] (n = 85)	Cross-sectional study Adult with HL compared with 88 adults with testicular cancer	Interview	POMS CES-D SCL-90 SAS	1–7.5	88	Physical functioning Psychological distress Social outcome
van Tulder et al. 1994[54] (n = 81)	Cross-sectional study Adult survivors of HL compared with 160 hospital visitors	SAQ	SF36 NV (insurance, sexuality)	14 (10–18)	92	Psychosocial adaptation Sexuality Insurance
Ferrel et al. 1995[99] (n = 687)	Cross-sectional study Long-term adult survivors: 43% breast, 17% lymphoma and HL, 8% ovarian	SAQ	QOL-CS FACT-G	—	57	Physical, psychological adaptation Social outcome Spiritual well-being

(Continued)

TABLE 27.1

CONTINUED

Author	Study type, population	Survey modality	Instruments used	FU (yrs)	PR (%)	Areas explored
Joly et al. 1996[53] (n = 93)	Cross-sectional study Adult survivors of HL compared with 186 healthy men	SAQ	QLQ-C30 NV (insurance, work situation, medical consumption)	10 (4–17)	91	Physical, psychological adaptation Social outcome Insurance
Norum & Wist 1996[31] (n = 42)	Cross-sectional study Adult survivors of HL	SAQ	QLQ-C30 IES VAS QoL	5 (1–12)	86	Physical, psychological adaptation Social outcome Insurance QALY
Kornblith et al. 1998[100] (n = 273)	Cross-sectional study Adult survivors from 13 CALGB trials 1966–1988: HL compared with 206 acute leukaemia patients	Telephone interview	PAIS BSI CNVI NSI NV (insurance, employment, sexuality)	5–9	—	Psychosocial adjustment Employment Insurance Sexuality
Flechtner et al. 1998[37] (n >800)	Longitudinal studies after treatment completion EORTC H8 trial &GHSG HL8 trial	SAQ	QLQ-C30 MFI-20 Sexuality	—	—	Physical, psychological adaptation Social outcome Sexuality Fatigue
Loge et al. 1999[69] (n = 459)	Cross-sectional study Adult survivors of HL compared with normative data from the general Norwegian population	SAQ	FQ SF 36 HADS	12 (6–18)	82	Physical, psychological adaptation Social outcome Fatigue
Greil et al. 1999[101] (n = 126)	Cross-sectional study Adult survivors of HL	SAQ	QLQ-C30	9.1 (2–17)	65	Physical, psychological adaptation Social outcome
Van Schaik et al. 1999[102] (n = 33)	Cross-sectional study Childhood HL survivors	SAQ	NV (15 items connected to the HUI)	—	75	Health status
Torbjornsen et al. 2000[103] (n = 107)	Cross-sectional study Adult survivors of HL	SAQ	NV (religiosity, beliefs, QoL)	1–6	58	Religious beliefs and attitudes QoL
Van Agthoven et al. 2001[104] (n = 91)	Cross-sectional study PBSCT compared with ABMT for refractory or relapsed HL and non-HL lymphoma	SAQ	EuroQol RSCL SF-36	3 mo	58	Physical, psychological adaptation Social outcome
Cameron et al. 2001[105] (n = 273)	Cross-sectional study Adult survivors of HL	SAQ	NV (retrospective report on symptoms and QoL)	1–20	—	Physical, psychological adaptation Symptoms
Knobel et al. 2001[106] (n = 116)	Cross-sectional study Adult survivors of HL	SAQ	FQ	9 (6–12)	—	Fatigue
Ganz et al. 2003[107] (n = 247)	Longitudinal study Adults with HL from randomized SWOG trial 9133	SAQ	SDS CARES SF-36 (Vitality Scale) NV (work, family, health perception)	Baseline, 6 mo, 1y, 2 y	—	Physical, psychological adaptation Symptoms Social outcome
Gil-Fernández et al. 2003[108] (n = 46)	Cross-sectional study Adult survivors of HL compared with 46 healthy controls	SAQ	QLQ-C30 HADS	7–6 (1–22)	69	Physical, psychological adaptation Social outcome
Geffen et al. 2003[109] (n = 44)	Cross-sectional study Adult survivors of HL (n = 8) and non-HL (n = 36) compared with 44 controls	SAQ	SF-36 PTSD Inventory	>2	—	Physical, psychological adaptation Social outcome PTSD

(Continued)

TABLE 27.1

CONTINUED

Author	Study type, population	Survey modality	Instruments used	FU (yrs)	PR (%)	Areas explored
Wettergren et al. 2003[110] (n = 121)	Cross sectional study Adult survivors of HL compared with 236 healthy controls	Interview	SEIQoL-DW	14 (6–26)	62	Physical, psychological adaptation Social outcome Important life areas
Mounier et al. 2003[85] (n = 563)	Longitudinal study after treatment completion GELA patients from EORTC H8 trial	SAQ	QLQ-C30 Global QoL Score	3	—	Q-TWiST model (Global analysis QoL)
Rueffer et al. 2003[111] (n = 863)	Cross-sectional study Adult survivors of HL from the GHSG trials HL1-6 (1981–1993) compared with 935 healthy controls	SAQ	QLQ-C30 MFI 20 Sexuality LSQ	5–2	61	Physical, psychological adaptation Social outcome Sexuality Fatigue Important life areas
Glossmann et al. 2003[112] (n = 60)	Longitudinal randomized study Salvage treatment after relapse	SAQ	QLQ-C30 MFI 20 Sexuality	—	—	Physical, psychological adaptation Symptoms Social outcome Sexuality Fatigue
Wettergren et al. 2004[113] [113] (n = 121)	Cross-sectional study Adult survivors of HL compared with 236 healthy controls	Interview SAQ	SEIQoL-DW HADS SF-12 SOC	14 (6–26)	62	Physical, psychological adaptation Social outcome Coping Important life areas
Holzner et al. 2004[114] (n = 126)	Cross-sectional study Adult survivors of HL compared with 926 healthy controls	SAQ	FACT-G	9.1 (2–16)	—	Physical, psychological adaptation Social outcome Important life areas
Wettergren et al. 2005[115] (n = 121)	Cross sectional study Adult survivors of HL	Interview SAQ	SEIQoL-DW HADS SF-12	14 (6–26)	62	Physical, psychological adaptation Social outcome Important life areas
Hjermstad et al. 2005[71] (n = 476)	Cross-sectional study Adult survivors of HL Comparison with prior assessment from 1994 (n = 280)	SAQ	FQ	16 (4–36)	81	Fatigue
Kawiecka Dziembowska B et al. 2005[116] (n = 50)	Cross-sectional study Adults with HL	SAQ	WHOQOL HLRS ZSTS	—	—	Physical, psychological adaptation Social outcome Temperament
Hjermstad et al. 2006[72] (n = 475)	Cross-sectional study Adult survivors of HL compared with normative data from the general Norwegian population	SAQ	FQ SF-36	16 (4–36)	80	Physical, psychological adaptation Social outcome Fatigue

SAQ, self-administered questionnaire; NV, not validated questionnaire; HL, Hodgkin lymphoma; GHSG, German Hodgkin Study Group, EORTC, European Organization for the Research and Treatment of Cancer; GELA, Groupe D'Etude des Lymphomes de L'Adulte; FU, Follow-up; PR: Participation rate. BDS, Beck depression scale; BSI, Brief Symptoms Inventory; CARES, Cancer Rehabilitation Evaluation System - Short Form; CES-D, Center for Epidemiologic Studies Depression scale; CNVI, Conditioned Nausea and Vomiting triggered by treatment-related stimuli; DAQ, Death Anxiety Questionnaire; DSFI, Derogatis Sexual Functioning Inventory; FACT-G, Functional Assessment of Cancer Therapy-General; FES, Family Environment Scale; FKV 102, Freiburg Questionnaire of Coping with Chronic Illness; FLZ, Questionnaire for Life Satisfaction; GAS, Global Assessment Scale; HADS, Hospital Anxiety and Depression Scale; RS, Hamilton Depression Rating Scale; HUI, Health Utilities Index; IES, Impact of Events Scales; LSQ, Life Situation Questionnaire; MFI-20, Multidimensional Fatigue Inventory; NSI, Negative Socioeconomic Impact of Cancer Index; PAIS, Psychosocial Adjustment to Illness Scale; POMS, Profile of mood states; QLQ-C30, EORTC Quality of life core questionnaire; QOL-CS, Quality of Life Cancer Survivors; Q-TWiST, Quality-adjusted Time Without Symptoms and Toxicity; RSCL, Rotterdam Symptom Checklist; RSES, Rosenberg Self-Esteem Scales; SAS, Social Activities Scale; SCL-90, 90-item Symptoms Checklist; SDS, Symptom Distress Scale; SEIQoL-DW, Schedule for the Evaluation of the Individual Quality of Life – Direct Weighting; SF-12, 12- item Short Form health survey; SF-36, 36-item Short Form health survey; SOC, Sense of Coherence Scale; STAI, State-Trait Anxiety Inventory; VAS, Visual Analogue Scale; WHOQOL, WHO Quality of Life Scale; ZSTS, Zawadzki and Strelau Temperament Scale.

investigations over the last 20 years include a variety of findings from subjective and objective sources. Severe limitations in long-term outcome were found as well as nearly undisturbed re-adaptation to normal life.[93–116]

To Address the Need for Rehabilitation

Cancer and its treatment affect many aspects of quality of life in long-term survivors of malignancy.[117] Information from different questionnaires can help better understand the needs of patients and improve support after treatment. Most validated questionnaires only consider overall quality of life or contain a limited number of aspects of quality of life such as depression or anxiety.[118,119] Although, for example, assessment of sexuality is present in 34% of studies on quality of life of cancer survivors, spiritual (10.4%) and economic (12.3%) patient-specific outcomes are infrequently addressed.[102] Aspects of quality of life, including difficulties in family, professional, and social settings, in using medical resources, and in financial security (one recent population-based study found that patients had difficulties in obtaining banks loans), must be correlated with standard quality-of-life scales.[53,111,121] Several of the above questions have been included in a few validated questionnaires such as the CARES.[122] To cover all aspects of quality of life, multiple questionnaires will have to be used during each assessment, although this will entail some duplication.

Predictors of Outcome or Prognosis

Performance status has been shown to significantly predict survival for a number of tumors. Patients with good scores on quality-of-life measures have longer survival times.[123,124] One explanation for this is that patients with fewer effects of the tumor have either an earlier stage of disease and thus a better prognosis or are more likely to tolerate and benefit from effective treatment.[125] Quality-of-life measures performed prior to treatment are used as variables for stratification in randomized clinical trials.[92,126] Although this represents progress, such stratification usually is based on a single measure, while quality of life can be highly dependent on the time of assessment. Also, the use of only one score, which may have been arbitrarily selected for stratification or as a predictor, may be less than optimal, as multiple scores are provided that correspond to well-defined quality-of-life dimensions that cannot be used separately. Also, there are concerns that "the use of quality-of-life data as part of the characterization of patients raises the possibility that such data might also be used as a basis for discrimination."[127] Validated quality-of-life questionnaires have not been used as indicators for response to therapy, clinical outcome, or survival. Only very recently quality-of-life dimensions (e.g., "fatigue") have been included in the initial planning of clinical trials, in particular when reduction of treatment burden was the aim.[128,129]

End-Points in Evaluating Treatment Outcome

In evaluating treatment outcome, the purpose is not to identify problems for rehabilitation but to compare the quality of life across alternative treatments. Repeated quality-of-life data might be used as an end-point or outcomes measure in clinical trials in addition to more conventional end-points such as survival and time to relapse. Disease-specific measures are clinically sensible in that patients and clinicians intuitively find the items directly relevant. This increases the potential for compliance and is particularly compelling in the clinical trial setting. The disadvantages of this approach are the multiple comparisons and the lack of a unified scoring system that may lead to

difficulties in interpretation.[130] In clinical trials that have equivalent disease-free and overall survival results, quality-of-life assessment may help in selecting the best treatment arm. However, quality-of-life assessment should not be considered as a surrogate end–point.[131]

Generic Versus Specific Questionnaires

Generic questionnaires cover a broad range of quality-of-life dimensions in a single instrument. Their use facilitates comparisons among various individuals or diseases. This approach is particularly important for studies aimed at evaluating rehabilitation and long-term sequelae of treatment. Generic questionnaires can be applied to both normal volunteers and to patients. The use of both generic and specific questionnaires can improve quality-of-life assessment because items included in specific questionnaires relate more to a particular disease than do generic questionnaires. Therefore, the type of questionnaire used (generic, specific, or both) depends on the objectives of the study; during the time of therapy, disease-specific measures might be of greatest interest, whereas generic measures, because they permit comparisons across conditions and populations, are of greatest interest in post-treatment longitudinal studies or in cross-sectional studies in long-term survivors.[132]

Psychometric Versus Utility Measures

Utility measures of quality of life, another type of generic instrument, are derived from economic and decision theory.[133] Their use is particularly appropriate when choices exist between length of life or length of remission and quality of life. In this approach (e.g., Q-TWIST), the survival time is weighed by disease progression and adverse events of treatment. Q-TWIST can add complementary data to the standard evaluation of survival, as was demonstrated in post-menopausal patients with breast cancer.[134] In clinical trials where the major focus is patient benefit, the Q-TWIST can be integrated with a psychometric scale. The association of two such complementary approaches can be of great interest in trials comparing two treatment modalities with similar efficacy but different toxicity. This is particularly the case in clinical trials aiming at scaling down treatment modalities such as in early-stage Hodgkin lymphoma. Because the methodology in assessing quality of life is not yet perfected, the results of quality-of-life studies should be regarded as a process to facilitate discussion, and not merely a process of measurement.[85]

When Should Quality-of-Life Instruments Be Administered?

The timing of quality-of-life assessment and its frequency depend on the study aim, the expected sensitivity of the survey, and constraints from both patients and medical staff. In spite of growing knowledge from recent longitudinal studies, it is difficult to suggest a standard schedule.[135] The use of infrequent evaluations may miss transient effects that are likely to appear during and after therapy. On the other hand, repeated inquiries may increase patient stress or decrease compliance. In randomized clinical trials, a baseline quality-of-life assessment before initiation of treatment is necessary. Subsequent quality-of-life assessments, during or after treatment, may need to take into account any preexisting intra-group differences in baseline quality-of-life characteristics. This may help to assess whether or not observed changes can be attributed to treatment.

The impact of cumulative toxicity can be measured at two or more points during treatment, whereas disease-related impact on quality of life should be measured after acute toxicity has subsided, generally months or years following the end of therapy.[136] This quality-of-life assessment could be coupled with routine follow-up visits. Later quality-of-life assessment in long-term survivors would help in distinguishing the respective impacts of the treatment and the cancer. The number and the timing of follow-up quality-of-life assessments depend on whether it is desirable to measure long-term treatment and disease-related toxicity as well as the entire duration of the beneficial effects of therapy. Development of specific questionnaires on rehabilitation needs is particularly appropriate in long-term quality-of-life assessment. Short questionnaires should improve long-term compliance. Ideally long-term quality-of-life assessments should be prospective and continuous. If these are not possible, cross-sectional studies with comparison to a healthy population can facilitate understanding of patients' long-term difficulties.[53,111]

USE OF QUALITY-OF-LIFE INSTRUMENTS IN CLINICAL TRIALS

A review of the most important randomized clinical trials in Hodgkin lymphoma also reveals that quality of life is disregarded as a primary or even as a secondary outcome measure and only since the mid-90s have international study groups like the EORTC Lymphoma Group and the German Hodgkin Study Group (GHSG) adopted longitudinal quality-of-life assessment in their randomized trials and used quality of life as a therapy end-point.[37,128] However, retrospective analyses of long-term survivors of Hodgkin lymphoma have already shown that a substantial subgroup of patients has demonstrable effects of the disease and its treatment even years after the end of treatment (Table 27.1). It remains unclear when in the course of the disease one can distinguish patients with good coping mechanisms from those without. To more precisely characterize the difficulties in adjustment after treatment, quality-of-life assessment has to be included in prospective randomized clinical trials.

Most randomized clinical trials must be conducted by cooperative groups because of the low incidence of Hodgkin lymphoma. A major challenge to prospective multicenter trials using longitudinal data on quality of life is the completeness of data sets, as missing data limits the value of the results.[137] A high standard of data collection is essential for the trial to be successful.[132] To obtain completeness of data, quality-of-life assessments have to be a mandatory component of the clinical trial design and part of the inclusion criteria.[138] However, assurance of a complete data set will only be guaranteed by convincing the patient and the participating physicians and nurses of the importance of, and the future therapeutic impact of, quality-of-life assessment in randomized clinical trials.

The prognosis of Hodgkin lymphoma has dramatically improved over the last decades.[139] Today, over 80% of all patients are cured. In patients with early- and intermediate-stage Hodgkin lymphoma, future therapeutic efforts should aim at reducing early and late toxicity. In recent years, several advances in reducing treatment-related toxicity in early and intermediate stages have been achieved. For example, in the H6 twin study, the EORTC Lymphoma Cooperative Group demonstrated that diagnostic staging laparotomy is no longer warranted in the workup of patients with early-stage Hodgkin lymphoma, because overall survival was similar in patients with or without laparotomy. The advantage of more extensive staging was counterbalanced by the morbidity and mortality of the procedure.[140] A meta-analysis conducted by Specht and colleagues[141] demonstrated that combined-modality treatment consisting of chemotherapy and irradiation results in lower recurrence rates than radiation alone in early-stage Hodgkin lymphoma. The recently published H7 trial of the EORTC Lymphoma Cooperative Group showed that EBVP and involved-field RT can replace STNI as standard treatment in favorable patients, whereas EBVP was inferior to MOPP/ABV in the unfavorable subgroup. Furthermore, a prognostic factor-based treatment approach led to high overall survival rates in both favorable and unfavorable patients.[142]

This strategy, however, may have a substantial impact on early and late toxicity as well as on quality of life. Because late toxicities, such as cardiopulmonary toxicities or secondary neoplasia, occur years after treatment, long-term follow-up has to be performed.[19] Quality-of-life assessments can help in demonstrating advantages of new treatment strategies and thus, quality-of-life assessment has to be included in studies aiming at reducing treatment-related toxicity. Until recently, treatment results were not satisfactory for patients with advanced Hodgkin lymphoma. Present studies, however, suggest that dose-intensive chemotherapy regimens might induce cure rates comparable to those observed in patients with early- and intermediate-stage disease. With the introduction of the BEACOPP (bleomycin, etoposide, Adriamycin [doxorubicin], cyclophosphamide, Oncovin [vincristine], procarbazine, and prednisone) regimens, higher freedom-from-treatment failure and survival rates were achieved by the GHSG.[143] This improvement is accompanied by a considerable increase in acute toxicity such as myelosuppression and infections. Future efforts should concentrate on the search for the most effective regimen with the lowest toxicity and the least influence on quality of life.

Quality of Life as Primary or Secondary Outcome

Quality-of-life assessment in patients with Hodgkin lymphoma is not yet established as a standard part of clinical trials, and it remains unclear whether quality-of-life scales are able to detect relevant differences between treatment arms. In particular, the question of what score difference constitutes a clinically relevant difference for the patient has gained considerable attention.[144] Data are available from a number of quality-of-life studies that suggest that score differences of at least 8/100 but preferably above 15/100 would mean a clinically relevant change for the patient. Considering that it is unknown what amount of time is required before long-term disadvantages in quality of life become obvious, the length of time during which patients should be evaluated cannot be anticipated. The EORTC LG together with the GELA and the GHSG are including longitudinal quality-of-life assessment in ongoing trials, and it is hoped that these will contribute answers to the questions posed. Preliminary analyses suggest that 2 to 3 years after completion of therapy seems to be a crucial time period and a possible turning point for recovery or long-term limitations.[128,129] However, mechanisms and details remain subject to further analyses and investigation.

Under the mentioned circumstances, quality-of-life assessment is regarded usually as a secondary outcomes measure. Before it can be used as a primary outcome, quality-of-life assessment must fulfill various requirements and the method of assessment must be shown to be applicable in a multicenter setting. However, in a study aiming at reducing treatment-related toxicities, assessment of quality of life should be mandatory, at least as a secondary end-point.

Does QALY Add to the Final Treatment Decision?

Recently, there have been attempts to evaluate treatment outcome using surrogate parameters of overall survival or freedom from treatment failure. Efforts have been made to set up a correlation between life-years gained and the patients' self-reported quality of life. However, there is still a substantial debate on how to measure health-related quality of life.[145,146]

Norum and co-workers[86] have shown that the cost-benefit correlation for patients with Hodgkin lymphoma is very favorable in the Norwegian setting. The cost per gained life-year was estimated at 1,651 English pounds. Compared with other cancer entities, the cost appears to be very low.

In patients with curable disease, one can argue that curing the patient is more important than the consequences of treatment, especially when there is not much difference from one strategy to another. However, early data are available on loss of quality of life years after treatment. Should longitudinal assessment of quality of life demonstrate that a significant loss in quality of life is dependent on the type of treatment administered and that it varies with treatment modality, an evaluation using the QALY approach might help identify which treatment is associated with the optimal cost-benefit. Nevertheless, to compare several Hodgkin lymphoma treatment strategies, methods of measuring health-related quality of life remain to be standardized.[146]

GENERAL POPULATION COMPARISON

The Importance of Control Comparison

The aim of randomized clinical trials is usually to compare the efficacy of two or more treatments. When the compared treatments are expected to differ, quality of life can be considered as an additional end-point; when the treatments are expected to be equivalent, quality of life can be considered as the main end-point. Because in randomized clinical trials patient characteristics are similar in both treatment arms, it is not necessary to use a healthy control population. In contrast, the use of a control group is particularly important in epidemiologic studies where the objectives are to evaluate the incidence and the impact of the disease and/or its treatment on the patients' quality of life. In long-term cancer survivors, the use of a healthy population as control is fundamental to evaluate the respective impact of cancer and its treatment compared to baseline socioeconomic quality of life. This approach contains two difficult aspects: the choice of a questionnaire that can be administered to both cancer patients and controls, and the selection of a reference population.[147,148]

Quality-of-Life Reference Data

A number of questionnaires were developed for, and validated on, the healthy population. All of them are generic—for example, the NHP questionnaire,[56] the SIP questionnaire,[57] and the MOS SF-36 questionnaire.[58] The advantages of using such questionnaires include the following: (a) they can be applied to healthy and patient populations, (b) they are quick to administer and easy to complete, and (c) reference scores from healthy populations are available. Disadvantages include (a) limited exploration of quality of life in healthy population, (b) socioprofessional parameters in long-term survivors are not explored, and (c) specific aspects of disease and treatment

are not evaluated. Validated generic quality-of-life questionnaires have been used in various healthy population studies and the results published.[147–149] These studies provide data on quality of life for use as a comparison with questionnaires issued to patients with cancer. However, these control data have some limitations. First, comparison is effective only at the time of the study, because socioeconomic conditions may change and they are likely to influence the quality of life of healthy subjects as well as that of cancer survivors. Second, even for a particular group of individuals, it might not be possible to extrapolate the available data from one country to another, or from one area of a given country to another, because of potential cross-cultural biases. Third, information obtained is restricted to that explored by the generic questionnaire(s) used.

Case-Control Studies

Case-control studies can be used to avoid the potential biases of quality-of-life reference data. Their advantages are that controls can be matched to patients at the time of the study, and that other questionnaires can be added to the generic one to assess marital and familial issues, socioprofessional status, medical care, and so on (as in the LSQ). This information might be particularly relevant in long-term cancer survivor studies.

Patients to be Enrolled

The selection of cases is important; it can greatly affect the results of the study. In general population studies, patients obtained from cancer registry databases, where available, represent unbiased cases. This approach controls for the characteristics and the specificity of medical practice in a given area. In contrast, cases from hospital series are only representative of the recruitment and the clinical practice of the specific hospital.

Selection of Controls

The designation of the type of control group is the most difficult task in planning a case-control study.[150] The selection of the controls depends on the study-specific aims and circumstances. If the aim of the study is to evaluate the quality of life of long-term cancer survivors in comparison to that of a healthy population, a population-based series is the best choice because such controls are especially comparable with the cases. When a hospital-based series of cases is assembled, the use of population controls is also recommended, because multiple biases can occur in the selection of hospital controls. There are two main disadvantages associated with the use of the general population-based controls. First, the individuals selected are often not cooperative, and response tends to be worse than that from other types of controls and from cases.[151,152] Second, a substantial proportion of controls might present with a previously unknown cancer history. For example, in a study by Rieker and associates,[153] cases from a hospital series were matched to general population controls on sociodemographic characteristics, while in an investigation by Joly and co-workers,[53] both cases and controls issued from the general population. An alternative to the selection of a general population control group is that of controls from among cases' neighbors,[154] hospital visitors,[54] or cases' siblings.[155] This alternative, however, should be considered with caution because of multiple potential biases.

When the objective of the study is to explore the impact of site-specific outcomes, because of disease-specific treatment, controls should be selected among patients treated for another

TABLE 27.2

CASE-CONTROL STUDIES IN LONG-TERM SURVIVORS OF HODGKIN LYMPHOMA (N = 12)

Study	Cases (patients)	Controls	Instruments	FU (yrs)	Main results
Cella & Tross 1986[94]	60 male survivors	20 healthy males matched on age	Interview	0.5–10	Significant lower intimacy motivation, increasing avoidant thinking about illness, prolonged difficulty in returning to premorbid work status and illness-related concerns Cancer patients were significantly more appreciative of life than controls
Kornblith et al. 1992[98]	33 patients treated with ABVD	Patients treated with MOPP (n = 31) or MOPP-ABVD (n = 29) within a clinical trial	Interview SAQ	2.2 (1–5)	No significant long-term advantage in psychological adaptation or psychosexual function for survivors of HL treated with the less gonadally toxic ABVD regimen
Bloom et al. 1993[10]	85 males treated in 3 university hospitals	88 men with testicular cancer	Interview	1–7.5	More focused symptoms among controls (decrease in sexual enjoyment, poor health habits) More generalized symptoms among cases (fatigue, energy loss, work impairment) Similar levels of infertility and erectile dysfunction Most of these differences were site-related
van Tulder et al. 1994[54]	81 patients treated at a single institution	116 hospital visitors	SAQ	14 (10–18)	More physical, role, sexuality impairment and low perception of overall health among cases
Joly et al. 1996[53]	93 patients issued from the regional cancer registry	186 matched controls (age and sex) from the regional population registry	SAQ	10 (4–17)	More physical, role, and cognitive impairments among cases Major limitation in borrowing from banks remained the major problem in cases
Loge et al. 1999[69]	459 patients (1971–1991) treated at the Norwegian Radium Hospital	General Norwegian population	SAQ	12 (6–18)	Higher levels and longer lasting of fatigue among cases Disease stage predicted fatigue No association with treatment characteristics
Gil-Fernández et al. 2003[108]	46 patients treated at a single institution	46 matched controls (age, sex, social status) from the local medical faculty	SAQ	7 (1–22)	More physical and social impairments among cases Higher levels of anxiety in females Higher depression level in patients above 45 years No differences in global quality of life
Geffen et al. 2003[109]	8 HL patients and 36 non-HL patients treated at a single institution	44 controls with a trauma history	SAQ	>2	No significant difference in the number of cases with PTSD (32% lymphoma patients vs. 25% controls) Lower physical HRQoL in lymphoma patients Significant increase in the hyperarousal scale in lymphoma patients
Wettergren et al. 2003, 2004, 2005[110,113,115]	121 patients treated in Stockholm County (1972–1991)	236 matched controls (age and sex) from the regional population registry	Interview SAQ	14 (6–26)	Most important reported life areas were: family, personal health, work, relations to other people Lower physical health in patients No other differences in mentioned areas or quality of life indices between cases and controls

(Continued)

TABLE 27.2

CONTINUED

Study	Cases (patients)	Controls	Instruments	FU (yrs)	Main results
Rueffer et al. 2003[111]	836 patients from the GHSG trials HD1-6 (1981–1993)	935 matched controls (age, sex, living area) from regional population registries	SAQ	5	Higher levels of fatigue in cases Fatigue associated with: systemic symptoms, KPS, occurrence of relapse Time since end of treatment had no influence on the reported fatigue levels
Holzner et al. 2004[114]	126 patients treated at a single institution (1969–1994)	926 controls from the general Austrian population	SAQ	9 (2–16)	Higher functional, social well-being and total scores in cases compared to controls
Hjermstad et al. 2006[72]	475 patients (1971–1997) treated at the Norwegian Radium Hospital	General Norwegian population	SAQ	12 (6–18)	Higher levels of total fatigue (TF) in cases Persisting chronic fatigue (CF) was associated with B-symptoms at diagnosis and treatment period 50% of patients reporting CF in 1994 did not report CF 8 years later No correlation of fatigue levels with treatment variables (e.g., radiation fields)

MOPP, mechlorethamine, vincristine, procarbazine, prednisone ; ABVD, adriamycin, bleomycin, vinblastine, dacarbazine.
SAQ, self-administered questionnaire; NV, not validated questionnaire; HL,: Hodgkin lymphoma; GHSG, German Hodgkin Study Group; EORTC, European Organization for the Research and Treatment of Cancer; GELA, Groupe D'Etude des Lymphomes de L'Adulte; HRQoL, Health-related quality of life: KPS, Karnofsky Performance Scale.

type of cancer with a similar clinical outcome. This approach was used by Bloom and colleagues, who compared the psychosocial outcomes of patients treated for testicular cancer and patients treated for Hodgkin lymphoma.[10]

Short Review on Ongoing and Completed Research

Case-controls studies performed in Hodgkin lymphoma survivors are listed in Table 27.2. Only one study concerned cases derived from a population cancer registry. Seven studies involved healthy controls (three from regional population registries and three from the general population). One study compared quality of life in Hodgkin lymphoma survivors to that of testicular-cancer survivors, and another to controls with a trauma history. Four studies used an interview alone or in combination with self-administrated questionnaires, and eight studies employed questionnaires alone. Results depend largely on the choice of controls; the main results are given in Table 27.2.

CONCLUSIONS

The assessment of quality of life has become important, especially in the evaluation of treatment given to patients with a chronic illness such as cancer. Although overall survival and survival without disease have long been used as the end-points in clinical trials, evaluation of these end-points alone is no longer accepted because other characteristics are now considered as important as survival by both patients and physicians. Among these, treatment burden, treatment-related

toxicity, as well as their psychological and social impacts, are of great importance.

This change stems from the dramatic improvement in the efficacy of cancer treatments, particular those for Hodgkin lymphoma. Effective therapies, however, have several drawbacks that might limit their use. Chemotherapy as well as radiation therapy can induce severe acute and late toxicities that may lead to death long before what would otherwise be expected. Because most patients with Hodgkin lymphoma have a very long life expectancy after diagnosis and treatment, one should always keep in mind the distinction that exists between curing the disease and curing the patient. Several studies have highlighted the difficulties that survivors may experience long after treatment ends, such as general fatigue, health fragility, and social and financial problems. These findings have been demonstrated in studies where a quality-of-life approach has been used.

In this chapter, we have attempted to illustrate how difficult it is to properly study the quality of life of patients both in the clinical trial setting and in epidemiologic studies. Instruments, mainly questionnaires, have been developed specifically for the general population or for patients, although there are no instruments specific to Hodgkin lymphoma. Most of these instruments are validated, but they are not always available in multiple languages, which limits their use. Also, they generally do not include items on family and social issues, professional limitations, and medical care. Thus, several research teams have begun developing life-situation questionnaires, but reliability and validity remain to be demonstrated.

Like happiness, quality of life is an ambiguous concept, with various definitions. Therefore, it is difficult for a questionnaire to adequately summarize all aspects of quality of life even though patients have contributed to its production. Interviews are less impersonal than questionnaires. Their reliability, however, depends on the experience the interviewer has gained and on his or her fairness in analyzing the patient's responses. In Hodgkin lymphoma, there has been no analysis of the results of interviews and of generic or specific questionnaires administered to the same patients. Such a study would potentially help interpret the results of studies limited to the use of self-administered questionnaires.

Before starting a quality-of-life assessment, one should always consider the following questions: What is the question being asked? Will quality-of-life assessment help answer the question? What is the population to be studied? How many patients should be enrolled? What should the study design be (e.g., cross-sectional or longitudinal)? Do validated instruments exist that can be used to assess quality of life? Can they be used in a longitudinal study, that is, can they be repeated over time? What would an interview add to questionnaires? Is the study feasible? Are its time demands reasonable?

These questions are not very different from the questions researchers face before undertaking a clinical study. Quality-of-life assessment should benefit patients by defining issues that are important to them, even long after they have been cured. Quality-of-life assessment should not be considered an end in itself, but rather a way to help physicians evaluate the efficacy and toxicity of treatment and help in making medical decisions among treatment strategies with similar efficacy but different toxicity.

References

1. Ware JE. Conceptualization and measurement of health-related quality of life: comments on an evolving field. *Arch Phys Med Rehabil* 2003;84(suppl 2):43–51.
2. Karnofsky DA, Burchenal JH. The clinical evaluation of chemotherapeutic agents in cancer. In: MacLeod CM, ed. *Evaluation of chemotherapeutic agents.* New York: Columbia University Press; 1949:191–195.
3. Strain JJ. The evolution of quality of life evaluations in cancer therapy. *Oncology* 1990;4:22–26.
4. *Guidance for Industry. Patient-Reported Outcome Measures: Use in Medical Product Development to Support Labeling Claims. Draft Guidance.* Rockville, MD.: U.S. Department of Health and Human Services, Food and Drug Administration; 2006.
5. Osoba D. What has been learned from measuring health-related quality of life in clinical oncology. *Eur J Cancer* 1999;35:1565–1570.
6. Cella DF. Quality of life: concepts and definition. *J Pain Symptom Manage* 1994;9:186–192.
7. Ganz PA. Quality of life and the patient with cancer. Iindividual and policy implications. *Cancer* 1994;74(Suppl):1445–1452.
8. Gotay CC. Trial-related quality of life: using quality-of-life assessment to distinguish among cancer therapies. *J Natl Cancer Inst Monogr* 1996;20:1–6.
9. Osoba D. Measuring the effect of cancer on health-related quality of life. *Pharmacoeconomics* 1995;7:308–319.
10. Bloom JR, Fobair P, Gritz E, Wellisch D. Psychosocial outcomes of cancer: a comparative analysis of Hodgkin's disease and testicular cancer. *J Clin Oncol* 1993;11:979–988.
11. Bloom JR, Gorsky RD, Fobair P, et al. Physical performance at work and at leisure: validation of a measure of biological energy in survivors of Hodgkin's disease. *J Psychosoc Oncol* 1990;8:49–55.
12. Bloom JR, Hoppe RT, Fobair P, et al. Effects of treatment on the work experiences of long-term survivors of Hodgkin's disease. *J Psychosoc Oncol* 1989;6:65–71.
13. Fobair P, Hoppe RT, Bloom J, et al. Psychosocial problems among survivors of Hodgkin's disease. *J Clin Oncol* 1986;4:805–814.
14. Fobair P, Mages NL. Psychosocial morbidity among cancer patients survivors. In: Ahmed P, ed. *Coping with cancer.* New-York: Elsevierl 1981:285–291.
15. Bloom JR, Fobair P, Spiegel D, et al. Social supports and the social well-being of cancer survivors. In: Algrecht G, ed. *Advances in medical sociology,* vol 2. New-York: JAI Press; 1991:95–99.
16. Hannah MT, Gritz ER, Wellisch DK, et al. Changes in marital and sexual functioning in long- term survivors and their spouses: testicular cancer versus Hodgkin's disease. *Psychooncology* 1992;1:89–94.
17. Donovan K, Sanson-Fisher RW, Redman S. Measuring quality of life in cancer patients. *J Clin Oncol* 1989;7:959–968.
18. Draube A, Behringer K, Diehl V. German Hodgkin's Lymphoma Study Group trials: lessons from the past and current strategies. *Clin Lymphoma Myeloma* 2006;6:458–468.
19. Mauch P, Ng A, Aleman B, et al. Report from the Rockefeller Foundation sponsored international workshop on reducing mortality and improving quality of life in long-term survivors of Hodgkin's disease: July 9–16, 2003, Bellagio, Italy. *Eur J Haematol* 2005;66:68–76.
20. Ganz PA, Haskell CM, Figlin RA, et al. Estimating the quality of life in a clinical trial of patients with metastatic lung cancer using the Karnofsky performance status and the Functional Living Index-Cancer. *Cancer* 1988;61:849–856.
21. Coates A, Gebski V, Bishop JF. Improving the quality of life during chemotherapy for advanced breast cancer. A comparison of intermittent and continuous treatment strategies. *N Engl J Med* 1987;317:1490–1495.
22. Cella DF, Tulsky DS. Quality of life in cancer: definition, purpose, and method of measurement. *Cancer Invest* 1993;11:327–336.
23. Coates A, Dillenbeck CF, McNeil DR. On the receiving end. II. Linear analogue self-assessment (LASA) in evaluation of aspects of the quality of life of cancer patients receiving therapy. *Eur J Cancer Clin Oncol* 1983;19: 1633–1637.
24. Bernhard J, Hürny C, Bacchi M, et al. Initial prognostic factors in small-cell lung cancer patients predicting quality of life during chemotherapy. *Br J Cancer* 1996;74:1660–1667.
25. Aaronson NK, Bullinger M, Ahmedzai S. A modular approach to quality-of-life assessment in cancer clinical trials. *Recent Results Cancer Res* 1988;111:231–249.
26. van Dongen-Melman JEWM, Sanders-Woudstra JAR. Psychosocial aspects of childhood cancer: A review of the literature. *J Child Psychol Psychiat* 1986;27:145–180.
27. Eiser C. Children and cancer. *Pediatr Rehabil* 2002;5:187–189.
28. Ferrell BR, Dow K, Grant M. Measurement of the quality of life in cancer survivors. *Qual Life Res* 1995;4:523–531.
29. Flechtner H, Rüffer U, Eisenbarth M, et al. Quality of life and life situation after cure from Hodgkin's disease. *Psychooncology* 1996;5:10.
30. Kornblith AB, Anderson J, Cella DF, et al. Quality of life assessment of Hodgkin's disease survivors: a model for cooperative clinical trials. *Oncology* 1990;4:93–101.
31. Norum J, Wist EA. Quality of life in survivors of Hodgkin's disease. *Qual Life Res* 1996;5:367–374.
32. Flechtner H. Quality of life research in somatic medicine and psychiatry. *Pharmacopsychiatry* 1997;30:239.
33. Anderson RT, Aaronson NK, Wilkin D. Critical review of the international assessments of health-related quality of life. *Qual Life Res* 1993;2:369–395.
34. Sprangers MA, Cull A, Bjordal K, et al. The European Organization for Research and Treatment of Cancer approach to quality of life assessment: guidelines for developing questionnaire modules. *Qual Life Res* 1993;2: 287–295.
35. Aaronson NK, Ahmedzai S, Bergman B, et al. The European Organization for Research and Treatment of Cancer QLQ-C30: a quality-of-life instrument for use in international clinical trials in oncology. *J Natl Cancer Inst* 1993;85:365–376.
36. van Dis FW, Mols F, Vingerhoets AJ, et al.. A validation study of the Dutch version of the Quality of Life-Cancer Survivor (QOL-CS) questionnaire in a group of prostate cancer survivors. *Qual Life Res* 2006;15:1607–1612.
37. Flechtner H, Rueffer JU, Henry-Amar M, et al. Quality of life assessment in Hodgkin's disease: a new comprehensive approach. First experiences from the EORTC/GELA and GHSG trials. EORTC Lymphoma Cooperative Group, Groupe D'Etude des Lymphomes de l'Adulte, and German Hodgkin Study Group. *Ann Oncol* 1998;9:147–154.
38. Ware JE. Methodology in behavioral and psychosocial cancer research. Conceptualizing disease impact and treatment outcomes. *Cancer* 1984;53 (suppl):2316–2326.
39. de Haes JC, van Knippenberg FC. The quality of life of cancer patients: a review of the literature. *Soc Sci Med* 1985;20:809–815.
40. Spitzer WO, Dobson AJ, Hall J, et al. Measuring the quality of life of cancer patients. *J Chron Dis* 1981;34:585–597.
41. Kornblith AB, Holland JC. Model for quality-of-life research from the Cancer and Leukemia Group B: the telephone interview, conceptual approach to measurement, and theoretical framework. *NCI Monogr* 1996;20:55–62.
42. Dehmel A. *Quality of life and quality of experience in patients with Hodgkin's disease.* Diploma thesis in psychology. Cologne, Germany: University of Cologne, 1997.
43. Fayers P, Hays R, eds. *Assessing quality of life in clinical trials.* 2nd ed. Oxford: Oxford University Press; 2006.
44. Cronbach LJ. Coefficient alpha and the internal structure of tests. *Psychometrika* 1951;16:297–305.
45. Osoba D, Rodrigues G, Myles J, et al. Interpreting the significance of changes in health-related quality-of-life scores. *J Clin Oncol* 1998;16:139–144.
46. Ganz PA. Impact of quality of life outcomes on clinical practice. *Oncology* 1995;9:61–65.
47. Stead ML, Brown JM, Velikova G, et al. Development of an EORTC questionnaire module to be used in health-related quality-of-life assessment for patients with multiple myeloma. European Organization for Research and Treatment of Cancer Study Group on Quality of Life. *Br J Haematol* 1999;104:605–611.
48. Scott NW, Fayers PM, Bottomley A, et al. Comparing translations of the EORTC QLQ-C30 using differential item functioning analyses. *Qual Life Res* 2006;15:1103–1115.
49. Derogatis LR. *The SCL-90R.* Baltimore, MD: Clinical Psychometric Research; 1977.

50. Harrer ME, Mosheim R, Richter R, et al. Coping and life satisfaction in patients with Hodgkin's disease in remission. A contribution to the question of adaptive aspects of coping processes. *Psychother Psychosom Med Psychol* 1993;43:121–132.

51. Kornblith AB, Anderson J, Cella DF, et al. Hodgkin's disease survivors at increased risk for problems in psychosocial adaptation. *Cancer* 1992;70:2214–2224.

52. Yellen SB, Cella DF, Bonomi A. Quality of life in people with Hodgkin's disease. *Oncology (Williston Park)* 1993;7:41–46.

53. Joly F, Henry-Amar M, Arveux P, et al. Late psychosocial sequelae in Hodgkin's disease survivors: a French population-based case-control study. *J Clin Oncol* 1996;14:2444–2453.

54. van Tulder MW, Aaronson NK, Bruning PF. The quality of life of long-term survivors of Hodgkin's disease. *Ann Oncol* 1994;5:153–158.

55. Thaler-DeMers D. Endocrine and fertility effects in male cancer survivors. *Cancer Nurs* 2006;29(suppl):66–71.

56. Hunt SM, McEwen J, McKenna SP. *The Nottingham Health Profile user's manual*, 1981.

57. Bergner M, Bobbitt RA, Kressel S, et al. The sickness impact profile: conceptual foundation and methodology for the development of a health status measure. *Int J Health Serv* 1976;6:393–401.

58. Ware JE, Sherbourne CD. The MOS 36-item short form health survey (SF-36) I. Conceptual framework and item selection. *Med Care* 1992;30: 473–482.

59. The EuroQol Group. EuroQol—a new facility for the measurement of health-related quality of life. *Health Policy* 1990;16:199–206.

60. WHOQOL Group. Study protocol for the World Health Organization project to develop a quality of life assessment instrument (WHOQOL). *Qual Life Res* 1993;2:153–159.

61. Nelson E, Wasson J, Kirk J, et al. Assessment of function in routine clinical practice: description the COOP chart method and preliminary findings. *J Chron Dis* 1987;40:5562.

62. Cella DF, Tulsky DS, Gray G, et al. The Functional Assessment of Cancer Therapy scale: development and validation of the general measure. *J Clin Oncol* 1993;11:570–579.

63. Schipper H, Clinch J, McMurray A, et al. Measuring the quality of life of cancer patients. The functional living index-cancer: development and validation. *J Clin Oncol* 1984;2:472–483.

64. Coscarelli-Shag CA, Heinrich RL. Development of a comprehensive quality of life measurement tool: CARES. *Oncology* 1990;4:135–138.

65. Schag CA, Ganz PA, Heinrich RL. Cancer Rehabilitation Evaluation System-short form (CARES-SF). A cancer specific rehabilitation and quality of life instrument. *Cancer* 1991;68:1406–1413.

66. de Haes JC, van Knippenberg FC, Neijt JP. Measuring psychological and physical distress in cancer patients: structure and application of the Rotterdam Symptom Checklist. *Br J Cancer* 1990;62:1034–1038.

67. Cella DF, Bonomi AE, Lloyd SR, et al. Reliability and validity of the Functional Assessment of Cancer Therapy-Lung (FACT-L) quality of life instrument. *Lung Cancer* 1995;12:199–220.

68. Smets EMA, Garssen B, Schuster-Uitterhoeve, et al. Fatigue in cancer patients. *Br J Cancer* 1993;68:220–227.

69. Loge JH, Abrahamsen AF, Ekeberg O, et al. Reduced health-related quality of life among Hodgkin's disease survivors: a comparative study with general population norms. *Ann Oncol* 1999;10:71–77.

70. Flechtner H, Bottomley A. Fatigue and quality of life: lessons from the real world. *Oncologist* 2003;8:45–52.

71. Hjermstad MJ, Fossa SD, Oldervoll L, et al. Fatigue in long-term Hodgkin's disease survivors: a follow-up study. *J Clin Oncol* 2005; 23:6587–6595.

72. Hjermstad MJ, Oldervoll L, Fossa SD, et al. Quality of life in long-term Hodgkin's disease survivors with chronic fatigue. *Eur J Cancer* 2006;42:327–333.

73. Smets EMA, Garssen B, Bonke B, et al. The Multidimensional Fatigue Inventory (MFI): psychometric qualities of an instrument to assess fatigue. *J Psychosom Res* 1995;39:315–325.

74. Flechtner H, Bottomley A. Fatigue assessment in cancer clinical trials. *Expert Rev Pharmocoeconomics Oucomes Res* 2002;2:67–76.

75. Banthia R, Malcarne VL, Roesch SC, et al.. Correspondence between daily and weekly fatigue reports in breast cancer survivors. *J Behav Med* 2006;29:269–279

76. Cremeens J, Eiser C, Blades M. Characteristics of health-related self-report measures for children aged three to eight years: a review of the literature. *Qual Life Res* 2006;15:739–754.

77. Foltz LM, Song KW, Connors JM. Hodgkin's lymphoma in adolescents. *J Clin Oncol* 2006;24:2520–2526.

78. Robison LL, Green DM, Hudson M, et al. Long-term outcomes of adult survivors of childhood cancer. *Cancer* 2005;104(suppl):2557–2564.

79. Proctor SJ, Rueffer JU, Angus B, et al. Hodgkin's disease in the elderly: current status and future directions. *Ann Oncol* 2002;13:133–137.

80. Stromgren AS, Sjogren P, Goldschmidt D, et al. A longitudinal study of palliative care: patient-evaluated outcome and impact of attrition. *Cancer* 2005;103:1747–1755.

81. Fryback DG. QALYs, HYEs, and the loss of innocence. *Med Decis Making* 1993;13:271–276.

82. Coast J. Reprocessing data to form QALYs. *Br Med J* 1992;305:87–95.

83. Stout NK, Rosenberg MA, Trentham-Dietz A, et al. Retrospective cost-effectiveness analysis of screening mammography. *J Natl Cancer Inst* 2006;98:774–782.

84. Gelber RD, Goldhirsch A. A new endpoint for the assessment of adjuvant therapy in postmenopausal women with operable breast cancer. *J Clin Oncol* 1986;4:1772–1780.

85. Mounier N, Ferme C, Flechtner H, et al. Model-based methodology for analyzing incomplete quality-of-life data and integrating them into the Q-TWiST framework. *Med Decis Making* 2003;23:54–66.

86. Norum J, Angelsen V, Wist E, et al. Treatment costs in Hodgkin's disease: A cost-utility analysis. *Eur J Cancer* 1996;32A:1510–1517.

87. Blazeby JM, Avery K, Sprangers M, et al. Health-related quality of life measurement in randomized clinical trials in surgical oncology. *J Clin Oncol* 2006;24:3178–3186.

88. Turner S, Maher EJ, Young T, et al. What are the information priorities for cancer patients involved in treatment decisions? An experienced surrogate study in Hodgkin's disease. *Br J Cancer* 1996;73:22–29.

89. Spiegel D, Bloom JR, Kraemer HC, et al. Effect of psychosocial treatment on survival of patients with metastatic breast cancer. *Lancet* 1989;2:888–896.

90. Osborn RL, Demoncada AC, Feuerstein M. Psychosocial interventions for depression, anxiety, and quality of life in cancer survivors: meta-analyses. *Int J Psychiatry Med* 2006;36:13–34.

91. Coates A, Gebski V. On the receiving end. VI. Which dimensions of quality-of-life scores carry prognostic information? *Cancer Treat Rev* 1996; 22(suppl A):63–71.

92. Coates AS, Gebski V, Signorini D, et al. Prognostic value of quality-of-life scores during chemotherapy for advanced breast cancer. *J Clin Oncol* 1992;10:1833–1840.

93. Hoerni B, Zittoun R, Rojouan J, et al. Psychosocial repercussions of the treatment of Hodgkin's disease. Assessment by questionnaire with 150 patients. *Bull Cancer* 1986;73:620–626.

94. Cella DF, Tross S. Psychological adjustment to survival from Hodgkin's disease. *J Consult Clin Psychol* 1986;54:616–622.

95. Wasserman AL, Thompson EI, Wilimas JA, et al. The psychological status of survivors of childhood/adolescent Hodgkin's disease. *Am J Dis Child* 1987;141:626–631.

96. Devlen J, Maguire P, Phillips P, et al. Psychological problems associated with diagnosis and treatment of lymphomas: prospective study. *Br Med J* 1987;295:955–963.

97. Carpenter PJ, Morrow GR, Schmale AH. The psychosocial status of cancer patients after cessation of treatment. *J Psychosocial Oncol* 1989;7:95–103.

98. Kornblith AB, Anderson J, Cella DF, et al. Comparison of psychosocial adaptation and sexual function of survivors of advanced Hodgkin disease treated by MOPP, ABVD, or MOPP alternating with ABVD. *Cancer* 1992;70:2508–2514.

99. Ferrell BR, Dow KH, Leigh S, et al. Quality of life in long-term cancer survivors. *Oncol Nurs Forum* 1995;22:915–924.

100. Kornblith AB, Herndon JE, Zuckerman E, et al. Comparison of psychosocial adaptation of advanced stage Hodgkin's disease and acute leukemia survivors. Cancer and Leukemia Group B. *Ann Oncol* 1998;9:297–306.

101. Greil R, Holzner B, Kemmler G, et al. Retrospective assessment of quality of life and treatment outcome in patients with Hodgkin's disease from 1969 to 1994. *Eur J Cancer* 1999;35:698706.

102. van Schaik CS, Barr RD, Depauw S, et al. Assessment of health status and health-related quality of life in survivors of Hodgkin's disease in childhood. *Int J Cancer* 1999;12:32–38.

103. Torbjornsen T, Stifoss-Hanssen H, Abrahamsen AF, et al. Cancer and religiosity –a follow up of patients with Hodgkin's disease. *Tidsskr Nor Laegeforen* 2000;120:346–348.

104. van Agthoven M, Vellenga E, Fibbe WE, et al. Cost analysis and quality of life assessment comparing patients undergoing autologous peripheral blood stem cell transplantation or autologous bone marrow transplantation for refractory or relapsed non-Hodgkin's lymphoma or Hodgkin's disease. a prospective randomised trial. *Eur J Cancer* 2001;37:1781–1789.

105. Cameron CL, Cella D, Herndon JE, et al. Persistent symptoms among survivors of Hodgkin's disease: an explanatory model based on classical conditioning. *Health Psychol* 2001;20:71–75.

106. Knobel H, Havard Loge J, Brit Lund M, et al. Late medical complications and fatigue in Hodgkin's disease survivors. *J Clin Oncol* 2001;19: 3226–3233.

107. Ganz PA, Moinpour CM, Pauler DK, et al. Health status and quality of life in patients with early-stage Hodgkin's disease treated on Southwest Oncology Group Study 9133. *J Clin Oncol* 2003;21:3512–3519

108. Gil-Fernandez J, Ramos C, Tamayo T, et al. Quality of life and psychological well-being in Spanish long-term survivors of Hodgkin's disease: results of a controlled pilot study. *Ann Hematol* 2003;82:14–18.

109. Geffen DB, Blaustein A, Amir MC, et al. Post-traumatic stress disorder and quality of life in long-term survivors of Hodgkin's disease and non-Hodgkin's lymphoma in Israel. *Leuk Lymphoma* 2003;44:1925–1929.

110. Wettergren L, Bjorkholm M, Axdorph U, et al. Individual quality of life in long-term survivors of Hodgkin's lymphoma–a comparative study. *Qual Life Res* 2003;12:545–554.

111. Rueffer JU, Flechtner H, Tralls P, et al. Fatigue in long-term survivors of Hodgkin's lymphoma; a report from the German Hodgkin Lymphoma Study Group (GHSG). *Eur J Cancer* 2003;39:2179–2186.

112. Glossmann JP, Engert A, Wassmer G, et al. Recombinant human erythropoietin, epoetin beta, in patients with relapsed lymphoma treated with aggressive sequential salvage chemotherapy—results of a randomized trial. *Ann Hematol* 2003;82:469–475.

113. Wettergren L, Bjorkholm M, Axdorph U, et al. Determinants of health-related quality of life in long-term survivors of Hodgkin's lymphoma. *Qual Life Res* 2004;13:1369–1379.
114. Holzner B, Kemmler G, Cella D, et al. Normative data for functional assessment of cancer therapy–general scale and its use for the interpretation of quality of life scores in cancer survivors. *Acta Oncol* 2004;43:153–160.
115. Wettergren L, Bjorkholm M, Langius-Eklof A. Validation of an extended version of the SEIQoL-DW in a cohort of Hodgkin lymphoma' survivors. *Qual Life Res* 2005;14:2329–2333.
116. Kawiecka-Dziembowska B, Borkowska A, Zurawski B, et al. The assessment of temperament, quality of life and intensity of depressive symptoms in patients with Hodgkin's disease in different stages of the illness. *Psychiatr Pol* 2005;39:679–690.
117. Ferrell BR, Dow Hassey K. Quality of life among long-term survivors. *Oncology* 1997;11:565–563.
118. Aaronson NK, Cull A, Kaasa S, et al. The EORTC modular approach to quality of life. Assessment in oncology. *Int J Ment Health* 1994;23: 75–84.
119. Hamilton M. The assessment of anxiety states. *Br J Psychol* 1959;32: 50–58.
120. Curbow B. Quality of life among long-term survivors [Comments]. *Oncology* 1997;11:572–580.
121. Siegel K, Christ GH. Hodgkin's disease survivorship: psychosocial consequences. In: Lacher MD, Mortimer J, Redman JR, eds. *Hodgkin's disease: the consequences of survival*. Philadelphia: Lea & Febiger; 1989:383–390.
122. Schag CC, Heinrich RL, Ganz PA. Cancer inventory of problem situations: An instrument for assessing cancer patients' rehabilitation needs. *J Psychosoc Oncol* 1983;1:11–19.
123. Ganz PA, Lee JJ, Siau J. Quality of life assessment. An independent prognostic variable for survival in lung cancer. *Cancer* 1991;67:3131–3139.
124. McCarter H, Furlong W, Whitton AC, et al. Health status measurements at diagnosis as predictors of survival among adults with brain tumors. *J Clin Oncol* 2006;24:3636–3643.
125. Selby P. Measurement of quality of life in cancer patients. *J Pharm Pharmacol* 1993;45:384–392.
126. Kaasa S, Mastekaasa A, Lund E. Prognosis factors for patients with inoperable non-small cell lung cancer, limited disease: the importance of patient's subjective experience of disease and psychosocial well-being. *Radiother Oncol* 1989;15:235–243.
127. Till JE. Use (and some possible abuses) of quality-of life measures. In: Osoba D, ed. *Effect of cancer on quality of life*. Boca Raton, FL: CRC Press; 1991:137–145.
128. Flechtner H, Rüffer J.-U. The German Hodgkin Study Group—studies on quality of life. In: Diehl V, Josting A, eds. *25 Years German Hodgkin Study Group*. Munich: Urban & Fischer; 2004;147–164.
129. Heutte N, Mounier N, Flechtner H, et al. Results of a longitudinal survey on quality of life (QoL) in 935 patients with supradiaphragmatic early stage Hodgkin lymphoma (HL) enrolled in the EORTC-GELA H8 trial (# 20931). *ASCO Meeting Abstracts* 2006;24:8582.
130. Guyatt GH, Feeny DH, Patrick DL. Measuring health-related quality of life. *Ann Int Med* 1993;118:622–631.
131. McMillen Moinpour C, Feigl P, Metch B, et al. Quality of life end points in cancer clinical trials: review and recommendations. *J Natl Cancer Inst* 1989;81:485–494.
132. Bottomley A, Flechtner H, Efficac F, et al. Health related quality of life outcomes in cancer clinical trials. *Eur J Cancer* 2005;41:1697–1709.
133. Grant J, Cranston A, Horsman J, et al. Health status and health-related quality of life in adolescent survivors of cancer in childhood. *J Adolesc Health* 2006;38:504–510.
134. Gelber RD, Cole BF, Goldhirsch A, et al. Adjuvant chemotherapy plus tamoxifen compared with tamoxifen alone for postmenopausal breast cancer: meta-analysis of quality-adjusted survival. *Lancet* 1996;347: 1066–1075.
135. Cole BF, Bonetti M, Zaslavsky AM, et al. A multistate Markov chain model for longitudinal, categorical quality-of-life data subject to non-ignorable missingness. *Stat Med* 2005;24:2317–2334.
136. Osoba D. Rationale for the timing of health-related quality-of life assessments in oncological palliative therapy. *Cancer Treat Rev* 1996;22(suppl A):69–78.
137. Ross L, Thomsen BL, Boesen EH, et al. In a randomized controlled trial, missing data led to biased results regarding anxiety. *J Clin Epidemiol* 2004;57:1131–1137.
138. Bottomley A, Vanvoorden V, Flechtner H, et al. The challenge and achievements of implementation of Quality of Life Research in cancer clinical trials. On behalf of the EORTC Quality of Life Group and EORTC Data Center. *Eur J Cancer* 2003;39:275–285.
139. Diehl V, Klimm B, Re D. Hodgkin lymphoma: a curable disease: what comes next? *Eur J Haematol* 2005;66:6–13.
140. Carde P, Hagenbeek A, Hayat M, et al. Clinical staging versus laparotomy and combined modality with MOPP versus ABVD in early-stage Hodgkin's disease: the H6 twin randomized trials from the European Organization for Research and Treatment of Cancer Lymphoma Cooperative Group. *J Clin Oncol* 1993;11:2258–2265.
141. Specht L, Gray RG, Clark MJ, et al. Influence of more extensive radiotherapy and adjuvant chemotherapy on long-term outcome of early-stage Hodgkin's disease: a meta-analysis of 23 randomized trials involving 3888 patients. *J Clin Oncol* 1998;16:830–838.
142. Noordijk EM, Carde P, Dupouy N, et al. Combined-modality therapy for clinical stage I or II Hodgkin's lymphoma: long-term results of the European Organisation for Research and Treatment of Cancer H7 randomized controlled trials. *J Clin Oncol* 2006;24:3128–3135.
143. Diehl V, Behringer K. Could BEACOPP be the new standard for the treatment of advanced Hodgkin's lymphoma? *Cancer Invest* 2006;24: 461–465.
144. Guyatt GH, Osoba D, Wu AW, et al. Methods to explain the clinical significance of health status measures. *Mayo Clin Proc* 2002;77:371–383.
145. Morris J, Goddard M. Economic evaluation and quality of life assessment in cancer clinical trials: the CHART trial. *Eur J Cancer* 1993;5:766–775.
146. Fryback DG, Lawrence WF. Dollars may not buy as many QALYs as we think: a problem with defining quality-of-life adjustments. *Med Decis Making* 1997;17:276–275.
147. Rumpold G, Soellner W. Quality of life in a healthy population. An epidemiologic research. *Qual Life Res* 1997;6:711–718.
148. Hjermstad MJ, Fayers P, Bjordal K, et al. Health-related quality of life in the general Norwegian population assessed by the European Organization for Research and Treatment of Cancer Core Quality-of-Life questionnaire: the QLQ-C30 (+3). *J Clin Oncol* 1998;16:1188–1195.
149. Schwarz R, Krauss O, Hinz A. Fatigue in the general population. *Onkologie* 2003;26:140–144.
150. Breslow NE, Day NE. The analysis of case-control studies in: *Statistical methods in cancer research*. Vol.1. IARC scientific pub. no. 32. Lyon: International Agency for Research on Cancer; 1980:14–22.
151. Dorval M, Maunsell E, Deschênes L, et al. Long-term quality of life after breast cancer: comparison of 8-year survivors with population controls. *J Clin Oncol* 1998;16:487–496.
152. Ware JE, Brook RH, Davies AR, et al. Choosing measures of healthy status for individuals in general population. *Am J Public Health* 1981;71: 620–628.
153. Rieker P, Fitzgerald E, Kalish L, et al. Psychosocial factors, curative therapies, and behavioral outcomes. *Cancer* 1989;64:2399–2408.
154. Olweny C, Juttner C, Rofe P, et al. Long-term effects of cancer treatment and coonsequences of cures: cancer survivors enjoy quality of life similar to their neighbours. *Eur J Cancer* 1993;29A:826—832.
155. Byrne J, Fears T, Steinhorn S, et al. Marriage and divorce after childhood and adolescent cancer. *JAMA* 1989;262:2693–2701.

SPECIAL TOPICS

CHAPTER 28 ■ UNUSUAL SYNDROMES IN HODGKIN LYMPHOMA

PHILIP J. BIERMAN, FRANCO CAVALLI, AND JAMES O. ARMITAGE

Painless lymphadenopathy is the most common physical finding associated with Hodgkin lymphoma. However, a number of unusual manifestations of disease, unrelated to direct histologic involvement, may also be present at diagnosis or relapse. In some cases, these symptoms may be more distressing and life-threatening than Hodgkin lymphoma itself. Such manifestations may be present for long periods of time and lead to extensive evaluations before the underlying diagnosis of Hodgkin lymphoma is made. This chapter discusses some of the unusual syndromes associated with Hodgkin lymphoma.

SYSTEMIC SYMPTOMS

The presence of constitutional symptoms such as fever, weight loss, night sweats, pruritus, malaise, and weakness have been noted since the earliest descriptions of Hodgkin's disease. Early investigators recognized that these symptoms had prognostic significance and felt that their presence should be recorded in a systematic manner. The need for a standardized clinical staging system for Hodgkin's disease led to the development of the Rye staging system, which subclassified each stage as A or B to indicate the absence or presence of fever, night sweats, and pruritus.[1] Later reports demonstrated the adverse prognostic significance of fever, night sweats, and weight loss, but they failed to document any adverse prognosis associated with pruritus.[2] These findings led to the development of the commonly used Ann Arbor staging system, in which pruritus was no longer considered to be a B-symptom.[3] In this staging system, systemic symptoms consisted of (a) unexplained weight loss of more than 10% of body weight in the previous 6 months, (b) unexplained fever with temperatures above 38°C, and (c) night sweats.

Fever was noted at the time of of diagnosis of Hodgkin lymphoma in 27% of patients at Stanford University,[4] and it has been noted with higher frequency in other reports.[5] Fever may be present for long periods of time and lead to prolonged evaluations and multiple courses of empiric antibiotic treatment before Hodgkin lymphoma is diagnosed. This diagnosis should be considered in any patient with fever of unknown origin. Fevers may be continuous or intermittent. They may be low grade or may exceed 40°C. Tachycardia frequently accompanies fever. Patients may be asymptomatic, or fevers may be associated with a sensation of discomfort or extreme fatigue. The classic Pel-Ebstein fever (Fig. 28.1) consists of cyclic episodes of high fevers lasting for 1 or 2 weeks, followed by afebrile periods of similar duration.[6–8] This presentation is now rarely seen, but it may be the initial manifestation of relapse.[9] Fevers invariably remit with the institution of treatment for Hodgkin lymphoma, and failure of fever to remit in the presence of responding disease should prompt a search for other causes of fever. Fevers also remit with administration of nonsteroidal anti-inflammatory agents.[10] Termination of fever may be attributed to antibiotic therapy, leading to additional diagnostic confusion.[8] Night sweats may take the form of mild dampness around the neck, but they are generally considered to be significant only if drenching in nature.[4] Patients frequently report the need to change bedclothes or linens because of sweating. Night sweats may occur independently of other systemic symptoms but are usually accompanied by fevers.[11] The etiology of night sweats is presumably related to fever defervescence. A slight rise in body temperature has been reported in the 30 minutes before sweating in patients with Hodgkin lymphoma.[12]

The etiology of fever in Hodgkin lymphoma is uncertain and has been related to host immune response, lymph node necrosis, inflamation, and damaged stromal cells.[13] These factors are not always observed, however.[14] A variety of cytokines have been isolated from cell lines established from lymph nodes of patients with Hodgkin lymphoma,[15,16] from serum of patients with Hodgkin lymphoma,[17] and from Hodgkin lymphoma tissue.[18] Patterns of cytokine expression are highly variable, but those most frequently produced include interleukin-6 (IL-6), tumor necrosis factor-α (TNF-α), and TNF-β.[15,19] Cytokine expression may vary among different histologic subtypes of Hodgkin lymphoma.[18] Some investigators have failed to find high levels of TNF protein expression in lymph nodes from patients with Hodgkin lymphoma, although nodes showed high levels of lymphotoxin expression.[20] Variations in lymphokine expression, even among morphologically similar lymph nodes, have been noted by other investigators, although IL-1 (interleukin-1) expression correlated with systemic symptoms.[21] Some cytokines, such as interleukin-8, may be produced by reactive cells rather than Reed-Sternberg cells.[22] Although elevated levels of serum IL-1 have been noted in Hodgkin lymphoma, cytokine levels did not correlate with B-symptoms.[23] Elevated serum levels of IL-6 have been associated with adverse prognostic factors and clinical outcomes, although the relation to systemic symptoms has been variable.[17,24,25] Expression of IL-6 and interleukin-10 may be upregulated in Epstein-Barr virus (EBV)-associated Hodgkin lymphoma.[26,27] Elevated levels of soluble interleukin-2 receptors, along with interleukins-7 and -8, have also been identified in the serum of patients with Hodgkin lymphoma and have been correlated with the presence of systemic symptoms.[17]

The presence of B-symptoms is associated with adverse outcome[28] and continues to be included in newer staging systems.[29] Patients who have all three B-symptoms have poorer survival when compared to patients who have one or two

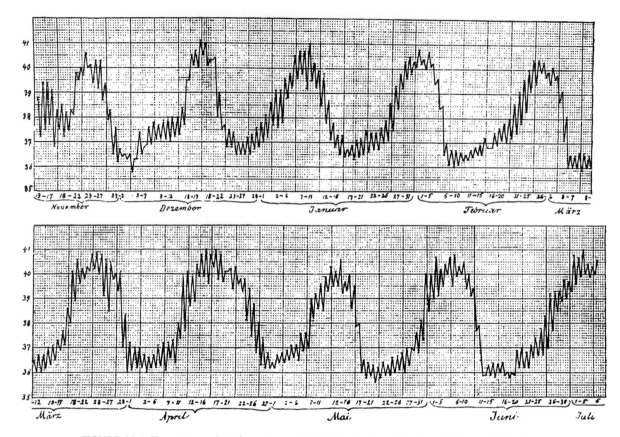

FIGURE 28.1. Temperature plot of a patient with Pel-Ebstein fever. (Reprinted with permission from Ebstein W. Das chronische Rückfallsfieber, eine neue Infectionskrankheit. *Berlin Klin Wochenschr* 1887;24:565.)

symptoms.[30] Night sweats may have less prognostic significance than the other systemic symptoms.[2,11,30]

PRURITUS

Pruritus may be a symptom of renal disease, cholestatic liver disease, diabetes, and thyroid disorders. It is also seen in patients with polycythemia vera and is frequently a manifestation of AIDS. Systemic disease is ultimately identified in 30% of patients with unexplained itching, and 1% to 11% will have malignancies.[31] Itching is one of the most common dermatologic manifestations of Hodgkin lymphoma.[32] Mild itching may be seen in 15% to 25% of patients with Hodgkin lymphoma, although severe itching is less common.[4,33] Itching has been reported to occur in as many as 85% of patients at some time in the course of disease.[5] Pruritus is generally more common in patients with advanced-stage disease and frequently accompanies other systemic symptoms.[4,33] Pruritis has been associated with other conditions such as generalized hyperhydrosis.[34] Itching may be more common in women.[4] Itching associated with Hodgkin lymphoma is usually generalized and may be severe enough that excoriations are produced from scratching. Itching may be the first manifestation of Hodgkin lymphoma, and patients may visit several physicians before lymphoma is diagnosed. It is not unusual for patients with unexplained itching to be referred to a psychiatrist before a diagnosis of Hodgkin lymphoma is made.[35] Patients with Hodgkin lymphoma may have itching related to cholestasis or to medications. In addition, various dermatologic manifestations of Hodgkin lymphoma may cause pruritus (see below). Finally, other causes of itching, such as scabies infection, which may mimic symptoms of active disease, should be

considered in the differential diagnosis of pruritus in patients with Hodgkin lymphoma.[36]

Although some early reports suggested that itching is not associated with poorer survival in patients with Hodgkin lymphoma,[2,4] others have suggested that patients with significant pruritus do have inferior overall survival and that the importance of pruritus is similar to that of other B-symptoms.[33,35] Nonspecific therapy for itching such as antihistamines is generally ineffective, although pruritus resolves when Hodgkin lymphoma is treated.[33,35] Return of itching in treated patients may be the initial symptom of relapse.[35]

The etiology of itching is poorly understood, although reports of resolution of itching accompanying spinal cord compression suggest that there may be a peripheral origin, with transmission of itching sensations through spinothalamic tracts.[37]

CUTANEOUS MANIFESTATIONS

Cutaneous manifestations of Hodgkin lymphoma may appear in several forms (Table 28.1). Primary cutaneous Hodgkin lymphoma in the absence of other sites is a rare disorder.[38] These patients may have an indolent course, and conservative treatment with excision or radiation may result in prolonged remission.[39,40] However, subsequent nodal Hodgkin lymphoma or other lymphoproliferative disorders may be seen. Lesions in these patients must be distinguished from those of other disorders, such as lymphomatoid papulosis, anaplastic large-cell lymphoma, and cutaneous T-cell lymphoma,[38,39,41] which may contain cells that are morphologically similar to Reed-Sternberg cells. Furthermore, lymphomatoid papulosis may be seen in patients who later develop Hodgkin lymphoma.

TABLE 28.1

CUTANEOUS MANIFESTATIONS OF HODGKIN LYMPHOMA

SPECIFIC SKIN LESIONS
Primary cutaneousa Hodgkin lymphoma
Lymphomatoid papulosis

NONSPECIFIC SKIN LESIONS
Paraneoplastic lesions
Infections (e.g., varicella-zoster)

From Milionis HJ, Elisaf MS. Psoriasiform lesions as paraneoplastic manifestation in Hodgkin's disease. *Ann Oncol* 1998;9:449.

Cutaneous involvement of Hodgkin lymphoma associated with nodal sites of disease occurs in 0.5% to 7.5% of cases.[42,43] Skin involvement in these patients is felt to be caused by obstruction of regional lymphatics, direct extension from underlying nodes, or hematogenous dissemination.[42] Lesions usually consist of erythematous nodules or papules, which may ulcerate. These lesions may be a direct extension of nodal areas of involvement or may appear at distant sites. Lesions are most common on the trunk but may appear anywhere on the body. Dermal involvement of Hodgkin lymphoma is often accompanied by extensive involvement at other sites and has been associated with a poor prognosis.[42]

A large number of nonspecific erythematous, urticarial, vesicular, and bullous cutaneous manifestations of Hodgkin lymphoma have been described,[44] mostly in case reports and small series. In some cases, these lesions are felt to represent a true paraneoplastic phenomenon, as they may be present at the time of diagnosis and remit with therapy. Reappearance of the lesions after treatment has heralded relapse. In other cases, the simultaneous appearance of skin lesions in association with Hodgkin lymphoma may be coincidental. It is postulated that cytokines secreted by tumor cells or accessory cells are responsible for the development of cutaneous paraneoplastic syndromes.[44]

Erythema nodosum consists of inflammatory nodules that appear most commonly on the anterior surface of the legs. These lesions are usually associated with infections, drugs, or inflammatory bowel disease, but they have also been described in association with Hodgkin lymphoma.[45,46] The lesions may be seen several months before relapse and respond to chemotherapy. Icthyosiform atrophy of the skin has also been associated with Hodgkin lymphoma and appears to respond to treatment for Hodgkin lymphoma.[47] Acrokeratosis paraneoplastica is a paraneoplastic dermatosis most commonly associated with carcinomas of the lung or upper gastrointestinal system. This disorder has also been described in Hodgkin lymphoma and is reported to respond to chemotherapy.[48] Granulomatous slack skin is a disorder associated with Hodgkin lymphoma as well as non-Hodgkin lymphoma.[49] Erythematous lesions gradually evolve into areas of pendulous skin. Although Hodgkin lymphoma responds to therapy, skin lesions do not usually regress. The multiple nevoid basal cell carcinoma is usually associated with solid tumors, although this syndrome has also been reported in association with Hodgkin lymphoma.[50] Other skin lesions reported to occur in association with Hodgkin lymphoma and that regress with therapy include icthyosis,[51,52] erythema annulare centrifugum,[53] granulomatous dermohypodermitis,[54] prurigo nodularis,[55] follicular mucinosis,[56] and alopecia areata.[57] The necrobiotic xanthogranuloma syndrome,[58] psoriasiform lesions,[44] and eczema craquele[59] have also been described in association with Hodgkin lymphoma.[59] Paraneoplastic

pemphigus is more commonly seen with non-Hodgkin lymphoma and chronic lymphocytic leukemia and is associated with a poor prognosis. This condition has been observed with Hodgkin lymphoma and may respond to therapy.[60]

In addition to cutaneous lesions, nail changes have also been described in patients with Hodgkin lymphoma. One such abnormality consists of transverse white lines, which may be associated with poor prognosis.[61] Hypertrophic osteoarthropathy has been reported to occur in patients with pulmonary and mediastinal Hodgkin lymphoma.[62,63]

NEUROLOGIC MANIFESTATIONS

Neurologic manifestations of Hodgkin lymphoma are unusual and may be caused by parenchymal disease, meningeal disease, spinal cord compression, therapy-induced leukoencephalopathy, or central nervous system infection. In addition, neuropathies may be seen with administration of vinca alkaloids and following radiation therapy. However, a number of paraneoplastic manifestations that are relatively specific for Hodgkin lymphoma have been described (Table 28.2).[64] These syndromes are usually associated with autoimmunity, and it is postulated that tumor cells express antigens that are similar to molecules on neurons.[65] It is thought that an autoimmune response arises against the tumor antigens and that this response spills over to attack normal neuronal tissue expressing similar antigens.

Paraneoplastic cerebellar degeneration is a condition associated with Hodgkin lymphoma and also with solid tumors, such as breast, lung, and ovarian carcinomas.[66–68] The abrupt or subacute onset of gait ataxia is generally the initial complaint. Other symptoms include dysarthria, nystagmus, and diplopia. The onset of symptoms may precede the diagnosis of Hodgkin lymphoma by months or years (Fig. 28.2). Male patients are predominantly affected. In some cases, the onset of symptoms may herald a recurrence of lymphoma. Treatment is generally ineffective, although disease may stabilize, and improvements with plasma exchange or treatment for Hodgkin lymphoma have been reported.[65,67–71] Neurologic improvement may be associated with a decrease in antibody titer.

The brains of patients with paraneoplastic cerebellar degeneration exhibit a diffuse loss of Purkinje cells throughout the cerebellar cortex.[67] Serum antibodies directed against human and rodent Purkinje cells may be identified in patients with Hodgkin lymphoma who have cerebellar degeneration, although many will not have detectable antibodies.[67,69] Paraneoplastic cerebellar degeneration in Hodgkin lymphoma is most commonly associated with anti-Tr antibodies, although circulating anti-mGluR1 antibodies have been described.[68,71] These antibodies are distinct from the anti-Yo and anti-Hu antibodies described in patients with breast, ovarian, and small-cell lung carcinomas. Anti-Tr antibodies from serum of

TABLE 28.2

PARANEOPLASTIC NEUROLOGIC MANIFESTATIONS OF HODGKIN LYMPHOMA

Subacute cerebellar degeneration
Limbic encephalitis
Subacute necrotic myelopathy
Subacute motor neuropathy

From Abate G, Corazzelli G, Ciarmiello A, et al. Neurologic complications of Hodgkin's disease: a case history. *Ann Oncol* 1997;8:593.

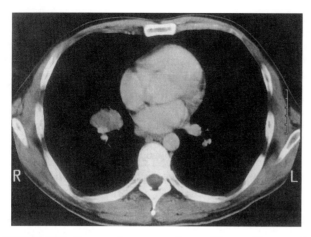

FIGURE 28.2. Computed tomogram from a 31-year-old man with subacute cerebellar degeneration. Progressive diplopia, dysarthria, and ataxia developed in this patient. Five months later, his serum was found to contain anti-Purkinje cell antibodies and a right hilar mass was identified. Biopsy revealed nodular-sclerosis Hodgkin lymphoma, and the patient achieved remission after combination chemotherapy. The patient continued in remission, although there was no improvement in his neurologic status.

patients with Hodgkin lymphoma reacts with cerebellar tissue, but is only rarely isolated from Hodgkin lymphoma tumor samples.[71] Antibody can also be detected in cerebrospinal fluid.[71] Antibody-negative patients may be slightly more likely to show neurologic improvement than patients with detectable anti-Purkinje cell antibodies in serum.[65,67]

Limbic encephalitis is a syndrome of memory loss and amnesia. Anti-Hu antibodies have been described in patients who exhibit this syndrome in association with small-cell lung carcinoma.[65] Limbic encephalitis has been described in association with Hodgkin lymphoma and may be reversible following chemotherapy.[72–74] The presence of anti-Tr antibodies has been noted in patients with Hodgkin lymphoma who have limbic encephalitis.[71] These antibodies have also been noted in patients with myorhythmia, a coarse alternating tremor.[75]

Subacute myelopathy has occasionally been associated with Hodgkin lymphoma.[76] Most cases have been identified at autopsy and have been associated with spinal cord necrosis.

Subacute motor neuropathy associated with Hodgkin lymphoma is characterized by progressive, painless lower motor neuron weakness.[77] The course of the disease is independent of Hodgkin lymphoma, and most patients stabilize or improve spontaneously. Motor neuron disease indistinguishable from amyotrophic lateral sclerosis has also been described in Hodgkin lymphoma.[64,78] Patients have normal findings on nerve conduction studies and no sensory loss. Postmortem examination demonstrates loss of motor neurons in the spinal cord, brainstem, and motor cortex. Neurologic improvement after treatment of Hodgkin lymphoma is unusual.

Hodgkin lymphoma may also be associated with neuropathies involving peripheral nerves[79–81] and cranial nerves.[79] These patients may respond to corticosteroids or Hodgkin lymphoma treatment. Other neurologic disorders that have been reported to occur in association with Hodgkin lymphoma include Guillain-Barré syndrome,[82,83] central pontine myelinolysis,[84] and diffuse encephalitis.[85] Stiff-man syndrome has also been described in patients with Hodgkin lymphoma.[65,86,87] This syndrome may be associated with autoantibodies and may remit after treatment of Hodgkin lymphoma.[65,87] Opsoclonus,[65] chorea,[88] and autonomic dysfunction leading to orthostatic hypotension[89] have also been reported as paraneoplastic complications of Hodgkin lymphoma.

RENAL MANIFESTATIONS

Autopsy series have demonstrated that Hodgkin lymphoma may directly involve the kidney in as many as 13% of cases.[90] Renal involvement may be unilateral or bilateral and may be present as diffuse involvement, discrete nodules, or microscopic disease. Renal involvement with Hodgkin lymphoma may go unrecognized, although parenchymal disease and ureteral obstruction may result in loss of function. Patients with Hodgkin lymphoma may also have renal dysfunction related to renal vein thrombosis, hypercalcemia, and hyperuricemia.

In addition to these direct and indirect effects on the kidney, Hodgkin lymphoma may be associated with glomerulonephritis. Although membranous nephropathy is generally associated with carcinomas, patients with Hodgkin lymphoma most commonly have minimal-change disease.[91] However, membranous glomerulonephritis, focal glomerulosclerosis, membranoproliferative glomerulonephritis, proliferative glomerulonephritis, crescentic glomerulonephritis, and glomerulonephritis secondary to IgA deposition have all been described in patients with Hodgkin lymphoma.[92–96] Glomerulonephritis may also be associated with antiglomerular basement membrane antibody[94] or immune complex deposition with immunoglobulin and C3.[97]

Nephrotic syndrome generally occurs early in the course of disease and may predate the diagnosis of Hodgkin lymphoma by many months.[92,97,98] Nephrotic syndrome in patients with Hodgkin lymphoma has also been described with other paraneoplastic disorders such as cerebellar degeneration.[99] Patients with Hodgkin lymphoma and nephrotic syndrome frequently have mixed-cellularity histology.[91] Nephrotic syndrome uniformly remits with successful treatment of Hodgkin lymphoma, even when radiation is used as the only means of therapy.[97] Proteinuria will often return in association with relapse of Hodgkin lymphoma; however, nephrotic syndrome associated with minimal-change disease or other glomerulopathies may occur following successful treatment of Hodgkin lymphoma without relapse.[100,101] In addition, minimal-change nephropathy may remit spontaneously in the face of Hodgkin lymphoma relapse.[102] Renal manifestations may occur at relapse even if they were not present initially.[96]

The etiology of minimal-change disease in the setting of Hodgkin lymphoma is unknown. It is postulated that humoral factors produced by neoplastic cells or infiltrating T-lymphocytes may increase vascular permeability, although these factors have not been identified.[96] Other investigators have suggested that disordered T-cell function may play a role in pathogenesis. The identity of the antigen associated with immune complex glomerulopathy is also unknown, although there is some evidence that virus-related antigens may play a role.[97]

In addition to glomerulonephritis, amyloidosis has been associated with nephrotic syndrome in patients with Hodgkin lymphoma.[92–94,96,97,103] Most cases appear to be associated with AA type amyloid.[96] Renal amyloidosis in Hodgkin lymphoma has generally occurred late in the course of disease. Although common in older series, this association appears to be decreasing in frequency, due to earlier diagnosis and treatment of Hodgkin lymphoma.

HEMATOLOGIC MANIFESTATIONS

A variety of hematologic abnormalities are associated with Hodgkin lymphoma. Myelosuppression in Hodgkin lymphoma may be caused by hypersplenism or bone marrow infiltration; however, some abnormalities have a clearly defined immunologic basis.

Anemia, leukocytosis, and lymphocytopenia occur frequently in Hodgkin lymphoma. These abnormalities are associated with poor prognosis and form the basis of several prognostic scores used in the management of Hodgkin lymphoma.[104–107] The etiology of these hematologic disorders appears to be related to excessive cytokine release.

A positive Coombs test result may be found at the time of diagnosis of Hodgkin lymphoma or at the time of relapse.[108,109] A positive Coombs test result may or may not be associated with overt hemolysis. Patients with a positive Coombs test frequently have advanced-stage disease and systemic symptoms, although prognosis may or may not be poor. Other patients may have a hemolytic anemia that has been present for months before diagnosis, and these patients may have limited-stage disease.[110,111] Cyclic hemolysis with exacerbations coinciding with Pel-Ebstein fever has been described.[112]

Chemotherapy results in the fall of antibody titers and resolution of hemolysis, although other modalities, such as splenectomy, may also be successful. Recurrence of hemolysis may accompany relapse.

The antibody in patients with autoimmune hemolytic anemia and Hodgkin lymphoma is usually reactive against immunoglobulin G and C3. In one study, antibodies with anti-It specificity were identified.[108]

Immune thrombocytopenia may accompany Hodgkin lymphoma in 1% to 2% of cases,[113] and it may occur in association with autoimmune hemolytic anemia. Thrombocytopenia may develop before, concurrently with, or after the diagnosis of Hodgkin lymphoma.[113,114] Immune thrombocytopenia may occur in patients with limited- or advanced-stage disease and with all histologic subtypes. Thrombocytopenia frequently occurs in patients in remission after Hodgkin lymphoma treatment, and the development of thrombocytopenia is not usually associated with relapse.[76,77] The simultaneous appearance of immune thrombocytopenia and Hodgkin lymphoma may represent a chance occurrence in these situations.

The treatment of immune thrombocytopenia in patients with Hodgkin lymphoma should be approached in the same manner as in patients without malignancy. The response to therapy is similar to that of other patients, although corticosteroids or splenectomy alone is less likely to be beneficial in the presence of active lymphoma.[114,115] Thrombotic thrombocytopenic purpura has also been described in Hodgkin lymphoma, and microangiopathic hemolytic anemia must be considered in any patient with Hodgkin lymphoma who has thrombocytopenia.[116]

Autoimmune neutropenia has also been described in patients with Hodgkin lymphoma.[117–119s] Neutropenia may occur before diagnosis and in patients who are apparently cured of lymphoma. This abnormality may resolve with Hodgkin lymphoma treatment or with the use of other modalities such as intravenous immune globulin.[120] Bone marrow aplasia and pure red cell aplasia have also been described in patients with Hodgkin lymphoma and may respond to therapy for Hodgkin lymphoma or immunosuppression.[121,122]

Eosinophilia is frequently associated with Hodgkin lymphoma. This complication was noted in 15% of patients who were entered in clinical trials conducted by the British National Lymphoma Investigation.[123] In the absence of general leukocytosis, eosinophilia was associated with improved survival. However, other series have failed to show improved prognosis associated with eosinophilia in Hodgkin lymphoma.[124] The presence of eosinophilia does not appear to be related to stage or histology.[125] In situ hybridization studies have demonstrated IL-5 production by Reed-Sternberg cells, which may explain the etiology of eosinophilia accompanying Hodgkin lymphoma.[126] Eosinophil-stimulating activity of serum from patients with Hodgkin lymphoma can be abolished with antibodies to IL-5.[127] Other cytokines implicated in the development of Hodgkin

lymphoma-associated eosinophila include interleukin-3 and GM-CSF.[124,128]

Hemophagocytic syndrome has also been described in patients with Hodgkin lymphoma.[129,130] This disorder may be the presenting symptom of disease.

Deficiencies of coagulation factors VII and XII in a patient with Hodgkin lymphoma have been reported.[131] Reduction of factor levels was associated with disease progression, and levels returned to normal following successful treatment with both radiation and chemotherapy.

Microcytosis also occurs in patients with Hodgkin lymphoma.[132,133] This abnormality may be related to unbalanced globin chain synthesis, and resolves with treatment of Hodgkin lymphoma. Iron deficiency and other causes of microcytic indices must be excluded in these patients.

ENDOCRINE AND METABOLIC MANIFESTATIONS

The most common endocrine abnormality associated with Hodgkin lymphoma is hypercalcemia.[134,135] The reported incidence of hypercalcemia in patients with Hodgkin lymphoma has ranged between 1% and 5%.[135] Hypercalcemia is frequently associated with advanced stage and poor prognostic features, although hypercalcemia may accompany limited-stage disease. Bone involvement is unusual in patients with hypercalcemia. Little information on the prognostic significance of hypercalcemia is available, although long-term survival has been described and serum calcium levels return to normal with treatment.

The etiology of hypercalcemia in Hodgkin lymphoma appears to be related to altered levels of $1,25\text{-}(OH)_2\text{-}D_3$ (calcitriol) levels in almost all cases.[134,135] Elevated calcitriol levels and hypercalcemia may be associated with relapses, and levels will return to normal following successful treatment.[136] Infiltrating nonmalignant macrophages are felt to be the source of excess calcitriol. In some cases, hypercalcemia may be related to excess production of parathyroid hormone related-peptide,[137] and reports of normalization of calcium levels with indomethacin suggest that prostaglandin synthesis may play a role in some cases of hypercalcemia.[138]

Two cases of hypoglycemia caused by insulin receptor antibodies in patients with Hodgkin lymphoma have been described.[139,140] In one case, immune hemolytic anemia had previously been described, and relapse of Hodgkin lymphoma was diagnosed after the onset of hypoglycemia.[140]

The development of lactic acidosis at the time of Hodgkin lymphoma relapse has been described.[141] Chemotherapy resolved the metabolic abnormality. Other metabolic abnormalities associated with Hodgkin lymphoma include hypouricemia[142] and syndrome of inappropriate secretion of antidiuretic hormone.[143]

ALCOHOL-INDUCED PAIN

One of the most unusual syndromes associated with Hodgkin lymphoma is alcohol-induced pain. This symptom has been reported to occur in less than 5% of cases,[4] and it may be less common than in the past.[144] The pain may begin within minutes of ingestion and usually occurs in areas of nodal enlargement. Pain may occur in the chest with radiation to the arms, back, and legs.[145] The pain may abate in minutes or rarely after several hours.[145,146] Patients will frequently discontinue alcohol because of the discomfort. Symptoms may be elicited after ingestion of even small amounts of alcohol.[145,147] The onset of alcohol-induced pain may be the presenting feature of disease and may precede the diagnosis of Hodgkin lymphoma by many months.[148–151] The pain diminishes with treatment of Hodgkin lymphoma and may recur before other signs or symptoms of relapse. In addition to pain, other symptoms, such as itching, flushing, nausea and vomiting, coughing, and dizziness may be associated with alcohol ingestion.[145] Although generally considered to be a syndrome that is relatively specific for Hodgkin lymphoma, alcohol-induced pain has been described in a wide variety of malignant conditions, as well as in nonmalignant conditions that may mimic Hodgkin lymphoma.[147] Alcohol-induced pain may be associated with systemic symptoms and other features of advanced disease.[152]

The mechanism of alcohol-induced pain is unknown, but edema of lesions, vasodilation, and release of histamine have been proposed as causes.[147] It is interesting that pain may be elicited by intravenous as well as oral alcohol.[145,146] Pain may also be blocked by administration of antihistamines.[147]

MISCELLANEOUS ABNORMALITIES

A variety of miscellaneous abnormalities, in addition to those previously described, have been seen in association with Hodgkin lymphoma. Jaundice in patients with Hodgkin lymphoma may result from hepatic involvement, extrahepatic obstruction, infections, drugs, or hemolysis. Unexplained cholestasis has been described in several patients with Hodgkin lymphoma.[153–157] This occurs in the absence of extrahepatic obstruction and liver biopsies reveal cholestasis. In some cases this syndrome has been associated with idiopathic ductopenia or vanishing bile duct syndrome. Liver function may normalize following radiation or chemotherapy, along with histologic improvement. In other cases cholestasis has persisted following radiation or chemotherapy. Cholestasis and acute hepatic failure have been described when Hodgkin lymphoma involves the liver.[158–161] In other cases of hepatic failure, liver involvement could not be identified.[162] High bilirubin levels in this situation have also been associated with renal failure.[159] Hodgkin lymphoma has also been described in association with fulminant steatohepatitis.[163] Esophageal Hodgkin lymphoma may present with tracheoesophageal fistula.[164,165]

Patients with Hodgkin lymphoma frequently have noncaseating granulomas in uninvolved tissues as well as in those containing lymphoma.[166] This finding may be associated with improved survival. Granulomatous angiitis of the brain[167] has been described in association with Hodgkin lymphoma, as has granulomatous angiitis of the spinal cord.[168] A case of granulomatous uveitis in a patient with noncaseating splenic granulomas has also been reported.[169] Uveitis persisted after successful lymphoma treatment.

Both polymyositis and scleroderma have been associated with Hodgkin lymphoma.[170] These conditions responded poorly to therapy. Hodgkin lymphoma has been associated with aortitis[171] and hypertension.[172] Blood pressure normalized when chemotherapy was initiated and then rose when Hodgkin lymphoma recurred. Lymphoma-associated retinopathy has been described in association with Hodgkin lymphoma.[173] Antibodies from the patient's serum reacted with bovine and monkey retina tissue.

References

1. Rosenberg SA. Report of the committee on the staging of Hodgkin's disease. *Cancer Res* 1966;26:1310.
2. Tubiana M, Attié E, Flamant R, et al. Prognostic factors in 454 cases of Hodgkin's disease. *Cancer Res* 1971;31:1801.
3. Carbone PP, Kaplan HS, Musshoff K, et al. Report of the committee on Hodgkin's disease staging classification. *Cancer Res* 1971;31:1860.
4. Kaplan HS. *Hodgkin's disease.* Cambridge, MA: Harvard University Press, 1972.
5. Ultmann JE, Cunningham JK, Gellhorn A. The clinical picture of Hodgkin's disease. *Cancer Res* 1966;26:1047.
6. Ebstein W. Das chronische Rückfallsfieber, eine neue Infectionskrankheit. *Berlin Klin Wochenschr* 1887;24:565.
7. Pel PK. Pseudoleukaemie oder chronisches Rückfallsfieber? *Berlin Klin Wochenschr* 1887;24:644.
8. Talbot TR. Cases from the Osler Medical Service at Johns Hopkins University. *Am J Med* 2002;112:312
9. Racchi O, Rapezzi D, Ferraris AM, et al. Unusual bone marrow relapse of Hodgkin's disease with typical Pel-Ebstein fever. *Ann Hematol* 1996;73:39.
10. Chang JC, Gross HM. Neoplastic fever responds to the treatment of an adequate dose of naproxen. *J Clin Oncol* 1985;3:552.
11. Gobbi PG, Cavalli C, Gendarini A, et al. Reevaluation of prognostic significance of symptoms in Hodgkin's disease. *Cancer* 1985;56:2874.
12. Gobbi PG, Pieresca C, Ricciardi L, et al. Night sweats in Hodgkin's disease: a manifestation of preceding minor febrile pulses. *Cancer* 1990;65:2074.
13. Ree HJ. Stromal macrophage-histiocytes in Hodgkin's disease. Their relation to fever. *Cancer* 1987;60:1479.
14. Ree HJ, Pezzullo JC. Inflammation and/or necrosis of tumors cannot account for fever in most febrile patients with Hodgkin's disease. *Cancer* 1987;60:1787.
15. Klein S, Jücker M, Diehl V, et al. Production of multiple cytokines by Hodgkin's disease derived cell lines. *Hematol Oncol* 1992;10:319.
16. Gruss HJ, Herrmann F, Drexler HG. Hodgkin's disease: a cytokine-producing tumor-a review. *Crit Rev Oncog* 1994;5:473.
17. Gorschlüter M, Bohlen H, Hasenclever D, et al. Serum cytokine levels correlate with clinical parameters in Hodgkin's disease. *Ann Oncol* 1995;6:477.
18. Teruya-Feldstein J, Tosato G, Jaffe ES. The role of chemokines in Hodgkin's disease. *Leuk Lymphoma* 2000;38:363.
19. Tabibzadeh SS, Poubouridis D, May LT, et al. Interleukin-6 immunoreactivity in human tumors. *Am J Pathol* 1989;135:427.
20. Sappino A-P, Seelentag W, Pelte M-F, et al. Tumor necrosis factor/cachectin and lymphotoxin gene expression in lymph nodes from lymphoma patients. *Blood* 1990;75:958.
21. Perfetti V, Dragani TA, Paulli M, et al. Gene expression of pyrogenic cytokines in Hodgkin's disease lymph nodes. *Haematologica* 1992;77:221.
22. Foss HD, Herbst H, Gottstein S, et al. Interleukin-8 in Hodgkin's disease. Preferential expression by reactive cells and association with neutrophil density. *Am J Pathol* 1996;148:1229.
23. Blay J-Y, Farcet J-P, Lavaud A, et al. Serum concentrations of cytokines in patients with Hodgkin's disease. *Eur J Cancer* 1994;30A:321.
24. Kurzrock R, Redman J, Cabanillas F, et al. Serum interleukin 6 levels are elevated in lymphoma patients and correlate with survival in advanced Hodgkin's disease and with B symptoms. *Cancer Res* 1993;53:2118.
25. Seymour JF, Talpaz M, Hagemeister FB, et al. Clinical correlates of elevated serum levels of interleukin-6 patients with untreated Hodgkin's disease. *Am J Med* 1997;102:21.
26. Herbst H, Samol J, Foss HD, et al. Modulation of interleukin-6 expression in Hodgkin and Reed-Sternberg cells by Epstein-Barr virus. *J Pathol* 1997;182:299.
27. Herbst H, Foss HD, Samol J, et al. Frequent expression of Interleukin-10 by Epstein-Barr virus-harboring tumor cells of Hodgkin's disease. *Blood* 1996;87:2918.
28. Longo DL, Young RC, Wesley M, et al. Twenty years of MOPP therapy for Hodgkin's disease. *J Clin Oncol* 1986;4:1295.
29. Lister TA, Crowther D, Sutcliffe SB, et al. Report of a committee convened to discuss the evaluation and staging of patients with Hodgkin's disease: Cotswolds meeting. *J Clin Oncol* 1989;7:1630.
30. Crnkovich MJ, Hoppe RT, Rosenberg SA. Stage IIB Hodgkin's disease: the Stanford experience. *J Clin Oncol* 1986;4:472.
31. Kurzrock R, Cohen PR. Mucocutaneous paraneoplastic manifestations of hematologic malignancies. *Am J Med* 1995;99:207.
32. Rubenstein M, Divic M. Cutaneous manifestations of Hodgkin's disease. *Int J Dermatol* 2006;45:251.
33. Gobbi PG, Attardo-Parrinello G, Lattanzio G, et al. Severe pruritus should be a B-symptom in Hodgkin's disease. *Cancer* 1983;51:1934.
34. Stadie V, Marsch WCH. Itching attacks with generalized hyperhydrosis as initial symptoms of Hodgkin's disease. *JEADV* 2003;17:559.
35. Feiner AS, Mahmood T, Wallner SF. Prognostic importance of pruritus in Hodgkin's disease. *JAMA* 1978;240:2738.
36. Seymour JF. Splenomegaly, eosinophilia, and pruritus: Hodgkin's disease, or . . .? *Blood* 1997;90:1719.
37. Olsson H, Brandt L. Relief of pruritus as an early sign of spinal cord compression in Hodgkin's disease. *Acta Med Scand* 1979;206:319.
38. Kadin ME. Lymphomatoid papulosis, Ki-1+ lymphoma, and primary cutaneous Hodgkin's disease. *Semin Dermatol* 1991;10:164.
39. Guitart J, Fretzin D. Skin as the primary site of Hogkin's disease: A case report of primary cutaneous Hodgkin's disease and review of its relationship with non-Hodgkin's lymphoma. *Am J Dermatopahtol* 1998;20:218.
40. Jurišić V, Bogunović M, Čolovic N, et al. Indolent course of cutaneous Hodgkin's disease. *J Cutan Pathol* 2005;32:176.

41. Davis TH, Morton CC, Miller-Cassman R, et al. Hodgkin's disease, lymphomatoid papulosis, and cutaneous T-cell lymphoma derived from a common T-cell clone. *N Engl J Med* 1992;326:1115.
42. White RM, Patterson JW. Cutaneous involvement in Hodgkin's disease. *Cancer* 1985;55:1136.
43. Tassies D, Sierra J, Montserrat E, et al. Specific cutaneous involvement in Hodgkin's disease. *Hematol Oncol* 1992;10:75.
44. Milionis HJ, Elisaf MS. Psoriasiform lesions as paraneoplastic manifestation in Hodgkin's disease. *Ann Oncol* 1998;9:449.
45. Simon S, Azevedo SJ, Byrnes JJ. Erythema nodosum heralding recurrent Hodgkin's disease. *Cancer* 1985;56:1470.
46. Pileckyte M, Griniūte R. Erythema modosum association with malignant lymphoma. *Medicine (Kaunas)* 2003;39:438.
47. Ronchese F, Gates DC. Ichthyosiform atrophy of the skin in Hodgkin's disease. *N Engl J Med* 1956;255:287.
48. Lucker GPH, Steijlen PM. Acrokeratosis paraneoplastica (Bazex syndrome) occurring with acquired ichthyosis in Hodgkin's disease. *Br J Dermatol* 1995;133:322.
49. Noto G, Pravatà G, Miceli S, et al. Granulomatous slack skin: report of a case associated with Hodgkin's disease and a review of the literature. *Br J Dermatol* 1994;131:275.
50. Potaznik D, Steinherz P. Multiple nevoid basal cell carcinoma syndrome and Hodgkin's disease. *Cancer* 1984;53:2713.
51. Ghislain PD, Roussel S, Marot L, et al. Acquired ichthyosis disclosing Hodgkin's disease. Simultaneous recurrence. *Presse Med* 2002;31:1126.
52. Rizos E, Milionis HJ, Pavlidis N, et al. Acquired ichthyosis: a paraneoplastic skin manifestation of Hodgkin's disease. *Lancet Oncol* 2002;3:727.
53. Leimert JT, Corder MP, Skibba CA, et al. Erythema annulare centrifugum and Hodgkin's disease. *Arch Intern Med* 1979;139:486.
54. Benisovich V, Papadopoulos E, Amorosi EL, et al. The association of progressive, atrophying, chronic, granulomatous dermohypodermitis with Hodgkin's disease. *Cancer* 1988;62:2425.
55. Shelnitz, LS, Paller AS. Hodgkin's disease manifesting as prurigo nodularis. *Pediatr Dermatol* 1990;7:136.
56. Ramon DR, Jorda E, Molina I, et al. Follicular mucinosis and Hodgkin's disease. *Int J Dermatol* 1992;31:791.
57. Mlczoch L, Attarbaschi A, Dworzak M, et al. Alopecia areata and multifocal bone involvement in a young adult with Hodgkin's disease. *Leuk Lymphoma* 2005;46:623.
58. Reeder CB, Connolly SM, Windelmann RK. The evolution of Hodgkin's disease and necrobiotic xanthogranuloma syndrome. *Mayo Clin Proc* 1991;66:1222.
59. Sparsa A, Liozon E, Boulinguez S, et al. Generalized eczema craquele as a presenting feature of systemic lymphoma: report of seven cases. *Acta Derm Venereol* 2005;85:333.
60. Dega H, Laporte JL, Joly P, et al. Paraneoplastic pemphigus associated with Hodgkin's disease. *Br J Dermatol* 1998;138:188.
61. Shahani RT, Blackburn EK. Nail anomalies in Hodgkin's disease. *Br J Dermatol* 1973;89:457.
62. Adler JJ, Sharma OP. Hypertrophic osteoarthropathy with intrathoracic Hodgkin's disease. *Am Rev Respir Dis* 1970;102:83.
63. Peck B. Hypertrophic osteoarthropathy with Hodgkin's disease in the mediastinum. *JAMA* 1977;238:1400.
64. Abate G, Corazzelli G, Ciarmiello A, et al. Neurologic complications of Hodgkin's disease: a case history. *Ann Oncol* 1997;8:593.
65. Dropcho EJ. Neurologic paraneoplastic syndromes. *J Neurol Sci* 1998;153:264.
66. Hammack J, Kotanides H, Rosenblum MK, et al. Paraneoplastic cerebellar degeneration. II. Clinical and immunologic findings in 21 patients with Hodgkin's disease. *Neurology* 1992;42:1938.
67. Dropcho EJ. Autoimmune central nervous system paraneoplastic disorders: mechanisms, diagnosis, and therapeutic options. *Ann Neurol* 1995;37(suppl 1):S102.
68. Shams'ili S, Grefkens J, de Leeuw B, et al. Paraneoplastic cerebellar degeneration associated with antineuronal antibodies: analysis of 50 patients. *Brain* 2003;126:1409.
69. Cehreli C, Payzin B, Undar B, et al. Paraneoplastic cerebellar degeneration in association with Hodgkin's disease: a report of two cases. *Acta Haematol* 1995;94:210.
70. Taniguchi Y, Tanji C, Kawai T, et al. A case report of plasmapheresis in paraneoplastic cerebellar ataxia associated with anti-Tr antibody. *Ther Apher Dial* 2006;10:90.
71. Bernal F, Shams'ili S, Rojas I, et al. Anti-Tr antibodies as markers of paraneoplastic cerebellar degeneration and Hogkin's disease. *Neurology* 2003;60:230.
72. Carr I. The Ophelia syndrome: memory loss in Hodgkin's disease. *Lancet* 1982;1:844.
73. Bernard P, Vinzio S, Talamin F, et al. Hodgkin's disease manifesting as paraneoplastic limbic-encephalitis. *Rev Med Interne* 2003;24:257.
74. Shinohara T, Kojima H, Nakamura N, et al. Pathology of pure hippocampal sclerosis in a patient with dementia and Hodgkin's disease: the Ophelia syndrome. *Neuropathology* 2005;25:353.
75. Wiener V, Honnorat J, Pandolfo M, et al. Myorhythmia associated with Hodgkin's lymphoma. *J Neurol* 2003;250:1382.
76. Dansey RD, Hammond-Tooke GD, Lai K, et al. Subacute myelopathy: an unusual paraneoplastic complication of Hodgkin's disease. *Med Pediatr Oncol* 1988;16:284.
77. Schold SC, Cho E-S, Somasundaram M, et al. Subacute motor neuropathy: a remote effect of lymphoma. *Ann Neurol* 1979;5:271.
78. Gordon PH, Rowland LP, Younger DS, et al. Lymphoproliferative disorders and motor neuron disease: an update. *Neurology* 1997;48:1671.
79. Vickers SM, Niederhuber JE. Hodgkin's disease associated with neurologic paraneoplastic syndrome. *South Med J* 1997;90:839.
80. Lachance DH, O'Neill BP, Harper CM, et al. Paraneoplastic brachial plexopathy in a patient with Hodgkin's disease. *Mayo Clin Proc* 1991;66:97.
81. Oh BC, Lim YM, Kwon YM, et al. A case of Hodgkin's lymphoma associated with sensory neuropathy. *J Korean Med Sci* 2004;19:130.
82. Hughes RAC, Britton T, Richards M. Effects of lymphoma on the peripheral nervous system. *J R SocMed* 1994;87:326.
83. Scully RE, Mark EJ, McNeely WF, et al. Case records of the Massachusetts Hospital. Case 39-1990. Presentation of case. *N Engl J Med* 1990;323:895.
84. Chintagumpala MM, Mahoney DH, McClain K, et al. Hodgkin's disease associated with central pontine myelinolysis. *Med Pediatr Oncol* 1993;21:311.
85. Epaulard O, Courby S, Pavese P, et al. Paraneoplastic acute diffuse encephalitis revealing Hodgkin's disease. *Leuk Lymphoma* 2004;45:2509.
86. Grimaldi LME, Martino G, Braghi S, et al. Heterogeneity of autoantibodies in stiff-man syndrome. *Ann Neurol* 1993;34:57.
87. Ferrari P, Federico M, Grimaldi LM, et al. Stiff-man syndrome in a patient with Hodgkin's disease. An unusual paraneoplastic syndrome. *Haematologica* 1990;75:570.
88. Batchelor TT, Platten M, Palmer-Toy DE, et al. Chorea as a paraneoplastic complication of Hodgkin's disease. *J Neurooncol* 1998;36:185.
89. Levy Y, Barron SA, Shahin S, et al. Sympathetic dysautonomia as a remote effect of Hodgkin's lymphoma. *Am J Med* 1993;95:340.
90. Richmond J, Sherman RS, Diamond HD, et al. Renal lesions associated with malignant lymphomas. *Am J Med* 1962;32:184.
91. Fer MF, McKinney TD, Richardson RL, et al. Cancer and the kidney: renal complications of neoplasms. *Am J Med* 1981;71:704.
92. Dabbs DJ, Striker LMM, Mignon F, et al. Glomerular lesions in lymphomas and leukemias. *Am J Med* 1986;80:63.
93. Yum MN, Edwards JL, Kleit S. Glomerular lesions in Hodgkin's disease. *Arch Pathol* 1975;99:645.
94. Ma KW, Golbus SM, Kaufman R, et al. Glomerulonephritis with Hodgkin's disease and herpes zoster. *Arch Pathol Lab Med* 1978;102:527.
95. Bergmann J, Buchheidt D, Waldherr R, et al. IgA nephropathy and hodgkin's disease: a rare coincidence. Case report and literature review. *Am J Kidney Dis* 2005;45:e16.
96. Ronco PM. Paraneoplastic glomerulopathies: New insights into an old entity. *Kidney Int* 1999;56:355.
97. Eagen JW, Lewis EJ. Glomerulopathies of neoplasia. *Kidney Int* 1977;11:297.
98. Bhatt N. Nephrotic syndrome preceding Hodgkin's lymphoma by 13 months. *Clin Nephrol* 2005;64:228.
99. Spyridonidis A, Fischer K-G, Glocker FX, et al. Paraneoplastic cerebellar degeneration and nephrotic syndrome preceding Hodgkin's disease: case report and review of the literature. *Eur J Haematol* 2002;68:318.
100. Shapiro CM, Vander Laan BF, Jao W, et al. Nephrotic syndrome in two patients with cured Hodgkin's disease. *Cancer* 1985;55:1799.
101. Delmez JA, Safdar SH, Kissane JM. The successful treatment of recurrent nephrotic syndrome with the MOPP regimen in a patient with a remote history of Hodgkin's disease. *Am J Kidney Dis* 1994;23:743.
102. Korzets Z, Golan E, Manor Y, et al. Spontaneously remitting minimal change nephropathy preceding a relapse of Hodgkin's disease by 19 months. *Clin Nephrol* 1992;38:125.
103. Pérez EE, Arguiñano JM, Gastearena J. Successful treatment of AA amyloidosis secondary to Hodgkin's disease with 4′-iodo-4′-deoxydoxorubicin. *Haematologica* 1999;84:93.
104. Hasenclever D, Diehl V. A prognostic score for advanced Hodkin's disease. *N Engl J Med* 1998;339:1506.
105. Straus DJ, Gaynor JJ, Myers J, et al. Prognostic factors among 185 adults with newly diagnosed advanced Hodgkin's disease treated with alternating potentially noncross-resistant chemotherapy and intermediate-dose radiation therapy. *J Clin Oncol* 1990;8:1173.
106. Proctor SJ, Taylor P, Mackie MJ. A numerical prognostic index for clinical use in identification of poor-risk patients with Hodgkin's disease at diagnosis. The Scotland and Newcastle Lymphoma Group (SNLG) Therapy Working Party. *Leuk Lymphoma* 1992;7(suppl):17.
107. Vaughan Hudson B, Maclennan KA, Bennett MH, et al. Systemic disturbance in Hodgkin's disease and its relation to histopathology and prognosis (BNLI report no. 30). *Clin Radiol* 1987;38:257.
108. Levine AM, Thornton P, Forman SJ, et al. Positive Coombs test in Hodgkin's disease: significance and implications. *Blood* 1980;55:607.
109. Ozdemir F, Yilmaz M, Akdogan R, et al. Hodgkin's disease and autoimmune hemolytic anemia: a case report. *Med Princ Pract* 2005;14:205.
110. Björkholm M, Holm G, Merk K. Cyclic autoimmune hemolytic anemia as a presenting manifestation of splenic Hodgkin's disease. *Cancer* 1982;49:1702.
111. Majumdar G. Unremitting severe autoimmune haemolytic anaemia as a presenting feature of Hodgkin's disease with minimum tumour load. *Leuk Lymphoma* 1995;20:169.
112. Ranlöv P, Videbaek A. Cyclic haemolytic anaemia synchronous with Pel-Ebstein fever in a case of Hodgkin's disease. *Acta Med Scand* 1963;174:583.

113. Xiros N, Binder T, Anger B, et al. Idiopathic thrombocytopenic purpura and autoimmune hemolytic anemia in Hodgkin's disease. *Eur J Haematol* 1988;40:437.

114. Kirshner JJ, Zamkoff KW, Gottlieb AJ. Idiopathic thrombocytopenic purpura and Hodgkin's disease: report of two cases and a review of the literature. *Am J Med Sci* 1980;280:21.

115. Sonnenblick M, Kramer MR, Hershko C. Corticosteroid responsive immune thrombocytopenia in Hodgkin's disease. *Oncology* 1986;43:349.

116. Linklater D, Voth A. Thrombocytopenic purpura. Importance of early diagnosis. *Can Fam Physician* 1996;42:1985.

117. Heyman MR, Walsh TJ. Autoimmune neutropenia and Hodgkin's disease. *Cancer* 1987;59:1903.

118. Fernández O, Morales E, Toledo J. Autoimmune processes terminating 24 years later in Hodgkin's disease. *Br J Haematol* 1992;81:308.

119. Hunter JD, Logue GL, Joyner JT. Autoimmune neutropenia in Hodgkin's disease. *Arch Intern Med* 1982;142:386.

120. Schoengen A, Fembacher PM, Schulz PC. Immunoglobulin therapy for autoimmune neutropenia in Hodgkin's disease. *Acta Haematol* 1995;94:36.

121. Johnston PG, Ruscetti FW, Connaghan DG, et al. Transient reversal of bone marrow aplasia associated with lymphocyte depleted Hodgkin's disease after combination chemotherapy. *Am J Hematol* 1994;46:48.

122. Reid TJ, Mullaney M, Burrell LM, et al. Pure red cell aplasia after chemotherapy for Hodgkin's lymphoma: in vitro evidence for T cell mediated suppression of erythropoiesis and response to sequential cyclosporin and erythropoietin. *Am J Hematol* 1994;46:48.

123. Vaughan Hudson B, Linch DC, MacIntyre EA, et al. Selective peripheral blood eosinophilia associated with survival advantage in Hodgkin's disease (BNLI report no 31). *J Clin Pathol* 1987;40:247.

124. Axdorph U, Porwit-MacDonald A, Grimfors G, et al. Tissue eosinophilia in relation to immunopathological and clinical characteristics in Hodgkin's disease. *Leuk Lymphoma* 2001;42:1055.

125. Desenne JJ, Acquatella G, Stern R, et al. Blood eosinophilia in Hodgkin's disease. A follow-up of 25 cases in Venezuela. *Cancer* 1992;69:1248.

126. Samoszuk M, Nansen L. Detection of interleukin-5 messenger RNA in Reed-Sternberg cells of Hodgkin's disease with eosinophilia. *Blood* 1990; 75:13.

127. Di Biagio E, Sánchez-Borges M, Desenne JJ, et al. Eosinophilia in Hodgkin's disease: a role for interleukin 5. *Int Arch Allergy Immunol* 1996;110:244.

128. Pinto A, Aldinucci D, Gloghini A, et al. Human eosinophils express functional CD30 ligand and stimulate proliferation of a Hodgkin's disease cell line. *Blood* 1996;88:3299.

129. Kojima H, Takei N, Mukai HY, et al. Hemophagocytic syndrome as the primary clinical symptom of Hodgkin's disease. *Ann Hematol* 2003; 82:53.

130. Dawson L, den Ottolander GJ, Kluin PM, et al. Reactive hemophagocytic syndrome as a presenting feature of Hodgkin's disease. *Ann Hematol* 2000;79:322.

131. Slease RB, Schumacher HR. Deficiency of coagulation factors VII and XII in a patient with Hodgkin's disease. *Arch Intern Med* 1977;137:1633.

132. Fahey JL, Rahbar S, Farbstein MJ, et al. Microcytosis in Hodgkin disease associated with unbalanced globin chain synthesis. *Am J Hematol* 1986; 23:123.

133. Shoho AR, Go RS, Tefferi A. 22 year-old woman with severe microcytic anemia. *Mayo Clin Proc* 2000;75:861.

134. Rieke JW, Donaldson SS, Horning SJ. Hypercalcemia and vitamin D metabolism in Hodgkin's disease. *Cancer* 1989;63:1700.

135. Seymour JF, Gagel RF. Calcitriol: the major humoral mediator of hypercalcemia in Hodgkin's disease and non-Hodgkin's lymphomas. *Blood* 1993;82:1383.

136. Mercier RJ, Thompson JM, Harman GS, et al. Recurrent hypercalcemia and elevated 1,25-dihydroxyvitamin D levels in Hodgkin's disease. *Am J Med* 1988;84:165.

137. Kremer R, Shustik C, Tabak T, et al. Parathyroid-hormone-related peptide in hematologic malignancies. *Am J Med* 1996;100:406.

138. Laforga JB, Vierna J, Aranda FI. Hypercalcaemia in Hodgkin's disease related to prostaglandin synthesis. *J Clin Pathol* 1994;47:567.

139. Braund WJ, Williamson DH, Clark A, et al. Autoimmunity to insulin receptor and hypoglycaemia in a patient with Hodgkin's disease. *Lancet* 1987;1:237.

140. Walters EG, Denton RM, Tavare JM, et al. Hypoglycaemia due to an insulin-receptor antibody in Hodgkin's disease. *Lancet* 1987;1:241.

141. Nadiminti Y, Wang JC, Chou S-Y, et al. Lactic acidosis associated with Hodgkin's disease. *N Engl J Med* 1980;303:15–17.

142. Bennett JS, Bond J, Singer I, et al. Hypouricemia in Hodgkin's disease. *Ann Intern Med* 1972;76:751.

143. Eliakim R, Vertman E, Shinhar E. Case report: syndrome of inappropriate secretion of antidiuretic hormone in Hodgkin's disease. *Am J Med Sci* 1986;291:126.

144. Bichel J. Is the alcohol-intolerance syndrome in Hodgkin's disease disappearing? *Lancet* 1972;1:1069.

145. Bichel J. The alcohol-intolerance syndrome in Hodgkin's disease. *Acta Med Scand* 1959;164:105.

146. James AH. Hodgkin's disease with and without alcohol-induced pain. *Q J Med* 1960;113:47.

147. Custodi P, Cerutti A, Bagnato R, et al. Alcohol-induced pain in tuberculous adenitis. *Haematologica* 1993;78:416.

148. Pinson P, Joos G, Praet M, et al. Primary pulmonary Hodgkin's disease. *Respiration* 1992;59:314.

149. Bobrove AM. Alcohol-related pain and Hodgkin's disease. *West J Med* 1983;138:874.

150. Callahan BC, Coe R, Place HM. Hodgkin disease of the spine presenting as alcohol-related pain. A case report and review of the literature. *J Bone Joint Surg Am* 1994;76:119.

151. Homan R, Lechner K, Neumann E, et al. Primary Hodgkin's disease of the lung. Case report and review of the literature. *Blut* 1983;47:231.

152. Atkinson K, Austin DE, McElwain TJ, et al. Alcohol pain in Hodgkin's disease. *Cancer* 1976;37:895.

153. Perera DR, Greene ML, Fenster LF. Cholestasis associated with extrabiliary Hodgkin's disease. *Gastroenterology* 1974;67:680.

154. Rodriguez-Gil FJ, Rincón-Fuentes JP, García-Pérez B, et al. Idiopathic cholestasis associated with bloody diarrhea as the first manifestation of Hodgkin's lymphoma. *Gastroenterol Hepatol* 2006;29:240.

155. Jansen PL, Van der Lelie H. Intrahepatic cholestasis and biliary cirrhosis associated with extrahepatic Hodgkin's disease. *Neth J Med* 1994;44:99.

156. Crosbie OM, Crown JP, Nolan NP, et al. Resolution of paraneoplastic bile duct paucity following successful treatment of Hodgkin's disease. *Hepatology* 1997;26:5.

157. de Medeiros BC, Lacerda MA, Telles JE, et al. Cholestasis secondary to Hodgkin's disease: report of 2 cases of vanishing bile duct syndrome. *Haematologica* 1998;83:1038.

158. Vardareli E, Dündar E, Aslan V, et al. Acute liver failure due to Hodgkin's lymphoma. *Med Princ Pract* 2004;13:372.

159. Kiewe P, Korfel A, Loddenkemper C, et al. Unusual sites of Hodgkin's lymphoma: case 3. Cholemic nephrosis in Hodgkin's lymphoma with liver involvement. *J Clin Oncol* 2004;22:4230.

160. Nohgawa M, Yonetani N, Sugiyama T. Hodgkin's disease presenting with progressive liver failure. *Rinsho Ketsueki* 2002;43:857.

161. Thompson DR, Faust TW, Stone MJ, et al. Hepatic failure as the presenting manifestation of malignant lymphoma. *Clin Lymphoma* 2001;2:123.

162. Dourakis SP, Tzemanakis E, Deutsch M, et al. Fulminant hepatic failure as a presenting paraneoplastic manifestation of Hodgkin's disease. *Eur J Gastroenterol Hepatol* 1999;11:1055.

163. Kosmidou IS, Aggarwal A, Ross JJ, et al. Hodgkin's disease with fulminant non-alcoholic steatohepatitis. *Dig Liver Dis* 2004;36:691.

164. Bernal AB, Rochling FA, DiBaise JK. Lymphoma and tracheoesophageal fistula: indication for a removable esophageal stent. *Dis Esophagus* 2005;18:57.

165. Munshi A, Pandey MB, Kumar L, et al. A case of Hodgkin's disease presenting with recurrent laryngeal nerve palsy and tracheoesophageal fistula. *Med J Malaysia* 2006;61:97.

166. Sacks EL, Donaldson SS, Gordon J, et al. Epithelioid granulomas associated with Hodgkin's disease. *Cancer* 1978;41:562.

167. Younger DS, Hays AP, Brust JC, et al. Granulomatous angiitis of the brain. *Arch Neurol* 1988;45:514.

168. Inwards DJ, Piepgras DG, Lie JT, et al. Granulomatous angiitis of the spinal cord associated with Hodgkin's disease. *Cancer* 1991;68:1318.

169. Mosteller MW, Margo CE, Hesse RJ. Hodgkin's disease and granulomatous uveitis. *Ann Ophthalmol* 1985;17:787.

170. Kedar A, Khan AB, Mattern QA, et al. Autoimmune disorders complicating adolescent Hodgkin's disease. *Cancer* 1979;44:112.

171. Fraumeni JF Jr, Herweg JC, Kissane JM. Panaortitis complicating Hodgkin's disease. *Ann Intern Med* 1967;67:1242.

172. Singh AP, Charan VD, Desai N, et al. Hypertension as a paraneoplastic phenomenon in childhood Hodgkin's disease. *Leuk Lymphoma* 1993;11:315.

173. To KW, Thirkill CE, Jakobiec FA, et al. Lymphoma-associated retinopathy. *Ophthalmology* 2002;109:2149.

CHAPTER 29 ■ THE MANAGEMENT OF HODGKIN LYMPHOMA DURING PREGNANCY

CAROL S. PORTLOCK AND JOACHIM YAHALOM

Since 1911, when the first case of Hodgkin's disease complicated by pregnancy was reported,[1] the management of Hodgkin lymphoma during pregnancy has presented difficult choices that are not always supported by a solid body of data. Pregnancy is more common in patients with Hodgkin lymphoma than in those with non-Hodgkin lymphoma because the period of peak incidence of Hodgkin lymphoma coincides with the female reproductive years. Nevertheless, this association remains sufficiently rare (3.2% of all cases of Hodgkin lymphoma at the M. D. Anderson Cancer Center)[2] that only a few large series have examined the many aspects of patient presentation, management, the interaction of malignancy and pregnancy, and the effects of treatment on the developing fetus and delivered infant.[3]

Ultimately, the collection of limited data from pregnant women with a variety of malignancies must form the basis for individual management decisions made in the care of a pregnant patient with Hodgkin lymphoma. The incidence of pregnancy associated with Hodgkin lymphoma is difficult to estimate accurately. Stewart and Monto[4] reported 3 cases within a period of 10 years at the Henry Ford Hospital, where about 18,000 deliveries were handled during the same period. Palacios Costa and associates reported 5 cases of Hodgkin lymphoma associated with 30,000 pregnancies, a similar incidence of 1 case in 6,000 pregnancies.[5] Smith and co-workers reported an incidence of 0.05 per 1,000 deliveries in a retrospective review of more than 3 million deliveries in California from 1992 to 1997.[46]

Initially, the influence of pregnancy on the course of Hodgkin lymphoma was controversial.[4,7] However, later studies suggested no significant effect of pregnancy on the course of the disease.[7,8] Barry and colleagues[9] reviewed all cases of Hodgkin lymphoma diagnosed at Memorial Sloan-Kettering Cancer Center from 1910 until 1960. Female patients between the ages of 18 and 40 were chosen for the study, resulting in the identification of 347 patients of child-bearing age with Hodgkin lymphoma. One age-corrected control group was established from the cases in which no pregnancy following Hodgkin lymphoma had occurred. Of the 347 patients, 84 became pregnant and yielded a total of 112 pregnancies following the treatment of Hodgkin lymphoma. The survival curve and median survival time of 90 months were similar in both groups. Survival statistics were similar for patients whose pregnancy was aborted and for patients whose pregnancy was allowed to continue. Hennessy and Rottino[8] reviewed 35 patients whose Hodgkin lymphoma was associated with pregnancy and reached the same conclusions. Stewart and Monto[4] were able to show that Hodgkin lymphoma did not affect the obstetric course of pregnancy and that women affected with

Hodgkin lymphoma did well during pregnancy, parturition, and puerperium. Only a single case report[10] suggests a possible "transmission" from a mother with Hodgkin lymphoma to her newborn, who died at the age of 5 months with disseminated Hodgkin lymphoma.

PRESENTATION

Lishner and associates[11] have reported the largest recent series, comprising 48 women with 50 pregnancies occurring during active Hodgkin lymphoma; they used the Princess Margaret Hospital (Toronto, Canada) database for 1958 to 1984. Each pregnant patient was matched with three non-pregnant controls. The analysis revealed a median age of 26 (range, 18–38 years). A similar age distribution was reported in a literature review by Yahalom.[3] In the 50 pregnancies in the Toronto series, the diagnosis of Hodgkin lymphoma was made in 12 patients before conception, in 27 patients within 9 months after delivery or termination of pregnancy, and in only 10 patients (20%) during pregnancy. Hodgkin lymphoma was treated during pregnancy in 22 patients. The stage of disease at diagnosis did not appear to differ significantly from that of nonpregnant controls in the Lishner series: stage I, 25%; stage II, 45.8%; stage III, 16.7%; and stage IV, 12.5%.

Several American series appear to reflect similar age and stage distribution.[2,3,12,13] An exception to these data in regard to stage was reported by Aviles et al. of the Mexican National Medical Center[14]; of 14 pregnant patients, 5 had stage II, 3 stage III, and 6 stage IV disease. Eight of the 14 patients had Hodgkin lymphoma of the mixed-cellularity subtype, and the other 6 had nodular-sclerosing Hodgkin lymphoma. These distributions most likely reflect the background of these women, residents of a developing country, in contrast to the distributions of their North American counterparts.

The most carefully evaluated pathology analysis of pregnancy-associated Hodgkin lymphoma was reported by Gelb and associates.[13] The Stanford investigators reviewed 17 cases, classifying 13 of them as nodular-sclerosis Hodgkin lymphoma and 3 as mixed-cellularity Hodgkin lymphoma; 1 case was unclassified. Nodal tissue was obtained from peripheral sites in 14 patients, the mediastinum in 1, and lung in 1 (unknown site in 1). In an earlier Stanford series, Jacobs and colleagues[12] found 14 of 15 patients with nodular-sclerosis Hodgkin lymphoma; similarly, the investigators from M. D. Anderson[2] reported that 16 of 16 patients had nodular-sclerosis Hodgkin lymphoma.

FETAL GROWTH AND DEVELOPMENT

Treatments for Hodgkin lymphoma, whether radiation therapy or chemotherapy, are potentially teratogenic. The risk for fetal malformation or death depends on the stage of fetal development, fetal susceptibility, the agent used, and the fetal dose of that agent.[15–17]

The first trimester is the most critical period for agent exposure, as implantation (the first 2 weeks) and embryogenesis (weeks 3–8) proceed. Spontaneous abortion is the most likely consequence of treatment exposure during implantation, whereas major morphologic abnormalities can be a consequence during weeks 3 to 8 of embryogenesis. Some structures, such as the limbs and palate, are vulnerable during limited periods of embryogenesis, whereas the central nervous system may be affected throughout all phases of embryogenesis and fetal development.

With radiation therapy, another consideration related to possible fetal toxicity is the increasing uterine fundal height, as it influences total dose exposure from internal radiation scatter.[2] The closer the fetus is to the diaphragm, the greater the possible whole-body fetal dose when the mother receives radiation above the diaphragm.

With chemotherapy, the placenta plays a pivotal role in drug transfer.[16] It is of interest that the placenta has a multidrug-resistant phenotype,[17] which may help to prevent or reduce the transfer of such natural products as doxorubicin, vinblastine, and vincristine to the fetus. However, case reports regarding the efficiency of placental transfer of doxorubicin are inconclusive.

A consideration of fetal drug metabolism and excretion must also take into account the recirculation of amniotic fluid.[16] This feature helps to explain the marked teratogenicity of the folate antagonists aminopterin and methotrexate when fetal doses are within the therapeutic range.

Finally, during the second and third trimesters, effects on the fetus may be more subtle.[3,15] Low birth weight, intrauterine growth retardation, premature birth, stillborn fetus, impaired functional development, mental retardation, and diminished learning capability are all possible effects of therapy for Hodgkin lymphoma.

TABLE 29.1

STAGING STUDIES IN THE PREGNANT PATIENT WITH HODGKIN LYMPHOMA

History and physical examination
Routine blood work
Chest assessment
   Single-view chest roentgenogram with adequate abdominal
     shielding (see text)
   Magnetic resonance imaging (as indicated)
   Computed tomography (rarely indicated)
Abdominal assessment (see text)
   Ultrasound (as indicated)
   Magnetic resonance imaging (as indicated)
   Computed tomography (rarely indicated)
Bone marrow biopsy (as indicated)
Not indicated:
   Gallium scanning
   PET scan
   Bone scan

PET, positron emission tomography.

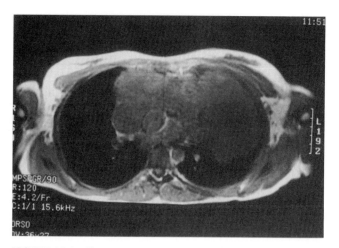

FIGURE 29.1. Chest magnetic resonance image in a pregnant patient reveals a large mediastinal mass.

STAGING DURING PREGNANCY

Hodgkin lymphoma presenting during pregnancy is a rare event. Most patients in North American series present without B-symptoms,[2,3,12,13] whereas the Aviles et al. series[14] from Mexico reveals a predominance of B-symptoms in 10 of 14 patients. A peripheral lymph node is usually the site of biopsy.[13]

Recommended staging studies have evolved with changing technology and therapeutic options (Table 29.1). A single posteroanterior chest roentgenogram with adequate abdominal shielding, blood work (complete blood count, tests of hepatic and renal function, sedimentation rate, and alkaline phosphatase and lactic dehydrogenase levels), and selected bone marrow biopsy continue to be indicated. More recently, magnetic resonance imaging (MRI) has been used, with the advantage that it can be used to evaluate nodes, liver, and spleen with good accuracy (Fig. 29.1). Although it is thought that MRI is probably safe in pregnant patients, no data are yet available to support this assumption. Abdominal ultrasonography is much less sensitive than MRI but may be adequate to screen for involvement with bulky disease, and it does permit serial examinations when needed in follow-up (Fig. 29.2). Gallium scanning and positron emission tomography (PET) are contraindicated. Computed axial tomography (CT) is rarely indicated if abdominal ultrasonography and MRI are available.

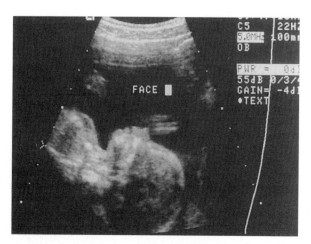

FIGURE 29.2. Abdominal ultrasonogram of a pregnant patient reveals a healthy fetus and no abdominal adenopathy.

As precise pathologic staging in Hodgkin lymphoma (with laparotomy) has been supplanted by clinical staging and therapy, the need for more careful definition in the pregnant patient has diminished. Moreover, it is acknowledged that Hodgkin lymphoma in most patients is a relatively indolent neoplasm that may often be monitored safely during pregnancy until fetal development and growth are adequate to permit a safe delivery.

TREATMENT

Radiation Therapy

Many series have documented the effectiveness of radiation therapy for the treatment of Hodgkin lymphoma during pregnancy.[1,3,11,12] Several principles are conducive to a successful outcome: delay irradiation until the second or third trimester, limit the whole-body fetal dose to 0.1 Gy or less, and realistically consider radiotherapy during pregnancy to be a holding or partial therapy rather than a definitive therapy.

The details of radiotherapy are limited in some reports, but compilations of radiotherapy experience in pregnant patients with Hodgkin lymphoma are available.[2,18] Data on estimated dose to the embyo are available from work on simulated phantoms and measurements in patients are available. Estimations of radiation dose from several sources are summarized in Table 29.2. Mazonakis and associates[19] used a humanoid phantom to simulate pregnancy at the first trimester of gestation. Embryo dose was measured for a 6-MV photon beam using three different field sizes. A shielding device consisting of 5 cm of lead was used to reduce the embryo dose. Dose measurements were carried out using thermoluminescent dosimeters. Local field irradiation in the regions of neck or axilla resulted in embryo doses below 0.1 Gy. For local field irradiation in the region of neck-mediastinum and for mantle treatment, the radiation dose to a shielded embryo was 0.028 to 0.19 Gy and 0.04 to 0.24 Gy depending upon the distance from the field isocenter and the field size used, respectively. The corresponding dose for an unshielded embryo exceeded 0.1 Gy. All of the above embryo doses were obtained for a tumor dose of 40 Gy. This study

showed that local field irradiation in the regions of neck or axilla may be safely performed even without uterus shielding. For local field irradiation in the region of neck-mediastinum and for mantle radiotherapy, the extent of the irradiated area, the distance separating the embryo from the field isocenter, and the tumor dose are the factors determining whether the radiation dose to a shielded embryo may possibly be reduced below 0.1 Gy.

Woo and associates[2] have provided a complete analysis of 16 pregnant patients with clinical stage (CS) I or IIA treated at the M. D. Anderson Cancer Center. Involved-field irradiation was administered to the neck (35 Gy) in 2 cases, extended-field to the neck and mediastinum (40 Gy) in 3 cases, and full-mantle irradiation to the remaining 11 patients (40 Gy). Uterine shielding was maximized by using 4 to 5 half-value layers of lead. The dose to the fetus was estimated in 9 patients and was 0.014 to 0.055 Gy with 6-MV photons and 0.1 to 0.136 Gy with cobalt-60. After delivery, 10 patients underwent lymphangiography and 5 underwent staging laparotomy (2 with positive findings). Eight patients subsequently had additional radiation therapy and/or chemotherapy. All offspring were reported to be physically and mentally normal, and the 10-year survival of the patients was 83%.

In a review of 47 patients with Hodgkin lymphoma during pregnancy from several series, 23 patients received supradiaphragmatic radiation therapy (5 in the first trimester), with no apparent harm to the fetus. Seventy-four percent of the patients remained without evidence of Hodgkin lymphoma at the time of the report.[3]

The Stanford group[12] reported the details of radiation therapy in 9 patients. Involved or mantle fields were used and doses were generally low (≤33 Gy in 6, full dose only in 3 who became pregnant during preplanned radiotherapy). Full staging and therapy were completed after delivery. These investigators recommended treatment delay whenever possible if Hodgkin lymphoma is detected during the last half of the second or during the third trimester. If radiation therapy is recommended, limited fields and dose should be considered.

Fetal outcome following radiotherapy depends on gestational age at radiation therapy, whole-body fetal dose, and maternal health. Although one would expect a higher frequency of spontaneous abortions and congenital anomalies, this has not been clearly evident from the literature. The M. D.

TABLE 29.2

ESTIMATED RADIATION DOSE TO THE FETUS AS PERCENTAGE OF THE TOTAL MANTLE[a] DOSE IN DIFFERENT STUDIES (PHANTOM MEASUREMENTS)

Study (ref.)	Energy	Trimester 1	Trimester 2	Trimester 3
Zucali et al. (20)[a]	Co-60	0.21	0.45	3.0
Zucali et al. (20)[a]	6 MV	0.15	0.34	2.0
Covington and Baker (21)	6 MV	0.19–0.4	0.9–1.4	3.7–7.1
Sharma et al. (23)	10 MV	0.4[c]–0.8[d]	0.6[c]–1.1[d]	1.2[c]–2.2[d]
Wong et al. (22)[b]	10 MV	1.3[c]–1.4[d]	1.9[c]–2.0[d]	4.3[c]–5.0[d]
Woo et al. (2)	6 MV		0.2–0.5	0.32–0.42
Woo et al. (2)	Co-60		0.48–0.82	
Yahalom (3)	6 MV	0.23	0.1–0.83	3.2

[a]Supraclavicular field 11 × 11 cm and opposed mediastinal fields 13 × 13 cm.
[b]Distances from the lower border of the field are slightly smaller than in Sharma et al.
[c]With shielding LMR-13 Toshiba accelerator.
[d]Without shielding Clinac 18.
MV, megavolt; Co-60, cobalt isotope.

Anderson series[2] had 16 full-term infants; the Stanford series[12] had 1 spontaneous abortion in a patient irradiated during the first trimester and 6 normal infants (3 therapeutic abortions). The Princess Margaret Hospital case-control study[11] of 50 pregnancies associated with Hodgkin lymphoma included 13 patients treated with radiation therapy (6 during and 7 after the first trimester). Interestingly, for the entire cohort of 50 pregnancies, there were no significant differences in gestational age, number of preterm births, birthweight, malformations, or number of stillbirths in comparison with matched controls. Unfortunately, the analysis did not assess the impact of radiation therapy alone in these cases.

In all reported series, it is obviously impossible to assess the confounding factor of therapeutic abortion in improving pregnancy outcome in the data. The general recommendation has been to terminate pregnancy in patients requiring radiotherapy during the first trimester, although this has not been consistently applied.[3]

Chemotherapy

Like radiation therapy, combination chemotherapy offers potentially curative treatment of Hodgkin lymphoma. However, because of concern regarding possible immediate and delayed side effects to the offspring, conventional combination chemotherapy has seldom been administered to pregnant patients.

In a comprehensive review of antineoplastic agents and pregnancy by Doll and co-workers,[16] the incidence of fetal malformations was approximately 15% with exposure during the first trimester. Alkylating agents and antimetabolites had the most consistent risk. Vinblastine was associated with the least risk, with only 1 abnormality among 14 patients treated in the first trimester. Similar data were reported elsewhere.[3] No data were available for vincristine alone.

During the second and third trimesters, chemotherapy is associated with a low risk for fetal malformation (1.3% of 150 exposed patients), probably not significantly different from that in the normal population (3.1%).[26] However, as emphasized by Doll and colleagues,[16] the relative lack of anomalies should not be interpreted as fetal safety, as delayed effects remain a significant concern.

Both MOPP (Mustargen [mechlorethamine], Oncovin [vincristine], procarbazine, prednisone) and ABVD (Adriamycin [doxorubicin], bleomycin, vinblastine, dacarbazine) have been administered to pregnant patients with Hodgkin lymphoma. The largest series is that of Aviles and colleagues,[14] in which 14 patients were treated, 5 during the first trimester and 9 during the second and third trimesters. All patients completed successful pregnancies (at 34–40 weeks), with no congenital anomalies noted. Eleven patients remain in complete remission 3 to more than 17 years after treatment. These authors have also reported their experience with CHOP (cyclophosphamide, hydroxydaunomycin, Oncovin [vincristine], prednisone) or its variants in 18 pregnant patients with non-Hodgkin lymphomas, with 9 treated during the first trimester and 9 during the second and third trimesters. Similarly, no congenital malformations were noted, and all fetuses were successfully delivered at 35 to 40 weeks.

In other reports,[16] procarbazine appears to be the most teratogenic agent in these drug combinations. During the first trimester, 1 congenital malformation occurred with single-agent procarbazine therapy, and 4 of 7 cases exposed to MOPP had malformations. Case reports regarding the apparent safety of rituximab and (peg)filgrastim during pregnancy are available; however, these agents should be administered with individualized consideration. All are considered group C drugs in the FDA use-in-pregnancy ratings (risk cannot be ruled out).

The timing of chemotherapy may also be important before delivery. The ability of a neonate to metabolize and excrete drugs is diminished.[15] Reynoso and associates[24] reported that 5 of 15 infants born to leukemic mothers who received chemotherapy within 30 days of delivery were cytopenic. Aviles and co-workers[14] noted no cytopenia in the infants of mothers treated for Hodgkin lymphoma, whereas 3 of 18 infants whose mothers were treated for non-Hodgkin lymphoma experienced transient cytopenia.

MONITORING DURING PREGNANCY

Because of concern regarding the possible teratogenic effects of therapy, many authors have recommended no active treatment of Hodgkin lymphoma during pregnancy. The eligibility criteria for this strategy are poorly defined but would include the following:

- "Limited" CS IA or IIA presenting during the late second and third trimester
- Stable, "nonurgent" presentations of disease diagnosed after 20 weeks of gestation

Few data are available to assess the application of these criteria. The Stanford group[12,13,30] has reported 5 cases of delayed therapy: 3 with CS IIA Hodgkin lymphoma, all in continuous complete remission following successful therapy after delivery, and 2 with infradiaphragmatic Hodgkin lymphoma, both of whom died of disease despite therapy after delivery. As emphasized by Jacobs and associates,[12] the decision to treat or monitor the pregnant patient must be individualized. Clearly, it is important that the site(s) of disease can be easily assessed if this strategy is to be undertaken.

DELIVERY

The timing of delivery must be a joint decision between the obstetrician and oncologist. Whenever possible, the fetus should be carried to term without compromising the health of mother or infant. Cesarean section is not necessary unless obstetrically indicated. Staging laparotomy performed in conjunction with delivery is not warranted.

If the pregnant patient has received therapy for Hodgkin lymphoma before delivery, it is important to keep in mind that the blood counts of both mother and infant may be adversely affected. Ideally, no potentially myelosuppressive therapy should be administered within 3 weeks of delivery.

MANAGEMENT AFTER DELIVERY

Staging assessment after delivery may proceed as in the nonpregnant patient. It is recommended that breast-feeding be discontinued once staging and therapy have begun. There is a risk that agents used for contrast and nuclear imaging, chemotherapeutic drugs, and ancillary, supportive medications may concentrate in breast milk. Lactating breasts show intense uptake on gallium scan, again suggesting possible concentration in breast milk (although data are unavailable on this point).

During and after gallium scanning, it is advisable not to hold the infant for 1 week. For PET, a 1-day wait is advisable.

PROGNOSIS OF PREGNANT PATIENTS WITH HODGKIN LYMPHOMA

The outcomes of patients with Hodgkin lymphoma presenting during pregnancy appear to be similar to those of their non-pregnant counterparts.[3,8,9] Smith and co-workers reported no increased risk of cesarean section, or postpartum maternal death, among 172 deliveries.[6] Lishner and associates[11] noted that when the cause-specific survival of 33 pregnant patients was compared with that of 67 case-matched controls,. approximately 70% of both groups were alive at 25 years, with no significant effect of age or stage at diagnosis on outcome.

Among 17 patients managed at Stanford,[12] only one died of disease after delivery, with more than 90% alive at 5 years. Similarly, among 16 patients with CS IA and IIA disease treated with radiotherapy at M. D. Anderson,[2] the cause-specific survival was 83% at 10 years. The National Medical Center of Mexico series[14] of 14 patients treated with combination chemotherapy (MOPP in 4 patients, ABVD in 7, and MOPP/ABVD in 3) for stages II (5 patients), III (3 patients), and IV (6 patients) revealed 11 patients in complete remission 3 to more than 17 years after treatment and 2 disease-related deaths; 1 patient was lost to follow-up.

OUTCOME OF OFFSPRING OF PREGNANCIES ASSOCIATED WITH HODGKIN LYMPHOMA

As discussed in detail by Garber,[25] the late manifestations of in utero exposure to antineoplastic agents may include impaired growth, diminished neurologic and/or intellectual function, decreased gonadal and reproductive function, mutagenesis of germline tissue, and carcinogenesis. Unfortunately, very few data are available regarding these critical questions. Aviles and colleagues[14] reported the status of 43 Mexican children exposed to chemotherapy during pregnancy (14 mothers and children had MOPP and/or ABVD). Their ages ranged from 3 to 19 years. All were examined, blood work was obtained, and intelligence testing was performed. A case-control group of 25 children was also evaluated. In this comprehensive evaluation, all children were normal in regard to routine blood work, lymphocyte function, immunoglobulins, cytogenetics, bone marrow aspirate and biopsy, school performance, neurologic testing, and medical histories. Sexual development appeared normal. A follow-up study of 84 children born to mothers with hematologic malignancies (including 26 with Hodgkin lymphoma and 29 with non-Hodgkin lymphoma) confirmed these findings.[32]

Reynoso and associates[24] reported the long-term follow-up of 8 children, ages 1 to 17 years, who were exposed in utero to antileukemic therapy. All but one child appeared normal. A male fraternal twin in whom neuroblastoma and thyroid cancer developed in childhood had congenital malformations and a low intelligence quotient. Of interest, his female fraternal twin was normal. Both had been exposed to cyclophosphamide and prednisone throughout gestation.

RECOMMENDATIONS FOR MANAGEMENT DURING PREGNANCY

How should the above data affect routine recommendations for the therapy of pregnant patients with Hodgkin lymphoma?

1. Risks to the fetus are greatest during the first trimester, and so it is reasonable to delay therapy during the first trimester whenever possible.
2. Based on the available data, it appears unreasonable to delay appropriate therapy for patients with symptomatic, bulky, subdiaphragmatic, or progressive Hodgkin lymphoma after the first trimester.
3. Treatment options include supradiaphragmatic radiotherapy (involved field or mantle field) for early-stage disease and single-agent vinblastine or combination chemotherapy with ABVD for bulky or subdiaphragmatic disease, as well as for symptomatic or advanced-stage presentations.
4. Radiation fields should be designed to decrease the fetal dose by allowing for the maximal distance between the inferior border of the field and the uterus. The uterus should be protected during radiotherapy with 10 half-value layer shielding. The maximal dose to the fetus should be calculated before treatment, and the dose to the fetus should be monitored during treatment.
5. One should not be reluctant to use combination chemotherapy when it is clearly indicated during the second or third trimester.
6. All pregnant patients with Hodgkin lymphoma should be managed as high-risk pregnancies by an obstetrician. Early delivery may not be required if the patient has received, or is receiving, adequate therapy.
7. Termination of pregnancy is rarely medically indicated in cases of newly diagnosed Hodgkin lymphoma; combination chemotherapy has been successfully administered during the first trimester, and vinblastine is even safer during embryogenesis.
8. Termination of pregnancy is often medically indicated in cases of relapsed Hodgkin lymphoma following combination chemotherapy, as high-dose chemoradiotherapy with stem-cell support is then usually indicated. If relapse occurs after radiotherapy alone, the pregnant patient may be satisfactorily managed with chemotherapy (as discussed above), and termination of the pregnancy is not required.
9. All women of child-bearing age receiving therapy for Hodgkin lymphoma should undergo pregnancy testing before treatment and should be counseled regarding birth control measures during therapy.

PREGNANCY AFTER TREATMENT

Ovarian function is usually maintained in women of child-bearing age successfully treated for Hodgkin lymphoma. Pelvic shielding with primary irradiation, oophoropexy for those requiring pelvic radiotherapy, and use of combination chemotherapy regimens not containing MOPP have all contributed to the preservation of fertility. Fertility preservation research is ongoing into the role of gonadotropin-releasing hormone agonists in conjunction with chemotherapy and oocyte/ovarian tissue cryopreservation prior to treatment.[31] Reports of pregnancy outcome among patients previously treated for Hodgkin lymphoma are also generally favorable (Table 29.3). In 1993, Aisner and associates[33] found that 35 of 43 premenopausal women (81%) who desired children had successful pregnancies. The median treatment-free interval to the birth of a child after treatment was 5.5 years (range, 0.6–14 years), and the median age at delivery was 30 years (range, 16–35 years). In this group of 35 women, 54 pregnancies resulted in delivery of 42 children, 1 spontaneous and 9 elective abortions, and 2 stillbirths. No major birth defects were reported in the 42 children, whose median birthweight was 6 lb 4 oz and whose 5-minute Apgar score was within normal range.

TABLE 29.3

FEMALE SURVIVORS OF HODGKIN LYMPHOMA: OUTCOME OF PREGNANCIES BEGUN AFTER THERAPY

Prior therapy	Pregnancies	Live births/ stillborn	Spontaneous/ therapeutic abortions	Congenital prior therapy anomalies	Reference
Radiation	36[a]	34/0	2[a]/0	1	27
	11	9/0	0/2	0	33
	22	16/3	0/3	1	32
Totals	69[a]	59/3	2[a]/5	2	
Chemotherapy with/without irradiation	16	14/0	0/1	2	27
	17[a]	15[a]/0	0/3	0	33
	11	8/1	2/0	1	32
Totals	44[a]	37[a]/1	2/4	3	

[a]One pregnancy with twins.

The pregnancy rate among premenopausal survivors of Hodgkin lymphoma now appears similar to that of the normal female population (85%). The probability of a successful pregnancy, as reported by Horning and associates,[34] is related to menopausal status and age at Hodgkin lymphoma therapy. This study, published in 1981, reported a 50% probability of pregnancy for Hodgkin lymphoma survivors who were treated as teenagers, in contrast to a probability approaching zero for those survivors treated at age 30. Pelvic irradiation with or without MOPP-containing combination chemotherapy most likely accounts for this low probability of fertility. ABVD is unlikely to result in permanent amenorrhea among women younger than 35 years.

Guidelines for planning subsequent pregnancy are empirically derived but based on the following observations:

1. Most relapses of Hodgkin disease occur within 2 to 3 years of definitive therapy (see Chapters 16 to 18).
2. Follow-up imaging is performed less frequently after years 2 to 3 and can safely be delayed in the pregnant patient (see Chapter 9).
3. Chemotherapy-induced menstrual irregularity is often transient and resolves within 1 to 2 years after therapy (see Chapter 26).
4. The risk for congenital abnormalities in children conceived after treatment for Hodgkin disease (and also other malignancies) does not appear to be greater than that in the general population. The largest study reported to date of children born to survivors of prior cancer treatment is that of Byrne and associates.[27] Among 2,198 offspring of survivors of pediatric and adolescent cancer treated before 1976, genetic disease was not significantly increased (3.4% in offspring of cancer survivors versus 3.1% in 4,544 control children). Moreover, the kinds of genetic abnormalities noted (simple malformations, single-gene defects, and cytogenetic syndromes) were not significantly different from those of controls. A similar population-based study has examined the incidence of cancer among offspring of 14,652 survivors of childhood and adolescent cancer. Using data from patients in Scandinavian countries in whom disease was diagnosed after 1940, Sankila and associates[28] report no evidence of a significantly increased risk for nonhereditary cancers based on offspring follow-up of 86,780 person-years (standardized incidence ratio of 1:3).

RECOMMENDATIONS FOR MANAGEMENT OF PREGNANCY CONCEIVED AFTER TREATMENT

Based on these observations, it is generally recommended that women be encouraged to delay pregnancy for 2 years after all treatment. Practical precautions that may be considered include the following:

1. Follow-up imaging should be performed before the patient attempts to conceive.
2. Thyroid function should be assessed and closely monitored among patients at risk for hypothyroidism (e.g., prior mantle irradiation). Hypothyroidism during pregnancy can result in hypertension, preterm delivery, and prematurity.[26] Moreover, thyroid replacement needs may increase during pregnancy.
3. A Hodgkin lymphoma-related physical examination should be performed at least once during pregnancy.
4. The patient should receive high-risk obstetric care.
5. Infertility should be evaluated promptly if conception is not achieved within 6 to 12 months.
6. No imaging is necessary while the patient is pregnant unless it is indicated by physical findings or symptoms.

References

1. Davis AB. Report of a case of Hodgkin's disease complicated by pregnancy. *Bull Lying-in Hosp N Y* 1911;7:151–158.
2. Woo SY, Fuller LM, Cundiff JH, et al. Radiotherapy during pregnancy for clinical stages IA–IIA Hodgkin's disease. *Int J Radiat Oncol Biol Phys* 1992; 23:407–412.
3. Yahalom J. Treatment options for Hodgkin's disease during pregnancy. *Leuk Lymphoma* 1990;2:151–161.
4. Stewart HL, Monto RW. Hodgkin's disease and pregnancy. *Am J Obstet Gynecol* 1952;63:570–578.
5. Palacios Costa N, Chavanne FC, Zebel Fernanccdez D. *An de ateneo.* Buenos Aires:1945:127.
6. Smith LH, Dalrymple JL, Leiserowitz GS, et al. Obstetrical deliveries associated with maternal malignancy in California, 1992 through 1997. *Am J Obstet Gynecol* 2001;184:1504–1513.
7. Bichel J. Hodgkin's disease and pregnancy. *Acta Radiol* 1950;33:427–434.
8. Hennessy JP, Rottino A. Hodgkin's disease in pregnancy. *Am J Obstet Gynecol* 1963;87:851–853.
9. Barry RM, Diamond HD, Carver LF. Influence of pregnancy on the course of Hodgkin's disease. *Am J Obstet Gynecol* 1962;84:445–454.

10. Priesel A, Winkelbauer A. Placentare ubertagung des lymphogranulomas. *Virchows Arch* 1926;262:749–796.
11. Lishner M, Zemlickis D, Degendorfer P, et al. Maternal and foetal outcome following Hodgkin's disease in pregnancy. *Br J Cancer* 1992;65:114–117.
12. Jacobs C, Donaldson SS, Rosenberg SA, et al. Management of the pregnant patient with Hodgkin's disease. *Ann Intern Med* 1981;95:669–675.
13. Gelb AB, Van de Rijn M, Warnke RA, et al. Pregnancy-associated lymphomas. A clinicopathologic study. *Cancer* 1996;78:204–210. See comments.
14. Aviles A, Diaz-Maqueo JC, Talavera A, et al. Growth and development of children of mothers treated with chemotherapy during pregnancy: current status of 43 children. *Am J Hematol* 1991;36:243–248.
15. Barnicle MM. Chemotherapy and pregnancy. *Semin Oncol Nurs* 1992; 8:124–132.
16. Doll DC, Ringenberg QS, Yarbro JW. Antineoplastic agents and pregnancy. *Semin Oncol* 1989;16:337–346.
17. Cordon-Cardo C, O'Brien JP, Casals D, et al. Multidrug-resistance gene (P-glycoprotein) is expressed by endothelial cells at blood-brain barrier sites. *Proc Natl Acad Sci USA* 1989;86:695–698.
18. Kal HB, Struikmans H. Radiotherapy during pregnancy: fact and fiction. *Lancet Oncol* 2005;6:328–333
19. Mazonakis M, Varveris H, Fasoulaki M, et al. Radiotherapy of Hodgkin's disease in early pregnancy: embryo dose measurments. *Radiother Oncol* 2003;66:333–339
20. Zucali R, Marchesini, R, DePalo O. Abdominal dosimetry for supradiaphragmatic irradiation of Hodgkin's disease in pregnancy. Experimental data and clinical considerations. *Tumori* 1981;67:203–208.
21. Covington EE, Baker AS. Dosimetry of scattered radiation to the fetus. *JAMA* 1969;209:414–415.
22. Wong PS, Rosemark PJ, Exler MC, et al. Doses to organs at risk from mantle field radiation therapy using 10 MV x-rays. *Mt Sinai J Med* 1985;52:216–220.
23. Sharma SC, Williamson JF, Khan FM, et al. Measurement and calculation of ovary and fetus dose in extended field radiotherapy for 10 MV x-rays. *Int J Radiat Oncol Biol Phys* 1981;7:843–846.
24. Reynoso EE, Shepherd FA, Messner HA, et al. Acute leukemia during pregnancy: the Toronto Leukemia Study Group experience with long-term follow-up of children exposed *in utero* to chemotherapeutic agents. *J Clin Oncol* 1987;5:1098–1106.
25. Garber JE. Long-term follow-up of children exposed *in utero* to antineoplastic agents. *Semin Oncol* 1989;16:437–444.
26. Montoro MN. Management of hypothyroidism during pregnancy. *Clin Obstet Gynecol* 1997;40:65–80.
27. Byrne J, Rasmussen SA, Steinhorn SC, et al. Genetic disease in offspring of long-term survivors of childhood and adolescent cancer. *Am J Hum Genet* 1998;62:45–52.
28. Sankila R, Olsen JH, Anderson H, et al. Risk of cancer among offspring of childhood cancer survivors. *N Engl J Med* 1998;338:1339–1344.
29. Holmes GE, Holmes FF. Pregnancy outcome of patients treated for Hodgkin's disease: a controlled study. *Cancer* 1978;41:1317–1322.
30. Ortin TT, Shostak CA, Donaldson SS. Gonadal status and reproductive function following treatment for Hodgkin's disease in childhood: the Stanford experience. *Int J Radiat Oncol Biol Phys* 1990;19:873–880.
31. Lobo RA. Potential options for preservation of fertility in women. *N. Engl J Med* 2005;353:64–73.
32. Aviles A, Neri N. Hematological malignancies and pregnancy: a report of 84 children who received chemotherapy in utero. *Clin Lymphoma* 2001;2:173–177.
33. Aisner J, Wiernik PH, Pearl P. Pregnancy outcome in patients treated for Hodgkin's disease. *J Clin Oncol* 1993;11:507–512.
34. Horning SJ, Hoppe RT, Kaplan HS, et al. Female reproductive potential after treatment for Hodgkin's disease. *N Eng J Med* 1981;304:1377–1382.

CHAPTER 30 ■ HODGKIN LYMPHOMA IN DEVELOPING COUNTRIES: AN AFRICAN PERSPECTIVE WITH A NOTE ON ASIA AND LATIN AMERICA

PETER JACOBS, LUCILLE WOOD, AND PAUL RUFF

Facts from Africa and parts of Asia and Latin America regarding Hodgkin lymphoma and other lymphomas are generally sketchy. This is in part a reflection of the priorities in underdeveloped lands, where imperatives are typically basic survival rather than nuances of exacting disease classification. Information-gathering by registries, and attempts to treat these cancers of the immune system in a consistent and acceptable manner, are often hampered by a shortage of resources and political interference. Specific examples are lack of trained staff and inadequate facilities for investigation, further aggravated by limited supplies of cytotoxic drugs or poor access to equipment for radiotherapy.

Not always appreciated are the vast ethnic and cultural differences on these continents. It is impossible to give a comprehensive picture of differences in natural history and outcome, especially when the diversity that includes black, white, and those of mixed ancestry together with others of Eurasian, Indian, and Mediterranean stock are considered. Finally, and not to be underestimated, usable records exist in relatively few centers in the north and south of Africa, with huge gaps in central regions, making generalization even more complicated. A similar caveat applies to parts of the Far East and South America.

Despite these daunting limitations it has been possible to assemble an overview of this entity as it has emerged during the last four decades and is presently seen by practitioners where there is access to hematology or oncology services. With such shortcomings in mind, five aspects are nevertheless sufficiently documented for analysis: (a) epidemiologic differences, if any, by race or geographic region; (b) patterns of presentation; (c) childhood variations; (d) the presence of retroviral or other infections; and (e) prevailing management programs. On this basis, some global comments emerge.

First there are notable differences in the demography between populations. In Africa, these neoplasms appear to be less common in blacks, most strikingly in the tropics but also at both extremities of this huge land mass. In addition, blacks have the lowest mean age at diagnosis, with those of mixed ancestry occupying an intermediate position, and with whites having the highest mean age at diagnosis. Also histopathology varies, with nodular sclerosis predominating in Caucasians whereas mixed cellularity and lymphocyte depletion are found with greater frequency in other ethnic groups. Late referral is more usual among poorer and less educated classes. This may, however, be caused more by perceptions and lack of medical care than by unique or disparate tumor biology. Penultimately

the coexistence of tuberculosis has long been recognized, and the time-honored observation that it follows like a shadow remains true, reflecting the severity and persistence of cell-mediated immunity in these cases. Finally, there is the immense impact of the acquired immunodeficiency epidemic that continues to further distort the course and survival in all affected individuals. Indeed, the last two decades have witnessed a profound impact on adults and children with mortality reducing life expectancy by 10 to 15 years.[1] Notably this excess is attributable to opportunistic microorganisms and neoplasms, of which Kaposi sarcoma and primary CNS lymphoma are now regarded as AIDS-defining.[2] In contrast to the impact of industrialization, the introduction of highly active antiretroviral drugs as well as other effective preventative or curative therapies has been delayed, and each year this situation remains responsible for over two million deaths in Africa.[1] Matching analyses from the other two continents are true to a greater or lesser extent.

Attempts to reach rational conclusions about this entity in geographical context inevitably attract equation with findings from comparable economically underdeveloped categories that include African Americans. Such exercises provide a chance to examine genetic influences that parallel the slave routes of yesteryear and also to explore any differences attributable to the environment. To this end, we have been able to review outcome in the northern and southern part of Africa and briefly to relate our findings with what is reported from other parts of the developing world. Thus it emerges that, stage for stage, there are no fundamental clinical disparities either where first seen or following therapy. The constellation of locally prevailing adverse prognostic markers, which culminate in dissemination and high bulk at initial consultation, seems to be a major determinant that impacts negatively on end result, rather than any genetic or ethnic differences in host or response mounted against the cancer.

The way in which these variables exert their influence has led to a perspective of poorly nourished people who delay seeking medical attention for prolonged periods of time and, consequently, appear with extensive spread. Superimposed on this is the high level of microbial co-morbidity. Also, there is a lack of disciplined protocol management, except in a few centers where first-world standards prevail. These circumstances combine to generate figures for emerging nations that range from appallingly poor response to those commensurate with developed countries. The extent to which such arguments can be extrapolated to other presumed similar regions has been difficult to define precisely. Accordingly, the focus and reference point for this research project remains the African experience, with commentary, where appropriate, from China, India, Malaysia, Brazil, Columbia, and Peru.

BACKGROUND

During the last four decades, research in Hodgkin lymphoma and other lymphomas in Africa concentrated largely on epidemiology with clinical descriptions outlined by race and region. Pioneering studies, such as those of Henre Falkson, focused on what was seen in white South Africans before the era of effective chemotherapy.[3] Only more recently has information emerged on black and other ethnic majorities.

In the past 20 years there has been a worldwide reorganization in the spectrum of lymphoproliferative disorders.[4] This was occasioned, in part, by emerging consensus in revised nomenclature[5] that now includes immunophenotyping and molecular genetics.[6] Such ever-expanding knowledge extends to all the many variants and has led to better, often quite definitive, understanding of these entities. Wherever feasible, even given persisting limitations, the newer concepts are finding expression in clinicopathologic case profiles.[7,8] Another change, having arguably even greater impact, came understandably from introduction of active drugs that led rapidly to the development of combination chemotherapy with resultant high complete remission rates.[9,10]

Consequently, cure is now possible in many, if not most, given that they are precisely diagnosed, correctly staged, and treated early with attention to risk stratification.[4-6] These ideals, however, are seldom realized in emancipating communities, where a major impediment to improving prognosis remains high-bulk lymphadenopathy and extensive extranodal involvement when patients are first seen. To reiterate, this phenomenon appears to be explicable by environmental forces that are characteristic of social deprivation rather than there being some unique or continent-specific difference in the malignant process itself. Superimposed are the adverse consequences of rampant malnutrition, compounded by the ravages of HIV and tuberculosis. To try to gain perspective of prevailing status, five topics have been singled out, and in each, a brief commentary highlights differences from the experience in more affluent westernized societies. Furthermore, where possible, findings have been matched to those in blacks from other parts of the world, because it is here that the opportunity exists to see if any distinction is present within a relatively uniform genetic pool that might then be modified by life under vastly different conditions or impacted by access to widely ranging levels of medical sophistication.

EPIDEMIOLOGY, WITH GEOGRAPHY AND RACE AS INDEPENDENT VARIABLES

Westernized Societies

Numerous publications, mostly from the developed or first world, show little variation when geographic areas are compared. There are two well-defined age peaks, the first at 25 and the other at 70 years.[11] Typically North America figures have parallels in Denmark and the Netherlands but they are distinct from Japanese, Singaporean, or Indian reports.[12]

One hypothesis advanced to explain this distribution is that the pathogenesis may differ with age. In young adults, there can be seen similarities to a chronic granulomatous or inflammatory process with an extensive host reaction but paucity of malignant cells. By contrast, in the elderly, truly neoplastic behavior is more the norm. This concept has precedent in the model for paralytic poliomyelitis. Here, infection with a virus of low virulence at an early age confers life-long immunity, but without such exposure, the subsequent manifestations are much more severe.[13] Such a postulate, however, fails to deal adequately with this lymphoma in childhood. Specifically, there is a greater frequency in Africa than elsewhere, and the predominant histopathology appears to be mixed cellularity with a relatively high proportion of neoplastic Reed-Sternberg cells having retinoblastoma protein detected in most cases independent of Epstein-Barr viral expression.[14] Another option for the bimodal age occurrence emanates from Colombian studies, which suggest a rather uniform cause but that different clinical syndromes reflect alternative host and environment interaction.[15]

African Experience

Whatever the explanation ultimately turns out to be, regional and socioeconomic differences exist in age, distribution of histopathology, and outcome. Some characteristics have precedent in, for example, the United Kingdom, with monotypic relationships demonstrable between mixed cellularity and the Townsend deprivation score supporting the involvement of environmental factors such as unemployment and household overcrowding in etiology.[16] In much the same way, the interaction between genetics, viruses, and immunity signpost directions for future research.[17] Interestingly, geographical and temporal variations are identifiable in childhood but may reflect improvements in case assertainment.[18] What remains unclear is how to interpret the impact of relocation to other parts of the world as, for example, Japanese moving at an early age to Hawaii, where this quite differently modifies later expression.[19]

Using such well-organized reference points as cancer incidence in five continents and the United States surveillance, epidemiology, and end-results program,[18] attention can be turned to seeking parallels, and perhaps more importantly distinctions, across the length and breadth of continents with their own set of often-unique challenges. As already noted, there is an increase from the equator to more temperate zones, whereas little if any information is available on possible relationships with tropical fevers like malaria,[20] chronic inflammation as suggested in Italy,[21] or increase of coccidiosis either spontaneously or in response to chemotherapy.[22] Also, there is a problem disentangling the exclusive effect of climate, because this may influence fauna and flora as natural vectors for parasites spanning the range of potential pathogens. There is, for example, a consistent association between Epstein-Barr virus and children in Kenya, with both type I and type II viral sequences having been found,[23] as well as in Tunisia and South Africa.[24]

Dominating literally every aspect of life, including the entire spectrum of lymphoproliferative disorders, has been the ongoing—and in many areas still uncontrolled—pandemic of rampant HIV dissemination. In western Europe there was a peak in 1995, with a relative risk for Hodgkin lymphoma of 10, indolent lymphomas of 14, but of over 300 for those with high-grade histopathology.[25] Inexplicably, despite the still-expanding volume of affected individuals in South Africa, an impact on cancer awaits clarification.[26] Thus, in the report from the national cancer registry and the epidemiology research group, excessive risks were found for Kaposi sarcoma, lymphocytic tumors, and vulvar as well as cervical cancer but did not include Hodgkin lymphoma cases. More challenging, but currently unexplained, is why these risks are substantially lower than those found in the West.[6] Of relevance is the observation that seroconversion results in a 20-fold increase, but specific figures for this lymphoma are not available at least in the report from Uganda and Zimbabwe.[27] Also notable is that in resource-poor areas there is an earlier onset in children compared to industrialized societies, and, as in adults, they have more aggressive and lymphocyte-depleted forms, typically extranodal, and males more than females.[28]

Exhaustive efforts to superimpose these observations on the map of Africa and so reveal the current status has proven impossible. In a major part there are simply no registry data but only vague generalization about mycobacterial or pneumocystis isolates and little reliable correlation with tumor pathogenesis. Where such comments are possible, they emanate from few centers, and even here acquisition is unreliable because inclusion of rural clinics, or villages, is almost always absent. In addition, there has been a huge delay, at least in South Africa, in accepting the elsewhere long-recognized viral causation for AIDS. Therefore, for the present there is at best considerable uncertainty of a causative role in these cases, which contrasts with a more confident incrimination for the other lymphomas and solid tumors.[2,25-27]

With this caveat it is noted that age standardized rates for men and women recorded from the Kampala Cancer Registry between 1964 and 1968[29] fell below those from Europe and North America, perhaps due to some underreporting. Numbers in Ugandan males probably exceed those from Britain at least for the first 10 years of life, but there is an unexplained failure to show a peak in young adults, and this remains small even in the fifth and sixth decades. Although poor-histology subtypes predominated,[29] accounts from elsewhere in this tropical zone, typically from single institutions or academic centers in large regional hospitals, again document a low prevalence except in childhood when compared to other malignancies. Uniquely, the Ibadan Province of Western Nigeria approaches what is generally encountered in the northern hemisphere, again loaded by unfavorable subtypes leading to the impression of a rapid and fulminating course.[30] This may reflect intraregional variation related to undefined local conditions. However, relatively low frequencies are reported from Zambia,[31] Kenya,[32] and Zimbabwe.[33] Other sources from the sub-Sahara, such as Mali, Uganda, and Gambia, show rates less than 0.8 per 100 000.[34,35]

Further regional consideration highlights some uniformity, and in places differences, that exist; but always with the reservation that reporting is patchy and interpretations inevitably biased. Algeria, with the regional register at Setif, has rates of 2.4/100 000 in adults and 0.7/100 000 in male and 0.4/100 000 in female children, respectively.[34] In North Africa, there appears to be a different and specific distribution of the Epstein-Barr viral strains between nasopharyngeal epithelial lesions and Hodgkin lymphoma arising in this same anatomic site, leading to speculation of other explanations for tumorogenesis.[36]

The Insitut Pasteur in Tunisia noted epidemiology going back to 1950[37-39] and added classification, stage, and outcome from 1969, when the Institut Salah Azaiz (ISA) was founded as a national cancer center[40] (Tables 30.1 and 30.2). Notably there is a high prevalence of Epstein-Barr viral infection in this drainage area.[41,42] There does not seem to be much difference between Algeria and Tunisia, but subtle, even important, variations may be obscured since no uniform repository exists. The ISA figures show the disease to comprise 4% of all cancers in adults and 11% of those in children,[40] with this lymphoma accounting for 7.43% in both sexes.[40] In Morocco, the corresponding rate was 10.1% of total malignancies.[43] Correspondingly a report from Rabat, with an age range of 2 to 15 years, shows about a quarter of the patients to be younger than 5, with a male-to-female ratio of 5 to 1.[44] Notably, there was a delay to diagnosis of 6

months despite cervical lymphadenopathy being present in about 90% of the individuals, constitutional complaints, mediastinal mass, and abdominal nodal enlargement in roughly half. Similarities are seen to Turkish and Indian studies. However, confidence and interpretation is weakened because of 49% loss to follow-up.[44]

TABLE 30.1

HODGKIN LYMPHOMA IN TUNISIA AND ALGERIA: DEMOGRAPHIC DATA

	Tunisia		Algeria	
	No. patients	%	No. patients	%
Total	113	100	262	100
Age				
0–15	34	30	80	31
16–25	18	16	62	23.5
26–40	37	33	83	31.5
>40	24	21	35	13.5
Histology				
LP	7	6	30	11.5
NS	55	49	105	40
MC	45	40	66	25
LD	4	4	7	3
Unclassified	2	1	56	21.5
Sex				
Male	70	62	180	68
Female	43	38	84	32
Median age (y)	28.5		—	
M/F ratio	1.6:1		2:1	

LP, lymphocyte predominant; NS, nodular sclerosis; MC, mixed cellularity; LD, lymphocyte depleted.
From Ben Abdallah M. Epidemiologie des cancers en Tunisie: registre de l'Institut Salah Azaiz. Tunis, 1997.

TABLE 30.2

HODGKIN LYMPHOMA IN TUNISIA AND ALGERIA: CLINICAL CHARACTERISTICS

	Tunisia		Algeria	
	No. patients	%	No. patients	%
Stage				
I–I	58	51.5	139	53
III–IV	55	48.5	123	47
B-symptoms	77	68	—	—
Mediastinal involvement				
None	80	71	—	—
Bulky	25	22	—	—
ESR (mm/hour)				
<40	34	30	—	—
>40	79	70	—	—

ESR, erythrocyte sedimentation rate.
From Ben Abdallah M. Epidemiologie des cancers en Tunisie: registre de l'Institut Salah Azaiz. Tunis, 1997.

North African migrants to France primarily from Algeria, Tunisia, Morocco, and Egypt have unusual and quite distinctive patterns of neoplasia, but specific data on Hodgkin lymphoma are not available.[45]

In the Maghreb, children and young adults are prominently affected, with those under the age of 15 accounting for almost one-third of cases.[37–40,43] In childhood the male-to-female ratio approximates 3 to 1, in contrast to adults, where it is greater than 2 to 1. Among the latter, nodular sclerosis predominates. The distribution between stage I and II versus III and IV is about equal. Delayed diagnosis is not unusual, with this occurring after 6 months from first signs in more than 40% of cases and thereby perhaps explaining the extensive initial involvement. In children from this region most have nodular sclerosing or mixed cellularity with stages III and IV predominating.

Egypt has the advantage of studies conducted in ten different cancer centers that are attached to various universities. Major contributors are the Egyptian National Cancer Institute (ENCI) and the Cairo University Hospital Oncology Centre known as NEMROCK. As a generalization, lymphoreticular disorders and leukemias constitute between 11.8% and 15.9% of documented neoplasms. In a survey of 557 cases, high-grade histopathology, designated in past years as of reticulum cell origin, was followed by Hodgkin lymphoma with a peak in the second decade and a male-to-female ratio of 3 to 1. Mixed cellularity was seen most often, while nodular sclerosis was rare.[46] In another report, Egyptian men had a greater frequency of these tumors than their counterparts from the Gaza strip, whereas the inverse situation was found in women. The authors noted that careful consideration of this kind of discrepancy may provide improved approaches for determining risks in causation and advocate increased cooperation among participating national registries.[47]

An analysis from the Egyptian and National Cancer Institute of 4,382 newly diagnosed individuals all reviewed by a single pathologist yielded 526 cases of malignant lymphoma or 7%, but only 193 cases of Hodgkin lymphoma or 2.57%.[48] Mixed cellularity was found in 50.71%, lymphocyte predominance in 23.78%, nodular sclerosis in 17%, and lymphocyte depletion in 8.29% of the patients. Unfortunately, age and sex distribution within the histologic variants was not recorded. In addition, at the Cairo University Hospital Oncology Centre, 7,325 consecutive adults were reviewed between 1990 and 1995, and 420 or 5.7% of the total number had non-Hodgkin lymphoma, 107 or 1.5% had Hodgkin lymphoma, and a further 5.7% had other variants, giving a ratio of 3.8 to 1,[49] which is largely comparable to the Egyptian National Cancer Institute, with 42% of patients having mixed cellularity and again the male-to-female ratio was equal. Lymphocyte predominant was only 5.6% and lymphocyte depleted 7.4%, but both were found largely among males. There were 48 examples of nodular sclerosing in this cohort of 107 patients over the age of 15 years, and a male-to-female ratio of around 2 to 1.

Clinical staging in the Cairo University Hospital series[49] showed that 12% were in stage I, mostly asymptomatic; 43% were in stage II, with half having weight loss or other evidence of systemic involvement; 35% had stage III; and 10% stage IV and, with dissemination, two-thirds to three-quarters became symptomatic. There was supradiaphragmatic localization in 73% with the mediastinum involved in 20%, but liver spread was noted in one-third and only sporadically was this demonstrable in bone marrow, skin, or nasopharynx.[49]

The characterization of changing distribution in cancer consequent upon cross-border migration provides useful insight into changes that follow relocation.[19] When Egyptian-born settlers were compared to indigenous French, with adjustment for such things as social status and areas of residence, there was a trend for higher risk of lymphoma in the new arrivals, although Hodgkin lymphoma is not specifically referred to.[46]

In Namibia (Annelle Zietsman, personal communication) this entity was the 28th most common cancer, and has moved up to 7th place in parallel with escalation of the AIDS epidemic. Thirty-nine patients were studied over the past 10 years of whom 27 were male, 17 were black, 14 were white, and 8 were of mixed ancestry. Eight were under 20 years of age, 16 between 20 and 45, and the remaining 15 over 45. Lymphocyte predominance existed in 5, nodular sclerosing in 16, mixed cellularity in 9, and lymphocyte depletion in 7, with the information missing in 2. Seven tested positive for the retrovirus, of whom 5 have died and 2 are alive on highly active therapy. When given standard chemotherapy, including radiotherapy as indicated, 22 remain alive. In keeping with what occurs in much of the third world, the patients are typically indigent and treated in state hospitals, although with the increasing availability of an active private sector, 8 benefitted from access to such facilities. It is noteworthy that most of the patients tested positive for Epstein-Barr virus and tuberculosis was seen widely, but documentation is incomplete. Jordan is an instructive model to further highlight this latter association. When viewed against North America, worldwide discrepancies become even more striking. Thus this ranges from less than 30% in Sweden to over 100% in Kenya. Here there are parallels with the situation in the United States, with rates being low to intermediate versus other parts of the world.[50]

The uniqueness of Africa is exemplified by the report from Dakar drawing attention to pulmonary parenchyma as a target and emphasizing the perspective predicated by the common finding of tuberculosis in the Senegal.[51] Western Ethiopia was the site of an illuminating retrospective regional study based in the Gondar College of Medical Sciences including the Amhara and Tigrai regions. Consecutive review of 83 examples over the years 1988 to 1999, with ages ranging from 4 to 79 years, showed roughly one-quarter to have Hodgkin lymphoma. Here about one-third had lymphocyte predominance and another 33% had mixed cellularity, with the highest frequency being in the first and second decades. This set the stage to undertake further prospective studies.[52] Again, from Burkina Faso comes the recognition of coexisting tuberculosis, and because both diseases are curable, emphasis was placed upon early diagnosis and treatment.[53] Twenty-two years of follow-up in 62 individuals treated in the Côte D'Ivoire showed an impressive 66% complete remission rate, but the precarious living conditions given the true event-free survival was difficult to define reliably.[54]

South of the equator, the findings in Zimbabwe are largely reflective of those further north, although the age split is slightly different. Thus, one-third of cases are seen before 20 years, with a male-to-female ratio of 1.8 to 1 and most comprise the mixed-cellularity variant (Table 30.3).[55,56]

Throughout South Africa regional trends can be traced, as when the Gauteng area, the old Pretoria and Johannesburg, are compared to the Western Cape.[57] Pathologists examined biopsy data in the two major race groups for frequency, age, and sex distribution and, insightfully, included American blacks and whites as well as examples from Nigeria and Uganda. Not surprisingly, there was a high frequency of mixed-cellularity and lymphocyte-depleted categories as well as childhood disease, with males predominating in all subtypes including nodular sclerosis. Whites had a low occurrence in this age range, an increased rate in young adults, relatively high frequency of nodular sclerosing, and an excess of females. Both ethnic groups fell into the intermediate pattern II, with a bias to pattern I in black patients judged to reflect poorer social circumstances in contrast to pattern III in the more affluent white patients.[57] Conversely, country-wide

TABLE 30.3

HODGKIN LYMPHOMA IN ZIMBABWE: DEMOGRAPHIC AND STAGE CHARACTERISTICS

	Number	Percent
Total	170	100
Age by decile		
0–9	4	2.4
10–19	48	28.2
20–29	40	23.5
30–39	37	21.8
40–49	21	12.3
50–59	8	4.7
60–69	9	5.3
70–79	3	1.8
Histology		
LP	7	4.1
NS	30	17.7
MC	92	54.1
LD	41	24.1
Sex		
Male	109	64
Female	61	36
Stage		
I–II	35	20.6
III–IV	135	79.4
Median age	28 years	
M/F ratio	1.8	

LP, lymphocyte predominant; NS, nodular sclerosis; MC, mixed cellularity; LD, lymphocyte depleted.
Data from L Levy (unpublished).

analysis has generously been provided thanks to the National Cancer Registry (Nokuzola Mqoqi, personal communication) The 10-year graphs from 1990 to 1999 show that for males and for females there was no evidence of a declining trend in the age-standardized incidence when examined by linear regression, with the observed fall of 1.9% annually not being significant (95% CI: −6.33, 2.81) and 0.4 (95% CI: −4.21, 3.58), respectively. In males aged 40 to 64 there was a significant decrease over this period, at a rate of 4.9% (95% CI: −9.46, 0.13) annually (Fig. 30.1). In a previous review, an age-adjusted rate of 0.81 for black women and 1.42 for their white counterparts was consistent over time, as was the 0.95 and 3.27 for respective groups of men (Fig. 30.2)[58] The apparently lower frequency in the blacks may in part be related to underreporting because this is a pathology database. Nevertheless, these figures are consistent with those described earlier for this region.[57]

There is also a marked difference between the histopathology found between groups in South Africa. In blacks, mixed cellularity or lymphocyte depletion predominates, whereas nodular sclerosing is most common among whites. This is illustrated by the Gauteng figures (Table 30.4), but also occurs in Natal and in the Free State. The Western Cape, however, has greater ethnic diversity. In the past there was predominance of white or mixed ancestry but more recently there has been substantial black influx. These shifting patterns may explain changes that in bygone era had conformed to northern Europe but now show a perceptible trend towards that more frequently seen in Africa since 1994. In the last 10 years, histology, race, and age have been nationally updated (Tables 30.5 to 30.7) (Nokuzola Mqoqi and Patricia Kellett, personal communication, 2005).

Especially instructive are findings in children. The investigators from St Jude Children's Research Hospital [59] confirm that the great majority of these cases, at least in the United States, differed from South American examples in having only 30% to 40% Epstein-Barr virus demonstrated as opposed to 100% from Latin America, and so drew

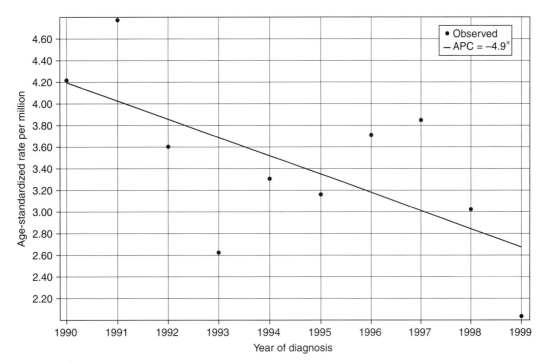

FIGURE 30.1. Hodgkin lymphoma in males age 40 to 64 from 1990 to 1999. APC, Annual percent change.

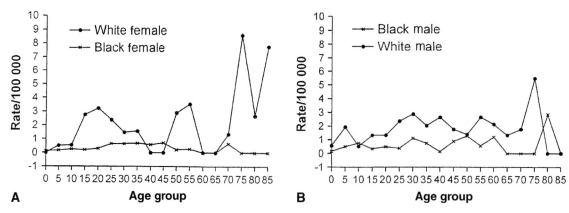

FIGURE 30.2. Distribution by age at diagnosis of Hodgkin lymphoma in black and white female (A) and male (B) South Africans. (Adapted from Sitas F, Blaauw D, Terblanche M, et al. *Cancer in South Africa 1988. National Cancer Registry of South Africa: incidence of histologically diagnosed cancer in South Africa, 1992.* Johannesburg: South African Institute for Medical Research; 1997:46–51.)

attention to the relationship with Burkitt lymphoma in equatorial Africa. The investigators then proceeded to examine pediatric cases of Hodgkin lymphoma from Brazil and the United States and postulated a multiple-etiology hypothesis for this entity.

Extrapolation to Southern Africa by the pediatric team at Stellenbosch University—Tygerberg Academic Hospital, acknowledging that blacks and those of mixed ancestry had less favorable socio-economic backgrounds, noted a 74% incidence of cervical lymphadenopathy, with 50% being symptomatic when first seen. There was again the recognized difference between racial groups, with localized as opposed to disseminated disease when whites are compared to blacks. Epidemiologically, the former were generally type I and the latter type III.[60] Another study from children documents a pattern intermediate between industrialized and nonindustrialized sites, emphasizing the poor prognosis and nondetection of Epstein-Barr viral products in the South African children.[24] A 22-year follow-up perhaps surprisingly revealed a large degree of concordance between adults and children, with late relapses and adverse events improved after shifting to the German Austrian Pediatric Study Group treatment regimen.[61]

Asia and South America

Regarded as a rare entity in the Far East, it follows that sparseness of information has hindered efforts to explore contributions from environment and heredity.[12] Better understanding is provided from population-based data comparing Chinese, Japanese, Filipinos, and Asian Indians living in the United States to two lands of origin where the incidence is low but, perhaps surprisingly, approximately double that for those living in North America. Of interest are the conclusions drawn from this discrepancy suggesting genetic resistance to disease development possibly associated with human leukocyte antigen typing and implication of environmental influences in etiology. In a clinicopathologic overview of 304 cases in the Sichuan province of China, 160 had Hodgkin lymphoma, with a male to female ratio of 5.7 to 1 and a greater prevalence in

TABLE 30.4

DISTRIBUTION OF HODGKIN LYMPHOMA BY AGE GROUP AND HISTOLOGIC SUBTYPE IN SOUTH AFRICA: CRUDE RATES BASED ON PATHOLOGIC DIAGNOSIS

Histologic subtype	Ethnic group, black: age range							Ethnic group, white: age range						
	10–14	15–24	25–34	35–44	45–54	>55	Total	10–14	15–24	25–34	35–44	45–54	>55	Total
LP	1	0	1	1	4	0	7	0	2	2	2	0	0	6
NS	2	4	7	6	2	7	28	2	6	5	3	0	5	21
MC	5	4	1	4	2	2	18	3	1	1	1	4	3	13
LD	1	5	4	2	1	4	17	0	1	0	1	1	4	7
NOS	9	15	20	17	6	15	82	3	8	16	10	9	18	64
Total	18	28	33	30	15	28	152	8	18	24	17	14	30	111

LP, lymphocyte predominant; NS, nodular sclerosis; MC, mixed cellularity; LD, lymphocyte depleted; NOS, not otherwise specified.
From Sitas F, Blaauw D, Terblanche M, et al. *Cancer in South Africa 1988. National Cancer Registry of South Africa: incidence of histologically diagnosed cancer in South Africa, 1992.* Johannesburg: South African Institute for Medical Research; 1997:46–51. Courtesy of National Cancer Registry of South Africa.

TABLE 30.5

HODGKIN LYMPHOMA IN SOUTH AFRICA, 1990–1999: HISTOLOGIC TYPES

Histotype	Total%
Malignant lymphoma, not otherwise specified	1,506 (49.54)
Nodular sclerosis	718 (23.62)
Mixed cellularity	532 (17.50)
Lymphocytic predominance	159 (5.23)
Lymphocytic depletion	109 (3.59)
Other	16 (0.53)
Total	3,040 (100)

Data from National Cancer Registry of South Africa (Nokuzola Mqoqi and Patricia Kellett, personal communication, 2005).

TABLE 30.6

HODGKIN LYMPHOMA IN SOUTH AFRICA, 1990–1999 (N = 3040)

Race	Female %	Male %	Total %
Asian	32 (2.9)	64 (3.8)	96 (3.5)
Black	538 (49)	965 (57.9)	1,503 (54.3)
Colored	99 (9.0)	133 (7.9)	232 (8.4)
White	429 (39.1)	507 (30.4)	936 (33.8)
Total	1,098 (100)	1,667 (100)	2,767 (100)
Unknown race/sex	273		
Average cases/year	304		
Mean age	33.7 ±18.3		
Median age	32		
Female: male ratio	1:1.5		

Data from National Cancer Registry of South Africa (Nokuzola Mqoqi and Patricia Kellett, personal communication, 2005).

TABLE 30.7

HODGKIN LYMPHOMA IN SOUTH AFRICA, 1990–1999

Age group	Female %	Male %	Total %
0–14	100 (9.4)	305 (18.9)	405 (15.1)
15–34	489 (45.8)	608 (37.8)	1,097 (41)
35–54	302 (28.3)	484 (30.1)	786 (29.4)
55–64	92 (8.6)	124 (7.7)	216 (8.1)
65+	85 (9)	89 (5.5)	174 (6.5)
Total	1,068 (100)	1,610 (100)	2,678 (100)
Female: male ratio	1:1.5		

Data from National Cancer Registry of South Africa (Nokuzola Mqoqi and Patricia Kellett, personal communication, 2005).

children between ages 5 and 9. One is again struck by the high incidence of the mixed-cellularity variant, found in 62.5% of the cases.[62] When such a childhood experience is compared to adults, it emerges that there is a low incidence of only 9.2% in Hong Kong, for which there is no current explanation. Nevertheless, it is pertinent that treatment outcome with advanced-stage or unfavorable subtypes is comparable to that in Caucasians.[63] In a large cohort from the hematolymphoreticular group of the Korean Society of Pathologists, cases over a 2-year period from 23 institutions were reviewed using the revised European-American classification, and again strikingly lower rates of this subtype emerged compared to the West, with the discrepancy that nodular sclerosis was higher compared to the previous study and the affirmation that the pattern of these lymphomas in the Republic of Korea is distinct from that in industrialized parts of the western world and parallel other patterns in the Far East. Also it is observed that over time, there have been changes in the relative rates for some of these subtypes, part of which is attributable to refined criteria for diagnosis.[64] A study from Kuala Lumpur in Malaysia illustrated the difficulty of reliable data capture. Of 98 biopsies from 92 patients, only 14 had Hodgkin lymphoma, of which 6 were mixed cellularity and 4 nodular sclerosing, with odd examples of lymphocyte-rich, lymphocyte-depleted, and lymphocyte-predominant histopathologies. The other non-Hodgkin lymphomas were approximately 4.7 times as frequently encountered, but the investigators observed that data may be skewed by lower use of this hospital service by the ethnic Chinese.[65] In another large series reported from Bangkok, a striking increase of 158.9% was noted over time, but almost paradoxically there was a decrease in Hodgkin lymphoma, from 28.9% to 8.5%, leading to the conclusion that the high frequency of intermediate- to high-grade tumors was largely attributable to those of B-cell phenotype; why this should occur is still puzzling.[66]

Indian scientists acknowledge the importance of the lymphomas and stress, as we have noted, that few reports describe this experience when compared to documentation from developed regions. Using a population-based registration from Bangalore, India, 1,397 cases from the cancer registry gave an age-adjusted incidence of 7.7 for males and 4.8 per 100 000 for females. Excellent follow-up provided mortality and survival information on 1,267 or 90.7% of the cases. Although lymphoid and hematopoietic malignancies were combined, the observed 5-year survival was 26%, with the demonstration that this was lower in all categories compared to matching outcome from developed countries.[67] Follow-up from greater Bombay showed the lymphatic malignancies to account for only 5% of the total registered, with, again, a rising trend in the incidence of all types of lymphoma in both sexes. To explore possible causes, epidemiologic studies are in progress, but data are currently not available.[68]

Turning now to Brazil, the case-control interview study conducted in Sao Paulo compared 70 cases of the lymphoma to an equal number of subjects matched for age and sex and 128 siblings of the patients. The major epidemiologic finding was a high incidence among children and a relative predominance of mixed cellularity and, perhaps surprisingly, high social status associated with an increased risk for this lymphoma. Tantalizingly, and suggested previously, has been correlation with a prior tonsillectomy, with the caveat that other variables such as sibship size, marital status, occupational exposure, and viral illnesses appear not to be determinants of risk.[69] From the Department of Hematology at the National Medical Centre in Mexico City, a retrospective analysis was conducted covering 264 patients over 15 years. In an instructive and rational approach, three therapeutic periods were compared. From 1974 to 1976, the focus was on staging procedures, and yielded 81 patients with 5- and 10-year survivals of 67% and 60%, respectively. In the second study, from 1977 to 1980 there was predominant use of combination chemotherapy and radiotherapy, and here 87 patients had an improved survival of 75% and 72% in each category. The last interval, from 1981 to 1984, was characterized by increasing relevance of prognostic factors in the alternating use of MOPP and ABVD. Ninety-six patients had 96% survival at 4 years. Instructively better results have been associated with increasing awareness of the high number of late complications due to therapy.[70] In this general context, a report from Monterrey, Mexico reemphasizes the value of bone marrow trephine biopsy as a staging procedure.[71]

Points of Contrast

In Africa, prominent differences are identified when this entity is compared to North America. In the terminology recommended by the International Union Against Cancer,[72] four categories have emerged. Type I, primarily in children, was associated with less favorable histopathology. Type III was mostly found in developed lands and prevailing in young adults, where a better outcome correlates with the lymphocyte- predominant and nodular-sclerosing variants. Type II is intermediate and type IV largely limited to Asia and not discussed further here. Viewed in this way, type I is dominant in the central part of Africa.[29–33] Further studies deserve mention, although in general they were of insufficient power for inclusion in our main analysis of geographic pathology. In Zambia, Hodgkin lymphoma was seen as 18.6% of lymphoma with 44% of the cases occurring in the first two decades of life; most were in an advanced stage and were of mixed-cellularity or lymphocyte-depletion subtypes.[31] Comparable experience comes from Nigeria,[73–76] Kenya,[32,77–79] Uganda,[80–83] Gabon,[84] and Zimbabwe.[55,56,85] From Uganda,[81] there is a single description of a bimodal age-specific curve approximating the classical type III, and this may result from intraregional variation.

Throughout the North African littoral and South Africa most cases are intermediate or type II,[7,86] approximating what was seen in North America during the 1950s and 1960s,[87–89] with occurrence less in blacks than whites, where there was aggressive histology and advanced stage. These findings were considered to be environmental rather than attributable to genetic predisposition. In this regard, there are indications that there has been a shift during the last 25 to 30 years among the North American blacks, but race remains a significant predictor for outcome[90] to more closely approximate type III. From such inferential reasoning it may be concluded that the intermediate pattern seen in South Africa reflects a transitional phase in epidemiology. However, this postulate needs to be confirmed to establish whether HLA or immune response-linked gene frequencies or other molecular aberrations might still play a major role in this regard.

It might also be debated whether there is a drift in what was seen typically over the years, from a lower to a higher overall frequency albeit to one with better prognostic factors, that could be interpreted as a step forward in cancer control. It may rather be argued that the available studies have not as yet provided any real clues to suggest a strategy of prevention for this entity in any population group.

Asian populations, even following relocation to the United States, have lower rates than American populations,[12] and there is weighting towards less favorable mixed-cellularity subtypes, although overall incidence appears to be increasing. Data from the National Cancer Registry Program in India, although having a relatively low incidence, report lower 5-year survival rates than from more industrialized reference points.

South American epidemiologic studies highlight the association with prior tonsillectomy.[69] In Sao Paolo, a strong association with Epstein-Barr infection emerges. The geographical differences reflect histologic subtype and age distribution.[91] A particularly telling point is made by the Hematopathology Committee of the Brazilian Society for Pathology, which was concerned about these apparently differing results, and so undertook a multicenter study. They then issued a definitive statement, derived from a large number of cases, to confirm the predominance of the nodular-sclerosing subtype and a high proportion of patients in their first two decades of life.[92] The interpretation is that the previous controversy regarding frequency of subtypes may be related to small numbers of cases, and this current study presents a picture close to the situation that parallels increasing industrialization.

CLINICAL PRESENTATION, STAGING, AND PROGNOSTIC FACTORS

Westernized Societies

The clinical features from North America in both adults and children provide a convenient orientation against which to examine intercontinental differences. Although, predictably, attention is drawn to this diagnosis by the finding of enlarged nodes, with confirmation dependent on biopsy in both developed and emerging societies, there are nevertheless quite striking contrasts.

African Experience

Overall, on this continent, the original Ann Arbor staging classification system,[93–95] with modifications that emerged from follow-up meetings in the Cotswolds,[96,97] is recommended and remains in general use. The problem of applying this essential step to individuals is organizational rather than methodological. Large numbers of people are in rural areas served by few centers that offer sophisticated evaluation such as CT, MRI, and nuclear medicine techniques such as gallium imaging or PET. However, imaging facilities are available along the North African littoral, to a limited extent in Zimbabwe, and increasingly in South Africa as well as in Kenya in East Africa, Nigeria, Ghana, and the francophone neighboring countries. However, because these are potentially curable cases, it is felt that no compromise should be considered but rather that all should be referred to available specialist establishments where full and adequate management can be carried out.

The substantial frequency of chronic bacterial and parasitic infestations throughout Africa, which are capable of giving rise to granulomatous or other processes that may coexist with the lymphoma, needs to be taken into account when evaluating lesions detected either clinically or radiologically.[98] Such complications include, for example, tuberculosis with its associated enlarged glands or the still rapidly rising occurrence of HIV, amebic abscesses, lymphogranuloma inguinale, hydatid cysts, syphilitic gummas, and schistosomiasis. Delay in diagnosis and empiric medication for typical and atypical mycobacterial lymphadenopathy, especially among those from rural areas, constitutes a major cause of delay in diagnosing the underlying Hodgkin lymphoma. Although these disorders usually demonstrate subtleties that are sufficiently distinctive for separation from an immunoproliferative disorder, this requires considerable judgment as well as a high index of suspicion.

The absence of pulmonary involvement by typical tuberculous changes should alert the clinician that glandular swelling might have an alternative explanation. Ultimately, however, the diagnostic problem can only be resolved by appropriate investigation. Access to, and provision of, laboratories that have well-standardized microbiologic and histologic services to establish the presence of this chronic inflammatory state, rather than reliance on empiric drug administration, is a high priority in this as other parts of the third world.

Enlarged spleens from endemic malaria give rise to the tropical splenomegaly syndrome. Here the question of staging laparotomy and surgical removal of this organ has been defined by a number of studies. The risk of this and other infections on the one hand, and the fact that most have stage IIB or more advanced stages on the other, make such a procedure largely inappropriate and, not surprisingly, has led to discontinuing it since 1985.

Initial disease extent and other prognostic pointers have been examined in some detail in northern and southern Africa. Tunisia and Algeria (Tables 30.1 and 30.2) show striking similarities, with nearly half of the cases being disseminated having fever, weight loss, sweating, elevated erythrocyte sedimentation rate, and a long delay in time to diagnosis. In addition, the relatively large numbers lost to follow-up or receiving suboptimal management, highlighted by ISA, is unfortunately repeated throughout the rest of the continent with as many as 20% of each cohort falling into these categories. For example, Zimbabwe shows an even more striking bias in favor of stage III and IV (Table 30.3). Little is known about the corresponding status in equatorial Africa because there are few publications to draw on.

Egyptian reports overlap with those from other areas in North Africa such as Algeria, Morocco, and Tunisia. However, when migration is taken into account, differences appear to exist, but interpretation is limited by relatively small numbers and lack of follow-up.[45] In South Africa, again as elsewhere, prognosis is multifactorial and not all the predictors are included in the anatomically based staging systems.[95,96] Although the impact of histology as an independent variable remains controversial, there is general agreement that mixed-cellularity and lymphocyte-depleted variants are usually associated with more advanced stage and the presence of B-symptoms when first seen (Tables 30.4 and 30.5) Proctor and co-workers developed a numerical index[99] that included stage of disease, age, hemoglobin level, lymphocyte count, and bulk. This could be applied to discriminate for good prognosis, with a failure-free survival over 80% at 10 years, and those with less satisfactory outcome, for whom the corresponding figure was only 59% in the same period. The predictive effect that some of these elements exert has been confirmed in another international analysis, where seven indices (Table 30.8) were identified, each of which reduced bulk control by 7% to 8% at 5 years.[100]

TABLE 30.8

INTERNATIONAL STUDY OF PROGNOSTIC FACTORS IN HODGKIN LYMPHOMA: FACTORS IDENTIFIED AS LEADING TO A SIGNIFICANT REDUCTION IN FAILURE-FREE SURVIVAL

Age ≤45 years

Male sex

Stage IV disease

Albumin <40 g/L

Hemoglobin <10.5 g/dL

Total WBC ≤1.5 × 10^9/L

Lymphocyte count <0.6 × 10^9/L or <8% of WBC

WBC, white blood cell count.
From Hasenclever D, Diehl V. A prognostic score for advanced Hodgkin's disease. International Prognostic Factors Project on Advanced Hodgkin's Disease. *N Engl J Med* 1998;339:1506–1514.

There are few corresponding studies from African investigators, although analysis from Johannesburg[101] confirmed the ability of the Newcastle Prognostic Index[99] to segregate good from poor outcome in Caucasians (Fig. 30.3). The frequency distribution by histology and other observations was not different from those reported from elsewhere in the world (Table 30.9).[102] However, this system proved less effective in blacks (Fig. 30.4).

Asia and South America

Here the incidence, as from Africa, which is roughly comparable to what occurs elsewhere as noted above, using the same diagnostic, staging, and prognostic criteria, gave conclusions that, probably because of inadequate numbers, are unreliable and in need of more critical testing.[92] Largely, however, it seems that as with the rest of the world, cases continue to increase, but whether this represents better documentation or true escalation requires further testing.

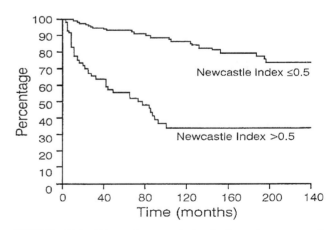

FIGURE 30.3. Disease-free survival of chemotherapy-treated (MOPP/ABVD) white patients with Hodgkin lymphoma, stratified according to the Newcastle Prognostic Index (*p* = 0.001). (Adapted from Bezwoda WR, MacPhail AP, Dawey R, et al. Hodgkin's disease in sub-Saharan Africa. Cambridge medical reviews. In: Armitage J, Newland A, Keating A, et al., eds. *Hematological oncology.* Vol. 4. Cambridge: Cambridge University Press; 1995:21–40.)

TABLE 30.9

DISTRIBUTION OF HISTOLOGIC SUBTYPE AMONG 494 ADULT BLACK AND WHITE PATIENTS WITH HODGKIN LYMPHOMA (OVERALL $x^2 = 60.52; p < 0.001$)

Age (decile)	Lymphocyte predominant		Nodular sclerosis		Mixed cellularity		Lymphocyte depleted		p Value
	Black	White	Black	White	Black	White	Black	White	
10–19	2	6	12	24	12	10	5	0	NS
20–29	2	13	13	51	26	12	15	5	$x^2 = 16.8$
30–39	0	9	18	24	27	22	12	2	$x^2 = 19.2$
40–49	2	2	12	20	10	10	3	3	NS
50–59	1	4	3	33	4	13	3	1	<0.3 $x^2 = 15.5$
60–69	—	—	0	9	4	8	1	1	NS
>70	—	12	—	10	—	10	—	3	NS
Total	7	36	58	171	83	85	39	15	

NS, not signigicant.
From Donaldson SS. Hodgkin's disease in children. *Semin Oncol* 1990;17:736–748.

Points of Contrast

Striking confirmation of these differences comes from updates (Table 30.10) that show significance to persist in the relative frequency distribution among components of the prognostic index, notably histology and age, between black and white. Despite the former being younger, with this providing substantial weighting toward good prognosis using the Newcastle criteria, the overall figures continue to more closely match those having adverse outcome among Caucasians. One consideration, which may be major in assessing the relative impact of prognostic indicators on end-results of Hodgkin lymphomas between blacks and whites, is that economic and educational level might be more predictive than ethnicity. However, here there may be correlations with race, making independent assessment difficult. Additionally, education and improving infrastructure will, it is hoped, improve this situation in the future. Precisely these arguments are applicable to other developing zones that, by definition, include those in Asian and South American specific aspects in children.

SPECIFIC ASPECTS IN CHILDREN

Westernized Societies

Occurrence in children is less frequent following industrialization and outcome is steadily improving.[103–106] Even when recurrent or refractory, many will have a successful result.[107] These publications outline standards of practice to be aimed for everywhere.

African Experience

An analysis of 242 consecutive children treated at the National Cancer Institute in Cairo between 1975 and 1980 showed a male to female ratio of 3 to 1, with mixed cellularity accounting for 60.74% of disease. Stages III and IV comprised 63.2% and typically were associated with high bulk. Not unexpectedly, staging laparotomy, which had been carried out in 154 instances, revealed more infradiaphragmatic localization than was clinically expected. Here there appeared to be a correlation with schistosomal hepatic fibrosis but this may have been coincidental.[108] From South Africa comes the suggestion that the frequency is lower in black children, irrespective of age, relative to whites[58] (Fig. 30.2).

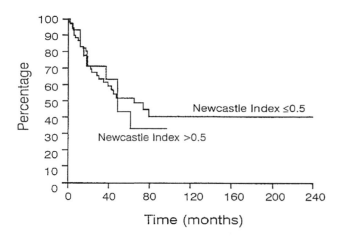

FIGURE 30.4. Disease-free survival of chemotherapy-treated (MOPP or MOPP/ABVD) black patients with Hodgkin lymphoma, stratified according to the Newcastle Prognostic Index. (Adapted from Bezwoda WR, MacPhail AP, Dawey R, et al. Hodgkin's disease in sub-Saharan Africa. Cambridge medical reviews. In: Armitage J, Newland A, Keating A, et al., eds. *Hematological oncology*. Vol. 4. Cambridge: Cambridge University Press; 1995:21–40.)

TABLE 30.10

RELATIVE DISTRIBUTION OF FACTORS CONSIDERED TO BE IMPORTANT IN PREDICTING OUTCOME OF TREATMENT FOR HODGKIN LYMPHOMA AMONG ADULT BLACK AND WHITE PATIENTS TREATED WITH COMBINATION THERAPY

	Black		White		
	Number	%	Number	%	*p* Value
Stage					
I and II	32	17	171	56	0.001
III and IV	155	83	136	44	
Symptoms					
A	29	11	95	31	<0.001
B	158	89	212	69	
Age					
<50	171	91	203	66	0.001
≥50	16	9	104	34	
Hemoglobin					
≥10	129	69	280	91	0.001
<10	58	31	27	9	
Disease bulk					
Bulky (≥10 cm)	90	48	98	32	0.02
Nonbulky (<10 cm)	97	52	209	68	
Lymphocyte count					
<1.0 × 10⁹/L	87	47	85	28	0.01
>1.0 × 10⁹/L	100	53	222	72	
Newcastle index					
≤0.5	109	76	212	76	NS
>0.5	35	24	67	24	

Bezwoda WR, MacPhail AP, Dawey R, et al. Hodgkin's disease in sub-Saharan Africa. Cambridge medical reviews. In: Armitage J, Newland A, Keating A, et al., eds. *Hematological oncology*. Vol. 4. Cambridge: Cambridge University Press; 1995:21–40.

In figures from the Western Cape, including 39 children under 15 years of age, there were 7 blacks, 12 whites, and 20 children of mixed ancestry (Tables 30.11 and 30.12).[109,110] The male-to-female ratio was 2.9:1, and the median ages were 147, 124, and 199 months in children of white, mixed, and black ancestry, respectively, the latter two having underprivileged backgrounds. Nodular sclerosis was present in 59% of whites, mixed cellularity in 40% of mixed-ancestry children, and lymphocyte depletion in 43% of blacks. Among all consecutive entries, 5% had clinical stage I, 41% stage II, 28% stage III, and 26% stage IV. By contrast, the majority of white children had localized disease.

TABLE 30.11

CHILDHOOD HODGKIN LYMPHOMA IN THE WESTERN CAPE: DISTRIBUTION OF HISTOLOGY BY ETHNIC GROUP

Histology	Black		Mixed		White	
	No. patients	%	No. patients	%	No. patients	%
MC	0	0	8	40	4	33
NS	2	29	7	35	7	59
LD	3	43	4	20	1	8
LP	1	14	0	0	0	0
Other	1	14	1	5	0	0
Total	7		20		12	

From Hesseling PB, Wessels G, van Riet FA. The Tygerberg Hospital Children's Tumour Registry 1983–1993. *Eur J Cancer* 1995;31A:1471–1475; and Jacobson RJ, Klappenbach RS, Clinton C, et al. Hodgkin's disease in South African children. *S Afr Med J* 1981;59:133–137.

TABLE 30.12

CHILDHOOD HODGKIN LYMPHOMA IN THE WESTERN CAPE: DISTRIBUTION OF STAGE BY ETHNIC GROUP

	Whole group		Black		Mixed		White	
Stage	No.	%	No.	%	No.	%	No.	%
I	2	5	0	0	1	5	1	9
II	16	41	2	29	8	40	6	50
III	11	28	2	29	4	20	5	41
IV	10	26	3	42	7	35	0	0
Total	39		7		20		12	

From Hesseling PB, Wessels G, van Riet FA. The Tygerberg Hospital Children's Tumour Registry 1983–1993. *Eur J Cancer* 1995;31A:1471–1475; and Jacobson RJ, Klappenbach RS, Clinton C, et al. Hodgkin's disease in South African children. *S Afr Med J* 1981;59:133–137.

Asia and South America

Occurrence is most common between 5 and 9 years of age, with male predominance and typically with cervical lymphadenopathy, but extranodal involvement was not seen. Mixed cellularity was common and these lymphomas, as a group, did better than other lymphoproliferative disorders.[62] Results encountered in Malaysian children were similar, but the numbers are too small for meaningful comment.[65] Bimodal age-specific incidence curves were reported from Brazil, with the relevance of tonsillectomy noted where there was a relative risk of 2.5 compared to those who have not undergone the operation.[69] In a prospective and nonrandomized study in 86 children with previously untreated disease, 70 out of the cohort did not relapse with conventional chemotherapy,[111] and when relapse did occur, salvage appeared to be readily achieved as is the experience in the Western Cape with actuarial, overall, and relapse-free survival at 5 years 100% and 90% for localized and 81% and 60%, respectively, for clinical IIIB and IV. This leads to the conclusion that in resource-poor communities most of the children with disease defined by noninvasive diagnostic techniques can be cured with chemotherapy alone. This has important implications, because of the limited availability of radiation therapy equipment.[111] In contrast, and unexplained, is a report from Campinas, Brazil,[112] where the distribution of histologic subtypes and stage is similar to that reported in developed countries, but outcome was less satisfactory, with the conclusion that this was not related to the histopathology.

Points of Contrast

A series in children under 13 years from Johannesburg[101] (Table 30.13) emphasizes the Cape Town situation (Table 30.11 and 30.12). Here, of the 91 children, 61 were black and 30 were white, with a clear demonstration of a difference in distribution of poor predictive values in late stages and lower hemoglobin levels in black children as compared to their white counterparts.

Supportive observations are derived from Namibia[113] and recently updated (Annelle Zietsmann, personal communication, 2005). Of note was increase in risk of tuberculosis sufficient to lead to the suggestion that prophylactic therapy was

reasonable in all children with malignancy being treated in the third world.[114]

As with other experiences in the younger age groups, the features are those with similarity rather than contrast when Africa, Asia, and Latin America are compared to the first world.

THE ROLE OF EPSTEIN-BARR VIRUS

Westernized Societies

Numerous studies have examined this association (see Chapter 3).[115,116] Although initial serologic methods were unable to show any clear relationship with this lymphoma, the advent of in situ hybridization studies revealed an integrated genome in the Reed-Sternberg cells in 35% of cases.[117] Furthermore, at least one gene product, the latent membrane protein or LMP-1, can be found on the surface where it may function as a target for cytotoxic T-lymphocytes and so facilitate host control. Conversely, if this surveillance mechanism is lost, the same molecule appears to have the capacity to enhance proliferation of the infected cells, leading to the emergence of a histologically aggressive neoplasm.[115-117] Such apparently opposing effects might underlie differences in the course of this lymphoid malignancy and raise the speculation that prevention may be achieved by means of vaccination.

African Experience

Regional comparisons[118,119] reveal differences in the expression of Epstein-Barr virus frequency, as between Kenya and Italy.[120] Biopsy material from children in ten different parts of the world was examined in one study. LMP-1 was found in 50% to 100% of cases, with the highest rate in those from underdeveloped countries. In this definitive study examining the role of Epstein-Barr virus, the model was childhood Hodgkin lymphoma using immunohistochemical staining and in situ hybridization to define latent membrane protein and small nuclear nontranscribed RNA or EBR-1 respectively. By a sensitive polymerase chain reaction–based procedure, the type I strain predominated in children from the United Kingdom,

TABLE 30.13

CLINICAL AND PATHOLOGIC FEATURES AMONG 91 CHILDREN WITH
HODGKIN LYMPHOMA FROM JOHANNESBURG (GAUTENG)

	Black		White		
	Number	%	Number	%	p Value
Sex					
Male	47	52	22	24	
Female	14	15	8	9	
Histologic subtype					
LP	1	1	3	3	
NS	20	22	12	13	
MC	39	43	14	16	
LD	1	1	1	1	
Stage					
I and II	18	20	19	21	
III and IV	43	47	11	12	0.001
Symptoms					
A	25	27	20	21	
B	36	40	10	12	<0.03
Hemoglobin					
≤10	24	26	18	20	
<10	37	41	12	13	0.06
Lymphocyte count					
≤1.0	50	55	18	19	
<1.0	11	12	12	12	<0.03
Disease bulk					
Bulky	31	34	5	5	<0.03
Nonbulky	30	33	25	27	
Age					
Mean ± SD	8.2 ± 3.1		9.4 ± 4.1		

From Bezwoda WR, MacPhail AP, Dawey R, et al. Hodgkin's disease in sub-Saharan Africa. Cambridge medical reviews. In: Armitage J, Newland A, Keating A, et al., eds. *Hematological oncology*. Vol. 4. Cambridge: Cambridge University Press; 1995:21–40.

South Africa, Australia, and Greece, whereas type II was most frequent in Egypt.[118] Dual presence was reported from the United Kingdom, Costa Rica, and Kenya, with the frequency again being highest where the population was poorest. The authors speculated that this specific latter occurrence might reflect relatively poor local conditions, leading to malnutrition-induced immunologic impairment.[118]

Asia and South America

In two studies China was defined as a developing country.[121,122] Using the same molecular characterization, one report documented frequent association with this virus and similar frequency as seen in the West.[121] In the follow-up study, however, EBNA–1 sequence variation explored possible geographical polymorphisms examining primarily nasopharyngeal carcinoma but comparing these to Hodgkin lymphoma. It transpired that the valine variant did not target the oral component but rather represented a dominant Asian subtype being found in the general population.[122] Further work by this group[123] in pediatric cases emphasized the etiologic heterogeneity and led to the proposal that this should now be regarded as a distinctive Epstein-Barr virus–related lymphoma.[121] Similarly in Thailand most of the cases of classical

Hodgkin lymphoma again document a strong association, especially with mixed cellularity.[124] Also in 100 consecutive cases undertaken as part of a larger study comparing it to other lymphomas that included both B- and T-lymphoproliferative disorders, it was noted that the EBV-encoded RNA was detected in nearly half of those with reactive lymphoid hyperplasia. Perhaps more revealing is how the data support strong association, once again, with Hodgkin lymphoma.[125]

From Korea there is confirmation of a low incidence of Hodgkin lymphoma, a strong correlation with the Epstein-Barr virus, and a high incidence of the mixed-cellularity subtype as well as the other variants. This extended to all age groups but was more frequent in children, suggesting a lowered immune surveillance or perhaps a different pathophysiology in youth.[126] A further study of this common herpesvirus[127] expanded the confidence of the relationship with type I, having a 73% incidence in Hodgkin lymphoma with the DF genotype. In Taiwan, the virus was isolated across subtypes and ages but, as anticipated, had a low endemic incidence, again focusing on the possibility that there may be other factors active in pathogenesis.[128] Instructive studies from Kuala Lumpur in Malaysia explored the association in a multiethnic population. A third were under 15 years of age and infection correlated strongly with the lymphoma—especially childhood cases where the figure was 93%.[129] In adults, mixed cellularity (86%)

was more frequent than nodular sclerosis (22%). Previously, although comparing Malaysian to Danish peripheral T-cell rather than Hodgkin lymphoma, there was the conclusion that specific deletions and single-base mutations occur independently during the evolution of the viral strains. Whether this has relevance as a pathogenetic role in carcinogenesis is uncertain, although it is noted that these constitute an advantage in some of the viral associated diseases.[130] From South India comes the report that the latent membrane protein-1 was found in 82% of the lymphomas and 96% of childhood cases.[131]

South American has supportive results implicating this virus in 80% to 100% of Hodgkin lymphoma cases, as opposed to only 30% to 40% in the United States or other industrialized countries.[59] Viewed against malignancies related to the Epstein–Barr virus that are thought to have geographical localization, such as nasopharyngeal carcinoma in South China and Burkitt lymphoma in equatorial Africa, comes the proposal that age and histologic subtype rather than geographical region are the major determinants of this association. In systematically exploring this possibility and using pediatric cases from South Brazil as the model, after adjustment for histopathology and age, the association remained independent of geography but remained more common in children under 10 years of age, supporting the multiple etiology hypothesis in pathogenesis.[59] Among 78 Brazilians the latent membrane protein-1 detected by immunohistochemistry and the EBV-encoded RNA or EBER by in situ hybridization, was similar to that in other developing regions, thereby reinforcing a relationship with community status and strong correlation between survival and expression of LMP-1.[132] Data from Medellin, Columbia showed an unusually high incidence of LMP-1 in children, with the characteristic bimodal peak between 5 and 10 years and (somewhat lower) between 15 and 25 years. Males predominate in children by ratio of 4.5 to 1. Again the epidemiologic pattern was type 1 found among the poor, but strangely a high frequency of nodular sclerosis and unusual anatomic localization with severe clinical manifestations.[15] In a further report, the same molecular technology was used to confirm the high percentage positivity and draw attention to a probable relationship with treatment outcome.[133] Contrasting the United States, Mexico City, and Costa Rica,[134] it was shown that the viral DNA was abundant and monoclonal in the infected Reed-Sternberg cells, being strongly and independently linked to mixed cellularity and Hispanic ethnicity. This type of finding provides impetus for novel approaches to tumor prevention or therapy. Subsequently, the general theme continued to explore Hodgkin lymphoma in the context of wealth and status, with the geography and ethnic heritage less important.[135] In Mexico an instructive study found an association between virus and lymphoma across all ages, reaching 92% in mixed-cellularity and lymphocyte-depleted subtypes and establishing this level to be greater than that found in the United States and other developed countries.[136] Similarly, typing of the virus led to the conclusion of this being the highest incidence for both the latent membrane protein-1 deletion variant and infection by type B reported so far worldwide.[137] Similar high prevalence was documented in Peru.[138]

Points of Contrast

Across the spectrum of underdeveloped countries the pattern is uniform, with Epstein-Barr virus being isolated in from 80% to 100% of Hodgkin lymphoma cases versus one-third to one-half of this incidence in the wake of industrialization. These observations appear independent of geography, of greater frequency in children, and support more than one causative factor in lymphogenesis.[59] Significantly, expression of the latent membrane protein-1 seems to predict better overall survival.[132] The challenge is to use the differences in geographical pathology to design tumor-prevention therapy.[134]

THE IMPACT OF HUMAN IMMUNODEFICIENCY VIRUS

Westernized Societies

The possible role of HIV as a predisposing factor in Hodgkin lymphoma is attracting increasing attention and a number of recent publications from Europe and the United States have supported its association with developing Hodgkin's disease.[139–145] Thus, those at risk are characteristically homosexual men with AIDS or intravenous drug abusers with low CD4 counts and other evidence of suppressed immune integrity.

African Experience

Already high rates continue to spiral out of control in many areas and the clinical syndrome is still widely regarded as of epidemic proportions throughout Africa. A causal relationship would logically therefore exert a major impact on lymphomagenesis including the Hodgkin category. Seropositivity rates of 7% to 10% have been recorded among antenatal clinic attendees in South Africa,[146] and in some circumstances this may be even higher.

However, perhaps surprisingly, no more such cases are yet being seen in the cancer registries. In a recent case-control study involving 913 blacks with cancer conducted in Johannesburg,[147] a notable correlation between HIV infection and neoplasia was observed only for patients with Kaposi sarcoma, with 27 of 35 cases being seropositive, giving an odds ratio of 61.8 (95% CI: 19.7–94.2). The corresponding figures for non-Hodgkin variants were 27 of 40 testing positive for HIV, with an odds ratio of 4.8 (95% CI: 1.5–14.8.) These statistics match those from several other sub-Saharan African communities[148–150] with high viral isolation rates, although the odds ratio was lower than reported in developed countries. The reasons for these findings are not clear but may include early mortality from tuberculosis in African HIV cases. This complication occurs at higher CD4 counts, in the region of 300 to 400/μL, than with the other lymphoproliferative disorders. Notably, as with Hodgkin lymphoma, carcinomas arising from liver, vagina, penis, esophagus, cervix, or the oropharynx, all of which may have an infectious etiology, correlated with the presence of this retrovirus. The Johannesburg cohort had a HIV seropositivity rate of 10.8% in those with Hodgkin lymphoma, giving an odds ratio of 2.0 (95% CI: 0.6–6.6).

Although there was no demonstrable correlation between HIV infection and Hodgkin lymphoma, they clearly coexist, likely because both are found in younger people. Of the 37 patients who were HIV positive, information is available on 28, thus allowing some observations to be made regarding clinical aspects of such cases among blacks. Of note are median CD34 counts of $488 \pm 195 \times 10^9$/L, which was not different from that found in a matched control group without demonstrable viral infection (Table 30.14).[108] There seem, therefore, to be no reliable predictors that identify those with coexistent human immunodeficiency viral infections and Hodgkin lymphoma. Accordingly there is no reason not to treat them on standard therapeutic approaches provided they are not, in addition, suffering from the advanced syndrome. Even here there is increasing evidence of fall in viral copies and reversal of immunologic status provided appropriate therapies are given, and this argues strongly in favor of properly designed protocols that provide current treatments for both diseases simultaneously.[151–154] Data

TABLE 30.14

PRESENTING CLINICAL AND LABORATORY FEATURES IN 28 BLACK HIV-POSITIVE PATIENTS WITH HODGKIN LYMPHOMA

	Number	%
Histologic subtype		
NS	8	29
MC	13	46
LD	7	25
Stage		
IIB	4	14
IIIA	1	4
IIIB	19	68
IVB	4	14
Male	18	64
Female	10	36
Bulky disease (>10 cm)	11	39
Nonbulky disease (<10 cm)	17	61
Hemoglobin (g/dL)	10.3 ± 1.2^a	
Lymphocytes ($\times 10^9$/L)	0.849 ± 0.102^a	
Age (y)	20.9 ± 4.2^a	

^{a}Mean $\pm$ SD.
NS, nodular sclerosis; MC, mixed cellularity; LD, lymphocyte depleted.
From Beral V. The epidemiology of cancer in AIDS patients. *AIDS* 1991;5(suppl 2):S99–S104.

TABLE 30.15

HODGKIN LYMPHOMA AND HIV IN ZIMBABWE: 89 PATIENTS OF KNOWN HIV STATUS

	HIV positive		HIV negative	
	Number	%	Number	%
Histologic subtype				
LP	0	0	5	8.9
NS	3	9.1	13	23.3
MC	24	72.7	25	44.6
LD	6	18.2	13	23.2
Age				
Median	34		25	
Range	17–70		9–70	
Stage				
I–II	3		16	
III–IV	30		40	
Sex				
M:F ratio	3.7:1		1.3:1	

LP, lymphocyte predominant; NS, nodular sclerosis; MC, mixed cellularity; LD, lymphocyte depleted; M, male; F, female.
Data from LM Levy (unpublished data).

from Zimbabwe collected between 1988 and 1996 (Table 30.15) for 105 new patients showed that of 89 tested, 37% were seropositive. These figures need to be seen in the context of an even higher frequency of infection in that country than in South Africa. Again, clinical features were similar, irrespective of retroviral status.

Asia and South America

Relatively little information is available on the correlation of Hodgkin lymphoma with the HIV-infected individual in these regions. The co-morbidity with tuberculosis, *Pneumocystis carinii* pneumonia, and cryptococcosis are well established. Economic loss is enormous, and the widely recognized importance of counseling and testing are difficult targets to achieve.[155] As in other poor areas, the pandemic proceeds with the focus on Kaposi sarcoma, non-Hodgkin and Burkitt lymphoma increasing in incidence, with the magnitude of the problem far from defined.[156] In China there has been a dramatic increase,[157] with ever-increasing public awareness focusing on prevention programs exemplified by the Thai experience.[158,159] Equally chilling concerns have been described for India.[160] In looking at all the currently available information, little useful data emerges for characterization of the associated lymphoreticular malignancies, with a focus still largely on the challenge of HIV disease control and associated inflammatory infections.

In Latin America and the Caribbean the picture is essentially similar.[161,162] However, from Brazil there is useful information on the social geography[163] but again relatively little information on related lymphomas, although when an association does occur it appears to be primarily with Epstein-Barr virus.[164]

Points of Contrast

The status in Africa provides the best counterpoint to what occurs in the first world but, while the relationship is increasingly being clarified, the impact of HIV infection, influence of highly active retroviral therapy, and a number of malignancies including Hodgkin and other lymphomas is far from clearly defined.[156] Whether vaccination will alter the natural history of this infectious disease globally is uncertain and creates a number of scientific challenges,[165] with an insightful analysis describing the problems in the third world with comparative information on Asia and the Pacific, Latin America, and northern, western and eastern Europe.[162,166,167]

What is to be made of all this?

The singular most striking observation is that, in contrast to much of Europe and North America, infection resulting in AIDS continues to run rampant through the developing world. Accurate reporting is virtually unknown, and the effective delivery of antiretroviral therapy, often also poorly supplied, is frequently nothing more than a political football! Against this emerges a clear need to favor immunologic reconstitution and reduction of viral load through appropriate medication, coupled with a further shift from managing only the AIDS-defining infections, to achieve clarity on the existing occurrence of lymphoreticular malignancies, including Hodgkin lymphoma. There is a unique opportunity to use the historical data to document changes in the incidence and subtypes of neoplastic processes correlated with this retroviral infection. Apart from the obvious benefits of improving survival, this is a rich area for international collaborative research to define the potential and possible clinical benefits of vaccination therapy both as a principle and, specifically, in these patients. Unfortunately the notoriously efficient mutations that characterize these viruses adds a further dimension to such scientific problems to be faced by those committed to solving what is one of the world's dominant problems for health delivery and, indeed in many parts of the undeveloped world, survival itself.

TREATMENT OUTCOMES

Westernized Societies

Evidence from an expanding literature clearly demonstrates that Hodgkin lymphoma can be cured. Here cardinal determinants are a reliable diagnosis, accurate staging, and management in well-tested multimodality programs that comprise combination chemotherapy with or without irradiation.[9,10,168] As experience has accumulated, a number of salvage programs have become widely accepted and culminate in either autologous or allogeneic hematopoietic stem-cell transplantation.[169,170]

There has been a major shift from the early days, when clinical assessment was converted to pathologic staging by surgery.[171,172] Currently favored are less-invasive methods that center on technological advances. These include high-resolution imaging procedures so that contemporary management can capitalize on the greater sensitivity and specificity of computerized axial and positron-emission tomography.[173–175]

Despite the favorable outcome for most individuals treated with conventional but risk-stratified approaches, there are still a number of problems. The first of these is refractory disease, slow response, or relapse, and here salvage is effective with high-dose chemotherapy and myeloprotection using stem-cell transplantation and progenitor cells.[169,170] Equally important is the ever-increasing appreciation that, although the use of optimum first-line therapy has curative capacity in those who are chemotherapy sensitive, late complications arise and adversely affect results, and this includes cardiomyopathy, breast cancer,[176] and myelodysplasia.[177] Safer but equally effective regimens are needed, and these are currently the focus of collaborative studies within the European Organization for Research and Treatment in Cancer,[178] the German Hodgkin Study Group,[179] and collaborative programs in the United States.[180,181]

African Experience

Management has been modified to keep abreast of new advances. Major impediments are limited budgets for state or provincial facilities on the one hand and the reluctance of managed health care organizations to approve funding for clinical trials in privately based academic centers on the other hand. In summarizing contemporary practice, radiation and chemotherapy have been somewhat artificially isolated, and children are considered separately.

Adults: Radiation Therapy

In a report from Johannesburg[101] the outcome after laparotomy for stage I to IIIA treated between 1976 and 1986 with total nodal irradiation was much poorer for blacks than whites. However, in this retrospective analysis, the difference disappeared in those with stage I and nonbulky stage II having a normal hemoglobin level and using the same regimens. These results suggest that radiotherapy can play an important role on this continent, as elsewhere, provided diagnosis is prompt and referral appropriate. One problem is, however, access to centers with the necessary equipment and staffed with experienced radiation oncologists. To this end the World Health Organization, in collaboration with the International Atomic Energy Commission, has embarked on a project of installing suitable cobalt sources or linear accelerators and providing oncology training in Ghana, Zambia, Kenya, and Ethiopia.

Adults: Chemotherapy

Systemic programs have long taken their lead from the traditional MOPP combinations. With few exceptions, the response rates in blacks are poorer than those observed with matching regimens from other parts of the world.[182–185] Also, a number of long-term follow-up studies across racial and ethnic gradients show racial disparities that do not disappear in the first world, and can be interpreted as blacks having a poorer prognosis.[90,186,187]

Evidence now suggests that the prognosis of patients is better for patients treated with six or even eight cycles of multidrug therapy combining MOPP, or its variant, with one or another form of ABVD than following MOPP alone.[188–192] A higher dose intensity is achieved with the hybrid regimens.[193–195] There have, however, been no randomized studies to determine whether this observation applies equally across a racial or ethnic divide. Our retrospective analysis shows a trend towards improved outcome in blacks when the MOPP-ABVD era from 1985 to 1995 is compared to the preceding 15 years spanning 1970 to 1985, when MOPP alone was used (Figs. 30.4 and 30.5). However, despite some improved outcome, the discrepancy between black and white patients, equivalently treated, remains evident (Fig. 30.5). Although costs are somewhat higher for regimens containing anthracycline, such as ABVD, these have increasingly become more widely used due to the limited availability of nitrogen mustard and procarbazine.

Results from the Cairo University Centre are instructive. The overall and event survival is shown in Fig. 30.6. Survival appears, in general, to be inferior by 10% to 15% to that reported for Western series, except in stage I treated with mantle or inverted-Y radiation therapy, where survival exceeds 88% at 5 years. The corresponding figures are 48% for stage II, 39% for stage III, and 33% for stage IV. As elsewhere, the explanation may be related to irregular cycles, with 47% being delayed more than 2 weeks because of social circumstances.[49]

Of note is the dose–response relationship for those with favorable results receiving high-dose chemotherapy supported by autologous bone-marrow transplantation for recurrence.[169,170,196,197] Because both dose intensification and improved compliance may be achieved using high-dose chemotherapy with autologous grafting for cases of advanced and therefore poor prognosis, a trial was initiated in Johannesburg using this as the initial approach. Twenty-six individuals received melphalan (140 mg/m^2 IV) combined with etoposide (VP16, 2.5 g/m^2) and hematologic rescue accomplished using non-cryopreserved autologous marrow ($n = 4$) or GCSF-stimulated peripheral blood stem and progenitor cells

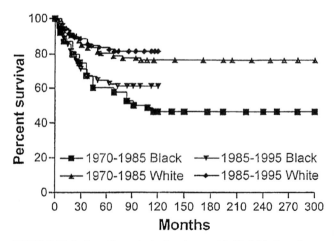

FIGURE 30.5. Overall survival of patients with Hodgkin lymphoma treated from 1970 to 1985 (MOPP alone) and from 1985 to 1995 (MOPP/ABVD). The difference between the survival curves for black and white patients was statistically significant ($p < 0.01$) for both time periods

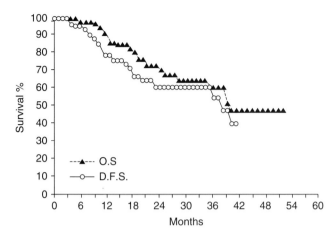

FIGURE 30.6. Actuarial 5-year survival for 107 adults with Hodgkin lymphoma. (O.S., overall survival; D.F.S., disease-free survival.) (Adapted from Azim HA, Moussa M, Hamada E, et al. Adult Hodgkin's disease: clinical presentation and results of treatment in NEMROCK (1992-1995). Dissertation, Cairo University, 1998.)

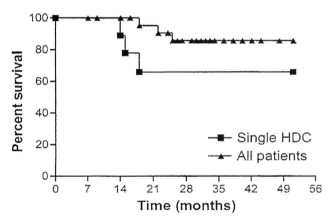

FIGURE 30.7. Disease-free survival of patients with Hodgkin lymphoma treated with primary high-dose chemotherapy using melphalan and etoposide supported by autologous hematopoietic rescue. (Adapted from Seymour LK, Dansey RD, Bezwoda WR. Single high-dose etoposide and melphalan with non-cryopreserved autologous marrow rescue as primary therapy for relapsed, refractory and poor-prognosis Hodgkin's disease. *Br J Cancer* 1994;70:526–530.)

($n = 22$). Not having to freeze and store the rescue products has made the whole procedure technically simpler and cheaper. Reconstitution to greater than $1.0 \times 10^9/L$ neutrophils and greater than $40 \times 10^9/L$ platelets, without transfusion dependence, occurred with the median recovery time of 17 days. Median hospitalization time was 19 days. Twenty-four of the 26 achieved complete remission following a single cycle with only one having a partial response and another failing, giving an overall complete response rate of 92% (24 of 26). The first 6 participants underwent only one single course of high-dose chemotherapy. There were 3 recurrences (at 18, 22, and 25 months).[198] Subsequently the induction cycle was repeated and then followed by the same autograft support with the second cycle, at an interval of 4 to 6 weeks. Time to hematologic recovery was not different following this modification. Among those given double high-dose chemotherapy with peripheral blood stem-cell rescue ($n = 20$), the complete remission rate was 100%. At a median follow-up of 30 months, there were no recurrences from this cohort. (Fig. 30.7)[199]

Although not randomized, it is of interest to note that one course of chemotherapy has an inadequate cure rate, even though the lymphoma is chemotherapy sensitive. The efficacy of a double induction regimen remains to be established. However, if successful, this approach is likely to provide an acceptable method, because there is a reduction in total time needed for completing treatment in those with poor prognosis whether this is in Africa or any other under-sourced area.

Children

Although reported series are small, they suggest an outcome superior to that achieved in adults.[200,201] Exceptionally good results have been reported with MOPP for children on this continent, as elsewhere, with initial complete response rates of 85% to 100%.[109,110,202,203] This outcome is noticeably better than that achieved in adults using the same therapeutic regimen. In a series reported from the Tygerberg Academic Hospital, those under 15 years of age (Tables 30.11 and 31.12) were treated with MOPP, its equivalent ChlVPP, or the MOPP/ABVD hybrid followed by 20 to 30 Gy involved-field radiotherapy to mediastinal bulk[110]; they had a projected survival at 10 years of 85% for stage I and II and 82% and 48% at 5 and 10 years, respectively, for stage III and IV (Fig. 30.8). Survival in children was identical irrespective of chemotherapy type (Fig. 30.9). Side effects did arise and include tuberculosis, which, in the Western Cape, caused morbidity, with one-third of the individuals requiring anti-mycobacterial medication.[114] Varicella was encountered in 6 cases. It is probably

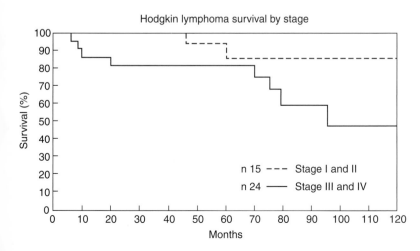

FIGURE 30.8. Disease-free survival of children (< 15 years) with Hodgkin lymphoma treated at Tygerberg Hospital (Western Cape). (Adapted from Hesseling PB, Wessels G, Van Jaarsveld D, et al. Hodgkin's disease in children in southern Africa: epidemiological characteristics, morbidity and long-term outcome. *Ann Trop Paediatr* 1997;17:367–373.)

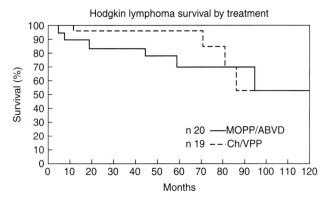

FIGURE 30.9. Disease-free survival of children with Hodgkin lymphoma analyzed by type of chemotherapy. (Adapted from Hesseling PB, Wessels G, Van Jaarsveld D, et al. Hodgkin's disease in children in southern Africa: epidemiological characteristics, morbidity and long-term outcome. *Ann Trop Paediatr* 1997;17:367–373.)

noteworthy that 2, who had undergone staging splenectomy, developed overwhelming sepsis and died, at 7 months and 8 years. Three deaths were related to treatment from marrow failure, tuberculous bronchiectasis and osteitis, and a second malignancy.

The survival of children in the Gauteng area more closely approximated that seen in the west (Fig. 30.10), with an observed 10-year event-free survival rate in excess of 80%. Most came from urban communities and attended a clinic with intensive support services; all were treated only with chemotherapy in the form of MOPP or the MOPP/ABVD hybrid. Compliance was excellent in that over 85% received the optimal dose as scheduled. The spectrum of infectious complications was markedly less, with only one recorded case of tuberculosis. These results emphasize the importance of the environmental elements, and adequacy of standardized management protocols, as the major influence of outcome in the individuals. Although the results in black children appear somewhat better than in adult counterparts, there was nevertheless still a demonstrable difference compared to white children.[101]

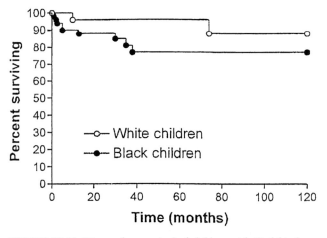

FIGURE 30.10. Disease-free survival of children with Hodgkin lymphoma in Gauteng (*p* = 0.03). (Adapted from Bezwoda WR, MacPhail AP, Dawey R, et al. Hodgkin's disease in sub-Saharan Africa. Cambridge medical reviews. In: Armitage J, Newland A, Keating A, et al., eds. *Hematological oncology*. Vol. 4. Cambridge: Cambridge University Press; 1995:21–40.)

Asia and South America

The experience detailed from Africa is broadly applicable to other matching parts of the world. For example, in India children treated with conventional programs established as standards of practice in the first world have 7-year event-free and actuarial survival rates of 73% and 64%, respectively.[204] Essentially similar data were reported from the same institution a decade later.[205] Furthermore, in Nicaragua, again using childhood as the model but without radiotherapy, results were equally good, with the caveat that a high prevalence with the mixed-cellularity subtype does not predicate poorer prognosis. It is relevant that patient tolerability is high, leading to the recommendation that this would be appropriate for low-income regions where radiotherapy facilities are scarce or unavailable. This leaves the challenge to precisely define this modality in the emerging world.[206]

Points of Contrast

These are related to the questions detailed in the introduction: specifically, and given the scanty reliable information available, a need to define differences in population and histologic subtypes. In this context are problems created by differences in wealth, education, and sanitary conditions that carry with them many life-threatening infections exemplified by tuberculosis, and this has particular relevance in those with Hodgkin lymphoma. It is entirely appropriate to reflect on the important role of infection with the Epstein-Barr virus, but perhaps more important is the astronomical challenge of the all-pervasive onslaught of HIV. Superimposed upon this are simple logistic constraints. For example, how do patients know that they have Hodgkin lymphoma? If the diagnosis is made, are they treated by local healers or will they find their way to hematologists or oncologists who have the knowledge and wherewithall to treat them? What is the outcome in these individuals, because registries and data reporting are seldom a priority in parts of the world where the challenges of daily living supercede all else.

It is this experience with Hodgkin lymphoma in Africa, Asia, and Latin America that offers such a rich mosaic of interrelated scientific questions that make it absolutely ideal for ongoing data collection and a coordinated research by the international scientific community. Goals are first to define those guidelines that will be optimally effective in most patients coupled with fewer side effects. Secondly, to overcome cultural and other bias or prejudice, based on good faith and patient acceptance of a westernized approach, to consider and if possible accept what is often a completely different therapeutic imperative.

CONCLUSION

Hodgkin lymphoma, as seen among children and adults over the face of Africa, creates a sense of déjà vu among investigators working in first-world centers. Indeed, precisely this focus is reflected in underdeveloped parts of Asia and Latin America. Our understanding of the available evidence is that there is a single causative pathophysiologic process, but the impact of environmental forces is much more profound than evident in the more uniform societies that generally evolved in the wake of industrialization. For example, the presenting characteristics and clinical course are profoundly and adversely influenced by malnutrition and the rampant, escalating HIV pandemic with its strong links to tuberculosis, often with resistant organisms. Logic would dictate that, if such compounding factors could be corrected, little difference would be seen between blacks and whites on this or other continents when compared with more affluent societies elsewhere on the globe. Based on currently available evidence, this target appears to be unattainable and even receding. Perhaps the most frightening reality to be faced is a widespread deterioration in medical standards, with reduction and restriction of available resources that range from unavailability of chemotherapy drugs to the nondelivery of irradiation for want of functional therapy equipment. If this is the truth, as seems to be the case, Africa and other under-resourced communities will continue to provide a model for the stark contrast between affluent and poor. This is a chilling scenario, and the antithesis of what all dedicated doctors and health care professionals strive toward. The goal must be improvement in each and every aspect of diagnosis and management of these people. Only in this way can the outcome be elevated to levels that in the future will not differ from the standard-setting academic centers in Europe, the United States of America, the Middle and Far East, and Australasia.

Acknowledgments

Supported by the Haematological Research Trust, Chairman's Fund of the Anglo-American Corporation, the Anthony Taberer, Louis Shill and Margaret Ward Foundations. Werner Bezwoda and Dalila Sellami contributed to the first version; the authors wish to thank them and many other colleagues in Africa who provided data for this chapter. Included are Annelle Zietsmann from the Department of Medical Oncology, Cancer Care Centre, Namibia; Lorraine Levy, Associate Professor, Department of Medicine at University of Zimbabwe and the Zimbabwean Cancer Registry; Dr. Hamdy Azim, of the Cairo Oncology Centre; Peter Hesseling, Professor and Head of the Department of Paediatrics and Child Health, University of Stellenbosch; Gary Culligan, Professor, Medical University of Southern Africa; Dr. Coenrad F. Slabber from the Department of Medical Oncology, University of Pretoria; Mr. Sedick Isaacs from the University of Cape Town, Groote Schuur Hospital; Dr. Ellen Bolding and Dr. Kathy Taylor, Pathcare; also particularly Miss Nokuzola Mqoqi and Ms. Patricia Kellet from the South African National Cancer Registry; Mrs. Christine Dölling for providing invaluable bibliographic assistance; Mrs. Sharon Smith prepared and impeccably typed drafts including the final manuscript.

References

1. UNAIDS. *Report on the global AIDS epidemic 2004.* Geneva: UNAIDS; 2004.

2. Sissolak G, Mayaud P. AIDS-related Kaposi's sarcoma: epidemiological, diagnostic, treatment and control aspects in sub-Saharan Africa. *Trop Med Intern Health* 2005;10:981–992.

3. Falkson HC. The value of N-isopropyl-alpha-(2-methyl-hydrazino)-p-toluamide hydrochloride relative to ionizing radiations in the treatment of Hodgkin's disease. Dissertation, University of Pretoria, 1965.

4. Jacobs P, Wood L, Armitage JO. Lymphoma: the immune system in disarray. *Specialist Forum* 2004;4:16–24.

5. The Non-Hodgkin's Lymphoma Classification Project. A clinical evaluation of the International Lymphoma Study Group classification of non-Hodgkin's lymphoma. *Blood* 1997;89:3909–3918.

6. Jacobs P, Wood L. Lymphoma—the immune system in disarray. Theme for the 11th Congress of the South African Lymphoma Study Group meeting. *Transfus Apheresis Sci* 2005;32:21–23

7. Omoti CE, Halim NKD. Adult lymphomas in Edo state, Niger Delta region of Nigeria— clinicopathological profile of 205 cases. *Clin Lab Haematol* 2005;27:302–306.

8. Jaffe ES, Harris NL, Stein H, et al., eds. World Health Organization of tumours. Pathology and genetics of tumours of haematopoietic and lymphoid tissues. Lyon: IARC; 2001.

9. DeVita VT Jr, Serpick AA, Carbone PP. Combination chemotherapy in the treatment of advanced Hodgkin's disease. *Ann Intern Med* 1970;73: 881–895.

10. van Spronsen DJ, Dijkema IM, Vrints LW. Improved survival of Hodgkin's disease patients in south-east Netherlands since 1972. *Eur J Cancer* 1997;33:436–441.

11. MacMahon B. Epidemiology of Hodgkin's disease. *Cancer Res* 1966;26: 1189–1200.

12. Glaser SL, Hsu JL. Hodgkin's disease in Asians: incidence patterns and risk factors in population-based data. *Leuk Res* 2002;26:261–269.

13. Newell GR, Mills PK, Johnson DE. Epidemiologic comparison of cancer of the testis and Hodgkin's disease among young males. *Cancer* 1984;54: 11171123.

14. Chetty R, Bickhoo A. Retinoblastoma protein and Epstein-Barr virus (EBV) expression in South African Hodgkin's disease. *Hematol Oncol* 1997;15: 191–195.

15. Bedoya V. Hodgkin's disease in Medellin, Colombia. *Z Krebsforsch Klin Onkol Cancer Res Clin Oncol* 1977;89:297–310.

16. McNally RJ, Alston RD, Cairns DP, et al. Geographical and ecological analyses of childhood acute leukaemias and lymphomas in north-west England. *Br J Haematol* 2003;123:60–65.

17. Cartwright RA, McKinney PA, Barnes N. Epidemiology of the lymphomas in the United Kingdom: recent developments. *Baillieres Clin Haematol* 1987;1:59–76.

18. Breslow NE, Langholz B. Childhood cancer incidence: geographical and temporal variations. *Int J Cancer* 1983;32:703716.

19. Weiss NS. Geographical variations in the incidence of the leukemias and lymphomas. *Natl Cancer Inst Monogr* 1979;53:139–142.

20. Kasili EG, Shah TS. Lymphoreticular disease in Kenya: pathological pattern of the superficial lymphadenopathies. *Trop Geogr Med* 1974;26: 242–256.

21. Tavani A, La Vecchia C, Franceschi S, et al. Medical history and risk of Hodgkin's and non-Hodgkin's lymphomas. *Eur J Cancer Prev* 2000;9: 59–64.

22. Rezk H, El-Shazly AM, Soliman M, et al. Coccidiosis among immuno-competent and–compromised adults. *J Egypt Soc Parasitol* 2001;31:823–834.

23. Weinreb M, Day PJ, Niggli F, et al. The consistent association between Epstein-Barr virus and Hodgkin's disease in children in Kenya. *Blood* 1996;87:3828–3826.

24. Engel M, Essop MF, Close P, et al. Improved prognosis of Epstein-Barr virus associated childhood Hodgkin's lymphoma: study of 47 South African cases. *J Clin Pathol* 2000;53:182–186.

25. Franceschi S, Dal Maso L, La Vecchia C. Advances in the epidemiology of HIV-associated non-Hodgkin's lymphoma and other lymphoid neoplasms. *Int J Cancer* 1999;83:481–485.

26. Sitas F, Pacella-Norman R, Carrara H, et al. The spectrum of HIV-1 related cancers in South Africa. *Int J Cancer* 2000;88:489–492.

27. Cook-Mozaffari P, Newton R, Beral V, Burkitt DP. The geographical distribution of Kaposi's sarcoma and of the lymphomas in Africa before the AIDS epidemic. *Br J Cancer* 1998;78:1521–1528.

28. Mueller BU. Cancers in children infected with the human immunodeficiency virus. *The Oncologist* 1999;4:309–317.

29. Wright DH. Epidemiology and histology of Hodgkin's disease in Uganda. *Natl Cancer Inst Monogr* 1973;36:25–30.

30. Edington GM, Osunkoya BO, Hendrickse M. Histologic classification of Hodgkin's disease in the Western State of Nigeria. *J Natl Cancer Inst* 1973;50:1633–1637.

31. Naik KG, Bhagwandeen SB. Hodgkin's disease in Zambia. *East Afr Med J* 1976;53:459–467.

32. Kung'u A. Hodgkin's disease in Kenya: a histopathological and epidemiological study. *East Afr Med J* 1983;60:416–427.

33. Emanuel DJ, Gelfand M. A survey into the clinical presentation of Hodgkin's disease at Harare Hospital, Salisbury, Rhodesia. *J Trop Med Hyg* 1975;78:44–46.

34. Hamdi Cherif M, Sekfali N, Benlatrech K. Algeria. In: Parkin DM, Muir CS, Whelan SL, et al., eds. *Cancer incidence in five continents.* Vol. 6. IARC Scientific Publication no. 120. Lyon: IARC; 1992:182–185.

35. Parkin DM, Muir CS, Whelan SL, et al. *Cancer incidence in five continents.* Vol. 6. IARC Scientific Publication no. 120. Lyon: IARC; 1992:186–193.

36. Bouzid M, Sheng W, Buisson M, et al. Different distribution of H1–H2 Epstein-Barr virus variant in oropharyngeal virus and in biopsies of Hodgkin's disease and in nasopharyngeal carcinoma from Algeria. *Int J Cancer* 1998;77:205–210.

37. Chadli A, Philippe E. La physionomie du cancer en Tunisie. *Arch Inst Pasteur* 1960;37:391–392.

38. Chadli A, Rethers L Landreat A, et al. La physionomie du cancer en Tunisie (II): etude de 7.959 cancers primitives. *Arch Inst Pasteur* 1976;53:318–323.

39. Cosset JM. Etude anatomo-pathologique et clinique de 112 cas de maladies de Hodgkin vus a l'Institut Salah Azaiz de Tunis du 01.01.1969 au 31.12.1972. These de medecine, Universite de Paris XI, 1975.

40. Ben Abdallah M. Epidemiologie des cancers en Tunisie: registre de l'Institut Salah Azaiz. Tunis, 1997.

41. Korbi S, Trimeche M, Sriha B, et al. Epstein-Barr virus in Hodgkin's disease: the example of central Tunisia. *Ann Pathol* 2002;22:96–101.

42. Trimeche M, Korbi S, Ziadi S, et al. Molecular characterization of Epstein-Barr virus associated with classical Hodgkin's lymphoma in

Tunisia: prevalence of the LMP1 oncogene deletions and A and B viruses strains. *Ann Biol Clin* 2005;63:193–199.

43. Chaouki N, El Gueddari B. Epidemiological descriptive approach of cancer in Morocco through the activity of the National Institute of Oncology, 1986–1987. *Bull Cancer* 1991;78:603–609.

44. Hessissen L, Oulhiane N, El Khorassani M, et al. Pediatric Hodgkins disease in Morocco. *Pediatr Blood Cancer* 2005;44:199.

45. Bouchardy C, Parkin DM, Wanner P, Khlat M. Cancer mortality among north African migrants in France. *Int J Epidemiol* 1996;25:5–13.

46. Nasr ALA, Tawfik HN, El-Einen AE. Lymphoreticular tumors and leukemias in Egypt. *J Natl Cancer Inst* 1973;50:1619–1621.

47. Kahan E, Ibrahim AS, El Najjar K, et al. Cancer patterns in the Middle East—special report from the Middle East Cancer Society. *Acta Oncol* 1997;36:631–636.

48. El-Boulkainy MN. *General pathology of cancer.* Cairo: Al-Asdekaa Graphic Ctr; 1991.

49. Azim HA, Moussa M, Hamada E, et al. Adult Hodgkin's disease: clinical presentation and results of treatment in NEMROCK (1992–1995). Dissertation, Cairo University, 1998.

50. Vasef MA, Ubaidat MA, Khalidi HS, et al. Association between Epstein-Barr virus and classic Hodgkin lymphoma in Jordan: a comparative study with Epstein-Barr virus-associated Hodgkin lymphoma in North America. *South Med J* 2004;97:273–277.

51. Ndiaye M, Hane AA, Diop AK, et al. Respiratory manifestations of malignant lymphomas: report of 5 cases. *Dakar Med* 2001;46:32–35.

52. Getachew A. Malignant lymphoma in western Ethiopia. *East Afr Med J* 2001;78:402–404.

53. Ouedraogo M, Ouedraogo SM, Cisse R, et al. Active tuberculosis in a patient with Hodgkin's disease: a case report. *Rev Pneumol Clin* 2000;56: 33–35.

54. Koffi KG, Sanogo I, Djigbenou D, et al. Results of treatment of 62 cases of Hodgkin's disease in Cote d'Ivoire. *Bull Soc Pathol Exot* 2000;93:55–57.

55. French TJ, Ross M. Hodgkin's disease at Harare Hospital. *Cent Afr J Med* 1976;22:237–241.

56. Levy LM. Hodgkin's disease in black Zimbabweans: a study of epidemiologic, histologic, and clinical features. *Cancer* 1988;61:189–194.

57. Cohen C, Hamilton DG. Epidemiologic and histologic patterns of Hodgkin's disease: comparison of the black and white populations of Johannesburg, South Africa. *Cancer* 1980;46:186–189.

58. Sitas F, Blaauw D, Terblanche M, et al. *Cancer in South Africa 1988. National Cancer Registry of South Africa: incidence of histologically diagnosed cancer in South Africa, 1992.* Johannesburg: South African Institute for Medical Research; 1997:46–51.

59. Razzouk BI, Gan YJ, Mendonca C, et al. Epstein-Barr virus in pediatric Hodgkin disease: age and histiotype are more predictive than geographic region. *Med Pediatr Oncol* 1997;28:248–254.

60. Hesseling PB, Wessels G, Van Jaarsveld D, et al. Hodgkin's disease in children in southern Africa: epidemiological characteristics, morbidity and long-term outcome. *Ann Trop Paediatr* 1997;17:367–373.

61. Wessels G, Hesseling PB. Perspectives of the management of childhood lymphoma: experience at Tygerberg Hospital, Western Cape, South Africa. *Transfus Apheresis Sci* 2005;32:27–31.

62. Zhang S, Du L, Li G, et al. Malignant lymphomas in childhood Sichuan province—a clinicopathological analysis of 304 cases. *Hua Xi Yi Ke Da Xue Xue Bao* 1994;25:94–97.

63. Chim CS, Kwong YL, Lie AKW, et al. Advanced stage and unfavourable Hodgkin's disease in the Chinese—a 20-year experience. *Am J Hematol* 1999;61:159–163.

64. Ko YH, Kim CW, Park CS, et al. REAL classification of malignant lymphomas in the Republic of Korea: incidence of recently recognized entities and changes in clinicopathologic features. The Hematolymphoreticular Study Group of the Korean Society of Pathologists. Revised European-American lymphoma. *Cancer* 1998;83:806–812.

65. Peh SC, Kim LH, Thanaletchimy N, et al. Spectrum of malignant lymphomas in Klang Hospital, a public hospital in Malaysia. *Malays J Pathol* 2000;22:13–20.

66. Sukpanichnant S, Sonakul D, Piankijagum A, et al. Malignant lymphoma in Thailand: changes in the frequency of malignant lymphoma determined from a histopathologic and immunophenotypic analysis of 425 cases at Siriraj Hospital. *Cancer* 1998;83:1197–1204.

67. Nandakumar A, Anantha N, Venugopal T, et al. Descriptive epidemiology of lymphoid and haemopoietic malignancies in Bangalore, India. *Int J Cancer* 1995;63:37–42.

68. Yeole BB, Jussawalla DJ. Descriptive epidemiology of lymphatic malignancies in greater Bombay. *Oncol Rep* 1998;5:771–777.

69. Kirchhoff LV, Evans AS, McClelland KE, et al. A case-control study of Hodgkin's disease in Brazil. I. Epidemiologic aspects. *Am J Epidemiol* 1980;112:595–608.

70. Aviles A, Diaz-Maqueo JC, Torras V, et al. Hodgkin's disease: a historical perspective. *Arch Invest Med* 1991;22:27–33.

71. Gomez-Almaguer D, Ruiz-Arguelles GJ, Lopez-Martines B, et al. Role of bone marrow examination in staging Hodgkin's disease: experience in Mexico. *Clin Lab Haematol* 2002;24:221–223.

72. Correa P, O'Conor GT. Geographic pathology of lymphoreticular tumors: summary of survey from the Geographic Pathology Committee of the International Union Against Cancer. *J Natl Cancer Inst* 1973;50: 1609–1617.

73. Edington GM, Hendrickse M. Incidence and frequency of lymphoreticular tumors in Ibadan and the Western State of Nigeria. *J Natl Cancer Inst* 1973;50:1623–1631.

74. Williams CK. Influence of life-style on the pattern of leukaemia and lymphoma subtypes among Nigerians. *Leuk Res* 1985;9:741–745.

75. Adedeji MO. The malignant lymphomas in Benin City, Nigeria. *East Afr Med J* 1989;66:134–140.

76. Okpala IE, Akang EE, Okpala UJ. Lymphomas in University College Hospital, Ibadan, Nigeria. *Cancer* 1991;68:1356–1360.

77. Kasili EG. Leukaemia and lymphoma in Kenya. *Leuk Res* 1985;9:747–752.

78. Kinuthia DM, Kasili EG. Hodgkin's disease in Kenyan children: a six-year report on management. *East Afr Med J* 1980;57:769–780.

79. Riyat MS. Hodgkin's disease in Kenya. *Cancer* 1992;69:1047–1051.

80. Dhru R, Templeton AC. Post-mortem findings in Ugandans with Hodgkin's disease. *Br J Cancer* 1972;26:331–334.

81. Amsel S, Nabembezi JS. Two-year survey of hematologic malignancies in Uganda. *J Natl Cancer Inst* 1974;52:1397–1401.

82. Tumwine LK, Wabinga H, Odida M. Haematoxylin and eosin staining in the diagnosis of Hodgkin's disease in Uganda. *East Afr Med J* 2003;80: 119–123.

83. Tumwine LK. Immunohistochemical analysis of Hodgkin's disease in Kampala, Uganda. *East Afr Med J* 2004;81:384–387.

84. Walter PR, Klotz F, Alfy-Gattas T, et al. Malignant lymphomas in Gabon (equatorial Africa): a morphologic study of 72 cases. *Hum Pathol* 1991;22: 1040–1043.

85. Levy LM. The pattern of haematological and lymphoreticular malignancy in Zimbabwe. *Trop Geogr Med* 1988;40:109–114.

86. Viana NJ, Thind IS, Louria DB, et al. Epidemiologic and histologic patterns of Hodgkin's disease in blacks. *Cancer* 1977;40:3133–3139.

87. Glaser SL. Hodgkin's disease in black populations: a review of the epidemiologic literature. *Semin Oncol* 1990;17:643–659.

88. Glaser SL. Black-white differences in Hodgkin's disease incidence in the United States by age, sex, histology subtype and time. *Int J Epidemiol* 1991; 20:68–75.

89. Hooper WC, Holman RC, Strine TW, et al. Hodgkin disease mortality in the United States: 1979–1988. *Cancer* 1992;70:1166–1171.

90. Zaki A, Natarajan N, Mettlin CJ. Early and late survival in Hodgkin disease among whites and blacks living in the United States. *Cancer* 1993;72: 602–606.

91. Elgui de Oliveira D, Bacchi MM, Abreu ES, et al. Hodgkin disease in adult and juvenile groups from two different geographic regions in Brazil: characterization of clinicopathologic aspects and relationship with Epstein-Barr virus infection. *Am J Clin Pathol* 2002;118:25–30.

92. Vassallo J, Pinto Paes R, Augusto Soares F, et al. Histological classification of 1,025 cases of Hodgkin's lymphoma from the State of Sao Paulo, Brazil. *Sao Paulo Med J* 2005;123:134–136.

93. Lukes RJ, Craver LF, Hall TC, et al. Report of the Nomenclature Committee. *Cancer Res* 1966;26:1310.

94. Rosenberg SA. Report of the Committee on the Staging of Hodgkin's Disease. *Cancer Res* 1971;26:1310.

95. Carbone PP, Kaplan HS, Musshoff K, et al. Report of the Committee on Hodgkin's Disease Staging Classification. *Cancer Res* 1971;31: 1860–1861.

96. Lister TA, Crowther D, Sutcliffe SB, et al. Report of a committee convened to discuss the evaluation and staging of patients with Hodgkin's disease: Cotswolds meeting. *J Clin Oncol* 1989;7:1630–1636.

97. Crowther D, Lister TA. The Cotswolds report on the investigation and staging of Hodgkin's disease. *Br J Cancer* 1990;62:551–552.

98. Stanford JL, Grange JM, Pozniak A. Is Africa lost? *Lancet* 1991;338: 557–558.

99. Proctor SJ, Taylor P, Mackie MJ, et al. A numerical index for clinical use in identification of poor-risk patients with Hodgkin's disease at diagnosis. The Scotland and Newcastle Lymphoma Group (SNLG) Therapy Working Party. *Leuk Lymphoma* 1992;7 (suppl):17–20.

100. Hasenclever D, Diehl V. A prognostic score for advanced Hodgkin's disease. International Prognostic Factors Project on Advanced Hodgkin's Disease. *N Engl J Med* 1998;339:1506–1514.

101. Bezwoda WR, MacPhail AP, Dawey R, et al. Hodgkin's disease in sub-Saharan Africa. Cambridge medical reviews. In: Armitage J, Newland A, Keating A, et al., eds. *Hematological oncology.* Vol. 4. Cambridge: Cambridge University Press; 1995:21–40.

102. Donaldson SS. Hodgkin's disease in children. *Semin Oncol* 1990;17: 736–748.

103. Thomson AB, Wallace WHB. Treatment of paediatric Hodgkin's disease: a balance of risks. *Eur J Cancer* 2002;38:468–477.

104. Donaldson SS. Pediatric Hodgkin's disease—up, up, and beyond. *Int J Radiat Oncol Biol Phys* 2002;54:1–8.

105. Donaldson SS. A discourse: the 2002 Wataru W. Sutow lecture Hodgkin disease in children—perspectives and progress. *Med Pediatr Oncol* 2003; 40:73–81.

106. Burkhardt B, Zimmermann M, Oschlies I, et al. The impact of age and gender on biology, clinical features and treatment outcome of non-Hodgkin lymphoma in childhood and adolescence. The BFM Group. *Br J Haematol* 2005;131:39–49.

107. Lieskovsky YYE, Donaldson SS, Torres MA, et al. High-dose therapy and autologous hematopoietic stem-cell transplantation for recurrent or refractory pediatric Hodgkin's disease: results and prognostic indices. *J Clin Oncol* 2004;22:4532–4540.

108. Gad-el-Mawla N, El-Deeb BB, Abu-Gabal A, et al. Pediatric Hodgkin's disease in Egypt. *Cancer* 1983;52:1129–1131.

109. Hesseling PB, Wessels G, van Riet FA. The Tygerberg Hospital Children's Tumour Registry 1983-1993. *Eur J Cancer* 1995;31A:1471–1475.

110. Jacobson RJ, Klappenbach RS, Clinton C, et al. Hodgkin's disease in South African children. *S Afr Med J* 1981;59:133–137.

111. Lobo-Sanahuja F, Garcia I, Barrantes JC, et al. Pediatric Hodgkin's disease in Costa Rica: twelve years' experience of primary treatment by chemotherapy alone, without staging laparotomy. *Med Pediatr Oncol* 1994;22:398–403.

112. Faria SL, Vassallo J, Cosset JM, et al. Childhood Hodgkin's disease in Campinas, Brazil. *Med Pediatr Oncol* 1996;26:90–94.

113. Wessels G. Paediatric cancer in Namibia (1983–1990). Dissertation, University of Stellenbosch, 1994.

114. Wessels G, Hesseling PB, Gie RP, et al. The increased risk of developing tuberculosis in children with malignancy. *Ann Trop Paediatr* 1992;12:277–281.

115. Pallesen G, Hamilton-Dutoit SJ, Rowe M, et al. Expression of Epstein-Barr virus latent gene products in tumour cells of Hodgkin's disease. *Lancet* 1991;337:320–322.

116. Pallesen G, Sandvej K, Hamilton-Dutoit SJ, et al. Activation of Epstein-Barr virus replication in Hodgkin and Reed-Sternberg cells. *Blood* 1991;78:1162–1165.

117. Knecht H, Odermatt BF, Bachmann E, et al. Frequent detection of Epstein-Barr virus DNA by the polymerase chain reaction in lymph node biopsies from patients with Hodgkin's disease without genomic evidence of B- or T-cell clonality. *Blood* 1991;78:760–767.

118. Weinreb M, Day PJR, Niggli F, et al. The role of Epstein-Barr virus in Hodgkin's disease from different geographical areas. *Arch Dis Child* 1996;74:27–31.

119. Geser A, de The G, Lenoir G, et al. Final case reporting from the Uganda prospective study of the relationship between EBV and Burkitt's lymphoma. *Int J Cancer* 1982;29:397–400.

120. Leoncini L, Spina D, Nyong'o A, et al. Neoplastic cells of Hodgkin's disease show differences in EBV expression between Kenya and Italy. *Int J Cancer* 1996;65:781–784.

121. Zhou XG, Hamilton-Dutoit SJ, Yan QH, et al. The association between Epstein-Barr virus and Chinese Hodgkin's disease. *Int J Cancer* 1993;55:359–363.

122. Sandvej K, Zhou XG, Hamilton-Dutoit S. EBNA-1 sequence variation in Danish and Chinese EBV-associated tumours: evidence for geographical polymorphism but not for tumour-specific subtype restriction. *J Pathol* 2000;191:127–131.

123. Zhou XG, Sandvej K, Li PJ, et al. Epstein-Barr virus (EBV) in Chinese pediatric Hodgkin disease: Hodgkin disease in young children is an EBV-related lymphoma. *Cancer* 2001;92:1621–1631.

124. Hemsrichart V, Pintong J. Association of the Epstein-Barr viruses with Hodgkin lymphoma: an analysis of pediatric cases in Thailand. *J Med Assoc Thai* 2005;88:782–787.

125. Mitarnum W, Pradutkanchana J, Ishida T. Epstein-Barr virus-associated nodal malignant lymphoma in Thailand. *Asian Pac J Cancer Prev* 2004;5:268–272.

126. Huh J, Park C, Juhng S, et al. A pathologic study of Hodgkin's disease in Korea and its association with Epstein-Barr virus infection. *Cancer* 1996;77:949–955.

127. Kim I, Park ER, Park SH, et al. Characteristics of Epstein-Barr virus isolated from the malignant lymphomas in Korea. *J Med Virol* 2002;67:59–66.

128. Liu SM, Chow KC, Chiu CF, et al. Expression of Epstein-Barr virus in patients with Hodgkin's disease in Taiwan. *Cancer* 1998;83:367–371.

129. Peh SC, Looi LM, Pallesen G. Epstein-Barr virus (EBV) and Hodgkin's disease in a multi-ethnic population in Malaysia. *Histopathology* 1997;30:227–233.

130. Sandvej K, Peh SC, Andresen BS, et al. Identification of potential hot spots in the carboxy-terminal part of the Epstein-Barr virus (EBV) BNLF-1 gene in both malignant and benign EBV-associated diseases: high frequency of a 30-bp deletion in Malaysian and Danish peripheral T-cell lymphomas. *Blood* 1994;84:4053–4060.

131. Karnik S, Srinivasan B, Nair S. Hodgkin's lymphoma: immunochistochemical features and its association with EBV LMP-1: experience from a south Indian hospital. *Pathology* 2003;35:207–211.

132. Vassallo J, Metze K, Traina F, et al. Expression of Epstein-Barr virus in classical Hodgkin's lymphomas in Brazilian adult patients. *Haematologica* 2001;86:1227–1228.

133. Quijano S, Saavedra C, Fiorentino S, et al. Epstein-Barr virus presence in Colombian Hodgkin lymphoma cases and its relation to treatment response. *Biomedica* 2004;24:163–173.

134. Gulley ML, Eagan PA, Quintanilla-Martinez L, et al. Epstein-Barr virus DNA is abundant and monoclonal in the Reed-Sternberg cells of Hodgkin's disease: association with mixed cellularity subtype and Hispanic American ethnicity. *Blood* 1994;83:1595–1602.

135. Monterroso V, Zhou Y, Koo S, et al. Hodgkin's disease in Costa Rica: a report of 40 cases analyzed for Epstein-Barr virus. *Am J Clin Pathol* 1998;109:618–624.

136. Zarate-Osorno A, Roman LN, Kingma DW, et al. Hodgkin's disease in Mexico: prevalence of Epstein-Barr virus sequences and correlations with histologic subtype. *Cancer* 1995;75:1360–1366.

137. Dirnhofer S, Angeles-Angeles A, Ortiz-Hidalgo C, et al. High prevalence of a 30-base pair deletion in the Epstein-Barr virus (EBV) latent membrane protein 1 gene and of strain type B EBV in Mexican classical Hodgkin's disease and reactive lymphoid tissue. *Hum Pathol* 1999;30:781–787.

138. Chang KL, Albujar PF, Chen YY, et al. High prevalence of Epstein-Barr virus in the Reed-Sternberg cells of Hodgkin's disease occurring in Peru. *Blood* 1993;81:496–501.

139. Tirelli U, Vaccher E, Rezza G, et al. Hodgkin disease and infection with the human immunodeficiency virus (HIV) in Italy. *Ann Intern Med* 1988;108:309–310.

140. Beral V. The epidemiology of cancer in AIDS patients. *AIDS* 1991;5 (suppl 2):S99–S104.

141. Pelstring RJ, Zellmer RB, Sulak LE, et al. Hodgkin's disease in association with human immunodeficiency virus infection: pathologic and immunologic features. *Cancer* 1991;67:1865–1873.

142. Rabkin CS, Blattner WA. HIV infection and cancers other than non-Hodgkin lymphoma and Kaposi's sarcoma. *Cancer Surv* 1991;10:151–160.

143. Rabkin CS, Biggar RJ, Horm JW. Increasing incidence of cancers associated with the human immunodeficiency virus epidemic. *Int J Cancer* 1991;47:692–696.

144. Hessol NA, Katz MH, Liu JY, et al. Increasing incidence of Hodgkin's disease in homosexual men with HIV infection. *Ann Intern Med* 1992;117:309–311.

145. Tirelli U, Serraino D, Carbone A. Hodgkin disease and HIV. *Ann Intern Med* 1993;118:313.

146. *Fifth national HIV survey attending antenatal clinics of the public health services in South Africa 1995.* Pretoria: Dept of Health; 1996.

147. Sitas F, Bezwoda WR, Levin V, et al. Association between human immunodeficiency virus type 1 infection and cancer in the black population of Johannesburg and Soweto, South Africa. *Br J Cancer* 1997;75:1704–1707.

148. Wabinga HR, Parkin DM, Wabwire-Mangen F, et al. Cancer in Kampala, Uganda, in 1989-91: changes in incidence in the era of AIDS. *Int J Cancer* 1993;54:26–36.

149. Bassett MT, Chokunonga E, Mauchaza B, et al. Cancer in the African population of Harare, Zimbabwe, 1990–1992. *Int J Cancer* 1995;63:29–36.

150. Newton R, Grulich A, Beral V, et al. Cancer and HIV infection in Rwanda. *Lancet* 1995;345:1378–1379.

151. Schooley RT. Starting highly active antiretroviral therapy for HIV infection: is it WIHS to wait? *Ann Intern Med* 2004;140:305–306.

152. Bonnet F, Lewden C, May T, et al. Malignancy-related causes of death in human immunodeficiency virus-infected patients in the era of highly active antiretroviral therapy. *Cancer* 2004;101:317–324.

153. Stevens W, Kaye S, Corrah T. Antiretroviral therapy in Africa. *BMJ* 2004;328:280–282.

154. Sidley P. Sharp rise in deaths in South Africa is largely due to AIDS. *BMJ* 2005;330:438.

155. Ratanasuwan W, Anekthananon T, Techasathit W, et al. Estimated economic losses of hospitalized AIDS patients at Siriraj hospital from January 2003 to December 2003: time for aggressive voluntary counseling and HIV testing. *J Med Assoc Thai* 2005;88:335–339.

156. Orem J, Otieno MW, Remick SC. AIDS-associated cancer in developing nations. *Curr Opin Oncol* 2004;16:468–476.

157. Portsmouth S, Stebbing J, Keyi X, et al. HIV and AIDS in the People's Republic of China: a collaborative review. *Int J STD AIDS* 2003;14:757–761.

158. Ainsworth M, Beyrer C, Soucat A. AIDS and public policy: the lessons and challenges of "success" in Thailand. *Health Policy* 2003;64:13–37.

159. Pancharoen C, Thisyakorn U. Preventive strategies of perinatal HIV-1 transmission: an experience from Thailand. *Expert Opin Pharmacother* 2003;4:179–182.

160. Dandona L. Enhancing the evidence base for HIV/AIDS control in India. *Natl Med J India* 2004;17:160–166.

161. Caceres CF. Interventions for HIV/STD prevention in Latin America and the Caribbean: a review of the regional experience. *Cad Saude Publica* 2004;20:1468–1485.

162. Cahn P, Belloso WH, Murillo J, et al. AIDS in Latin America. *Infect Dis Clin North Am* 2003;14:185–209.

163. Bastos FI, Barcellos C. The social geography of AIDS in Brazil. *Rev Saude Publica* 1995;29:52–62.

164. Bacchi CE, Bacchi MM, Rabenhorst SH, et al. AIDS-related lymphoma in Brazil: histopathology, immunophenotype, and association with Epstein-Barr virus. *Am J Clin Pathol* 1996;105:230–237.

165. Esparza J, Osmanov S. HIV vaccines: a global perspective. *Curr Mol Med* 2003;3:183–193.

166. Ayoubzadeh S, Ben-Abdallah T, Engelhard P, et al. AIDS and the third world. *Environ Afr* 1987;1:140.

167. Mertens TE, Low-Beer D. HIV and AIDS: where is the epidemic going? *Bull World Health Org* 1996;74:121–129.

168. Henry-Amar M, Somers R. Survival outcome after Hodgkin's disease: a report from the International Data Base on Hodgkin's Disease. *Semin Oncol* 1990;17:758–768.

169. Lavoie JC, Connors JM, Phillips GL, et al. High-dose chemotherapy and autologous stem cell transplantation for primary refractory or relapsed Hodgkin lymphoma: long-term outcome in the first 100 patients treated in Vancouver. *Blood* 2005;106:1473–1478.

170. Horning SJ, Chao NJ, Negrin RS, et al. High-dose therapy and autologous hematopoietic progenitor cell transplantation for recurrent or refractory Hodgkin's disease: analysis of the Stanford University results and prognostic indices. *Blood* 1997;89:801–813.

171. Munker R, Stengel A, Stabler A, et al. Diagnostic accuracy of ultrasound and computed tomography in the staging of Hodgkin's disease: verification by laparotomy in 100 cases. *Cancer* 1995;76:1460–1466.

172. Green DM, Ghoorah J, Douglass HO Jr, et al. Staging laparotomy with splenectomy in children and adolescents with Hodgkin's disease. *Cancer Treat Rev* 1983;10:23–38.

173. Burton C, Ell P, Linch D. The role of PET imaging in lymphoma. *Br J Haematol* 2004;126:772–784.

174. Munker R, Glass J, Griffeth LK, et al. Contribution of PET imaging to the initial staging and prognosis of patients with Hodgkin's disease. *Ann Oncol* 2004;15;1699–1704.

175. Keresztes K, Lengyel Z, Devenyi K, et al. Mediastinal bulky tumour in Hodgkin's disease and prognostic value of positron emission tomography in the evaluation of post-treatment residual masses. *Acta Haematol* 2004;112:194–199.

176. Yahalom J. Breast cancer after Hodgkin disease: hope for a safer cure. *JAMA* 2003;290:529–531.

177. Josting A, Wiedenmann S, Franklin J, et al. Secondary myeloid leukemia and myelodysplastic syndromes in patients treated for Hodgkin's disease: a report from the German Hodgkin's Lymphoma Study Group. *J Clin Oncol* 2003;21:3440–3446.

178. Eghbali H, Raemaekers J, Carde P. The EORTC strategy in the treatment of Hodgkin's lymphoma. *Eur J Haematol* 2005;75(suppl 66):135–140.

179. Eich HT, Star S, Gossmann A, et al. The HD12 panel of the German Hodgkin Lymphoma Study Group (GHSG): a quality assurance program based on a multidisciplinary panel reviewing all patients' imaging. *Am J Clin Oncol* 2004;27:279–284.

180. Ganz PA, Moinpour CM, Pauler DK, et al. Health status and quality of life in patients with early-stage Hodgkin's disease treated on Southwest Oncology Group Study 9133. *J Clin Oncol* 2003;21:3512–3519.

181. Gisselbrecht C, Mounier N, Andre M, et al. How to define intermediate stage in Hodgkin's lymphoma? *Eur J Haematol* 2005;75(suppl 66):111–114.

182. Olweny CLM, Ziegler JL, Berard CW, et al. Adult Hodgkin's disease in Uganda. *Cancer* 1971;27:1295–1301.

183. Olweny CLM, Katongole-Mbidde E, Kiire C, et al. Childhood Hodgkin's disease in Uganda: a ten year experience. *Cancer* 1978;42:787–792.

184. Oluboyede OA, Esan GJ. The therapy of Hodgkin's disease in Nigeria: a five year study. *Afr J Med Med Sci* 1976;5:201–207.

185. Williams CK. Prospective studies on Hodgkin's disease in Ibadan—a preliminary report. *Afr J Med Med Sci* 1985;14:37–43.

186. Clarke CA, Glaser SL, Keegan TH, et al. Neighborhood socioeconomic status and Hodgkin's lymphoma incidence in California. *Cancer Epidemiol Biomarkers Prev* 2005;14:1441–1447.

187. Briggs NC, Levine RS, Hall HI, et al. Occupational risk factors for selected cancers among African American and white men in the United States. *Am J Public Health* 2003;93:1748–1752.

188. Canellos GP, Anderson JR, Propert KJ, et al. Chemotherapy of advanced Hodgkin's disease with MOPP, ABVD, or MOPP alternating with ABVD. *N Engl J Med* 1992;327:1478–1484.

189. Longo DL, Duffey PL, DeVita VT Jr, et al. Treatment of advanced-stage Hodgkin's disease: alternating noncrossresistant MOPP/CABS is not superior to MOPP. *J Clin Oncol* 1991;9:1409–1420.

190. Somers R, Carde P, Henry-Amar M, et al. A randomized study in stage IIIB and IV Hodgkin's disease comparing eight courses of MOPP versus an alternation of MOPP with ABVD: a European Organization for Research and Treatment of Cancer Lymphoma Cooperative Group and Groupe Pierre-et-Marie-Curie controlled clinical trial. *J Clin Oncol* 1994;12:279–287.

191. Radford JA, Crowther D, Rohatiner AZ, et al. Results of a randomized trial comparing MVPP chemotherapy with a hybrid regimen, ChlVPP/EVA, in the initial treatment of Hodgkin's disease. *J Clin Oncol* 1995;13:2379–2385.

192. Viviani S, Bonadonna G, Santoro A, et al. Alternating versus hybrid MOPP and ABVD combinations in advanced Hodgkin's disease: ten-year results. *J Clin Oncol* 1996;14:1421–1430.

193. Carde P, MacKintosh FR, Rosenberg SA. A dose and time response analysis of the treatment of Hodgkin's disease with MOPP chemotherapy. *J Clin Oncol* 1983;1:146–153.

194. Longo DL, Young RC, Wesley M, et al. Twenty years of MOPP therapy for Hodgkin's disease. *J Clin Oncol* 1986;4:1295–1306.

195. Bezwoda WR, Dansey R, Bezwoda MA. Treatment of Hodgkin's disease with MOPP chemotherapy: effect of dose and schedule modification on treatment outcome. *Oncology* 1990;47:29–36.

196. Jagannath S, Armitage JO, Dicke KA, et al. Prognostic factors for response and survival after high-dose cyclophosphamide, carmustine, and etoposide with autologous bone marrow transplantation for relapsed Hodgkin's disease. *J Clin Oncol* 1989;7:179–185.

197. Kessinger A, Nademanee A, Forman SJ, et al. Autologous bone marrow transplantation for Hodgkin's and non-Hodgkin's lymphoma. *Hematol Oncol Clin North Am* 1990;4:577–587.

198. Seymour LK, Dansey RD, Bezwoda WR. Single high-dose etoposide and melphalan with non-cryopreserved autologous marrow rescue as primary therapy for relapsed, refractory and poor-prognosis Hodgkin's disease. *Br J Cancer* 1994;70:526–530.

199. Bezwoda WR, Dansey R. High dose chemotherapy with bone marrow rescue for treatment of relapsed and refractory Hodgkin's disease. *Leuk Lymphoma* 1989;1:71–76.

200. Martin J, Radford M. Current practice in Hodgkin's disease. The United Kingdom Children's Cancer Study Group. In: Kamps WA, Humphrey GB, Poppema S, eds. *Hodgkin's disease in children: controversies and current practice.* Boston: Kluwer; 1989:263–275.

201. Hunger SP, Link MP, Donaldson SS. ABVD/MOPP and low-dose involved-field radiotherapy in pediatric Hodgkin's disease: the Stanford experience. *J Clin Oncol* 1994;12:2160–2166.

202. Oberlin O, Leverger G, Pacquement H, et al. Low-dose radiation therapy and reduced chemotherapy in childhood Hodgkin's disease: the experience of the French Society of Pediatric Oncology. *J Clin Oncol* 1992;10:1602–1608.

203. Sankila R, Garwicz S, Olsen JH, et al. Risk of subsequent malignant neoplasms among 1,641 Hodgkin's disease patients diagnosed in childhood and adolescence: a population-based cohort study in the five Nordic countries. The Association of the Nordic Cancer Registries and the Nordic Society of Pediatric Hematology and Oncology. *J Clin Oncol* 1996;14: 1442–1446.

204. Kapoor G, Advani SH, Dinshaw KA, et al. Treatment results of Hodgkin's disease in Indian children. *Pediatr Hematol Oncol* 1995;12:559–569.

205. Laskar S, Gupta T, Vimal S, et al. Consolidation radiation after complete remission in Hodgkin's disease following six cycles of doxorubicin, bleomycin, vinblastine, and dacarbazine chemotherapy: is there a need? *J Clin Oncol* 2004;22:62–68.

206. Baez F, Ocampo E, Conter V, et al. Treatment of childhood Hodgkin's disease with COPP or COPP-ABV (hybrid) without radiotherapy in Nicaragua. *Ann Oncol* 1997;8:247–250.